D0173938

DOWNLOAD

CLINICAL DRUG DATA *11th Edition*

FOLLOW THESE INSTRUCTIONS TO DOWNLOAD:

1) Use your Web browser to go to:
   http://www.mhprofessional.com/clinicaldrugdata/

2) Register now

3) Fill in the required fields

4) Enter your unique registration code below

5) Download the file and sync into your handheld device *fb89a8*

   Code Listed Here

   ℓG

NOTE: BOOK IS NOT RETURNABLE ONCE SCRATCH-OFF IS REMOVED

Scratch off coating above to reveal your unique code
to download your mobile device file.

See above for complete directions.

If you have any problems accessing your download,
please email: techsolutions@mhedu.com

P/N 9780071626873
0071626875
part of set
ISBN 978-0-07-162688-0
MHID 0-07-162688-3

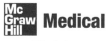

Mc Graw Hill Medical

mcgraw-hillmedical.com

Clinical
Drug Data

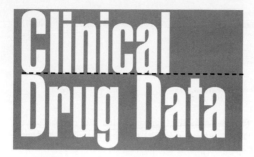

Clinical Drug Data

eleventh edition

EDITORS

Kelly M. Smith, PharmD, BCPS, FASHP, FCCP
Associate Dean, Academic and Student Affairs Practice
Associate Professor, Pharmacy Practice and Science
University of Kentucky College of Pharmacy
Lexington, Kentucky

Daniel M. Riche, PharmD, BCPS, CDE
Assistant Professor
University of Mississippi Schools of Pharmacy and Medicine
University of Mississippi Medical Center
Jackson, Mississippi

Nickole N. Henyan, PharmD
Clinical Pharmacist
Shore Health System
University of Maryland Medical System
Easton, Maryland

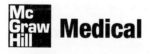 **Medical**

New York   Chicago   San Francisco   Lisbon   London   Madrid
Mexico City   Milan   New Delhi   San Juan   Seoul   Singapore
Sydney   Toronto

Clinical Drug Data, Eleventh Edition

1 2 3 4 5 6 7 8 9 0   DOC/DOC   14 13 13 11 10

Set ISBN 978-0-07-162688-0; MHID 0-07-162688-0
Book ISBN 978-0-07-162685-9; MHID 0-07-162685-9
Bind-in-Card ISBN 978-0-07-162687-3; MHID 0-07-162687-5

This book was set in Times Roman at Aptara, Inc.
The editors were Michael Weitz and Regina Y. Brown.
The production supervisor was Sherri Souffrance.
Project management provided by Deepa Krishnan, Aptara, Inc.
The cover designer was Malvina D'Alterio.
RR Donnelley was printer and binder.

This book is printed on acid-free paper.

Cataloging-in-Publication is on file for this title at the Library of Congress.

International Edition Set ISBN 978-0-07-174845-2; MHID 0-07-174845-8
International Edition Book ISBN 978-0-07-174844-5; MHID 0-07-174844-X
International Bind-in-Card ISBN 978-0-07-162687-3; MHID 0-07-162687-5

Contents

Contributors

Philip O. Anderson, PharmD, FCSHP, FASHP
Health Sciences Clinical Professor of Pharmacy
Skaggs School of Pharmacy and Pharmaceutical Sciences
University of California, San Diego
La Jolla, California

Phil Ayers, PharmD, BCNSP
Clinical Team Leader
Department of Pharmacy
Clinical Specialist, Nutrition Support
Mississippi Baptist Medical Center
Clinical Assistant Professor
University of Mississippi School of Pharmacy
Jackson, Mississippi

Danial E. Baker, PharmD, FASHP, FASCP
Professor of Pharmacotherapy
Washington State University College of Pharmacy
Spokane, Washington

Christopher Betz, PharmD, BCPS
Associate Professor
Sullivan University College of Pharmacy
Louisville, Kentucky

Toy S. Biederman, PharmD
Assistant Professor of Pharmacy Practice
University of Findlay College of Pharmacy
Findlay, Ohio

Gina C. Biglane, PharmD
Assistant Professor
University of Louisiana at Monroe College of Pharmacy
Monroe, Louisiana

Paula J. Biscup-Horn, PharmD, BCPS, CACP
Clinical Pharmacist, Anticoagulation Management
Allegheny General Hospital (West Penn Allegheny Health System)
Pittsburgh, Pennsylvania

Jessica Helmer Brady, PharmD, BCPS
Clinical Assistant Professor
University of Louisiana at Monroe College of Pharmacy
Monroe, Louisiana

Courtney M. Brown, PharmD, BCPS
PGY2 Pharmacy Resident, Pediatrics
Nationwide Children's Hospital
Columbus, Ohio

David J. Caldwell, PharmD, AAHIVE
Assistant Professor
University of Louisiana at Monroe College of Pharmacy
Monroe, Louisiana

R. Keith Campbell, RPh, BPharm, MBA, CDE
Distinguished Professor in Diabetes Care
Washington State University College of Pharmacy
Pullman, Washington

F. Lee Cantrell, PharmD, DABAT
Director
California Poison Control System
San Diego Division
Associate Professor of Clinical Pharmacy
University of California, San Francisco School of Pharmacy
San Diego, California

Juliana Chan, PharmD
Assistant Director of Pharmacy Clinical Services
Clinical Assistant Professor
Department of Pharmacy Practice, College of Pharmacy
Department of Medicine, Sections of Digestive Diseases & Nutrition and
    Section of Hepatology
University of Illinois at Chicago
Chicago, Illinois

John D. Cleary, PharmD, FCCP
Professor
University of Mississippi School of Pharmacy
Associate Professor
University of Mississippi School of Medicine
Jackson, Mississippi

Timothy M. Clifford, PharmD, BCPS
Transplant Clinical Specialist
University of Kentucky HealthCare

Adjunct Assistant Professor, Pharmacy Practice and Science
University of Kentucky College of Pharmacy
Lexington, Kentucky

Paul G. Cuddy, PharmD, MBA
Senior Associate Dean
University of Missouri-Kansas City School of Medicine
Kansas City, Missouri

William E. Dager, PharmD, FCSHP, FCCP
Pharmacist Specialist
UC Davis Medical Center
Clinical Professor of Pharmacy
University of California, San Francisco School of Pharmacy
Clinical Professor of Medicine
UC Davis School of Medicine
Sacramento, California

George A. Davis, PharmD, BCPS
Adjunct Associate Professor, Pharmacy Practice and Science
University of Kentucky College of Pharmacy
Lexington, Kentucky

Heather F. DeBellis, PharmD
Assistant Professor, Pharmacy Practice
South University School of Pharmacy
Savannah, Georgia

Robert J. DiDomenico, PharmD
Cardiovascular Clinical Pharmacist
University of Illinois Medical Center at Chicago
Associate Professor
University of Illinois at Chicago
Chicago, Illinois

Betty J. Dong, PharmD, FASHP, FCCP
Professor of Clinical Pharmacy
Clinical Pharmacist, Thyroid Clinic
Departments of Clinical Pharmacy and Medicine
University of California, San Francisco
San Francisco, California

Linda M. Farho, PharmD, BCPS
Assistant Professor, Pharmacy Practice
University of Nebraska Medical Center College of Pharmacy
Omaha, Nebraska

Catherine E. Ferara, PharmD
Clinical Pharmacist
Shore Health System
University of Maryland Medical System
Easton, Maryland

John Garofalo, PharmD
Associate Director, Clinical Pharmacy Services
University of Illinois Medical Center
Clinical Assistant Professor
Department of Pharmacy Practice
University of Illinois at Chicago College of Pharmacy
Chicago, Illinois

Mary Gauthier-Lewis, PharmD
Assistant Dean and Associate Professor
University of Louisiana at Monroe College of Pharmacy
Baton Rouge, Louisiana

Aaron P. Gibson, PharmD, MS
Assistant Professor of Pharmacy Practice
The University of New Mexico
Albuquerque, New Mexico

Emily R. Hajjar, PharmD, BCPS, CGP
Assistant Professor
Jefferson School of Pharmacy
Thomas Jefferson University
Philadelphia, Pennsylvania

Brett H. Heintz, PharmD, BCPS
Assistant Professor of Clinical Pharmacy
University of California, San Francisco School of Pharmacy
San Francisco, California
Pharmacist Specialist, Infectious Diseases
Department of Pharmaceutical Services
University of California, Davis Health System
Sacramento, California

Shirley Hogan, PharmD
Clinical Associate Professor
Department of Pharmacy Practice
University of Mississippi School of Pharmacy
Affiliate Assistant Professor in Pediatrics
University of Mississippi School of Medicine
Jackson, Mississippi

Mark T. Holdsworth, PharmD, BCOP
Associate Professor of Pharmacy & Pediatrics
Pharmacy Practice Department Chair
University of New Mexico College of Pharmacy
Albuquerque, New Mexico

John R. Horn, PharmD, FCCP
Professor of Pharmacy Practice
University of Washington School of Pharmacy
Associate Director of Pharmacy Services
University of Washington Medical Center
Seattle, Washington

Mikael D. Jones, PharmD, BCPS
Clinical Assistant Professor
University of Kentucky College of Pharmacy
Lexington, Kentucky

Michael P. Kane, PharmD, FCCP, BCPS
Professor
Department of Pharmacy Practice
Albany College of Pharmacy and Health Sciences
Clinical Pharmacy Specialist
The Endocrine Group, LLP
Albany, New York

Amber P. Lawson, PharmD, BCOP
Hematology/Oncology Clinical Specialist
University of Kentucky HealthCare
Lexington, Kentucky

Davey P. Legendre, PharmD, BCPS
Associate Director of Clinical Pharmacy
Health Management Associates
Atlanta, Georgia

Melanie Mabins, PharmD
Clinical Assistant Professor, Pharmacy Practice and Science
University of Kentucky College of Pharmacy
Lexington, Kentucky

Scott S. Malinowski, PharmD
Clinical Pharmacy Manager
University of Mississippi Medical Center
Clinical Assistant Professor of Pharmacy Practice
University of Mississippi School of Pharmacy
Jackson, Mississippi

T. Joseph Mattingly II, PharmD, MBA
Pharmacist
The Kroger Company
Louisville, Kentucky

Gary R. Matzke, PharmD, FCP, FCCP, FASN, DPNAP
Professor and Associate Dean for Clinical Research and Public Policy
School of Pharmacy
Virginia Commonwealth University-MCV Campus
Richmond, Virginia

Annette T. McFarland, PharmD
Assistant Professor of Pharmacy Practice, Drug Information
Butler University College of Pharmacy and Health Sciences
Indianapolis, Indiana

Andrea L. McKeever, PharmD, BCPS
Associate Professor
Department of Pharmacy Practice
South University School of Pharmacy
Savannah, Georgia

Renee-Claude Mercier, PharmD
Associate Professor and Regents' Lecturer, Pharmacy Practice
University of New Mexico College of Pharmacy
Albuquerque, New Mexico

Katherine D. Mieure, PharmD, BCPS
Clinical Pharmacist Specialist, Critical Care
University of Chicago Medical Center
Chicago, Illinois

April D. Miller, PharmD, BCPS
Assistant Professor
South Carolina College of Pharmacy-USC Campus
Columbia, South Carolina

Trenika R. Mitchell, PharmD, BCPS
Clinical Assistant Professor, Pharmacy Practice and Science
University of Kentucky College of Pharmacy
Lexington, Kentucky

William E. Murray, PharmD
Rady Children's Hospital, San Diego
Clinical Assistant Professor of Pharmacy
University of California, San Francisco
San Diego Program
San Diego, California

James J. Nawarskas, PharmD, BCPS
Associate Professor of Pharmacy
University of New Mexico College of Pharmacy
Albuquerque, New Mexico

Amy Sutton Peak, PharmD
Director of Drug Information Services
Butler University College of Pharmacy and Health Sciences
Indianapolis, Indiana

Peggy Piascik, PhD
Associate Professor of Pharmacy Practice and Science
University of Kentucky College of Pharmacy
Lexington, Kentucky

Kurt Reinhart, PharmD
Assistant Professor of Pharmacy
Wingate University School of Pharmacy
Wingate, North Carolina

Krista Dale Riche, PharmD, BCPS
Pharmacy Clinical Specialist
Mississippi Baptist Health Systems
Jackson, Mississippi

Daniel M. Riche, PharmD, BCPS, CDE
Assistant Professor
University of Mississippi Schools of Pharmacy and Medicine
Jackson, Mississippi

Treavor T. Riley, PharmD, BCPS
Assistant Professor
University of Louisiana at Monroe College of Pharmacy
Baton Rouge, Louisiana

Frank Romanelli, PharmD, MPH, BCPS
Associate Dean and Associate Professor of Pharmacy and Medicine
University of Kentucky
Lexington, Kentucky

Laura L. Sanders, PharmD, BCNSP
Clinical Assistant Professor, Department of Pharmacy Practice
University of Mississippi School of Pharmacy
Clinical Pharmacy Specialist
Baptist Memorial Hospital-North Mississippi
Baptist Memorial Health Care Corporation
Oxford, Mississippi

Heather M. Schumann, PharmD
Emergency Medicine Clinical Pharmacist
Clinical Assistant Professor
Department of Pharmacy Practice
University of Illinois at Chicago College of Pharmacy
Chicago, Illinois

Stephen M. Setter, PharmD, DVM, CGP, CDE
Associate Professor
Department of Pharmacotherapy
College of Pharmacy
Washington State University/Elder Services
Spokane, Washington

Sachin A. Shah, PharmD
Assistant Professor of Pharmacy Practice
Thomas J. Long School of Pharmacy and Health Sciences
University of the Pacific
Stockton, California

Kelly M. Smith, PharmD, BCPS, FASHP, FCCP
Associate Dean, Academic and Student Affairs
Associate Professor, Pharmacy Practice and Science
University of Kentucky College of Pharmacy
Lexington, Kentucky

Roxie L. Stewart, PharmD
Assistant Professor
University of Louisiana at Monroe College of Pharmacy
Monroe, Louisiana

Kayla R. Stover, PharmD
Assistant Professor
University of Mississippi School of Pharmacy
Jackson, Mississippi

Stephanie Dixon Sutphin, PharmD, BCOP
Hematology/Oncology Clinical Specialist
University of Kentucky HealthCare
Adjunct Assistant Professor, Pharmacy Practice and Science
University of Kentucky College of Pharmacy
Lexington, Kentucky

Gary D. Theilman, PharmD
Associate Professor of Pharmacy Practice
University of Mississippi School of Pharmacy
Jackson, Mississippi

Andrea N. Traina, PharmD
Endocrine Specialty Pharmacy Resident
The Endocrine Group, LLP
Instructor, Department of Pharmacy Practice
Albany College of Pharmacy and Health Sciences
Albany, New York

William R. Vincent III, PharmD, BCPS
Assistant Professor of Pharmacy Practice
Arnold & Marie Schwartz College of Pharmacy and Health Sciences
Long Island University
Clinical Pharmacy Educator, Critical Care
The Brooklyn Hospital Center
Brooklyn, New York

Kristina E. Ward, BS, PharmD, BCPS
Clinical Assistant Professor of Pharmacy Practice
Director, Drug Information Services
University of Rhode Island College of Pharmacy
Kingston, Rhode Island

C. Michael White, PharmD, FCP, FCCP
Professor of Pharmacy Practice
School of Pharmacy
University of Connecticut
Connecticut
Director
Hartford Hospital Evidence-based Practice Center
Hartford

John R. White Jr., PA, PharmD
Professor
Department of Pharmacotherapy
College of Pharmacy
Washington State University
Spokane, Washington

P. Shane Winstead, PharmD
Medical ICU Clinical Specialist
University of Kentucky HealthCare
Adjunct Assistant Professor, Pharmacy Practice and Science
University of Kentucky College of Pharmacy
Lexington, Kentucky

James M. Wooten, PharmD
Associate Professor
University of Missouri-Kansas City School of Medicine
Kansas City, Missouri

Krysta A. Zack, PharmD
Clinical Pharmacist, Emergency Medicine
The Nebraska Medical Center
Adjunct Faculty
University of Nebraska Medical Center
Omaha, Nebraska

Preface

After years of absence, *Clinical Drug Data* returns with this—the 11th edition. Users of past editions of what was the *Handbook of Clinical Drug Data* will find a familiar approach to the style, formatting, and organization of the 11th edition. Entries are arranged by focused content area in three parts. Part I features drug monographs, while Parts II and III include therapeutic overviews and clinically relevant appendices.

There are a number of notable changes with this edition, however. Perhaps the most expected is the inclusion of US market drug changes since the last edition, in addition to the seemingly continuous information about drug safety profiles and unique medication uses. Some monograph categories have been relocated to different chapters, while other new chapters have been developed (e.g., Viral Hepatitis, Tyrosine Kinase Inhibitors, and Inflammatory Bowel Disease). An exciting new feature is the PDA download option, further contributing to the goal of providing portable, clinically relevant, well-referenced drug information compiled by expert clinicians. We also boast a balanced grouping of both new and long-standing authors of whom we are proud to count as members of the team.

Changes in the team extend to the editor level. We as new editors pay our regards to the extraordinary legacy of Drs. Philip Anderson, James Knoben, and William Troutman. These outstanding colleagues worked tirelessly to establish the outstanding reputation and import of this title and have paved the way for us to continue that excellence. As your new editors, we pledge to uphold the signature style and value with which this publication has always been linked, and we thank our predecessors for their dedicated assistance during the editorial transition.

Given the rate of new drug approvals, the explosion of biological agents, and the advent of pharmacogenomics, users can expect a greater update frequency of content moving forward. That will translate to a new edition approximately every 3 years. As always, our editorial and author team is committed to providing users the most clinically focused, well-referenced drug information handbook around.

Kelly M. Smith
Daniel M. Riche
Nickole N. Henyan
March 2010

How to Use This Book

Part I of this book is organized around 10 major drug categories, which have been subdivided into common therapeutic groups. Within these therapeutic groups, drug information is alphabetically presented in three formats: ***Monographs, Minimonographs,*** and ***Comparison Charts***. Monographs and Comparison Charts are *grouped together* to ensure that related drugs are easy to *compare* and *contrast*. Charts are located after the monographs to which they relate. Drug antagonists are grouped together with agonists to simplify organization and accessibility.

Monographs are used for drugs of major importance and prototype agents.

Minimonographs are used for drugs similar to prototype drugs, those of lesser importance within a therapeutic class, and promising investigational agents. Minimonographs contain only selected subheadings of information rather than all subheadings contained in the full monographs.

Comparison Charts are used to present clinically useful information on members of the same pharmacologic class and different drugs with a similar therapeutic use, as well as to present clinically relevant information on certain other topics.

The preferred method to gain access to complete information on a *particular brand* or *generic drug* is to use the index at the end of the book. The index may also direct the user to *other pertinent information* on the drug.

MONOGRAPH FORMAT

CLASS INSTRUCTIONS

This is an optional heading at the beginning of each drug class. It consists of patient instructions that apply to more than one of the drug monographs in this subcategory. If all drugs are not identical in their instructions, only the common information is found here. The Patient Instructions section of each monograph that is affected states, *"See Class Instructions"* as the opening phrase.

GENERIC DRUG NAME   Brand Name(s)

The *nonproprietary (generic)* name is listed on the left, followed by common brand names listed on the right. Brand-name products listed are not necessarily superior or preferable to other brand-name or generic products; *"Various"* indicates the availability of additional brand and/or generic products.

Pharmacology. A description of the chemistry, major mechanisms of action, and human pharmacology of the drug in clinical application.

Administration and Adult Dosage. Route of administration, indications, and usual adult dosage range are given for the most common labeled uses. Dosages correspond to those in the product labeling or in standard reference sources. "Dose" refers to a single administration and "dosage" to a cumulative amount (e.g., daily dosage).

Special Populations. Dosages in patient populations other than the typical adult are listed:

Pediatric Dosage (given by age or weight range)

Geriatric Dosage (given by age range)

Other Conditions (renal failure, hepatic disease, obesity, etc.)

Dosage Forms. The most commonly used dosage forms and available strengths are listed, as well as popular combination product dosage forms. Prediluted IV piggyback or large-volume parenteral containers are not listed unless this is the only commercially available product.

Patient Instructions. Key information that should be provided to the patient when prescribing or dispensing medication is presented. When introductions apply to an entire drug category, see "Class Instructions" at the beginning of that subcategory.

Missed Doses. What the patient should do if one or more doses are missed.

Pharmacokinetics. Data are presented as the mean ± the standard deviation. Occasionally the standard error of the mean (SE) is the only information available on variability, and it is identified as such.

Onset and Duration (time course of the pharmacologic or therapeutic effect)

Serum Levels (therapeutic and toxic plasma concentrations are given)

Fate (The course of the drug in the body is traced. Pharmacokinetic parameters are generally provided as total body weight normalized values. The volume of distribution is either a V_d in a one-compartment system or V_c and $V_{d\beta}$ or V_{dss} in a two-compartment system.)

$t_{1/2}$ (terminal half-life is presented)

Adverse Reactions. Reactions known to be dose related are usually given first, then other reactions in decreasing order of frequency. Reaction frequency is classified into three ranges. However, percentages of reactions may be provided for reactions that occur more frequently than 1%.

frequent	(>1/100 patients)
occasional	(1/100 to 1/10,000 patients)
rare	(<1/10,000 patients)

Contraindications. Those listed in product labeling are given. "Hypersensitivity" is not listed as a contraindication because it is understood that patients should usually not be given a drug to which they are allergic or hypersensitive—exceptions are noted.

Precautions. Warnings for use of the drug in certain disease states and/or patient populations, together with any cross-sensitivity with other drugs. Part II, Section 2, "Drug Use in Special Populations," should be consulted for more information, particularly regarding pregnancy and breastfeeding.

Drug Interactions. The most important drug interactions are listed.

Parameters to Monitor. Important clinical signs and/or laboratory tests to monitor to ensure safe and effective use are presented. The frequency of monitoring may also be given; however, for many drugs the optimal frequency has not been determined.

Notes. Distinguishing characteristics, therapeutic usefulness, or relative efficacy of the drug are presented, as well as unique or noteworthy physicochemical properties, handling, storage, or relative cost.

PART I

Drug Monographs

Principal Editors: Daniel M. Riche and Nickole N. Henyan

Analgesic and Anti-Inflammatory Drugs

1

Daniel M. Riche

Chapter 1

Antimigraine Drugs

Toy S. Biederman

DIHYDROERGOTAMINE MESYLATE	D.H.E. 45, Migranal, Various

Pharmacology. Dihydroergotamine (DHE) is a semisynthetic ergot alkaloid that is hypothesized to exert its antimigraine effect via its agonist activity at the serotonin 5-HT$_{1D}$ receptor, resulting in vasoconstriction of intracranial blood vessels and inhibition of inflammatory neuropeptide release.[1] The drug also binds with high affinity to adrenergic and dopamine receptors; however, the antimigraine effect of these events is unknown. Compared with ergotamine, DHE is a weaker vasoconstrictor, is less active as an emetic, and is less oxytocic.

Administration and Adult Dosage. **IM, SQ for migraine and cluster headache**— 1 mg initially, then 1 mg every h as needed, to a maximum of 3 mg/d or 6 mg/wk. **IV for migraine and cluster headache** (for rapid effect)—0.5–1 mg, may repeat in 1 h to a maximum of 2 mg/d or 6 mg/wk. Consider administering metoclopramide 10 mg IV before DHE to treat nausea caused by migraine and prevent nausea caused by the drug.[2] **Intranasal for migraine**—1 spray (0.5 mg) into each nostril; may repeat in 15 min to a maximum of 2 mg over 24 h. The safety of doses greater than 3 mg/d or 4 mg/wk has not been established.[3]

Special Populations. *Pediatric Dosage.* Safety and efficacy not established.

Geriatric Dosage. Same as adult dosage.

Dosage Forms. **Inj** 1 mg/mL; **Nasal spray** 4 mg/mL.

Patient Instructions. This drug can cause numbness and tingling in fingers, toes, or face. Notify your physician if you are pregnant or have heart disease or high blood pressure. Do not exceed the maximum dosage. The nasal spray can cause local irritation. Do not reuse the applicator; use the solution right after opening and discard after 8 h. Review training materials with your health care provider and report the use of all cold or allergy medications and all over-the-counter (OTC) medications.

3

Pharmacokinetics. Onset is under 5 min IV, within 15–30 min after IM or intranasal spray; duration 3–4 h. Intranasal 50%–70% of patients respond in 4 h.

Fate. The drug is absorbed directly into the systemic circulation when administered intranasally, but it undergoes extensive first-pass metabolism if given orally. Bioavailability of the nasal spray is 38% ± 16%, variable depending on self-administration technique.[4] Protein binding is 93%. After administration of 1 mg, peak levels are 1 ± 0.4 μg/L (intranasal) and 4.4 μg/L (IM), occurring at 0.9 ± 0.6 h (intranasal) and 0.4 ± 0.3 h (IM).[4] After IM administration, V_c is 12 ± 4 L/kg and $V_{dβ}$ is 33 ± 0.2 L/kg, suggesting distribution into deep tissue compartments. Clearance is 1.6 ± 0.17 L/h/kg. The drug is metabolized to at least 4 metabolites, 3 of which are active. The major route of excretion for DHE and its metabolites is in the feces via the bile.[1] **Half-life** α phase (intranasal) 1 ± 0.5 h, (IM) 0.9 ± 0.3 h; β phase (intranasal) 7.9 ± 4 h, (IM) 7.2 ± 2.2 h.[4]

Adverse Reactions. The most frequently reported adverse events with intranasal administration are rhinitis, pharyngitis, altered sense of taste, application site reactions, nausea, vomiting, and dizziness. With all routes of administration, nausea, vomiting, diarrhea, and localized edema occur frequently.[2,3] Numbness and tingling of fingers and toes, muscle pain in extremities, weakness in legs, pruritus, rash, and infection occur occasionally. Pleural and retroperitoneal fibrosis occurs rarely with prolonged use.

Contraindications. Pregnancy and lactation; peripheral vascular disease; coronary artery disease; ischemic heart disease; hemiplegic or basilar migraine; sepsis; recent history of vascular surgery; severely impaired hepatic or renal function; hypersensitivity to ergot alkaloids. Any formulation of DHE is contraindicated with potent CYP 3A4 inhibitors (ritonavir, nelfinavir, indinavir, fosamprenavir, erythromycin, clarithromycin, troleandomycin, ketoconazole, itraconazole) because of vasospasm, which causes cerebral ischemia and ischemia of the extremities (black box warning). DHE should not be used within 24 h of other ergot-type medications, methysergide, or serotonin agonists/triptans.[1]

Precautions. Pregnancy category C. Use caution to avoid overuse by patients with chronic vascular headaches. Patients with risk factors for coronary artery disease should undergo periodic cardiovascular and cerebrovascular evaluation.

Drug Interactions. (*See* Contraindications and Ergotamine Tartrate.) DHE can antagonize the antianginal effects of nitrates. The risk of bleeding with warfarin (e.g., wound hematoma, anemia, hematuria) is worsened with coadministration of DHE. Macrolides including erythromycin can increase the risk of ergot toxicity. Sumatriptan can exacerbate coronary artery vasospasm and should not be taken within 24 h of DHE. SSRIs can cause weakness, hyperreflexia, or incoordination.

Notes. IV DHE is used when oral agents have failed to abort migraine and for terminating cluster or migraine headache in an emergency setting. It is not intended for prophylaxis or the management of hemiplegic or basilar migraine. The intranasal preparation is a noninvasive option for outpatients. Intranasal administration also results in improved bioavailability over the oral form because it does not undergo a first-pass effect in the liver. DHE does not cause physical dependence and is associated with a more favorable side effect profile than ergotamine, especially with regard to GI and peripheral vascular effects. In one study, SQ administered **sumatriptan** appeared to be more effective than DHE nasal spray; however, DHE was better tolerated.[5]

ERGOTAMINE TARTRATE
Ergomar

Pharmacology. Ergotamine is an ergot alkaloid that is hypothesized to exert its antimigraine effects via its agonist activity at the serotonin $5-HT_{1D}$ receptor, resulting in vasoconstriction of intracranial blood vessels and inhibition of inflammatory neuropeptide release. The drug also binds with high affinity to adrenergic receptors; however, the antimigraine effect of this binding is unknown. The mechanism in migraine is thought to be vasoconstriction of cranial blood vessels, with a concomitant decrease in the amplitude of pulsations as well as depression of serotonergic neurons that mediate pain.

Administration and Adult Dosage. SL for migraine and vascular headache— 2 mg initially, then 2 mg every 30 min as needed, to a maximum of 6 mg/d or 10 mg/wk.[6] Titrate the dosage during several attacks gradually, then administer the minimum effective dosage with subsequent attacks. Patients who routinely require over 2 mg/headache can be given the total effective dosage at the onset of the headache.

Special Populations. *Pediatric Dosage.* Safety and efficacy not established. (>12 years) 1 mg initially, then 1 mg every 30 min as needed, to a maximum of 3 mg/attack.

Other Conditions. Decrease dosage by 50% in patients receiving methysergide as prophylaxis.

Dosage Forms. SL Tab 2 mg.

Patient Instructions. Initiate therapy at the first signs of an attack. Take only as directed and do not exceed recommended dosages. Report tingling or pain in extremities immediately.

Pharmacokinetics. *Serum Levels.* 200 ng/L (176 pmol/L) or greater appears to be therapeutic; a high frequency of adverse reactions has been associated with levels >1.8 μg/L (1.5 nmol/L).[7] Onset (oral) 5 h.[7]

Fate. Bioavailability 1%–2% orally, 5% rectally; relative bioavailability decreases in the following order: PR > PO > SL.[7,8] Peak serum level after 2 mg rectally is 454 ± 407 ng/L (390 ± 350 pmol/L), 50 + 43 min after the dose. Peak serum level after 2 mg with caffeine 100 mg orally is 21 ± 12 ng/L (18 ± 11 pmol/L), 69 ± 191 min after the dose.[8] V_d is 1.9 ± 0.8 L/kg; clearance is 0.68 ± 0.24 L/h/kg.[7] The drug is extensively metabolized in the liver, with 90% of metabolites excreted in the bile. Half-life 1.9 ± 0.3 h; apparent half-life is 3.4 ± 1.9 h after rectal administration because of slow absorption.[5,6]

Adverse Reactions. Nausea, vomiting, visual disturbance, and muscle weakness occur frequently. Signs and symptoms of ergotamine intoxication include weakness in legs, coldness and muscle pain in extremities, numbness or tingling of fingers and toes, precordial pain, transient tachycardia or bradycardia, and localized edema; these rarely develop with recommended dosages. Frequent or worsening headaches can occur with frequent, long-term, or excessive dosages. Ergotamine dependence can result in withdrawal symptoms occurring within 24–48 h after drug discontinuation.[5]

Contraindications. Pregnancy category X; peripheral vascular disease; coronary artery disease; hypertension; hepatic or renal impairment; sepsis; severe pruritus, concomitant potent inhibitors of cytochrome P450 3A. (*See* Dihydroergotamine.)

Precautions. Lactation; avoid excessive dosage or prolonged administration because of the potential for ergotism and gangrene.

Drug Interactions. Dopamine and epinephrine can cause increased vasoconstriction and increased risk of peripheral ischemia or hypertension. β-Blockers, specifically propranolol, have been reported to potentiate the vasoconstrictive action of ergotamine tartrate/caffeine tablets by blocking the vasodilating property of epinephrine. The macrolides (especially erythromycin and troleandomycin), triazole antifungals, and protease inhibitors can inhibit the metabolism of ergot alkaloids.

Notes. The stimulant action of oral and rectal preparations containing **caffeine** (**Cafergot** tablets; **Migergot** suppositories) can keep patients from the beneficial effects of sleep. Caffeine, however, can improve dissolution of the oral formulation. Ergotamine is commonly used for abortive therapy of migraine and provides relief in 50%–90% of patients.[7] **Aspirin** (650 mg) or **naproxen** (750–1250 mg/d) might be effective in aborting migraine headache in mild cases or in patients who cannot take ergotamine. OTC products containing aspirin, **acetaminophen**, and caffeine (Excedrin Migraine) or **ibuprofen** (Advil Migraine, Motrin Migraine) have approval for mild to moderate migraine. Prescription combination products, such as **Midrin** and **Fiorinal**, might be useful, but overuse of any antimigraine combination product can lead to rebound headache. **NSAIDs** are useful for prophylaxis against menstrual-related migraines when taken during the perimenstrual period. **Butorphanol** spray might be beneficial for patients with infrequent, severe headaches who cannot tolerate ergot products or triptans, but frequent use can cause dependency. The β-blockers **propranolol** and **timolol** are approved for migraine prophylaxis, but other β-blockers without intrinsic sympathomimetic activity (e.g., **atenolol, nadolol**) are also useful. **Verapamil** can prevent migraines in some patients but can take several months to reach maximum effectiveness. **Tricyclic antidepressants** (e.g., **amitriptyline, nortriptyline**) have been more successful in migraine prophylaxis than SSRIs. **Divalproex** and **topiramate** are approved for migraine prophylaxis. (*See* Anticonvulsants.) Consider frequency of attacks (more than 2 attacks/mo), comorbid conditions, and side effects when choosing prophylactic therapy. Effective doses for migraine prophylaxis drugs are usually lower than those used for other indications.[9]

SUMATRIPTAN SUCCINATE   Imitrex

Pharmacology. Sumatriptan is a serotonin (5-HT) analogue and a selective agonist at 5-HT$_{1D}$ receptors in cerebral vascular smooth muscle. Receptor activation results in migraine relief by vasoconstriction of intracranial blood vessels and attenuation of the release of vasoactive peptides responsible for inflammation of sensory nerves.[10] (*See* Selective Serotonin Agonists Comparison Chart.)

Administration and Adult Dosage. **PO for migraine**—25–100 mg; a second dose of up to 100 mg may be administered in 2 h, if response is unsatisfactory. A 100-mg dose may not provide any greater effect than a 50-mg dose. If headache returns, additional doses may be given every 2 h, up to 200 mg in a 24-h period. **SQ for**

migraine and cluster headache—6 mg; a second 6 mg injection may be administered 1 h after the initial dose, but limited to no more than 2 injections within a 24-h period. Controlled studies have not verified a beneficial effect of a second dose. **Intranasal for migraine**—5–20 mg in one nostril or 5 mg in each nostril; may repeat in 2 h to a maximum of 40 mg/d.

Special Populations. *Pediatric Dosage.* (<18 years) Safety and efficacy not established. Trials of oral and nasal sumatriptan in adolescents have not shown efficacy compared with placebo.[11]

Geriatric Dosage. Not recommended due to the higher risk of coronary artery disease and more pronounced blood pressure increases, and due to the decreased hepatic function in this population.[11]

Dosage Forms. **Tab** 25, 50, 100 mg; **Inj** 4 mg/0.5 mL, 6 mg/0.5 mL; **Nasal spray** 5, 20 mg.

Patient Instructions. Sumatriptan is used for relief of migraine and not for the prevention of a migraine attack. Do not take this drug if you are pregnant without consulting with your physician. Inform your physician if you have high blood pressure, diabetes, seizures, heart, liver, or kidney disease, or if you are a smoker. Report pain or tightness in chest, shortness of breath, wheezing, or rash immediately. **PO**—do not take more than 200 mg within 24 h and allow at least 2 h after the first tablet.[11] **SQ injection**—do not take more than 2 injections within 24 h and allow at least 1 h between injections. Pain or redness at injection site lasts less than 1 h.[10] **Nasal spray**—if 1 dose does not provide adequate relief, you may take another dose after 2 h. Do not take more than 40 mg in 1 day.[12]

Pharmacokinetics. PO—50%–62% of patients respond in 2 h; peak 1.5 h.[11] SQ—73% of patients respond within 1 h and 70% within 2 h; peak 12 min.[10] Intranasal—50%–64% of patients respond in 2 h.[12]

Fate. Oral bioavailability is 14% ± 3% owing to presystemic metabolism and erratic absorption. Absorption is delayed by approximately 0.5 h if taken with food. After a 100-mg oral dose, a peak of 54 μg/L (180 nmol/L) occurs in approximately 1.5 h. SQ bioavailability is 97% ± 16%; a peak of 74 μg/L (250 nmol/L) occurs in 12 min after a 6-mg SQ dose. After a 20-mg intranasal dose, the mean peak is 16 μg/L (54 nmol/L). Plasma protein binding is 14%–21%. V_d is 2.7 L/kg; clearance is 0.96 ± 0.12 L/h/kg. Hepatic metabolism is carried out by MAO-A to an indole acetic acid, followed by glucuronidation and renal elimination. Approximately 40% is found in the feces and 60% is excreted renally, 22% unchanged, and 40% as the active indole acetic acid metabolite.[13,14] **Half-life** 1.9 ± 0.3 h.[10]

Adverse Reactions. Frequent side effects are pain and redness at SQ injection site, tingling, hot flushes, dizziness, and chest tightness or heaviness. With the nasal spray, throat discomfort and unusual taste occur frequently. With all routes of administration, occasional weakness, myalgia, burning sensation, tightness in chest, transient hypertension, drowsiness, headache, numbness, neck pain, abdominal discomfort, mouth/jaw discomfort, and sweating occur. Rarely, cardiac arrhythmias, myocardial ischemia, polydipsia, dehydration, dyspnea, skin rashes, dysuria, and dysmenorrhea occur. Sumatriptan can accumulate in melanin-rich tissues such as the eye with long-term use. Several cases of ischemic colitis have been reported after sumatriptan use.

Contraindications. IV administration; history or symptoms of ischemic cardiac, cerebrovascular, or peripheral vascular disease; Prinzmetal's angina; uncontrolled hypertension; concurrent administration of MAO inhibitors or within 2 weeks of discontinuation; within 24 h of an ergotamine-containing drug or ergot derivative such as DHE or another serotonin agonist; hemiplegic or basilar migraine; severe hepatic impairment; hypersensitivity to sumatriptan or any component of the product. Sumatriptan is not recommended for anyone at high risk of undiagnosed coronary artery disease (e.g., hypertension, hypercholesterolemia, smoker, postmenopausal women, men older than 40 years).[10]

Precautions. Pregnancy. Use with caution in those with impaired hepatic function, seizure disorder, or neurologic lesion. Sumatriptan is not recommended for anyone at high risk of undiagnosed coronary artery disease due to the presence of risk factors (hypertension, hypercholesterolemia, smoker, postmenopausal women, men older than 40 years).

Drug Interactions. Nonselective MAO inhibitors or MAO-A inhibitors can increase the systemic availability of sumatriptan (especially after oral administration). Theoretically, ergot alkaloids and sumatriptan can cause prolonged vasospastic reactions if used together. (*See* Contraindications.) SSRIs may cause weakness, hyperreflexia, incoordination, and other symptoms of serotonin syndrome when given with sumatriptan and other triptans.

Parameters to Monitor. The manufacturer encourages registration of pregnant patients (Sumatriptan Pregnancy Registry) to monitor fetal outcomes of women exposed to sumatriptan (800) 336–2176.[10]

Notes. Available in combination with naproxen (Treximet).

SELECTIVE SEROTONIN AGONISTS COMPARISON CHART

DRUG	DOSAGE FORMS	ADULT DOSAGE	ONSET (h)	HALF-LIFE (h)	COMMENTS
Almotriptan Axert	Tab 6.25, 12.5 mg	PO 6.25–12.5 mg; may repeat in 2 h, to maximum of 25 mg/d	1–2	3–4	Low headache recurrence rate. Similar efficacy to oral sumatriptan, but better tolerated. No propranolol interaction. AUC increased by CYP3A4 inhibitors. Use lower dose in severe renal impairment.
Eletriptan Relpax	Tab 20, 40 mg	PO 20–40 mg; may repeat in 2 h, to maximum of 80 mg/d	1–2	4	Do not use within 72 h of potent CYP3A4 inhibitors: ketoconazole, itraconazole, nefazodone, troleandomycin, clarithromycin, ritonavir, nelfinavir.
Frovatriptan Frova	Tab 2.5 mg	PO 2.5 mg; may repeat in 2 h, to a maximum of 7.5 mg/d	2–4	26	Lowest recurrence rate. AUC increased 30% by oral contraceptives, 24%–60% by propranolol; decreased 25% by ergotamine. AUC increased 50%–100% in elderly.
Naratriptan Amerge	Tab 1, 2.5 mg	PO 1–2.5 mg may repeat once in 4 h, to a maximum of 5 mg/d	1–3	6	Low headache recurrence rate. More specific than other agents for 5HT$_{1B}$. Smoking increases and oral contraceptives decrease clearance. Contraindicated in severe renal or hepatic impairment.
Rizatriptan Maxalt Maxalt-MLT	Tab and dissolving Tab 5, 10 mg	PO 5–10 mg; may repeat in 2 h, to a maximum of 30 mg/d	0.5–2	2–3	Onset of rapidly dissolving tablet is slightly *slower* than conventional. Reduce dose when used with propranolol (5 mg initially; 15 mg/d maximum). Contraindicated in patients taking MAO inhibitors.

(continued)

9

SELECTIVE SEROTONIN AGONISTS COMPARISON CHART (*continued*)

DRUG	DOSAGE FORMS	ADULT DOSAGE	ONSET (h)	HALF-LIFE (h)	COMMENTS
Sumatriptan Imitrex	Inj 6 mg Tab 25, 50, 100 mg Nasal spray 5, 20 mg/spray	SQ 6 mg; may repeat once in 1 h, to a maximum of 12 mg/d PO 25–100 mg; may repeat every 2 h, to a maximum of 200 mg/d Nasal 5–20 mg; may repeat once in 2 h, to a maximum of 40 mg/d	0.2 (SQ) 0.5–1 (PO) <1 (nasal)	2.5	Headache recurrence rate of 40%; relatively high (5%) frequency of chest pain and tightness. Maximum oral dose 100 mg if patient received initial SQ dose. Contraindicated in patients taking MAO inhibitors.
Sumatriptan/Naproxen Treximet	85 mg (as 119 mg sumatriptan succinate) with naproxen sodium 500 mg	1 tablet; may repeat in 2 h, to a maximum of 2 tablets/d	0.5–1	2.5	*See monograph.*
Zolmitriptan Zomig Zomig-ZMT	Tab and dissolving Tab 2.5, 5 mg Nasal spray 5 mg/spray	PO 2.5–5 mg Spray 5 mg; may repeat once (tablet or spray) in 2 h, to a maximum of 10 mg/d	0.5–2	3	Onset of rapidly dissolving tablet is slightly *slower* than conventional. Cimetidine or oral contraceptives increase AUC by 50%. Contraindicated in patients taking MAO-A inhibitors.

From Refs. 9 and 12–14 and product information.

■ REFERENCES

1. Product Information: D. H.E.45®, Dihydroergotamine mesylate. East Hanover, NJ: Novartis Pharmaceuticals Corporation; 2001.
2. Bigal MJ, Tepper SJ. Ergotamine and dihydroergotamine: a review. *Curr Pain Headache Rep*. 2003;7:55-62.
3. Product Information: Migranal®, Dihydroergotamine mesylate. Aliso Viejo, CA: Valeant Pharmaceuticals North America; 2007.
4. Humbert H et al. Human pharmacokinetics of dihydroergotamine administered by nasal spray. *Clin Pharmacol Ther*. 1996;60:265-275.
5. Touchon J et al. A comparison of subcutaneous sumatriptan and dihydroergotamine nasal spray in the acute treatment of migraine. *Neurology*. 1996;47:361-365.
6. Perrin VL. Clinical pharmacokinetics of ergotamine in migraine and cluster headache. *Clin Pharmacokinet*. 1985;10:334-352.
7. Sanders SM et al. Pharmacokinetics of ergotamine in healthy volunteers following oral and rectal dosing. *Eur J Clin Pharmacol*. 1986;30:331-334.
8. Ibraheem JJ et al. Kinetics of ergotamine after intravenous and intramuscular administration to migraine sufferers. *Eur J Clin Pharmacol*. 1982;23:235-240.
9. Rapoport AM. Acute and prophylactic treatments for migraine: present and future. *Neurol Sci*. 2008;29:S110-S122.
10. Product Information: Imitrex Injection®, sumatriptan succinate. Research Triangle Park, NC: GlaxoSmithKline; 2007.
11. Product Information: Imitrex tablets®, sumatriptan succinate. Research Triangle Park, NC: GlaxoSmithKline; 2007.
12. Product Information: Imitrex Nasal Spray®, sumatriptan. Research Triangle Park, NC: GlaxoSmithKline; 2007.
13. Fowler PA et al. The clinical pharmacology, pharmacokinetics and metabolism of sumatriptan. *Eur Neurol*. 1991;31:291-294.
14. Dixon CM et al. Disposition of sumatriptan in laboratory animals and humans. *Drug Metab Dispos Biol Fate Chem*. 1993;21:761-769.

Chapter 2

Antirheumatic Drugs

Danial E. Baker and Stephen M. Setter

ABATACEPT   Orencia

Pharmacology. Abatacept inhibits T cell (T lymphocyte) activation by binding to CD80 and CD86, thereby blocking interaction with CD28. By modulating this activity, the costimulatory signal necessary for full activation of T lymphocytes is not available. In vitro, abatacept decreases T lymphocyte product and inhibits the production of cytokines [e.g., TNF alpha (TNFα), interferon-γ, and interleukin-2]. Abatacept is indicated for the treatment of adult rheumatoid arthritis alone or concomitantly with disease-modifying antirheumatic drugs (DMARDs) other than TNF antagonists and children (6 years of age and older) with moderately to severely active polyarticular juvenile arthritis alone or concomitantly with methotrexate.

Administration and Adult Dosage. **IV for rheumatoid arthritis**—dosing is weight based. Administration is 30 min. The dose of adult patients weighing <60 kg is 500 mg; 60–100 kg is 750 mg; and >100 kg is 1000 mg.

Special Populations. *Pediatric Dosage.* Children <75 kg are given 10 mg/kg and those weighing 75 kg or more should be dosed using the adult recommendations, not to exceed a maximum dose of 1000 mg. All children should be 6 years and older.

Geriatric Dosage. Same as adult dosage.

Dosage Forms. **Inj** 250 mg vials.

Patient Instructions. Prior to starting treatment they should be evaluated and tested for tuberculosis. Once therapy is started they should seek medical attention if they develop persistent cough, wasting, weight loss, low-grade fever; signs and symptoms of infection; or pregnancy.

Missed Doses. Give a missed dose as soon as possible and resume usual schedule.

Pharmacokinetics. *Fate.* Mean clearance is 0.22 mL/h/kg. **Half-life** 13.1 days.

Adverse Reactions. Headache, upper respiratory tract infections, nasopharyngitis, and nausea occurred in at least 10% of the patients treated with abatacept.[1] More serious adverse effects, such as infectious disease and acute exacerbation of COPD, also commonly occur. Cancer risk is approximately 1.3%.

Contraindications. None.

Precautions. Serious infection, hypersensitivity, anaphylaxis, and anaphylactoid reactions, history of recurrent infections or underlying conditions, predisposing to infections may experience more infections, COPD patients may develop more frequent respiratory adverse events, and patients with juvenile idiopathic arthritis should be brought up to date with all immunizations prior to therapy.

Parameters to Monitor. Monitor patients closely for infection. Discontinue treatment if serious infection or hypersensitivity reaction occurred.

Drug Interactions. Live vaccines should not be given concurrently with or within 3 months of abatacept administration. The effectiveness of some immunizations may be blunted by abatacept effects on the immune system. Concurrent administration of a TNF antagonist with abatacept has been associated with an increased risk of serious infections and no significant additional efficacy over use of the TNF antagonists alone. Concurrently with other biologic RA therapy, such as anakinra, it is not recommended until more safety and efficacy data are available. Abatacept infusion can interfere with the readings of blood glucose monitors that use test strips with glucose dehydrogenase pyrroloquinolinequinone (GDH-PQQ) on the day administration.

Notes. Abatacept must be refrigerated at 2°C–8°C (38°F–46°F) and protected from light.[1]

ADALIMUMAB   Humira

Pharmacology. Adalimumab binds to TNFα and blocks its interaction with p55 and p75 TNF receptors on the cell surface. This reduces the signs and symptoms of various arthritic conditions. It is indicated for adults with moderately to severely active rheumatoid arthritis, alone or in combination with methotrexate or other disease-modifying antirheumatic drugs; juvenile idiopathic arthritis; ankylosing spondylitis; Crohn's disease; and plaque psoriasis.

Administration and Adult Dosage. SQ for rheumatoid arthritis, psoriatic arthritis, and ankylosing spondylitis—40 mg every other week. SQ for Crohn's disease—160 mg initially (given as four 40 mg injections in 1 day or as two 40 mg injections/d for 2 consecutive days), followed by 80 mg in 2 weeks (day 15). Subsequent injections beginning on day 29—40 mg every other week should be given. SQ for plaque psoriasis—initial dose is 80 mg, followed by 40 mg every other week (use beyond 1 year had not been evaluated).

Special Populations. *Pediatric Dosage.* SQ for juvenile idiopathic arthritis. Weight-based dosing in children 4–17 years of age (15–30 kg = 20 mg every other week; ≥30 kg = 40 mg every other week).

Geriatric Dosage. Same as adult dosage.

Dosage Forms. Inj pen 40 mg; prefilled syringe 20 mg and 40 mg.

Patient Instructions. This drug may be self-administered. Instruct patient on proper injection preparation and subcutaneous injection technique along with appropriate syringe and needle disposal methods. Rotate injection sites and avoid areas where the skin is tender, bruised, red, or hard. Prior to starting treatment, patients should be evaluated and tested for tuberculosis. Once therapy is started, patients should seek medical attention if they develop persistent cough, wasting, weight loss, low-grade fever, or signs and symptoms of infection.

Missed Doses. Give a missed dose as soon as possible and resume usual schedule.

Pharmacokinetics. *Fate.* Bioavailability with SQ injection is 64%, with peak plasma concentrations achieved within 131 ± 56 h.[2] Mean clearance is 12 mL/h.[2] **Half-Life** 2 weeks (ranges from 10 to 20 days).[2]

Adverse Reactions. Injection site reactions may involve erythema, itching, hemorrhage, pain, or swelling (20% vs. 14% with placebo).[2] Other adverse reactions include clinical flare, rash, infections, tuberculosis and opportunistic infections, malignancies, autoantibodies, and immunogenicity.

Contraindications. None.

Precautions. Serious infection, sepsis, tuberculosis, and cases of opportunistic infections have been reported in patients treated with TNF-blocking agents. Treatment should not be initiated in patients with active infections.

Parameters to Monitor. Monitor patients closely for infection and hematologic abnormalities during therapy. Discontinue treatment if serious infection, sepsis, or hematologic abnormality develops.

Drug Interactions. Concurrent use with anakinra is not recommended because there is an increased risk of serious infections and neutropenia with no additional therapeutic benefit associated with the combination. Live vaccines should be avoided. Methotrexate may decrease the clearance of adalimumab.

Notes. Adalimumab must be refrigerated at 2°C–8°C (38°F–46°F) and protected from light; do not freeze.[2]

ANAKINRA   Kineret

Pharmacology. Anakinra is a recombinant, nonglycosylated form of the human interleukin-1 receptor antagonist (IL-1Ra). It blocks the biologic activity of IL-1 at the interleukin-1 type I receptor and results in a reduction in inflammatory and immunological responses. It is indicated for the reduction in signs and symptoms and slowing the progression of structural damage in moderately to severely active rheumatoid arthritis, in patients 18 years of age or older who have failed 1 or more DMARDs. It can be used alone or in combination with DMARDs other than TNF-blocking agents.

Administration and Adult Dosage. **SQ for rheumatoid arthritis**—100 mg/d. Higher doses do not demonstrate any improvement in the response rate.

Special Populations. *Pediatric Dosage.* Not recommended. The prefilled syringes do not permit accurate dosing lower than 100 mg and safety and efficacy has not been established in this patient population. The dose proven safe in an investigational trial for the treatment of polyarticular course juvenile rheumatoid arthritis (ages 2–17 years) was 1 mg/kg SQ daily, up to a maximum dose of 100 mg.[3]

Geriatric Dosage. Same as adult dosage; elderly patients may be at a higher risk of infection and the dose may need to be altered based on the patient's renal function.

Renal Impairment. Patients who have severe renal insufficiency or end-stage renal disease ($Cl_{Cr} < 30$ mL/min) may be given 100 mg every other day.

Dosage Forms. Single-use, prefilled syringes—0.67 mL (100 mg) of anakinra.

Patient Instructions. This drug may be self-administered. Instruct patient on proper injection preparation and subcutaneous injection technique along with appropriate syringe and needle disposal methods. Rotate injection sites (outer area of the upper arms, abdomen, front of the middle thighs, and upper outer areas of the buttocks) and avoid areas where the skin is tender, bruised, red, or hard.

Patients should consult their prescriber if they develop signs and symptoms of a serious infection.

Missed Doses. Give a missed dose as soon as possible and resume usual schedule.

Pharmacokinetics. *Fate.* Bioavailability with SQ injection is 95% with peak plasma concentrations achieved within 3–7 h. **Half-life** 4–6 h.[4] Clearance is influenced by renal function. Adjustments in the dosing schedule may be necessary in patients with severe renal insufficiency or end-stage renal disease.

Adverse Reactions. Injection site reactions are the most common adverse reactions; may include redness, swelling, bruising, itching, and stinging. Most injection site reactions are mild and last approximately 2–4 weeks. Other common adverse reactions include infections, worsening of their arthritis, headache, nausea, diarrhea, sinusitis, arthralgia, and abdominal pain.

Contraindications. Hypersensitivity to *Escherichia coli*-derived proteins, anakinra, or any components of the product.

Precautions. Infections—drug should be discontinued if the patient develops a serious infection and therapy should not be initiated in patients with active infections. Concomitant use with any TNF antagonist is not recommended because there is an increased risk of serious infections. Impact on active and/or chronic infections and the development of malignancies is unknown.

Parameters to Monitor. Monitor patients closely for infection and hematologic abnormalities during therapy. Discontinue treatment if serious infection, sepsis, or hematologic abnormality develops.

Drug Interactions. Concurrent use of anakinra with any TNF antagonist is not recommended because there is an increased risk of infections and neutropenia with no additional therapeutic benefit. Live vaccines should be avoided and information on the impact of anakinra on other types of vaccines is unknown.

Notes. Anakinra must be refrigerated at 2°C–8°C (36°F–46°F) and protected from light; do not freeze OR shake.[4]

ETANERCEPT	Enbrel

Pharmacology. Etanercept is a dimeric fusion protein that binds to tumor necrosis factor (TNFα and β) and blocks its interaction with TNF receptors on the cell surface. This reduces the signs and symptoms of rheumatoid arthritis and delays joint damage in adults with moderate to severe rheumatoid arthritis. It is indicated for reducing signs and symptoms, inducing major clinical response, inhibiting the progression of structural damage, or improving physical function in patients with moderately to severely active rheumatoid arthritis, active rheumatoid arthritis, and psoriatic arthritis. It can be initiated in combination with methotrexate or used alone. It is indicated for reducing signs and symptoms of moderately to severely active polyarticular juvenile idiopathic arthritis in patients aging 2 years and older. It is also approved for reducing signs and symptoms in patients with active ankylosing spondylitis and in the treatment of adult patients with chronic moderate to severe plaque psoriasis who are candidates for systemic therapy or phototherapy.

Administration and Adult Dosage. **SQ for rheumatoid arthritis, psoriatic arthritis, or ankylosing spondylitis**—50 mg/wk. **SQ for plaque psoriasis**—50 mg twice weekly (administered 3 or 4 days apart) for 3 months followed by a mainte-nance dose of 50 mg/wk; starting dose may be 25–50 mg/wk.

Special Populations. *Pediatric Dosage.* **SQ for polyarticular-course juvenile idiopathic arthritis**—ages ≥2 years—0.8 mg/kg/wk up to a maximum of 50 mg/wk.

Geriatric Dosage. Same as adult dosage.

Dosage Forms. **Inj** 25 mg, 50 mg; single-use prefilled syringe, prefilled autoin-jector, and multidose vials.

Patient Instructions. This drug may be self-administered. Instruct patient on proper injection preparation and subcutaneous injection technique along with appropriate syringe and needle disposal methods. Rotate the injection sites and give injections at least 1 in. from an old site. Avoid tender, bruised, red, or hard areas. Inform your physician immediately of any persistent fever, bruising, bleed-ing, or pallor. Prior to starting treatment patients should be evaluated and tested for tuberculosis. Once therapy is started they should seek medical attention if they develop persistent cough, wasting, weight loss, low-grade fever, or signs and symptoms of infection. (*See* Notes.)

Missed Doses. Injections should be given 3 or 4 days apart. Give a missed dose as soon as possible and resume usual schedule.

Pharmacokinetics. *Fate.* Bioavailability with SQ injection is 58%, with peak plasma concentrations achieved within 48–96 h. Clearance is 160 mL/h. **Half-life** 102 ± 30 h.

Adverse Reactions. Injection site reactions that involve mild to moderate ery-thema, itching, pain, or swelling occur in approximately 37% of patients. Upper respiratory infections, headache, rhinitis, dizziness, pharyngitis, and cough occur frequently. Etanercept is well tolerated in children with juvenile rheumatoid arthritis with adverse reactions similar to those experienced by adults. Rare cases of CNS demyelinating disorders, malignancies, and pancytopenia have been reported.

Contraindications. Sepsis or known hypersensitivity to etanercept or any of its components.

Precautions. Serious infection, sepsis, tuberculosis, reactivation of hepatitis B virus, and cases of opportunistic infections have been reported in patients treated with TNF-blocking agents. Treatment should not be initiated in patients with active infections. Do not administer to patients with active infections or children with significant exposure to varicella virus. In patients with juvenile rheumatoid arthritis exposed to varicella zoster, temporarily discontinue etanercept and give varicella zoster immunoglobulin. Update vaccinations before initiating etanercept therapy. Do not give live vaccines during etanercept therapy. The needle cover provided with the diluent syringe contains latex and should not be handled by those with latex allergy. Administer with caution to patients with recent history of CNS demyelinating disorders.

Parameters to Monitor. Monitor patients closely for infection and hematologic abnormalities during therapy. Discontinue treatment if serious infection, sepsis, or hematologic abnormality develops.

Drug Interactions. Risk of serious infections may be increased when used concomitantly with anakinra. Concurrent use with cyclophosphamide is not recommended because of a potential increase in the incidence of noncutaneous solid malignancies. A decrease in mean neutrophil count may occur with concurrent use of sulfasalazine.

Notes. Etanercept sterile powder must be refrigerated at 2°C–8°C (38°F–46°F); do not freeze. Reconstitute 25 mg vial with 1 mL of bacteriostatic sterile water (included); inject diluent slowly to avoid foaming. Administer the solution as soon as possible after reconstitution; however, the solution may be stored under refrigeration for up to 6 h in the vial. Prefilled syringes and devices may not be useful in pediatric patients weighing <31 kg. Etanercept may be used concurrently with other rheumatoid arthritis therapies such as analgesics, NSAIDs, salicylates, corticosteroids, or methotrexate.[5,6]

INFLIXIMAB	Remicade

Pharmacology. Infliximab is a chimeric monoclonal antibody that binds to soluble and transmembrane forms of TNFα, thereby neutralizing the activity of TNFα and inhibiting TNFα binding to its receptor sites. It has no effect on lymphotoxin (TNFβ).[5] Infliximab induces proinflammatory cytokines including interleukins 1 and 6 and increases endothelial cell permeability by enhancing leukocyte migration. It is indicated for reducing signs and symptoms, inhibiting the progression of structural damage, and improving physical function in patients with moderately to severely active rheumatoid arthritis; reducing signs and symptoms and inducing and maintaining clinical remission in adult and pediatric patients with moderately to severely active Crohn's disease who have had an inadequate response to conventional therapy; reducing signs and symptoms in patients with active ankylosing spondylitis; reducing signs and symptoms of active arthritis, inhibiting the progression of structural damage, and improving physical function in patients with psoriatic arthritis; treatment of adult patients with chronic severe (i.e., extensive and/or disabling) plaque psoriasis who are candidates for systemic therapy and when other systemic therapies are medically less appropriate; and reducing signs and symptoms, inducing and maintaining clinical remission and mucosal healing, and eliminating corticosteroid use in patients with moderately to severely active ulcerative colitis who have had an inadequate response to conventional therapy.

Administration and Adult Dosage. **IV for rheumatoid arthritis**—2-h infusion of 3 mg/kg, with repeat infusions at weeks 2 and 6, then every 8 weeks thereafter; should be used with concomitant methotrexate. Dose may be increased up to 10 mg/kg OR administered as often as every 4 weeks. **IV for moderately to severely active or fistulizing Crohn's disease, psoriatic arthritis, plaque psoriasis, and ulcerative colitis**—induction regimen–5 mg/kg IV infusion at 0, 2, and 6 weeks followed by maintenance dose of 5 mg/kg every 8 weeks. **IV for ankylosing spondylitis**—5 mg/kg at 0, 2, and 6 weeks followed by 5 mg/kg every 6 weeks. (*See* Notes.)

Special Populations. *Pediatric Dosage.* **IV for moderately to severely active Crohn's disease**—5 mg/kg infusion at 0, 2, and 6 weeks followed by 5 mg/kg every 8 weeks.

Geriatric Dosage. Same as adult dosage.

Dosage Forms. Inj 100 mg.

Patient Instructions. Infliximab is administered intravenously by your health care professional. Notify your physician if chest pain, fever, chills, facial flushing, itching, hives, or difficult breathing occurs within a few hours of administration. Prior to starting treatment, patients should be evaluated and tested for tuberculosis. Once therapy is started they should seek medical attention if they develop persistent cough, wasting, weight loss, low-grade fever, or signs and symptoms of infection.

Pharmacokinetics. *Fate.* Infliximab is distributed primarily within the vascular compartment. Direct and linear relationship between dose, maximum serum concentration, and AUC. Age and weight do not affect Cl or V_d. No systemic accumulation of infliximab occurs. **Half-life** 7.7–9.5 days.

Adverse Reactions. Serious infections have been reported. Infusion-related reactions such as fever, chills, pruritus, urticaria, chest pain, hypotension, hypertension, and dyspnea have occurred during or within the 2-h postinfusion period. If these reactions occur, slow the infusion rate. Reactions occurring in ≥5% of patients include headache, nausea, abdominal pain, fatigue, fever, pharyngitis, vomiting, pain, dizziness, bronchitis, rash, rhinitis, chest pain, coughing, pruritus, sinusitis, myalgia, and back pain. Hypersensitivity reactions to infliximab can occur and antibodies to infliximab develop in 10%–15% of patients. Patients most likely to experience infusion-related reactions are those who developed antibodies.[5] Have medications (e.g., acetaminophen, antihistamine, corticosteroid, and epinephrine) available for immediate use in the event of a hypersensitivity reaction. Lupus-like syndrome and lymphoproliferative disorders rarely occur.[6]

Contraindications. Hypersensitivity to murine proteins; presence of serious infection.

Precautions. Serious infection, sepsis, tuberculosis, reactivation of hepatitis B virus, and cases of opportunistic infections have been reported in patients treated with TNF-blocking agents. Treatment should not be initiated in patients with active infections. Women should use adequate contraception for the duration of and at least 6 months after therapy.[5] Avoid use in patients with known GI luminal strictures.[5]

Parameters to Monitor. Monitor patients closely for adverse effects, especially for infusion-related reactions during or within the 2-h postinfusion period and for infection during therapy. (Crohn's disease) Observe for improvement in abdominal cramping and in bowel consistence and rectal bleeding.

Drug Interactions. None known.

Notes. Dilute the total volume of the reconstituted infliximab solution dose to 250 mL with 0.9% NaCl. Gently mix. Administer over at least 2 h through a nonpyrogenic, low protein-binding filter with a pore size of ≤1.2 μm.

LEFLUNOMIDE	Arava

Pharmacology. Leflunomide's active metabolite (M1) inhibits dihydroorotate dehydrogenase, thereby inhibiting pyrimidine biosynthesis. M1 exhibits immunomodulating and anti-inflammatory effects. It is indicated for the treatment of active rheumatoid arthritis to reduce signs and symptoms, inhibit structural damage, and improve physical function alone or in combination with NSAIDs, corticosteroids, or aspirin.

Administration and Adult Dosage. **PO for rheumatoid arthritis**—100 mg/d for 3 days, then 20 mg/d. If 20 mg/d is not tolerated, reduce dose to 10 mg/d.

Special Populations. *Pediatric Dosage.* Safety and efficacy not been fully established. It has been used to treat children with polyarticular course juvenile rheumatoid arthritis. The drug was useful in improving the signs and symptoms of the disease, but the response was less robust in those patients weighing <40 kg.

Geriatric Dosage. Same as adult dosage.

Dosage Forms. **Tab** 10, 20, 100 mg.

Patient Instructions. Do not use if you are pregnant or planning to become pregnant. Men should use condoms because leflunomide can cause birth defects. Also, men planning on fathering children should discontinue leflunomide therapy and consult with their physicians. If you experience any major medical problems while on therapy, notify your physician. Avoid alcohol because this medication with alcohol can increase the risk of liver damage. Avoid immunizations unless approved by your physician.

Missed Doses. Take a missed dose as soon as you remember; if it is near the time for next dose, skip the dose; do not take a double dose.

Pharmacokinetics. *Fate.* Leflunomide is 80% bioavailable, with peak plasma levels achieved in 6–12 h. Because of its long half-life, an oral loading dosage is given over 3 days. Leflunomide is metabolized to a primary active M1, with the parent drug rarely detectable in plasma. The specific site of metabolism is unknown; however, hepatic cytosolic and microsomal cellular fractions have been identified. V_{dss} of M1 is 0.13 L/kg; 99.3% is bound to albumin. M1 is eliminated by renal and biliary routes. Approximately 45% is eliminated as glucuronide and oxanilic acid metabolites in the urine and 48% as M1 in the feces. **Half-life** M1— 18 ± 9 days.

Adverse Reactions. Diarrhea, dyspepsia, hypertension, headache, rash, alopecia, and elevated liver function tests occur frequently. (*See* Notes.)

Contraindications. Immunocompromised patients; those positive for hepatitis B or C; preexisting hepatic impairment; women planning to conceive or who are not using reliable contraception; known hypersensitivity to the drug or any of the other components.

Precautions. Caution in patients with renal insufficiency. Do not give live vaccines to patients receiving leflunomide. Patients developing new onset or worsening pulmonary symptoms (e.g., cough and dyspnea) with or without associated fever should be evaluated for interstitial lung disease and possible drug discontinuation. Rare cases of Stevens-Johnson syndrome and toxic epidermal necrolysis have been reported.

Drug Interactions. Potentially hepatotoxic medications such as methotrexate can increase risk of hepatotoxicity. Rifampin increases peak plasma levels of M1. M1 inhibits CYP2C9. Plasma-free fraction of NSAIDs and tolbutamide levels might be increased. Increased INR may occur with warfarin. Coadministration with cholestyramine or activated charcoal decreases M1 levels.

Parameters to Monitor. Monitor ALT at baseline and then monthly during the first 6 months. If ALT levels are stable, then every 6–8 weeks. Platelet, white blood cell count, and hemoglobin or hematocrit monitored at baseline and monthly for 6 months following initiation of therapy and every 6–8 weeks thereafter. Patients receiving concomitant methotrexate and other immunosuppressants should be screened for bone marrow suppression monthly.

Notes. If toxicity develops or if plasma levels must be decreased quickly, follow this drug elimination protocol: administer cholestyramine 8 g 3 times daily for 11 days. Verify that plasma levels are <0.02 mg/L by 2 separate tests at least 14 days apart. Without this procedure, drug elimination can take up to 2 years. Leflunomide is equally or more effective than traditional antirheumatic agents such as methotrexate, sulfasalazine, injectable gold, and cyclosporine.[5,6]

ANTIRHEUMATIC DRUGS COMPARISON CHART

DRUG	DOSAGE FORMS	ADULT DOSAGE	ADVERSE EFFECTS	LABORATORY MONITORING
Abatacept Orencia	Inj 250 mg	*See monograph.*	Headache, upper respiratory tract infections, nasopharyngitis, and nausea.	TB infection.
Adalimumab Humira	Inj Pen 40 mg Prefilled syringe 20 mg and 40 mg	*See monograph.*	Injection site reactions may involve erythema, itching, hemorrhage, pain, or swelling; clinical flare, rash, infections, tuberculosis and opportunistic infections, malignancies, autoantibodies, and immunogenicity.	TB and HBV infection.
Anakinra Kineret	Inj 100 mg	100 SC mg/d.	Injection site reactions (redness, swelling, bruising, itching, and stinging), infections, worsening of their arthritis, headache, nausea, diarrhea, sinusitis, arthralgia, and abdominal pain.	Infections Neutrophil counts monthly for 3 mo followed by quarterly for 1 yr.
Auranofin Ridaura	Cap 3 mg	PO 3–9 mg/d (3 mg as a single dose and 6 and 9 mg/d as 2 and 3 divided doses, respectively).	Loose stools, diarrhea, abdominal pain or cramping, rash, pruritus, stomatitis.	CBC, platelets, urinalysis monthly.
Aurothioglucose Solganal	Inj 50 mg/mL	IM 10 mg first dose, 25 mg second and third dose, 50 mg subsequent doses; 25–50 mg at 3–4 wk intervals.	Cutaneous reactions, stomatitis, gingivitis, glossitis, hematologic toxicity, nephrotoxicity, hepatotoxicity.	CBC and platelets every 2 wk; urinalysis before each injection.

(continued)

ANTIRHEUMATIC DRUGS COMPARISON CHART (*continued*)

DRUG	DOSAGE FORMS	ADULT DOSAGE	ADVERSE EFFECTS	LABORATORY MONITORING
Azathioprine Imuran	Tab 50, 75, 100 mg	PO 1–2.5 mg/kg/d; single or twice daily.	Myelosuppression, nausea, vomiting, anorexia, diarrhea, hepatotoxicity.	CBC, platelets weekly first month, twice monthly for second and third month, then monthly.
Cyclosporine Neoral[a]	Cap 25, 100 mg Soln 100 mg/mL	PO 1.2–7.5 mg/kg/d in divided doses.	Nephrotoxicity, hypertension, tremor, hirsutism, gingival hyperplasia, diarrhea, nausea, vomiting.	Cyclosporine levels periodically; BUN, serum creatinine, serum bilirubin, ALT; serum lipids, magnesium, and potassium; CBC and ALT monthly, if used with methotrexate.
Etanercept Enbrel	Inj 25, 50 mg	Most indications: IV 25–50 mg twice weekly; 50 mg twice weekly maintenance for plaque psoriasis.	Erythema, itching, pain, swelling at injection site; headache, rhinitis, dizziness, cough.	TB and HBV infection.
Gold Sodium Thiomalate Aurolate	Inj 10, 25, 50 mg/mL	IM 25–50 mg q 2 wk for 2–20 wk (may increase interval to 3–4 wk if stable).	*See Aurothioglucose.*	*See Aurothioglucose.*
Hydroxychloroquine Sulfate Plaquenil	Tab 200 mg	PO 200–800 mg/d; once or twice daily.	Retinopathy, nausea, vomiting, diarrhea, pruritus.	CBC periodically.
Infliximab[b] Remicade	Inj 100 mg	IV (over 2 h) 3–5 mg/kg, repeat at wk 2 and 6 and then 5 mg/kg every 8 wk. Can be given to patients on methotrexate.	Infusion reactions, headache, nausea, fatigue, myalgia, rhinitis, pain, pruritus, urticaria, hypo- or hypertension, chest pain, vomiting, dyspnea.	TB and HBV infection.

(continued)

ANTIRHEUMATIC DRUGS COMPARISON CHART (*continued*)

DRUG	DOSAGE FORMS	ADULT DOSAGE	ADVERSE EFFECTS	LABORATORY MONITORING
Leflunomide Arava	Tab 10, 20, 100 mg	100 mg/d for 3 days, then 20 mg once daily.	Diarrhea, respiratory infection, headache, nausea, rash, liver enzyme elevations, dyspepsia, alopecia, hypertension, teratogenicity.	Monitor ALT at baseline and then monthly during the first 6 mo. If ALT levels are stable, then every 6–8 wk. Platelet, white blood cell count, and hemoglobin or hematocrit monitored at baseline and monthly for 6 mo following initiation of therapy and every 6–8 wk thereafter.
Methotrexate Mexate-AQ Rheumatrex Various	Tab 2.5, 5, 7.5, 10, 15 mg Inj 25 mg/mL	PO 7.5–25 mg (as a single dose or 3 divided doses) once weekly; or SC or IM 7.5–25 mg once weekly.	Myelosuppression, stomatitis, abdominal distress, diarrhea, nausea, vomiting, hepatotoxicity, pulmonary toxicity.	CBC, platelets, urinalysis, AST, serum albumin, serum creatinine every 4–8 wk.
Penicillamine Cuprimine Depen	Cap 125, 250 mg Tab 250 mg	PO 530–750 mg/d as a single daily dose (up to 500 mg) or in divided doses if >500 mg.	Sensitivity reaction with skin rash, renal and hematologic toxicity.	CBC, platelet count, urine analysis every 2 wk until dosage is stable, then every month.
Rituximab Rituxan	Inj 100 mg/10 mL, 500 mg/50 Ml	Two 1 g IV infusions separated by 2 wk in combination with methotrexate; pretreatment with methylprednisoone 100 mg IV or equivalent glucocorticoid recommended 30 min to infusion.	Hypertension, nausea, upper respiratory tract infection, arthralgia, pruritus, pyrexia, infusion reactions, serious infections, tumor lysis syndrome.	HBV infection CBC and platelet counts regular intervals and more frequently in patients who develop cytopenias.
Sulfasalazine Azulfidine Various	Tab 500 mg	PO 2 g/c in 2 divided doses.	Nausea, vomiting, heartburn, dizziness, headache, hypersensitivity, skin rash, leukopenia.	CBC and ALT every 2 wk for first 3 mo monthly for 3 mo, and then every 3 mo.

[a]Neoral, a nonaqueous liquid formulation forms an emulsion in aqueous fluids and has a higher oral bioavailability than conventional formulations (e.g., Sandimmune, which is not indicated for rheumatoid arthritis). Do not use these products interchangeably.
[b]Approved for use in patients taking methotrexate.
Adapted from Refs. 5, 7, and 8 and product information.

■ REFERENCES

1. Orencia [package insert]. Princeton, NJ: Bristol-Myers Squibb Company; April 2008.
2. Humira [package insert]. North Chicago, IL: Abbott Laboratories; December 2008.
3. Ilowite N et al. Anakinra in the treatment of polyarticular-course juvenile rheumatoid arthritis: safety and preliminary efficacy results of a randomized multicenter study. *Clin Rheumatol.* 2009;28:129-137.
4. Kineret [package insert]. Thousand Oaks, CA: Amgen, Inc; 2006.
5. Donahue KE et al. Systematic review: comparative effectiveness and harms of disease-modifying medications for rheumatoid arthritis. *Ann Intern Med.* 2008;148:124-134.
6. Saag KG et al. American College of Rheumatology 2008 recommendations for the use of nonbiologic and biologic disease-modifying antirheumatic drugs in rheumatoid arthritis. *Arthritis Rheum.* 2008;59:762-784.
7. Horton S et al. Use of cyclosporine in rheumatoid arthritis. *Ann Pharmacother.* 1993;27:44-46.
8. Schuna AA et al. Rheumatoid arthritis. In: DiPiro JT et al., eds. *Pharmacotherapy: A Pathophysiologic Approach.* 4th ed. Stamford, CT: Appleton & Lange; 1999:1427-1440.

Chapter 3

Chronic Gout Therapy

Daniel M. Riche

Gout is a common chronic arthritis that can be diagnosed with certainty, has a known cause, and can be cured with appropriate therapy.[1] Hypouricemic agents that reduce uric acid concentrations by inhibiting uric acid production or enhancing uric acid excretion are used to prevent gout.[1] Acute gout attacks can lead to significant disability. For acute gout attacks, a nonsteroidal anti-inflammatory drug (NSAID) or a corticosteroid (systemically or intra-articularly) is the preferred therapy. Commonly used NSAIDs include indomethacin, ibuprofen, ketorolac, naproxen, and celecoxib. Preferred corticosteroids include prednisone, methylprednisolone, triamcinolone, and corticotropin. Doses and pharmacological properties of these medications are detailed in another section of *Clinical Drug Data*. (*See* Nonsteroidal Anti-Inflammatory Drugs and Adrenal Hormones.) This section concentrates on gout prophylaxis.

Several medications are currently available for gout prophylaxis, and though not much had changed over the past 40 years, there are some interesting therapies worth mentioning and one new drug approval, febuxostat (Uloric).[2] Rasburicase (Elitek), a recombinant form of the enzyme urate oxidase which oxidizes uric acid to allantoin, is also under investigation for the treatment of hyperuricemia in patients with chronic gout.[3] Rasburicase is currently approved for the treatment of hyperuricemia associated with tumor lysis syndrome; and, though not approved, rasburicase has already been used successfully in a patient with allopurinol allergy.[4] Benzbromarone, a uricosuric drug that blocks renal tubular reabsorption of uric acid, had its approval withdrawn due to reports of hepatotoxicity. Sulfinpyrazone, an analogue of phenylbutazone with a mechanism resembling probenecid, has also been withdrawn from the market.[5]

ALLOPURINOL
Zyloprim, Aloprim, Various

Pharmacology. Allopurinol, a structural analogue of the purine base hypoxanthine, competitively inhibits xanthine oxidase. Allopurinol reduces serum and urinary uric acid levels by blocking the conversion of hypoxanthine and xanthine to uric acid and decreasing urine synthesis.[5–7]

Administration and Adult Dosage. **PO for maintenance of mild gout**—100 mg/d initially, increasing in 100 mg/d increments at weekly intervals until a serum uric acid level of ≤6 mg/dL is attained. 200–300 mg/d in single or divided doses is typically required in mild cases. **PO for maintenance of moderate-severe gout**—400–600 mg/d, to a maximum of 800 mg/d for resistant cases. Give dosages that exceed 300 mg/d in divided doses. **PO for hyperuricemia associated with malignancy or tumor lysis syndrome**—600–800 mg/d for 2–3 days is advisable with a high fluid intake and then reduce to 300 mg/d. Start at least 2–3 days (preferably 5 days) before initiation of chemotherapy. Discontinue when the potential for uric acid overproduction is no longer present.[8,9] IV should be used only in those who do not tolerate PO allopurinol. **IV for hyperuricemia associated with tumor lysis syndrome**—200–400 mg/m^2/d 1–2 days prior to initiation of chemotherapy as a single infusion OR in equally divided infusions at twice daily to 4 times daily intervals, to a maximum dose of 600 mg/d. **PO for recurrent calcium oxalate calculi in hyperuricosuria**—200–300 mg/d in single or divided doses, to a maximum of 300 mg/dose and 800 mg/d.

Special Populations. *Pediatric Dosage.* **PO for hyperuricemia associated with malignancy and tumor lysis syndrome**—(<6 years) 150 mg/d in 1–3 divided doses; (6–10 years) 300 mg/d in 1–3 divided doses. **IV for hyperuricemia associated with tumor lysis syndrome**—200 mg/m^2/d as a single infusion OR in equally divided twice to 4 times daily infusions, to a maximum of 600 mg/d. Start at least 2–3 days (preferably 5 days) before chemotherapy.[8] Evaluate response 48 h after cancer therapy is started and adjust dosage as needed.

Geriatric Dosage. Lower dosage might be required in some patients because of the age-related decrease in renal function.

Other Conditions. In renal impairment, reduce initial dosage as follows: (Cl$_{Cr}$ 80–99 mL/min) 250 mg/d; (Cl$_{Cr}$ 60–79 mL/min) 200 mg/d; (Cl$_{Cr}$ 40–59 mL/min) 150 mg/d; (Cl$_{Cr}$ 20–39 mL/min) 100 mg/d; (Cl$_{Cr}$ 10–19 mL/min) 100 mg every 2 days; (Cl$_{Cr}$ <10 mL/min) 100 mg every 3 days.[1,10] Base subsequent dosage adjustment on serum uric acid levels.

Special Instructions. Give prophylactic colchicine 0.5–1.2 mg/d AND/OR an NSAID before starting allopurinol and continuing for several months after initiation of therapy due to an initial increased risk of gouty attacks with mobilization of urate crystals from established tophi.[5–7,11] A fluid intake sufficient to yield a daily urinary output of at least 2 L and the maintenance of a neutral or slightly alkaline urine are desirable. In transferring from a uricosuric agent to allopurinol, reduce the uricosuric dosage over several weeks while gradually increasing the dosage of allopurinol.

Dosage Forms. **Tab** 100 and 300 mg; **Inj** 500 mg/30 mL.

Patient Instructions. This drug may be taken with food, milk, or an antacid to minimize stomach upset. Adults should drink at least 10–12 full glasses (each containing 8 fluid ounces) of fluid each day. Avoid large amounts of alcohol (can increase uric acid in blood) or vitamin C (can increase the possibility of kidney stones by making the urine more acidic). Report any skin rash, painful urination, blood in urine, eye irritation, swelling of lips or mouth, itching, chills, fever, sore throat, nausea, or vomiting while taking this drug.

Missed Doses. Take this drug at regular intervals. If you miss a dose, take it as soon as you remember. Do not double the dose or take an extra dose.

Pharmacokinetics. *Onset and Duration.* A measurable decrease in uric acid occurs in 2–3 days; normal serum uric acid is achieved in 1–3 weeks.

Fate. Well absorbed orally (67%–81%), but rectal absorption is poor (0%–6% of oral bioavailability). Rapidly oxidized to oxypurinol, an active, but less potent, inhibitor of xanthine oxidase. Protein binding of allopurinol or oxypurinol is negligible.[12] Allopurinol V_d is 1.5 ± 0.7 L/kg, clearance is 0.77 ± 0.22 L/h/kg;

oxypurinol V_d is approximately 1.6 L/kg.[12,13] Oxypurinol and allopurinol are excreted unchanged in urine in a ratio of approximately 10:1.[12] **Half-life** (allopurinol) 1.4 ± 0.4 h; (oxypurinol) 19.7 ± 7.3 h with normal renal function, 5–10 days in renal failure.[12]

Adverse Reactions. A mild maculopapular skin rash occurs in approximately 2% of patients, but the percentage increases to approximately 20% with concurrent ampicillin. These rashes might not recur, if allopurinol is stopped and restarted at a lower dosage and oral desensitization to minor rashes from allopurinol in patients has been effective.[7,14,15] Exfoliative, urticarial, purpuric, and erythema multiform lesions also are reported occasionally. These more severe reactions require drug discontinuation because severe hypersensitivity reactions such as vasculitis, toxic epidermal necrolysis, Stevens-Johnson syndrome, renal impairment, and hepatic damage can result. An occasional hypersensitivity syndrome (frequently referred to as DRESS [drug rash (or reaction) with eosinophilia and systemic symptoms] syndrome marked by fever, rash, hepatitis, renal failure, and eosinophilia) has a mortality rate reportedly as high as 27%. It can begin 1 day or up to 2 years (on average approximately 6 weeks) after start of therapy and appears related to pre-existing renal dysfunction, elevated oxypurinol serum levels, or concurrent thiazide or other diuretic therapy.[10,16,17] Occasionally, nausea, vomiting, and abdominal pain occur. Rarely, alopecia, cataract formation, hepatotoxicity, bone marrow depression, leukopenia, leukocytosis, or renal xanthine stones occur.[18]

Contraindications. Patients who have developed severe reactions or have documented hypersensitivity. (*See* Adverse Reactions.)

Precautions. Pregnancy and lactation. Use with caution and in reduced dosage in renal impairment. Adjust dosage conservatively in patients with impaired renal function who are on a diuretic concomitantly.[10,17]

Drug Interactions. Diuretics can theoretically contribute to allopurinol toxicity, although a cause and effect relationship has not been established. Allopurinol markedly increases the toxicity of oral azathioprine and mercaptopurine. Dose reductions of azathioprine and mercaptopurine to one-third or one-fourth of the usual dose are required. Allopurinol can increase the risk of hypersensitivity reactions to captopril and enalapril, ampicillin and amoxicillin skin rashes, bone marrow suppression caused by cyclophosphamide, neurotoxicity of vidarabine, and nephrotoxicity of cyclosporine. Allopurinol also can increase the effect of some oral anticoagulants, but not that of warfarin. Large doses (600 mg/d) of allopurinol can increase theophylline serum levels. Concurrent use of salicylate for its antirheumatic effect does not compromise the action of allopurinol. Uricosuric agents can increase the excretion and decrease the effect of oxypurinol.

Parameters to Monitor. Monitor serum uric acid levels; pretreatment 24-h urinary uric acid excretion.[5–7] Periodically determine liver function (particularly in patients with preexisting liver disease). Monitor renal function tests and CBC, especially during the first few months of therapy. Renal function is particularly important in patients on concurrent diuretic therapy.[10,17]

Notes. Allopurinol is the drug of choice for gout in patients with impaired renal function who respond poorly to uricosuric agents; however, these patients should be monitored closely because of increased frequency of adverse reactions.[5–7,10,11]

Current data do not support the routine treatment of asymptomatic hyperuricemia in patients not receiving chemotherapy for malignancies OR documented marked overexcreters.[5-7] Allopurinol has been used investigational to reduce tissue damage during coronary artery bypass surgery, for organ transplantation storage solutions, in the treatment of both leishmaniasis and malaria, and as an adjunct in schizophrenia.[19] Because of limited studies showing very poor to no absorption of extemporaneously compounded allopurinol suppositories, this dosage form is not recommended.[12] Although preliminary reports indicated that extemporaneously prepared allopurinol mouthwash might be effective in protecting against fluorouracil-induced mucositis, one well-controlled clinical trial found it ineffective for this indication, and it is not recommended.[20]

COLCHICINE   Various

Pharmacology. Colchicine is an anti-inflammatory agent relatively specific for gout, with activity probably because of the impairment of leukocyte chemotaxis, mobility, adhesion and phagocytosis, and a reduction of the lactic acid production resulting from a decrease in urate crystal deposition.[7]

Administration and Adult Dosage. **PO for acute gout**—0.5–1.2 mg initially at the first warning of an attack, then 0.5–0.6 mg every hour OR 1.0–1.2 every 2 h until pain is relieved or GI toxicity occurs (e.g., nausea, vomiting, stomach pain, and especially diarrhea), to a typical total dosage of 4 mg and a maximum dose of 8 mg/attack. Pain and swelling typically abate within 12 h and usually are gone in 1–2 days. An interval of 3 days is advised, if a second course is required. **PO for prophylaxis in chronic gout**—<1 attack/y 0.5–0.6 mg daily OR every other day; >1 attack/y <1 attack/y 1.5–1.8 mg daily depending on severity; divided doses are preferred with higher dosages. **PO for surgical prophylaxis in patients with gout**—0.5–0.6 mg 3 times daily, 3 days before and after surgery. **IV for acute gout.** (*See* Notes for availability.) (If patient cannot take oral preparation) 1–2 mg initially, diluted (if desired) in nonbacteriostatic NS, over 2–5 min, then 0.5 mg every 6–24 h as needed, to a maximum of 4 mg/24 h, or a maximum 4 mg for a single course of treatment.[7,21] Some clinicians recommend a single IV dose of 3 mg over 5 min; others recommend an initial dose of ≤1 mg, then 0.5 mg 1–2 times daily as needed. If pain recurs, give IV 1–2 mg/d for several days; however, no more colchicine should be given by any route for at least 7 days after a full course (4 mg) of IV therapy.[7,21] IV colchicine is very irritating and extravasation should be avoided to prevent tissue and nerve damage; change to oral therapy as soon as possible. Do not administer by SQ or IM routes.

Special Populations. *Pediatric Dosage.* Safety and efficacy not established.

Geriatric Dosage. Reduce the maximum IV colchicine dosage to 2 mg, with at least 3 weeks between courses, and lower the dosage further, if previously maintained on oral colchicine.

Other Conditions. Reduce the total dosage of colchicine in renal impairment in proportion to the remaining renal function.[21,22] The dosage of prophylactic colchicine should not exceed 0.5 mg/d with $Cl_{Cr} \leq 50$ mL/min, because of increased risk of peripheral neuritis and myopathy.[23] Not recommended in patients who require hemodialysis.[23]

Dosage Forms. **Tab** 500 (with probenecid) and 600 μg; **Inj** 500 μg/mL. (*See* Notes for availability.)

Patient Instructions. You should always have a supply of this drug on hand, and you should take it promptly at the earliest symptoms of a gout attack. Relief of gout pain or occurrence of nausea, vomiting, stomach pain, or diarrhea indicates that the full therapeutic dosage has been attained and no more drugs should be taken. After treatment of an attack, do not take any more colchicine for at least 3 days. Immediately report black tarry stools or bright red blood in the stools, which can indicate gastrointestinal bleeding. Report any tiredness, weakness, numbness, or tingling. Also, immediately report sore throat, fever, oral lesions, or unusual bleeding that can be an early sign of a severe, but rare, blood disorder.

Missed Doses. If you are taking this drug at regular intervals, such as daily, and you miss a dose, take it as soon as you remember. If it is about time for the next dose, take that dose only. Do not double the dose or take an extra dose.

Pharmacokinetics. *Fate.* Rapidly, but variably absorbed after oral administration (healthy young adults, 44% ± 17%; elderly, 45% ± 19%), with partial hepatic deacetylation. Plasma protein binding is approximately 50%; extensive leukocyte uptake occurs with levels found for up to 9 days. Distribution after IV administration is triphasic; V_d of the terminal phase is 6.7 ± 1.4 L/kg for healthy young adults and 6.3 ± 2.3 L/kg for the elderly. Clearance is 0.15 ± 0.02 L/h/kg for healthy young adults and 0.12 ± 0.01 L/h/kg for the elderly. Urinary (approximately 10% unchanged), biliary, and fecal elimination occur.[22,24,25] **Half-life** (healthy young adults) 2nd phase 1.2 ± 0.2 h; terminal phase 30 ± 6 h; (elderly) 2nd phase 1.2 ± 0.1 h; terminal phase 34 ± 8 h.[24]

Adverse Reactions. Nausea, vomiting, stomach pain, and particularly diarrhea are frequent and can occur several hours after oral or IV drug administration; discontinue the drug upon symptoms. Prolonged administration occasionally can cause bone marrow depression with agranulocytosis, thrombocytopenia, aplastic anemia, and purpura. Peripheral neuritis and myopathy with characteristically elevated creatine kinase occur occasionally. This reaction is associated with standard (unadjusted) dosage in renal insufficiency and usually resolves in 3–4 weeks after drug withdrawal.[7,21–23] Alopecia, reversible malabsorption of vitamin B_{12}, and reversible azoospermia occur. Tissue and nerve damage can occur with IV extravasation. Overdosage can cause hemorrhagic gastroenteritis, vascular damage leading to shock, nephrotoxicity, and paralysis. As little as 7 mg has proved fatal, but much larger dosages have been survived.[22,26–28]

Contraindications. Serious gastrointestinal, renal, hepatic, or cardiac disorders; combined hepatic and renal dysfunction; blood dyscrasias.[22,23]

Precautions. Use with great caution in elderly or debilitated patients, especially those with early manifestations of hepatic, renal, gastrointestinal, or heart disease symptoms. Reduce dosage if weakness, anorexia, nausea, vomiting, stomach pain, or diarrhea occurs.[22,29]

Drug Interactions. Macrolides and grapefruit juices may increase risk of colchicines toxicity. Hypolipidemics (statins and gemfibrozil) may increase risk of myopathy/rhabdomyolysis.

Notes. Products containing colchicine for IV use had been marketed without approval. The FDA accounts 50 reported adverse events associated with IV colchicine use, including 23 deaths through June 2007. As of February 2008, all IV colchicine formulations will require full FDA approval prior to be reinstated on the market. There are no IV formulations currently available. Colchicine is most effective when used early in the attack before most WBC chemotaxis takes place.[5-7] Daily colchicine often is given for prophylaxis against recurrent gout attacks before and during the first several months of allopurinol or uricosuric treatment.[5-7] Continuous prophylactic colchicine therapy can be effective in suppressing the acute attacks and renal dysfunction of familial Mediterranean fever in adults and children.[22,28] Colchicine therapy also might be effective for primary biliary cirrhosis and certain inflammatory dermatoses.[22,28,29]

FEBUXOSTAT   Uloric

Pharmacology. Febuxostat is a nonpurine, selective xanthine oxidase inhibitor.[2] Febuxostat reduces serum uric acid levels by blocking the conversion of hypoxanthine and xanthine to uric acid and decreasing urine synthesis.[2]

Administration and Adult Dosage. **PO for chronic gout**—40 mg once daily, may increase to 80 mg once daily in 2 weeks if serum uric acid ≥ 6 mg/dL.[30]

Special Populations. *Pediatric Dosage.* Safety and efficacy not established.

Geriatric Dosage. Same as adult dosage.

Other Conditions. No dosing adjustments are required for mild-to-moderate renal or hepatic impairment. Pregnancy category C. Cautioned in breastfeeding.

Special Instructions. If a gout flare occurs during treatment, febuxostat need not be discontinued. Prophylactic therapy (e.g., NSAID or colchicine) may be beneficial upon initiation of treatment and for up to 6 months.[30] (*See* Precautions.)

Dosage Forms. Tab 40 and 80 mg.

Patient Instructions. This drug may be taken without regard for food or an antacid to minimize stomach upset. Be sure to have your liver function tests measured by the provider. There is potential for adverse cardiovascular events after initiation of febuxostat therapy, monitor for signs and symptoms of myocardial infarction and stroke. Concomitant prophylaxis with an NSAID or colchicine for gout flares may be considered. (*See* Special Instructions.)

Missed Doses. If you miss a daily dose, take it as soon as you remember. If it is about time for the next dose, take that dose only. Do not double the dose or take an extra dose.

Pharmacokinetics. *Fate.* 50% absorbed, reaching maximum plasma concentrations between 1 and 1.5 h. Though there is an 18% decrease in AUC following a high-fat meal, there is no clinically significant change in serum uric acid concentration reduction between the fed and fasting states. The steady state V_d is approximately 50 L. Protein binding is 99.2% (primarily to albumin). Extensively metabolized by both conjugation via uridine diphosphate glucuronosyltransferase enzymes and oxidation via cytochrome P450 (CYP) enzymes including CYP1A2, 2C8 and 2C9, and non-P450 enzymes. In urine and feces, both acyl glucuronide (approximately 35% of the dose) and oxidative (approximately 35% of the dose) appear to be the major metabolites of febuxostat in vivo. Febuxostat and its metabolites are recovered in the urine (approximately 49%) and feces (approximately 45%). **Half-life** 5–8 h.[30]

Adverse Reactions. The most frequent adverse effect is liver function test abnormalities, while nausea, arthralgia, and rash are also common.[30] Numerous rare but serious adverse effects have been reported.[30]

Contraindications. Concomitant use of azathioprine, mercaptopurine, or theophylline.

Precautions. Use with caution in patients with severe renal or hepatic impairment. An increase in gout flares is frequently observed during initiation of antihyperuricemic agents, including febuxostat. A higher rate of cardiovascular thromboembolic events was observed in patients treated with febuxostat than allopurinol in clinical trials.[30]

Drug Interactions. Concomitant administration with xanthine oxidase substrate medications (e.g., azathioprine, mercaptopurine, or theophylline) may lead to increased levels and severe toxicity. Studies have not been performed to evaluate interactions with cytotoxic chemotherapy medications.[30] There is no clinically significant interaction with colchicine, naproxen, indomethacin, hydrochlorothiazide, warfarin, or desipramine.[30]

Parameters to Monitor. Serum uric acid may be performed as early as 2 weeks following initiation.[30] Monitor liver function tests periodically. Monitor for signs and symptoms of myocardial infarction and stroke.

Notes. Febuxostat is not recommended for the treatment of asymptomatic hyperuricemia or hyperuricemia associated with malignancy or tumor lysis syndrome.[30] Upon the initial FDA submission, there were concerns about the cardiovascular safety of febuxostat. Long-term cardiovascular safety studies demonstrated no statistical difference between febuxostat, allopurinol, and placebo, although event rates were higher in the febuxostat group versus the allopurinol group.[30]

PROBENECID   Various

Pharmacology. Probenecid, a sulfonamide, is an organic acid that inhibits renal tubular reabsorption of urate, thereby increasing the urinary excretion of uric acid and lowering serum urate. Probenecid also interferes with renal tubular secretion of many drugs, causing an increase or prolongation in their serum levels. (*See* Notes.)

Administration and Adult Dosage. PO for chronic gout—250 mg twice daily for 1 week, then 500 mg twice daily (not to be started during an acute attack), and increase by 500 mg/4 wk if symptoms persist OR urate excretion <700 mg, to a maximum of 2 g/d. Decrease daily dosage by 500 mg every 6 months if no acute attacks occur, adjusted to maintain normal serum uric acid levels. **PO to prolong penicillin or cephalosporin action**—2 g/d in 4 divided doses, except with known renal impairment. **PO with procaine penicillin G for uncomplicated gonorrhea**—1 g as a single dose prior to penicillin OR ampicillin.[31]

Special Populations. *Pediatric Dosage.* (<2 years) Contraindicated. **PO to prolong penicillin or cephalosporin action**—(<50 kg) 25 mg/kg initially, then maintain at 40 mg/kg/d or 1.2 g/m^2/d in 4 divided doses; (>50 kg) same as adult dosage.

Geriatric Dosage. Same as adult dosage unless renal impairment is present.

Other Conditions. Reduce dosage for prolonging penicillin or cephalosporin action in patients with renal impairment.

Special Instructions. *Colchicine*—0.5–1.2 mg/d OR an NSAID should be started before and continued for the first several months after initiation of uricosuric treatment diminishes exacerbation of uricosuric-induced gouty attacks.[5–7] To prevent hematuria, renal colic, costovertebral pain, and urate stone formation, liberal fluid intake and alkalinization of the urine with 3–7.5 g/d sodium bicarbonate or 7.5 g/d potassium citrate are recommended, at least until serum uric acid levels normalize and tophaceous deposits disappear. If an acute gout attack is precipitated during therapy, increase the dosage of colchicine OR add a corticosteroid OR an NSAID to control the attack.[5–7] (*See* Precautions.)

Dosage Forms. Tab 500 mg.

Patient Instructions. This drug may be taken with food, milk, or an antacid to minimize stomach upset. Drink a large amount (10–12 full glasses) of fluids each day and avoid the use of aspirin- or salicylate-containing products unless directed otherwise.

Missed Doses. If you are taking this drug at regular intervals, such as daily, and you miss a dose, take it as soon as you remember. If it is about time for the next dose, take that dose only. Do not double the dose or take an extra dose.

Pharmacokinetics. *Fate.* Rapidly and completely absorbed from the GI tract; 74%–99% plasma protein bound (decreasing with increasing dose), mostly to albumin.[32] V_d is 0.17 ± 0.03 L/kg.[33] Probenecid is extensively metabolized or conjugated, exhibiting Michaelis-Menten elimination; approximately 40% is excreted in urine as the monoacylglucuronide, <5% as unchanged drug, and the remainder as hydroxylated metabolites, which can have uricosuric activity.[34,35] **Half-life** dose dependent (increases with increasing dose): 4.5 ± 0.6 h with 0.5 g; 12 h with 2 g.[33,36]

Adverse Reactions. Headache, nausea, vomiting, urinary frequency, rash, and dizziness occur frequently. Exacerbation of gout, hematuria, renal colic, costovertebral pain, and uric acid stones can occur. Nephrotic syndrome, hepatic necrosis, aplastic anemia, pancytopenia, hemolytic anemia (possibly related to G-6-PD deficiency), and severe allergic reactions occur rarely.

Contraindications. Children <2 years old; known blood dyscrasias or uric acid kidney stones; initiation during an acute gout attack; coadministration of salicylates; Cl_{Cr} <50 mL/min.

Precautions. Hypersensitivity reactions require drug discontinuation. Use with caution in patients with histories of sulfonamide allergy, peptic ulcer disease, or G-6-PD deficiency.

Drug Interactions. Salicylates and pyrazinamide antagonize the uricosuric action of probenecid. Probenecid can increase the serum concentration of many drugs, including acyclovir, benzodiazepines, some β-lactams, clofibrate, dapsone, methotrexate, NSAIDs, penicillamine, sulfonamides, sulfonylureas, thiopental, and zidovudine. NSAID clearance may be decreased by competitively inhibiting formation or renal excretion of acylglucuronide metabolites.[37]

Parameters to Monitor. Serum uric acid weekly until stable when treating hyperuricemia; pretreatment 24-h urinary uric acid excretion. If alkali is administered, periodically determine acid–base balance.

Notes. Current data do not support the treatment of patients with asymptomatic hyperuricemia caused by *undersecretion* of uric acid.[5,7,11] Probenecid is most useful in symptomatic patients with reduced urinary excretion of urate: <800 mg/d on an unrestricted diet or <600 mg/d on a purine-restricted diet.[5] Probenecid is ineffective in prolonging the half-life of β-lactams that do not undergo renal tubular secretion (e.g., ceftazidime and ceftriaxone).[38]

■ REFERENCES

1. Stamp LK et al. Emerging therapies in the long-term management of hyperuricaemia and gout. *Intern Med J.* 2007;37:258-266.
2. Bruce SP. Febuxostat: a selective xanthine oxidase inhibitor for the treatment of hyperuricemia and gout. *Ann Pharmacother.* 2006;40:2187-2194.
3. Vogt B. Urate oxidase (rasburicase) for treatment of severe tophaceous gout. *Nephrol Dial Transplant.* 2005;20:431-433.
4. Richette P, Bardin T. Successful treatment with rasburicase of a tophaceous gout in a patient allergic to allopurinol. *Nat Clin Pract Rheumatol.* 2006;2:338-342.
5. Star VL, Hochberg MC. Prevention and management of gout. *Drugs.* 1993;45:212-222.
6. Conaghan PG, Day RO. Risks and benefits of drugs used in the management and prevention of gout. *Drug Safety.* 1994;11:252-258.
7. Emmerson BT. The management of gout. *N Engl J Med.* 1996;334:445-451.
8. Conger JD. Acute uric acid nephropathy. *Med Clin North Am.* 1990;74:859-871.
9. Smalley RV et al. Allopurinol: intravenous use for prevention and treatment of hyperuricemia. *J Clin Oncol.* 2000;18:1758-1763.
10. Hande KR et al. Severe allopurinol toxicity: description and guidelines for prevention in patients with renal insufficiency. *Am J Med.* 1984;76:47-56.
11. Campbell SM. Gout: how presentation, diagnosis, and treatment differ in the elderly. *Geriatrics.* 1988;43(11):71-77.
12. Murrell GAC, Rapeport WG. Clinical pharmacokinetics of allopurinol. *Clin Pharmacokinet.* 1986;11:343-353.
13. Walter-Sack I et al. Disposition and uric acid lowering effect of oxypurinol: comparison of different oxypurinol formulations and allopurinol in healthy individuals. *Eur J Clin Pharmacol.* 1995;49:215-220.
14. Fam AG et al. Desensitization to allopurinol in patients with gout and cutaneous reactions. *Am J Med.* 1992;93:299-302.
15. Tanna SB et al. Desensitization to allopurinol in a patient with previous failed desensitization. *Ann Pharmacother.* 1999;33:1180-1183.
16. Roujeau JC, Stern RS. Severe adverse cutaneous reactions to drugs. *N Engl J Med.* 1994;331:1272-1285.
17. Arellano F, Sacristán JA. Allopurinol hypersensitivity syndrome: a review. *Ann Pharmacother.* 1993;27: 337-343.
18. Pascual E. Gout update: from lab to the clinic and back. *Curr Opin Rheumatol.* 2000;12:213-218.
19. Day RO. New uses for allopurinol. *Drugs.* 1994;48:339-344.
20. Loprinzi CL et al. A controlled evaluation of an allopurinol mouthwash as prophylaxis against 5-fluorouracil-induced stomatitis. *Cancer.* 1990;65:1879-1882.
21. Wallace SL, Singer JZ. Review: systemic toxicity associated with the intravenous administration of colchicine—guidelines for use. *J Rheumatol.* 1988;15:495-499.
22. Levy M et al. Colchicine: a state-of-the-art review. *Pharmacotherapy.* 1991;11:196-211.
23. Wallace SL et al. Renal function predicts colchicine toxicity: guidelines for the prophylactic use of colchicines in gout. *J Rheumatol.* 1991;18:264-269.
24. Rochdi M et al. Pharmacokinetics and absolute bioavailability of colchicine after IV and oral administration in healthy human volunteers and elderly subjects. *Eur J Clin Pharmacol.* 1994;46:351-354.
25. Jusko WJ, Gretch M. Plasma and tissue protein binding of drugs in pharmacokinetics. *Drug Metab Rev.* 1976;5:43-140.
26. Hood RL. Colchicine poisoning. *J Emerg Med.* 1994;12:171-177.
27. Mullins ME et al. Fatal cardiovascular collapse following acute colchicine ingestion. *Clin Toxicol.* 2000;38:51-54.
28. Ben-Chetrit E, Levy M. Colchicine: 1998 update. *Semin Arthritis Rheum.* 1998;28:48-59.
29. Sullivan TP et al. Colchicine in dermatology. *J Am Acad Dermatol.* 1998;39:993-999.
30. Uloric [package insert]. Deerfield, Illinois: Takeda Pharmaceuticals America, Inc.; February 2009.

31. Anon. Drugs for sexually transmitted infections. *Med Lett Drugs Ther.* 1999;41:85-90.
32. Emanuelsson BM et al. Non-linear elimination and protein binding of probenecid. *Eur J Clin Pharmacol.* 1987;32:395-401.
33. Benet LZ et al. Design and optimization of dosage regimens; pharmacokinetic data. In: Hardman JG et al, eds. *Goodman and Gilman's the Pharmacological Basis of Therapeutics.* 9th ed. New York: McGraw-Hill; 1996:1707-1792.
34. Israili ZH et al. Metabolites of probenecid. Chemical, physical, and pharmacological studies. *J Med Chem.* 1972;15:709-713.
35. Perel JM et al. Identification and renal excretion of probenecid metabolites in man. *Life Sci I.* 1970;9:1337-1343.
36. Dayton PG et al. The physiological disposition of probenecid, including renal clearance, in man, studied by an improved method for its estimation in biological material. *J Pharmacol Exp Ther.* 1963;140:278-286.
37. Smith PC et al. Effect of probenecid on the formation and elimination of acyl glucuronides: studies with zomepirac. *Clin Pharmacol Ther.* 1985;38:121-127.
38. Brown GR. Cephalosporin-probenecid drug interactions. *Clin Pharmacokinet.* 1993;24:289-300.

Chapter 4

Nonsteroidal Anti-Inflammatory Drugs

Stephen M. Setter and Danial E. Baker

ACETAMINOPHEN Tylenol, Various

Pharmacology. Acetaminophen possesses analgesic and antipyretic activities with few anti-inflammatory effects. It has the same effectiveness as aspirin in inhibiting brain prostaglandin synthetase but very little activity as a peripheral prostaglandin inhibitor. This difference from aspirin and other nonsteroidal anti-inflammatory drugs (NSAIDs) might explain its relative lack of effectiveness as an anti-inflammatory, antirheumatic agent. Acetaminophen does not inhibit normal platelet action, prothrombin activity, or adversely affect gastrointestinal (GI) mucosal health.

Administration and Adult Dosage. **PO for pain, dysmenorrhea, headache, or fever** (non-SR)—325–1000 mg every 4–6 h, to a maximum of 4 g/d; (SR tablet)—1300 mg every 8 h. **Rectally for pain, dysmenorrhea, headache, or fever**—650 mg every 4–6 h, to a maximum of 4 g/d.

Special Populations. *Pediatric Dosage.* **PO for pain, dysmenorrhea, headache, or fever**—10–15 mg/kg every 4–8 h, may repeat dose every 4 h, not to exceed 5 doses/day; or (up to 3 months) 40 mg/dose, (4–11 months) 80 mg/dose, (12–23 months) 120 mg/dose, (2–3 years) 160 mg/dose, (4–5 years) 240 mg/dose, (6–8 years) 320 mg/dose, (9–10 years) 400 mg/dose, (11 years) 480 mg/dose, (12–14 years) 640 mg/dose, (>14 years) 650 mg/dose. **Rectally for pain, dysmenorrhea, headache, or fever**—(3–11 months) 80 mg every 6 h, (1–3 years) 80 mg every 4 h, (3–6 years) 120–125 mg every 4–6 h, to a maximum of 720 mg/d; (6–12 years) 325 mg every 4–6 h, to a maximum of 2.6 g/d; (>12 years) Same as adult dosage.

Geriatric Dosage. Same as adult dosage.

Dosage Forms. **Cap** 325, 500 mg; **Gelcap** 500 mg; **Chew Tab** 80, 160 mg; **SR Tab** 650 mg; **Tab** 160, 325, 500, 650 mg; **Drp** 48, 100 mg/mL; **Elxr** 16, 24, 26, 32, 65 mg/mL; **Syrup** 32 mg/mL; **Supp** 80, 120, 125, 300, 325, 650 mg.

Patient Instructions. Do not exceed the maximum recommended daily dosage of 4 g (2 g in alcoholics). Report unresponsive fever or continued pain persisting for more than 3–5 days to your physician. Do not use with other anti-inflammatory agents unless directed by your physician.

Missed Doses. If you take this drug on a regular schedule, take a missed dose as soon as you remember. If it is about time for the next dose, take that dose only; do not double the dose or take extra.

Pharmacokinetics. *Serum Levels.* (analgesia, antipyresis)—10–20 mg/L (66–132 μmol/L). Serum concentrations >300 mg/L (2 mmol/L) at 4 h or 45 mg/L (300 μmol/L) at 12 h after acute overdosage are associated with severe hepatic damage, whereas toxicity is unlikely if levels are <120 mg/L (800 μmol/L) at 4 h or 30 mg/L (200 μmol/L) at 12 h.[1] (*See* Notes and Adverse Reactions.)

Fate. Rapid absorption from the GI tract, with peak plasma concentrations being achieved within 0.5–2 h. Absorption of liquid preparations is more rapid. Unbound to plasma proteins at therapeutic doses; 20%–50% bound in overdose. Extensively metabolized in the liver to inactive conjugates of glucuronic and sulfuric acids and cysteine (saturable) and to a hepatotoxic intermediate metabolite (first order) by CYP1A2 and CYP2E1. The intermediate is detoxified by glutathione (saturable). V_d is 0.95 ± 0.12 L/kg; clearance is 0.3 ± 0.084 L/h/kg, decreased in hepatitis and increased in hyperthyroidism, pregnancy, and obesity; 2%–3% excreted unchanged in urine.[1] **Half-life** 2 ± 0.5 h, decreased in hyperthyroidism and pregnancy, and increased in hepatitis and neonates.[1]

Adverse Reactions. Nontoxic at therapeutic doses. In acute overdose (single dose equaling or exceeding 10 g or 7.5–10 g daily for 1–2 days), potentially fatal hepatic necrosis and possible renal tubular necrosis can occur, but clinical and laboratory evidence of hepatotoxicity might be delayed for several days. (*See* Serum Levels.) Toxic hepatitis also has been associated with long-term ingestion of 5–8 g/d for several weeks or 3–4 g/d for a year. Occasionally, maculopapular rash or urticarial skin reactions occur; methemoglobinemia, neutropenia, and thrombocytopenic purpura are rarely reported. Analgesic nephropathy has been associated with the consumption of 1–15.3 kg of acetaminophen over 3–23 years.[2]

Contraindications. G-6-PD deficiency; chewable tablets in patients with phenylketonuria PKU.

Precautions. Use with caution in chronic alcoholics (not to exceed 2 g/d) and patients with phenylalanine hydroxylase deficiency (phenylketonuria) or G-6-PD deficiency. Some formulations contain aspartame, which is metabolized to phenylalanine; therefore, do not use these products in patients with phenylketonuria. Also, some products contain sulfites.

Drug Interactions. Chronic alcoholics might be at increased risk for hepatic toxicity.[3] The risk of hepatotoxicity also is increased by long-term use of other enzyme inducers (e.g., barbiturates, carbamazepine, phenytoin, rifampin, sulfinpyrazone) and acetaminophen's efficacy also can be decreased by these agents. Coadministration with isoniazid increases the risk of hepatotoxicity; therefore, avoid acetaminophen in persons on isoniazid. Acetaminophen may increase the anticoagulant effect of warfarin at higher doses; therefore, monitor INR closely when adding, increasing, or discontinuing long-term acetaminophen use.[4]

Notes. Pregnancy category A. Management of acute overdosage includes emesis and/or gastric lavage, if no more than a few hours have elapsed since ingestion. Supportive measures such as respiratory support and fluid and electrolyte therapy are recommended in addition. Administration of activated charcoal is not recommended because it can interfere with the absorption of acetylcysteine, which is used in the treatment of severe acute overdosage. Potentially dangerous acetaminophen levels (*see* Serum Levels) can be managed by the administration of 140 mg/kg acetylcysteine diluted 1:3 in a soft drink or plain water; follow with 70 mg/kg every 4 h for 17 doses. If administered within 8–16 h of ingestion, this therapy has been shown to minimize the expected hepatotoxicity, but treatment is still indicated as late as 24 h after ingestion, with some data showing effectiveness up to 36 h postingestion.[5] For the short-term treatment of osteoarthritis of the knee, acetaminophen 2.6 and 4 g/d are comparable to **naproxen** 750 mg/d and **ibuprofen** 1.2–2.4 g/d, respectively.[6]

ASPIRIN   Various

Pharmacology. Aspirin is an analgesic, antipyretic, and anti-inflammatory agent. Anti-inflammatory properties are related to the inhibition of prostaglandin biosynthesis. Aspirin nonselectively inhibits cyclooxygenase-1 (Cox-1), which is associated with GI and renal effects and inhibition of platelet aggregation, and cyclooxygenase-2 (Cox-2), which is associated with the inflammatory response. Unlike other NSAIDs, its antiplatelet effect is irreversible and permanent (because of transacetylation of platelet Cox for the life of the platelet (8–11 days). Salicylates without acetyl groups (e.g., **sodium salicylate**) have essentially no antiplatelet effect but retain analgesic, antipyretic, and anti-inflammatory activities. Low dosages (1–2 g/d) decrease urate excretion; high dosages (>5 g/d) induce uricosuria.[7]

Administration and Adult Dosage. **PO or rectally for fever, headache, pain, arthritis, and rheumatic conditions**—325–1000 mg every 4–6 h, to a maximum of 4 g/d. **PO for migraine**—1000 mg once per 24 h. **PO for acute rheumatic fever**—5–8 g/d in divided doses. **PO for treatment and prevention of TIA**—50–100 mg/d. **PO for percutaneous coronary intervention and primary prevention of myocardial infarction**—75–100 mg/d; 81–325 mg/d. **PO for secondary myocardial infarction risk reduction and stroke treatment**—162–325 mg/d. **PO for unstable and chronic stable angina**—75–325 mg/d. **PO for prevention of coronary artery bypass graft occlusion**—75–325 mg/d started 6 h postoperatively and continued indefinitely. **PO for nonrheumatic atrial fibrillation**—75–325 mg/d. The optimum dosage for platelet inhibition has not been determined for all medical conditions. Aspirin is used in combination with clopidogrel or dipyridamole for the prevention of vascular events.[8–11]

Special Populations. *Pediatric Dosage.* **PO for juvenile rheumatoid arthritis**—60–130 mg/kg/d in 4 divided doses. **PO for fever** (>12 years old)—same as adult dosage. **PO for Kawasaki disease**—80–100 mg/kg/d in 4 divided doses; decrease to 5 mg/kg/d after fever resolves. (*See* Precautions.) **PO as an analgesic/antipyretic**—10 mg/kg/dose every 4 h, to a maximum of 60 mg/kg/d. Alternatively, (2–3 years) 162 mg every 4 h; (4–5 years) 243 mg every 4 h; (6–8 years) 325 mg every 4 h; (9–10 years) 405 mg every 4 h; (11 years) 486 mg every 4 h; (≥12 years) 650 mg every 4 h. (*See* Precautions.)

Geriatric Dosage. Use minimal effective dosages; elderly are more susceptible to GI bleeding and acute renal insufficiency.

Other Conditions. Uremia or reduced albumin levels are likely to produce higher unbound drug levels that can increase pharmacologic or toxic effects. Dosage reduction might be required in these patients (e.g., kidney disease, malnutrition).

Dosage Forms. **Chew Tab** 81 mg; **EC Tab** 81, 165, 325, 500, 650, 975 mg; **Effervescent Tab** 81 mg; **gum** 227 mg; **SR Tab** 650, 800 mg; **Supp** 60, 125, 200, 325, 650 mg; **Tab** 81, 325, 500 mg.

Patient Instructions. Children and teenagers (<16 years) should not use aspirin-containing medications for chickenpox or flu symptoms because of the association with Reye's syndrome, a rare but serious illness. Take this drug with food, milk, or a full glass of water to minimize stomach upset; report any symptoms of GI ulceration or bleeding. Contact your physician if ringing in the ears or GI pain occurs. Do not crush or chew enteric-coated or sustained-release preparations. Avoid other products containing aspirin or NSAIDs.

Missed Doses. If you take this drug on a regular schedule and you miss a dose, take it as soon as you remember. If it is about time for the next dose, take that dose only. Do not double the dose or take an extra dose.

Pharmacokinetics. *Onset and Duration.* PO onset of analgesia 30 min.[1]

Serum Levels. (Salicylate)—150–300 mg/L (1.1–2.2 mmol/L) for rheumatic diseases, often accompanied by mild toxic symptoms. Tinnitus occurs at 200–400 mg/L (1.5–2.9 mmol/L), hyperventilation at >350 mg/L (2.6 mmol/L), acidosis at >450 mg/L (3.3 mmol/L), and severe or fatal toxicity at >900 mg/L (6.6 mmol/L) 6 h after acute ingestion.[12,13]

Fate. Rapidly absorbed from the GI tract; oral bioavailability of aspirin is 80%–100%. Enteric coating does not adversely affect absorption.[14] A single analgesic/antipyretic dose produces peak salicylate levels of 30–60 mg/L (0.22–0.44 mmol/L). Aspirin is 49% plasma protein bound, decreased in uremia; V_d is 0.15 ± 0.03 L/kg; clearance is 0.56 ± 0.07 L/h/kg. Aspirin is rapidly hydrolyzed to salicylate, which also is pharmacologically active. Salicylate is metabolized primarily in the liver to 4 metabolites (salicyluric acid, gentisic acid, phenolic and acyl glucuronides). Salicylate plasma protein binding is dose dependent, 95% at 15 mg/L and 80% at 300 mg/L, and decreased in uremia, hypoalbuminemia, neonates, and pregnancy; V_d is 0.17 ± 0.03 L/kg; clearance is dose dependent, 0.012 L/h/kg at 134–157 mg/L, and decreased in hepatitis and neonates. Only 1% of a dose of aspirin is excreted unchanged in the urine. **Half-life** Aspirin—0.25 ± 0.03 h.[1] (Salicylate) dose dependent—2.4 h with 0.25 g, 5 h with 1 g, 6.1 h with 1.3 g, 19 h with 10–20 g.[15]

Adverse Reactions. Hearing impairment, GI upset, and occult bleeding frequently occur, while acute hemorrhage from gastric erosion also likely. As with other NSAIDs, aspirin can cause renal dysfunction, particularly in those with preexisting renal disease or heart failure. Rare hepatotoxicity occurs, primarily in children with rheumatic fever or rheumatoid arthritis and adults with systemic lupus erythematosus (SLE) or preexisting liver disease;[16] the syndrome of asthma, angioedema, and nasal polyps can be provoked in susceptible patients.[17] A single analgesic dose can suppress platelet aggregation and prolong bleeding time for up to 1 week; large dosages can prolong PT.[18]

Contraindications. Bleeding disorders; hypersensitivity to other NSAIDs or tartrazine dye.

Precautions. Use with caution in patients with renal disease, gastric ulcer, bleeding tendencies, hypoprothrombinemia, or **history of asthma,** or during anticoagulant therapy. Because of the association with Reye's syndrome, the use of salicylates in children and teenagers with flu-like symptoms or chickenpox is not recommended.[19,20] Those developing bronchospasm with aspirin can develop similar reactions to other NSAIDs.[17] Sodium salicylate and other nonacetylated salicylates (except diflunisal) are usually well tolerated in these patients.[19,21]

Drug Interactions. Alkalinizing agents (e.g., acetazolamide, antacids) can reduce salicylate levels; acetazolamide also can enhance central nervous system (CNS) penetration of salicylate. Corticosteroids can reduce serum salicylate levels. Large doses of salicylates can increase oral anticoagulant effect; even small doses can increase risk of bleeding with oral anticoagulants or heparin because of the antiplatelet effect of aspirin. Alcohol and salicylate increase the risk of GI blood loss. Salicylates can cause an increased response to sulfonylureas, especially chlorpropamide. Salicylate decreases the uricosuric effect of uricosuric agents (e.g., probenecid, sulfinpyrazone). Salicylate, especially in large doses, can decrease renal elimination of methotrexate and displace it from plasma protein binding sites.

Parameters to Monitor. Monitor for abnormal bleeding or bruising and occult GI blood loss (periodic hematocrit) in patients who ingest salicylates regularly. Serum salicylate level determinations are recommended with higher dosage regimens because of the wide variation among patients in serum levels produced. Monitor renal function and hearing changes (tinnitus); however, using tinnitus as an index of maximum salicylate tolerance is NOT recommended.[12]

Notes. Available in combination with butalbital/caffeine, codeine phosphate, dipyridamole, meprobamate, oxycodone, and pravastatin.

CELECOXIB   Celebrex

Pharmacology. Inhibition of the Cox-2 enzyme isoform is thought to be responsible for the anti-inflammatory effects of NSAIDs, whereas inhibition of Cox-1 results in GI and possibly other side effects. A relatively selective Cox-2 inhibitor should combine anti-inflammatory, analgesic, and antipyretic efficacies equivalent to older, nonselective NSAIDs with improved safety.[22,23]

Administration and Adult Dosage. **PO for osteoarthritis**—100 mg twice daily OR 200 mg daily. **PO for rheumatoid arthritis**—100–200 mg twice daily. **PO for familial adenomatous polyposis**—400 mg twice daily with food. **PO for ankylosing spondylitis**—200 mg once daily or 100 mg twice daily and if no effect after 6 weeks, the dose can be increased to 400 mg/d and reevaluate within 6 weeks. **PO for acute pain and primary dysmenorrhea**—400 mg initially followed by 200 mg as needed on day one and 200 mg twice daily as needed thereafter.

Special Populations. *Pediatric Dosage.* (<18 years) Safety and efficacy not established.

Geriatric Dosage. Dosage adjustment is usually not necessary; however, use the lowest effective dose; (<50 kg) initiate therapy at the lowest recommended dose. Patients with moderate hepatic dysfunction should receive 50% of the recommended dose and the drug should be avoided in those with severe hepatic impairment.

Dosage Forms. **Cap** 100, 200, 400 mg.

Patient Instructions. This drug can cause headache, upset stomach, or diarrhea. Report edema, rash, unusual weight gain, or signs and symptoms of GI bleeding to your physician. Avoid products that contain aspirin and NSAIDs unless otherwise directed. Take without regard to meals (unless 400 mg twice daily, then take with food).

Missed Doses. If you take this drug on a regular schedule, take a missed dose as soon as you remember. If it is about time for the next dose, take that dose only; do not double the dose or take an extra dose.

Pharmacokinetics. *Fate.* Absolute bioavailability not studied, but celecoxib has rapid systemic absorption. Peak plasma levels occur in 3 h. With high-fat meals, peak levels are delayed 1–2 h with accompanying increases in total absorption of 10%–20%; 97% plasma protein bound. Predominantly metabolized hepatically by CYP2C9 to inactive metabolites with <3% excreted unchanged in urine or feces. **Half-life** 11 h.

Adverse Reactions. Indication specific. Celecoxib can cause GI toxicity, dyspepsia, abdominal pain, nausea, vomiting, and diarrhea at a rate similar to placebo and less than conventional NSAIDs. Renal, cardiovascular and liver effects are equivalent to other NSAIDs.[24,25]

Contraindications. History of aspirin- or NSAID-induced asthma, urticaria, or allergic type reactions or allergy to sulfonamides; treatment of pain in the setting of coronary artery bypass graft surgery.

Precautions. Use celecoxib cautiously in patients with preexisting asthma, renal or hepatic impairment, fluid retention, hypertension, or heart failure. Some patients may exhibit hypertension, congestive heart failure, edema, GI ulceration, bleeding, perforation, decreased renal function, anaphylactoid reactions, skin reactions (e.g., exfoliative dermatitis, Stevens-Johnson syndrome, toxic epidermal necrolysis), and an increased risk of cardiovascular thrombotic events.

Drug Interactions. NSAIDs can diminish the effects of ACE inhibitors, furosemide, and thiazide diuretics and increase lithium plasma levels. Concurrent use with anticoagulants can increase the risk of bleeding. Inhibitors of CYP2C9 (e.g., fluconazole) can increase serum concentrations of celecoxib. Increased prothrombin time may occur in some patients using concurrent warfarin therapy.

Parameters to Monitor. Monitor for weight gain, renal function during long-term use, and occult blood loss if on concomitant aspirin or anticoagulant therapy.

Notes. Celecoxib 100 or 200 mg twice daily is as effective as **naproxen** 500 mg twice daily for the treatment of osteoarthritis and produces fewer gastroduodenal ulcers than naproxen, **diclofenac**, or **ibuprofen**.[24,25]

IBUPROFEN   Advil, Motrin, Nuprin, Various

Pharmacology. Ibuprofen is an NSAID with analgesic and antipyretic properties. It is a nonselective inhibitor of Cox-1 and Cox-2 and reversibly alters platelet function and prolongs bleeding time.

Administration and Adult Dosage. **PO for mild to moderate pain**—200–400 mg every 4–6 h as needed, maximum 1200 mg/d. **PO for primary dysmenorrhea**—400 mg every 4 h as needed. **PO for rheumatoid arthritis and osteoarthritis**—400–800 mg 3–4 times daily, to a maximum of 3.2 g/d. **PO for migraine**—400 mg once daily up to 10 days. **PO for adult fever** (over the counter)—200–400 mg every 4–6 h as needed, to a maximum of 1200 mg/d, not to exceed 10 days unless directed by physician. **PO for headache**—200–400 mg every 4–6 h as needed, to a maximum of 1200 mg/24 h.

Special Populations. *Pediatric Dosage.* **PO for fever**—(6 months to 12 years) 5 mg/kg for fever <102.5°F OR 10 mg/kg for fever >102.5°F given every 6–8 h, to a maximum of 40 mg/kg/d. **PO for pain**—(6 months to 12 years) 10 mg/kg every 6–8 h as needed, to a maximum of 40 mg/kg/d. **PO for juvenile arthritis**—30–40 mg/kg/d in 3 or 4 divided doses; 20 mg/kg/d in milder disease. **PO for headache**—variable dosing based on age and weight.

Geriatric Dosage. Use minimal effective dosages because the elderly are more susceptible to GI bleeding and acute renal insufficiency.

Dosage Forms. **Cap** 200 and 400 mg; **Chew Tab** 50 and 100 mg; **Tab** 100, 200, 400, 600, and 800 mg; **Susp** 20 and 40 mg/mL.

Patient Instructions. This drug may be taken with food, milk, or antacid to minimize stomach upset. Report any symptoms of GI ulceration or bleeding, skin rash, weight gain, or edema. Dizziness can occur; until the extent of this effect is known, use appropriate caution.

Missed Doses. If you take this drug on a regular schedule and you miss a dose, take it as soon as you remember. If it is about time for the next dose, take that dose only. Do not double the dose or take an extra dose.

Pharmacokinetics. *Serum Levels.* 10 mg/L (48 μmol/L) for antipyretic effect.[1] Serum concentrations over 200 mg/L (971 mmol/L) 1 h after acute overdosage may be associated with severe toxicity (e.g., apnea, metabolic acidosis, and coma).[26]

Fate. Rapidly absorbed from the GI tract with bioavailability over 80%.[1] Peak serum levels in children of 17–42 mg/L (82–204 μmol/L) after a dose of 5 mg/kg and 25–53 mg/L (121–257 μmol/L) after a dose of 10 mg/kg are achieved in 1.1 ± 0.3 h.[27] Greater than 99% plasma protein bound; metabolized to at least 2 inactive metabolites; V_d is 0.15 ± 0.02 L/kg, increased in cystic fibrosis; clearance is 0.045 ± 0.012 L/h/kg, increased in cystic fibrosis. Less than 1% is excreted unchanged in the urine.[1] **Half-life** 2 ± 0.5 h.[1]

Adverse Reactions. Gastric distress, blood loss, diarrhea, vomiting, dizziness, and skin rash occur occasionally; GI ulceration (for all NSAIDs there is a greater risk in the elderly and with higher dosages) and fluid retention have been reported.[28] Ibuprofen occasionally causes renal dysfunction, particularly in those with preexisting renal disease, heart failure, or cirrhosis.[29] Higher doses of NSAIDs, except naproxen, may be associated with increased risk of cardiovascular disease (e.g., MI).[30] A slight rise in the bleeding time, elevation of liver enzymes, lymphopenia, agranulocytosis, aplastic anemia, and aseptic meningitis have been reported rarely.[31,32]

Contraindications. Syndrome of nasal polyps; angioedema; bronchospastic reactivity to aspirin or other NSAIDs, treatment of perioperative pain in setting of coronary artery bypass graft surgery; bleeding, especially those with active intracranial hemorrhage or GI bleeding; coagulation defects. (IV formulation for preterm infants) congenital heart disease in whom patency of the ductus arteriosus is necessary for satisfactory pulmonary or systemic blood flow; hypersensitivity to ibuprofen; untreated proven or suspected infection; necrotizing enterocolitis; renal function impairment; thrombocytopenia.

Precautions. Pregnancy category D. Use with caution in patients with preexisting renal disease, heart failure, asthma, or hepatic impairment;[29] a history of ulcer disease or bleeding; or risk factors associated with peptic ulcer disease (e.g., advanced age, high-dose NSAIDs, concomitant steroids, or anticoagulants) or cardiovascular disease.

Drug Interactions. NSAIDs may inhibit the antihypertensive response to ACE inhibitors, β-blockers, diuretics, and hydralazine, and the natriuretic effect of diuretics. Possible GI bleeding and the antiplatelet effect of NSAIDs can increase the risk of serious bleeding during anticoagulant therapy. NSAIDS plus selective serotonin reuptake inhibitors may increase the risk of upper GI bleeding and hemorrhage.[33] NSAIDs can decrease renal lithium clearance. NSAIDs, including ibuprofen, can increase methotrexate levels and cause toxicity.

Parameters to Monitor. Monitor for symptomatic improvement, complete blood count, blood loss, weight gain, liver, and renal function during long-term use.

Notes. Do not take the over-the-counter ibuprofen longer than 10 days, unless directed by a physician. **Misoprostol** is effective in preventing NSAID-associated GI ulceration. Histamine H2-receptor antagonists, however, prevent duodenal but not gastric ulcerations and may mask the signs and symptoms of NSAID-induced GI ulceration. Proton pump inhibitors (e.g., omeprazole) are effective in treating NSAID-related dyspepsia and preventing NSAID-induced ulcers.[34] Available in combination with oxycodone and hydrocodone. Ibuprofen lysine is approved in children from 500 to 1500 g and <32 weeks gestational age for treatment of patent ductus arteriosus.

INDOMETHACIN   Indocin, Various

Pharmacology. Indomethacin is an indoleacetic acid NSAID that is one of the most potent nonselective inhibitors of cyclooxygenase available. In addition to its anti-inflammatory effects, indomethacin has prominent analgesic and antipyretic properties. It also has been used to suppress uterine activity and prevent premature labor.

Administration and Adult Dosage. **PO for rheumatoid arthritis, rheumatoid (ankylosing) spondylitis, and osteoarthritis**—25 mg 2–3 times daily initially. Increase in 25 mg/d increments at weekly intervals until satisfactory response or to a maximum of 150–200 mg/d. Alternatively, up to 100 mg of the daily dosage may be given at bedtime for persistent night or morning stiffness. **PO for acute gouty arthritis**—50 mg 3 times daily until resolved. **SR capsule**—75 mg 1–2 times/d can be substituted for all uses except gouty arthritis, based on non-SR dosage.

Pediatric Dosage. (<14 years) Safety and efficacy not established; **IV for pharmacologic closure of persistent patent ductus arteriosus in premature infants**—0.2 mg/kg, followed by 2 additional IV doses of 0.1–0.25 mg/kg (depending on age) at 12- to 24-h intervals.

Dosage Forms. **Cap** 25, 50 mg; **SR Cap** 75 mg; **Supp** 50 mg; **Susp** 5 mg/mL; **Inj** (powder for reconstitution) 1 mg.

Pharmacokinetics. Indomethacin is rapidly and well absorbed from the GI tract, with a bioavailability of 98%. Peak serum levels are reached within 2 h with effective concentrations in the range of 0.3–3 mg/L (0.8–8 μmol/L). It is 90% plasma protein bound and has extensive O-demethylation and N-deacylation to inactive metabolites; V_d is 0.29 ± 0.04 L/kg; clearance is 0.084 ± 0.012 L/h/kg, lower in premature infants, neonates, and the aged; 15% ± 8% is excreted unchanged in the urine. The half-life of the drug is 2.4 ± 0.4 h, higher in premature infants, neonates, and the aged.

Adverse Reactions. Adverse effects are frequent, and approximately 20% of patients cannot tolerate the drug. Frontal lobe headache, drowsiness, dizziness, mental confusion, and GI distress are frequent, especially with dosages >100 mg/d; occasional peripheral neuropathy, occult bleeding, and peptic ulcer occur. Pancreatitis, corneal opacities, hepatotoxicity, aplastic anemia, agranulocytosis, thrombocytopenia, aggravation of psychiatric disorders, and allergic reactions are reported rarely. The syndrome of asthma, angioedema, and nasal polyps may be provoked in susceptible patients. Precautions, drug interactions, and monitoring are similar to other NSAIDs. (*See* Ibuprofen.)

Notes. The maximum oral OR rectal daily dose is 200 mg, and the lowest dose for the shortest duration is recommended. An alternative to the above IV regimen for pharmacologic closure of persistent patent ductus arteriosus in premature infants includes 0.3 mg/kg as a single dose OR 1 or more doses of 0.1 mg/kg as a retention enema or orogastric tube.[1,18]

NAPROXEN	Naprosyn, Various
NAPROXEN SODIUM	Aleve, Anaprox, Various

Pharmacology. *See* Ibuprofen.

Administration and Adult Dosage. **PO for mild to moderate pain, dysmenorrhea, or acute tendinitis or bursitis**—(naproxen) 500 mg, followed by 250 mg every 6–8 h, maximum 1250 mg/d; (naproxen sodium)—550 mg, followed by 275 mg every 6–8 h, maximum 1375 mg/d. **PO for rheumatoid arthritis, osteoarthritis, and ankylosing spondylitis**—(naproxen) 250–500 mg twice daily initially, maximum 1500 mg/d for limited periods; (naproxen sodium)—275–550 mg twice daily OR 275 mg every morning and 550 mg every evening initially, maximum 1650 mg/d for limited periods. If no improvement has occurred after 4 weeks of therapy, consider other drug therapy. **PO for acute gout**—(naproxen) 750 mg, followed by 250 mg every 8 h until resolved; (naproxen sodium)—825 mg, followed by 275 mg every 8 h until resolved. **PO (over the counter) for pain, fever, and headache**—200–400 mg initially, followed by 200 mg every 8–12 h as needed, maximum 600 mg/24 h.

Special Populations. *Pediatric Dosage.* **PO for juvenile arthritis**—10 mg/kg/d in 2 divided doses. **PO** (over the counter) **for pain, fever, and headache**—same as adult dosage.

Geriatric Dosage. Use minimal effective dosages because the elderly are more susceptible to GI bleeding and acute renal insufficiency.

Dosage Forms. **Tab** (naproxen) 250, 375, 500 mg; (naproxen sodium) 220, 275, 550 mg; **EC Tab** (naproxen) 375, 500 mg; **SR Tab** (naproxen sodium) 375, 500, 750 mg; **Susp** (naproxen) 25 mg/mL.

Patient Instructions. *See* Ibuprofen.

Pharmacokinetics. *Serum Levels.* Trough concentrations >50 mg/L (>217 μmol/L) are associated with response in rheumatoid arthritis.[1]

Fate. Rapidly absorbed from the GI tract with a bioavailability of approximately 99%. Greater than 99.7% plasma protein bound, saturable with increasing dosage, increased with uremia, cirrhosis, and in the elderly, and decreased in rheumatoid arthritis and hypoalbuminemia; V_d is 0.16 ± 0.02 L/kg, increased in uremia, cirrhosis, and rheumatoid arthritis. Clearance is 0.0078 ± 0.0012 L/h/kg, increased in rheumatoid arthritis, and decreased in uremia; less than 1% is excreted unchanged in urine.[1] **Half-life** 14 ± 1 h, increased in the elderly.[1]

Adverse Reactions. Naproxen can occasionally cause renal dysfunction, particularly in those with preexisting renal disease, heart failure, or hepatic impairment. Interstitial nephritis and nephrotic syndrome have been reported.[35,36] (*See* Ibuprofen.) Contraindications, precautions, drug interactions, and monitoring are similar to other NSAIDs. (*See* Ibuprofen.)

Notes. Available in combination with lansoprazole and sumatriptan. The lowest dose for the shortest duration is recommended.

OXICAMS	
MELOXICAM	Mobic, Various
PIROXICAM	Feldene, Various

The oxicam class of medications are NSAID with analgesic properties. It is generally accepted that these medications inhibit prostaglandin synthetase. Generally, this class is similar to other NSAIDs.

Pharmacology. *See* Ibuprofen.

Administration and Adult Dosage. (piroxicam) **PO for osteoarthritis and rheumatoid arthritis**—20 mg/d in 1–2 divided doses; (meloxicam) **PO for osteoarthritis and rheumatoid arthritis**—7.5–15 mg/d.

Special Populations. *Pediatric Dosage.* (Piroxicam) safety and efficacy not established; (meloxicam) (2 years and older) **PO for juvenile arthritis**—0.125 mg/kg once daily, to a maximum of 7.5 mg/d.

Geriatric Dosage. (piroxicam) 10 mg once daily. Doses >20 mg/d are associated with significant increase in GI toxicity and ulceration.

Other Conditions. **Renal Impairment.** (meloxicam) (Cl_{Cr} <15 mL/min) Not recommended.

Dosage Forms. (piroxicam) **Cap** 10 and 20 mg; (meloxicam) **Tab** 7.5 and 15 mg, **Susp** 7.5 mg/5 mL.

Patient Instructions. *See* Ibuprofen.

Pharmacokinetics. *Fate.* Rapid GI absorption, 3–5 h to peak concentration, with approximately 90% bioavailability. 99% protein binding. V_d 0.14 L/kg. Extensively hepatically metabolized via hydroxylation, conjugation, cyclodehydration, hydrolysis, decarboxylation, ring contraction and N-demethylation. Approximately 5% unchanged via renal excretion (0.28 mL/h/kg). **Half-life** (piroxicam) 50 h; (meloxicam) 20 h with adjustments based on age, hepatic, and renal function.

Adverse Reactions. *See* Ibuprofen.

NONSTEROIDAL ANTI-INFLAMMATORY DRUGS COMPARISON CHART

CLASS AND DRUG	DOSAGE FORMS	ADULT DOSAGE	HALF-LIFE (h)	COMMENTS
ACETIC ACIDS				
Diclofenac				
Cataflam	Tab (diclofenac potassium) 50 mg	PO (pain, dysmenorrhea) (Cataflam). 50 mg 3 times daily	1.1 ± 0.2	Although it is unclear whether the risk of hepatotoxicity is any greater than with other NSAIDs, careful monitoring of symptoms and liver function tests is recommended.
Voltaren	Tab (diclofenac sodium)	PO (arthritis) 100–200 mg/d in 2 doses.		
Various	50, 75 mg plus misoprostol 200 μg (Arthrotec)	PC, SR 100 mg once or twice daily (dosage expressed as diclofenac)		
Solaraze	SR Tab (diclofenac sodium) 25, 50, 75, 100 mg	Solaraze: actinic kertoses—affected area twice daily		
Voltaren	Gel (diclofenac sodium) 1% and 3%	Voltaren: pain of osteoporosis–affected area 4 times daily		
Flector	Patch 1.3% diclofenac epolamine	Acute strains, sprains, contusions: apply one patch to painful area twice daily.		
Etodolac				
Lodine	Cap 200, 300, mg	PO (pain) 200–400 mg every 6–8 h;	7.3 ± 4	Recommended for treatment of osteoarthritis; not as effective as other NSAIDs for rheumatoid arthritis.
Various	Tab 400, 500 mg	PO (arthritis) 600–1200 mg/d in 2–3		
	SR Tab 400, 500, 600 mg	divided doses. Maximum dose 1200 mg/d or if ≤60 kg, 20 mg/kg/d.		
Indomethacin				
Indocin	Cap 25, 50 mg	PO (gouty arthritis) 100 mg, then	2.4 ± 0.4 (higher in premature infants, neonates, and the aged).	See monograph. Associated with a high frequency of CNS effects such as drowsiness, dizziness, mental confusion, and frontal lobe headache.
Various	SR Cap 75 mg	50 mg 3 times daily;		
	Susp 5 mg/mL	PO or PR (arthritis) 50–200 mg/d		
	Supp 50 mg	in 3 divided doses.		
	Inj 1 mg	SR in 1–2 doses, can substitute for equal daily dosage of non-SR (75 mg daily to twice daily).		

(continued)

NONSTEROIDAL ANTI-INFLAMMATORY DRUGS COMPARISON CHART (continued)

CLASS AND DRUG	DOSAGE FORMS	ADULT DOSAGE	HALF-LIFE (h)	COMMENTS
Ketorolac Toradol Various	Tab 10 mg Inj 15, 30, 60 mg	PO (pain, short-term) 10 mg every 4–6 h PRN, to a maximum of 40 mg/d for 5 days (including IM/IV) IM or IV (short-term management of pain) 30 or 60 (IM only) mg once, then 15–30 mg every 6 h.	4.5	For short-term (up to 5 days) use only. Do not exceed 60 mg/d parenterally in patients 65 y or older, under 50 kg, or with elevated serum creatinine.
Sulindac Clinoril	Tab 150, 200 mg	PO (arthritis) 150 mg/d twice daily. Bursitis, tendinitis, acute gout: 200 mg twice daily.	15 ± 4 (active sulfide metabolite)	Purported "renal-sparing" effect has been questioned. Because the active sulfide metabolite has a relatively long half-life, renal effects may not be observed for several days.
Tolmetin Tolectin Various	Cap 400 mg Tab 200, 600 mg	PO (arthritis) 0.6–1.8 g/d in 3–4 divided doses.	4.9 ± 0.3	Higher frequency of anaphylactoid reactions than other NSAIDs.
ANTHRANILIC ACIDS (FENAMATES) *Meclofenamate* Meclomen Various	Cap 50, 100 mg	PO (pain) 50 mg every 4–6 h (Maximum 400 mg/d); PO (arthritis) 200–400 mg/d in 3–4 divided doses.	3	The fenamates as a group are more toxic than other NSAIDs and associated with headache, dizziness, and hemolytic anemia.
Mefenamic Acid Ponstel	Cap 250 mg	PO (pain, dysmenorrhea) 500 mg initially, then 250 mg q 6 h for up to 1 wk PEDS >14 y: use adult dose.	3	Not recommended; see Meclofenamate comments.

(continued)

NONSTEROIDAL ANTI-INFLAMMATORY DRUGS COMPARISON CHART (continued)

CLASS AND DRUG	DOSAGE FORMS	ADULT DOSAGE	HALF-LIFE (h)	COMMENTS
NONACIDIC COMPOUNDS				
Nabumetone Relafen	Tab 500, 750 mg	PO (arthritis) 1–2 g/d in 1–2 doses.	23 ± 4 (active 6-MNA metabolite)	Reported to have less GI toxicity than other NSAIDs.
OXICAMS				
Meloxicam Mobic	Tab 7.5 mg, 15 mg Susp 7.5 mg/5 mL	PO (arthritis) 7.5–15 mg once daily. PEDS: JRA: ≥2 y: 0.125 mg/kg daily to maximum of 7.5 mg.	20	Less mucosal damage than with piroxicam.
Piroxicam Feldene Various	Cap 10, 20 mg	PO (arthritis) 20 mg/d in 1–2 doses.	48 ± 8	Elderly patients may be at increased risk of renal and GI adverse events.
PROPIONIC ACIDS				
Fenoprofen Nalfon	Cap 200, 300 mg Tab 600 mg	PO (pain) 200 mg every 4–6 h; PO (arthritis) 1.2–2.4 g/d in 3–4 divided doses.	2.5 ± 0.5	Similar to ibuprofen.
Flurbiprofen Ansaid	Tab 50, 100 mg	PO (arthritis) 200–300 mg/day in 2–4 divided doses.	3.8 ± 1.2	Similar to ibuprofen.
Ibuprofen Advil Motrin Nuprin Various	See monograph	PO (pain, dysmenorrhea) 400 mg every 4–6 h. PO (arthritis) 1.2–3.2 g/d in 3–4 divided doses.	2 ± 0.5	See monograph.

(continued)

NONSTEROIDAL ANTI-INFLAMMATORY DRUGS COMPARISON CHART (*continued*)

CLASS AND DRUG	DOSAGE FORMS	ADULT DOSAGE	HALF-LIFE (h)	COMMENTS
Ketoprofen Actron Orudis Orudis KT Oruvail Various	Cap 25, 50, 75 mg Tab 12.5 mg SR Cap 100, 150, 200 mg	PO (pain) 25–50 mg every 6–8 h; PO (arthritis) 150–300 mg/d in 3 divided doses. PO SR 200 mg/d in 1 dose.	1.8 ± 0.3	Similar to ibuprofen.
Naproxen Aleve Anaprox Naprelan Naprosyn Various	Tab (naproxen sodium) 220, 275, 550 mg Tab (naproxen) 250, 375, 500 mg EC Tab (naproxen) 375, 500 mg SR Tab (naproxen) 375, 500, 750 mg Susp (naproxen) 25 mg/mL	PO (pain) 500 mg, then 250 mg every 6–8 h; PO (arthritis) 0.5–1.5 g/d in 2 divided doses; PO (acute gout) 750 mg, then 250 mg every 8 h. (Doses expressed as naproxen.)	14 ± 1	*See monograph.* Equal in efficacy and safety to ibuprofen.
Oxaprozin Daypro	Caplet, tablet 600 mg	PO (arthritis) 1.2 g/d in 1 dose. Maximum dose 1.8 g/d or 26 mg/kg/d, whichever is lower.	50–60	Similar to other NSAIDs.
SALICYLATES **Aspirin** Various	*See monograph*	PO (pain) 325–1000 mg every 4 h; PO (arthritis) 3.6–5.4 g/d in 3–4 divided doses.[a]	0.25 ± 0.03 (aspirin) 2–19 (salicylate, dose dependent)	*See monograph.*

(continued)

NONSTEROIDAL ANTI-INFLAMMATORY DRUGS COMPARISON CHART (*continued*)

CLASS AND DRUG	DOSAGE FORMS	ADULT DOSAGE	HALF-LIFE (h)	COMMENTS
Choline Magnesium Trisalicylate Trilisate	Tab 500, 750 mg, 1 g Liquid 100 mg/mL	PO (pain, arthritis) 1.5–3 g/d in 1–2 divided doses.[a] PEDS: JRA 50 mg/kg/d (up to 37 kg) PO divided twice daily.	2–19 (salicylate, dose dependent)	Salicylate is only a weak inhibitor of cyclooxygenase. It therefore has no antiplatelet effect and can usually be administered safely to individuals with aspirin sensitivity. See also Aspirin monograph.
Diflunisal Dolobid Various	Tab 250, 500 mg	PO (arthritis) 500–1000 mg divided bid. Maximum dose 1.5 g/d.	11 ± 2 (dose dependent)	Similar to other NSAIDs.
Magnesium Salicylate Doan's Various	Tab 500, 545, 600 mg	PO (pain, arthritis) 3.6–4.8 g/d in 3–4 divided doses.[a]	2–19 (salicylate, dose dependent)	*See* Choline Magnesium Trisalicylate comments and Aspirin monograph.
Salsalate Disalcid Various	Tab 500, 750 mg	PO (arthritis) 3 g/d in 2–3 divided doses.[a]	2–19 (salicylate, dose dependent)	*See* Choline Magnesium Trisalicylate comments and Aspirin monograph.
SELECTIVE COX-2 INHIBITORS				
Celecoxib Celebrex	Cap 50, 100, 200, 400 mg	PO for osteoarthritis 100 mg twice daily or 200 mg/d; PO for rheumatoid arthritis 100–200 mg twice daily; PEDS: JRA 2–17 y 10–25 kg: 50 mg twice daily; >25 kg: 100 twice daily PO for familial adenomatous polyposis 400 mg twice daily with food.	11	Equal efficacy to other NSAIDs with improved GI safety profile. (*See* monograph.)

[a]Long-term dosage for arthritis should be guided by serum salicylate levels. *See* Aspirin monograph.
Adapted from Refs. 1, 18, and 35–45 and product information.

■ REFERENCES

1. Dahlof C. The ideal 5-HT1D agonist. In: Olesen J, Tfelt-Hansen P, eds. *Headache Treatment: Trial Methodology and New Drugs.* Philadelphia, PA: Lippincott-Raven; 1997:243-251.

2. Segasothy M et al. Paracetamol: a cause for analgesic nephropathy and end-stage renal disease. *Nephron.* 1988;50:50-54.

3. Zimmerman HJ, Maddrey WC. Acetaminophen (paracetamol) hepatotoxicity with regular intake of alcohol: analysis of instances of therapeutic misadventure. *Hepatology.* 1995;22:767-773.

4. Shek KL et al. Warfarin-acetaminophen drug interaction revisited. *Pharmacotherapy.* 1999;19:1153-1158.

5. Buckley NA et al. Oral or intravenous N-acetylcysteine: which is the treatment of choice for acetaminophen (paracetamol) poisoning? *J Toxicol Clin Toxicol.* 1999;37:759-767.

6. Towheed TE, Hochberg MC. A systematic review of randomized controlled trials of pharmacological therapy in osteoarthritis of the knee, with an emphasis on trial methodology. *Semin Arthritis Rheum.* 1997;26:755-770.

7. Hirsh J et al. Aspirin and other platelet-active drugs. The relationship among dose, effectiveness, and side effects. *Chest.* 1995;108:247S-257S.

8. Bowry ADK et al. Meta-analysis of the efficacy and safety of clopidogrel plus aspirin as compared to antiplatelet monotherapy for the prevention of vascular events. *Am J Cardiol.* 2008;101:960-966.

9. Berger JS et al. Low-dose aspirin in patients with stable cardiovascular disease: a meta-analysis. *Am J Med.* 2008;121:43-49.

10. Verro P et al. Aspirin plus dipyridamole versus aspirin for prevention of vascular events after stroke or TIA: a meta-analysis. *Stroke.* 2008;39:1358-1363.

11. Hennekens CH et al. Dose of aspirin in the treatment and prevention of cardiovascular disease: current and future directions. *J Cardiovasc Pharmacol Ther.* 2006;11:170-176.

12. Mongan E et al. Tinnitus as an indication of therapeutic serum salicylate levels. *JAMA.* 1973;226:142-145.

13. Done AK. Aspirin-overdosage: incidence, diagnosis, and management. *Pediatrics.* 1978;62(suppl):890-897.

14. Lanza FL et al. Endoscopic evaluation of the effects of aspirin, buffered aspirin, and enteric-coated aspirin on gastric and duodenal mucosa. *N Engl J Med.* 1980;303:136-138.

15. Levy G. Pharmacokinetics of salicylate elimination in man. *J Pharm Sci.* 1965;54:959-967.

16. Tolman KG. Hepatotoxicity on non-narcotic analgesics. *Am J Med.* 1998;105(1B):13S-19S.

17. Stevenson DD, Mathison DA. Aspirin sensitivity in asthmatics. When may this drug be safe? *Postgrad Med.* 1985;78:111-119.

18. Bonica JJ, ed. *The Management of Pain.* 2nd ed. Philadelphia, PA: Lea & Febiger; 1990.

19. Rahwan GL, Rahwan RG. Aspirin and Reye's syndrome: the change in prescribing habits of health professionals. *Drug Intell Clin Pharm.* 1986;20:143-145.

20. Pinsky PF et al. Reye's syndrome and aspirin: evidence for a dose-response effect. *JAMA.* 1988;260:657-661.

21. Housholder GT. Intolerance to aspirin and the nonsteroidal anti-inflammatory drugs. *J Oral Maxillofac Surg.* 1985;43:333-337.

22. Chen YF et al. Cyclooxygenase-2 selective non-steroidal anti-inflammatory drugs (etodolac, meloxicam, celecoxib, rofecoxib, etoricoxib, valdecoxib, and lumiracoxib) for osteoarthritis and rheumatoid arthritis: a systematic review and economic evaluation. *Health Technol Assess.* 2008;12:1-278, iii.

23. Laine L et al. Cox-2 selective inhibitors in the treatment of osteoarthritis. *Semin Arthritis Rheum.* 2008;38:165-187.

24. Solomon SD et al. Cardiovascular risk of celecoxib in 6 randomized placebo-controlled trials: The cross trial safety analysis. *Circulation.* 2008;117:2104-2113.

25. Zhang J et al. Adverse effects of cyclooxygenase 2 inhibitors on renal and arrhythmia events: meta-analysis of randomized trials. *JAMA.* 2006;296:1619-1632.

26. Hall AH et al. Ibuprofen overdose—a prospective study. *West J Med.* 1988;148:653-656.

27. Nahata MC et al. Pharmacokinetics of ibuprofen in febrile children. *Eur J Clin Pharmacol.* 1991;40:427-428.

28. Hollander D. Gastrointestinal complications of nonsteroidal anti-inflammatory drugs: prophylactic and therapeutic strategies. *Am J Med.* 1994;96:274-281.

29. Whelton A et al. Renal effects of ibuprofen, piroxicam, and sulindac in patients with asymptomatic renal failure. *Ann Intern Med.* 1990;112:568-576.

30. Hennekens CH, Borzak S. Cyclooxygenase-2 inhibitors and most traditional nonsteroidal anti-inflammatory drugs cause similar moderately increased risks of cardiovascular disease. *J Cardiovasc Pharmacol Ther.* 2008;13:41-50.

31. Stempel DA, Miller JJ. Lymphopenia and hepatotoxicity with ibuprofen. *J Pediatr.* 1977;90:657-658.

32. Bernstein RF. Ibuprofen-related meningitis in mixed connective tissue disease. *Ann Intern Med.* 1980;92:206-207.

33. Look YK et al. Meta-analysis: gastrointestinal bleeding due to interaction between selective serotonin uptake inhibitors and non-steroidal anti-inflammatory drugs. *Aliment Pharmacol Ther.* 2008;27:31-40.

34. Bhatt DL et al. ACCF/ACG/AHA 2008 expert consensus document on reducing the gastrointestinal risk of antiplatelet therapy and NSAID use: a report of the American College of Cardiology Foundation Task Force on Clinicial Expert Consensus Documents. *Circulation.* 2008;118:1894-1909.

35. Maniglia R et al. Non-steroidal anti-inflammatory nephrotoxicity. *Ann Clin Lab Sci.* 1988;18:240-252.

36. Marsh CC et al. A review of selected investigational nonsteroidal anti-inflammatory drugs of the 1980s. *Pharmacotherapy.* 1986;6:10-25.

37. Riendeau D et al. Comparison of the cyclooxygenase-1 inhibitory properties of nonsteroidal anti-inflammatory drugs (NSAIDs) and selective Cox-2 inhibitors, using sensitive microsomal and platelet assays. *Can J Physiol Pharmacol.* 1997;75:1088-1095.

38. Furst DE. Meloxicam: selective Cox-2 inhibition in clinical practice. *Semin Arthritis Rheum.* 1997;26(suppl 1):21-27.

39. Wallace JL. Nonsteroidal anti-inflammatory drugs and gastroenteropathy: the second hundred years. *Gastroenterology.* 1997;112:1000-1016.

40. Vane JR, Botting RM. Mechanism of action of aspirin-like drugs. *Semin Arthritis Rheum.* 1997;26(suppl 1):2-10.

41. Litvak KM, McEvoy GK. Ketorolac, an injectable nonnarcotic analgesic. *Clin Pharm.* 1990;9:921-935.

42. Brooks PM, Day RO. Nonsteroidal anti-inflammatory drugs—differences and similarities. *N Engl J Med.* 1991;324:1716-1725.

43. Helfgott SM et al. Diclofenac-associated hepatotoxicity. *JAMA.* 1990;264:2660-2662.

44. Middleton E Jr et al., eds. *Allergy Principles and Practice.* 3rd ed. St. Louis, MO: CV Mosby; 1988.

45. Quercia RA, Ruderman M. Focus on nabumetone: a new chemically distinct nonsteroidal anti-inflammatory agent. *Hosp Formul.* 1991;26:25-34.

Chapter 5

Opioids

Mark T. Holdsworth

Class Instructions. These medications can cause drowsiness. Until the extent of this effect is known, use caution when driving, operating machinery, or performing other tasks requiring mental alertness. Avoid excessive concurrent use of alcohol and other drugs that cause drowsiness. Prolonged use of this medication can cause constipation, and concurrent use of a laxative with prolonged use would likely be necessary.

For moderate to severe pain (pain rating >5 on a 0–10 scale), you must take doses at regular intervals around the clock to anticipate and prevent pain. When the drug is taken at the correct interval and pain relief does not last for this period, use additional "rescue" doses of a short-acting drug to maintain pain relief. When more than 4 rescue doses are frequently used daily, contact the prescriber to increase the dosage. Addiction does not occur when these drugs are used for legitimate painful conditions. Dependence, a condition in which withdrawal may occur if the medication is suddenly discontinued, can occur with prolonged usage but can be managed by slowly decreasing the dosage when no longer needed.

Missed Doses. If you miss a dose, take it as soon as you remember. If it is about time for the next dose, take that dose only. Do not double the dose or take an extra dose. Take subsequent doses at the same interval previously established for pain relief.

CODEINE SALTS   Various

Pharmacology. Codeine is 3-methoxymorphine, a phenanthrene opioid with very low affinity for opioid receptors. Its analgesic activity appears to result from conversion to morphine. Poor metabolizers of debrisoquine/sparteine (approximately 7% of the Caucasian population) cannot convert appreciable amounts of codeine to morphine or obtain analgesia from codeine but are still subject to the same adverse effects.[1-4] (*See* Morphine Sulfate.)

Administration and Adult Dosage. **PO, SQ, or IM for analgesia**—15–60 mg every 4–6 h. **PO or SQ for antitussive action**—10–20 mg every 4–6 h, to a maximum of 120 mg/d. IV not recommended. (*See* Precautions.)

Special Populations. *Pediatric Dosage.* **PO, SQ, or IM for analgesia**—(≥1 year) 0.5 mg/kg every 4–6 h, to a maximum of 60 mg/dose. **PO for antitussive action**—(2–6 years) 2.5–5 mg every 4–6 h, to a maximum of 30 mg/d; (6–12 years) 5–10 mg every 4–6 h, to a maximum of 60 mg/d; (>12 years) Same as adult dosage. (*See* Notes.)

Geriatric Dosage. Same as adult dosage.[5]

Other Conditions. Reduce initial dosage in debilitated patients or those with hypoxia or hypercapnia.

Dosage Forms. **Tab** 15, 30, 60 mg; **Inj** 15, 30, 60 mg/mL; **oral liquid** 2, 2.4, 3 mg/mL in various combinations. Formulated as phosphate or sulfate salt.

Patient Instructions. (*See* Opioids Class Instructions.)

Pharmacokinetics. *Onset and Duration.* PO, SQ onset 15–30 min; IM peak analgesia 0.5–1 h; duration (all routes) 4–6 h.[6]

Fate. Systemic availability averages 40% but with a wide range (12%–84%), reflecting large variability in hepatic enzyme activity.[7] A single PO 15-mg dose produces serum levels of 26–33 μg/L (82–104 nmol/L) in 2 h and 13–22 μg/L (41–69 nmol/L) in 5 h.[8] The drug is 7% plasma protein bound. V_d is 2.6 $\pm$ 0.3 L/kg; clearance is 0.66 $\pm$ 0.12 L/h/kg.[9] Metabolized in the liver to codeine-6-glucuronide, N-demethylated to norcodeine, and O-demethylated to morphine by genetic polymorphic CYP2D6. Codeine-6-glucuronide is the major metabolite, while norcodeine and morphine are minor metabolites, each accounting for approximately 10% of the dose.[3] Accumulation of morphine occurs with repeated administration, resulting in a morphine:codeine AUC ratio of 0.29:1.[10] Variation in the reported rates of codeine conversion to morphine may be related to the assays used, with much higher concentrations of morphine reported with radioimmunoassays than with HPLC or GC-MS.[7] Primarily urinary excretion of inactive forms; 3% 16% is excreted unchanged in urine.[11] **Half-life** 2.9 $\pm$ 0.7 h.[9]

Adverse Reactions. Sedation, dizziness, nausea, vomiting, constipation, and respiratory depression occur frequently. Dose-related signs of intoxication are miosis, drowsiness, decreased rate and depth of respiration, bradycardia, and hypotension. Dose-related adverse reactions in children are somnolence, ataxia, miosis, and vomiting at 3–5 mg/kg/d and respiratory depression at >5 mg/kg/d. Because hepatic glucuronidation is incomplete in infants, they are at particular risk for dose-related adverse effects.[12]

Precautions. Because of severe hypotension, do not administer codeine phosphate IV.[13,14]

Drug Interactions. Potent CYP2D6 inhibitors (e.g., quinidine and fluoxetine) can abolish the conversion to morphine and the pharmacologic effects of codeine.[5,15]

Notes. Codeine is no more effective than placebo in suppressing nighttime cough in children. The American Academy of Pediatrics recommends that parents be educated about the lack of proven antitussive effects and the potential risks of codeine-containing products because overdosage has been reported.[12] Available in different combinations with guaifenesin, aspirin, acetaminophen, and promethazine.

FENTANYL
Duragesic, Fentanyl, Oralet, Sublimaze, Various

Pharmacology. Fentanyl is a phenylpiperidine opioid agonist with predominant effects on the mu opioid receptor and is approximately 50–100 times more potent as an analgesic than morphine. Other related compounds are **sufentanil** (Sufenta), which is 5–7 times more potent than fentanyl; **alfentanil** (Alfenta), which is less potent than fentanyl but acts more rapidly and has a shorter duration of action; and **remifentanil** (Ultiva), which is more potent than fentanyl and is extremely short acting because of its rapid ester hydrolysis.[1,2] (*See* Morphine Sulfate.)

Administration and Adult Dosage. **IV patient-controlled analgesia (PCA)**—
20–100 μg per activation with 3–10 min lockout period, both titrated to patient
response. (*See* Patient-Controlled Analgesia Guidelines Chart.) **Epidurally for
analgesia**—25–150 μg as an intermittent bolus dose OR 25–150 μg/h as a continuous infusion, titrated to patient response.[6] (*See* Notes and Intraspinal Narcotic
Administration Guidelines Chart.) **Transdermal for analgesia**—calculate the previous 24-h analgesic requirement and convert this amount to the equal analgesic
oral morphine dosage from the Opioid Analgesics Comparison Chart. A short-acting opioid OR the fentanyl lozenge (Actiq) must be used for control of breakthrough pain until sufficient transdermal fentanyl is absorbed to achieve adequate
analgesia. Use Transdermal Fentanyl Comparison Chart to determine the fentanyl
transdermal dosage from the daily equivalent oral morphine dosage.

TRANSDERMAL FENTANYL COMPARISON CHART

24-HR ORAL MORPHINE DOSAGE[a] (mg/d)	FENTANYL TRANSDERMAL DOSAGE (μg/h)
60–134	25
135–224	50
225–314	75
315–404	100
405–494	125
495–584	150
585–674	175
675–764	200
765–854	225
855–944	250
945–1034	275
1035–1124	300

[a]Assumes morphine 10 mg IM is equivalent to morphine 60 mg orally; however, equivalent dosages
can vary among patients because of individual variability. These conversion dosages are conservative,
and approximately 50% of patients are likely to require a dosage increase after initial application.
(*See* Opioid Analgesics Comparison Chart.)

Initiate treatment using the recommended transdermal fentanyl dosage and
increase based on response no more frequently than every 3–6 days. Multiple
transdermal patches can be used to achieve appropriate dosage (do not cut patches
for a partial dosage). To change treatment to another opioid, discontinue the transdermal patch for 12–18 h and start treatment with the new opioid at about one-half
the equivalent analgesic dosage. **IV for induction and maintenance anesthesia**—
loading: 4–20 μg/kg, Maintenance: 2–10 μg/kg/h, Additional Bolus: 25–100 μg.[16]
IV for postoperative (recovery room) pain control—50–100 μg every 1–2 h as
needed. **Lozenge (Oralet) for anesthesia premedication or induction of conscious sedation**—5 μg/kg (provides effects similar to 0.75–1.25 μg/kg given IM),
to a maximum of 400 μg. **Lozenge for the management of breakthrough cancer**

pain (Actiq) in patients already receiving >60 mg of oral morphine/d or >50 μg/h of transdermal fentanyl—initial dose of 200 μg. Until the appropriate dose is reached, an additional dose can be used to treat an episode of breakthrough pain. Readministration can start 15 min after the previous lozenge has been completed. Do not give >2 units for a breakthrough pain episode while a patient is in the titration phase. Evaluate each new dose in the titration period over several breakthrough pain episodes. If >4 units/d are needed, increase the dosage of the long-acting opioid.

Special Populations. *Pediatric Dosage.* IV for sedation in neonates—9–20 μg/kg/h; tolerance limits its usefulness for prolonged sedation.[17] **IV for induction and maintenance anesthesia**—(2–12 years) 2–3 μg/kg initially, followed by 1–5 μg/kg/h.[16] **Lozenge for anesthesia premedication or induction of conscious sedation**— (<15 kg) contraindicated; (≥15 kg) 5–15 μg/kg, to a maximum of 400 μg.

Geriatric Dosage. **Lozenge for anesthesia premedication or induction of conscious sedation**—(>65 years) 2.5–5 μg/kg, to a maximum of 400 μg. Altered pharmacodynamics rather than pharmacokinetics appear to be responsible for increased sensitivity in elderly patients.[18]

Other Conditions. In patients with head injury, cardiovascular, pulmonary, or hepatic disease, consider a lower dosage of 2.5–5 μg/kg, to a maximum of 400 μg.

Dosage Forms. **Inj** 50 μg/mL; **SR patch** 12.5, 25, 50, 75, 100 μg/h; **lozenge for anesthesia (Oralet)** 100, 200, 300, 400 μg; **lozenge (on a stick) for breakthrough cancer pain (Actiq)** 200, 400, 600, 800, 1200, 1600 μg.

Patient Instructions. (*See* Opioids Class Instructions.) (Actiq) Once an effective dosage is determined; limit consumption to ≤4 units/d.

Pharmacokinetics. *Onset and Duration.* IM—onset 7–15 min; duration 1–2 h. Epidural onset 5 min; duration 4–6 h.[6] Transdermal—onset 6–8 h; peak 24–72 h; duration after a single application 72 h.[19,20] More than 17 h are required for serum levels to fall by one-half after patch removal.

Serum Levels. Analgesia—1–3 μg/L (3–9 nmol/L);[19,20] balanced anesthesia— 6–20 μg/L (18–60 nmol/L).[16]

Fate. Bioavailability is 52% with lozenge. Of the fentanyl released by the transdermal system, 92% is absorbed, but overall systemic bioavailability of the transdermal preparation is approximately 30%. The drug is 84% ± 2% plasma protein bound; it is metabolized rapidly primarily by the liver to norfentanyl and other inactive metabolites; V_d is 4 ± 0.4 L/kg; clearance is 0.78 ± 0.12 L/h/kg, decreased in the elderly and increased in neonates and children. Pharmacokinetics are not altered in renal insufficiency or compensated hepatic cirrhosis. Less than 10% is excreted unchanged in the urine.[1,18–21] **Half-life** 6.1 ± 2 h;[21] 7.1–11 h during cardiopulmonary bypass surgery.[16]

Adverse Reactions. (*See* Morphine Sulfate.) Unlike other opioids, fentanyl, alfentanil, remifentanil, and sufentanil are not associated with histamine release and may be preferable when cardiovascular stability is an issue.[16] The frequency of pruritus is lower than morphine, but not as low as meperidine.[22,23] PCA fentanyl produces less depression of postoperative cognitive function in elderly patients than does PCA morphine.[24] Development of withdrawal reactions after use for sedation in neonates and infants is likely with a total dosage >2.5 mg/kg or duration of infusion >9 days.[25]

Contraindications. (*See* Morphine Sulfate.) Fentanyl SR patch—acute or postoperative pain, including outpatient surgery; patients <12 years or <50 kg; pain that can be managed by conventional analgesics; and doses >25 μg/h at the initiation of opioid therapy. Oralet—management of acute and chronic pain. Actiq—management of acute or postoperative pain.

Precautions. (*See* Morphine Sulfate.) Analyses of fentanyl transdermal systems after 3 days of continuous application demonstrated a considerable amount of remaining drug (28%–84%), which is a potentially lethal dose (up to 1036 μg) for a 70 kg individual.[26] Cutting the membrane-controlled fentanyl transdermal system to achieve a different dosage is not recommended because it can damage the integrity of the semipermeable membrane. Placing a piece of impermeable material (e.g., adhesive bandage) on the skin proportionate in surface area to the intended reduction in dosage may be effective.[27]

Drug Interactions. (*See* Morphine Sulfate.) The effects of fentanyl may be potentiated by other CNS depressant drugs (e.g., barbiturates, general anesthetics, narcotics, and tranquilizers) and ritonavir, the latter by inhibition of CYP2D6.[28] Carbamazepine may decrease fentanyl's effect during anesthesia for craniotomy.

Parameters to Monitor. Monitor vital signs and pain ratings routinely.

Notes. Epidural administration has not been shown to be more advantageous than IV administration during surgery.[29] Lack of rapid titration precludes the usefulness of the transdermal fentanyl system for pain control in patients with rapidly changing analgesic requirements. Transdermal fentanyl for cancer pain causes a lower frequency of constipation than SR morphine.[30] IV is the parenteral route of choice after major surgery. This route is suitable for titrated bolus or continuous administration, but requires close monitoring because of a great risk of respiratory depression with superoptimal doses.[31]

MEPERIDINE HYDROCHLORIDE   Demerol, Various

Pharmacology. Meperidine is a phenylpiperidine opioid agonist with important antimuscarinic activity and negative inotropic effects on the heart. Its major metabolite, normeperidine, has excitant effects that can precipitate tremors, myoclonus, or seizures. Meperidine's antimuscarinic activity might negate the miosis that occurs with other opioids.[2] (*See* Morphine Sulfate.)

Administration and Adult Dosage. **PO, IV, or SQ for analgesia**—50–150 mg every 3–4 h. (*See* Notes.) Oral doses are about one-half as effective as parenteral doses. **IM or SQ for obstetric pain**—50–100 mg every 1–3 h. IM not recommended.[31] (*See* Notes.)

Special Populations. *Pediatric Dosage.* **PO, IV, or SQ for analgesia**—1–1.8 mg/kg every 3–4 h, to a maximum of 100 mg/dose. IM painful and should not be used in children.[32] (*See* Notes.)

Geriatric Dosage. Same as adult dosage.

Dosage Forms. **Syrup** 10 mg/mL; **Tab** 50, 100 mg; **Inj** 10, 25, 50, 75, 100 mg/mL.

Patient Instructions. *See* Opioids Class Instructions.

Pharmacokinetics. *Onset and Duration.* PO—onset approximately 15 min; duration 2–3 h. SQ or IM—onset approximately 10 min; peak analgesia 0.5–1 h; duration 2–3 h.[6,9]

Serum Levels. 500–700 g/L (2–2.8 μmol/L) appear to be required for analgesia.[19]

Fate. Oral bioavailability is approximately 52% ± 3%, increasing to 80%–90% in cirrhosis caused by decreased first-pass metabolism.[9,33] After a single 100-mg IM dose, mean serum levels of 670 μg/L (2.7 μmol/L) and 650 μg/L (2.6 μmol/L) are attained in 1 and 2 h, respectively;[34,35] 58% ± 9% plasma protein bound, largely to $α_1$-acid glycoprotein; decreased in the elderly and in uremia.[9,36] V_d is 4.4 ± 0.9 L/kg, increased in the elderly and premature infants; clearance 1.02 ± 0.3 L/h/kg, reduced by 25% in surgical patients and 50% in cirrhosis, and reduced in acute viral hepatitis.[9] Hydrolyzed and metabolized in the liver to normeperidine (an active metabolite), which is also hydrolyzed. An average of 2% unchanged drug and 1%–21% (average 6%) normeperidine are excreted in urine.[36] **Half-life** (Meperidine) α phase 12 min, β phase 3.2 h, increasing to 7 h in patients with cirrhosis or acute liver disease and 14–21 h in patients with moderate to severe renal dysfunction.[35,37,38] (Normeperidine) 14–21 h, increasing to 35 h in renal failure.[39]

Adverse Reactions. (*See* Morphine Sulfate.) Factors that can predispose to normeperidine-induced seizures are dosage >400–600 mg/d, renal failure, history of seizures, long-term administration to cancer patients, and coadministration of agents that increase N-demethylation to normeperidine.[40] (*See* Drug Interactions.) Local irritation and induration occur with repeated SQ injection.

Contraindications. MAO inhibitors within the past 14–21 days; chronic pain.

Precautions. (*See* Morphine Sulfate.) Avoid in patients with reduced renal function and avoid continuous administration for more than a few days. The combination of meperidine with promethazine and chlorpromazine for painful procedures is not recommended because it has poor efficacy compared with alternative approaches and is associated with a high frequency of adverse effects.[31]

Drug Interactions. (*See* Morphine Sulfate.) Concurrent use with an MAO inhibitor can cause marked blood pressure alterations, sweating, excitation, and rigidity. Barbiturates, chlorpromazine, and phenytoin can decrease meperidine serum concentrations and increase normeperidine, reducing analgesia and increasing the risk of stimulation and seizures.[41] Ritonavir can increase meperidine AUC via CYP2D6 inhibition.[28] Reduce dosage when given concomitantly with a phenothiazine or other drugs that potentiate the depressant effects of meperidine.

Parameters to Monitor. Monitor vital signs and pain scores at regular intervals. Jerking and twitching movements may be signs of normeperidine accumulation and impending toxicity.[42]

Notes. All opioids including meperidine and morphine increase biliary tract pressure. Sphincter of Oddi spasm may be less with meperidine than with morphine, but there is little evidence that this has clinical relevance. Unlike other opioids, 25–50 mg of meperidine is useful in treating the shaking and shivering associated with general anesthesia or amphotericin B administration.[40] Because of its low therapeutic index, reserve meperidine for very brief courses in otherwise healthy patients who have demonstrated untoward effects during treatment with other opioids, such as morphine or hydromorphone.[31] Because of the unreliable absorption and breakthrough pain when meperidine is administered IM, more rapid and predictable routes (e.g., IV) are recommended.[32,43,44] Oral meperidine is not recommended for cancer pain because the high dosage required to relieve severe pain increases the risk of CNS toxicity.[32]

| **METHADONE HYDROCHLORIDE** | Dolophine, Various |

Pharmacology. Methadone is a phenylheptylamine opioid agonist qualitatively similar to morphine but with a chemical structure unrelated to the alkaloid-type structures of the opium derivatives. Analgesic activity of (*R*)-methadone is 8–50 times that of (*S*)-methadone, and (*R*)-methadone has a 10-fold higher affinity for opioid receptors. Methadone is lipophilic and has considerable tissue distribution; plasma concentrations during long-term treatment are sustained by this peripheral reservoir. It does not share cross-tolerance with other opioids, and the dosage required to achieve analgesia in opioid-tolerant patients is much lower than predicted by opioid conversion tables and single-dose studies. Unlike other opioids, methadone does not have active or toxic metabolites that are associated with CNS toxicity (e.g., myoclonus, seizures).[45,46] Because methadone is a long-acting opioid, it can be substituted for short-acting opioids for analgesia maintenance and detoxification. Methadone abstinence syndrome is similar to morphine; however, onset is slower and duration is longer. (*See* Morphine Sulfate.)

Administration and Adult Dosage. **PO, IV, IM, or SQ for pain**—5–80 mg/d in 1–3 divided doses. Dosage escalation is slower than with other opioids and averages approximately 2%/d.[45] **PO for maintenance and detoxification treatment**—the minimum effective dosage for reducing illicit heroin use is approximately 60 mg/d, and the optimum dosage range is 80–120 mg/d. Premature termination of treatment and use of suboptimal dosages remain common problems. If tapering is attempted, taper gradually over 4–12 months or longer.[47]

Special Populations. *Pediatric Dosage.* Though safety and efficacy not established in patient <18 years. 0.1–0.2 mg/kg every 6–8 h have been used for treatment of pain.[32]

Geriatric Dosage. Same as adult dosage.

Dosage Forms. **Tab** 5, 10 mg; **Dispersible Tab** 40 mg; **Sol** 1, 2, 10 mg/mL; **Inj** 10 mg/mL; **Pwdr** 50, 100, 500, 1000 g.

Patient Instructions. (*See* Opioids Class Instructions.) Increase dosage cautiously with the assistance of your clinician.

Pharmacokinetics. *Onset and Duration.* (analgesia) Onset SQ—10–20 minutes, PO—30–60 min; peak SQ 0.5–1 h; duration PO, SQ, or IV—4–5 h after a single dose, 8–48 h with multiple doses.[19,45,46]

Serum Levels. Best rehabilitation in methadone maintenance patients has been associated with serum levels >211 μg/L (682 nmol/L).[48] There is no good correlation between serum levels and analgesia.[46]

Fate. Oral bioavailability is 92% ± 21%; 89% plasma protein bound. Pharmacokinetics are best described by a 2-compartment model. $V_{d\beta}$ is 3.8 ± 0.6 L/kg; clearance is 0.084 ± 0.03 L/h/kg. Both $V_{d\beta}$ and clearance are greater for (*R*)-methadone.[46] Extent of metabolism may increase with long-term therapy, resulting in a 15%–25% decline in serum levels, although this has also been attributed to poor compliance. Metabolized in the liver to inactive metabolites via N-demethylation; metabolites are excreted in urine and bile.[45] The drug is 24% ± 10% excreted unchanged in the urine, increased by urine acidification.[9,48,49] **Half-life** β phase 35 ± 12 h;[9] (*R*)-methadone has a longer half-life (37.5 h) than (*S*)-methadone (28.6 h).[48]

Adverse Reactions. (*See* Morphine Sulfate.) Because of its long half-life and lack of cross-tolerance, patients receiving methadone are at greater risk for toxicity when inappropriate dosage increases are made.

Precautions. (*See* Morphine Sulfate.) Pregnancy category C. The process of switching from another opioid to methadone is complex and should only be attempted by an experienced clinician in an inpatient setting over 3–6 days. (*See* Administration and Adult Dosage.)[45] The recent increased use of methadone as an analgesic has been associated with substantial increases in morbidity and mortality.[50]

Drug Interactions. (*See* Morphine Sulfate.) Carbamazepine, phenytoin, rifampin, and other drugs that induce CYP3A4 can decrease methadone serum levels and result in withdrawal symptoms in patients on methadone maintenance programs. Diazepam, erythromycin, fluvoxamine, ritonavir, and possibly other enzyme inhibitors can increase methadone levels and effects.[41,51]

Parameters to Monitor. During analgesia, monitor vital signs and pain ratings routinely. During methadone maintenance, monitor for signs of withdrawal, which include lacrimation, rhinorrhea, diaphoresis, yawning, restlessness, insomnia, dilated pupils, and piloerection.[47]

Notes. To convert from another opioid decrease the previous opioid dosage by one-third over 24 h and replace it with methadone using a dosage ratio of 1 mg oral methadone = 10 mg oral morphine. During day 2, attempt another one-third decrease in the dosage of the previous opioid while maintaining the previous dosage of methadone; on day 3, the final one-third of the dosage of the previous opioid may be discontinued. Maintain the patient on an 8-h schedule with approximately 10% of the daily methadone dosage as an extra dose for breakthrough pain.[33] For treatment of opioid addiction in detoxification or maintenance programs, methadone may be dispensed only by approved pharmacies. Maintenance therapy (treatment for longer than 3 weeks) may be undertaken only by approved methadone programs; this does not apply to addicts hospitalized for other medical conditions.

MORPHINE SULFATE   Various

Pharmacology. Morphine and other opioids interact with stereospecific opiate receptors in the CNS and other tissues. (*See* Opioid Receptor Specificity Comparison Chart.) Opioid analgesia is caused by actions at several CNS sites. Morphine and other mu opioid agonists inhibit nociceptive reflexes through inhibition of neurotransmitter release, have inhibitory actions on neurons conveying nociceptive information to higher brain centers, and enhance activity in descending pathways that exert inhibitory effects on the processing of nociceptive information in the spinal cord. Mu receptors are responsible for analgesia, respiratory depression, miosis, decreased GI motility, and euphoria. Stimulation of kappa receptors results in analgesia, less intense miosis and respiratory depression, dysphoria, and psychotomimetic effects. It is unclear what the consequences of delta receptor stimulation are in humans.[1] The relief of pain is fairly specific; other sensory modalities are essentially unaffected, and mental processes are not impaired (unlike anesthetics), except when given in large doses or to opiate-naive individuals. These drugs also have antitussive effects, usually at dosages less than those required for analgesia.

Administration and Adult Dosage. With the exception of transdermal fentanyl, there is no ceiling or maximum dosage for morphine or other opioid agonists, and very large doses may be required for severe pain.[32] **PO for analgesia**—8–20 mg every 4 h; **SR tablet, 12-h**—(opioid-naive patients) 30 mg every 8–12 h initially; (opioid-tolerant patients) Total daily oral morphine dosage equivalent in 2 divided doses every 12 h; **SR capsule, 24-h**—(opioid-naive patients) 20 mg every 24 h initially; (opioid-tolerant patients) Total daily oral morphine dosage equivalent every 24 h; **SQ for analgesia**—5–15 mg every 4 h (10 mg/70 kg is the optimal initial dose); **PR for analgesia**—10–20 mg every 4 h; **IV for analgesia**—4–10 mg, dilute and inject slowly over a 2–3-min period. **IV infusion**—1–10 mg/h;[52] Some patients with chronic pain may require a dosage as high as 95 mg/h or more.[53] **IV PCA**—1 mg per activation initially with 5–20 min lockout period, both titrated to patient response.[54,55] Continuous infusion combined with PCA is effective in chronic cancer pain.[56] **Epidural for analgesia (unpreserved solution)**—(intermittent) 5 mg initially, may repeat with 1–2 mg after 1 h; (continuous infusion) 0.05–0.1 mg/kg loading dose, then 0.005–0.01 mg/kg/h.[57] **IT for cancer pain (unpreserved solution)** 0.4–8.3 mg/d (average 1–23 mg/d).[58] **IT for cesarean section (unpreserved solution)** 0.1 mg.[59] **Intraventricular (unpreserved solution)**—0.1–2 mg, repeated approximately every 24 h.[60] **Inhalation for dyspnea**—5–15 mg in 2 mL sterile water or NS via nebulizer every 4 h;[61] **IM**—painful and is not recommended.[32]

Special Populations. *Pediatric Dosage.* **PO**—0.3 mg/kg every 3–4 h. **IV**—0.05–0.2 mg/kg every 4 h. **IV infusion**—0.01–0.04 mg/kg/h. **Epidural**—0.05–0.08 mg/kg. **IT**—0.01–0.03 mg/kg.[32,62,63]

Geriatric Dosage. Reduce initial dosage in elderly patients and make smaller percentage incremental increases in total daily dosage (e.g., 25%) than in younger patients.

Other Conditions. Reduce initial dosage in debilitated patients.

Dosage Forms. **Cap** 30 mg; **Sol** 2, 4, 20 mg/mL; **Supp** 5, 10, 20, 30 mg; **Tab** 10, 15, 30 mg; **SR Tab** (8, 12 h) 15, 30, 60, 100, 200 mg; **SR Cap (24 h)** 10, 20, 30, 45, 50, 60, 75, 80, 90, 100, 120, 200 mg; **Inj** (unpreserved solution) 0.5, 1, 4, 5, 8, 10, 15, 25, 50 mg/mL; (preserved solution) 2, 3, 4, 5, 8, 10, 15, 25, 50 mg/mL; **epidural** (liposome suspension) 10 mg/mL.

Patient Instructions. *See* Opioids Class Instructions.

Pharmacokinetics. *Onset and Duration.* Analgesia—onset IM 10–30 min; peak 0.5–1 h; duration 3–5 h.[19] *Serum Levels.* It is speculated that moderate analgesia requires serum levels of at least 50 µg/L (88 nmol/L).

Fate. Well absorbed from the GI tract, but first-pass conjugation is extensive, reducing oral bioavailability to 24% ± 12%.[9,64] Nebulized morphine by inhalation has a low bioavailability, 5% ± 3%, but a rapid peak at 10 min.[64] After an IM dose of 10 mg, peak morphine levels of approximately 56 µg/L (98 nmol/L) are reached within 20 min. The drug is 35% ± 2% plasma protein bound and decreased in acute viral hepatitis, cirrhosis, and hypoalbuminemia.[9] V_d is 2.12 L/kg in young normals and 1.16 L/kg in elderly patients; clearance is 2.02 L/h/kg in young normals and 1.66 L/h/kg in elderly patients.[52] Morphine clearance reaches adult level by age 6 months to 2.5 years.[65] Inactivated in the liver, primarily by conjugation to morphine-6-glucuronide (active) and morphine-3-glucuronide (inactive or antagonistic)[9,66] Decreased clearance of glucuronide metabolites has been demonstrated in patients with renal insufficiency.[67] Greater plasma concentrations of morphine-6-glucuronide are present with oral than with parenteral administration.[68] Mostly excreted in urine; 14% ± 7% as the active morphine-6-glucuronide and 3.4% (oral) to 9% (parenteral) of a dose is excreted unchanged.[9,66,69] **Half-life** 1.9 ± 0.5 h, increased in neonates and premature infants.[9]

Adverse Reactions. Respiratory and circulatory depression and constipation are major adverse effects. Patients with renal failure are more prone to develop adverse reactions.[70] Dose-related signs of intoxication are miosis, drowsiness, decreased rate and depth of respiration, bradycardia, and hypotension. Sedation, dizziness, nausea, vomiting, sweating, and constipation occur frequently. Euphoria, dysphoria, dry mouth, biliary tract spasm, postural hypotension, syncope, tachy- or bradycardia, urinary retention, and myoclonus occur occasionally. Myoclonus appears to be somewhat dose related and has been described after large doses via IV or intraspinal routes. Myoclonus can be managed by changing to another opioid or with a **benzodiazepine** or **dantrolene**.[71,72] Frequent adverse effects from epidural administration are urinary retention and pruritus; the latter can be managed with **naloxone** or **butorphanol**.[57] Possible allergic-type reactions are reported occasionally. Most allergic-type reactions consist of skin rash and wheal and flare over a vein, which can occur with IV injection; these are caused by direct stimulation of histamine release, are not allergic, and are not a sign of a more serious reaction. True allergy is rare. Confusion and disorientation have been linked to phenol and formaldehyde preservatives in epidural infusions, and seizures have been associated with high-dose IV infusions containing sodium bisulfite.[73,74]

Precautions. Use with caution and in reduced dosage when giving concurrently with other CNS-depressant drugs. Use with caution in pregnancy; the presence of head injury, other intracranial lesions, or preexisting increase in intracranial pressure; patients having an acute asthmatic attack; COPD or cor pulmonale; decreased respiratory reserve; preexisting respiratory depression, hypoxia, or hypercapnia; patients whose ability to maintain blood pressure is already compromised; patients with atrial flutter or other supraventricular tachycardias; patients with prostatic hypertrophy or urethral stricture; elderly or debilitated patients; and patients with acute abdominal pain, when administration of the drug might obscure the diagnosis or clinical course. Use with caution in the elderly and neonates and in patients with renal dysfunction or elevated bilirubin or LDH levels.[65,67,68,70] Infants older than 1 month eliminate morphine efficiently and are unlikely to be unusually sensitive to the respiratory depressant effects but may require longer dosage intervals.[65] Do not administer IV, IT, or epidurally to opiate-naive patients unless an opioid antagonist and facilities for assisted or controlled respiration are immediately available.

Drug Interactions. Concurrent use of opioids with other CNS depressants (e.g., alcohol, antipsychotics, general anesthetics, heterocyclic antidepressants, and sedative-hypnotics) can cause respiratory depression. Cimetidine can increase serum concentration and duration of effect of the opioids.[41]

Parameters to Monitor. Monitor for pain control and signs of respiratory or cardiovascular depression.

NALOXONE HYDROCHLORIDE	Narcan, Various

Pharmacology. Naloxone, an N-allyl derivative of oxymorphone, is an opioid antagonist that competitively binds at opiate receptors. Naloxone is essentially free of opioid agonist properties and is used to reverse the effects of opioid agonists and drugs with partial agonist properties.[75]

Administration and Adult Dosage. **IV (preferred) or SQ for known or suspected opioid overdose**—0.1–0.2 mg as a first dose, then progressively double the dose every 2–3 min OR 0.4 mg diluted in 9 mL saline and injected in 1-mL increments every 30–60 s, until respiration and consciousness have become normal OR until 10 mg has been given. If response occurs, to prevent recurrent toxicity caused by short naloxone half-life, IV infusion at an hourly rate equal to the initial dose required for arousal, with a possible repeat bolus of 50% required 20–30 min after start of infusion.[76,77] If a total of 10 mg has been given and there is no response, the diagnosis of opioid overdose should be questioned. The frequency of repeat doses is based on clinical evaluation of the patient. **IV for postoperative opioid respiratory depression**—0.1–0.2 mg initially, may repeat every 2–3 min until desired level of reversal is reached. Subsequent doses might be needed if the effect of the opioid outlasts the action of naloxone. (*See* Notes.) **PO for septic shock**—Optimal dosing as an adjunct not defined.

Special Populations. *Pediatric Dosage.* **IV for known or suspected opioid overdose**—0.01 mg/kg, may repeat as needed. **IV for postoperative opioid depression**—0.005–0.01 mg initially, may repeat every 2–3 min until desired level of reversal is reached. **IV (preferred) or SQ for opioid depression**—(neonates) 0.01 mg/kg initially, may repeat every 2–3 min until desired level of reversal is reached. Endotracheal and intratracheal administration not recommended in neonates.

Geriatric Dosage. Same as adult dosage.

Dosage Forms. **Inj** 0.02, 0.4, 1 mg/mL.

Pharmacokinetics. *Onset and Duration.* Onset IV within 2–3 min, up to 15 min when given IM or SQ; duration variable but usually 1 h or less.[78,79]

Fate. From 59% to 67% metabolized by hepatic conjugation and renal elimination of the conjugated compound.[80] V_d is approximately 2–3 L/kg;[9,81] clearance is approximately 1.3 L/h/kg.[9] **Half-life** 64 ± 12 min in adults,[82] 71 ± 36 min in neonates.[83]

Adverse Reactions. Naloxone administration has been occasionally associated with life-threatening complications such as pulmonary edema, seizures, hypertension, arrhythmias, and violent behavior within 10 min of parenteral administration.[76,77]

Contraindications. None known.

Precautions. Administration to opioid-dependent persons (including neonates of dependent mothers) might precipitate acute withdrawal symptoms.

Drug Interactions. None known except for opioid antagonism.

Parameters to Monitor. Respiratory rate, pupil size (might not be useful in mixed-drug or opioid partial agonist overdoses), heart rate, blood pressure, and symptoms of acute opioid withdrawal syndrome.

Notes. Naloxone is effective when administered endotracheally to patients with difficult venous access.[84] It is routinely used in the initial treatment of patients with coma of unknown origin. Also used IV for epidural opioid-induced pruritus (0.005–0.01 mg/kg either in incremental doses or as an hourly infusion)[57] and PO for opioid-induced constipation (4–12 mg not more often than every 6 h; more frequent administration might precipitate withdrawal). Give at a daily dose of approximately 20% of the 24-h morphine dose. Initial doses should not exceed 5 mg.[85,86] Its use in **clonidine** overdose has produced mixed results; use in septic and hemorrhagic shock has been disappointing.[75] Also available in combination with buprenorphine and pentazocine.

OPIOID PARTIAL AGONISTS

Pharmacology. These agents can be classified based on their effects on the opioid receptors. Opioid partial agonists have analgesic effects but are characterized by an analgesic ceiling, such that, beyond a certain point, further increases in dosage do not result in additional analgesia but might produce adverse effects.[1,32] **Tramadol** is partly metabolized by CYP2D6, thereby producing an active metabolite (M1) that binds to mu opioid receptors. Patients who are poor metabolizers of debrisoquine and sparteine have negligible M1 production and reduced analgesia, although some pain relief remains because of activation of monoaminergic antinociceptive pathways from tramadol enantiomers.[1,87]

Administration, Dosage, and Dosage Forms. *See* Opioid Analgesics Comparison Chart.

Patient Instructions. *See* Opioids Class Instructions.

Pharmacokinetics. *See* Opioid Analgesics Comparison Chart.

Adverse Reactions. Sedation, sweating, dizziness, nausea, vomiting, euphoria, dysphoria (agents with delta receptor activity), and hallucinations are most frequent. Occasionally, insomnia, anxiety, anorexia, constipation, dry mouth, syncope, visual blurring, flushing, decreased blood pressure, and tachycardia are reported. After parenteral use, diaphoresis, sting on injection, respiratory depression, transient apnea in the newborn from administration to the mother during labor, shock, urinary retention, and alterations in uterine contractions during labor occur rarely. Other rarely reported effects are muscle tremor and toxic epidermal necrolysis. Local skin reactions and ulceration and fibrous myopathy at the injection site have been reported with long-term parenteral use of pentazocine.[1] **Tramadol** adverse reactions include seizures (some after the first dose) with recommended and excessive dosages. Seizure risk is increased in patients taking concomitant medications that can reduce the seizure threshold (e.g., heterocyclic antidepressants, selective serotonin reuptake inhibitors, MAO inhibitors, neuroleptics) and with certain medical conditions (e.g., epilepsy, head trauma, metabolic disorders, alcohol and drug withdrawal, or CNS infection). In addition, **naloxone** administration for tramadol overdose can increase the risk of seizure. Anaphylactoid reactions also have been described in tramadol postmarketing surveillance.[88–90] Dependence/addiction and major psychological disturbances have been reported with **butorphanol** nasal spray.[91]

Contraindications. (Tramadol) prior allergy to any opiate; acute intoxication with alcohol, hypnotics, centrally acting analgesics, opioids, or psychotropic drugs. (*See* Notes.)

Precautions. (*See* Morphine Sulfate.) Also, use cautiously in MI patients because **pentazocine** and **butorphanol** increase cardiac workload. All of these agents can produce dependence and withdrawal symptoms after extended use.

Drug Interactions. (*See* Morphine Sulfate.) With the possible exception of tramadol, these agents can precipitate acute withdrawal in opioid-dependent individuals.[92]

Notes. Because of their ceiling effect, risk of precipitating opiate withdrawal, and marked adverse effects, these agents are not recommended for the management of cancer pain.[32] Effects of pentazocine are antagonized by naloxone. Naloxone in Talwin NX tablets is not absorbed orally but theoretically prevents parenteral abuse of the oral dosage form; however, IV abuse of Talwin Nx plus tripelennamine has been reported.[93]

OPIOID RECEPTOR SPECIFICITY COMPARISON CHART

DRUG	RECEPTOR TYPE		
	Mu	*Kappa*	*Delta*
Buprenorphine	Partial agonist–antagonist	Unknown	Minimal activity
Butorphanol	Partial agonist–antagonist	Agonist	Unknown
Dezocine	Partial agonist–antagonist	Agonist	Minimal agonist activity
Morphine	Agonist	Minimal agonist activity	Unknown
Nalbuphine	Antagonist	Agonist	Agonist
Pentazocine	Partial agonist–antagonist	Agonist	Unknown
Tramadol[a]	Partial or pure agonist[b]	Minimal activity	Unknown

[a]Also blocks norepinephrine and serotonin reuptake.
[b]Not a classic agonist–antagonist; has little or no antagonist properties but appears to have partial Mu receptor agonist activity.

PATIENT-CONTROLLED ANALGESIA (PCA) GUIDELINES CHART[a]

DRUG	IV BOLUS DOSE (mg)	LOCKOUT INTERVAL (min)
Buprenorphine	0.03–0.2	10–20
Fentanyl	0.02–0.1	3–10
Hydromorphone	0.1–0.5	3–15
Meperidine[b]	5–30	5–15
Methadone	0.5–3	10–20
Morphine[a]	0.5–3	5–20
Nalbuphine	1–5	5–15
Oxymorphone	0.2–0.8	5–15
Pentazocine	5–30	5–15
Sufentanil	0.003–0.015	3–10

[a]Some clinicians recommend combining PCA with a basal continuous infusion of the narcotic. The hourly dosage is determined by the patient's previous narcotic dose requirements and adjusted every 8–24 h based on the dose of PCA bolus administered, basal continuous infusion, and pain response. A typical starting hourly basal continuous infusion rate for morphine in a 70-kg adult is 0.5–3 mg/h.
[b]Use with caution (preferably avoid) for PCA and consider factors that might predispose to seizures, which include dosage over 100 mg every 2 h for longer than 24 h, renal failure, or history of seizure disorder.
From Refs. 6, 54, and 56.

INTRASPINAL NARCOTIC ADMINISTRATION GUIDELINES CHART[a]

ROUTE AND DRUG	INTRASPINAL BOLUS DOSE (mg)	ONSET (min)	DURATION (h)
EPIDURAL			
Alfentanil	0.7–2[b]	Rapid	1.5–1.7[c]
Fentanyl	0.025–0.15	5	2–4
Hydromorphone	1–2	15	10–16
Methadone	1–10	10	6–10
Morphine	1–10	30	6–24
Sufentanil	0.015–0.05	15	4–6
INTRATHECAL (SUBARACHNOID)			
Morphine	0.1–0.5	15	8–24

[a]Use only preservative-free preparations for intraspinal narcotic administration.
[b]Based on a 70-kg adult body weight (e.g., 10–30 μg/kg).
[c]Very short duration of action; requires epidural infusion to obtain prolonged analgesia. Like fentanyl, prolonged epidural infusions produce high systemic concentrations and appear to have little advantage over IV infusion.
From Refs. 6 and 16.

OPIOID ANALGESICS COMPARISON CHART

DRUG AND SCHEDULE[a]	DOSAGE FORMS	EQUIVALENT PARENTERAL DOSAGE[b] (mg)	EQUIVALENT ORAL DOSAGE[c] (mg)	PARENTERAL/ ORAL EFFICACY RATIO	DURATION OF ANALGESIA (h)	PARTIAL ANTAGONIST ACTIVITY
Alfentanil (C-II) Alfenta	Inj 500 µg/mL	1	—	—	<1	N
Buprenorphine (C-V) Buprenex Subutex[d]	Inj 0.324 mg/mL SL Tab 2, 8 mg	0.3–0.6 (0.4–0.8[d,e])	—	—	6–8	Y
Butorphanol Stadol (NC) Stadol NS (C-IV)	Inj 1, 2 mg/mL Nasal spray 10 mg/mL (1 mg/spray)[f]	2	—	1/16	3–4	Y
Codeine (C-II) Various	Inj 30, 60 mg/mL Sol 3 mg/mL Tab 15, 30, 60 mg	120	30	1/2–2/3	4–6	N
Dezocine (NC) Dalgan	Inj 5, 10, 15 mg/mL	10–15	—	—	3–4	Y
Fentanyl (C-II) Actiq Duragesic Ionsys Oralet Sublimaze Various	Inj 50 µg/mL SR patch 12.5, 25, 50, 75, 100 µg/h Iontophoretic transdermal system 40 µg/dose (80 doses/system) Lozenge 100, 200, 300, 400 µg Lozenge on a stick 200, 400, 600, 800, 1200, 1600 µg Buccal Tab 100, 200, 400, 600, 800 µg	0.1	—	1/5	1–2 (patch, 72)	N

(continued)

OPIOID ANALGESICS COMPARISON CHART (continued)

DRUG AND SCHEDULE[a]	DOSAGE FORMS	EQUIVALENT PARENTERAL DOSAGE[b] (mg)	EQUIVALENT ORAL DOSAGE[c] (mg)	PARENTERAL/ ORAL EFFICACY RATIO	DURATION OF ANALGESIA (h)	PARTIAL ANTAGONIST ACTIVITY
Hydrocodone and Acetaminophen (C-III) Vicodin Various	Tab 5, 7.5, 10 mg with acetaminophen 400 mg; 2.5, 5, 7.5 mg with acetaminophen 500 mg; 7.5 mg with acetaminophen 400, 500, 650, 750 mg; 10 mg with acetaminophen 325, 400, 500, 650, 660 mg Cap 5 mg with acetaminophen 500 mg Sol 0.5 mg with acetaminophen 33 mg/mL	—	5	—	4–6	N
Hydromorphone (C-II) Dilaudid Palladone Various	Inj 1, 2, 4, 10 mg/mL Tab 2, 4, 8 mg Sol 1 mg/mL Supp 3 mg	1.5	1	1/5–1/2	3–5	N
Levorphanol (C-II) Levo-Dromoran	Inj 2 mg/mL Tab 2 mg	2	—	1/2	4–6	N
Meperidine (C-II) Demerol Various	Inj 10, 25, 50, 75, 100 mg/mL Tab 50, 100 mg Syrup 10 mg/mL	75–100	50	1/3–1/2	2–4	N
Methadone (C-II) Dolophine Various	Inj 10 mg/mL Tab 5, 10 mg Dispersible Tab 40 mg Sol 1, 2, 10 mg/mL	9	9	1/2	8–48	N

(continued)

67

OPIOID ANALGESICS COMPARISON CHART (continued)

DRUG AND SCHEDULE[a]	DOSAGE FORMS	EQUIVALENT PARENTERAL DOSAGE[b] (mg)	EQUIVALENT ORAL DOSAGE[c] (mg)	PARENTERAL/ ORAL EFFICACY RATIO	DURATION OF ANALGESIA (h)	PARTIAL ANTAGONIST ACTIVITY
Morphine (C-II) Various	Inj 0.5, 1, 2, 4, 5, 8, 10, 15, 25, 50 mg/mL Tab 15, 30 mg Cap 15, 30 mg Sol 2, 4, 20 mg/mL SR Cap 20, 30, 50, 60, 80, 90, 100, 120, 200 mg SR Tab 15, 30, 60, 100, 200 mg Supp 5, 10, 20, 30 mg	10	5	1/3	3–5	N
Nalbuphine (NC) Nubain Various	Inj 10, 20 mg/mL	10	—	1/6	3–6	Y
Oxycodone (C-II) Oxycontin Roxicodone Various	Cap 5 mg Tab 5, 15, 30 mg Tab 2.5, 5 mg with acetaminophen 325 mg; 5 mg with acetaminophen 500 mg; 7.5 mg with acetaminophen 500 mg; 10 mg with acetaminophen 650 mg Sol 1, 20 mg/mL SR Tab 10, 20, 40, 80 mg	—	5	—	3–4	N

(continued)

OPIOID ANALGESICS COMPARISON CHART (continued)

DRUG AND SCHEDULE[a]	DOSAGE FORMS	EQUIVALENT PARENTERAL DOSAGE[b] (mg)	EQUIVALENT ORAL DOSAGE[c] (mg)	PARENTERAL/ ORAL EFFICACY RATIO	DURATION OF ANALGESIA (h)	PARTIAL ANTAGONIST ACTIVITY
Oxymorphone (C-II) Numorphan	Inj 1 mg/mL Tab 5, 10 mg SR Tab 5, 10, 20, 40 mg	1–1.5	—	1/6	4–5	N
Pentazocine (C-IV) Talwin Talwin Nx Various	Inj 30 mg/mL Tab 50 mg with naloxone 0.5 mg Tab 12.5 mg with aspirin 325 mg; 25 mg with acetaminophen 650 mg	30–60	25	1/3	2–3	Y
Propoxyphene (C-IV) Darvocet Darvon Various	Cap (HCl) 65 mg Tab (HCl) 65 mg with acetaminophen 650 mg Tab (napsylate) 50, 100 mg Tab (napsylate) 50 mg with acetaminophen 325 mg; 100 mg with acetaminophen 650 mg Susp (napsylate) 10 mg/mL	—	65 (HCl); 100 (napsylate)	—	4–6	N
Remifentanil (C-II) Ultiva	Inj 1, 2, 5 mg	0.1	—	—	<0.5	N

(continued)

OPIOID ANALGESICS COMPARISON CHART (*continued*)

DRUG AND SCHEDULE[a]	DOSAGE FORMS	EQUIVALENT PARENTERAL DOSAGE[b] (mg)	EQUIVALENT ORAL DOSAGE[c] (mg)	PARENTERAL/ ORAL EFFICACY RATIO	DURATION OF ANALGESIA (h)	PARTIAL ANTAGONIST ACTIVITY
Sufentanil (C-II)						
Sufenta	Inj 50 µg/mL	0.01	—	—	2.5–3.5	N
Tramadol (NC)						
Ultracet	Tab 50 mg	—	25	—	4–6	—
Ultram	SR Tab 100, 200, 300 mg					
Various	Tab 50 mg with acetaminophen (Ultracet)					

[a]Controlled Substance Schedule designated after each drug (in parentheses); NC = not controlled.
[b]Parenteral dose equivalent to 10 mg morphine.
[c]Oral dose equivalent to 30 mg codeine. Not for SR products.
[d]Subutex and Suboxone (buprenorphine plus naloxone) are used in treating addiction.
[e]Equivalent sublingual dose.
[f]Recommended dosage is one spray in one nostril, repeated as needed in 60–90 min; this cycle may then be repeated every 3–4 h as needed for pain.
[g]See Pharmacology and Notes in Methadone monograph.
From Refs. 1, 6, 16, 19, 20, 33, and 94–97 and product information.

■ REFERENCES

1. Reisine T, Pasternak G. Opioid analgesics and antagonists. In: Hardman JG et al., eds. *Goodman and Gilman's the Pharmacological Basis of Therapeutics.* 9th ed. New York: McGraw-Hill; 1996:521-555.

2. Way WL. Opioid analgesics and antagonists. In: Katzung BG, ed. *Basic and Clinical Pharmacology.* 6th ed. Norwalk, CT: Appleton & Lange; 1995:460-475.

3. Poulsen L et al. Codeine and morphine in extensive and poor metabolizers of sparteine: pharmacokinetics, analgesic effect and side effects. *Eur J Clin Pharmacol.* 1995;51:289-295.

4. Eckhardt K et al. Same incidence of adverse drug events after codeine administration irrespective of the genetically determined differences in morphine formation. *Pain.* 1998;76:27-33.

5. Özdemir V et al. Pharmacokinetic changes in the elderly. Do they contribute to drug abuse and dependence? *Clin Pharmacokinet.* 1996;31:372-385.

6. Bonica JJ, ed. *The Management of Pain.* 2nd ed. Philadelphia, PA: Lea & Febiger; 1990.

7. Persson K et al. The postoperative pharmacokinetics of codeine. *Eur J Clin Pharmacol.* 1992;42:663-666.

8. Schmerzier E et al. Gas chromatographic determination of codeine in serum and urine. *J Pharm Sci.* 1966;55:155-157.

9. Benet LZ et al. Design and optimization of dosage regimens: pharmacokinetic data. In: Hardman JG et al., eds. *Goodman and Gilman's the Pharmacological Basis of Therapeutics* 9th ed. New York: McGraw-Hill; 1996:1707-1792.

10. Guay DR et al. Pharmacokinetics of codeine after single- and multiple-oral-dose administration to normal volunteers. *J Clin Pharmacol.* 1987;27:983-987.

11. Way EL, Adler TK. The pharmacologic implications of the fate of morphine and its surrogates. *Pharmacol Rev.* 1968,12:383-446.

12. American Academy of Pediatrics Committee on Drugs. Use of codeine- and dextromethorphan-containing cough remedies in children. *Pediatrics* 1997;99:918-920.

13. Cox RG. Hypoxaemia and hypotension after intravenous codeine phosphate. *Can J Anaesth.* 1994;41:1211-1213.

14. Parke TJ et al. Profound hypotension following intravenous codeine phosphate. Three case reports and some recommendations. *Anaesthesia.* 1992;47:852-854.

15. Caraco Y et al. Pharmacogenetic determination of the effects of codeine and prediction of drug interactions. *J Pharmacol Exp Ther.* 1996;278:1165-1174.

16. Bowdle TA et al., eds. *The Pharmacologic Basis of Anesthesiology.* New York: Churchill Livingstone; 1994.

17. Arnold JH et al. Changes in the pharmacodynamic response to fentanyl in neonates during continuous infusion. *J Pediatr.* 1991;119:639-643.

18. Scholz J et al. Clinical pharmacokinetics of alfentanil, fentanyl and sufentanil. An update. *Clin Pharamacokinet.* 1996;31:275-292.

19. Donnelly AJ. Pharmacology of pain management agents. *Anesthesia Today.* 1989;1:6-10.

20. Gourlay GK et al. The transdermal administration of fentanyl in the treatment of postoperative pain: pharmacokinetics and pharmacodynamic effects. *Pain.* 1989;37:193-202.

21. Varvel JR et al. Absorption characteristics of transdermally administered fentanyl. *Anesthesiology.* 1989;70:928-934.

22. Smith AJ et al. A comparison of opioid solutions for patient-controlled epidural analgesia. *Anaesthesia.* 1996;51:1013-1017.

23. Woodhouse A et al. A comparison of morphine, pethidine and fentanyl in the postsurgical patient-controlled analgesia environment. *Pain.* 1996;64:115-121.

24. Herrick IA et al. Postoperative cognitive impairment in the elderly. Choice of patient-controlled analgesia opioid. *Anaesthesia.* 1996;51:356-360.

25. Jacqz-Aigrain E, Burtin P. Clinical pharmacokinetics of sedatives in neonates. *Clin Pharmacokinet.* 1996;31:423-443.

26. Marquardt KA et al. Fentanyl remaining in a transdermal system following three days of continuous use. *Ann Pharmacother.* 1995;29:969-971.

27. Lee HA, Anderson PO. Giving partial doses of transdermal patches. *Am J Health Syst Pharm.* 1997;54:1759-1760.

28. Michalets EL. Update: clinically significant cytochrome P-450 drug interactions. *Pharmacotherapy.* 1998;18:84-112.

29. Guinard J-P et al. Epidural and intravenous fentanyl produce equivalent effects during major surgery. *Anesthesiology.* 1995;82:377-382.

30. Ahmedzai S, Brooks D. Transdermal fentanyl versus sustained-release oral morphine in cancer pain: preference, efficacy, and quality of life. *J Pain Symptom Manage.* 1997;13:254-261.

31. Acute Pain Management Guideline Panel. *Acute pain management: operative or medical procedures and trauma. Clinical practice guideline.* AHCPR Publication No. 92-0032. Rockville, MD: Agency for Health Care Policy and Research, Public Health Service, Department of Health and Human Services; February 1992.

32. Jacox A et al. *Management of cancer pain. Clinical practice guideline no. 9.* AHCPR Publication No. 94-0592. Rockville, MD: Agency for Health Care Policy and Research, Public Health Service, Department of Health and Human Services; March 1994.

33. Edwards DJ et al. Clinical pharmacokinetics of pethidine: 1982. *Clin Pharmacokinet*. 1982;7:421-433.

34. Fochtman FW, Winek CL. Therapeutic serum concentrations of meperidine (Demerol). *J Forensic Sci*. 1969;14:213-218.

35. Klotz U et al. The effect of cirrhosis on the disposition and elimination of meperidine in man. *Clin Pharmacol Ther*. 1974;16:667-675.

36. Julius HC et al. Meperidine binding to isolated alpha1-acid glycoprotein and albumin. *DICP*. 1989;23:568-572.

37. McHorse TS et al. Effect of acute viral hepatitis in man on the disposition and elimination of meperidine. *Gastroenterology*. 1975;68:775-780.

38. Chan K et al. Pharmacokinetics of low-dose intravenous pethidine in patients with renal dysfunction. *J Clin Pharmacol*. 1987;27:516-522.

39. Tang R et al. Meperidine-induced seizures in sickle cell patients. *Hosp Formul*. 1980;15:764-772.

40. Clark RF et al. Meperidine: therapeutic use and toxicity. *J Emerg Med*. 1995;13:797-802.

41. Quinn DI, Day RO. Drug interactions of clinical importance. An updated guide. *Drug Saf*. 1995;12:393-452.

42. Geller RJ. Meperidine in patient-controlled analgesia: a near-fatal mishap. *Anesth Analg*. 1993;76:655-657.

43. Erstad BL et al. Site-specific pharmacokinetics and pharmacodynamics of intramuscular meperidine in elderly postoperative patients. *Ann Pharmacother*. 1997;31:23-28.

44. Isenor L, Penny-MacGillivray T. Intravenous meperidine infusion for obstetric analgesia. *J Obstet Gynecol Neonatal Nurs*. 1993;22:349-356.

45. Ripamonti C et al. An update on the clinical use of methadone for cancer pain. *Pain*. 1997;70:109-115.

46. Kristensen K et al. Stereoselective pharmacokinetics of methadone in chronic pain patients. *Ther Drug Monit*. 1996;18:221-227.

47. Moolchan ET, Hoffman JA. Phases of treatment: a practical approach to methadone maintenance treatment. *Int J Addict*. 1994;29:135-160.

48. Holmstrand J et al. Methadone maintenance: plasma levels and therapeutic outcome. *Clin Pharmacol Ther*. 1978;23:175-180.

49. Berkowitz BA. The relationship of pharmacokinetics to pharmacological activity: morphine, methadone and naloxone. *Clin Pharmacokinet*. 1976;1:219-230.

50. Sims SA et al. Surveillance of methadone-related adverse drug events using multiple public health data sources. *J Biomed Inform*. 2007;40:382-389.

51. Geletko SM, Erickson AD. Decreased methadone effect after ritonavir initiation. *Pharmacotherapy*. 2000;20:93-94.

52. Beauclair TR, Stoner CP. Adherence to guidelines for continuous morphine sulfate infusions. *Am J Hosp Pharm*. 1986;43:671-676.

53. Holmes AH. Morphine IV infusion for chronic pain. *Drug Intell Clin Pharm*. 1978;12:556-557.

54. White P. Use of patient-controlled analgesia for management of acute pain. *JAMA*. 1988;259:243-247.

55. Baumann TJ et al. Patient-controlled analgesia in the terminally ill cancer patient. *Drug Intell Clin Pharm*. 1986;20:297-301.

56. Kerr IG et al. Continuous narcotic infusion with patient-controlled analgesia for chronic cancer pain in outpatients. *Ann Intern Med*. 1988;108:554-557.

57. Lutz LJ, Lamer TJ. Management of postoperative pain: review of current techniques and methods. *Mayo Clin Proc*. 1990;65:584-596.

58. Gestin Y et al. Long-term intrathecal infusion of morphine in the home care of patients with advanced cancer. *Acta Anaesthesiol Scand*. 1997;41:12-17.

59. Milner AR et al. Intrathecal administration of morphine for elective Caesarean section. A comparison between 0.1 mg and 0.2 mg. *Anaesthesia*. 1996;51:871-873.

60. Lobato RD et al. Intraventricular morphine for intractable cancer pain: rationale, methods, clinical results. *Acta Anaesthesiol Scand*. 1987;31(suppl 85):68-74.

61. Farncombe M, Chater S. Clinical application of nebulized opioids for treatment of dyspnoea in patients with malignant disease. *Support Care Cancer*. 1994;2:184-187.

62. Dews TE et al. Intrathecal morphine for analgesia in children undergoing selective dorsal rhizotomy. *J Pain Symptom Manage*. 1996;11:188-194.

63. Pounder DR, Steward DJ. Postoperative analgesia: opioid infusions in infants and children. *Can J Anaesth*. 1992;39:969-974.

64. Masood AR, Thomas SHL. Systemic absorption of nebulized morphine compared with oral morphine in healthy subjects. *Br J Clin Pharmacol*. 1996;41:250-252.

65. Saarenmaa E et al. Morphine clearance and effects in newborn infants in relation to gestational age. *Clin Pharmacol Ther*. 2000;68:160-166.

66. Glare PA, Walsh TD. Clinical pharmacokinetics of morphine. *Ther Drug Monit*. 1991;13:1-23.

67. Davies G et al. Pharmacokinetics of opioids in renal dysfunction. *Clin Pharmacokinet*. 1996;31:410-422.

68. Tiseo PJ et al. Morphine-6-glucuronide concentrations and opioid-related side effects: a survey in cancer patients. *Pain*. 1995;61:47-54.

69. Stanski DR et al. Kinetics of intravenous and intramuscular morphine. *Clin Pharmacol Ther.* 1978;24:52-59.

70. Chan GLC, Matzke GR. Effects of renal insufficiency on the pharmacokinetics and pharmacodynamics of opioid analgesics. *Drug Intell Clin Pharm.* 1987;21:773-783.

71. Mercadante S. Dantrolene treatment of opioid-induced myoclonus. *Anesth Analg.* 1995;81:1307-1308.

72. Holdsworth MT et al. Continuous midazolam infusion for the management of morphine-induced myoclonus. *Ann Pharmacother.* 1995;29:25-29.

73. Du Pen SL et al. Chronic epidural morphine and preservative-induced injury. *Anesthesiology.* 1987;67:987-988.

74. Meisel SB, Welford PK. Seizures associated with high-dose intravenous morphine containing sodium bisulfite preservative. *Ann Pharmacother.* 1992;26:1515-1517.

75. Chamberlain JM, Klein BL. A comprehensive review of naloxone for the emergency physician. *Am J Emerg Med.* 1994;12:650-660.

76. Hoffman RS, Goldfrank LR. The poisoned patient with altered consciousness. Controversies in the use of a 'coma cocktail.' *JAMA.* 1995;274:562-569.

77. Osterwalder JJ. Naloxone—for intoxications with intravenous heroin and heroin mixtures—harmless or hazardous? A prospective clinical study. *J Toxicol Clin Toxicol.* 1996;34:409-416.

78. Longnecker DE et al. Naloxone for antagonism of morphine-induced respiratory depression. *Anesth Analg.* 1973;52:447-453.

79. Evans JM et al. Degree and duration of reversal by naloxone of effects of morphine in conscious subjects. *Br Med J.* 1974;2:589-591.

80. Fishman J et al. Disposition of naloxone-7,8-3H in normal and narcotic-dependent men. *J Pharmacol Exp Ther.* 1973;187:575-580.

81. Vozeh S et al. Pharmacokinetic drug data. *Clin Pharmacokinet.* 1988;15:254-282.

82. Ngai SH et al. Pharmacokinetics of naloxone in rats and in man: basis for its potency and short duration of action. *Anesthesiology.* 1976;44:398-401.

83. Stile IL et al. The pharmacokinetics of naloxone in the premature newborn. *Dev Pharmacol Ther.* 1987;10:454-459.

84. Tandberg D, Abercrombie D. Treatment of heroin overdose with endotracheal naloxone. *Ann Emerg Med.* 1982;11:443-445.

85. Culpepper-Morgan JA et al. Treatment of opioid-induced constipation with oral naloxone: a pilot study. *Clin Pharmacol Ther.* 1992;52:90-95.

86. Sykes NP. An investigation of the ability of oral naloxone to correct opioid-related constipation in patients with advanced cancer. *Palliat Med.* 1996;10:135-144.

87. Poulsen L et al. The hypoalgesic effect of tramadol in relation to CYP2D6. *Clin Pharmacol Ther.* 1996;60:636-644.

88. Spiller HA et al. Prospective multicenter evaluation of tramadol exposure. *J Toxicol Clin Toxicol.* 1997;35:361-364.

89. Kahn LH et al. Seizures reported with tramadol. *JAMA.* 1997;278:1661. Letter.

90. Nightingale SL. From the Food and Drug Administration. Important new safety information for tramadol hydrochloride. *JAMA.* 1996;275:1224.

91. Fisher MA, Glass S. Butorphanol (Stadol): a study in problems of current drug information and control. *Neurology.* 1997;48:1156-1160.

92. Strain EC et al. Precipitated withdrawal by pentazocine in methadone-maintained volunteers. *J Pharmacol Exp Ther.* 1993;267:624-634.

93. Reed DA, Schnoll SH. Abuse of pentazocine-naloxone combination. *JAMA.* 1986;256:2562-2564.

94. Gourlay GK, Cousins MJ. Strong analgesics in severe pain. *Drugs.* 1984;28:79-91.

95. Miller RR. Evaluation of nalbuphine hydrochloride. *Am J Hosp Pharm.* 1980;37:942-949.

96. Ameer B, Salter FJ. Drug therapy reviews: evaluation of butorphanol tartrate. *Am J Hosp Pharm.* 1979;36:1683-1691.

97. Dayer P et al. The pharmacology of tramadol. *Drugs.* 1994;47(suppl 1):3-7.

Antimicrobial Drugs | 2

Daniel M. Riche

Chapter 6

Aminoglycosides

Renée-Claude Mercier

AMINOGLYCOSIDES

Pharmacology. Aminoglycosides are aminocyclitol derivatives that have concentration-dependent bactericidal activity against gram-negative aerobic bacteria via binding to the interface between the 30S and 50S ribosomal subunits; anaerobic bacteria are universally resistant because aminoglycoside transport into cells is oxygen dependent. Dibasic cations (e.g., magnesium and calcium) and acidic conditions decrease the in vitro action of aminoglycosides. Streptomycin and kanamycin have poor activity against some gram-negative bacteria, especially *Pseudomonas aeruginosa*. Some gram-positive organisms (e.g., streptococci) are relatively resistant to all aminoglycosides; however, in combination with some bacterial cell wall inhibitors, such as penicillins or vancomycin, these organisms are often synergistically inhibited or killed. Aminoglycosides have a postantibiotic effect against gram-negative bacteria, which can be exploited by using less frequent dosage intervals. Resistance is caused by transferable plasmid-mediated enzymatic modification or decreased drug uptake.[1,2] (*See* Notes.)

Administration and Adult Dosage. IM or IV by slow intermittent infusion over **30–60 min**—although 15-min infusions are safe, high dose once-daily regimens combine the usual daily dosage into a **single IV infusion administered over 60 min**.[3,4] This method takes advantage of the concentration-related bactericidal effects and postantibiotic effect of aminoglycosides and may result in less toxicity.[2–4] **Intrathecal (IT) or intraventricular administration** is usually necessary to achieve therapeutic cerebrospinal fluid (CSF) levels. (*See* Aminoglycosides Comparison Chart.)

Special Populations. *Pediatric Dosage.* *See* Aminoglycosides Comparison Chart.

Geriatric Dosage. Same as adult dosage, but adjust for age-related reduction in renal function.

75

Other Conditions. Use of ideal body weight (IBW) for determining the mg/kg dosage appears to be more accurate than dosage based on total body weight (TBW). In morbid obesity, dosage requirement may best be estimated using a dosing weight of IBW + 0.4 (TBW − IBW).[1,2] With conventional dosage methods, serum drug levels should be in the range of 3–10 mg/L; high peaks (e.g., >6 mg/L with gentamicin and tobramycin) may be associated with better outcome in bacteremia, pneumonia, and other systemic infections.[1,2] Critically ill patients with serious infections or in disease states known to markedly alter aminoglycoside pharmacokinetics (e.g., cystic fibrosis, burns, or major surgery) often have variable distribution and excretion of the drugs.[1,2] When the drug is administered once daily, higher peak concentrations (e.g., >10–20 mg/L with gentamicin and tobramycin) are targeted based on the patient's disease state and pharmacokinetic parameters.[3–5] (*See* Aminoglycosides Comparison Chart.) Adjust dosage based on renal function. Individualization is critical because these agents have a low therapeutic index. In renal impairment, the following guidelines may be used to determine initial dosage:[6]

1. Select loading dose in mg/kg (IBW or dosing weight as above) to provide peak serum levels in the range listed below for the desired aminoglycoside.

AMINOGLYCOSIDE	USUAL CONVENTIONAL LOADING DOSE (mg/kg)	EXPECTED PEAK SERUM LEVEL (mg/L)
Tobramycin	1–2	3–10
Gentamicin	1–2	3–10
Amikacin	5–7.5	15–30

2. Select maintenance dose (as percentage of chosen loading dose) to continue peak serum levels indicated above, according to desired dosage interval and the patient's corrected Cl_{Cr}.

PERCENTAGE OF LOADING DOSE REQUIRED FOR DOSAGE INTERVAL SELECTED

Cl_{Cr} (mL/min)	HALF-LIFE[a] (h)	8 HOURS	12 HOURS	24 HOURS
90	3.1	84%	−	−
80	3.4	80	91%	−
70	3.9	76	88	−
60	4.5	71	84	−
50	5.3	65	79	−
40	6.5	57	72	92%
30	8.4	48	63	86
25	9.9	43	57	81
20	11.9	37	50	75
17	13.6	33	46	70
15	15.1	31	42	67

(continued)

Cl$_{Cr}$ (mL/min)	HALF-LIFE[a] (h)	8 HOURS	12 HOURS	24 HOURS
12	17.9	27	37	61
10[a]	20.4	24	34	56
7[b]	25.9	19	28	47
5[b]	31.5	16	23	41
2[b]	46.8	11	16	30
0[b]	69.3	8	11	21

[a]Alternatively, 50% of the chosen loading dose can be given at an interval approximately equal to the estimated half-life.
[b]Use measured serum levels to adjust dosage for patients with Cl$_{Cr}$ <10 mL/min. Give supplemental doses of 50%–75% of the loading dose after each hemodialysis period.

These guidelines are based on population data; serum levels in individual patients might deviate from guideline estimates. No guidelines have been developed for streptomycin.

Dosage Forms. *See* Aminoglycosides Comparison Chart.

Patient Instructions. Report any dizziness or sensations of ringing or fullness in the ears.

Pharmacokinetics. *Serum Levels. See* Parameters to Monitor and Aminoglycosides Comparison Chart.

Fate. Absorption after oral or rectal administration is approximately 0.2%–2%; absorption across denuded skin can reach 5%. Irrigation of vascularized areas (e.g., peritoneal cavity) results in absorption approximating IM use.[7] IM administration is followed by rapid and complete absorption, with peak serum levels occurring after 0.5–1.5 h. IV infusions over 0.5–1 h produce serum levels similar to equal IM doses. Binding of aminoglycoside to plasma proteins is low. These agents distribute rapidly into the extracellular fluid compartment with a V_d of about 0.3 ± 0.08 L/kg, which is increased by fever, edema, ascites, and fluid overload, and in neonates.[8] Aminoglycosides accumulate markedly in some tissues, especially the renal cortex, to levels many times those found in the serum,[2,8] particularly with frequent dosage intervals compared with the same dosage given at less frequent intervals.[2,3] Levels in the cerebrospinal fluid of patients with meningitis generally do not exceed 25% of serum levels, except in neonates;[2,8] penetration into the eye is inadequate for treatment of intraocular infections. Penetration into lung tissues and sputum is low, and large doses might be necessary to optimally treat pneumonia with relatively insensitive organisms (e.g., *P. aeruginosa*). Distribution of aminoglycosides into the peritoneal cavity of patients with peritonitis is therapeutically adequate.[7,8] Elimination is via glomerular filtration of unchanged drug;[1,2] clearance is approximately 90% of Cl$_{Cr}$. After discontinuation, low levels of aminoglycoside can be detected in the urine for several days caused by excretion of drug that had accumulated in deep tissue compartments.[2,8] **Half-life** α phase 5–15 min; β phase (adults) about 2 ± 0.4 h with normal renal function (1.5–9 h in neonates <1 week and 3 h in older infants); can be more variable in certain groups (e.g., obstetric and burn patients) despite normal renal function; 50–70 h in anuria. A prolonged γ elimination phase is observed when concentrations fall to the lower range of detectability, representing egress from deep tissue compartments and subsequent renal elimination; the half-life of this phase is 60–350 h (usually 150–200 h).[2–8] β phase half-life is most important for use in calculating individualized dosage, but the γ phase may account for the gradual rise of serum levels and apparent increase in half-life with continued therapy, despite stable renal function.[2,8]

Adverse Reactions. Aminoglycoside-induced nephrotoxicity is usually mild and reversible; progression to severe renal disease and dependence on dialysis is rare. Nephrotoxicity is manifested by elevations in serum creatinine, BUN, and aminoglycoside concentrations and appearance of renal tubular casts, enzymes, and β_2-microglobulin and occurs in 5%–30% of patients, depending on the criteria used and the population risk factors present.[1,2,9] Duration of therapy, prior aminoglycoside therapy, advanced age, preexisting renal disease, liver disease, volume depletion, and female sex have been identified as risk factors for nephrotoxicity.[1,2] Concomitant use of nephrotoxic drugs also increases the risk of nephrotoxicity. Elevated trough levels are NOT a risk factor but often a result of nephrotoxicity.[2,10] There is no evidence that there are clinically important differences in nephrotoxicity between gentamicin, tobramycin, netilmicin, and amikacin.[9] Depletion of magnesium and other minerals caused by increased renal excretion occurs. Occasional, but often permanent, vestibular toxicity is reported, usually in association with streptomycin. Subclinical vestibular disturbances can be detected in 1%–11% or more of patients receiving aminoglycosides.[1,2,9,11,12] Early cochlear damage can be detected only by sequential audiometric examination because hearing loss in conversational frequencies is a sign of advanced auditory impairment. Furthermore, early auditory damage is not as apparent in the elderly or others with preexisting high-tone deficits. Risk factors for ototoxicity are duration of therapy, bacteremia, hypovolemia, peak temperature, and liver disease.[1,2,12] Elevated serum concentrations apparently are not associated with increased ototoxicity risk[10]; however, there are apparent differences between gentamicin, tobramycin, netilmicin, and amikacin.[9,11] The pooled incidence of vestibular toxicity is 10.9% for gentamicin, 7.4% for amikacin, 3.5% for tobramycin, and 1.1% for netilmicin.[11] Oral aminoglycosides, primarily neomycin, have been associated with a sprue-like malabsorption syndrome.[1,2] Neuromuscular blockade with respiratory failure is rare, except in predisposed patients. (*See* Precautions.)

Precautions. Pregnancy category D due to reports of irreversible bilateral deafness in infants born to mother who received streptomycin; enters the breast milk in small amount (American Academy of Pediatrics rates as compatible); preexisting renal impairment; vestibular or cochlear impairment; myasthenia gravis; hypocalcemia; postoperative or other conditions that depress neuromuscular transmission.

Drug Interactions. Concurrent or sequential use of other nephro- or ototoxic agents can increase the risk of aminoglycoside toxicities. Concurrent use of aminoglycosides with neuromuscular blocking agents can potentiate neuromuscular blockade and cause respiratory paralysis.[2] The action of oral anticoagulants can be potentiated by oral neomycin, presumably via reduced absorption or synthesis of vitamin K. Ticarcillin and acylampicillins can degrade aminoglycosides in vitro, resulting in artificially low levels; the extent of degradation is dependent on time, temperature, and β-lactam concentration.[8,13,14] Amikacin is the aminoglycoside least susceptible to β-lactam inactivation.[8,13]

Parameters to Monitor. Renal function tests before and every 2–3 days during therapy. Audiometry and electronystagmography may be performed in patients able to cooperate. Monitor aminoglycoside serum concentrations carefully, especially in the elderly, those with renal impairment, hemodynamically unstable patients, and those requiring high peak serum concentrations or prolonged (>10 days) therapy. In adults receiving conventional therapy, monitor serum levels after steady state is achieved. With once-daily therapy targeting high peaks and undetectable troughs, obtain levels after the first dose. Obtain follow-up levels if renal function changes.[2–5] In neonates or other patients with rapidly changing renal function, obtain serum drug concentrations initially and every 2–3 days until stable. However, with once or twice-daily dosage and in pediatric patients, trough serum levels are often undetectable and other sampling strategies are necessary.[3–5,15] (*See* Special Populations, Other Conditions.)

Notes. Of the available aminoglycosides, gentamicin, tobramycin, and amikacin are the most clinically useful. **Streptomycin** use is largely restricted to the treatment of enterococcal endocarditis (in combination with ampicillin), tuberculosis, brucellosis, plague, and tularemia; it is currently available only for compassionate use from the manufacturer. Amikacin is often used as part of a combination regimen for treatment of *Mycobacterium avium* complex infection. **Neomycin** is much more toxic than the other aminoglycosides when given parenterally. It is restricted to oral use for hepatic encephalopathy, as it reduces the ammonia forming bacteria in the intestinal tract and topical use for minor infections. Neomycin combined with polymyxin B is sometimes used as a solution for urinary bladder irrigation. Resistance among gram-negative organisms, especially *P. aeruginosa*, has virtually eliminated the systemic use of **kanamycin.** Tobramycin is roughly equivalent to gentamicin therapeutically, although it is about 2–4 times more active against *P. aeruginosa* than is gentamicin, is often active against gentamicin-resistant *P. aeruginosa*, and may be preferred because of a superior peak-to-MIC ratio.[16] Resistance of gram-negative bacilli is lowest with amikacin, and amikacin use does not appear to result in increased resistance to the drug.[1,2]

AMINOGLYCOSIDES COMPARISON CHART

DRUG	DOSAGE FORMS	ADULT DOSAGE[a]	PEDIATRIC DOSAGE[a]	USUAL THERAPEUTIC SERUM LEVELS (mg/L)[b] Peak[c]	Trough
Amikacin Sulfate Amikin	Inj 50, 250 mg/mL	IM or IV 15–20 mg/kg/d in 2 equally divided doses; Intrathecal 5–20 mg/d.	IM or IV (<1 wk) 12–15 mg/kg every 36–48 h; IM or IV (infants >1 wk) 12 mg/kg every 24 h; IM or IV (children) same as adult mg/kg dosage.	20–35	≤10
Gentamicin Sulfate Various	Inj 10, 40 mg/mL Ophth Oint 3 mg/g Ophth Soln 0.3% Top Crm 0.1% Top Oint 0.1%	IM or IV 5–6 mg/kg/d in equally divided doses every 8–12 h or in a single-dose IV every 24 h;[d] IM or IV for less serious infections or infective endocarditis[d] 3–5 mg/kg/d in equally divided doses every 8–12 h OR in a single-dose IV every 24 h IT 4–8 mg every 24 h.	IM or IV (<1 wk) 4–5 mg/kg every 36–48 h; IM or IV (infants >1 wk) 4 mg/kg every 24 h; IM or IV (children) 6–7.5 mg/kg/d (7–10 mg/kg/d in cystic fibrosis) in 3–4 equally divided doses every 6–8 h intrathecal 1–2 mg every 24 h.	6–12	≤2
Streptomycin Sulfate Various	Inj 1 g	IM[e] 15–25 mg/kg/d (usually 1–2 g/d) in 2 equally divided doses every 12 h; IM for TB 12–15 mg/kg/d to a maximum of 1 g or 25–30 mg/kg to a maximum of 1.5 g 2–3 times/wk.	IM (neonates) 20–30 mg/kg/d in 2 equally divided doses every 12 h IM (children) 20–40 mg/kg/d in 2 equally divided doses every 12 h IM for TB 20–40 mg/kg/d 2–3 times/wk OR 25–30 mg/kg.	15–30	≤5

(continued)

AMINOGLYCOSIDES COMPARISON CHART (continued)

DRUG	DOSAGE FORMS	ADULT DOSAGE[a]	PEDIATRIC DOSAGE[a]	USUAL THERAPEUTIC SERUM LEVELS (mg/L)[b]	
				Peak[c]	Trough
Tobramycin Sulfate	Inj 10, 40 mg/mL	IM or IV same as gentamicin; IV for	IM or IV same as gentamicin;	6–12	≤2
AKTob	Inj 1.2 g	cystic fibrosis 10 mg/kg/d; Inhalation for	IV for cystic fibrosis 10 mg/kg/d;		
Tobrex	Ophth Oint	cystic fibrosis 300 mg every 12 h for	Inhalation for cystic fibrosis 300 mg		
TOBI	3 mg/g Ophth	28 days; Intrathecal 4–8 mg every 24 h.	every 12 h for 28 days.		
Various	Soln 0.3%				
	Nebulizer Soln				
	60 mg/mL				

[a]For systemic infections; UTIs are adequately treated with lower dosages.

[b]Based on divided doses given every 8–12 h; higher peaks and lower (or undetectable) troughs are seen when less frequent dosage intervals are used.

[c]As seen 30 min after a 30-min IV infusion or approximately 1 h after IM administration of a usual adult dose. Uncomplicated UTIs can be treated with smaller doses that produce much lower serum levels; however, serious infections, such as gram-negative bacteremia, pneumonia, or endocarditis might require doses resulting in serum levels in the higher part of the range. Clinical efficacy appears to increase as the ratio of the peak serum level to the MIC of the pathogen increases.[13]

[d]These doses conform to those used in published clinical trials, but higher dosages might be necessary in certain patient populations. Patients with infective endocarditis require only low dose 1 mg/kg every 8 h when gram-positive organisms are suspected.

[e]IV administration not recommended however has been administered intravenously over 30–60 min.

■ REFERENCES

1. Lortholary O et al. Aminoglycosides. *Med Clin North Am*. 1995;79:761-787.
2. Gilbert DN. Aminoglycosides. In: Mandell GL et al., eds. *Principles and Practice of Infectious Diseases*. 6th ed. Philadelphia, PA: Elsevier Churchill Livingstone; 2005:328-356.
3. Preston SL, Briceland LL. Single daily dosing of aminoglycosides. *Pharmacotherapy*. 1995;15:297-306.
4. Nicolau DP et al. Experience with a once-daily aminoglycoside program administered to 2184 patients. *Antimicrob Agents Chemother*. 1995;39:650-655.
5. Blaser J et al. Monitoring serum concentrations for once-daily netilmicin dosing regimens. *J Antimicrob Chemother*. 1994;33:341-348.
6. Sarubbi FA, Hull JH. Amikacin serum concentrations, predictions of levels and dosage guidelines. *Ann Intern Med*. 1978;89:612-618.
7. Walshe JJ et al. Crossover pharmacokinetic analysis comparing intravenous and intraperitoneal administration of tobramycin. *J Infect Dis*. 1986;153:796-799.
8. Schentag JJ et al. Aminoglycosides. In: Burton ME et al., eds. *Applied Pharmacokinetics & Pharmacodynamis. Principles of Therapeutic Drug Monitoring*. Vol 14. 4th ed. Baltimore, MD: Lippincott Williams & Wilkins; 2006:285-327.
9. Kahlmeter G, Dahlager JI. Aminoglycoside toxicity—a review of clinical studies published between 1975 and 1982. *J Antimicrob Chemother*. 1984;13(suppl A):9-22.
10. McCormack JP, Jewesson PJ. A critical reevaluation of the "therapeutic range" of aminoglycosides. *Clin Infect Dis*. 1992;14:320-329.
11. Ariano RE, Zelenitsky SA, Kassum DA. Aminoglycoside-induced vestibular injury: maintaining a sense of balance. *Ann Pharmacother*. 2008;42:1282-1289.
12. Selimoglu E. Aminoglycoside-induced ototoxicity. *Curr Pharm Des*. 2007;13:119-126.
13. Pickering LK et al. Effect of concentration and time upon inactivation of tobramycin, gentamicin, netilmicin, and amikacin by azlocillin, carbenicillin, mecillinam, mezlocillin, and piperacillin. *J Pharmacol Exp Ther*. 1981;217:345-349.
14. Thompson MI et al. Gentamicin inactivation by piperacillin or carbenicillin in patients with end-stage renal disease. *Antimicrob Agents Chemother*. 1982;21:268-273.
15. Erdmay SM et al. An updated comparison of drug dosing methods. Part III. Aminoglycoside antibiotics. *Clin Pharmacokinet*. 1991;20:374-388.
16. Moore RD et al. Clinical response to aminoglycoside therapy: importance of the ratio of peak concentration to minimum inhibitory concentration. *J Infect Dis*. 1987;155:93-99.

Chapter 7

Antifungal Drugs

John D. Cleary and Kayla R. Stover

AMPHOTERICIN B	Fungizone
AMPHOTERICIN B CHOLESTERYL SULFATE	Amphotec
AMPHOTERICIN B LIPID COMPLEX	Abelcet
LIPOSOMAL AMPHOTERICIN B	AmBisome

Pharmacology. Amphotericin B is a polyene macrolide antifungal drug isolated from the bacteria *Streptomyces nodosus*. Drug binding to ergosterol constituents within the cytoplasmic membrane of fungi, with subsequent disruption of membrane integrity and function, is the pharmacologic mechanism of action for amphotericin B. Resistance to amphotericin B has occurred in patients taking long-term therapy; and, though infrequent, resistance of *Candida* species such as *C. lusitaniae* and *C. guilliermondii* has occurred.[1] Sensitivity of fungi to amphotericin B is related to the concentration of ergosterol present in the cytoplasmic membrane.[2,3]

Indications and Adult Dosage. IV for severe fungal infections. (*See* Amphotericin B Formulations Comparison Chart.) Therapy is generally initiated at 0.25 mg/kg daily and titrated upward to 1.0 mg/kg daily or 1.5 mg/kg daily if using an alternate day schedule. Maximum dose is 1.5 mg/kg daily. Overdose may result in cardiac and/or respiratory arrest. Initiate therapy with the full treatment dose for patients with life-threatening fungal disease. Some advocate initiation of amphotericin B at a fraction of the therapeutic dose with daily incremental increases to achieve the desired therapeutic dosage in less critically ill patients. Although it has not been evaluated in a controlled manner, the intent of this approach is improvement of patient tolerance to infusion-related adverse effects.[2,4] Monitor pulse and respiratory rate, temperature, and blood pressure in patients closely for up to 2 h after the test dose.[2] **Long-term suppressive or maintenance therapy for the immunocompromised**—conventional amphotericin B and amphotericin B lipid complex can be given every other day or Monday, Wednesday, and Friday in an attempt to attenuate renal dysfunction.[2,5] **IV for prophylaxis after bone marrow transplantation**—(conventional amphotericin B) 0.1 mg/kg or 5–10 mg daily has been used.[6] **Infusion time**—the frequency and severity of infusion-related adverse effects is similar with administration of amphotericin B over 1–2 h and 4–6 h.[4] **Duration of therapy** with amphotericin B is not well defined. Patients with life-threatening mycotic disease must receive amphotericin B until resolution of clinical and microbiologic evidence of fungal infection or until unacceptable drug-induced toxicity occurs. The cumulative total dosage of amphotericin B is generally 10–20 mg/kg.[2,4] **Topical** apply to affected area 2–4 times daily for 1–4 weeks. **IM or PO administration** is not recommended for injectable amphotericin B.

Alternative routes of administration of extemporaneously prepared amphotericin B for injection are infrequently used to facilitate drug availability to a sanctuary site or minimize systemic toxicity. Use of alternative routes of amphotericin B administration is based primarily on case reports, and the safety and efficacy of extemporaneously prepared amphotericin B administered by alternative routes have not been evaluated in a controlled manner. Subsequently, administration of amphotericin B by an alternative route should not replace standard therapy. **Inhaled for prophylaxis or treatment of pulmonary fungal infections**—10 mg 3–4 times daily or 50 mg daily in 3 divided doses via nebulization has been reported.[7,8] **Intra-articular for fungal arthritis**—5–50 mg every 2–7 days. The dose of intra-articular amphotericin B is determined by the size of the infected joint.[9] **Intracavitary for pulmonary aspergillomas**—5–50 mg in D5W daily or 2–3 times weekly has been used in patients unable to undergo surgical resection.[10] **Inhalation for prophylaxis against *Aspergillus* spp. after bone marrow transplantation**—0.15% in D5W nebulized to deliver 10 mg/d in 2 divided doses.[11] **Intranasal for prophylaxis in bone marrow transplant recipients**—amphotericin B 0.5% in sterile water 10 mg/d in divided doses.[12] **Intraperitoneal for the treatment of fungal peritonitis** has been used in patients receiving peritoneal dialysis.[2] Instillation is problematic because amphotericin B is physically incompatible with ionic solutions such as dialysate. **Intrathecal** administration of conventional amphotericin B 0.5–1 mg 2–3 times/wk or 0.3 mg/d has been reported. The intrathecal dosage of conventional amphotericin B is generally started at 0.025–0.05 mg/dose, with subsequent doses increased at 0.025–0.05 mg/d increments to the desired therapeutic or maximum tolerated dosage. **CNS administration** is generally via an Ommaya reservoir. Although an Ommaya reservoir is not mandatory for intrathecal administration of amphotericin B, the device facilitates repeated drug administration with more precise drug delivery, improved patient tolerance, and clarified CSF diagnostic quality. Amphotericin B administration by lumbar puncture and intracisternal injection has been reported.[2] **Bladder irrigation for the treatment of uncomplicated fungal cystitis**—infuse 50 mg/L in sterile water over 24 h.[2] **Topical ocular for the treatment of keratomycosis**—amphotericin B 0.15% (0.1%–0.25%) in preservative-free sterile water has been given concurrently with atropine ophthalmic drops every 30–60 min for the initial 48–72 h of treatment; subsequent to subjective improvement and ocular reepithelization, the dosage interval may be changed to 4 times daily for at least 1 month.[2,13] **Intravitreal for fungal keratomycosis**—5 μg/0.1 mL preservative-free sterile water has been used.[14] **Subtenonian injection for the treatment of postoperative fungal endophthalmitis**—500 μg/d for 8 doses has been used.[2]

Special Populations. *Pediatric Dosage.* IV—same as adult dosage for conventional amphotericin B, amphotericin B colloidal dispersion, amphotericin B lipid complex, and liposomal amphotericin. **IV for prophylaxis after bone marrow or solid organ transplantation**—(liposomal amphotericin B) 1 mg/kg/d has been used.[15] **PO**—same as adult dosage. **Topical**—same as adult dosage for cream, lotion, and ointment.

Geriatric Dosage. Same as adult dosage for conventional amphotericin B, amphotericin B colloidal dispersion, amphotericin B lipid complex, and liposomal amphotericin. Long-term intravenous administration is more likely to be limited by renal impairment. Comorbid conditions might reduce patient tolerance to ancillary medications used for management of infusion-related adverse effects (e.g., corticosteroid induced sodium retention).

Other Conditions. (All products) with preexisting chronic renal dysfunction, no dosage adjustment is necessary, but the duration of the infusion must be 4–h to prevent drug-related hyperkalemia. In acute renal dysfunction, interrupt treatment or extend dosage interval or decrease dosage to reduce exacerbation of renal impairment, as patient's clinical condition allows.[4] For patients 1.3 times IBW, calculate dose based on IBW or dosing weight of IBW + 0.4 × (TBW − IBW).[16]

Dosage Forms. **Inj** *See* Amphotericin B Formulations Comparison Chart.

Patient Instructions. Amphotericin B is used to treat fungal infections. Infusion reactions such as shaking, chills, fever, nausea, and other symptoms can occur when this medication is being given. Although uncomfortable, these effects are transient. Certain medications (acetaminophen or meperidine) reduce infusion reactions for most people. Amphotericin B might affect your kidneys. If this occurs, you may need to take mineral supplements by mouth.

Pharmacokinetics. Preclinical and phase I testing of conventional amphotericin B preceded development of high-performance liquid chromatography and refinement of pharmacokinetic methodology. Pharmacokinetic parameters quoted in tertiary literature might actually reflect drug concentration analysis using microbiologic assays.

Serum Concentrations. A correlation between serum concentrations and therapeutic or toxic drug effects has not been identified or defined for any commercially available amphotericin B formulation.

Fate. (Conventional amphotericin B) poor oral and IM absorption. End of infusion serum concentration was 0.984 ± 0.056 mg/L after 0.25 mg/kg to 8 normal healthy volunteers.[2] V_{dss} is 0.74 ± 0.13 L/kg.[17] Extensively bound (>90%) to plasma lipoproteins.[2] Accumulation into hepatic, splenic, pulmonary, and renal tissue has been observed.[16] V_{dss} of 4 ± 0.3 L/kg is derived from bioanalysis of serum from 2 patients completing chronic therapy with amphotericin B.[2] Clearance is 0.01 ± 0.001 L/h/kg.[17] Metabolites of amphotericin B have not been identified.[2] Urinary elimination is 3%–8%.[2,17] Amphotericin B lipid complex has a V_{dss} of 3.9 ± 0.3 L/kg; clearance is 0.08 ± 0.02 L/h/kg; AUC is 2.76 ± 0.25 mg/L/h.[17] Liposomal amphotericin B has a V_{dss} is 0.37 L/kg; clearance is 0.023 L/h/kg; AUC is 423 mg/L/h.[18] **Half-life** Conventional amphotericin B: β phase 24 h and γ phase 15 days;[2,17] amphotericin B lipid complex β phase 45 ± 6.3 h;[17] liposomal amphotericin B: β phase 1.74 h; γ phase 23.6 h.[18]

Adverse Reactions. Frequent adverse effects include infusion-related reactions, nephrotoxicity, normochromic normocytic anemia, and phlebitis. Infusion reactions ordinarily include rigors, chills, and fever. Less common infusion-related reactions include nausea, tachycardia, tachypnea, hypotension, hypertension, bradycardia, myalgia, and arthralgia. Symptoms generally occur during or within 60–90 min after completion of the infusion. Symptoms decrease with ancillary medications and repeated administration. **Meperidine**—25–50 mg IV reduces the duration and intensity of rigors and chilling. **Acetaminophen**—325–650 mg PO reduces hyperpyrexia, and is often administered as premedication. **Diphenhydramine**—25–50 mg PO or IV is often included as a premedication, however, no data support its use. **Hydrocortisone**, which reduces fever, chills, and nausea, is reserved for patients with infusion reactions refractory to other ancillary medications. Although premedication with **ibuprofen** reduces the rigors and chills, the combination with amphotericin B formulations may increase the risk for nephrotoxicity.[2,4] The prevalence of infusion reactions is greater with conventional amphotericin B or amphotericin B cholesteryl sulfate than with amphotericin B lipid complex or liposomal amphotericin. Rapid infusion (<60 min) of amphotericin B can cause hyperkalemia and cardiovascular collapse in anephric or hyperkalemic patients.[4] Amphotericin B cholesteryl sulfate, amphotericin B lipid complex, and liposomal amphotericin are each less nephrotoxic than conventional amphotericin B. However, the lipid-based formulations are not devoid of nephrotoxicity. Nephrotoxicity is generally reversible. Permanent renal impairment can occur, particularly in patients receiving conventional amphotericin B at doses over 1 mg/kg/d or that have preexisting renal impairment, prolonged therapy, sodium depletion, or concurrent nephrotoxic agents. Signs of nephrotoxicity are increased BUN and S_{Cr}, hypomagnesemia, hypokalemia, and renal tubular acidosis. Nephrotoxicity can be reduced with infusion of 0.9% NaCl 250–1000 mL over 30–45 min immediately before amphotericin B. The saline infusion may be repeated immediately after amphotericin B administration. The patient's body size and cardiovascular status must be considered when selecting the volume and rate of 0.9% NaCl infusion. Normochromic normocytic anemia, which is secondary to amphotericin B-induced nephrotoxicity, is mild and transient and rarely requires intervention. Phlebitis is secondary to chronic peripheral administration of amphotericin B formulations. Some advocate adding heparin 1 IU/mL to minimize phlebitis.[2,4] Rare adverse effects reported with amphotericin B are anorexia, emesis, diarrhea, cramping epigastric pain, premature ventricular contraction, bradycardia, dilated cardiomyopathy, hypertension, diffuse alveolar hemorrhage, rhabdomyolysis, and parkinsonian syndrome.[2,4,19–22] Intrathecal administration of amphotericin B causes headache, nausea, vomiting, abdominal pain, urinary retention, tinnitus, visual changes, ventriculitis, paresthesias, numbness, mono- or paraparesis, arachnoiditis, focal neurologic defects, and chemical or bacterial meningitis. Life-threatening brain puncture and hemorrhage can occur with intracisternal injection.[2]

Precautions. Pregnancy category B; lactation. Impaired renal function. Avoid rapid infusions (<4 h) in patients with Cl_{Cr} <20 mL/min, hyperkalemia, elderly or reduced ability to excrete potassium.[4] Separate from neutrophil infusions by at least 6 h.[23] Complete infusion at least 2 h before platelet transfusions.[24]

Drug Interactions. Additive nephrotoxicity can occur with cyclosporine, tacrolimus, aminoglycosides, loop diuretics, or other nephrotoxic agents. Corticosteroids can enhance potassium loss.

Parameters to Monitor. Monitor infusion-related adverse effects with first 3 doses, then as indicated by severity of reactions. Monitor serum creatinine, BUN, magnesium, and potassium before therapy, and at least twice weekly during therapy. Monitor patients at great risk for renal dysfunction daily. Monitor hemoglobin at least weekly. Monitor microbiologic, radiographic, and clinical signs of fungal infection. Ancillary use of hydrocortisone, acetaminophen, or aspirin might mask fevers.

Notes. To ensure even lipid complex distribution, invert admixtures of amphotericin B lipid complex several times immediately before starting the infusion and every 2h thereafter. Because amphotericin B has a propensity to precipitate, avoid admixture or Y-site administration of all amphotericin B formulations with IV fluids (except dextrose solution), other intravenous drugs, or blood products. Avoid admixture of conventional amphotericin B with lipid emulsion. Physical incompatibility of this admixture evolves >10 μm particles and phase separation.[25] Acronyms for the various amphotericin B formulations are as follows: conventional amphotericin B, DAmB; amphotericin B cholesteryl sulfate, ABCD; amphotericin B lipid complex, ABLC; liposomal amphotericin B, L-AmB. Amphotericin B cholesteryl sulfate is also known as amphotericin B colloidal dispersion and Amphocil. Abbreviations: DMPC, dimyristoylphosphatidyl choline; DMPG, dimyristoylphosphatidyl glycerol; DSPC, distearoylphosphatidyl choline; HSPC, hydrogenated soy phosphatidyl choline.

AMPHOTERICIN B PRODUCTS COMPARISON CHART

	CONVENTIONAL AMPHOTERICIN B	AMPHOTERICIN B CHOLESTERYL SULFATE	AMPHOTERICIN B LIPID COMPLEX	LIPOSOMAL AMPHOTERICIN B
	Fungizone	*Amphotec*	*Abelcet*	*AmBisome*
LIPID CHEMISTRY				
Lipid component	Deoxycholate	Cholesteryl sulfate	DMPG, DMPC	HSPC, DSPC
Diameter (nm)	35	120–140	1600–11,000	80–120
Configuration	Micelle	Discoid	Ribbon-like	Spherical liposome
PHARMACEUTICAL CHARACTERISTICS				
Vial size (mg)	50	50, 100	100	50
Storage conditions	2°C–8°C	2°C–8°C	2°C–8°C	2°C–8°C
ADMINISTRATION AND DOSAGE				
Daily dosage (mg/kg)	0.5–1	3–4	2.5–5	1–3
Susceptible fungi	1–1.5	6	5	3–6
Less-susceptible fungi	1–6 (≤50 mg/h)	2–4	2	1–2
Infusion duration (h)	Not recommended	Do not filter	Do not filter	May use if pore size ≥1 μ
In-line filter	D5W	D5W	D5W	D5W
Compatible IV fluids	0.5–0.25	0.16–0.83	1–2	1–2
Admixture concentration (mg/mL)	Determined by lack of preservative	24 h at 2°C–8°C	48 h at 2°C–8°C, 6 h at room temperature	6 h at 2°C–8°C or at room temperature SWFI: 24 h at 2°C–8°C

(continued)

AMPHOTERICIN B PRODUCTS COMPARISON CHART (continued)

	CONVENTIONAL AMPHOTERICIN B	AMPHOTERICIN B CHOLESTERYL SULFATE	AMPHOTERICIN B LIPID COMPLEX	LIPOSOMAL AMPHOTERICIN B
	Fungizone	*Amphotec*	*Abelcet*	*AmBisome*
PHARMACOKINETICS				
V_{tiss} (L/kg)	1.1	4.3	43	0.1⁻
Clearance (mL/h/kg)	28	11	211	121
AUC (mg/L/h)	36	43	9.5	555
Half-life (h)	24–50	27–28	173[a]	6–11

DMPC, dimyristoylphosphatidyl choline; DMPG, dimyristoylphosphatidyl glycerol; DSPC, distearoylphosphatidyl choline; HSPC, hydrogenated soy phosphatidyl choline.

[a]Terminal elimination half-life.
From Ref. 50 and product information.

ANIDULAFUNGIN
Eraxis

Pharmacology. Anidulafungin is an echinocandin antifungal derived from *Aspergillus nidulans* that is a specific noncompetitive inhibitor of β-(1,3)-glucan synthetase in fungal cell membranes. This action leads to a weakened cell wall and eventual cell lysis and death. It has good activity against *Candida* spp., *Aspergillus* spp., and *Pneumocystis jiroveci.* Therapeutic response is directly related to achieving a good C_{max}:MIC ratio (i.e., 20–30).[26,27]

Indications and Adult Dosage. **IV for candidemia and other forms of** *Candida* infections and for refractory invasive aspergillosis—200 mg on day 1, then 100 mg/d. Infuse doses over 1 h. Infusion rate should not exceed 1.1 mg/min to avoid infusion-related adverse reactions. Recommended duration of therapy is 14 days after the last positive culture. Reconstitute with companion diluent only. May be further diluted with D5W or NS. No experience exists suggesting dosage reductions are required in mild to severe hepatic impairment. Safety and efficacy not established in patients who are younger than 18 years.

Dosage Forms. **Inj** 50 mg and 100 mg.

Patient Instructions. Anidulafungin treats infections caused by a fungus. This medication is given into the vein. Report any infusion-related reactions including rash, itching, flushing, fever, or chills to health care provider.

Pharmacokinetics. Anidulafungin is approximately 97% plasma protein bound and is distributed to free body water. It is slowly metabolized by hydrolysis (autodegradation). Metabolites are not microbiologically active. Less than 10% is excreted unchanged in urine. The principle half-life is 24–26 h. This agent does not appear to be impacted by hepatic insufficiency or renal insufficiency (including renal dialysis).[28]

Adverse Reactions. Anidulafungin has been well tolerated in licensing studies, with headache, fever, nausea, vomiting, flushing, pruritus, rash, and infusion vein complications most commonly reported. Some effects may be related to histamine release and infusion rate greater than 1.1 mg/min. The reported rates for these reactions are the lowest for all the echinocandins released to date. Elevation of liver function tests has been reported, especially with concurrent cyclosporine. Hepatitis and worsening hepatic failure have also been reported.

Precautions. Pregnancy category C, lactation. Because of the large structure of the echinocandins, no significant penetration into breast milk is anticipated. However, little data is available at this time.[28]

Drug Interactions. Anidulafungin does not inhibit the CYP450 enzymes and is not a substrate or inducer of CYP3A4. No significant drug interactions have been observed except with cyclosporine. Minor increases (22%) in anidulafungin concentrations are observed with cyclosporine coadministration; no dosage adjustment is necessary.[28]

Parameters to Monitor. Hepatic enzymes, signs and symptoms of a histamine release reaction.[28]

CASPOFUNGIN ACETATE
Cancidas

Pharmacology. Caspofungin is an echinocandin antifungal derived from the fungi *Glarea lozoyensis* that is a specific noncompetitive inhibitor of β-(1,3)-glucan synthetase in fungal cell membranes. This action leads to a weakened cell wall and eventual cell lysis and death. It has good activity against *Candida* spp., *Aspergillus* spp., and *Pneumocystis jiroveci*. Therapeutic response is directly related to achieving a good C_{max}:MIC ratio (e.g., 20–30).[26,27]

Indications and Adult Dosage. **IV for refractory invasive aspergillosis, *Candidemia*, and empiric therapy for neutropenic fever**—70 mg on day 1, then 50 mg/d. Infuse doses over 1 h. Do not mix with dextrose-containing solutions. Some evidence supports a 70 mg/d dose in patients unresponsive to 50 mg/d or in patients taking medications that increase antifungal clearance (rifampin). For treatment of Esophageal candidiasis, 50 mg/d is recommended with no loading dose. In moderate hepatic impairment, give 35 mg/d after the 70 mg loading dose; no experience exists in severe hepatic impairment.

Special Populations. *Pediatric Dosage.* 3 months to 17 years. 70 mg/m² loading dose on day 1, followed by 50 mg/m² daily. Do not exceed 70 mg daily, regardless of calculated dose.[29]

Dosage Forms. Inj 50 mg and 70 mg.

Patient Instructions. Caspofungin treats infections caused by a fungus. This medication is given into the vein. Report any infusion-related reactions including rash, itching, flushing, fever, or chills.

Pharmacokinetics. Caspofungin is approximately 97% plasma protein bound and distributed in free body water. It is slowly metabolized by hydrolysis and N-acetylation. Less than 2% is excreted unchanged in urine. The principle half-life is 9–11 h.[28]

Adverse Reactions. Caspofungin has been well tolerated in limited studies, with diarrhea, pyrexia, chills, headache, fever, nausea, vomiting, flushing, pruritus, rash, increases in serum alkaline phosphatase, decreases in serum potassium, decreased hemoglobin and hematocrit, and infusion vein complications most commonly reported. Some effects may be related to histamine release. Elevation of liver function tests has been reported, especially with concurrent cyclosporine.

Precautions. Pregnancy category C, lactation. Because of the large structure of the echinocandins, no significant penetration into breast milk is anticipated. However, little data is available at this time. Hepatic impairment.

Drug Interactions. Caspofungin can reduce tacrolimus concentrations by approximately 20%. Cyclosporine increases caspofungin AUC by 35% and causes transient increases in ALT and AST. Concomitant use of cyclosporine and caspofungin is not recommended unless no safer alternative is available. Caspofungin does not inhibit any P450 enzymes, is not a substrate for these enzymes and does not induce CYP3A4. Some inducers of drug metabolism (i.e., rifampin) appear to decrease caspofungin concentrations; consider using the 70 mg/d dosage in patients who do not respond while on an inducer.[26]

Parameters to Monitor. Serum transaminase concentrations, hemoglobin, hematocrit, signs and symptoms of a histamine release reaction.[27]

CLOTRIMAZOLE   Gyne-Lotrimin, Lotrimin, Mycelex

Pharmacology. Clotrimazole is an imidazole used for local therapy of fungal infections. The topical formulations are equivalent to other topical antifungals in the treatment of *Candida* spp. or dermatophyte skin infections.[30] (*See* Topical Antifungals Comparison Chart.)

Indications and Adult Dosage. **Topical for tinea infections**—apply to affected area twice daily. **Vaginal tablet for vulvovaginal candidiasis**—100 mg/d at bedtime for 7 days; or 2–100 mg tablets once daily at bedtime for 3 days; or 1–500 mg tablet once at bedtime. **Vaginal cream for vulvovaginal candidiasis**—1 applicatorful (50 mg) at bedtime for 6–14 days. **PO to treat oropharyngeal candidiasis**—dissolve 10 mg troche in the mouth 5 times/d. **PO for prophylaxis of oral candidiasis in patients receiving immunosuppressive drugs**—dissolve 10 mg troche in the mouth 3 times daily.

Special Populations. *Pediatric Dosage.* Topical same as adult dosage. Troche (<3 years) safety and efficacy not established; (≤3 years) same as adult dosage. Vaginal cream, tablet (<12 years) safety and efficacy not established; (≤12 years) same as adult dosage.

Dosage Forms. **Top Crm, Top Lot, Top Soln** 1%; **Vag Crm** 1% and 2%; **troche** 10 mg; **Vag Tab** 100 and 200 mg. Combination packages (Gyne-Lotrimin 3) **Vag Supp** 200 mg (#3) and 1%; (Gyne-Lotrimin 7) **Vag Supp** 100 mg (#7) and **Top Crm** 1%.

Patient Instructions. Clotrimazole is used to treat fungal infections. For topical forms, wash and dry area before applying medication. Apply a thin layer to affected area, avoiding the eyes. For vaginal forms, refrain from intercourse during therapy and avoid use of tampons and douches. Vaginal forms may compromise the integrity of condoms and diaphragms. Burning and irritation may occur.

Adverse Reactions. Nausea, vomiting, bad taste, and mildly abnormal liver function tests have occurred with oral troche. Vulvovaginal burning, itching, and irritation have been reported with vaginal products. Skin rash occurs occasionally with vaginal or topical use.

Contraindications. Concomitant use with ergot alkaloids.

Precautions. Pregnancy category C; lactation; hepatic impairment; concomitant use with tacrolimus, sirolimus, trimetrexate, and fentanyl.

Drug Interactions. CYP3A4 inhibitor, substrate. Clotrimazole may increase the ergotism of ergot alkaloids resulting in nausea, vomiting, and vasospastic ischemia. Clotrimazole may decrease the clearance of tacrolimus, sirolimus, trimetrexate, and fentanyl; monitoring of these drugs for increased toxicity is warranted.

Parameters to Monitor. Liver function tests, signs and symptoms of skin reactions.

FLUCONAZOLE   Diflucan

Pharmacology. Fluconazole is a triazole antifungal agent that is highly water soluble and active in vivo against many fungal species (especially *Cryptococcus* spp.). The drug has good activity against many yeasts including *Candida* sp., *Cryptococcus* spp., *Blastomyces dermatitidis, Coccidioides immitis*, and *Histoplasma capsulatum*. Antifungal effects are caused by inhibition of fungal cytochrome P450-dependent enzymes that prevent conversion of lanosterol to ergosterol.[31–33]

Indications and Adult Dosage. **PO or IV for oropharyngeal or esophageal candidiasis**—200 mg on day 1, then 100 mg/d for 10–14 days. Severe esophageal candidiasis may require up to 400 mg/d.[31,34] **PO or IV for systemic candidiasis**—6–12 mg/kg/d. **PO or IV for cryptococcal meningitis:** (short-term therapy)—400 mg/d for 6–10 weeks. **PO or IV for cryptococcal meningitis in patients with HIV**—400 mg on Day 1, then 200–400 mg once daily for 10–12 weeks after negative CSF culture, then 200 mg once daily for suppression. In patients with concomitant HIV, flucytosine should be added if there is altered mental status; maintenance therapy in patients with AIDS 200 mg/d indefinitely.[35] Dosages up to 12 mg/kg/d have been used for cryptococcal meningitis. Combination therapy with fluconazole and flucytosine for treatment of cryptococcal meningitis appears to be superior to single-agent therapy[31]; further studies of this combination and of fluconazole plus amphotericin B are needed. Fluconazole-resistant *Candida albicans* has been clinically demonstrated; increased use of prophylactic fluconazole increases the likelihood of the emergence of resistant strains such as *Candida krusei* (intrinsic) or *Candida glabrata* (acquired).[34] **PO for uncomplicated vaginal candidiasis**—150 mg as a single dose.[33] **PO or IV for prophylaxis of candidiasis in bone marrow transplantation**—400 mg/d and continued for 7 days after granulocyte count exceeds 1000/L. Initiate therapy several days before onset of neutropenia.[34]

Special Populations. *Pediatric Dosage.* **PO or IV for candidiasis**—6 mg/kg once, then 3 mg/kg/d for at least 2 weeks for oropharyngeal candidiasis and at least 3 weeks (or 2 weeks after symptom resolution) for esophageal candidiasis; dosages up to 12 mg/kg/d have been used. **PO or IV for systemic candidiasis**—6–12 mg/kg/d. **PO or IV for treatment or prophylaxis of cryptococcal meningitis**—12 mg/kg once, then 6 mg/kg/d; continue treatment for at least 10–12 weeks after negative CSF cultures. Prophylaxis in HIV-infected children continues indefinitely.

Geriatric Dosage. (>65 years). Although half-life is prolonged, dosage adjustment appears unnecessary, unless renal impairment is severe.[32] (*See* Other Conditions.)

Other Conditions. Reduce dosage in impaired renal function: for Cl_{Cr} of 20–50 mL/min, give the usual dose q48h; Cl_{Cr} of 10–19 mL/min, 50–200 mg q48h; Cl_{Cr} <10 mL/min, 50–100 mg q48h. Give a full dose after hemodialysis on dialysis days. Patients on chronic ambulatory peritoneal dialysis may receive 50–200 mg/d. Alternative renal dosing recommended by the manufacturer is Cl_{Cr} >50, give 100% of dose, Cl_{Cr} <50 (no dialysis) give 50% of dose, dialysis: give 100% of dose after each dialysis.

Dosage Forms. **Tab** 50, 100, 150, 200 mg; **Susp** 10, 40 mg/mL; **Inj** 2 mg/mL.

Patient Instructions. Fluconazole is used to treat fungal infections. Tell health care provider if taking terfenadine, cisapride, a "statin" for cholesterol, medications for diabetes or seizures, or warfarin. Take with a meal if stomach upset occurs. Report signs of allergic reaction (itching, rash, swelling, difficulty breathing), changes in appetite, dark urine, or light stools.

Pharmacokinetics. *Fate.* Rapidly and well absorbed (90%) orally, unaffected by gastric pH. Peak concentrations of 1.8–2.8 mg/L (5.9–9 μmol/L) achieved 2 h after administration of 100–150 mg orally. Plasma protein binding is 11%–12%; penetrates well into CSF (>60% of simultaneous serum concentrations). V_d is 0.65 ± 0.2 L/kg; Cl is 0.015 ± 0.006 L/h/kg. Approximately 64% of a dose is excreted unchanged in urine.[32] **Half-life** 22 ± 4 h; 37 h in patients older than 65 years; up to 125 h in patients with renal impairment.[32]

Adverse Reactions. Occasional nausea, vomiting, diarrhea, abdominal pain, or elevations of liver transaminases occur. Severe hepatitis or exfoliative skin reactions occur rarely.[31,34]

Contraindications. Concomitant use with terfendaine or cisapride.

Precautions. Pregnancy category C. Observe patients who develop significant elevations (>3-fold) in liver transaminases for worsening of hepatic function and signs of liver failure and rash for worsening of the lesions. Discontinue the drug if necessary.

Drug Interactions. CYP 3A4 inhibitor (major). Prolongation of the QTc interval may occur with terfenadine or cisapride; use with fluconazole is contraindicated. Low doses of fluconazole have been shown to increase the serum concentrations of tolbutamide, glipizide, glyburide, and possibly other sulfonylureas. This could lead to a greater hypoglycemic effect, and dosage reduction might be necessary.[34] Fluconazole increases serum concentration of phenytoin, cyclosporine, theophylline, and astemizole; monitoring of serum drug concentrations is recommended. Fluconazole increases serum concentrations of warfarin and may result in bleeding events; monitoring of prothrombin time is recommended. Fluconazole increases serum concentrations of midazolam and possibly other benzodiazepines; consider decrease in benzodiazepine dose. Rifampin induces the metabolism of fluconazole and can lead to clinical failure; consider increasing dose of fluconazole. Use with tacrolimus may cause nephrotoxicity; monitoring for renal dysfunction is recommended. Risk of rhabdomyolysis is increased with use of statins.

Parameters to Monitor. Liver function tests weekly initially, then monthly. Monitor renal function tests weekly if abnormal at outset of therapy. (*See* Precautions). Monitor patients with elevated transaminases more carefully for hepatitis.

FLUCYTOSINE   Ancobon

Pharmacology. Flucytosine (5-FC) is a fluorinated cytosine analogue that appears to be deaminated to the cytotoxic antimetabolite fluorouracil by cytosine deaminase, an enzyme present in fungal but not in human cells. It has a narrow spectrum of activity and is used with other antifungals because resistance develops rapidly when used alone in *Candida* and *Cryptococcus* sp. infections.[30]

Indications and Adult Dosage. **PO for treatment of candidiasis or cryptococcosis**—50–150 mg/kg/d in 4 divided doses at 6-h intervals; the use of higher dosages has been suggested to prevent the emergence of resistance. Duration of therapy must be guided by the severity of infection and response to therapy. Flucytosine may be synergistic with **amphotericin B**, depending on the organism involved; the combination is useful in treating cryptococcal meningitis in AIDS and non-AIDS patients,[36] although the superiority of the combination in AIDS patients has not been established. Flucytosine might be additive or synergistic with **fluconazole** for the treatment of cryptococcal meningitis; however, further experience in clinical trials is needed before this combination can be recommended.[37]

Special Populations. *Pediatric Dosage.* **PO**—same as adult dosage in mg/kg for patients with HIV.

Geriatric Dosage. Same as adult dosage but adjust for age-related reduction in renal function, (*See* Other Conditions).

Other Conditions. Reduce dosage in impaired renal function. An approximate dosage reduction can be determined by administering doses at intervals in hours equal to 4 times the serum creatinine. Alternative regimens such as reduced doses at 6-h intervals have been recommended. In patients on maintenance hemodialysis, every 48–72 h, give 20–50 mg/kg after each dialysis.[30,38] Use normal dosage in liver disease.

Dosage Forms. Cap 250, 500 mg.

Patient Instructions. Flucytosine is used to treat fungal infections. Take the capsules required for a single dose over a 15-min period with food to minimize stomach upset.

Pharmacokinetics. *Fate.* Rapidly and well absorbed (approximately 90%), with peak about 1–2 h after administration of a 500-mg dose to adults averaging 8–12 mg/L (62–93 mol/L) in patients with normal renal function. Negligible binding to plasma proteins; V_d is 0.7 L/kg. Widely distributed throughout the body, including the CSF and eye. Eliminated almost entirely (average 90%) in the urine by glomerular filtration unchanged, with urine concentrations many times greater than serum concentrations. High serum concentrations of **fluorouracil** have been found in patients taking flucytosine and may be responsible for hematologic toxicity.[30,38] Toxicity is most likely >100 mg/L (780 μmol/L). (See also Precautions.) **Half-life** 6 ± 0.6 h; up to 100 h or greater with renal impairment.[30,38]

Adverse Reactions. Most common effects are gastrointestinal and include nausea, vomiting, and diarrhea. Occasional rash, urticaria, photosensitivity, peripheral neuropathy, elevated S_{Cr} and BUN, and elevated liver function tests (usually asymptomatic and rapidly reversible).[30,38] Infrequent but serious reactions include bone marrow suppression (leukopenia and thrombocytopenia after the first 2–4 weeks of therapy, especially when serum drug concentrations exceed 100 mg/L and with concomitant amphotericin B use; often dose-limiting in HIV patients); cardiac arrest, ventricular dysfunction including QTc prolongation and torsades, toxic epidermal necrolysis, gastrointestinal perforation or bleeding, seizure, and hallucination.

Contraindications. Concomitant use with levomethadyl.

Precautions. Pregnancy category C, lactation; severe renal impairment (elimination is highly variable and monitoring of serum concentrations is recommended; keep peak concentrations <100 mg/L); impaired hepatic function; hematologic disorders, including bone marrow depression or history of concomitant therapy with myelosuppressive drugs (e.g., zidovudine, ganciclovir, cancer chemotherapy) or radiation.[30,38]

Drug Interactions. Use with levomethadyl is contraindicated due to potential for QTc prolongation. Use with amphotericin B or zidovudine can increase the hematologic toxicity of flucytosine; dose reduction of flucytosine may be needed.

Parameters to Monitor. Before and frequently during therapy, monitor BUN, serum creatinine, Cl_{Cr}, complete blood counts, and liver function tests. (*See also* Precautions.)

GRISEOFULVIN
Fulvicin, Grifulvin V, Grisactin

Pharmacology. Griseofulvin is a fungistatic agent that appears to affect mitosis in fungal cells. It has good activity against dermatophytes but is not useful in the treatment of yeast or other fungal infections.[30]

Indications and Adult Dosage. PO for tinea infections of the skin, hair, and nails—(microsize) 0.5–1 g/d in a single or 2–4 divided doses; (ultramicrosize) 375–750 mg/d in 1–2 divided doses. Therapy usually must be continued for at least 3 weeks; infections of the palms or soles require 4–8 weeks of therapy; nail infections usually require 6–12 months of therapy.

Special Populations. *Pediatric Dosage.* (microsize) 10–20 mg/kg/d; (ultramicrosize) 7.3 mg/kg/d, given as for adults.

Dosage Forms. (Microsize) **Cap** 250 mg **Tab** 500 mg; **Susp** 25 mg/mL; (ultramicrosize) **Tab** 125, 250, 330 mg.

Patient Instructions. Griseofulvin is used to treat fungal infections. Take with meals high in fat to enhance absorption and avoid stomach upset. May cause sensitivity to sunlight; avoid prolonged sun exposure and wear sunscreen or protective clothing. Use of alcohol while taking this medication may result in a severe reaction including nausea, vomiting, diarrhea, flushing, fast heart rate, and a drop in blood pressure. Do not take if pregnant. May decrease the effect of oral contraceptives; additional contraceptive methods should be used during and 1 month after therapy (6 months for males).

Adverse Reactions. Adverse reactions include occasional headache (up to 15%), diarrhea, nausea, and vomiting. Photosensitivity reactions, peripheral neuritis, and pancytopenia are rare. The drug can exacerbate acute intermittent porphyria and lupus erythematosus. Disulfiram-like reaction may occur with concomitant alcohol use.

Contraindications. Porphyria and hepatocellular failure; pregnancy during and within 1 month of discontinuation of therapy.

Precautions. Additional contraceptive precautions during and 1 month after discontinuing therapy (males should not father a child for 6 months following discontinuation of therapy); penicillin allergy; photosensitivity.

Drug Interactions. Griseofulvin may decrease the efficacy of oral contraceptives (*See* Precautions) and of warfarin; dose adjustments of warfarin may be needed. Disulfiram-like reaction with concomitant use of alcohol. High-fat meals increase griseofulvin absorption 50%–100%.

ITRACONAZOLE
Sporanox

Pharmacology. Itraconazole is a synthetic triazole antifungal agent that is more active than ketoconazole or fluconazole against certain fungi, notably *Aspergillus* spp. It also has activity against *Coccidioides, Cryptococcus, Candida, Histoplasma, Blastomyces,* and *Sporotrichosis* spp. Itraconazole inhibits fungal cytochrome P450-dependent enzymes. This inhibition blocks ergosterol biosynthesis, creating disturbances in membrane function and membrane-bound enzymes and affecting fungal cell growth and viability.[34,39]

Indications and Adult Dosage. PO for systemic fungal infections—200–600 mg/d, depending on site and severity of infection. Give dosages over 200 mg/d in 2–3 divided doses. **PO for vulvovaginal candidiasis**—200 mg twice daily for 1 day or 200 mg/d for 7 days. **PO for dermatomycoses**—100 mg/d for 15 days or 200 mg/d for 7 days. **PO for pityriasis versicolor**—200 mg/d for 7 days. **PO for plantar tinea pedis and palmar tinea manuum**—100 mg/d for 30 days or 200 mg twice daily for 7 days. **PO for onychomycosis**—200 once daily for 3 months.[40] **IV for blastomycosis, histoplasmosis, or aspergillosis**—200 mg twice daily for 4 doses, then 200 mg/d.

Special Populations. *Pediatric Dosage.* Limited data exists but PO doses of 5 mg/kg/d for 2 weeks for age 6 months–12 years and 100 mg/d for ages 3–16 years have been used. For age 5 and older with systemic fungal infections, 2.5 mg/kg twice daily can be used.

Other Conditions. Dosage reduction in patients with hepatic impairment might be necessary, but guidelines are not established. No dosage adjustment is necessary in renal impairment. However, the manufacturer recommends that the injection not be used in patients with Cl_{Cr} <30 mL/min.

Dosage Forms. Cap 100 mg; Soln 10 mg/mL; Inj 10 mg/mL.

Patient Instructions. Itraconazole is used to treat fungal infections. Take this drug with food to ensure maximal absorption. Do not take within 2 h of taking medications that decrease stomach acid (e.g., antacids, histamine H2-receptor antagonists, omeprazole). Report any medications you are taking, including statins for cholesterol and the blood thinner warfarin. Report symptoms of fatigue, loss of appetite, nausea, vomiting, yellowing of the skin, dark urine, or pale stools.

Pharmacokinetics. *Fate.* Relative oral bioavailability of the capsules compared with an oral solution is >70%.[34] The solubility of itraconazole is aided by an acidic environment, and food increases absorption. Peak serum concentration occurs in 4 h; peak concentration is 20 μg/L (28 nmol/L) after a single 100-mg oral dose during fasting, increasing to 180 μg/L (0.26 μmol/L) when taken with food.[39] The drug is >99% protein bound, primarily to albumin, with only 0.2% available as free drug.[39] It is highly lipid soluble, and concentrations are much higher in tissues than in serum. Itraconazole is metabolized in the liver and exhibits dose-dependent elimination.[34] One metabolite, hydroxyl-itraconazole, has antifungal activity, and serum concentrations are double those of itraconazole at steady state. *Serum concentrations*. Itraconazole concentrations <5 mg/L (<7 μmol/L) are associated with prophylaxis failure in Aspergillus infections.[41] **Half-life** 24–42 h; possibly longer with large daily dosages.[34]

Adverse Reactions. Itraconazole is generally well tolerated with long-term use. It has a negative inotropic effect and rarely is reported to worsen heart failure. Occasional rash, pruritus, nausea, vomiting, abdominal discomfort, headache, dizziness, decreased libido, hypertriglyceridemia[42] and hypertension occur. Mild transient elevations of transaminases occur frequently. Hepatotoxicity is rare, but deaths have occurred. Hearing loss, transient or permanent may occur, especially in the elderly. There are no apparent adverse effects on testicular or adrenal steroidogenesis.[34,39]

Contraindications. Pregnancy; Coadministration with drugs metabolized through CYP3A4 such as astemizole, cisapride, oral midazolam, pimozide, quinidine, dofetilide, triazolam, HMGCoA reductase inhibitors, and calcium channel blockers.

Precautions. Lactation; hepatic impairment; treatment of onychomycosis in patients with ventricular dysfunction (e.g., heart failure).

Drug Interactions. Itraconazole inhibits CYP3A3/4 resulting in increased concentrations of drugs metabolized through these enzymes. Cardiovascular events such as QTc prolongation, torsades, and ventricular tachycardia can occur. Itraconazole inhibits metabolism of certain drugs such as cyclosporine and warfarin. (*See* Contraindications.) Warfarin dosage reduction might be necessary during concurrent use. Cyclosporine dosage might need to be reduced by 50% with itraconazole dosages over 100 mg/d. Avoid concurrent use with antiretrovirals, carbamazepine, phenytoin, or rifampin because they can induce the metabolism of itraconazole and dramatically reduce its serum concentration.[41,43] Histamine H2-receptor antagonists, antacids, and probably proton pump inhibitors (e.g., omeprazole, lansoprazole) might reduce itraconazole oral absorption.

Parameters to Monitor. Closely monitor prothrombin time in patients on concurrent warfarin and cyclosporine concentrations in patients taking these drugs. Monitor liver function tests in patients with preexisting hepatic impairment. Monitoring serum drug concentrations can be helpful if poor absorption or increased metabolism of itraconazole is suspected. Monitor heart failure patients for worsening of symptoms.

KETOCONAZOLE Nizoral

Pharmacology. Ketoconazole is an imidazole antifungal agent that exerts its antifungal effects through inhibition of the synthesis of ergosterol (a fungal cell wall component) by inhibiting fungal cytochrome P450. It is used primarily for mucocutaneous fungal infections, including candidiasis, and in tinea versicolor unresponsive to topical therapy. It is used to treat blastomycosis, histoplasmosis, and paracoccidioidiomycosis in immunocompetent patients. Because of its poor CSF penetration, ketoconazole is not recommended for fungal infections of the CNS.[37,39] Because of its effects on steroid synthesis (*see* Adverse Reactions), the drug has been used in prostatic cancer, skin disorders (dermatitis) and Cushing syndrome.

Indications and Adult Dosage. **PO**—200–400 mg daily or twice daily, depending on site and severity of infection. **Topical**—apply once daily or twice daily for dermatophytoses, superficial mycoses, or seborrheic dermatitis. **Topical for dandruff**—apply shampoo twice weekly to wet hair (leave for 5 min, then rinse) for up to 8 weeks, then as needed for dandruff control.

Special Populations. *Pediatric Dosage.* PO (<2 years) not established; (>2 years) 3.3–6.6 mg/kg/d in 1 or 2 divided doses. The drug is bioavailable when tablets are crushed and mixed in applesauce or juice. Topical (<12 years) not established; (12 years and older) apply once daily.

Other Conditions. Limited data suggest that dosage adjustment is unnecessary in patients with hepatic impairment; however, definitive studies are needed. No adjustment is necessary in renal dysfunction.

Dosage Forms. Tab 200 mg; Crm, foam, gel 2%; shampoo 1, 2%.

Patient Instructions. Ketoconazole is used to treat fungal infections. This drug is best absorbed if taken on an empty stomach, but may be taken with meals if stomach upset occurs. Do not take within 2 h of taking medications that decrease stomach acid (e.g., antacids, histamine H2-receptor antagonists, omeprazole). Use of alcohol while taking this medication may result in a severe reaction including nausea, vomiting, diarrhea, flushing, fast heart rate, and a drop in blood pressure. Topical formulations may cause stinging or itching of the skin. Report symptoms of fatigue, loss of appetite, yellowing of the skin, dark urine, or pale stools. Taking this drug with an acidic beverage (e.g., a cola drink) can increase the absorption substantially. If using concomitant 0.1 N HCl to promote absorption, the solution should be sipped through a straw to avoid damaging the teeth.

Pharmacokinetics. Bioavailability is approximately 75% and is dose dependent. An acidic environment is necessary for dissolution and absorption. Bioavailability appears to be decreased by 20%–40% when the drug is administered with food and is even more markedly reduced if gastric pH is elevated. Poor absorption can occur in AIDS patients because of achlorhydria and other pathologic changes in the GI track. Achlorhydric patients may be given concomitant glutamic acid hydrochloride or 0.1 N HCl (using a drinking straw) to increase absorption.[44] An acidic drink (e.g., a cola) also may be used to increase ketoconazole absorption by approximately 65% in achlorhydria.[45] Peak serum concentrations of 3.4 ± 0.3 mg/L (6.4 ± 0.6 μmol/L) are attained after a 200 mg dose taken with a meal. The drug is 93%–96% plasma protein bound. V_d is estimated to be 0.36 ± 0.1 L/kg with a single dose, increasing to 2.4 ± 1.6 L/kg during long-term therapy; Cl is estimated to be 0.5 ± 0.25 L/h/kg during long-term therapy. Ketoconazole is extensively metabolized by the liver to inactive metabolites, with only 2%–4% of a dose excreted unchanged in urine.[30,44,46] **Half-life** 8.7 ± 0.2 h after a single dose, decreasing to 3.3 ± 1 h during long-term therapy.[30,46]

Adverse Reactions. Generally well tolerated, with the most frequent side effects being nausea, vomiting, pruritus, and abdominal discomfort. Hepatotoxicity, including massive hepatic necrosis, occurs occasionally, but mild elevations of transaminases occur frequently. Gynecomastia occurs, probably caused by ketoconazole-induced suppression of testosterone synthesis. Ketoconazole also blocks cortisol production; however, clinically apparent hypoadrenalism occurs rarely. Irritation, pruritus, and stinging can occur with topical use. Disulfiram-like reaction with concomitant alcohol use has been reported.

Contraindications. Concomitant use with astemizole, cisapride, triazolam, or terfenadine.

Precautions. Pregnancy category C; concomitant use with alcohol.

Drug Interactions. Ketoconazole inhibits CYP3A4 resulting in increased concentrations of drugs metabolized through these enzymes. Cardiovascular events such as QTc prolongation, torsades, and ventricular tachycardia can occur. Ketoconazole also inhibits metabolism of certain drugs such as cyclosporine, methylprednisolone, and warfarin. (*See* Contraindications.) Warfarin dosage reduction may be necessary during concurrent use. Histamine H2-receptor antagonists, antacids, and probably proton pump inhibitors (e.g., omeprazole, lansoprazole) might reduce ketoconazole oral absorption. Disulfiram-like reaction with concomitant alcohol use.

Parameters to Monitor. Monitor liver function tests before starting therapy and often during therapy. Closely monitor prothrombin time in patients on concurrent warfarin and cyclosporine concentrations in patients taking this drug.

MICAFUNGIN   Mycamine

Pharmacology. Micafungin is an echinocandin antifungal derived from the fungi *Coleophoma empetri* that is a specific noncompetitive inhibitor of β-(1,3)-glucan synthetase in fungal cell membranes. This action leads to a weakened cell wall and eventual cell lysis and death. It has good activity against *Candida* spp., *Aspergillus* spp., and *Pneumocystis jiroveci*. Echinocandins are dose dependent anti-infectives. Therapeutic response is directly related to achieving a good C_{max}:MIC ratio (i.e., 20–30).[26,27]

Indications and Adult Dosage. IV for candidemia and empiric therapy for neutropenic fever—100–150 mg/d. Infuse doses over 1 h. May be both reconstituted and diluted with D5W or NS. **IV for esophageal candidiasis**—150 mg/d. **IV for fungal (*Candida*) prophylaxis in stem cell transplant patient**—50 mg/d.

Dosage Forms. Inj 50 mg and 100 mg.

Pharmacokinetics. Micafungin is approximately 98% plasma protein bound and distributed in free body water. It is slowly metabolized by hydrolysis and COMT activity in the liver. Less than 2% is excreted unchanged in urine. The principle half-life is 11–21 h.[28]

Adverse Reactions. Micafungin has been well tolerated in licensing studies, with headache, fever, nausea, vomiting, flushing, pruritus and infusion vein complications most commonly reported. Some effects may be related to histamine release. The reported rates for these reactions are low. Elevated liver function tests and elevations in serum creatinine and BUN have been reported with low incidence.

Precautions. Pregnancy category C; lactation. Because of the large structure of the echinocandins, no significant penetration into breast milk is anticipated. However, little data is available at this time. Use with caution in patients with severe hepatic and renal dysfunction.[26]

Drug Interactions. No significant drug interactions have been observed with micafungin. Micafungin may increase sirolimus, nifedipine, and itraconazole concentrations, and these patients should be monitored for toxicity.[28]

Parameters to Monitor. Hepatic and renal function, signs and symptoms of a histamine release reaction.

Notes. IV is not currently approved for refractory invasive aspergillosis.

MICONAZOLE NITRATE   M-Zole, Micatin, Monistat, Various

Pharmacology. Miconazole is an imidazole antifungal agent available in topical preparations.[30] (*See* Topical Antifungals Comparison Chart.)

Indications and Adult Dosage. Topical for tinea infections.—apply twice daily. **Vaginal suppository for vulvovaginal candidiasis**—100 mg at bedtime for 7 days, 200 mg at bedtime for 3 days, or 1200 mg once. **Vaginal cream for vulvovaginal candidiasis**—5 g at bedtime for 7 days.

Special Populations. *Pediatric Dosage.* Topical same as adult dosage; vaginal cream, suppository (<12 years) safety and efficacy not established; (≤12 years) same as adult dosage.

Dosage Forms. IV form has been discontinued and is no longer available from the manufacturer. **Top Crm, Topical Oint, Top spray, Top Pwdr, Top effervescent Tab** 2%, **Top tincture** 2%, **Vag Crm** 2%, **Vag Supp** 100 and 200 mg. Combination packages (Monistat 7 Combination Package) **Vag Supp** 100 mg (#7) and **Vag Crm** 2%; (Monistat-3 Combination Package) **Vag Supp** 200 mg (#3) and **Vag Crm** 2%; (Monistat-1) **Vag Supp** 1200 mg and **Vag Crm** 2%.

Patient Instructions. Miconazole is used to treat fungal infections. For topical forms, wash and dry area before applying medication. Apply a thin layer to affected area, avoiding the eyes. For vaginal forms, refrain from intercourse during therapy and avoid use of tampons and douches. Vaginal forms may compromise the integrity of condoms and diaphragms. Burning and irritation may occur.

Adverse Reactions. Topical formulations may cause burning, allergic contact dermatitis, and maceration. Vaginal formulations may cause abdominal cramps, burning, irritation, and itching.

Notes. Vaginal and topical effects are similar to those of clotrimazole.

NYSTATIN   Mycostatin, Nilstat, Various

Pharmacology. Nystatin is a polyene antifungal agent very similar to amphotericin B, but, too toxic for parenteral use. Oral absorption is negligible, and there is no absorption through intact skin or mucous membranes.[30] (*See* Topical Antifungals Comparison Chart.)

Indications and Adult Dosage. PO for oral candidiasis—(suspension) 400,000–600,000 units 4 times daily (as a "swish and swallow"); (troches) 200,000–400,000 units 4–5 times/d. Treat for at least 48 h after oral symptoms have cleared and cultures have returned to normal. Immunocompromised patients require longer therapy (e.g., 10–14 days). The vaginal tablet has been successfully used orally in place of the oral suspension; its slow dissolution allows prolonged contact time. **PO for GI candidiasis**—500,000–1,000,000 units 3 times daily. **Vaginal for candidiasis**—100,000 units daily or twice daily for 2 weeks. **Topical for cutaneous candidiasis**—apply 2–3 times daily.

Special Populations. *Pediatric Dosage.* **PO for candidiasis**—(suspension) (infants) 200,000 units 4 times daily; (children) 400,000–600,000 units 4 times daily. Topical same as adult dosage.

Dosage Forms. PO Tab 500,000 units; **troche** 200,000 units; **Susp** 100,000 units/mL; **Top Crm, Oint, Pwdr** 100,000 units/g; **Vag Tab** 100,000 units.

Patient Instructions. Nystatin is used to treat fungal infections. For topical forms, wash and dry area before applying medication. Apply a thin layer to affected area, avoiding the eyes. When using liquid form in infants, apply half of the dose to each side of the mouth and avoid food for 5–10 min. In children and adults, swish liquid in mouth for as long as possible, and then swallow. Allow lozenges to dissolve in the mouth completely. May cause stomach upset. For vaginal forms, refrain from intercourse during therapy and avoid use of tampons and douches. Vaginal forms may compromise the integrity of condoms and diaphragms.

Adverse Reactions. Nontoxic by oral, topical, and vaginal routes. Nausea and vomiting may occur with higher doses (5,000,000 units daily). Allergic sensitization occurs rarely.

POSACONAZOLE   Noxafil

Pharmacology. Posaconazole is an azole antifungal that is a derivative of itraconazole. Posaconazole inhibits fungal cytochrome P450-dependent enzymes to block ergosterol biosynthesis and create disturbances in membrane function and membrane-bound enzymes, affecting fungal cell growth and viability. It has a broad spectrum of activity against yeasts and molds, including *Candida* and *Aspergillus,* and clinical efficacy against Zygomycetes. In vitro activity extends to *Scedosporium* spp., *Fusarium* spp., *C. neoformans, Coccidioides* spp., and *Histoplasma* spp.[26,27,34,39]

Indications and Adult Dosage. **PO for prophylaxis of invasive fungal infections**—PO 200 mg 3 times daily. **PO for oropharyngeal candidiasis**—loading dose of 100 mg/d twice daily for 1 day, then 100 mg/d for an additional 13 days is recommended. **PO for oropharyngeal candidiasis refractory to itraconazole or fluconazole**—400 mg twice daily is recommended. Off label, up to 800 mg/d has been used for treatment of difficult to eradicate molds and yeasts.

Dosage Forms. Susp 40 mg/mL.

Patient Instructions. Posaconazole is used to treat fungal infections. This drug can cause nausea, vomiting, diarrhea, and abdominal pain. It should be taken with a full meal or liquid nutritional supplement for best absorption. Report any medications you are taking, including those for cholesterol or seizures.

Pharmacokinetics. Bioavailability is extremely variable and is dose and food dependent. Bioavailability appears to be increased by administration with food or oral supplemental liquids. Splitting dosage from once daily to multiple times daily increases absorption. Absorption appears saturable above 800 mg/d. Patients who have gastrointestinal diseases (diarrhea, vomiting) may need to have serum drug concentrations closely monitored. Peak serum concentrations are highly variable. The drug appears highly plasma protein bound. V_d is estimated to be 343–1341 L. Posaconazole is predominately excreted in the feces and not renally dialyzed. No adjustment is needed for mild to severe renal dysfunction. Distribution into breast milk may occur during therapy. **Half-life** 25–31 h.[26]

Adverse Reactions. Most commonly associated with diarrhea, QTc prolongation or torsades de pointes, headache, dizziness, insomnia, fever, rash, hypokalemia. Occasional abdominal discomfort, anorexia, mucositis, neutropenia, anemia can occur. Rarely, adrenal insufficiency, hemolytic uremic syndrome, thrombotic thrombocytopenia purpura, and allergic reactions can occur. Mild transient elevations of transaminases occur frequently. Hepatotoxicity is rare.[28]

Contraindications. Coadministration of sirolimus, cisapride, and CYP3A4 substrates terfenadine, astemizole, pimozide, halofantrine, or quinidine.

Precautions. Pregnancy category C, lactation. Impaired renal (variable serum concentrations) or hepatic function. Use with caution in patients with prolonged QTc or at risk for arrhythmia, concomitant use with drugs known to cause QTc prolongation, concomitant use with drugs metabolized through CYP3A4.

Drug Interactions. Posaconazole concentrations can be reduced by cimetidine, rifabutin, and phenytoin and these combinations should be avoided. Posaconazole is a strong inhibitor of CYP3A4, and inhibits metabolism of drugs such as cyclosporine, tacrolimus, and phenytoin. Initial doses of these drugs should be reduced, and patients should be monitored for adverse reactions and serum concentrations.[28]

Parameters to Monitor. Monitor hepatic function prior to and during treatment. Monitor renal function, CBC, and electrolytes. Serum drug concentrations may need monitoring in patients with poor responses or questionable drug absorption.

TERBINAFINE   Lamisil

Pharmacology. Terbinafine is a synthetic allylamine antifungal agent that exerts its activity by inhibiting fungal ergosterol synthesis through inhibition of squalene epoxidase. Terbinafine is active orally and topically. It has demonstrated activity against dermatophyte infections but is less active than azole antifungals against yeast species.[30,47] (*See* Topical Antifungals Comparison Chart.)

Indications and Adult Dosage. PO for onychomycosis of fingernails—250 mg once daily for 6 weeks. **PO for onychomycosis of the toenails**—250 mg once daily for 12 weeks. Reduce dosage in severe hepatic or renal dysfunction. **Topical for tinea corporis or cruris, or cutaneous candidiasis**—apply cream twice daily for 1 week. **Topical for tinea pedis**—apply solution or spray twice daily for 1 week, cream may require therapy up to 4 weeks, especially for plantar infections. **Topical for tinea versicolor**—apply solution or spray twice daily for 1 week.

Special populations. *Pediatric Dosage.* **PO for tinea capitis**—(4 years and older) if <25 kg, 125 mg once daily; if between 25 and 35 kg, 187.5 mg daily; if >35 kg, 250 mg daily. Dose for 6 weeks. **Topical for tinea cruris or corporis**—(12 years and older) apply once daily for 1 week. **Topical for tinea pedis**—(12 years and older) same as adult dosage.

Other Conditions. Use is not recommended in patients with Cl_{Cr} of 50 mL/min or less.

Dosage Forms. **Crm** 1%; **gel** 1%; **Top spray** 1%; **Top Soln** 1%; **Tab** 250 mg; **oral packet** 125 and 187.5 mg.

Pharmacokinetics. Terbinafine is 70%–80% orally absorbed regardless of the presence of food. Peak concentrations after 250 and 500 mg oral doses are 0.9 mg/L (3.1 μmol/L) and 2 mg/L (6.9 μmol/L), respectively, within 2 h. Terbinafine is highly lipophilic and is widely distributed with a V_d of 13.5 L/kg. It is extensively metabolized to inactive metabolites, and its plasma elimination half-life is 11–16 h; however, an additional elimination phase of 200–400 h may reflect the gradual release of terbinafine from adipose tissue.

Adverse Reactions. Dyspepsia, abdominal pain, diarrhea, skin reactions, headache, abnormal color vision, taste disturbance, and erectile dysfunction occur frequently during oral therapy. Rare but serious skin reactions have occurred including Stevens-Johnson syndrome, toxic epidermal necrolysis, cutaneous lupus erythematosus, and erythema multiforme. Blood dyscrasias including agranulocytosis, neutropenia, and pancytopenia have occurred. Hepatic failure has been reported rarely with the treatment of onychomycoses. Avoid in patients with liver disease.

Precautions. Pregnancy category B; lactation; chronic or active liver disease (use of terbinafine is not recommended); renal impairment; immunodeficiency.

Drug Interactions. Terbinafine can inhibit CYP2D6 and increase concentrations of drugs metabolized by this route. Its clearance is increased 100% by rifampin and decreased 33% by cimetidine.

Parameters to Monitor. Baseline liver function tests; repeat if symptoms of hepatotoxicity occur, signs and symptoms of skin reactions.

VORICONAZOLE	Vfend

Pharmacology. Voriconazole is an triazole antifungal. Voriconazole inhibits fungal cytochrome P450-dependent enzymes to block ergosterol biosynthesis and create disturbances in membrane function and membrane-bound enzymes, affecting fungal cell growth and viability. It has good activity against *Candida* and *Aspergillus*, with superior activity against *Candida albicans, C. krusei,* and *C. glabrata*. Activity also extends to *Pseudalescherii boydii, Fusarium* spp, and *Scedosporium asiosperium*.[27,48]

Indications and Adult Dosage. IV for invasive aspergillosis, candidemia/invasive candidiasis in nonneutropenic patients, scedosporiosis or fusariosis infections—loading dose 6 mg/kg every 12 h for 1 day, maintenance IV 4 mg/kg every 12 h or PO 200 mg twice daily. Infuse at a maximum rate of 3 mg/kg/h over 1 or 2 h. **PO for systemic fungal infections PO for esophageal candidiasis**—200 mg twice daily for patients weighing 40 kg or more; 100 mg twice daily for patients weighing <40 kg.

Dosage Forms. Tab 50, 200 mg; **Susp** 40 mg/mL; **Inj** 200 mg.

Patient Instructions. This drug may cause visual changes, which may impair the ability to drive or work. Effects usually begin 30 min after the dose is administered and last for 30 min, and tend to last only for the first few days of therapy. Voriconazole may also cause skin rash or photosensitivity. Sun exposure should be avoided, and a physician should be contacted if a rash develops.[26]

Pharmacokinetics. Oral bioavailability is 58% and decreased by high-fat meals. Steady-state plasma concentrations are 2.1–4.8 mg/L with an oral dosage of 200 mg twice daily. The drug is 51%–67% plasma protein bound; V_d is 4.6 L/kg. Peak concentrations after multiple 200 mg (3.0 μg/mL) and 300 mg (4.66 μg/mL) oral doses appear **nonlinear in accumulation.** After multiple parenteral doses (3 mg/kg every 12 h) including a loading dose (6 mg/kg every 12 h × 2 doses), peak values are 4.7 μg/mL on day 1 and 3.06 μg/mL on day 14. It is metabolized by the liver, primarily by CYP2C9 and 3A4. Elimination half-life is about 6 h, but the drug can be detected in urine and feces for several days after prolonged therapy. Less than 2% of unchanged drug appears in urine.[48,49]

Adverse Reactions. Reversible mild to moderate dose-related visual disturbances, elevations in hepatic enzymes, and skin rashes occur frequently. Rare but serious reactions include prolongation of QTc and torsades, Stevens-Johnson syndrome, toxic epidermal necrolysis, erythema multiforme, pancreatitis, hepatic failure, and renal failure. Cases of photosensitivity have also been reported.[48]

Contraindications. Concomitant use of carbamazepine, CYP3A4 substrates, ergot alkaloids, long-acting barbiturates, rifamycins, ritonavir in high doses (400 mg every 12 h), sirolimus, or St. John's wort.

Precautions. Pregnancy category D, lactation. Because of the large structure of the echinocandins, no significant penetration into breast milk is anticipated. However, little data is available at this time.[28] Impaired renal or hepatic function. Concomitant use of strong P450 inducers; proarrhythmic disorders; lactose intolerance.

Drug Interactions. Voriconazole is a substrate for CYP2C19, 2C9, and 3A4, and interacts with drugs that affect or are metabolized by this system, including cyclosporine, tacrolimus, carbamazepine, phenytoin, and warfarin. Initial doses of these drugs should be reduced, and patients should be monitored for adverse reactions and toxicities.[26] In cases of significant renal dysfunction, accumulation of the cyclodextran may occur with the parenteral formulation. The significance of this accumulation is still being debated, however, it may lead to neurotoxicity. Hemodialysis removes both voriconazole and cyclodextran.

Parameters to Monitor. Hepatic enzymes, including alkaline phosphatase and total bilirubin; renal function; electrolytes; visual function prior to and during therapy; and signs and symptoms of a histamine release reaction.[26]

TOPICAL ANTIFUNGALS COMPARISON CHART

CLASS AND DRUG	DOSAGE FORMS	ADULT DOSAGE[a]	COMMENTS
ALLYLAMINES AND BENZYLAMINES			
Butenafine HCl Mentax, Mentax TC, Lotrimin Ultra	Top Crm 1%	Top (tinea pedis) apply daily for 1–4 wk.	A benzylamine similar to the allylamines.
Naftifine HCl Naftin	Top Crm 1% Topical gel 1%	Top (tinea) apply twice daily for 4 wk.	First agent of allylamine class; response is faster than with imidazoles.
Terbinafine HCl Lamisil	Top Crm 1% Top Soln 1% Top gel 1% Top spray 1%	Top (tinea cruris or corporis) apply once to twice daily for 1–4 wk; (tinea pedis) apply twice daily for up to 4 wk.	Allylamine; 10–100 times more potent than naftifine. Response is more rapid than imidazoles, and it has excellent penetration in tinea pedis.
IMIDAZOLES			
Butoconazole Nitrate Femstat Gynazole-1	Vag Crm 2%	Vag (nonpregnant) 2% Crm at bedtime for 3–6 days OR (Gynazole-1) 2% cream 1 applicatorful once (pregnant, second OR third trimester) 2% Crm at bedtime for 6 days.	None.
Clotrimazole Lotrimin AF Mycelex	Top Crm 1% Top Lot 1% Top Soln 1% Vaginal tablet 100 Vaginal cream 1%	Top (Candida, tinea) apply twice daily. Vag 100 mg suppository OR 1% Crm at bedtime for 7 days; 500 mg suppository at bedtime once.	Useful for first trimester Trichomonas vaginitis, but less effective than metronidazole.

(continued)

TOPICAL ANTIFUNGALS COMPARISON CHART (*continued*)

CLASS AND DRUG	DOSAGE FORMS	ADULT DOSAGE[a]	COMMENTS
Econazole Nitrate	Top Crm 1%.	Top (*Candida*) apply twice daily; (tinea) apply once daily.	None.
Ketoconazole Nizoral Extina Xolegel	Top Crm 2% Top shampoo 1% and 2% Top foam 2% Top gel 2%	Top (*Candida*, tinea) apply daily for 2–6 wk; (seborrhea) apply twice daily for 4 wk; (shampoo) twice weekly for 4 wk.	None.
Miconazole Nitrate Micatin Monistat Miconazol-3	Top Crm 2% Top Oint 2% Vag Crm 2% Vag Crm 4%	Top apply twice daily.	Less effective than some newer topical imidazoles.
Oxiconazole Nitrate Oxistat	Top Crm 1% Top Lot 1%	Top (tinea) apply once to twice daily for 2–4 wk.	Superior to tolnaftate in dermatomycoses.
Sulconazole Nitrate Exelderm	Top Crm 1% Top Soln 1%	Top (tinea) apply once to twice daily for 3–4 wk.	Superior to miconazole in dermatomycoses.
Terconazole Terazol	Vag Crm 0.4% and 0.8% Vag Supp 80 mg	Vag 0.4% Crm at bedtime for 7 days; 0.8% Crm OR 80 mg Supp at bedtime for 3 days.	None.
Tioconazole Vagistat-1	Vag Oint 6.5%	Vag at bedtime once.	More effective than older imidazoles; appears effective in vaginal trichomoniasis.

(continued)

TOPICAL ANTIFUNGALS COMPARISON CHART (*continued*)

CLASS AND DRUG	DOSAGE FORMS	ADULT DOSAGE[a]	COMMENTS
POLYENES			
Nystatin Mycostatin Nilstat	Top Crm 100,000 units/g Top Oint 100,000 units/g Top Pwdr 100,000 units/g Vag Tab 100,000 units	Top (*Candida*) apply 2–3 times daily. Vag 1 Tab at bedtime for 14 days.	Similar to amphotericin B.
MISCELLANEOUS			
Ciclopirox Olamine Loprox Penlac	Top Crm 0.77% Top Lot 0.77% Top gel 0.77% Top Susp 0.77% Nail lacquer 8%	Top Crm, Lot (*Candida*, tinea) apply twice daily. Top nail lacquer apply daily.	A hydroxypyridone. More effective than clotrimazole for tinea versicolor. Nail lacquer is inexpensive, but has poor efficacy rate.
Tolnaftate Tinactin Ting	Top Crm 1% Top gel 1% Top Soln 1% Pwdr 1% Spray Liquid 1% Spray Pwdr 1%	Top (tinea) apply twice daily for 2–6 wk.	A thiocarbamate. Less effective than imidazoles for dermatomycoses.

[a]The dosage for vaginal creams for *Candida* infections is one applicatorful at the interval shown. Tinea pedis should be treated at the maximum dosage (usually twice daily) for the longest time mentioned, usually 4 wk.
From product information.

■ REFERENCES

1. Alexander BD et al. Antifungal resistance trends towards the year 2000. Implications for therapy and new approaches. *Drugs*. 1997;54:657-678.

2. Gallis HA et al. Amphotericin B: 30 years of clinical experience. *Rev Infect Dis*. 1990;12:308-309.

3. Gary-Bobo CM. Polyene-sterol interaction and selective toxicity. *Biochimie*. 1989;71:37-47.

4. Kintzel PE et al. Practical guidelines for preparing and administering amphotericin B. *Am J Hosp Pharm*. 1992;49:1156-1164.

5. Kline S et al. Limited toxicity of prolonged therapy with high doses of amphotericin B lipid complex. *Clin Infect Dis*. 1995;21:1154-1158.

6. O'Donnell MR et al. Prediction of systemic fungal infection in allogeneic marrow recipients: impact of amphotericin B prophylaxis in high-risk patients. *J Clin Oncol*. 1994;12:827-834.

7. De Laurenzi A et al. Amphotericin B prophylaxis against invasive fungal infections in neutropenic patients: a single center experience from 1980 to 1995. *Infection*. 1996;24:361-366.

8. Gryn J et al. The toxicity of daily inhaled amphotericin B. *Am J Clin Oncol*. 1993;16:43-46.

9. Bennett JE. Antifungal drugs. In: Mandell GL et al., eds. *Principles and Practice of Infectious Diseases*. 3rd ed. New York: Churchill Livingstone; 1990:361-376.

10. Varkey B et al. Pulmonary aspergilloma. A rational approach to treatment. *Am J Med*. 1976;61:626-631.

11. Schwartz S et al. Aerosolized amphotericin B inhalations as prophylaxis of invasive aspergillus infections during prolonged neutropenia: results of a prospective randomized multicenter trial. *Blood*. 1999;93:3654-3661.

12. Trigg ME et al. Successful program to prevent aspergillus infections in children undergoing marrow transplantation: use of nasal amphotericin. *Bone Marrow Transplant*. 1997;19:43-47.

13. Gordon MA et al. Corneal allescheriosos. *Arch Ophthalmol*. 1959;62;758-763.

14. Perraut LE et al. Successful treatment of *Candida albicans* endophthalmitis with intravitreal amphotericin B. *Arch Ophthalmol*. 1981;99:1565-1567.

15. Ringden O et al. Prophylaxis and therapy using liposomal amphotericin B (AmBisome) for invasive fungal infection in children undergoing organ or allogeneic bone marrow transplantation. *Pediatr Transplant*. 1997;1:124-129.

16. Christiansen KJ et al. Distribution and activity of amphotericin B in humans. *J Infect Dis*. 1985;152:1037-1043.

17. Kan VL et al. Comparative safety, tolerance, and pharmacokinetics of amphotericin B lipid complex and amphotericin B desoxycholate in healthy male volunteers. *J Infect Dis*. 1991;164:418-421.

18. Heinemann V et al. Pharmacokinetics of liposomal amphotericin B (AmBisome) versus other lipid-based formulations. *Bone Marrow Transplant*. 1994;14(suppl 5):S8-S9.

19. Levy M et al. Amphotericin B–induced heart rate decrease in children, *Clin Pediatr*. 1995;34:358-364.

20. Le Y et al. Amphotericin B–associated hypertension. *Ann Pharmacother*. 1996;30:765-767.

21. Manley TJ et al. Reversible parkinsonism in a child after bone marrow transplantation and lipid-based amphotericin B therapy. *Pediatr Infect Dis J*. 1998;17:433-434.

22. Rossi MR et al. Severe rhabdomyolysis, hyperthermia and shock after amphotericin B colloidal dispersion in an allogeneic bone marrow transplant recipient. *Pediatr Infect Dis J*. 2000;19:172-173.

23. Wright DG et al. Lethal pulmonary reactions associated with the combined use of amphotericin B and leukocyte transfusions. *N Engl J Med*. 1981;304:1185-1189.

24. Hussein MA et al. Transfusing platelets 2 h after the completion of amphotericin-B decreases its detrimental effect on transfused platelet recovery and survival. *Transfus Med*. 1998;8:43-47.

25. Trissel LA. Amphotericin B does not mix with fat emulsion. *Am J Health Syst Pharm*. 1995;52:1463-1464.

26. Boucher HW et al. Newer systemic antifungal agents: pharmacokinetics, safety, and efficacy. *Drugs*. 2004;64:1997-2020.

27. Mohr J et al. Current options in antifungal pharmacotherapy. *Pharmacotherapy*. 2008; 28:614-645.

28. Juang P. Update on new antifungal therapy. *AACN Adv Crit Care*. 2007;18:253-260.

29. Cancidas [package insert]. Whitehouse Station, NJ: Merck and Co., Inc; revised 2008.

30. Hoy JF. Antifungal drugs. In: Kucers A et al., eds. *The Use of Antibiotics*. 5th ed. Oxford, UK: Butterworth-Heinemann; 1997:1245-1505.

31. Powderly WG. Fluconazole. *Infect Med*. 1995;12:257, 281-282.

32. Debruyne D, Ryckelynck J-P. Clinical pharmacokinetics of fluconazole. *Clin Pharmacokinet*. 1993;24:10-27.

33. Perry CM et al. Fluconazole. An update of its antimicrobial activity, pharmacokinetic properties, and therapeutic use in vaginal candidiasis. *Drugs*. 1995;49:984-1006.

34. Como JA, Dismukes WE. Oral azole drugs as systemic antifungal therapy. *N Engl J Med*. 1994;330:263-272.

35. Saag MS et al. Practice guidelines for the management of cryptococcal disease. *Clin Infect Dis*. 2000;30:710-718.

36. Bennett JE et al. A comparison of amphotericin B alone and combined with flucytosine in the treatment of cryptococcal meningitis. *N Engl J Med*. 1979;301:126-131.

37. Allendoerfer R et al. Combined therapy with fluconazole and flucytosine in murine cryptococcal meningitis. *Antimicrob Agents Chemother.* 1991;35:726-729.

38. Terrell CL, Hughes CE. Antifungal agents for deep-seated mycotic infections. *Mayo Clin Proc.* 1992;67:69-91.

39. Lyman CA, Walsh TJ. Systemically administered antifungal agents. A review of their clinical pharmacology and therapeutic applications. *Drugs.* 1992;44:9-35.

40. Haria M et al. Itraconazole. A reappraisal of its pharmacological properties and therapeutic use in the management of superficial fungal infections. *Drugs.* 1996;51:585-620.

41. Tucker RM et al. Interaction of azoles with rifampin, phenytoin, and carbamazepine: in vitro and clinical observations. *Clin Infect Dis.* 1992;14:165-174.

42. Tucker RM et al. Adverse events associated with itraconazole in 189 patients on chronic therapy. *J Antimicrob Chemother.* 1990; 26:561-566.

43. Ducharme MP et al. Itraconazole and hydroxyitraconazole serum concentrations are reduced more than tenfold by phenytoin. *Clin Pharmacol Ther.* 1995;58:617-624.

44. Barriere SL. Pharmacology and pharmacokinetics of traditional antifungal agents. *Pharmacotherapy.* 1990;10(suppl):134S-140S.

45. Chin TW et al. Effects of an acidic beverage (Coca-Cola) on absorption of ketoconazole. *Antimicrob Agents Chemother.* 1995;39:1671-1675.

46. Benet LZ et al. Design and optimization of dosage regimens: pharmacokinetic data. In: Hardman JG et al., eds. *Goodman and Gilman's the Pharmacological Basis of Therapeutics.* 9th ed. New York: McGraw-Hill; 1996:1707-1792.

47. Balfour JA, Faulds D. Terbinafine: a review of its pharmacodynamic and pharmacokinetic properties, and therapeutic potential in superficial mycoses. *Drugs.* 1992;43:259-284.

48. Sabo JA, Abdel-Rahman SM. Voriconazole: a new triazole antifungal. *Ann Pharmacother.* 2000;34:1032-1043.

49. Vfend [package insert]. New York, NY: Pfizer, Inc; revised 2008.

50. Lipp HP. Antifungal agents–clinical pharmacokinetics and drug interactions. *Mycoses.* 2008;51(suppl 1):7-18.

Chapter 8

Antimycobacterial Drugs

Gina C. Biglane and Jessica H. Brady

ETHAMBUTOL
Myambutol

Pharmacology. Ethambutol is a tuberculostatic agent that is only active against mycobacteria, including *Mycobacterium avium* complex (MAC). It does not directly enhance short-course (6–9 months) regimens of isoniazid, rifampin, and pyrazinamide (PZA). Ethambutol is recommended to be included as part of a 4-drug initial regimen if there is a possibility of drug resistance and should be continued for 12 months if isoniazid resistance is demonstrated. Ethambutol is also used in combination with clarithromycin to treat disseminated *Mycobacterium avium intracellulare* (MAI) infection in patients with AIDS.[1-5]

Administration and Adult Dosage. PO for treatment of active tuberculosis — 15–25 mg/kg/d as a single dose given in combination with isoniazid and/or rifampin and/or PZA. **PO for MAC** -15 mg/kg/d, to a maximum of 1 g/d, as a single dose in combination with clarithromycin or azithromycin.

Special Populations. *Pediatric Dosage.* Same as adult dosage, to a maximum of 1 g/d.

Other Conditions. Dosage may require reduction in patients with decreased renal function.[6] In patients with a $Cl_{Cr} \leq 30$ mL/min or receiving hemodialyisis, a dose of 15–25 mg/kg/dose 3 times/wk is recommended.[7]

Dosage Forms. Tab 100, 400 mg.

Pharmacokinetics. Ethambutol is approximately 80% absorbed from the GI tract with complex disposition characteristics. A peak serum concentration of 2–6 mg/L (8–25 μmol/L) 2 h after an oral 15–25 mg/kg dose is proposed as evidence of adequate absorption. Its half-life is 4–6 h, increasing to 32 h in severe renal impairment. Approximately 80% is excreted unchanged in urine, while an additional 8%–15% appears in the form of metabolites.[8]

Adverse Reactions. Rare with the recommended dosage of 15–25 mg/kg/d. Optic neuritis (decreased visual acuity, difficulty with red–green color discrimination, and restricted visual fields) occurs rarely with dosages of 15 mg/kg/d and is usually reversible with prompt drug discontinuation. Return of visual acuity generally occurs weeks to months after discontinuation. Hyperuricemia can occur because of impairment of uric acid excretion as well as hepatotoxicity.[7]

Precautions. Pregnancy category B; considered compatible with breast-feeding. Use with caution in children in whom visual acuity cannot be monitored.[9]

Drug Interactions. Coadministration of ethambutol and aluminum-containing antacids results in reduced ethambutol serum concentrations. Administration should be separated by at least 2–4 h.[6]

Parameters to Monitor. Measure baseline visual acuity and red–green color discrimination, and periodically reassess based on results of symptom assessment. Baseline and periodic liver function tests should also be monitored. Monitor uric acid levels and symptoms of gout flares.[6,9]

ISONIAZID   Various

Pharmacology. Isoniazid (INH) inhibits the synthesis of mycolic acid, a component of the mycobacterial cell wall. Its activity is limited to mycobacteria; it is tuberculostatic or tuberculocidal depending on concentration and reproductive rate of the organism. Resistance is uncommon in preventive therapy but can develop rapidly if used alone in active tuberculosis. Places with high-prevalence of HIV infection (e.g., hospitals and prisons) are having increased primary resistance.[1,2,4,10,11]

Administration and Adult Dosage. **PO for treatment of latent tuberculosis infection**—5 mg/kg/d (usually 300 mg/d) as a single-daily dose, to a maximum of 300 mg/d, given as a single agent for 6–9 months.[12] (*See* Notes, and Treatment of Latent Tuberculosis Infection Comparison Chart.) **PO for treatment of latent tuberculosis infection**—15 mg/kg/dose, to a maximum of 900 mg/dose, twice weekly by directly observed therapy (DOT) for 6–9 months.[12] **PO for treatment of active tuberculosis**—5 mg/kg/d (usually 300 mg/d) combined with rifampin 600 mg/d and PZA 15–30 mg/kg/d for 8 weeks, followed by 16 weeks of INH and rifampin. **PO for treatment of active tuberculosis with directly observed therapy (DOT)**—INH, rifampin, ethambutol, and PZA for 2 weeks, followed by INH 15 mg/kg (to a maximum of 900 mg), rifampin 600 mg, ethambutol 50 mg/kg (to a maximum of 2.5 g), and PZA 50–70 mg/kg (to a maximum of 4 g) in 2 or 3 divided doses twice weekly for a total of 6 weeks by DOT, then continue INH and rifampin twice weekly for 16 weeks by DOT.[3,4] In 3-times-a-week regimens, ethambutol dosage is 25–30 mg/kg/d (to a maximum of 2.5 g), with INH, rifampin, and PZA at the same doses as in the twice-weekly regimen, but continued for 6 months by DOT. If PZA cannot be taken, a 9-month course may be administered in which INH in the above dosage is combined with rifampin 600 mg/d; **IM or IV** (rarely used)—same as oral dosage.

Special Populations. *Pediatric Dosage.* **PO for treatment of latent tuberculosis infection**—10–20 mg/kg/d as a single dose, to a maximum of 300 mg/d, given as a single agent for 6–9 months.[12] Alternatively, give INH 20–40 mg/kg/dose (up to 900 mg) twice weekly by DOT for 6–9 months.[12] **PO for treatment of active tuberculosis**—same dosage as above, but combined with rifampin 10–20 mg/kg (to a maximum of 600 mg), and PZA 15–30 mg/kg/d (to a maximum of 2 g/d) in 2 or 3 divided doses for 8 weeks followed by 16 weeks of INH and rifampin. **PO for treatment of active tuberculosis with DOT**—daily doses of INH, rifampin, ethambutol, and PZA for 2 weeks, followed by INH 20–40 mg/kg (to a maximum of 900 mg), rifampin 10–20 mg/kg (to a maximum of 600 mg), ethambutol 50 mg/kg (to a maximum of 2.5 g), and PZA 50–70 mg/kg (to a maximum of 4 g) in 2 or 3 divided doses twice weekly for a total of 6 weeks by DOT, then continue INH and rifampin twice weekly for 16 weeks by DOT. In 3-times-a-week regimens, PZA dosage is 50–70 mg/kg/d (to a maximum of 3 g/d) in 2–3 divided doses. If PZA cannot be taken, a 9-month course may be administered in which INH in the above dosage is combined with rifampin 10–20 mg/kg (to a maximum of 600 mg).[3,4] **IM or IV** (rarely used)—same as oral dosage.

Geriatric Dosage. Same as adult dosage.

Other Conditions. In slow acetylators with renal impairment, a dosage of 150–200 mg/d is recommended.[13]

Dosage Forms. Tab 50, 100, 300 mg; **Syrup** 10 mg/mL; **Cap** 150 mg with rifampin 300 mg (Rifamate); **Tab** 50 mg with rifampin 120 mg and PZA 300 mg (Rifater); **Inj** 100 mg/mL.

Patient Instructions. Report any burning, tingling, or numbness in the extremities; unusual malaise; fever; dark urine; or yellowing of the skin or eyes. Take on an empty stomach.[8]

Missed Doses. Take at regular intervals. If you miss a dose, take it as soon as you remember. If it is almost time for your next dose, take that dose only and go back to your regular dosage schedule. Leave at least 12 h between doses. Do not double the dose or take extra.

Pharmacokinetics. *Serum Levels.* A peak serum level of 3–5 mg/L (22–36 μmol/L) 2 h after the dose is proposed as evidence of adequate absorption.[1]

Fate. Rapid and nearly complete oral absorption with peak serum concentrations of 1–5 mg/L (7–36 μmol/L) 1 h after a 5 mg/kg dose.[10] Food delays and reduces the absorption of INH. In particular, high-fat meals cause a 51% drop in C_{max}.[1] Widely distributed in body tissues including the CSF of normal patients and those with meningitis. Eliminated primarily by acetylation in the liver to inactive metabolites that are excreted in the urine. Specific pattern of elimination depends on acetylator phenotype of the individual.[13] **Half-life** Rapid acetylators 1.1 ± 0.1 h, slow acetylators 2.1 ± 1.1 h. Increased to 4 h with renal impairment and 6.7 h with liver disease.

Adverse Reactions. Pyridoxine-responsive peripheral neuropathy can occur, especially in alcoholics, diabetics, patients with renal failure, malnourished patients, slow acetylators, and with dosages >5 mg/kg/d.[13] Subclinical hepatitis is frequent (10%–20%) and characterized by usually asymptomatic elevations of AST and ALT, which can return to normal despite continued therapy; it might be more frequent with combined INH–rifampin therapy.[14] Clinical hepatitis is rare in those <20 years, but is strikingly related to age (rising to 2%–3% in 50- to 65-year-old patients). Rare cases of massive liver atrophy resulting in death usually appear in association alcoholism with or preexisting liver disease; most severe cases occur within the first 6 months.[14] With acute overdosage (usually 6–10 g), INH can produce severe CNS toxicity including coma and seizures as well as hypotension, acidosis, and occasionally death.[13]

Contraindications. Acute or chronic liver disease; previous INH-associated hepatitis.

Precautions. Pregnancy; lactation. Use with caution in daily users of alcohol, elderly, and those with a slow acetylator phenotype.

Drug Interactions. INH can inhibit the metabolism of carbamazepine and phenytoin, increasing the risk of toxicity, particularly of phenytoin in slow acetylators.

Mental changes can result from effects of INH and disulfiram on metabolism of adrenergic neurotransmitters; avoid the use of disulfiram in patients who must take INH. Aluminum-containing antacids can interfere with INH absorption. Rifampin can increase the metabolism of INH to hepatotoxic metabolites.

Parameters to Monitor. Monitor for signs of hepatitis (e.g., fever, malaise) and signs of peripheral neuropathy monthly during therapy. Baseline and monthly AST and ALT are recommended only in high-risk groups (>35 years, daily alcohol users, and a history of liver dysfunction).[14]

Notes. To prevent peripheral neuropathy, give **pyridoxine** in a dosage of 50 mg/d to adults receiving large dosages of INH (10 mg/kg/d or more) and those who are predisposed to peripheral neuritis (e.g., diabetic patients, HIV-infected patients, alcoholic patients). Pyridoxine IV in a dosage equal to the estimated amount of INH ingested is recommended for acute INH overdose.[15] Add **ethambutol** or **streptomycin** to the initial treatment regimen until drug susceptibility studies are available.[3,16] (*See* Second-Line Antituberculosis Agents Comparison Chart.)

PYRAZINAMIDE   Various

Pharmacology. PZA is a synthetic pyrazine analogue of nicotinamide that is only active against mycobacteria by unknown mechanism. The drug is most active at low pH and is active against intracellular organisms. Resistance develops rapidly when used alone, but no cross-resistance with isoniazid is observed.[3-5]

Adult Dosage. PO for treatment of latent tuberculosis infection—15–20 mg/kg/d (to a maximum of 2 g/d) in combination with rifampin 10 mg/kg/d (to a maximum of 600 mg/d) as a single-daily dose for 2 months. Alternatively, give PZA 50 mg/kg/dose (to a maximum of 4 g/dose) in combination with rifampin 10 mg/kg/dose (to a maximum of 600 mg/dose) twice weekly for a total of 2–3 months by DOT. (*See* Treatment of Latent Tuberculosis Infection Comparison Chart.) **PO for treatment of active tuberculosis.** (*See* Isoniazid Dosage).

Special Populations. *Pediatric Dosage.* **PO for treatment of active tuberculosis**—15–30 mg/kg/d, to a maximum of 2 g/d, OR 50 mg/kg/d twice weekly, to a maximum of 4 g/d.[7]

Other Conditions. **Renal and Hepatic impairment**—25–35 mg/kg/dose 3 times/wk is recommended in patients with a $Cl_{Cr} \leq 30$ mL/min or those receiving hemodialysis.[7]

Dosage Forms. **Tab** 500 mg; **Tab** 300 mg with isoniazid 50 mg and rifampin 120 mg (Rifater).

Patient Instructions. Notify a health care provider if darkened urine, flu-like symptoms, pain or swelling of the joints, or yellow discoloration of the eyes or skin occurs.[17]

Pharmacokinetics. The drug is well absorbed from the GI tract with serum concentrations of 40–50 mg/L (0.3–0.4 mmol/L) achieved about 2 h after a 1-g dose. A peak serum concentration of 20–60 mg/L (163–488 μmol/L) 2 h after an oral 1–2 g dose is proposed as evidence of adequate absorption. The parent compound and several metabolites are excreted in urine. **Half-life** 9–10 h but may be prolonged in patients with renal or hepatic dysfunction.[8]

Adverse Reactions. Frequent hyperuricemia, GI upset, and occasional dose-dependent hepatotoxicity occur. As many as 1%–5% of patients taking regimens including isoniazid, rifampin, and PZA develop laboratory evidence of hepatic damage. Nongouty polyarthralgia may occur in up to 40% of patients receiving daily doses of PZA.[7]

Contraindications. Persons with severe hepatic damage, those who have shown hypersensitivity to PZA, and those with acute gout.[9]

Precautions. Pregnancy; lactation. Use is not recommended due to lack of teratogenicity data.[9]

Drug Interactions. PZA may increase serum concentrations of cyclosporine.[9]

Parameters to Monitor. Baseline liver function studies and uric acid levels prior to therapy initiation. Repeat based on symptom assessment.[7,9]

RIFABUTIN
Mycobutin

Pharmacology. Rifabutin is derived from rifamycin–S and belongs to a group of antibiotics known as rifamycins.[18] These agents inhibit DNA-dependent RNA polymerase and initiation of transcription. The antimicrobial spectrum of rifabutin includes mycobacteria and many gram positive- and gram-negative organisms.

Administration and Adult Dosage. **PO for prophylaxis of MAI infections in patients with advanced HIV infection for primary prevention**—300 mg/d (as an alternative to macrolide-based regimen). **PO for prophylaxis of MAI infections in patients with advanced HIV infection for secondary prevention**—300 mg/d (added to macrolide/ethambutol regimen). **PO for treatment of disseminated MAI infection in patients with HIV infection**—300 mg/d added to macrolide/ethambutol regimen. **PO for treatment of active tuberculosis**—5 mg/kg as a single-daily dose in as part of a multidrug regimen, to a maximum of 300 mg/d.

Special Populations. *Pediatric dosage.* Safety and efficacy have not been established. Limited use in children has indicated no benefit for doses >5mg/kg.

Other conditions. In patients with Cl_{Cr} <30mL/min, 50% of the dose should be given.

Dosage Forms. Cap 150 mg.

Patient Instructions. May produce an orange–brown discoloration of body fluids, which may stain soft contact lenses, clothing, or skin.

Pharmacokinetics. Bioavailability is low and unpredictable, which may necessitate monitoring of plasma concentrations.[19] Rifabutin is lipophilic and widely distributed in the body.[20] It is 85% plasma protein bound and has an estimated V_d of 9.3 +/− 1.5 L/kg and clearance of 0.69 ± 0.32 L/h/kg.[21] Approximately 53% of the drug is excreted in the urine; 30% in the feces.[21] It induces its own metabolism. **Half-life** 45 h (range 16–69 h).[21]

Adverse Reactions. The most frequent adverse reactions are rash, taste alterations, GI upset, discoloration of body fluids, and uveitis (>300 mg/d).[21] For patients experiencing severe stomach upset, 150 mg twice daily may be administered.[21]

Precautions. Do not use for MAI prophylaxis in patients with active tuberculosis.

Drug Interactions. CYP3A subfamily enzyme inducer and metabolite.

Monitoring parameters. Neutropenia and, more rarely, thrombocytopenia.

Notes. Rifabutin can be substituted for rifampin in antituberculosis regimens.

RIFAMPIN
Rimactane, Rifadin, Various

Pharmacology. Rifampin is a synthetic rifamycin B derivative that inhibits the action of DNA-dependent RNA polymerase. It is highly active against mycobacteria, most gram-positive bacteria, and some gram-negative bacteria, most notably *Neisseria meningitidis*. It is also used to enhance bactericidal activity of other antistaphylococcal agents in refractory or chronic infections.[22] Antagonism with vancomycin is observed in vitro but is probably not clinically relevant. Primary resistance is uncommon, but resistance can develop rapidly if used alone.[20]

Administration and Adult Dosage. **PO or IV for treatment of tuberculosis infection**—10 mg/kg/d as a single-daily dose, to a maximum of 600 mg/d. **PO for prophylaxis of meningococcal meningitis**—600 mg twice daily for 2 days. **PO for staphylococcal infection**—600 mg/d as a single dose in combination with another antistaphylococcal agent.

Special Populations. *Pediatric Dosage.* **PO for treatment of tuberculosis—(>5 years)** 10–20 mg/kg/d as a single-daily dose, to a maximum of 600 mg/d. **PO for prophylaxis of meningococcal meningitis**—(<1 month) 5 mg/kg twice daily for 2 days. **PO for prophylaxis of meningococcal meningitis**—(1 month to 12 years) 10 mg/kg twice daily for 2 days, to a maximum of 600 mg/d.

Geriatric Dosage. Same as adult dosage.

Other Conditions. Accumulation is expected in patients with hepatic dysfunction or biliary obstruction, but dosage guidelines are not available. No dosage adjustment is necessary in patients with impaired renal function.

Dosage Forms. **Cap** 150, 300 mg; **Cap** 300 mg with isoniazid 150 mg (Rifamate); **Tab** 120 mg with isoniazid 50 mg and PZA 300 mg (Rifater); **Inj** 600 mg.

Patient Instructions. Take this medication with a full glass of water on an empty stomach (1 h before or 2 h after meals) for best absorption. It is important to take this medication regularly as directed because inconsistent use might increase its toxicity. This drug can cause harmless red–orange discoloration of bodily secretions, which can cause discoloration of skin, clothes and may permanently discolor soft contact lenses.

Missed Doses. Take this drug at regular intervals. If you miss a dose of this medicine, take it as soon as you remember. If it is almost time for your next dose, take that dose only and go back to your regular dosage schedule. Leave at least 12 h between doses. Do not double the dose or take an extra dose.

Pharmacokinetics. *Serum Levels.* A peak serum level of 8–24 mg/L is the targeted level following a 600-mg dose.[8]

Fate. Following an oral dose, absorption is rapid nearly complete, with a 600-mg dose producing a peak serum concentration of approximately 10 μg/L 1–3 h after administration.[22] Food delays absorption and can cause a decrease in peak serum concentration.[8] First-pass hepatic extraction is substantial but saturated with doses

>300–450 mg; thus, larger doses produce disproportionate increases in serum levels. Widely distributed throughout the body; however, useful amounts appear in the CSF only in the presence of inflamed meninges. Approximately 80% plasma protein bound; V_d is 0.97 ± 0.36 L/kg; clearance is 0.21 ± 0.1 L/h/kg. Eliminated primarily by deacetylation in the liver to a partially active metabolite that is extensively enterohepatically recirculated, producing very high biliary concentrations. Approximately 60%–65% of a dose is eventually excreted in the feces. Urinary excretion is variable and appears to increase with the dose. At usual dosages, up to 30% is excreted unchanged in the urine.[23] **Half-life** 2–3 h on an average, after repeated doses.[24] Half-life increases with higher doses but can become shorter over the first few weeks of treatment. Unchanged by renal impairment but increased unpredictably by liver disease or biliary obstruction.[22]

Adverse Reactions. Liver dysfunction, jaundice, hyperbilirubinemia may occur.[24] GI symptoms are frequent. Intermittent, high-dose administration is associated with more frequent adverse effects such as flulike syndrome, hematopoietic reactions, and hepatic toxicity.[24]

Contraindications. Hypersensitivity to any rifamycin derivative.

Precautions. Pregnancy; lactation. Use with caution in daily users of alcohol, those with preexisting liver disease, and those with a history of drug-associated hepatic damage (especially from antituberculars).

Drug Interactions. Rifampin accelerates the metabolism of many drugs because of potent inducing effects on CYP3A (e.g., oral contraceptives, HIV protease inhibitors, corticosteroids).[25] The dosage of these drugs may need to be increased during concurrent use. Rifampin can increase the metabolism of isoniazid to hepatotoxic metabolites. Patients using systemic hormonal contraceptives should switch to a nonhormonal or additional method of contraception.

Parameters to Monitor. Hepatic enzymes, bilirubin, serum creatinine, CBC, and platelet counts.[24]

Notes. Rifampin is a useful drug for tuberculosis but should be used only in combination regimens because of rapid emergence of resistant mutants of *Mycobacterium tuberculosis* when it is used alone. The recent emergence of multiple drug resistance among strains of *M. tuberculosis* in patients with AIDS includes high-level rifampin resistance. Oral rifampin may be used in conjunction with ciprofloxacin in the treatment of endocarditis due to *Staphylococcus aureus* in patients with a history of IV drug use who are unwilling to undergo parenteral therapy. For patients with endocarditis due to *S. aureus* in the presence of a prosthetic valve, rifampin may be used with either nafcillin, oxacillin, or vancomycin for 6 weeks, along with gentamicin for the first 2 weeks.[23]

RIFAPENTINE   Priftin

Pharmacology. Rifapentine belongs to the group of antibiotics known as rifamycins, similar to rifampin and rifabutin.

Administration and Adult Dosage. **PO for tuberculosis**—(initial phase) 600 mg twice weekly for 2 months with at least 72 h between doses. **PO for tuberculosis**—(continuation phase) 600 mg once weekly for 4 months.

Special Populations. *Pediatric dosage.* Safety in children <12 years is not established.[26] Doses of 600 mg administered to adolescents weighing >45 kg or 450 mg for those weighing <45 kg resulted in kinetics similar to those of healthy adults.[26]

Other Conditions. The disposition of rifapentine in patients with renal or hepatic impairment is not known.[26]

Dosage Forms. **Tab** 150 mg.

Patient instructions. Take with food or milk if stomach discomfort occurs. May produce a reddish-brown discoloration of body fluids, which may stain dentures, soft contact lenses, skin, or clothes.[26]

Pharmacokinetics. Rifapentine is approximately 70% bioavailable. Peak serum levels occur 4–5 h after an oral dose.[27] Food enhances the absorption.[26] Rifapentine is 97% bound to serum albumin. V_d is estimated to be 70.2 ± 9.1 L. The drug is hydrolyzed by an esterase to the active metabolite 25-desacetyl rifapentine.[28] Half-lives of the drug and metabolite are each about 13 h, which allows for less frequent dosing than rifampin.[26] Primarily excreted in the feces.[28]

Adverse Reactions. The most frequent side effects in combination regimens were hyperuricemia, neutropenia, leukopenia, anemia, increased liver enzymes, GI upset, arthralgias, hypertension, headache, and rash.[26]

Contraindications. Hypersensitivity to any rifamycin.

Precautions. Avoid use in patients with porphyria.[26]

Drug Interactions. Rifapentine induces hepatic isoenzymes CYP2C8/9 and 3A4 and can increase the metabolism of drugs metabolized by these pathways.[29] Use with caution in conjunction with protease inhibitors and other drugs metabolized by CYP2C8/9 or 3A4.[26]

Monitoring Parameters. Obtain baseline liver enzymes, bilirubin, CBC, and platelet count before starting therapy.[26] Routine laboratory monitoring during therapy is not necessary unless clinically indicated.[26]

TREATMENT OF LATENT TUBERCULOSIS INFECTION COMPARISON CHART

MEDICATION	DURATION (mo)	DOSAGE INTERVAL	RATING (EVIDENCE)[a]	
			HIV−	*HIV+*
Isoniazid	9	Daily	A (II)	A (II)
		Twice weekly	B (II)	B (II)
Isoniazid	6	Daily	B (I)	C (I)
		Twice weekly	B (II)	C (I)
Rifampin, pyrazinamide	2	Daily	B (II)	A (I)
	2–3	Twice weekly	C (II)	C (I)
Rifampin	4	Daily	B (II)	B (III)

[a]Rating: A, preferred; B, acceptable alternative; C, offer when A and B cannot be given. Evidence: I, randomized clinical trial data; II, data from clinical trials that are not randomized or were conducted in other populations; III, Expert opinion.
From Ref. 30.

SECOND-LINE ANTITUBERCULOSIS AGENTS COMPARISON CHART[a]

DRUG	DOSAGE FORMS	ADULT DOSAGE	PEDIATRIC DOSAGE	SERUM LEVELS[b] (mg/L)	HALF-LIFE		MAJOR ADVERSE EFFECTS
					NORMAL	RENAL IMPAIRMENT	
Aminosalicylic Acid Salts[c] Paser	Granules 4 g	PO 8–12 g/d in 2–3 divided doses (as the acid)	200–300 mg/kg/d in 2–4 divided doses, to a maximum of 10 g/d	20–60[d] (4 g)	1 h	–	GI intolerance; hepatitis; lupus-like syndrome. Rarely used.
Capreomycin Sulfate Capastat	Inj 1 g	Same as streptomycin	Same as streptomycin	Same as streptomycin	2.5 h	↑	Nephrotoxicity; ototoxicity.
Clofazimine Lamprene	Cap 50 mg	PO 100–200 mg/d	Not well established	0.5–2 (100–200 mg)	70 days	–	Brown–black discoloration of skin and bodily secretions; nausea; vomiting; GI pain because of deposition in GI tissues.
Cycloserine Seromycin	Cap 250 mg	PO 10–15 mg/kg/c to a maximum of 1 g in 2 doses, usually 500–750 mg/d in 2 doses	PO 10–15 mg/kg/d to a maximum of 1 g/d	20–35 (250–500 mg)	10 h	↑	CNS (drowsiness, dizziness, headache, depression, rare seizures, and psychosis).
Ethionamide Trecator	Tab 250 mg	PO 15–20 mg/kg/d (usually 500–750 mg/d in a single-daily dose or 2 divided doses) to a maximum of 1 g/d	PO 15–20 mg/kg/d to a maximum of 1 g/d	1–5 (250–500 mg)	3 h	–	GI intolerance; goiter; gynecomastia; alopecia; photodermatitis.

(continued)

119

SECOND-LINE ANTITUBERCULOSIS AGENTS COMPARISON CHART[a] (continued)

DRUG	DOSAGE FORMS	ADULT DOSAGE	PEDIATRIC DOSAGE	SERUM LEVELS[b] (mg/L)	HALF-LIFE		MAJOR ADVERSE EFFECTS
					NORMAL	RENAL IMPAIRMENT	
Kanamycin Sulfate Kantrex	Inj 37.5, 250, 333, 500 mg/mL	Same as streptomycin	Same as streptomycin	Same as streptomycin	2–3 h	80–90 h	Nephrotoxicity; ototoxicity.
Rifabutin Mycobutin	Cap 150 mg	PO 5 mg/kg to a maximum of 300 mg/d as a single dose	Not well established; (1 y) 15–25 mg/kg/d; (2–10 y) 4–19 mg/kg/d; (14–16 y) 2.8–5.4 mg/kg/d	—	45 (range 16–69)	—	See monograph.
Streptomycin Sulfate Various	Inj 400 mg/mL	IM 15 mg/kg/d to a maximum 1 g, and 10 mg/kg/d in persons older than 59 y to a maximum of 750 mg or 25–30 mg/kg to a maximum of 1.5 g 2–3 times/wk	IM 20–40 mg/kg/d to a maximum of 1 g or 20 mg/kg to a maximum of 1.5 g 2 times/wk	35–40 (12–15 mg/kg); 65–80 (22–25 mg/kg)	2–3 h	↑	Potential for nephrotoxicity, vestibular and cochlear ototoxicity

[a]Use only in combination with other effective antituberculars.

[b]Peak serum level 1 h (IV) or 2 h (PO) after the adult dose in parentheses that is evidence of adequate absorption.

[c]Sodium salt contains 73% aminosalicylic acid; increase dosage accordingly. Sodium content is 4.7 mEq/g.

[d]Peak serum level 6 h after a dose of Paser granules.

Adapted from Refs. 1, 3, 10, 13, and 30.

■ REFERENCES

1. Peloquin CA. Pharmacology of the antimycobacterial drugs. *Med Clin North Am.* 1993;77:1253-1262.
2. Brausch LM, Bass JB. The treatment of tuberculosis. *Med Clin North Am.* 1993;77:1277-1290.
3. Bass JB Jr et al. Treatment of tuberculosis and tuberculosis infection in adults and children. *Am J Resp Crit Care Med.* 1994;149:1359-1374.
4. American Thoracic Society. Initial therapy for tuberculosis in the era of multidrug resistance. *MMWR Morab Mortal Wkly Rep.* 1993;42 (RR-7):1-8.
5. Heifets LB. Antimycobacterial drugs. *Semin Respir Infect.* 1994;9:84-103.
6. Myambutol® (ethambutol) [product information]. Marietta, GA: Versa Pharm Incorporated; April 2005.
7. American Thoracic Society, CDC, Infectious Diseases Society of America. Treatment of tuberculosis. *Am J Respir Crit Care Med.* 2003;167:603-662.
8. Peloquin CA. Therapeutic drug monitoring in the treatment of tuberculosis. *Drugs.* 2002;62:2169-2183.
9. Guidelines for the management of adverse drug effects of antimycobacterial agents. Lawrence Flick Memorial Tuberculosis Clinic, Philadelphia Tuberculosis Control Program, November 1998.
10. van Scoy RE, Wilkowske CJ. Antituberculous agents. *Mayo Clin Proc.* 1992;67:179-187.
11. American Thoracic Society. Prevention and treatment of tuberculosis among patients infected with human immunodeficiency virus: principles of therapy and revised recommendations. *MMWR Morab Mortal Wkly Rep.* 2000;47(RR-20):36-42.
12. American Thoracic Society. Targeted tuberculin testing and treatment of latent tuberculosis infection. *MMWR Morab Mortal Wkly Rep.* 2000;49(RR-6):1-53.
13. Pratt WB, Fekety R. Drugs that act on mycobacteria. In: Pratt WB, Fekety R, eds. *The Antimicrobial Drugs.* New York: Oxford University Press; 1986:277-316.
14. Alexander MR et al. Isoniazid-associated hepatitis. *Clin Pharm.* 1982,1:148-153.
15. Holdiness MR. Neurological manifestations and toxicities of the antituberculosis drugs. A review. *Med Toxicol Adv Drug Exp.* 1987;2:33-51.
16. O'Brien RJ. Drug-resistant tuberculosis: etiology, management and prevention. *Semin Respir Infect.* 1994;9:104-112.
17. Pyrazinamide [product information]. Marietta, GA: VersaPharm Incorporated; April 2001.
18. Kunin C. Antimicrobial activity of rifabutin. *Clin Infect Dis.* 1996;22(suppl 1):S3-S14.
19. Skinner MH et al. Pharmacokinetics of rifabutin. *Antimicrob Agents Chemother.* 1989;33:1237-1241.
20. Thornsberry C et al. Rifampin: spectrum of antibacterial activity. *Rev Infect Dis.* 1983;5(suppl 3):S412-S417.
21. Mycobutin (rifabutin) casules [package insert]. New York, NY: Pfizer, 2007.
22. Vesely JJ et al. Rifampin, a useful drug for nonmycobacterial infections. *Pharmacotherapy.* 1998;18:345-357.
23. Baddour LM et al. Infective endocarditis: diagnosis, antimicrobial therapy, and management of complications: a statement for healthcare professionals from the committee on rheumatic fever, endocarditis, and Kawasaki disease, council on cardiovascular disease in the young, and the councils on clinical cardiology, stroke, and cardiovascular surgery and anesthesia, American Heart Association: endorsed by the infectious diseases society of America. *Circulation.* 2005;111:e394-e434.
24. Rifadin (rifampin) capsules and injection [package insert]. Bridgewater, New Jersey: Sanofi-Aventis; 2007.
25. Venkatesan K. Pharmacokinetic drug interactions with rifampicin. *Clin Pharmacokinet.* 1992;22:47-65.
26. Priftin (rifapentine) capsules [package insert]. Bridgewater, New Jersey. Sanofi-Aventis; 2006.
27. Rastogi N et al. Activity of rifapentine and its metabolite 25-O-desacetylrifapentine compared with rifampicin and rifabutin against Mycobacterium tuberculosis, Mycobacterium africanum, Mycobacterium bovis and M. bovis BCG. *J Antimicrob Chemother.* 2000;45:565-570.
28. Reith K et al. Disposition and metabolism of 14C-rifapentine in healthy volunteers. *Drug Metab Dispos.* 1998;26:733-738.
29. Jarvis B, Lamb H. Rifapentine. *Drugs.* 1998;56:607-616.
30. American Thoracic Society, CDC. Targeted tuberculin testing and treatment of latent tuberculosis infection. *Am J Respir Crit Care Med.* 2000;161:S221-S247.

Chapter 9

Antiparasitic Drugs

Kayla R. Stover

ALBENDAZOLE Albenza

Pharmacology. Albendazole is a benzimidazole drug similar to mebendazole that binds to the free β-tubulin, inhibiting polymerization and microtubule-dependent uptake of glucose. The newest agent in this class, albendazole has the broadest range of activity.[1]

Administration and Adult Dosage. **PO for hydatid disease, including echinococcosis**—(≥60 kg) 400 mg twice daily for 28 days, followed by a 14-day free interval. Repeat for a total of 3 cycles. **PO for neurocysticercosis**—(≥60 kg) 400 mg twice daily for 8–30 days, repeat as needed. **PO for** *Clonorchis sinensis*—10 mg/kg/d for 7 days. **PO for cutaneous larva migrans**—400 mg/d for 3 days. **PO for capillariasis**—400 g/d for 10 days. **PO for ascariasis, eosinophilic enterocolitis, hookworm, trichostrongylus, or trichuriasis**—400 mg once. **PO for pinworms**—400 mg once, then repeat in 2 weeks. **PO for microsporidiosis**—400 mg twice daily (ocular infections require the addition of **fumagillin**), typically for 21 days. **PO for trichinosis**—400 mg bid for 8–14 days. **PO for visceral larva migrans (toxocariasis)**—400 mg twice daily for 5 days.[2] (*See* Notes.)

Special Populations. *Pediatric Dosage.* Safety and efficacy not established. **PO for hydatid disease, including echinococcosis**—(<60 kg) 15 mg/kg/d (maximum of 800 mg/d) for 28 days, followed by a 14-day free interval. Repeat for a total of 3 cycles. **PO for neurocysticercosis**—(<60 kg) 15 mg/kg/d (maximum of 800 mg/d) in 2 divided doses for 8–30 days, repeat as needed. **PO for** *Camellia. sinensis*—10 mg/kg/d for 7 days. **PO for cutaneous larva migrans**—400 mg/d for 3 days. **PO for capillariasis**—400 g/d for 10 days. **PO for ancylostomiasis, ascariasis, eosinophilic enterocolitis, hookworm, necatoriasis, trichostrongylus, or trichuriasis**—400 mg once. **PO for eosinophilic enterocolitis**—400 mg once. **PO for pinworms**—400 mg once, then repeat in 2 weeks. **PO for trichinosis**—400 mg twice daily for 8–14 days. **PO for visceral larva migrans (toxocariasis)**—400 mg twice daily for 5 days.[2]

Geriatric Dosage. Same as adult dosage.

Dosage Forms. **Tab** 200 mg.

Missed Doses. Take this drug at regular intervals. If you miss a dose of this medicine, take it as soon as you remember. If it is almost time for your next dose, take that dose only and go back to your regular dosage schedule. Do not double the dose or take an extra dose.

Pharmacokinetics. Absorption is poor but enhanced by fat. Oral bioavailability of unchanged albendazole is negligible because of first-pass metabolism to albendazole sulfoxide, the active form of the drug. The sulfoxide has a peak serum level 2–3 h after a dose. CNS concentrations are 40% of serum levels; concentration in echinococcal cysts is approximately 25% of serum levels. The absorbed drug is excreted primarily in urine as metabolites.[3] **Half-life** (albendazole sulfoxide) 10–15 h.[3]

Adverse Reactions. Abdominal pain, nausea, vomiting, diarrhea, headache, and fever. Rarely, neutropenia, alopecia, Stevens-Johnson syndrome, or increased transaminases occur.[1,2]

Precautions. Pregnancy, lactation; liver dysfunction. May cause granulocytopenias.

Drug Interactions. Concurrent dexamethasone increases serum levels by 50%.[3]

Parameters to Monitor. Monitor hepatic transaminases and WBC count during prolonged therapy.

Patient Instructions. Take this drug with a fatty meal to increase absorption and improve effectiveness. The tablets may be crushed, chewed, or swallowed whole. For pinworms, purgation, enemas, or special dietary restrictions are unnecessary with this drug, which may be taken with food or beverages. To avoid reinfestation with pinworms, wash the perianal area thoroughly each morning. Change and wash nightclothes, undergarments, and bedclothes daily. Wash hands and under fingernails thoroughly after bowel movements and before eating. Treat all family members simultaneously and clean bedroom and bathroom floors thoroughly at the end of the course of treatment. To demonstrate a cure, no eggs must be found in the anal area at least 5 weeks after the end of treatment.

Notes. The only approved indications for albendazole is echinococcosis and neurocysticercosis. Doses and treatment of roundworm, hookworm, pinworm, filariasis, cutaneous larva migrans, toxocariasis, clonorchis, and capillariasis are NOT currently approved.

IVERMECTIN   Stromectol

Pharmacology. Ivermectin is a semisynthetic anthelmintic that binds to glutamate-gated chloride channels in invertebrate nerve and muscle cells, leading to increased cellular permeability, hyperpolarization of nerve cells, paralysis, and death.

Administration and Adult Dosage. PO for strongyloidiasis—200 μg/kg/d for 1–2 days, repeat if still present in 3 months. PO for onchocerciasis—150 μg/kg once, repeat in 3–12 months until asymptomatic. PO for *Mansonella streptocerca*—150 μg/kg once. PO for pediculosis (head or pubic lice) or scabies—200 μg/kg once. PO for cutaneous larva migrans—200 μg/kg/d for 1–2 days.[2] (*See* Notes.)

Special Populations. *Pediatric Dosage.* (<15 kg) Safety and efficacy not established; (>15 kg) same as adult dosage.

Geriatric Dosage. Same as adult dosage.

Dosage Forms. Tab 3 mg.

Pharmacokinetics. Ivermectin is absorbed orally. It does not enter the CNS. Most of the drug is metabolized hepatically, and the drug and metabolites are excreted in the feces. Less than 1% is excreted unchanged in urine. **Half-life** 18 h.

Adverse Reactions. Dizziness and pruritus are most common. In onchocerciasis, inflammation caused by dead and dying larvae can cause more severe and frequent cutaneous reactions, fever, lymph node swelling and tenderness, edema, and arthralgia; ocular effects include limbitis and punctate opacity (commonly referred to as Mazzotti reaction).[4]

Precautions. Pregnancy. May cause cutaneous AND/OR systemic reactions of varying severity (including fatal encephalopathy) and ophthalmologic reactions in patients with onchocerciasis.[4]

Drug Interactions. Ivermectin may cause an increased INR in patients taking warfarin.[4]

Monitoring parameters. Follow stool cultures. Obtain periodic ophthalmologic examinations.

Patient Instructions. Take on an empty stomach with water. Repeated follow-up, and retreatment is often necessary.

Notes. Ivermectin is the drug of choice for strongyloidiasis and onchocerciasis and an alternative for the other infestations listed, as these indications are not currently approved. Ivermectin has no activity against adult *Onchocerca volvulus* parasites in the subcutaneous nodules. This requires surgical nodulectomy to eliminate the microfilariae producing adult parasite.

MEBENDAZOLE Vermox

Pharmacology. Mebendazole is active against intestinal roundworms. It binds to helminth tubulin and inhibits glucose uptake in the parasite, with no effect on blood glucose concentrations in the host.[3]

Administration and Adult Dosage. PO for pinworms—100 mg once, repeat in 3 weeks if needed. **PO for ascariasis or hookworms**—100 mg twice daily for 3 days, repeat in 3 weeks if needed. **PO for capillariasis**—200 mg twice daily for 20 days. **PO for eosinophilic enterocolitis**—100 mg twice daily for 3 days. **PO for roundworms or whipworms**—100 mg twice daily for 3 days, repeat in 3 weeks if needed. **PO for tapeworm**—100 mg twice daily for 6 days. **PO for strongyloidiasis**—200 mg twice daily for 3 days.[2,5] (*See* Notes.)

Special Populations. *Pediatric Dosage.* (<2 years) Safety and efficacy not established. (>2 years) **PO for pinworms, ascariasis, capillariasis, roundworms, whipworms, eosinophilic enterocolitis, tapeworm, or hookworms**—same as adult dosage. **PO for strongyloidiasis**—100 mg twice daily for 3 days.[2,5]

Geriatric Dosage. Same as adult dosage.

Dosage Forms. Chew Tab 100 mg.

Pharmacokinetics. Poorly absorbed orally. Absorption increases when taken with food. Almost all eliminated unchanged in the feces, but up to 10% can be recovered in the urine 48 h after a dose, primarily as the decarboxylated metabolite.[3,5]

Adverse Reactions. Transient abdominal pain and diarrhea in cases of massive infestation and expulsion of worms. With high doses, allergic reactions, alopecia, transient neutropenia, agranulocytosis, and hypospermia may occur.[2,5]

Precautions. Pregnancy. Not recommended for use in children younger than 2 years old.

Drug Interactions. Carbamazepine, phenytoin, and antimalarials can reduce mebendazole serum levels.

Parameters to Monitor. When treating whipworm, take a stool sample for egg count 3 weeks after treatment to detect frequent (approximately 30%) persistent infestation requiring retreatment. When using high doses, monitor complete blood counts and hepatic transaminases.[5]

Patient Instructions. May chew, crush, or swallow tablets whole. For pinworms, purgation, enemas, or special dietary restrictions are unnecessary with this drug, which may be taken with food or beverages. To avoid reinfestation with pinworms, wash the perianal area thoroughly each morning. Change and wash nightclothes, undergarments, and bedclothes daily. Wash hands and under fingernails thoroughly after bowel movements and before eating. Treat all family members simultaneously and clean bedroom and bathroom floors thoroughly at the end of the course of treatment. To demonstrate a cure, no eggs must be found in the anal area at least 5 weeks after the end of treatment.[5]

Notes. Mebendazole is the agent of choice for whipworm, demonstrating approximately 70% cure rate with a single treatment. The cure rate is 90%–100% with roundworms, hookworms, and pinworms. Particularly useful in mixed infestations.[2,3] Doses and treatment of tapeworm and strongyloidiasis are NOT currently approved in pediatrics or adults.

PERMETHRIN	Acticin, Elimite, Nix, Rid, Various

Pharmacology. Permethrin is a pyrethroid that disrupts sodium channel currents in the arthropod nerve cell membranes to cause delayed polarization and paralysis. It is active against lice (including unhatched eggs) and mites (e.g., scabies).

Administration and Adult Dosage. **Topical for head lice**—apply 1% cream rinse to clean, towel-dried hair. Leave on for no longer than 10 min and rinse with water. If live lice are seen after 7 days, reapply as above. **Topical for scabies**—thoroughly massage 5% cream into the skin from the head to the soles of the feet. Remove by showering or bathing after 8–14 h. If live mites are seen after 14 days, reapply as above. (*See* Notes.)

Special Populations. *Pediatric Dosage.* **Topical for lice**—(<2 months) safety and efficacy not established; (>2 months) same as adult dosage. **Topical for scabies**—(>2 months) same as adult dosage. (*See* Notes.)

Geriatric Dosage. Same as adult dosage.

Dosage Forms. **Spray** 0.4% and 0.5%; **Top Lot** 1% (Nix, various); **Top Crm** 5% (Acticin, Elimite).

Pharmacokinetics. <2% absorbed after topical application. Permethrin is rapidly metabolized by ester hydrolysis to inactive metabolites, which are excreted in urine.[6]

Adverse Reactions. Burning, stinging, or tingling with use of 5% cream. Itching, edema, and erythema are often symptoms of scabies and can be exacerbated temporarily by treatment with permethrin. Intolerable burning and stinging can occur in patients with AIDS and scabies.[6] Itching and skin irritation can persist after successful treatment because of local allergic reactions to the dead mites. Allergic reactions are rare and might be caused by the formaldehyde preservative.

Contraindications. Documented allergy to any pyrethroid or vehicle component. Use of topical lotion is contraindicated in infants <2 months.

Precautions. Pregnancy, although animal studies indicate no teratogenicity. During lactation, discontinue nursing temporarily during treatment with 5% cream; use of 1% cream rinse poses little risk during breast-feeding. Avoid contact with eyes and mucous membranes. May worsen pruritus, edema, or erythema.

Drug Interactions. None known.

Parameters to Monitor. Observe for parasites 7–10 days after treatment of lice infestation or 14 days after treatment of scabies.

Patient Instructions. Lice—wash hair and towel dry. Apply enough cream rinse to saturate hair and scalp, especially behind the ears and on the nape of the neck. Use the comb provided with the product to remove nits. Wash all pillowcases, pajamas, and towels in hot, soapy water and dry using the hot cycle of a dryer for at least 20 min. Clothing and bedding that cannot be washed should be sealed in a plastic bag for 2 weeks or dry-cleaned. Soak combs in hot water for 5–10 min. If infestation of the eyebrows or eyelashes occurs, consult your health care provider. Scabies—itching, mild burning, or stinging can occur after application. Itching usually resolves by 4 weeks. If irritation persists, consult your health care provider.

Notes. Permethrin is the drug of choice for pediculosis and scabies. **Malathion** 0.5% lotion (Ovide) is an alternative for pediculosis. **Synergized pyrethrins** (pyrethrins and piperonyl butoxide) have efficacies similar to that of permethrin for head lice but are not as persistent as permethrin and require a repeat treatment after 1 week.[2] In scabies, permethrin is safer and more effective than **lindane** and more effective and easier to use than **crotamiton**.[6,8] Lindane is not recommended because resistance occurs frequently and lindane is a persistent environmental contaminant.[8] Spray formulation is typically used for bedding and furniture. Treatment of pubic lice in adults and scabies in neonates is NOT currently approved.[7–9] In neonates, cream should be applied from head to toe as with adults, but removed after 6 h.[7]

PRAZIQUANTEL	Biltricide

Pharmacology. Praziquantel causes a loss of intracellular calcium, resulting in paralysis and dislodgement of worms from sites of attachment. In higher dosages, it damages the parasite's surface membrane, allowing the host's immune response to destroy the worm.[1]

Administration and Adult Dosage. PO for schistosomiasis—(*Schistosoma haematobium* or *Schistosoma mansoni*) 20 mg/kg 2 times in 1 day, but heavy infestations require 60 mg/kg in 3 divided doses at 4- to 6-h intervals;[1,2] (*Schistosoma japonicum* or *Schistosoma mekongi*) 20 mg/kg 3 times in 1 day. **PO for flukes**—(e.g., clonorchiasis, opisthorchiasis) 25 mg/kg 3 times in 1 day at 4- to 6-h intervals; (paragonimiasis) 25 mg/kg 3 times daily for 2 days.[1,2] **PO for tapeworms**—(beef, dog, fish, pork) 5–10 mg/kg once; (dwarf tapeworm) 25 mg/kg once. **PO for neurocysticercosis**—15–20 mg/kg 3 times daily for 15 days.[1,2] (*See* Notes.)

Special Populations. *Pediatric Dosage.* (<4 years) Safety and efficacy not established. (>4 years) Same as adult dosage.[2]

Geriatric Dosage. Same as adult dosage.

Dosage Forms. **Tab** 600 mg.

Pharmacokinetics. The drug is 80% absorbed orally, but undergoes extensive first-pass metabolism. CSF concentrations are 14%–20% of serum levels. The drug is metabolized and metabolites are excreted primarily in urine. **Half-life** 1.1 ± 0.3 h.

Adverse Reactions. Dizziness, headache, malaise, abdominal discomfort, fever, eosinophilia, and rash. Drowsiness or fatigue might occur because of a structural similarity to benzodiazepines.[2] In patients treated for cysticercosis, an inflammatory response, presumably caused by dead and dying organisms, occurs that is manifested by headache, seizures, and increased intracranial pressure.

Contraindications. Ocular cysticercosis.

Precautions. Liver disease; pregnancy. Avoid breast-feeding for 72 h after the last dose.

Drug Interactions. Drugs that induce CYP3A3/4 (e.g., dexamethasone, carbamazepine, phenobarbital, phenytoin, rifampin) can increase clearance, decrease bioavailability, and cause treatment failure; drugs that inhibit CYP3A3/4 (e.g., cimetidine, erythromycin, ketoconazole) decrease clearance, increase serum levels, and lengthen half-life.[1,3]

Parameters to Monitor. Observe for CNS toxicity when treating cysticercosis.

Patient Instructions. Take with liquid during meals but do not chew tablets. Tablets should be taken at least 4 h apart, but should not be taken more than 6 h apart. This drug can cause dizziness or drowsiness. Use caution when driving, operating machinery, or performing other tasks requiring mental alertness.

Notes. Doses and treatment of tapeworms and neurocysticercosis are NOT currently approved. Concomitant corticosteroid therapy is recommended for patients treated for neurocysticercosis.

PYRANTEL PAMOATE
Ascarel, Pin-X, Various

Pharmacology. Pyrantel is a depolarizing neuromuscular blocker that produces spastic paralysis of the parasite with no similar effects on the host after oral use. It also inhibits acetylcholinesterases.[3]

Administration and Adult Dosage. **PO for pinworms and roundworms**—11 mg/kg once, maximum dose 1 g; (for pinworms) repeat in 2 weeks. **PO for moniliformis**—11 mg/kg once at 2-week intervals for 3 doses. **PO for hookworms and eosinophilic enterocolitis**—11 mg/kg/d for 3 days, maximum 1 g/d.[2] Doses are expressed as base equivalent. (*See* Notes.)

Special Populations. *Pediatric Dosages.* (<2 years) Safety and efficacy not established. (≥2 years) Same as adult dosage.[2]

Geriatric Dosage. Same as adult dosage.

Dosage Forms. **Tab** 180 mg (62.5 mg as pyrantel base); **Chew Tab** 720.5 mg (250 mg pyrantel base); **Susp** 144 mg/mL (50 mg/mL as pamoate base).

Pharmacokinetics. Slight oral absorption. More than 50% is excreted unchanged in feces, and less than 15% of the dose is excreted as parent drug and metabolites in the urine.[3]

Adverse Reactions. Occasional nausea, vomiting, headaches, dizziness, rash, and transient AST elevations.[2]

Precautions. Avoid during pregnancy. Use caution in patients with liver disease, anemia, or malnutrition.

Drug Interactions. Piperazine and pyrantel might be mutually antagonistic in ascariasis.

Patient Instructions. For pinworms, purgation, enemas, or special dietary restrictions are unnecessary with this drug, which may be taken with food or beverages. To avoid reinfestation with pinworms, wash the perianal area thoroughly each morning. Change and wash nightclothes, undergarments, and bedclothes daily. Wash hands and under fingernails thoroughly after bowel movements and before eating. Treat all family members simultaneously and clean bedroom and bathroom floors thoroughly at the end of the course of treatment. To demonstrate a cure, no eggs must be found in the anal area at least 5 weeks after the end of treatment. Shake suspension well. May mix with water, juice, or milk.

Notes. Except for pinworms and moniliformis, pyrantel is an alternative to other drugs.[2] Doses are given as the base, but dosage formulations are reported as the salt (1 mg of pyrantel base = 2.88 mg of pyrantel pamoate salt).

THIABENDAZOLE	Mintezol

Pharmacology. Thiabendazole is a benzimidazole drug that inhibits helminth-specific mitochondrial fumarate reductase.[10]

Administration and Adult Dosage. PO for ascariasis, strongyloidiasis, unicinaria, and trichuriasis—10 mg/lb (in 250-mg increments) twice daily for 2 days, maximum 3 g/d OR 50 mg/kg as a single dose. **PO for cutaneous larva migrans**—10 mg/lb (in 250-mg increments) twice daily for 2 days, maximum 3 g/d. **PO for visceral larva migrans**—10 mg/lb (in 250-mg increments) twice daily for 7 days, maximum 3 g/d. **PO for trichinosis**—10 mg/lb (in 250-mg increments) twice daily for 2–4 days, maximum 3 g/d.[10]

Special Populations. *Pediatric Dosages.* (<30 lb) Safety and efficacy not established. (≥30 lb) Same as adult dosage.[10]

Geriatric Dosage. Same as adult dosage.

Dosage Forms. Chew Tab 500 mg.

Pharmacokinetics. Rapidly absorbed, with peak plasma concentrations 1–2 h following oral administration. Approximately 90% is excreted unchanged in the urine, and 5% is excreted unchanged in feces.[10]

Adverse Reactions. Fatigue, dizziness, nausea, anorexia, headache, and rash, including Stevens-Johnson syndrome. Abnormal eye sensations, xanthopsia, and blurred vision have been described. Jaundice, cholestasis, and liver dysfunction occur in up to 34%. Rarely, liver damage leads to irreversible hepatic failure.[10,11]

Precautions. Lactation. Use caution in patients with renal or hepatic impairment. Discontinue use immediately with signs of hypersensitivity reactions such as Stevens-Johnson syndrome. Should not be used in patients with mixed infections with ascaris.[10]

Drug Interactions. Thiabendazole may increase the levels of theophylline.[10]

Parameters to Monitor. Hepatic transaminases and renal function.

Patient Instructions. Purgation or enemas are unnecessary with this drug, but drinking fruit juice aids in the expulsion of worms. To avoid reinfestation, change and wash nightclothes, undergarments, and bedclothes daily. Wash hands and under fingernails thoroughly after bowel movements and before eating. Treat all family members simultaneously and clean bedroom and bathroom floors thoroughly at the end of the course of treatment. Use caution while driving or operating machinery, as this drug may cause dizziness, fainting, or changes in vision. Report any itching or skin rash.

Notes. Thiabendazole should be used as an alternative to other agents due to the high incidence of adverse effects, particularly with single dose regimens. It is inappropriate as first-line therapy for pinworms, and should NOT be used for hookworm, trichuriasis, or ascariasis unless other therapy is unavailable or contraindicated. Thiabendazole tablets may be crushed and suspended in a vehicle for topical application for cutaneous larva migrans, but no comparative data are available for this unapproved dosage form.[12]

■ REFERENCES

1. Liu LX, Weller PF. Antiparasitic drugs. *N Engl J Med.* 1996;334:1178-1184.
2. Anon. Drugs for parasitic infections. *Med Lett Drugs Ther.* 2000 March:1-12. http://www.medicalletter.com/freedocs/parasitic.pdf
3. Jernigan JA, Pearson RD. Antiparasitic drugs. In: Mandell GL et al., eds. *Principles and Practice of Infectious Diseases.* 4th ed. New York: Churchill Livingstone; 1995:458-492.
4. Stromectol [package insert]. Whitehouse Station, NJ: Merck & Co., Inc; revised 2007.
5. ADCO-WORMEX [package insert]. Bryanston, South Africa: Adcock Ingram Limited; 2000.
6. Meinking TL, Taplin D. Safety of permethrin vs lindane for the treatment of scabies. *Arch Dermatol.* 1996;132:959-962.
7. Quarterman MJ, Lesher LJ Jr. Neonatal scabies treated with permethrin 5% cream. *Pediatr Dermatol.* 1994;11:264-266.
8. Brown S et al. Treatment of ectoparasitic infections: review of the English-language literature, 1982-9. *Clin Infect Dis.* 1995;20(suppl 1):S104-S109.
9. Kalter DC et al. Treatment of pediculosis pubis. *Arch Dermatol.* 1987;123:1315-1319.
10. Mintezol [package insert]. Whitehouse Station, NJ: Merck & Co., Inc; revised 2003.
11. Zaha O et al. Strongyloidiasis—progress in diagnosis and treatment. *Intern Med.* 2000;39:695-700.
12. Caumes E. Treatment of cutaneous larva migrans. *Clin Infect Dis.* 2000;30:811-814.

Chapter 10

Antiviral Drugs

David J. Caldwell

Class Instructions: Human Immunodeficiency Virus (HIV) Medications. Under-dosage, noncompliance, or partial compliance with dosing regimens for these medications may result in development of resistant strain(s) of HIV that will not be susceptible to treatment. Do not stop taking this medication unless told to do so by your health care provider. This drug should be used in combination with other anti-HIV medications. Currently available anti-HIV medications do not cure or prevent HIV infection. It is possible for a person taking this medication to transmit the virus to another. Opportunistic infections and other complications associated with HIV infection can continue to develop while you take this medication. Protease inhibitors and nonnucleoside reverse transcriptase inhibitors (NNRTI) have a potential for serious interactions with a large number of commonly prescribed medications. Always check with your health care provider before starting any new medication.

Missed Doses. Missing doses can result in the development of resistance that can lead to treatment failure. If you forget a dose, take it as soon as you remember. If it is almost time for your next scheduled dose (within 4 h), skip the missed dose. Do not double your dose.

ACYCLOVIR	Zovirax, Various
VALACYCLOVIR	Valtrex

Pharmacology. Acyclovir is an acyclic nucleoside analogue of deoxyguanosine that is selectively phosphorylated by the virus-encoded thymidine kinase to its monophosphate form. Cellular enzymes then convert the monophosphate to the active antiviral acyclovir triphosphate, which inhibits viral DNA synthesis by incorporation into viral DNA, resulting in chain termination. Acyclovir has potent activity against herpes simplex virus (HSV) I and II and herpes zoster virus (varicella-zoster virus [VZV]). Activity against cytomegalovirus, which lacks a specific virus-encoded thymidine kinase, is limited, but resistance can be overcome with high serum concentrations in some patient populations. Acyclovir inhibits Epstein-Barr virus but has not been found clinically useful. Human herpes virus 6 is resistant.[1-3] Valacyclovir is the L-valyl ester of acyclovir, which undergoes extensive first-pass hydrolysis to yield high serum acyclovir concentrations.[4]

Administration and Adult Dosage. **IV for severe localized HSV infection—** (acyclovir) 5 mg/kg every 8 h for 5 days for nonimmunocompromised patients OR 7–10 days for immunocompromised patients. **IV for VZV (chickenpox) infection in immunocompromised patients—**10 mg/kg every 8 h for 7–10 days. **IV for HSV encephalitis—**10 mg/kg every 8 h for 10–14 days. Dilute to 50–250 mL and infuse over at least 60 min; avoid bolus IV, SQ, or IM injections. Maintain minimum urine output of 500 mL/24 h for each gram of acyclovir administered. **PO for primary or recurrent genital HSV infection**—(acyclovir) 200 mg 5 times/d for 10 days; (valacyclovir, immunocompetent patients) 500 mg twice daily for 5 days. **PO for prevention of recurrent genital HSV infection**—(acyclovir) 400 mg twice daily or 200 mg 3–5 times/d; (valacyclovir in immunocompetent patients) 1 g/d or 500 mg twice daily. **PO for active VZV (chickenpox) or herpes zoster**—(acyclovir) 800 mg every 4 h 5 times/d for 5 days (chickenpox) OR 7–10 days (zoster). **PO for herpes zoster in immunocompetent patients**—(valacyclovir) 1 g every 8 h for 7 days. **Topical for initial genital HSV infection and limited non–life-threatening mucocutaneous HSV infections in immunocompromised patients**—(acyclovir) 0.5-in. ribbon to cover 4-square-inch affected skin area every 3 h 6 times/d for 7 days.

Special Populations. *Pediatric Dosage.* (All dosages apply to acyclovir.) **IV for HSV infection**—(neonates) 10 mg/kg every 8 h for 10–14 days;[2] (13 months to 11 years) 750 mg/m^2/d in 3 divided doses for 7 days. **IV for VZV (chickenpox) in immunocompromised children**—(13 months to 11 years) 1500 mg/m^2/d in 3 divided doses. **IV for HSV encephalitis**—(6 months to 11 years) 1500 mg/m^2/d in 3 divided doses for 10 days. Infuse over at least 60 min; avoid bolus IV, SQ, or IM injections. **PO for VZV (chickenpox)**—(acyclovir) (>2 years and <40 kg) 20 mg/kg/dose, to a maximum of 800 mg every 6 h for 5 days; (>40 kg) same as adult dosage; (valacyclovir) safety and efficacy not established.

Geriatric Dosage. Same as adult dosage, adjusted for renal function.

Other Conditions. (Acyclovir) in obesity, base dosage on IBW. In renal insufficiency, reduce parenteral and oral dosage: (Cl$_{Cr}$ 25–50 mL/min) usual dose every 12 h; (Cl$_{Cr}$ 10–25 mL/min) usual dose every 24 h; (Cl$_{Cr}$ 0–10 mL/min) 50% of the usual dose every 24 h. For patients on hemodialysis, give the usual daily dosage after dialysis. (Valacyclovir) in renal insufficiency, reduce the dosage: (Cl$_{Cr}$ 30–49 mL/min) 1 g every 12 h; (Cl$_{Cr}$ 10–29 mL/min) 1 g every 24 h; (Cl$_{Cr}$ <10 mL/min) 500 mg every 24 h.

Dosage Forms. (Acyclovir) **Cap** 200 mg; **Tab** 400, 800 mg; **Inj** 500 mg, 1 g; **Inj** 50 mg/mL; **Oint** 5%; **Susp** 40 mg/mL. (Valacyclovir) **Tab** 500 mg.

Patient Instructions. Use a finger cot or latex glove when applying acyclovir ointment. The ointment might cause transient burning or stinging.

Missed Doses. Take this (oral) medication at regular intervals. If you miss a dose of this medicine, take it as soon as you remember. If it is almost time for your next dose, take that dose only and go back to your regular dosing schedule. Leave at least 4 h between doses. Do not double the dose or take an extra dose.

Pharmacokinetics. *Fate.* Oral bioavailability of acyclovir is estimated to be 15%–30%; valacyclovir is well absorbed, with a bioavailability of 54%.[5] Valacyclovir is extensively converted to acyclovir after oral administration. After 200–600 mg of acyclovir orally, mean peak steady-state levels are 0.56–1.3 mg/L (2.5–5.9 μmol/L); levels after IV doses of 2.5–15 mg/kg are 5–24 mg/L (23–105 μmol/L). After an oral dose of 1 g of valacyclovir, mean peak steady-state acyclovir level is 5–6 mg/L (22–27 μmol/L).[6] CSF acyclovir concentrations are 25%–70% of simultaneous serum level. Decay is biphasic, with $V_{d\beta}$ of 0.69 ± 0.19 L/kg;

clearance is 0.21 ± 0.03 L/h/kg with normal renal function;[5] 86%–92% is excreted unchanged in urine; the remainder is metabolized to 9-carboxymethoxymethylguanine. Renal clearance is 75%–80% of total clearance and is markedly reduced by concomitant probenecid.[7] **Half-life** (acyclovir) 2.9 ± 0.8 h in adult patients, increasing to nearly 20 h in end-stage renal disease; 5.7 h on dialysis; approximately 4 h in neonates;[7] (valacyclovir) 2.5–3.3 h.

Adverse Reactions. (Acyclovir) nephrotoxicity, thought to be caused by precipitation of acyclovir crystals in the nephron, occurs in about 10% of patients if the drug is given by bolus (<10 min) injection. Phlebitis at injection site occurs frequently with IV infusion because of the high pH (9–11) of the product. Other reported side effects are CNS toxicity (e.g., headache, lethargy, tremulousness, delirium, seizures), nausea, vomiting, and skin rash. CNS toxicity occurs primarily in patients with underlying neurologic disease or end-stage renal disease, or with cancer chemotherapy and irradiation to the CNS, and might not be primarily caused by the drug. Topical application to herpes lesions can be painful.[1,2] (Valacyclovir) adverse reactions appear comparable to acyclovir. Nausea, vomiting, diarrhea, abdominal pain, and headache have been reported frequently with valacyclovir use. Thrombotic thrombocytopenic purpura/hemolytic-uremic syndrome has been reported in patients with advanced HIV disease and in bone marrow and renal transplant patients. This phenomenon has not been reported in immunocompetent patients.[6]

Contraindications. (Valacyclovir) allergy to the drug or to acyclovir.

Precautions. Use caution in renal impairment, dehydration, or preexisting neurologic disorders. Valacyclovir not indicated in immunocompromised patients.

Drug Interactions. Zidovudine and acyclovir can result in drowsiness and lethargy. Probenecid can increase oral bioavailability and half-life of acyclovir.

Parameters to Monitor. Monitor renal function and injection site for signs of phlebitis daily. Carefully monitor patients with underlying neurologic diseases for evidence of neurotoxicity. (*See* Adverse Reactions.)

Notes. Acyclovir-resistant strains of virus that are deficient in thymidine kinase have been isolated from patients after treatment. Although thought to be less virulent than sensitive strains, HSV strains resistant to acyclovir have been described in AIDS patients.[2]

CIDOFOVIR Vistide

Pharmacology. Cidofovir is a nucleotide analogue with potent in vitro and in vivo activities against cytomegalovirus (CMV) and other herpes viruses. Cidofovir contains a phosphonate group that enables it to bypass initial virus-dependent phosphorylation. Cellular enzymes convert cidofovir to cidofovir diphosphate, the active intracellular metabolite.[8–10]

Administration and Adult Dosage. IV induction for CMV retinitis—5 mg/kg infused over 1 h once weekly for 2 weeks, then **IV maintenance**—5 mg/kg once every other week. Reduce dosage to 3 mg/kg if serum creatinine increases by 0.3–0.4 mg/dL above baseline or if >2+ proteinuria occurs. It is essential to give the following with cidofovir: 2 g **probenecid PO**—3 h before administration and 1 L of NS IV over 1 h just before administration. If tolerated, give another liter of

NS with or after cidofovir administration; finally, give PO 1 g probenecid 2 h and 8 h after the end of cidofovir infusion. Cidofovir is also being investigated as an intravitreal injection for CMV retinitis.

Dosage Forms. **Inj** 75 mg/mL.

Pharmacokinetics. Peak serum cidofovir concentration averages 26.1 ± 3.2 mg/L (83 ± 10 μmol/L) after a 5 mg/kg IV infusion with concomitant probenecid and hydration. Cidofovir is not appreciably bound to plasma proteins; V_d averages 0.5 L/kg. Cidofovir is excreted almost entirely unchanged in the urine. The elimination half-life of cidofovir is 3–6 h when administered with probenecid. **Half-life** (intracellular) 17–65 h, which allows infrequent administration schedules of once weekly to once every other week.

Adverse Reactions. Nephrotoxicity is the most frequent adverse reaction, and high-dose probenecid (*see* Administration and Adult Dosage) must be used with administration of cidofovir. Probenecid decreases uptake of cidofovir in proximal renal tubular cells, decreasing the risk of nephrotoxicity. Other frequent adverse reactions are proteinuria, elevated serum creatinine, nausea, vomiting, fever, asthenia, neutropenia, rash, headache, diarrhea, alopecia, anemia, and abdominal pain. Ocular hypotony and decreased intraocular pressure have been reported occasionally. Nausea, vomiting, fever, rash, and chills are frequent reactions reported with probenecid.

ENFUVIRTIDE Fuzeon

Pharmacology. Enfuvirtide is a peptide inhibitor of gp41, a viral surface glycoprotein involved in the mechanism of HIV's entry into the host cell. By inhibiting the interaction between gp41 and host CD4, fusion of cellular membranes and, consequently, viral entry is prevented.[11]

Administration and Adult Dosage. SQ for treatment-experienced HIV—90 mg (1 mL) SQ twice daily.

Special Populations. *Pediatric Dosage.* SQ for treatment-experienced HIV— (<6 years) safety and efficacy not established; (6–16 years) reported as mg/dose (injection volume) to be given SQ twice daily; 11–15.5 kg: 27 mg (0.3 mL); 15.6–20 kg: 36 mg (0.4 mL); 20.1–24.5 kg: 45 mg (0.5 mL); 24.6–29 kg: 54 mg (0.6 mL); 29.1–33.5 kg: 63 mg (0.7 mL); 33.6–38 kg: 72 mg (0.8 mL); 38.1–42.5 kg: 81 mg (0.9 mL); ≥ 42.6 kg: 90 mg (1 mL).

Special Instructions. Injection should be given subcutaneously twice daily into the upper arm, anterior thigh, or abdomen. Injection sites should be rotated, and the solution should not be injected into moles, scar tissue, bruises, or the navel. After adding 1.1 mL of sterile water for injection to the vial, gently tap and roll the vial for 10 s to ensure all of the powder comes into contact with the liquid. The vial should then be allowed to rest as the powder goes into solution, a process that may take as long as 45 min. The product contains no preservatives and should therefore not be reconstituted >24 h before use. Decrease the risk and severity of injection site reactions, massage the injection site for 5–10 min before and after administration.

Dosage Forms. **Inj** (lyophilized) 108 mg (approximately 90 mg/mL when reconstituted).

Patient Instructions. Never use more than one dose from the same vial. After each dose, discard the remaining contents and vial. To save time, both vials for the two daily doses may be mixed at the same time. The unused vial may be stored in the refrigerator for up to 24 h before it must be discarded. Do not inject enfuvirtide into the same area as was used for the previous dose.

Missed Doses. Take this drug at regular intervals. If you miss a dose, take it as soon as you remember. Do not double the dose or take an extra dose.

Pharmacokinetics. Enfuvirtide is slowly but nearly completely absorbed following subcutaneous administration, resulting in relatively consistent plasma concentrations. Bioavailability is 84.3% and the half-life of the drug is 3.8 h, which supports the twice daily dosing. The volume of distribution, systemic clearance, and plasma protein binding level are 5.48 L, 1.4 L/h, and 92%, respectively. Enfuvirtide is primarily eliminated by catabolism to its amino acid residues.[12]

Adverse Reactions. More than 98% of patients who received enfuvirtide in clinical trials experience an injection site reaction. These reactions range from erythema (87.1%) and mild tenderness (49.7%) to induration (84.0%) and nodule and cyst formation (81.6%). No injection site reactions required hospitalization and <3% discontinued therapy due to these reactions. Infection, particularly bacterial pneumonia occurred more frequently in trials in the enfuvirtide group than placebo. Other reactions most frequently reported were diarrhea, nausea, and fatigue; these events occurred no more frequently than in the control arms.[13]

Contraindications. Hypersensitivity to enfuvirtide or any of its components.

Precautions. Injection site reactions are common and required nontopical analgesics or limiting of usual activity in 9% of patients in clinical trials. Carefully monitor for signs and symptoms of pneumonia and attempt to eliminate modifiable risk factors for pneumonia such as smoking and IV drug use.

Drug Interactions. None reported.

Parameters to Monitor. Patients receiving enfuvirtide should be periodically screened for signs and symptoms of injection site reactions and bacterial pneumonia, in addition to monitoring for appropriate virologic and immunologic response to the drug.

FAMCICLOVIR	Famvir
PENCICLOVIR	Denavir

Pharmacology. Famciclovir is the diacetyl, 6-deoxy ester of the antiviral guanosine analogue penciclovir. Famciclovir is absorbed rapidly and converted to penciclovir in the intestinal wall and liver. Viral thymidine kinase converts penciclovir to its monophosphate form. Cellular enzymes then convert the monophosphate to the active antiviral penciclovir triphosphate. The triphosphate inhibits viral DNA synthesis by incorporation into viral DNA, resulting in termination of the chain. Penciclovir has potent activity against HSV I and II and herpes zoster virus (VZV). Penciclovir also has some activity against Epstein-Barr virus and CMV but has not demonstrated clinical usefulness against infections with these agents.[14-16]

Administration and Adult Dosage. **PO for herpes zoster**—(famciclovir) 500 mg every 8 h for 7 days. **PO for recurrent genital HSV infection**—(famciclovir)

1000 mg twice daily for 1 day. **Topical for herpes labialis**—(penciclovir) apply to lesions every 2 h while awake for 4 days, starting as early as possible at the beginning of an outbreak.

Special Populations. *Pediatric Dosage.* Safety and efficacy not established.

Other Conditions. **Renal Impairment.** (Famciclovir) reduce the dosage for herpes zoster as follows: Cl_{Cr} 40–59 mL/min, 500 mg every 12 h; Cl_{Cr} 20–39 mL/min, 500 mg every 24 h; Cl_{Cr} <20 mL/min, 250 mg every 24 h; hemodialysis, 250 mg after each dialysis; reduce the dosage for genital HSV infection as follows: Cl_{Cr} 20–39 mL/min, 500 mg as a single dose; Cl_{Cr} <20 mL/min, 250 mg as a single dose; with hemodialysis, 250 mg as a single dose following dialysis.

Dosage Forms. **Crm** (penciclovir) 1%; **Tab** (famciclovir) 125, 250, 500 mg.

Pharmacokinetics. Topical penciclovir is virtually unabsorbed. The absolute bioavailability of penciclovir is 77% after a 500-mg oral dose of famciclovir. Peak serum concentrations are 0.84 ± 0.22 (3.3 ± 0.9 µmol/L) and 3.34 ± 0.58 mg/L (13 ± 2.3 µmol/L) 45 min after 125 and 500 mg oral doses of famciclovir, respectively. Penciclovir is <20% protein bound, and the V_d is approximately 1 L/kg. Penciclovir is eliminated primarily by renal excretion. The elimination half-life is approximately 2 h with normal renal function, increasing to over 13 h in patients with severely impaired renal function.

Adverse Reactions. Nausea, vomiting, diarrhea, and headache occur frequently with famciclovir. Pruritus, paresthesias, and fatigue occur occasionally. Penciclovir causes mild erythema occasionally.

Drug Interactions. Cimetidine might enhance the bioavailability of famciclovir and its conversion to penciclovir.

FOSCARNET SODIUM Foscavir

Pharmacology. Foscarnet sodium (phosphonoformic acid [PFA]) is a pyrophosphate analogue. Foscarnet actively inhibits viral DNA polymerases in its parent form and does not require phosphorylation for optimal antiviral activity. It has antiviral activity against HSV I and II, human CMV, Epstein-Barr virus, hepatitis B virus, VZV, and some retroviruses including HIV. Foscarnet sodium inhibits DNA synthesis in CMV and other herpes viruses by inhibiting viral DNA polymerase.[17]

Administration and Adult Dosage. **IV induction for CMV retinitis in AIDS patients**—60 mg/kg every 8 h OR 90 mg/kg every 12 h for 14–21 days.[18] **IV maintenance for CMV retinitis in AIDS patients**—90–120 mg/kg/d in 1 dose. **IV for acyclovir-resistant herpes virus infection**—40 mg/kg every 8 h OR 60 mg/kg every 12 h until clinical resolution.[18] **IV for acyclovir-resistant herpes simplex infection**—40 mg/kg every 8–2 h for 14–21 days or until clinical resolution.[19]

Special Populations. *Pediatric Dosage.* Safety and efficacy not established.

Geriatric Dosage. Same as adult dosage, but adjusted for renal function.

Other Conditions. **Renal Impairment.** (HSV induction equivalent to 40 mg/kg every 12 h) Cl_{Cr} >1.4 mL/min/kg, 40 mg every 12 h; Cl_{Cr} 1–1.4 mL/min/kg, 30 mg every 12 h; Cl_{Cr} 0.8–1 mL/min/kg, 20 mg every 12 h; Cl_{Cr} 0.6–0.8 mL/min/kg, 35 mg every 24 h; Cl_{Cr} >0.5–0.6 mL/min/kg, 25 mg every 24 h; Cl_{Cr} 0.4–0.5 mL/min/kg, 20 mg every 24 h; Cl_{Cr} 0.4 mL/min/kg, NOT recommended. (HSV induction equivalent to 40 mg/kg every 8 h) $Cl_{Cr} > 1.4$ mL/min/kg, 40 mg every 8 h; Cl_{Cr} 1–1.4 mL/min/kg, 30 mg every 8 h; Cl_{Cr} 0.8–1 mL/min/kg, 35 mg every 12 h; Cl_{Cr} 0.6–0.8 mL/min/kg, 25 mg every 12 h; Cl_{Cr} 0.5–0.6 mL/min/kg, 40 mg every 24 h; Cl_{Cr} 0.4–0.5 mL/min/kg, 35 mg every 24 h; $Cl_{Cr} < 0.4$ mL/min/kg, NOT recommended. (CMV induction equivalent to 60 mg/kg every 8 h) $Cl_{Cr} > 1.4$ mL/min/kg, 60 mg every 8 h; Cl_{Cr} 1–1.4 mL/min/kg, 45 mg every 8 h; Cl_{Cr} 0.8–1 mL/min/kg, 50 mg every 12 h; Cl_{Cr} 0.6–0.8 mL/min/kg, 40 mg every 12 h; Cl_{Cr} 0.5–0.6 mL/min/kg, 60 mg every 24 h; Cl_{Cr} 0.4–0.5 mL/min/kg, 50 mg every 24 h; $Cl_{Cr} < 0.4$ mL/min/kg, NOT recommended. (CMV induction equivalent to 90 mg/kg every 12 h) $Cl_{Cr} > 1.4$ mL/min/kg, 90 mg every 12 h; Cl_{Cr} 1–1.4 mL/min/kg, 70 mg every 12 h; Cl_{Cr} 0.8–1 mL/min/kg, 50 mg every 12 h; Cl_{Cr} 0.6–0.8 mL/min/kg, 80 mg every 24 h; Cl_{Cr} 0.5–0.6 mL/min/kg, 60 mg every 24 h; Cl_{Cr} 0.4–0.5 mL/min/kg, 50 mg every 24 h; $Cl_{Cr} < 0.4$ mL/min/kg, NOT recommended. (CMV maintenance equivalent to 90 mg/kg once daily) $Cl_{Cr} > 1.4$ mL/min/kg, 90 mg every 24 h; Cl_{Cr} 1–1.4 mL/min/kg, 70 mg every 24 h; Cl_{Cr} 0.8–1 mL/min/kg, 50 mg every 24 h; Cl_{Cr} 0.6–0.8 mL/min/kg, 80 mg every 48 h; Cl_{Cr} 0.5–0.6 mL/min/kg, 60 mg every 48 h; Cl_{Cr} 0.4–0.5 mL/min/kg, 50 mg every 48 h; $Cl_{Cr} < 0.4$ mL/min/kg, NOT recommended. (CMV maintenance equivalent to 120 mg/kg once daily) $Cl_{Cr} > 1.4$ mL/min/kg, 120 mg every 24 h; Cl_{Cr} 1–1.4 mL/min/kg, 90 mg every 24 h; Cl_{Cr} 0.8–1 mL/min/kg, 65 mg every 24 h; Cl_{Cr} 0.6–0.8 mL/min/kg, 105 mg every 48 h; Cl_{Cr} 0.5–0.6 mL/min/kg, 80 mg every 48 h; Cl_{Cr} 0.4–0.5 mL/min/kg, 65 mg every 48 h; $Cl_{Cr} < 0.4$ mL/min/kg, NOT recommended.

Dosage Forms. **Inj** 24 mg/mL.

Patient Instructions. Foscarnet is not a cure for CMV retinitis and progression of disease might continue during or after treatment. Regular eye examinations are important to monitor for disease progression. Report symptoms of tingling around the mouth or numbness in extremities, which might indicate a need for temporary discontinuation of foscarnet.

Missed Doses. Take this drug at regular intervals. If you miss a dose of this medicine, take it as soon as you remember. If it is almost time for your next dose, take that dose only and go back to your regular dosage schedule. Leave at least 12 h between doses. Do not double the dose or take an extra dose.

Pharmacokinetics. *Fate.* After twice-daily infusion of 90 mg/kg over 2 h, peak serum levels are 98 ± 27 mg/L (577 ± 161 μmol/L) and troughs are 6.4 ± 8.3 mg/L (38 ± 49 μmol/L).[18] Plasma protein binding is 14%–17%. CSF concentrations are 35%–103% of simultaneous serum levels. V_{dss} is 0.3–0.7 L/kg; clearance is 0.13 ± 0.05 L/h/kg. Foscarnet is not metabolized and is 70%–90% excreted unchanged in the urine.[18] **Half-life** α phase 1.4 ± 0.6 h, β phase 6.8 ± 5 h in patients receiving continuous or intermittent infusions. A terminal half-life of 36–196 h may represent release of the drug from binding sites in bone.[18]

Adverse Reactions. Abnormal renal function, including decreased Cl_{Cr} and acute renal failure, occurs in about one-third of patients. Electrolyte abnormalities such as hypocalcemia, hypophosphatemia, hyperphosphatemia, hypokalemia, and hypomagnesemia occur in 6%–16% of patients. Seizures have been reported in 10% of patients and might be related to electrolyte abnormalities or underlying disease. Other adverse reactions frequently reported are fever (65%), nausea (47%),

anemia (33%), diarrhea (30%), vomiting (26%), headache (26%), and granulocytopenia (14%). Local irritation, inflammation, and pain might occur at the injection
site with peripheral administration at a frequency of 1%–5%.[17-19]

Precautions. Use with extreme caution in patients with renal impairment of
nephrotoxic drugs, preexisting cytopenias, preexisting electrolyte abnormalities, or
underlying neurologic disorders.

Drug Interactions. Concurrent use of nephrotoxic drugs such as aminoglycosides
or radiologic contrast media can increase risk and severity of nephrotoxicity. IV
pentamidine can increase the risk of hypocalcemia; avoid this combination, if possible, although inhaled pentamidine does not seem to be a risk factor.[20]

Parameters to Monitor. Monitor serum creatinine 2 or 3 times/wk during induction therapy and weekly during maintenance therapy. Monitor serum calcium,
magnesium, potassium, and phosphorus at the same frequency as serum creatinine.
Symptoms of perioral tingling, numbness in extremities, or other paresthesias
might indicate electrolyte abnormalities and require more frequent monitoring and
a need to obtain ionized calcium levels.

GANCICLOVIR	Cytovene, Vitrasert
VALGANCICLOVIR	Valcyte

Pharmacology. Ganciclovir (DHPG) is a synthetic acyclic nucleoside analogue of
guanine. Antiviral activity is a result of its conversion to the triphosphate form,
which functions as an inhibitor of and faulty substrate for viral DNA polymerase.
Ganciclovir has antiviral activity against HSV I and II, human CMV, Epstein-Barr
virus, and VZV.[21] Valganciclovir is the valine ester prodrug that is hydrolyzed to
ganciclovir after oral administration.

Administration and Adult Dosage. Take all oral doses with food. **IV for CMV
retinitis (induction)**—5 mg/kg every 12 h for 14–21 days, then (**maintenance**)
5 mg/kg once daily for 7 d/wk OR 6 mg/kg once daily for 5 d/wk. **PO for CMV
retinitis (induction)**—(valganciclovir) 900 mg every 12 h for 21 days, then
(**maintenance**) 900 mg once daily. Induction may be repeated for patients who
experience disease progression. Oral ganciclovir should never be used for induction. **IV for prevention of CMV disease in transplant recipients**—5 mg/kg
every 12 h for 7–14 days, followed by 5 mg/kg once daily for 7 d/wk OR 6 mg/kg
once daily for 5 d/wk. Duration depends on duration and degree of immunosuppression. Dilute IV dose in 100 mL NS or D5W and infuse over 60 min. **PO for
CMV retinitis (maintenance after IV induction)**—(ganciclovir) 1 g every 8 h
OR (valganciclovir) 900 mg once daily. **PO for prophylaxis of CMV disease**—
(ganciclovir) 1 g every 8 h indefinitely; (valganciclovir) 900 mg once daily.

Special Populations. *Pediatric Dosage.* Same as the adult dosage in mg/kg.

Geriatric Dosage. Same as adult dosage, but adjusted for renal function.

Other Conditions. In renal insufficiency (ganciclovir). *Parenteral induction:* (Cl_{Cr}
50–69 mL/min) 2.5 mg/kg every 12 h; (Cl_{Cr} 25–49 mL/min) 2.5 mg/kg every 24 h;
(Cl_{Cr} <25 mL/min) 1.25 mg/kg every 24 h; (hemodialysis) 1.25 mg/kg 3 times/wk.
On hemodialysis days, give dose after hemodialysis. *Parenteral maintenance:*

(Cl$_{Cr}$ 50–69 mL/min) 2.5 mg/kg every 24 h; (Cl$_{Cr}$ 25–49 mL/min) 1.25 mg/kg every 24 h; (Cl$_{Cr}$ 10–24 mL/min) 0.625 mg/kg every 24 h; (hemodialysis) 0.625 mg/kg 3 times/wk after hemodialysis. *Oral maintenance:* (Cl$_{Cr}$ 50–69 mL/min) 1.5 g once daily or 500 mg tid; (Cl$_{Cr}$ 25–49 mL/min) 1 g/d in 1 or 2 doses; (Cl$_{Cr}$ 10–24 mL/min) 500 mg/d; (Cl$_{Cr}$ <10 mL/min) 500 mg 3 times/wk after hemodialysis. (Valganciclovir) *Oral induction:* (Cl$_{Cr}$ 40–59 mL/min) 450 mg every 12 h; (Cl$_{Cr}$ 25–39 mL/min) 450 mg/d; (Cl$_{Cr}$ 10–24 mL/min) 450 mg every 48 h; (hemodialysis) use ganciclovir. *Maintenance:* (Cl$_{Cr}$ 40–59 mL/min) 450 mg/d; (Cl$_{Cr}$ 25–39 mL/min) 450 mg every 48 h; (Cl$_{Cr}$ 10–24 mL/min) 450 mg twice weekly.

Dosage Forms. (Ganciclovir) **Cap** 250, 500 mg; **Inj** 500 mg; **Ocular Implant** 4.5 mg (nominal release). (Valganciclovir) **Tab** 450 mg.

Patient Instructions. This drug is not a cure for CMV retinitis and progression might continue during or after treatment. Concurrent use with zidovudine can result in severe reduction in white blood cell count; therefore, report any signs or symptoms of infection, such as fever, chills, or sweats. Take oral ganciclovir or valganciclovir with food.

Missed Doses. Take this drug at regular intervals. If you miss a dose of this medicine, take it as soon as you remember. If it is almost time for your next dose, take that dose only and go back to your regular dosage schedule. Leave at least 4 h between doses. Do not double the dose or take an extra dose.

Pharmacokinetics. Fate. Ganciclovir is absorbed poorly from the GI tract; oral bioavailability is 6% when taken with food (approximately 20% greater than when taken on an empty stomach). Average peak serum concentration of 0.34 ± 0.13 mg/L (1.3 ± 0.5 μmol/L) occurs 1–2 h after a single 1-g oral dose. Valganciclovir bioavailability is 61%. Mean peak and trough steady-state levels after IV doses of 5 mg/kg every 12 h in patients with normal renal function are 5.3 ± 2.8 mg/L (21 ± 11 μmol/L) and 1.1 ± 0.4 mg/L (4.3 ± 1.5 μmol/L), respectively. Ganciclovir is 1%–2% plasma protein bound; CSF concentration is 24%–67% of simultaneous serum level. V_c is 0.26 ± 0.08 L/kg; V_{dB} is 1.17 ± 0.54 L/kg; clearance is 0.25 ± 0.13 L/h/kg with normal renal function. The drug is 90%–99% excreted unchanged in the urine. Hemodialysis reduces serum levels by 53% ± 12%. Renal excretion occurs principally via glomerular filtration, although limited renal tubular secretion also can occur.[21,22] **Half-life** α phase 0.76 ± 0.67 h; β phase 3.6 ± 1.4 h in adult patients, increasing to 11.5 ± 3.9 h in renal insufficiency.[21,22]

Adverse Reactions. Granulocytopenia (ANC <1000/μL) occurs in 13%–67% of patients and is the most frequent dose-limiting adverse effect.[21] Thrombocytopenia (platelets <50,000/μL) occurs in 20% of patients. CNS toxicity (e.g., headache, lethargy, dizziness, confusion, seizure, coma) has been reported at a frequency of 5%–17%. Phlebitis, inflammation, and pain at the site of IV infusion occur frequently because of the high pH of the solution. Anemia, fever, rash, and abnormal liver function tests occur in about 2% of patients.[21,23]

Contraindications. Hypersensitivity to acyclovir or ganciclovir.

Precautions. Use with caution in renal impairment, preexisting cytopenias, or concurrent myelosuppressive drug therapy.

Drug Interactions. Didanosine AUC can be increased when given within 2 h of ganciclovir. Probenecid decreases the renal excretion of ganciclovir. Use extreme caution in combination with zidovudine because of additive myelosuppression. Concurrent nephrotoxic drugs can increase the nephrotoxicity of ganciclovir. Concurrent cytotoxic drugs increase the toxicity of ganciclovir. Seizures have been reported with concurrent use of ganciclovir and imipenem-cilastatin.

Parameters to Monitor. Monitor CBC and platelet counts twice weekly during induction treatment and at least weekly during maintenance. Monitor renal function at least every 2 weeks. Check injection site for phlebitis and infection daily.

Notes. Ganciclovir-resistant CMV strains have been isolated from patients during treatment.[24] Disease progression caused by these strains has been observed and might require changing therapy to an alternative antiviral (e.g., foscarnet).

MARAVIROC	Selzentry

Pharmacology. Maraviroc expresses antiviral activity by antagonizing CCR5 on CD4 cells.[25] HIV is unable to enter human CD4 cells without binding to two different receptors. The viral envelope glycoprotein, gp-120, binds to the CD4 receptor. Subsequently, a second glycoprotein, gp-41, binds to either CCR5 or CXCR4, depending upon mutations in the viral genome. If CCR5 is occupied by maraviroc, R5-tropic viruses are unable to gain entry into the host cell. Without being able to enter the cell, further replication is inhibited.

Administration and Adult Dosage. **PO for treatment-experienced R5-tropic HIV with a CYP3A4 inhibitor with or without a CYP3A4 inducer**—150 mg twice daily. **PO for treatment-experienced R5-tropic HIV–infected without a CYP3A4 inhibitor or inducer**—300 mg twice daily. **PO for treatment-experienced R5-tropic HIV–infected with a CYP3A4 inducer AND a strong CYP3A4 inhibitor**—600 mg twice daily.

Special Populations. *Pediatric Dosage.* Safety and efficacy not established.

Special Instructions. Because CYP3A4 is the major enzyme responsible for the metabolism of maraviroc, the presence of concomitant medications with inducing or inhibiting effects on that enzyme guide dosage selection. Strong CYP3A4 inhibitors such as protease inhibitors (except tipranavir/ritonavir), delavirdine, ketoconazole, itraconazole, clarithromycin, nefazodone, telithromycin, and others reduce the metabolism of maraviroc, requiring the lower dose, 150 mg twice daily. Other concomitant medications such as tipranavir/ritonavir, nevirapine, all nucleoside reverse transcriptase inhibitors (NRTIs), and enfuvirtide have little effect on CYP3A4, and maybe be given with maraviroc 300 mg twice daily. Strong CYP3A4 inducers such as carbemazepine, phenobarbital, phenytoin, efavirenz, and rifampin increase the metabolism of maraviroc and require the higher dose, 600 mg twice daily. If both an inhibitor and an inducer of CYP3A4 are administered with maraviroc, the inhibitor is considered to have the greater effect, and maraviroc 150 mg twice daily should be administered.

Dosage Forms. **Tab** 150 and 300 mg.

Patient instructions. This drug may be taken with or without food. Immediately report any signs or symptoms of allergic reaction to your physician.

Missed Doses. Take this drug at regular intervals. If you miss a dose, take it as soon as you remember. Do not double the dose or take an extra dose.

Pharmacokinetic. *Fate.* Maraviroc is absorbed with a T_{max} between 0.5 and 4 h in healthy individuals.[26] The T_{max} did not change with length of treatment. The half-life of maraviroc is between 9 and 14 h with some increase after repeated doses. Steady state occurs after approximately seven days of therapy using doses greater than 100 mg daily. The area under the curve (AUC) increases from day one to day twelve demonstrating some accumulation of the medication over the time period. Eighty percent of the dose is absorbed with a first-pass extraction rate of approximately 60%. The bioavailability of maraviroc is estimated to be 30% at the 300 mg dose and 23% with a 100-mg dose.[27] The mean volume of distribution is 194 L. Maraviroc is extensively metabolized through CYP3A4 and is a substrate of P-glycoprotein.[28] Oxidation and N-dealkylation reactions comprise the majority of the metabolism. A large number of other medications are processed through these systems, thus drug–drug interactions are expected.

Adverse Reactions. The majority of data regarding the safety of maraviroc have been derived from the MOTIVATE studies. The pooled 48-week results of MOTIVATE-1 and MOTIVATE-2 revealed comparable adverse effects across all arms, specifically diarrhea, nausea, headache, and fatigue at rates of greater than 10%. Rates of upper respiratory tract infection and cough were higher in the maraviroc arms than the placebo arm; however, the difference did not reach statistical significance.[29,30] Hepatotoxicity has been reported in both health volunteers and in phase III trials.[29–31] Orthostatic hypotension has been reported at higher doses, and may be more frequent when maraviroc is not adjusted appropriately to account for the boosting effect of strong CYP3A4 inhibitors.[31]

Contraindications. None reported.

Precautions. Because maraviroc blocks a receptor in the human immune system, immune function may be affected. In clinical trials, patients taking maraviroc experienced higher rates of upper respiratory tract and herpes virus infections versus patients not receiving maraviroc.[29,30] As with other antiretroviral agents, when initiating therapy with maraviroc, there is a possibility of the development of an immune-mediated inflammatory reaction to underlying opportunistic infections. The events may require timely diagnosis, evaluation, and treatment. Use with caution in hepatic and renal impairment.

Drug Interactions. *See* Special Instructions.

Parameters to Monitor. Patients receiving maraviroc should be periodically monitored for increases in liver function tests, orthostatic hypotension, and signs and symptoms of infection.

NONNUCLEOSIDE REVERSE TRANSCRIPTASE INHIBITORS	
DELAVIRDINE	Rescriptor
EFAVIRENZ	Sustiva, Atripla (with tenofovir DF and emtricitabine)
ETRAVIRINE	Intelence
NEVIRAPINE	Viramune

Pharmacology. NNRTIs block the action of viral reverse transcriptase in a noncompetitive fashion by binding to a location adjacent to the catalytic site. This induces a change in the stereochemistry of the protein that essentially inactivates the enzyme. Reverse transcriptase is responsible for the transcription of viral RNA to viral DNA, an essential step in the viral life cycle that must be completed before the viral is able to use the host cell machinery to manufacture additional viral copies.[32]

Administration and Adult Dosage. (*See* NNRTI Comparison Chart.) NNRTIs should generally be administered as part of a combination–drug therapy regimen including two NRTIs to form a regimen of at least three fully active agents. Etravirine is the exception to this, as it has been proven inferior to other therapies in combination with two NRTIs at achieving viral suppression in treatment-experienced patients.[33] Etravirine should be administered with at least two of the following agents: darunavir/ritonavir, saquinavir/ritonavir, lopinavir/ritonavir, enfuvirtide, maraviroc, and raltegravir.[34]

Special Populations. *See* NNRTI Comparison Chart.

Other Conditions. None of the NNRTIs require dosage adjustment in renal dysfunction; little data exists on the use of etravirine in renal dysfunction, though significant effects are unlikely.[34–38] Atripla, however, is a coformulated product containing two NRTIs that must be adjusted for renal impairment. Little data is available regarding the use of NNRTIs in patients with hepatic dysfunction. Use with caution.[34,37] Nevirapine specifically should be avoided in patients with mild to moderate hepatic impairment as this agent can be hepatotoxic.[37] Efavirenz is pregnancy category D and should be avoided in pregnancy.[36]

Dosage Forms. *See* NNRTI Comparison Chart.

Patient Instructions. *See* NNRTI Comparison Chart.

Pharmacokinetics. *See* NNRTI Comparison Chart.

Adverse Reactions. Adverse reactions associated with delavirdine are generally mild and include rash, increased aminotransferases, and headache.[35] Efavirenz has been associated with CNS symptoms such as sleep disturbance characterized by vivid or bizarre dreams, morning grogginess, and less frequently hallucinations, amnesia, euphoria, depression, suicidical ideation paranoia, and aggressive behavior.[39,40] Additional adverse reactions may include rash (rarely Stevens-Johnson syndrome), fat redistribution, lipid abnormalities, and hepatotoxicity.[36] The most common side effect associated with etravirine is mild, self-limiting rash, which clears after 1–2 weeks of continued dosing.[34] Nevirapine has been implicated in drug-related hepatotoxicity that seems to be related to patients' baseline CD4 count: counts >250 cells/mm^3 and >400 cells/mm^3 in women and men, respectively, increase the risk.[41]

Contraindications. Hypersensitivity to any of the agents or their components is a contraindication to that agent. Coadministration of any agents that are highly dependent on CYP450 metabolism (such as astemizole, bepredil, midazolam, pimozide, triazolam, or ergot derivatives) are contraindications to the use of delavirdine and efavirenz. See each products' package insert for complete lists of specific contraindicated agents.[35,36]

Precautions. *See* Adverse Reactions and NNRTI Comparison Chart.

Drug Interactions. Delavirdine is primarily a CYP3A4 inhibitor; therefore, the plasma levels of drugs relying primarily upon this isozyme for metabolism may be greatly increased. Delavirdine also requires an acidic environment for absorption, so coadministration with H2-antagonists or proton pump inhibitors may decrease plasma levels of this drug.[35] Efavirenz is a mixed inducer/inhibitor of CYP3A4 and an inhibitor of CYP2C9 and 2C19. Etravirine is an inducer of CYP3A4 and an inhibitor of CYP2C9 and 2C19. Nevirapine is an inducer and substrate of CYP3A4 and 2B6. (See NNRTI Drug Interactions Table and NNRTI Drug-Specific Interactions.)

Parameters to Monitor. Patients receiving any of the NNRTIs should be periodically screened for signs and symptoms, agent-specific adverse effects, lipodystrophy, and hyperlipidemia, in addition to monitoring for appropriate virologic and immunologic response to the drug.

Notes. Efavirenz may cause a false-positive urine test for cannabinoid use.[42]

NUCLEOS(T)IDE REVERSE TRANSCRIPTASE INHIBITORS	
ABACAVIR	Ziagen, Epzicom (with lamivudine), Trizivir (with lamivudine and zidovudine)
DIDANOSINE	Videx EC
EMTRICITABINE	Emtriva, Atripla (with tenofovir DF and efavirenz, Truvada (with tenofovir DF)
LAMIVUDINE	Epivir, Epzicom (with abacavir), Combivir (with zidovudine), Trizivir (with abacavir and zidovudine)
STAVUDINE	Zerit
TENOFOVIR DISOPROXIL FUMARATE	Viread, Atripla (with emtricintabine and efavirenz), Truvada (with emtricitabine)
ZIDOVUDINE	Retrovir, Combivir (with lamivudine)

Pharmacology. NRTIs block the action of viral reverse transcriptase by competing with endogenous nucleosides for incorporation into the growing proviral DNA chain. These agents require phosphorylation by various host enzymes to become active. Because of their lack of a 3′-hydroxyl group, incorporation into the proviral DNA chain results in termination of strand elongation.[43]

Administration and Adult Dosage. (See NRTI Comparison Chart.) The use of two NRTIs are typically recommended to provide the "backbone" of antiretroviral therapy in treatment-naïve patients. They should never be used as the only class of antiretroviral therapy, but rather should be used in combination with at least one agent from another class, such as the NNRTIs, protease inhibitors, entry inhibitors, or integrase inhibitors.[38]

Special Populations. See NRTI Comparison Chart.

Other Conditions. **Renal Impairment.** (See NRTI Comparison Chart.) Abacavir is the only NRTI that should be adjusted in hepatic impairment; in mild hepatic impairment the plasma concentration–time curve and elimination half-life were increased by 89% and 58%, respectively.[44,45] There is currently no data concerning the use of abacavir in higher degrees of hepatic impairment, and its use in such situations should therefore be avoided.

Dosage Forms. *See* NRTI Comparison Chart.

Patient Instructions. *See* NRTI Comparison Chart.

Pharmacokinetics. *See* NRTI Comparison Chart.

Adverse Reactions. (*See* NRTI Comparison Chart.) As a class, the NRTIs have affinity for mitochondrial DNA polymerase-gamma, the sole enzyme responsible for the replication of mitochondrial DNA. By inhibiting this enzyme, various levels of cellular activity are dysregulated that may lead to the adverse effects of myopathy, lipoatrophy, hepatic steatosis, hyperlactatemia/lactic acidosis, bone marrow suppression, neuropathy, and possibly pancreatitis.[46] Each agent has a different affinity for mitochondrial DNA polymerase-gamma, reflecting the propensity of certain agents to cause more adverse effects than other; didanosine > stavudine > zidovudine > lamivudine = tenofovir = abacavir.[47]

Contraindications. Hypersensitivity. Additionally, a positive HLA-B*5701 contraindicates the use of abacavir. (*See* NRTI Comparison Chart.)

Precautions. *See* Adverse Reactions and NRTI Comparison Chart.

Drug Interactions. None of the NRTIs are substrates or inducers/inhibitors of the CYP450 system, so no drug interactions exist by that mechanism. (*See* NRTI Drug Interactions Table.)

Parameters to Monitor. In addition to monitoring for appropriate virologic and immunologic response to the medication, patients receiving any of the NRTIs should be periodically screened for signs and symptoms agent-specific and class-specific adverse effects. (*See* Adverse Reactions and NRTI Comparison Chart.)

Notes. For additional information on lamivudine. (*See* Hepatitis Antiviral Drugs.)

PROTEASE INHIBITORS (HIV PROTEASE)	
ATAZANAVIR	Reyataz
DARUNAVIR	Prezista
FOSAMPRENAVIR	Lexiva
INDINAVIR	Crixivan
LOPINAVIR/RITONAVIR	Kaletra
NELFINAVIR	Viracept
RITONAVIR	Norvir
SAQUINAVIR	Invirase
TIPRANAVIR	Aptivus

Pharmacology. HIV-1 protease inhibitors prevent cleavage of viral protein precursors in acutely and chronically infected cells, preventing the formation of new mature, infectious virions.[48] Protease inhibitors are key components of several "preferred" antiretroviral regimens, as mentioned by the DHHS and IAS-USA treatment guidelines.[38,49] Similar to other antiretroviral agents, suboptimal adherence to protease inhibitors results in the development of viral resistance to individual agents and potentially cross-resistance to other agents in the class.[48,50]

Adult Dosage. *See* Protease Inhibitor Comparison Chart.

Dosage Forms. *See* Protease Inhibitor Comparison Chart.

Pharmacokinetics. *See* Protease Inhibitor Comparison Chart.

Adverse Reactions. *See* Protease Inhibitor Comparison Chart.

Drug Interactions. Drug–drug interactions are almost exclusively based on the cytochrome P450 characteristics of a specific PI. (*See* Protease Inhibitor Comparison Chart and PI Drug Interactions Table and PI Drug-Specific Interactions.)

RALTEGRAVIR   Isentress

Pharmacology. Raltegravir is an HIV-1 integrase inhibitor. Integrase is a viral enzyme that catalyzes the transfer of virally encoded DNA into the host chromosome. By inhibiting this step of viral replication, the virus is unable to use the host cell as a site for manufacturing additional viral particles.[51,52]

Administration and Adult Dosage. **PO for treatment of HIV-1 infection in adults and adolescents in treatment-naive, treatment-experienced or multi-agent resistant patients with evidence of multiagent resistance**—400 mg twice daily.

Special Populations. *Pediatric Dosage.* (<16 years) Safety and efficacy not established.

Geriatric Dosage. Dosage should be the same as that for healthy adults and adolescents, with consideration given to the greater likelihood of this population having reduced renal or hepatic function and higher numbers of concomitant medications.

Other Conditions. No dosage modifications are necessary for renal dysfunction or mild to moderate hepatic dysfunction. The effects of severe hepatic dysfunction on the pharmacokinetics of raltegravir have not been studied.

Special Instructions. This agent should be used in combination with two or more antiretroviral agents with documented susceptibility by genotypic or phenotypic testing. Monotherapy with raltegravir is not an appropriate therapeutic application.

Dosage Forms. **Tab** 400 mg.

Patient Instructions. This drug may be taken with or without food. Report any new-onset muscle pain or weakness to your physician immediately.

Missed Doses. Take this drug at regular intervals. If you miss a dose, take it as soon as you remember. Do not double the dose or take an extra dose.

Pharmacokinetics. *Fate.* Raltegravir is rapidly absorbed with a T_{max} in the fasting state ranging from 0.5 to 1.3 h. The absolute bioavailability of raltegravir has not been established. Raltegravir exhibits considerable inter- and intrapatient pharmacokinetic variability. Raltegravir is approximately 83% bound to plasma proteins. This agent is metabolized by uridinylglucuronosyltransferase (UGT) 1A1. The CYP450 enzyme system has no measureable effect on the metabolism of raltegravir.[53,54] **Half-life** α phase 1 h; β phase 7–12 h.

Adverse Reactions. The most common adverse effects in clinical trials were headache, diarrhea, nausea, and pyrexia. Creatine kinase elevations have been observed in patients receiving raltegravir. Patients at increased risk for myopathy or rhabdomyolysis should be cautioned about the potential of these effects.[55]

Contraindications. None reported.

Precautions. As with other antiretroviral agents, when initiating therapy with raltegravir, there is a possibility of the development of an immune-mediated inflammatory reaction to underlying opportunistic infections. The events may require timely diagnosis, evaluation, and treatment.

Drug Interactions. Because raltegravir is metabolized outside of the CYP450 system, it is free from many of the interactions associated with the other classes of antiretrovirals. However, several medications affect UGT1A1. Tipranavir and atazanavir induce and inhibit UGT1A1, respectively. At this time, however, there is no recommended dosage adjustment for raltegravir when coadministered with these agents. Rifampin is also a strong inducer of UGT1A1; when these two agents are given together, the dose of raltegravir should be increased to 800 mg twice daily.[56]

OSELTAMIVIR PHOSPHATE   Tamiflu

Pharmacology. Oseltamivir phosphate is the ethyl ester prodrug of oseltamivir carboxylate, which is a selective inhibitor of the enzyme neuraminidase.[57–59] (*See* Zanamivir.)

Administration and Adult Dosage. **PO for treatment of influenza virus A or B (start within 48 h of onset of symptoms)**—75 mg twice daily for 5 days; **PO for prophylaxis of influenza virus A or B (start within 48 h after exposure)**—75 mg daily for 10 days.

Special Populations. *Pediatric Dosage.* (<1 year) Safety and efficacy not established. (*See* Notes.) (<13 years) **PO for treatment of influenza virus A or B**—(≤33 lb) 30 mg twice daily for 5 days; (33–51 lb) 45 mg twice daily for 5 days; (51–88 lb) 60 mg twice daily for 5 days; (>88 lb) 75 mg twice daily for 5 days. **PO for prophylaxis of influenza virus A or B**—(≤33 lb) 30 mg daily for 10 days; (33–51 lb) 45 mg daily for 10 days; (51–88 lb) 60 mg daily for 10 days; (>88 lb) 75 mg daily for 10 days.

Geriatric Dosage. Same as adult dosage.

Other Conditions. **Renal Impairment.** (Cl_{Cr} 10–30 mL/min) reduce dose to 75 mg/d for 5 days. There is no dosage information for Cl_{Cr} <10 mL/min.

Dosage Forms. **Cap** 30, 45, 75 mg. **Pwdr for Susp** 12 mg/mL.

Patient Instructions. Begin treatment with oseltamivir within 2 days of initial flu symptoms. Oseltamivir is not a substitute for influenza vaccination.

Missed Doses. Take this drug at regular intervals. If you miss a dose of this medicine, take it as soon as you remember. If it is almost time for your next dose (within 2 h), take that dose only and go back to your regular dosage schedule. Leave at least 12 h between doses. Do not double the dose or take an extra dose.

Pharmacokinetics. *Fate.* Oseltamivir phosphate is extensively absorbed after oral ingestion and converted by hepatic esterases to the active oseltamivir carboxylate. Food does not affect overall systemic exposure to the oseltamivir carboxylate. Oral bioavailability of oseltamivir carboxylate is >75% after a 75-mg dose. The peak serum concentration is 348 ± 63 μg/L within 2–3 h after a 75-mg dose. Protein binding of oseltamivir carboxylate is approximately 3%. V_d is estimated to be 0.35 ± 0.02 L/kg. Oseltamivir is eliminated (>99%) by renal excretion.[57,58] **Half-life** 7.5 ± 0.7 h.[58]

Adverse Reactions. Nausea and vomiting are the most frequent adverse events, occurring in about 10% of patients. Bronchitis, insomnia, and vertigo occur occasionally.[58,60]

Drug Interactions. Oseltamivir is neither a substrate for nor does it affect cytochrome P450 isoenzymes. Coadministration of probenecid results in a 2-fold exposure to oseltamivir carboxylate; however, no dosage adjustments are recommended.[61]

Parameters to Monitor. Progression of influenza symptoms.

Notes. There are no data to support the safety or efficacy in patients who begin oseltamivir after 48 h of influenza symptom onset. Patients should continue to receive an annual influenza vaccination according to guidelines on immunization practices. Oseltamivir is also used for the treatment and prophylaxis of Avian influenza and Novel influenza A (H1N1) at similar dosage recommendations above. Oseltamivir can be given to children <1 year old for treatment and prophylaxis of Novel influenza A (H1N1) at reduced dosages.

ZANAMIVIR   Relenza

Pharmacology. Zanamivir is an inhibitor of the enzyme neuraminidase (sialidase), which is essential for the replication of type A and B influenza viruses. Neuraminidase catalyzes the viral cleavage of terminal sialic acid (N-acetylneuraminic acid), which allows release of budded virus from infected cells, such that virions do not aggregate at the cell surface or with each other, allowing viral spread to occur within the host.[57,60,62]

Administration and Adult Dosage. **Inhalation for treatment of influenza virus A or B (start within 48 h of onset of symptoms)**—10 mg (2 inhalations) twice daily for 5 days. **Inhalation for prophylaxis of influenza virus A or B (start within 48 h of onset of symptoms)**—10 mg (2 inhalations) daily for 10 days. Give the first dose under the supervision of an informed health care professional to observe correct use of the inhalation device.

Special Populations. *Pediatric Dosage.* (5–7 years) Prophylaxis: same as adult dosage. Treatment: safety and efficacy not established; (≥7 years) same as adult dosage.

Geriatric Dosage. Same as adult dosage.

Dosage Forms. **Dry Pwdr Inhal** 5 mg.

Patient Instructions. Read and follow carefully the accompanying Patient Instructions for Use with each Diskhaler device. Take 2 doses on the first day of treatment if they are given at least 2 h apart. Take doses on days 2 through 5 approximately 12 h apart and at the same time each day. To avoid the spread of infection, do not use the inhaler for more than one person. Zanamivir is not a substitute for influenza vaccination.

Missed Doses. Take this drug at regular intervals. If you miss a dose of this medicine, take it as soon as you remember. If it is almost time for your next dose, take that dose only and go back to your regular dosage schedule. Leave at least 12 h between doses. Do not double the dose or take an extra dose.

Pharmacokinetics. *Fate.* (Inhalation) the peak serum concentration is 39–54 g/μL within 1–2 h after a 10-mg inhaled dose. Oral bioavailability of inhaled zanamivir is 4%–17%. Protein binding is less than 10%. Zanamivir is excreted unchanged in the urine.[62] **Half-life** 3.6 ± 1.3 h.[62]

Adverse Reactions. Nasal and throat discomfort, cough, headache have occurred in 2%–3% of patients. This prevalence is similar to placebo and might be related to inhalation of the lactose vehicle. Bronchospasm has occurred occasionally in patients with asthma or COPD.[60]

Precautions. Use with extreme caution in patients with underlying airway diseases such as asthma or COPD because of the potential for causing bronchospasm. Instruct patients who use inhaled bronchodilators concurrently with zanamivir to use their bronchodilators before inhaling zanamivir.

Drug Interactions. Zanamivir is not a substrate and does not affect cytochrome P450 isoenzymes. There are no known clinically relevant drug interactions.

Parameters to Monitor. Inhalation technique, progression of influenza symptoms.

Notes. There are no data to support the safety or efficacy in patients who begin zanamivir treatment after 48 h of influenza symptom onset. Patients should continue to receive an annual influenza vaccination. Zanamivir is also used for the treatment and prophylaxis of Avian influenza and Novel influenza A (H1N1). Zanamivir can be given to children >7 years old for treatment and >5 years old for prophylaxis of Avian influenza and Novel influenza A (H1N1) at similar dosage recommendations above.

ANTIRETROVIRAL THERAPY FOR HIV

Many formidable hurdles stand in the way of effective HIV treatment, including patient adherence to dosage regimens, adverse effects, and drug–drug interactions. These hurdles interfere with quality of life and control of the viral burden and also contribute to the emergence of resistance. It is essential for health care providers and patients to appreciate the complexity of antiretroviral medication regimens to achieve harmony between goals of antiretroviral therapy and optimal patient care. General principals of treatment that guide contemporary treatment decisions are outlined below:

- Viral load monitoring is essential to guide decision making.
- Attaining and maintaining an undetectable HIV RNA in blood is the goal of therapy.
- Introduce effective antiretroviral therapy *before* extensive immune system damage has occurred.
- Three-drug combination therapy is the regimen most likely to achieve the goal of an undetectable HIV RNA level and provide a durable response.
- Compliance with the treatment regimen is critical to success and must be considered in initiating and choosing regimens.
- Change most or all drugs in a failing regimen simultaneously; use antiretroviral drug resistance testing to guide new antiretroviral regimen decisions.

For further information and clarification on appropriate uses of antiretroviral therapy, see US Public Health Service guidelines for the use of antiretroviral agents in pediatric HIV infection and HIV-infected adults and adolescents.[38,63]

ANTIVIRAL DRUGS FOR HIV INFECTION COMPARISON CHART

MEDICATION	DOSAGE FORMS	ADULT DOSAGE	PEDIATRIC DOSAGE	RENAL DOSING[a]	PHARMACOKINETICS	CYP450 ISOZYMES	ADVERSE REACTIONS	COMMENTS
HIV NUCLEOSIDE REVERSE TRANSCRIPTASE INHIBITORS								
Abacavir Ziagen	Tab 300 mg Soln 20 mg/mL	PO 300 mg twice daily, 600 mg once daily	PO (3 mo–16 y) 8 mg/kg, to a maximum of 300 mg twice daily.	No adjustment necessary.	Bioavailability 83%, no food effects; approximately 50% bound to plasma proteins; metabolized primarily by alcohol dehydrogenase and glucuronyl transferase; inactive metabolites excreted in feces and urine.	No effect.	Rash, asthenia, hypersensitivity reaction.	An HLA-B*5701 should be obtained prior to the use of abacavir to rule out potential hypersensitivity. Symptoms include rash, fever, GUI complaints, constitutional symptoms, and/or respiratory symptoms. Patients who have a hypersensitivity reaction must not take the drug; rechallenge could be fatal.
Didanosine Videx Videx EC	Pwdr for oral Soln (pediatric) 2, 4 g Cap 125, 200, 250, 400 mg	PO Cap (≥60 kg) 400 mg daily, (25–60 kg) 250 mg daily, (20–24 kg) 200 mg daily PO Pwdr for oral Soln (≥60 kg) 200 mg twice	PO Cap (≥60 kg) 400 mg daily, (25–60 kg) 250 mg daily, (20–24 kg) 200 mg daily. PO Pwdr for oral Soln (>8 mo) 120 mg/m^2	Cap (≥60 kg) Cl$_{Cr}$ ≥60, 400 mg daily; Cl$_{Cr}$ 30–59, 200 mg daily; Cl$_{Cr}$ <30, 125 mg daily. (<60 kg) Cl$_{Cr}$ >60, 250 mg daily; Cl$_{Cr}$	Rapidly absorbed, C$_{max}$ and AUC decreased 55% by food; protein binding <5%; 60% excreted unchanged in urine, remaining metabolized to ddATP, hypoxanthine, and uric acid.	No effect.	Neuropathy, pancreatitis, nausea, dysgeusia, diarrhea, hyperuricemia, headache, asthenia, seizures, pruritus.	Must be administered on empty stomach unless coadministered with tenofovir; dosage must be reduced with concomitant tenofovir; (≥60 kg, Cl$_{Cr}$ ≥60 mL/min) 250 mg daily, (<60 kg, Cl$_{Cr}$ ≥60 mL/min) 200 mg danile. Should not *(continued)*

ANTIVIRAL DRUGS FOR HIV INFECTION COMPARISON CHART (*continued*)

MEDICATION	DOSAGE FORMS	ADULT DOSAGE	PEDIATRIC DOSAGE	RENAL DOSING[a]	PHARMACOKINETICS	CYP450 ISOZYMES	ADVERSE REACTIONS	COMMENTS
		daily, (<60 kg) 125 mg twice daily	twice daily, (2 wk–8 mo) 100 mg/m^2 twice daily, (<2 wk) Not recommended.	<60, 125 mg daily. Pwdr for oral Soln (≥60 kg) Cl_{Cr} ≥60, 200 mg twice daily; Cl_{Cr} 30–59, 200 mg once daily or 100 mg twice daily; Cl_{Cr} 10–29, 150 mg once daily; Cl_{Cr} <10, 100 mg once daily. (<60 kg) Cl_{Cr} ≥60 125 mg twice daily; Cl_{Cr} 30–59, 150 mg once daily or 75 mg twice daily; Cl_{Cr} 10–29, 100 mg once daily; Cl_{Cr} <10, 75 mg once daily.				be coadmin stered with stavudine due to additive adverse effects.

(continued)

ANTIVIRAL DRUGS FOR HIV INFECTION COMPARISON CHART (*continued*)

MEDICATION	DOSAGE FORMS	ADULT DOSAGE	PEDIATRIC DOSAGE	RENAL DOSING[a]	PHARMACOKINETICS	CYP450 ISOZYMES	ADVERSE REACTIONS	COMMENTS
Emtricitabine Emtriva	Cap 200 mg Oral Soln 10 mg/mL	PO Cap 200 mg daily PO Soln 240 mg daily	(0–3 mo) PO Soln 3 mg/kg daily (3 mo–17 y) PO Soln 6 mg/kg NTE 240 mg daily PO Cap (>33 kg) 200 mg daily.	Cap $Cl_{cr} \geq 50$, 200 mg daily; Cl_{cr} 30–49, 200 mg every 48 h; Cl_{cr} 15–29, 200 mg every 72 h; Cl_{cr} <15, 200 mg every 96 h. Oral Soln Cl_{cr} ≥50, 240 mg daily; Cl_{cr} 30–49, 120 mg every 24 h; Cl_{cr} 15–29, 80 mg every 24 h; Cl_{cr} <15, 60 mg every 24 h.	Rapidly and extensively absorbed with no food effects; plasma protein binding <4%; majority excreted unchanged in urine.	No effect.	Minimal: headache, diarrhea, nausea, rash.	Active against HBV; potential for HBV flare if discontinued in coinfected patient or if virus becomes resistant.
Lamivudine Epivir	Tab 100, 150 mg Soln 5, 10 mg/mL	PO 150 mg twice daily, 300 mg daily	PO 150 (3 mo–16 y) 4 mg/kg every 12 h, to a	Cl_{cr} 30–49, 150 mg daily; Cl_{cr} 15–29, 150 mg once, then	Rapidly absorbed with no food effects; plasma protein binding <36%; majority	No effect.	Nausea, headache, fatigue, rash, anorexia; generally well	Active against HBV; potential for HBV flare if discontinued in coinfected patient or if virus becomes resistant. *(continued)*

ANTIVIRAL DRUGS FOR HIV INFECTION COMPARISON CHART (*continued*)

MEDICATION	DOSAGE FORMS	ADULT DOSAGE	PEDIATRIC DOSAGE	RENAL DOSING[a]	PHARMACOKINETICS	CYP450 ISOZYMES	ADVERSE REACTIONS	COMMENTS
			maximum of 150 mg every 12 h.	100 mg daily; Cl$_{Cr}$ 5–14, 150 mg once, then 50 mg daily; Cl$_{Cr}$ <5, 50 mg once, then 25 mg daily.	excreted unchanged in urine		tolerated, but pancreatitis is a risk in pediatric population but not in adults.	
Stavudine Zerit	Cap 15, 20, 30, 40 mg Soln 1 mg/mL	PO (<60 kg) 30 mg twice daily; PO (≥60 kg) 40 mg twice daily; reduce dosage for mild to moderate peripheral neuropathy (<60 kg) 15 mg twice daily, (≥60 kg) 20 mg twice daily	PO (≤30 kg) 1 mg/kg every 12 h.	≥60 kg: Cl$_{Cr}$ >50, 40 mg twice daily; Cl$_{Cr}$ 26–50, 20 mg twice daily; Cl$_{Cr}$ 10–25, 20 mg daily <60 kg: Cl$_{Cr}$ >50, 30 mg twice daily; Cl$_{Cr}$ 26–50, 15 mg twice daily; Cl$_{Cr}$ 10–25, 15 mg daily.	Rapidly absorbed with no food effects; negligible binding to serum proteins; metabolic fate not elucidated; renal excretion approximately 40%.	No effect.	Neuropathy, headache, nausea, asthenia, insomnia, elevated hepatic enzymes, elevated triglycerides, lipoatrophy.	Should not be coadminstered with didanosine due to additive adverse effects. Antagonistic with zidovudine.

(*continued*)

ANTIVIRAL DRUGS FOR HIV INFECTION COMPARISON CHART (*continued*)

MEDICATION	DOSAGE FORMS	ADULT DOSAGE	PEDIATRIC DOSAGE	RENAL DOSING[a]	PHARMACOKINETICS	CYP450 ISOZYMES	ADVERSE REACTIONS	COMMENTS
Tenofovir Disoproxil Fumarate (DF) Viread	Tab 300 mg	PO 300 mg daily	Not established.	300 mg/dose, interval changes; $Cl_{Cr} \geq 50$, every 24 h; Cl_{Cr} 30–40, every 48 h; Cl_{Cr} 10–29, every 72–96 h.	Oral bioavailability approximately 25%, food effects insignificant; binding to plasma or serum proteins <0.7% and 7.2%, respectively; eliminated by a combination of glomerular filtration and active tubular secretion.	No effect	Asthenia, diarrhea, depression, headache, nausea, pain, and rash.	May be associated with decline of renal function in patients with preexisting renal dysfunction; monitor renal function consistently. Active against HBV; potential for HBV flare if discontinued in coinfected patient or if virus becomes resistant.
Zidovudine Retrovir	Cap 100 mg Tab 300 mg Syrup 10 mg/mL Inj 10 mg/mL	PO 200 mg 3 times daily or 300 mg twice daily. (*See* monograph for other indications.)	PO (neonates) 2 mg/kg every 6 h; IV (neonates) 1.5 mg/kg every 6 h (infants and children) 480 mg/m² daily, 240 mg/m² twice daily.	Cl_{Cr} <15, 300 mg daily.	Rapidly absorbed with negligible food effects; primarily eliminated by hepatic metabolism.	No effect.	Bone marrow suppression (anemia, neutropenia), nausea, abdominal pain, elevated hepatic enzymes, headache, malaise, elevated CPK, myopathy, nail discoloration.	Should not be used with stavudine due to antagonism. Most patients become macrocytic on zidovudine; many become anemic; Hgb <10 mg/dL is not uncommon.

(*continued*)

ANTIVIRAL DRUGS FOR HIV INFECTION COMPARISON CHART (continued)

MEDICATION	DOSAGE FORMS	ADULT DOSAGE	PEDIATRIC DOSAGE	RENAL DOSING[a]	PHARMACOKINETICS	CYP450 ISOZYMES	ADVERSE REACTIONS	COMMENTS
Abacavir and Lamivudine Epzicom	Tab 600 mg (abacavir) PLUS 300 mg (lamivudine)	PO 1 Tab daily	Not established.	Use adjusted doses of individual components.	(See individual components.)	No effect.	(See individual components.)	Contains abacavir; precede use with HLA-B*5701. (See individual components.)
Tenofovir DF and Emtricitabine Truvada	Tab 300 mg (tenofovir) PLUS 200 mg (emtricitabine)	PO 1 Tab daily	Not established.	Use adjusted doses of individual components.	(See individual components.)	No effect.	(See individual components.)	(See individual components.)
Zidovudine and Lamivudine Combivir	Tab 300 mg (zidovudine) PLUS 150 mg (lamivudine)	PO 1 Tab twice daily.	Not recommended for children <12 y.	Use adjusted doses of individual components.	(See individual components.)	No effect.	(See individual components.)	(See individual components.)
Zidovudine, Lamivudine and Abacavir Trizivir	Tab 300 mg (zidovudine) PLUS 150 mg (lamivudine) PLUS 300 mg (abacavir)	PO 1 Tab twice daily.	Not recommending for children weighing <40 kg.	Use adjusted doses of individual components.	(See individual components.)	No effect	(See individual components.)	Contains abacavir; precede use with HLA-B*5701. (See individual components.)

(continued)

153

ANTIVIRAL DRUGS FOR HIV INFECTION COMPARISON CHART (*continued*)

MEDICATION	DOSAGE FORMS	ADULT DOSAGE	PEDIATRIC DOSAGE	PHARMACOKINETICS	CYP450 ISOZYMES	ADVERSE REACTIONS	COMMENTS
HIV NONNUCLEOSIDE REVERSE TRANSCRIPTASE INHIBITORS							
Delavirdine Rescriptor	Tab 100, 200 mg	PO 400 mg 3 times daily	Not established	Rapid absorption with no food effects; approximately 98% bound to plasma proteins, primarily albumin; primarily metabolized by CYP3A and 2D6 to a lesser degree.	*Inhibits* CYP2C9 CYP2C19 CYP3A4	Rash, headache, elevated hepatic enzymes.	Tablets may be dispersed in water to allow easier administration. Should separate doses from any antacids by >1 h.
Efavirenz Sustiva	Cap 50, 200 mg Tab 600 mg	PO 600 mg daily	(10–14 kg) 200 mg/d; (15–19 kg) 250 mg/d; (20–24 kg) 300 mg/d; (25–32.5 kg) 350 mg/d; (32.5–39 kg) 400 mg/d; (≥40 kg) 600 mg/d	AUC and C_{max} increased 28% and 79%, respectively, when administered with high-fat meal; approximately 99.5%–99.75% protein bound; metabolized by CYP3A4 and 2B6; majority of metabolites excreted in feces.	*Induces* CYP3A4 *Inhibits* CYP2C9 CYP2C19 CYP3A4	CNS symptoms, dizziness, rash, dysphoria, anxiety, nausea, insomnia, inability to concentrate.	Should be administered on an empty stomach or low-fat snack at bedtime. CNS symptoms frequently resolve within 2–4 wk of initiating therapy. Rash frequent in first 2 wk, but usually resolves in 2 mo. Pregnancy category D; should be avoided in pregnancy and women of child-bearing potential should use at least 2 forms of birth control.

(continued)

ANTIVIRAL DRUGS FOR HIV INFECTION COMPARISON CHART (*continued*)

MEDICATION	DOSAGE FORMS	ADULT DOSAGE	PEDIATRIC DOSAGE	PHARMACOKINETICS	CYP450 ISOZYMES	ADVERSE REACTIONS	COMMENTS
Nevirapine Viramune	Tab 200 mg Susp 10 mg/mL	PO 200 mg/d for 14 days, then 400 mg/d in 1 or 2 doses. (*See* comments.)	PO (2 mo–8 y) 4 mg/kg daily for 14 days, then 7 mg/kg twice daily; (>8 y) 2 mg/kg daily for 14 days, then 4 mg/kg twice daily	>90% absorbed with negligible food effects; approximately 60% bound to plasma proteins; primarily metabolized by CYP3A4 and 2B6.	*Induces* CYP3A4 and 2B6	Rash, hepatitis, fatigue, headache.	To reduce the frequency of rash, it is essential to increase the dosage over 14 days. Increase to full dosage only if no rash or other adverse effects occur. Risk of hepatotoxicity higher in females with baseline CD4 counts >250 cells/mm^3 and in males with baseline CD4 counts >400 mm^3. Avoid in this population.
Etravirine Intelence	Tab 100 mg	PO 200 mg twice daily	Not established	Absorption enhanced by food, always take with a meal; approximately 99.9% bound to plasma proteins; primarily metabolized by CYP3A4, 2C9 and 2C19.	*Induces* CYP3A4 *Inhibits* CYP2C9 and 2C19	Rash and GI upset.	Indicated for treatment-experienced patients with the K103N resistance mutation. Should not be administered with only two NRTIs. Should be administered with two or more of the following: darunavir, enfuvirtide, lopinavir/ritonavir, maraviroc, raltegravir, and saquinavir.

(continued) |

ANTIVIRAL DRUGS FOR HIV INFECTION COMPARISON CHART (*continued*)

MEDICATION	DOSAGE FORMS	ADULT DOSAGE	PEDIATRIC DOSAGE	PHARMACOKINETICS	CYP450 ISOZYMES	ADVERSE REACTIONS	COMMENTS
Efavirenz, Emtricitabine, and Tenofovir DF Atripla	Tab 600 mg (efavirenz) PLUS 200 mg (emtricitabine) PLUS 300 mg (tenofovir)	PO 1 Tab daily	Not recommended in patients <18 y	(*See* individual components.)	(*See* individual components.)	(*See* individual components.)	(*See* individual components.)
HIV PROTEASE INHIBITORS							
Atazanavir Reyataz[b]	Cap 100, 150, 200, 300 mg	PO 300 mg coadministered with ritonavir 100 mg as a single dose with food (usual dosage) or PO 400 mg as a single dose with food; (*See Atazanavir Dosing with Acid-Reducing Medications.*)	Treatment naïve (6–18 y): PO 8.5 mg/kg with ritonavir 4 mg/kg daily with food (15–20 kg): PO 7 mg/kg with ritonavir 4 mg/kg daily with food, NTE atazanavir 300 mg/d and ritonavir 100 mg/d (≥20 kg). Treatment-experienced (>25 kg):	Absorption enhanced and variability reduced by administration with food; 86% bound to serum proteins; metabolized by CYP3A	*Inhibits* CYP3A, CYP2C8, and UGT1A1	GI upset, potential jaundice, or scleral icterus, prolongation of QTc.	Absorption requires acidic environment; separation from histamine H2-receptor antagonists and proton pump inhibitors may be necessary. Coadministration with tenofovir requires 300 mg daily with ritonavir-boosting. Because of atazanavir's inhibition of UGT1A1, a benign indirect hyperbilirubinemia is commonly present.

(continued)

ANTIVIRAL DRUGS FOR HIV INFECTION COMPARISON CHART (*continued*)

MEDICATION	DOSAGE FORMS	ADULT DOSAGE	PEDIATRIC DOSAGE	RENAL DOSING[a]	CYP450 ISOZYMES	ADVERSE REACTIONS	COMMENTS
			PO 7 mg/kg with ritonavir 4 mg/kg daily with food, NTE atazanvir 300 mg/d and ritonavir 100 mg/d				
Darunavir Prezista[b]	Tab 75, 300, 400, 600 mg	Treatment-naïve: PO 800 mg with ritonavir 100 mg daily with food Treatment-experienced: PO 600 mg with ritonavir 100 mg twice daily with food	(6–18 y and 20–30 kg) PO 375 mg with ritonavir 50 mg twice daily, (30–40 kg) PO 450 mg with ritonavir 60 mg twice daily, (≥40 kg) 600 mg with ritonavir 100 mg twice daily.	Absolute bioavailability 37%–82%; C_{max} and AUC 30% higher with food; approximately 95% bound to plasma proteins; metabolized by CYP3A	*Inhibits* CYP3A4 and P-glycoprotein	Skin rash, GI upset.	Contains sulfonamide moiety; use with caution in patients with sulfa allergy. Must be administered with food.

(continued)

ANTIVIRAL DRUGS FOR HIV INFECTION COMPARISON CHART (*continued*)

MEDICATION	DOSAGE FORMS	ADULT DOSAGE	PEDIATRIC DOSAGE	RENAL DOSING[a]	CYP450 ISOZYMES	ADVERSE REACTIONS	COMMENTS
Fosamprenavir Lexiva[b]	Tab 700 mg Oral Susp 50 mg/mL	Treatment-naïve: PO 1400 mg twice daily, 1400 mg daily with ritonavir 200 mg daily, 1400 mg daily with ritonavir 100 mg daily, 700 mg twice daily plus ritonavir 100 mg twice daily Treatment-experienced: PO 700 mg twice daily with ritonavir 100 mg twice daily	Treatment-naïve: (2–5 y old) PO 30 mg/kg suspension twice daily NTE 1400 mg twice daily, (≥6 y old) PO 30 mg/kg suspension twice daily NTE 1400 mg twice daily OR 18 mg/kg twice daily with ritonavir 3 mg/kg twice daily NTE 700/100 twice daily. Treatment-experienced: (2–5 y old) Safety and efficacy not established, (≥6 y) 18 mg/kg twice daily with ritonavir 3 mg/kg twice daily NTE700/ 100 twice daily.	Absorption independent of food; approximately 90% bound to plasma proteins; converted to active amprenavir by hydrolysis in gut epithelium and metabolized by CYP3A4	*Induces/ Inhibits* CYP3A4	Skin rash, GI upset, headache.	Contains sulfonamide moiety; use with caution in patients with sulfa allergy.

(continued)

ANTIVIRAL DRUGS FOR HIV INFECTION COMPARISON CHART (*continued*)

MEDICATION	DOSAGE FORMS	ADULT DOSAGE	PEDIATRIC DOSAGE	RENAL DOSING	CYP450 ISOZYMES	ADVERSE REACTIONS	COMMENTS
Indinavir Mesylate Crixivan	Cap 100, 200, 333, 400 mg	PO 800 mg every 8 h. *Combinations:* PO 400 mg twice daily PLUS PO ritonavir 400 mg twice daily PO 800 mg twice daily PLUS PO ritonavir 200 mg twice daily[b]	Optimal dose not established. PO 500 mg/m² every 8 h is undergoing clinical trials).	Rapidly absorbed in the fasting state; administration with food decreases oral absorption by approximately 75%; 60% bound to human plasma proteins; primarily metabolized by CYP3A4 and <20% excreted unchanged in the urine; half-life 1.8 ± 0.4 h	*Inhibits* CYP3A4	Nausea, headache, abdominal pain, hyperbilirubinemia, insomnia, dizziness, nephrolithiasis.	Administer on an empty stomach 1 h before or 2 h after a meal (or can take with a light meal). Adequate hydration is required to minimize risk of nephrolithiasis.
Lopinavir and Ritonavir Kaletra[b]	Tab 100 mg (lopinavir) PLUS 25 mg (ritonavir), 200 mg (lopinavir) PLUS 50 mg (ritonavir) Oral Soln 80 mg (lopinavir) PLUS 20 mg (ritonavir) per mL	PO 400 mg (lopinavir) PLUS 100 mg (ritonavir) twice daily OR 800 mg (lopinavir) PLUS 200 mg (ritonavir) daily (treatment naïve only)	(7–15 kg) 12 mg/kg twice daily: (7–10 kg) 1.25 mL/dose; (10–15 kg) 1.75 mL/dose; (15–40 kg) 10 mg/kg twice daily: (15–20 kg) 2.25 mL/dose, (20–25 kg) 2.75 mL/dose; (25–30 kg) 3.5 mL/ dose; (30–35 kg) 4 mL/dose; (35–40 kg) 4.75 mL/dose; (>40 kg) 400 mg twice daily.	Lopinavir approximately 98%–99% bound to plasma proteins; lopinavir metabolized almost exclusively by CYP3A; <3% excreted unchanged in urine	*Inhibits* CYP3A	Nausea, diarrhea, vomiting.	Tablets may be taken with or without food. Oral Soln must be taken with food. Once-daily dosing should not be used in children <18 y.

(continued)

159

ANTIVIRAL DRUGS FOR HIV INFECTION COMPARISON CHART (*continued*)

MEDICATION	DOSAGE FORMS	ADULT DOSAGE	PEDIATRIC DOSAGE	RENAL DOSING[a]	CYP450 ISOZYMES	ADVERSE REACTIONS	COMMENTS
Nelfinavir Viracept	Tab 250 mg, 625 mg Pwdr 50 mg (nelfinavir) per level scoopful (1 g)	PO 750 mg 3 times daily OR 1250 mg twice daily with food	(<2 y) Safety and efficacy not established; (2–13 y) 45–55 mg/kg twice daily OR 25–35 mg/kg 3 times daily. (*See* Nelfinavir Dosing Table for Children Older Than 2 y.)	Absorption increased 2–3 fold when administered with food; peak 2–4 h after dose; plasma protein binding >98%; metabolized by CYP3A4 (minor substrate of 2C9, 2C19, 2D6); <2% excreted unchanged in urine	*Inhibits* CYP3A4	Diarrhea, nausea, abdominal pain and discomfort, dysphagia, rash.	Administer with food or light snack to increase absorption 2- to 3-fold. Diarrhea can be severe; oral calcium carbonate 500–1000 mg daily or bid has decreased prevalence in some patients.
Ritonavir Norvir	Cap 100 mg Soln[b] 80 mg/mL	PO 600 mg twice daily; however, used most often as a booster for other protease inhibitors	PO 400 mg/m² every 12 h, start at 250 mg/m² twice daily and increase by 50 mg/m² twice daily every 2–3 days.	Rapidly absorbed and increased by 15% with food; 98%–99% protein bound; serum concentrations decrease over time due to autoinduction of metabolizing enzymes, CYP3A, and 2D	*Inhibits* CYP3A4 CYP2C9 CYP2C19 CYP2D6	Nausea, vomiting, diarrhea, headache, circumoral and extremity paresthesias, asthenia, taste perversion, elevated serum triglycerides, hepatic transaminases CPK, uric acid.	Titrate dosage from 300 mg q12h to 600 mg q12h over 10–14 days to reduce adverse events. However, ritonavir rarely used as only protease inhibitor; used almost exclusively in low doses as adjunct to another protease inhibitor.

(continued)

ANTIVIRAL DRUGS FOR HIV INFECTION COMPARISON CHART (*continued*)

MEDICATION	DOSAGE FORMS	ADULT DOSAGE	PEDIATRIC DOSAGE	RENAL DOSING[a]	CYP450 ISOZYMES	ADVERSE REACTIONS	COMMENTS
Saquinavir Mesylate Invirase	Cap 200 mg Tab 500 mg	PO 1000 mg twice daily co-administered with ritonavir 100 mg twice daily	Not established.	Absorption is erratic; undergoes extensive first-pass metabolism; absolution bioavailability averages 4%; metabolized by CYP3A4	*Inhibits* CYP3A4	Nausea, headache, elevated hepatic transaminases.	Saquinavir must always be administered with ritonavir and within 2 h after a meal.
Tipranavir Aptivus	Cap 250 mg	PO 500 mg twice daily coadministered with ritonavir 200 mg twice daily	Not established.	Absorption is enhanced by food; >99.9% plasma protein bound; metabolized by CYP3A4	*Induces* CYP3A4 and P-glycoprotein	Rash, GI intolerance, severe hepatitis, intracranial bleed (rare).	Considering separating doses from acid-reducing agents. Use caution in patients with sulfonamide allergy.

[a]Cl$_{Cr}$ are reported as mL/min.
[b]Department of Health and Human Services preferred agents for antiretroviral-naïve patients.
From product information.

NELFINAVIR DOSING TABLE FOR CHILDREN OLDER THAN 2 YEARS

BODY WEIGHT		TWICE DAILY 45–55 mg/kg		TWICE DAILY 25–35 mg/kg	
Kg	*lb*	*Scoops of Powder (50 mg/kg)*	*Teaspoons of Powder*[a]	*Scoops of Powder (50 mg/kg)*	*Teaspoons of Powder*[a]
9 to <10.5	20 to <23	10	2.5	6	1.5
10.5 to <12	23 to <26.5	11	2.75	7	1.75
12 to <14	26.5 to <31	13	3.25	8	2
14 to <16	31 to <35	15	3.75	9	2.25
16 to <18	35 to ≥39.5	Not recommended[b]	Not recommended[b]	10	2.5
18 to <23	39.5 to <50.5	Not recommended[b]	Not recommended[b]	12	3
≥23	≥50.5	Not recommended[b]	Not recommended[b]	15	3.75

[a]If a teaspoon is used to measure nelfinavir oral powder, 1 level teaspoon contains 200 mg of nelfinavir (4 level scoops equals 1 level teaspoon).
[b]Use nelfinavir 250 mg tablet.
From product information.

ATAZANAVIR DOSING WITH ACID-REDUCING MEDICATIONS[a]

ACID-REDUCING MEDICATION	COMPARABLE MEDICATION/DOSAGE	DIRECTIONS
Treatment Naïve		
H2-antagonist	Famotidine 40 mg twice daily	Simultaneously or 10 h following H2-anatgonist: atazanavir/ritonavir 300/100 mg
Proton pump inhibitor	Omeprazole 20 mg daily	12 h following proton pump inhibitor: atazanavir/ritonavir 300/100 mg
Treatment Experienced[b]		
H2-antagonist	Famotidine 20 mg twice daily	Simultaneously or 10 h following H2-anatgonist: atazanavir/ritonavir 300/100 mg
H2-antagonist + NRTI	Famotidine 20 mg twice daily + tenofovir	Simultaneously or 10 h following H2-anatgonist: atazanavir/ritonavir 400/100 mg

[a]Unboosted atazanavir not appropriate with H2-antagonist or PPI.
[b]Atazanavir should not be coadministered with PPIs in treatment-experienced patients.

NNRTI DRUG INTERACTIONS TABLE

CONCOMITANT DRUG CLASS/NAME	NNRTI	EFFECT ON NNRTI OR CONCOMITANT DRUG CONCENTRATIONS	DOSING RECOMMENDATIONS AND CLINICAL COMMENT
Antifungals			
Fluconazole	DLV, EFV	No significant effect	
	ETR	$\uparrow$ ETR	No dosage adjustment necessary.
	NVP	NVP C_{max}, AUC, and C_{min} $\uparrow$ 100%	Increased risk of hepatotoxicity possible with this combination. Monitor NVP toxicity.
Itraconazole	DLV, NVP	No data, potential for bidirectional interactions	Consider monitoring NNRTI and itraconazole levels.
	EFV	Itraconazole and OH-itraconazole AUC, C_{max}, and C_{min} $\downarrow$ 35%–44%	Dose adjustments for itraconazole may be necessary. Monitor itraconazole level.
	ETR	$\uparrow$ ETR $\downarrow$ Itraconazole	Dose adjustments for itraconazole may be necessary. Monitor itraconazole level.
Ketoconazole	DLV	$\uparrow$ DLV	No dosage adjustment necessary.
	EFV	No data	

(continued)

NNRTI DRUG INTERACTIONS TABLE (*continued*)

CONCOMITANT DRUG CLASS/NAME	NNRTI	EFFECT ON NNRTI OR CONCOMITANT DRUG CONCENTRATIONS	DOSING RECOMMENDATIONS AND CLINICAL COMMENT
	ETR	↑ ETR ↓ Ketoconazole	Dose adjustment for ketoconazole may be necessary depending on other coadministered drugs.
	NVP	Ketoconazole ↓ 63%, NVP ↑ 15%–30%	**Coadministration not recommended.**
Posaconazole	DLV, NVP	No data	
	EFV	Posaconazole AUC ↓ 50%, C_{max} ↓45% EFV C_{max} ↑ 13%	Consider alternative antifungal if possible or consider monitoring posaconazole level if available
	ETR	↑ ETR	No dosage adjustment necessary.
Voriconazole	DLV	No data	Potential for bidirectional inhibition of metabolism. Monitor for toxicity.
	EFV	EFV ↑ 44% Voriconazole ↓ 77%	**Contraindicated at standard doses.** Dose: voriconazole 400 mg bid, EFV 300 mg daily
	ETR	↑ ETR ↑ Voriconazole	Dose adjustments for voriconazole may be necessary depending on other coadministered drugs. Monitor voriconazole level.
	NVP	No data	Potential for induction of voriconazole metabolism and inhibition of NVP metabolism. Monitor for toxicity and antifungal outcome.
Anticonvulsants **Carbamazepine** **Phenobarbital** **Phenytoin**	DLV	DLV C_{min} ↓ 90% by phenytoin, phenobarbital, and carbamazepine	**Contraindicated—do not coadminister.**
	EFV	Carbamazepine + EFV: AUCs ↓ 27% and 36%, respectively, when combined. EFV + phenytoin: ↓ EFV concentrations (case report)	Monitor anticonvulsant levels, or if possible, use alternative anticonvulsant.
	ETR	No data. Potential for ↓ ETR and anticonvulsant concentrations.	**Do not coadminister.** Consider alternative anticonvulsants.
	NVP	No data	

(continued)

NNRTI DRUG INTERACTIONS TABLE (*continued*)

CONCOMITANT DRUG CLASS/NAME	NNRTI	EFFECT ON NNRTI OR CONCOMITANT DRUG CONCENTRATIONS	DOSING RECOMMENDATIONS AND CLINICAL COMMENT
Antimycobacterials			
Clarithromycin	DLV	Clarithromycin ↑ 100% DLV ↑ 44%	Reduce clarithromycin dose by 50% in patients with Cl_{Cr} 30–60 mL/min and by 75% in patients with Cl_{Cr} <30 mL/min.
	EFV	Clarithromycin ↓ 39%	Monitor for efficacy or consider alternative agent, such as azithromycin, for MAC prophylaxis and treatment.
	ETR	ETR AUC ↑ 42%, clarithromycin AUC ↓ 39% and C_{min} ↓ 53%, OH-clarithromycin AUC ↑ 21%	Consider alternative agent, such as azithromycin, for MAC prophylaxis and treatment.
	NVP	NVP ↑ 26%, Clarithromycin ↓ 30%	Monitor for efficacy or use alternative agent.
Rifabutin	DLV	DLV ↓ 80% Rifabutin ↑ 100%	**Coadministration not recommended.**
	EFV	Rifabutin ↓ 35%	Dose: rifabutin 450–600 mg once daily or 600 mg 3 times/wk if EFV is not coadministered with a PI.
	ETR	ETR AUC ↓ 37% and C_{min} ↓ 35% Rifabutin AUC ↓ 17% and C_{min} ↓ 24%, 25-O-desacetylrifabutin AUC ↓ 17% and C_{min} ↓ 22%	Dose: rifabutin 300 mg once daily if ETR is not coadministered with a RTV-boosted PI. If ETR is coadministered with DRV/r or SQV/r and rifabutin is needed, consider alternative ARV agent to ETR. If ETR is coadministered with LPV/r, use rifabutin 150 mg qod or 3 times/wk. Acquired rifamycin resistance has been reported in patients with inadequate rifabutin levels while on 150 mg twice weekly and RTV-boosted PIs. Consider therapeutic drug monitoring and adjust dose accordingly.
	NVP	↓ NVP ↑ Rifabutin	No dosage adjustment necessary.

(continued)

NNRTI DRUG INTERACTIONS TABLE (*continued*)

CONCOMITANT DRUG CLASS/NAME	NNRTI	EFFECT ON NNRTI OR CONCOMITANT DRUG CONCENTRATIONS	DOSING RECOMMENDATIONS AND CLINICAL COMMENT
Rifampin	DLV	DLV ↓ 96%	**Contraindicated—do not coadminister.**
	EFV	↓ EFV 25%	Maintain efavirenz dose at 600 mg once daily and monitor for viral response. Some clinicians suggest EFV 800 mg dose in patients >60 kg.
	ETR	Potential for significant ↓ ETR levels	**Do not coadminister.**
	NVP	↓ NVP 20%–58%	**Do not coadminister.**
Benzodiazepines			
Alprazolam	DLV	No data May ↑ alprazolam	**Do not coadminister.** Consider alternative benzodiazepines, such as lorazepam, oxazepam, or temazepam.
	EFV, NVP, ETR	No data	Monitor for therapeutic efficacy of alprazolam.
Diazepam	DLV	No data May ↑ diazepam	Consider alternative benzodiazepines, such as lorazepam, oxazepam, or temazepam.
	EFV, NVP ETR	No data ↑ Diazepam	Decreased dose of diazepam may be necessary.
Lorazepam	DLV, ETR, NVP	No data	
	EFV	Lorazepam C_{max} ↑ 16%, no significant effect on lorazepam AUC	No dosage adjustment necessary.
Midazolam	DLV, EFV	No data May ↑ midazolam	**Do not coadminister with oral midazolam.** Parenteral midazolam can be used with caution as a single dose and can be given in a monitored situation for procedural sedation.
	ETR, NVP	No data	

(continued)

NNRTI DRUG INTERACTIONS TABLE (*continued*)

CONCOMITANT DRUG CLASS/NAME	NNRTI	EFFECT ON NNRTI OR CONCOMITANT DRUG CONCENTRATIONS	DOSING RECOMMENDATIONS AND CLINICAL COMMENT
Triazolam	DLV, EFV	No data May ↑ triazolam	**Do not coadminister.**
	ETR, NVP	No data	
Herbal Products			
St. John's wort	All NNRTIs	↓ NNRTI	Administration of St. John's wort with NNRTIs is not recommended.
Hormonal Contraceptives			
Hormonal Contraceptives	DLV	No data Potential for ↑ ethinyl estradiol levels.	Clinical significance unknown.
	EFV	↑ Ethinyl estradiol	Use alternative or additional methods. No data on other components.
	ETR	↑ Ethinyl estradiol No effect on norethindrone levels.	No dosage adjustment necessary.
	NVP	Ethinyl estradiol ↓ 20%.	Use alternative or additional methods.
HMG-CoA Reductase Inhibitors			
Atorvastatin	DLV	No data potential for inhibition of atorvastatin metabolism.	Use lowest possible dose and monitor for toxicity, or consider other HMG-CoA reductase inhibitors with less potential for interaction.
	EFV	Atorvastatin AUC ↓ 37%–43%.	Adjust atorvastatin according to lipid responses, not to exceed the maximum recommended dose.
	ETR	↓ Atorvastatin AUC 37%	Dose: standard, adjust dose according to response.
	NVP	No data potential for induction of atorvastatin metabolism	Dose: standard, adjust dose according to response
Fluvastatin	DLV, EFV, NVP	No data	
	ETR	↑ Fluvastatin	Dose adjustments for fluvastatin may be necessary.
Lovastatin Simvastatin	DLV	No data. Potential for large increase in statin levels.	**Avoid concomitant use.**
	EFV	Simvastatin AUC ↓ 68%	Adjust simvastatin dose according to lipid responses, not to exceed the maximum recommended dose.

(continued)

NNRTI DRUG INTERACTIONS TABLE (*continued*)

CONCOMITANT DRUG CLASS/NAME	NNRTI	EFFECT ON NNRTI OR CONCOMITANT DRUG CONCENTRATIONS	DOSING RECOMMENDATIONS AND CLINICAL COMMENT
	ETR	↓ Lovastatin ↓ Simvastatin	Adjust lovastatin or simvastatin dose according to lipid responses, not to exceed the maximum recommended dose. If used with RTV-boosted PI, simvastatin and lovastatin should be avoided.
Pravastatin **Rosuvastatin**	DLV, NVP EFV	No data Pravastatin AUC ↓ 44%.	Adjust pravastatin dose according to lipid responses, not to exceed the maximum recommended dose.
	ETR	No effect	Dose: standard.
Methadone **Methadone**	DLV	No effect on DLV Potential for ↑ methadone	Monitor for methadone toxicity and need for dose reduction
	EFV	Methadone ↓ 60%	Potential for opiate withdrawal; increased methadone dose often necessary.
	ETR	No effect	Dose: standard
	NVP	↓ Methadone No effect on NVP	Opiate withdrawal common; increased methadone dose often necessary.
Oral Anticoagulant **Warfarin**	DLV	No data	May increase warfarin levels. Monitor INR.
	EFV, NVP	No data	May increase or decrease warfarin levels. Monitor INR.
	ETR	↑ Warfarin	Monitor INR and adjust warfarin dose accordingly.

From Ref. 38.

NNRTI DRUG-SPECIFIC INTERACTIONS

NNRTI	CONCOMITANT DRUG CLASS/NAME	EFFECT ON NNRTI OR CONCOMITANT DRUG CONCENTRATIONS	DOSAGE RECOMMENDATIONS AND CLINICAL COMMENT
DLV	**Fluoxetine**	↑ DLV	No dosage adjustment necessary.
	Quinidine	No data. May increase quinidine levels	Monitor quinidine level and toxicities.
	Sildenafil **Vardenafil** **Tadalafil**	No data potential for increased phospho-diesterase inhibitor levels	Use cautiously. Start with reduced dose of sildenafil 25 mg q48h, vardenafil 2.5 mg q24h, and tadalafil 5 mg q72h.
ETR	**Antiarrhythmics**	↓ Antiarrhythmics	Use with caution with antiarrhythmic level monitoring if available.
	Dexamethasone	↓ ETR	Use systemic dexametha-sone with caution or con-sider alternative corticos-teroid for long-term use.
	Sildenafil	↓ Sildenafil	May need to increase sildenafil dose based on clinical effect. Levels: sildenafil AUC ↓ 57%.

From Ref. 38.

NRTI DRUG INTERACTIONS TABLE

CONCOMITANT DRUG CLASS/NAME	NRTI	EFFECT ON NRTI OR CONCOMITANT DRUG CONCENTRATIONS	CLINICAL COMMENT
Antivirals			
Ganciclovir (GCV) **Valganciclovir**	ddI	↑ ddI AUC ↑ 50%–111% ↓ GCV AUC ↓ 21% when ddI administered 2 h prior to oral GCV.	Appropriate doses for combination of ddI and GCV have not been established.
		No change in IV GCV concentrations.	Monitor for ddI associated toxicities.
	TDF	No data	Serum concentrations of these drugs and/or TDF may be increased. Monitor for dose-related toxicities.
	ZDV	No significant pharmacokinetic effects	Potential increase in hematologic toxicities.

(continued)

NRTI DRUG INTERACTIONS TABLE (*continued*)

CONCOMITANT DRUG CLASS/NAME	NRTI	EFFECT ON NRTI OR CONCOMITANT DRUG CONCENTRATIONS	CLINICAL COMMENT
Ribavirin	ddI	↑ Intracellular ddI	**Coadministration not recommended.** May cause ddI-related serious toxicities.
	ZDV	Ribavirin inhibits phosphorylation of ZDV.	Avoid coadministration if possible, or closely monitor virologic response and hematologic toxicities.
Methadone			
Methadone	ABC	↓ Methadone	Monitor for opiate withdrawal and titrate methadone as clinically indicated. May require ↑ methadone dose.
	d4T	↓ d4T	No dosage adjustment necessary.
	ZDV	↑ ZDV AUC 43%	Monitor for ZDV-related adverse effects.
NRTIs			
Didanosine	d4T	No significant effect	Avoid coadministration if possible. Peripheral neuropathy, lactic acidosis, and pancreatitis seen with this combination.
	TDF	↑ ddI-EC AUC and C_{max} 48%–60%	Dose if Cl_{Cr} >60 mL/min: ddI-EC 250 mg/d if patient weighs >60 kg and ddI-EC 200 mg if patient weighs <60 kg. Monitor for ddI-associated toxicity.
PIs			
Atazanavir (ATV)	ddI	Simultaneous ddI-EC + ATV (with food) ↓ ddI AUC 34%. ATV no change.	ATV with food should be administered 2 h before or 1 h after ddI.
	TDF	↓ ATV AUC 25% and C_{min} 23%–40% (higher C_{min} with RTV than without) ↑ TDF AUC 24%–30%	Dose: ATV/r 300/100 mg daily coadministered with TDF 300 mg daily. Avoid concomitant use without ritonavir. Monitor for TDF-associated toxicity.
	ZDV	↓ ZDV C_{min} 30%, no change in AUC	Clinical significance unknown.
Darunavir (DRV)	TDF	↑ TDF AUC 22%, C_{max} 24%, C_{min} 37%	Clinical significance unknown. Monitor for TDF toxicity.
Indinavir (IDV)	TDF	↑ IDV	No dosage adjustment necessary.
Lopinavir/ritonavir (LPV/r)	TDF	↓ LPV/r AUC 15% ↑ TDF AUC 34%	Clinical significance unknown. Monitor for TDF toxicity.

(continued)

NRTI DRUG INTERACTIONS TABLE (*continued*)

CONCOMITANT DRUG CLASS/NAME	NRTI	EFFECT ON NRTI OR CONCOMITANT DRUG CONCENTRATIONS	CLINICAL COMMENT
Tipranavir/ritonavir (TPV/r)	ABC	↓ ABC 35%–44% with TPV/r 1,250/100 mg bid	Appropriate doses for this combination have not been established.
	ddl	↓ ddl-EC 10% and ↓ TPV C_{min} 34% with TPV/r 1,250/100 mg bid	Separate doses by at least 2 h.
	TDF	↓ TPV AUC 9%–18% and C_{min} 12%–21% with TPV/r 1,250/100 mg bid	Clinical significance is unknown.
	ZDV	↓ ZDV AUC 31%–43% and C_{max} 46%–51% with TPV/r 1,250/100 mg bid	Appropriate doses for this combination have not been established.

From Ref. 38.

PI DRUG INTERACTIONS TABLE

CONCOMITANT DRUG CLASS/NAME	PROTEASE INHIBITOR (PI)	EFFECT ON PI OR CONCOMITANT DRUG CONCENTRATIONS	DOSING RECOMMENDATIONS AND CLINICAL COMMENTS
Acid Reducers			
Antacids	ATV + RTV	No data	↓ ATV concentrations expected when given simultaneously. Give ATV at least 2 h before or 1 h after antacids or buffered medications.
	FPV	APV AUC ↓ 18%; C_{min}: no significant change	Can be given simultaneously or separated at least 2 h before or 1 h after antacids.
	DRV/r, FPV/r, IDV + RTV, LPV/r, NFV, SQV/r	No data	
	TPV/r	↓ TPV approximately 30%	Give TPV at least 2 h before or 1 h after antacids.

(continued)

PI DRUG INTERACTIONS TABLE (*continued*)

CONCOMITANT DRUG CLASS/NAME	PROTEASE INHIBITOR (PI)	EFFECT ON PI OR CONCOMITANT DRUG CONCENTRATIONS	DOSING RECOMMENDATIONS AND CLINICAL COMMENTS
Histamine H2-receptor antagonists	**RTV-boosted PI** ATV/r	↓ ATV	Histamine H2-receptor antagonist dose should not exceed a dose equivalent to famotidine 40 mg bid in treatment-naïve patients or 20 mg bid in treatment-experienced patients. ATV 300 mg + RTV 100 mg should be administered simultaneously with and/or >10 h after the histamine H2-receptor antagonist. In treatment-experienced patients, if TDF is used with histamine H2-receptor antagonists, ATV 400 mg + RTV 100 mg should be used.
	DRV/r, LPV/r FPV/r, SQV/r, TPV/r	No effect No data	
	PIs without RTV ATV	↓ ATV	Histamine H2-receptor antagonist single dose should not exceed a dose equivalent of famotidine 20 mg or total daily dose equivalent of famotidine 20 mg bid in treatment-naïve patients. ATV should be administered >2 h before and/or >10 h after the histamine H2-receptor antagonist.
	FPV	APV AUC ↓ 30%; C_{min}: unchanged	Separate administration if coadministration is necessary. Consider boosting with RTV.
	IDV, NFV	No data	

(continued)

PI DRUG INTERACTIONS TABLE (*continued*)

CONCOMITANT DRUG CLASS/NAME	PROTEASE INHIBITOR (PI)	EFFECT ON PI OR CONCOMITANT DRUG CONCENTRATIONS	DOSING RECOMMENDATIONS AND CLINICAL COMMENTS
Proton Pump Inhibitors (PPIs)	ATV	↓ ATV	**PPIs are not recommended in patients receiving unboosted ATV.** In these patients, consider alternative acid-reducing agents, ritonavir-boosting, or alternative PIs.
	ATV/r	↓ ATV	PPIs should not exceed a dose equivalent to omeprazole 20 mg daily in treatment-naïve patients. PPIs should be administered >12 h prior to ATV/r. **PPIs are not recommended in treatment-experienced patients.**
	DRV/r, FPV + RTV, LPV/r	No effect	
	IDV + RTV	No data	
	NFV	NFV AUC ↓ 36% M8 AUC ↓ 92%	**Do not coadminister PPIs and NFV.**
	SQV/r	SQV AUC ↑ 82%	Monitor for SQV toxicities.
	TPV/r	↓ Omeprazole, TPV: no effect	May need to increase omeprazole dose.
Antifungals			
Fluconazole	**RTV-boosted PI**		
	ATV/r	No effect	
	DRV/r, FPV/r, IDV/r, LPV/r	No data	
	SQV/r	No data with RTV-boosting; SQV AUC ↑ 50%, C_{max} ↑ 56% with SQV 1200 mg tid	
	TPV/r	TPV AUC ↑ 50%, C_{max} ↑ 32%, C_{min} ↑ 69%	Fluconazole >200 mg daily not recommended.
	PIs without RTV		
	ATV, FPV, NFV	No data	
	IDV	No effect	

(continued)

PI DRUG INTERACTIONS TABLE (*continued*)

CONCOMITANT DRUG CLASS/NAME	PROTEASE INHIBITOR (PI)	EFFECT ON PI OR CONCOMITANT DRUG CONCENTRATIONS	DOSING RECOMMENDATIONS AND CLINICAL COMMENTS
Itraconazole	**RTV-boosted PI**		
	ATV/r, DRV/r, FPV/r, IDV/r, TPV/r	No data	Potential for bidirectional inhibition between itraconazole and PIs. Consider monitoring itraconazole level to guide dosage adjustments. High doses (>200 mg/d) are not recommended.
	LPV/r	↑ itraconazole	Consider not exceeding 200 mg itraconazole daily, or monitor itraconazole level.
	SQV/r	Bidirectional interaction has been observed.	Dose not established, but decreased itraconazole dosage may be warranted. Consider monitoring itraconazole level.
	PIs without RTV		
	ATV, FPV, NFV	No data	Potential for bidirectional inhibition between itraconazole and PIs. Consider monitoring itraconazole level to guide dosage adjustments.
	IDV	↑ IDV IDV 600 mg q8h + itraconazole 200 mg bid: AUC similar to IDV 800 mg q8h	Dose: IDV 600 mg q8h (without ritonavir); Do not exceed 200 mg itraconazole bid. Dosing of IDV when used with ritonavir and itraconazole not established.
Ketoconazole	**RTV-boosted PI**		
	ATV/r, FPV/r	↑ Ketoconazole levels	Use with caution. Do not exceed 200 mg ketoconazole daily.
	DRV/r	DRV AUC ↑ 42%, ketoconazole ↑ 3-fold	
	IDV/r	No data	
	LPV/r	May ↑ or ↓ LPV, ketoconazole ↑ 3-fold	Potential for bidirectional interaction between ketoconazole and IDV/r, SQV/r, TPV/r.
	SQV/r	SQV ↑ 3× (when ketoconazole used with unboosted SQV)	
	TPV/r	No data	

(*continued*)

PI DRUG INTERACTIONS TABLE (*continued*)

CONCOMITANT DRUG CLASS/NAME	PROTEASE INHIBITOR (PI)	EFFECT ON PI OR CONCOMITANT DRUG CONCENTRATIONS	DOSING RECOMMENDATIONS AND CLINICAL COMMENTS
	PIs without RTV		
	ATV, NFV		No dosage adjustment necessary.
	FPV	No data with FPV ↑ APV ↑ Ketoconazole	Consider ketoconazole dose reduction if dose is >400 mg/d. Presumably similar interaction as seen with APV: APV ↑ 31%; ketoconazole ↑ 44%
	IDV	↑ IDV	Dose: IDV 600 mg q8h. Levels: IDV ↑ 68% IDV dosage when used with ritonavir and ketoconazole has not been established.
Posaconazole Voriconazole	All PIs	No data	
	RTV-boosted PI		
	ATV/r, DRV/r, FPV/r, IDV/r, LPV/r, SQV/r, TPV/r	Voriconazole AUC ↓ 82% with RTV 400 mg bid and ↓ 39% with RTV 100 mg bid	Administration of voriconazole and RTV 100 mg once daily or bid is not recommended unless benefit outweighs risk. Consider monitoring voriconazole level. **Administration of voriconazole and RTV 400 mg bid or higher is contraindicated.**
	PIs without RTV		
	ATV FPV NFV	No data	Potential for bidirectional inhibition between voriconazole and PIs. Monitor for toxicities.
	IDV	No significant effect	No dose adjustment.
Anticonvulsants Carbamazepine Phenobarbital Phenytoin	**RTV-boosted PI**		
	ATV/r, DRV/r, IDV/r, LPV/r SQV/r, TPV/r	↑ Carbamazepine ↓ PI level	Consider alternative anticonvulsant or monitor levels of both drugs.
	FPV/r	↓ phenytoin ↑ APV	Monitor anticonvulsant level, and adjust dose accordingly. No change in FPV/r dose recommended.

(continued)

PI DRUG INTERACTIONS TABLE (*continued*)

CONCOMITANT DRUG CLASS/NAME	PROTEASE INHIBITOR (PI)	EFFECT ON PI OR CONCOMITANT DRUG CONCENTRATIONS	DOSING RECOMMENDATIONS AND CLINICAL COMMENTS
	LPV/r	↓ Phenytoin ↓ Phenobarbital ↓ LPV/r level May ↓ other PI levels	Consider alternative anticonvulsant or monitor levels of both drugs.
	PIs without RTV		
	ATV FPV NFV	No data May ↓ PI levels substantially NFV ↓ phenytoin	Monitor anticonvulsant level and virologic response. Consider alternative anticonvulsant, RTV boosting for ATV and FPV, and/or monitoring PI level.
	IDV	↓ IDV	Consider alternative anticonvulsant, RTV boosting, and/or monitoring IDV level.
Antimycobacterials			
Clarithromycin	ATV + RTV	Clarithromycin AUC ↑ 94%	May cause QTc prolongation. Reduce clarithromycin dose by 50%. Consider alternative therapy.
	DRV/r IDV + RTV LPV/r SQV/r TPV/r	DRV/r ↑ Clar AUC 57%; IDV ↑ Clar AUC 53%; LPV/r ↑ Clar AUC 77%; RTV ↑ Clar 77%; SQV ↑ Clar 45%; Clar ↑ SQV 177%; TPV/r ↑ Clar 19% and ↓ active Metabolite 97%; Clar ↑ TPV 66%	Reduce clarithromycin dose by 50% in patients with Cl$_{Cr}$ 30–60 mL/min. Reduce clarithromycin dose by 75% in patients with Cl$_{Cr}$ <30 mL/min.
	FPV	↑ APV	No dose adjustment.
	NFV	No data	
Rifabutin	**RTV-boosted PI**		
	ATV + RTV FPV/r DRV/r IDV/r LPV/r SQVr TPV/r	ATV ↑ rifabutin AUC 2.5-fold; FPV/r, DRV/r, IDV/r: no PK data, expect ↑ rifabutin; RTV (500 mg bid) ↑ rifabutin 4 times; LPV/r ↑ rifabutin AUC 3-fold, ↑ 25-O-desacetyl	Rifabutin 150 mg qod or 3 times/wk. Acquired rifamycin resistance has been reported in patients with inadequate rifabutin levels while on 150 mg twice weekly and RTV-boosted PIs.

(*continued*)

PI DRUG INTERACTIONS TABLE (*continued*)

CONCOMITANT DRUG CLASS/NAME	PROTEASE INHIBITOR (PI)	EFFECT ON PI OR CONCOMITANT DRUG CONCENTRATIONS	DOSING RECOMMENDATIONS AND CLINICAL COMMENTS
		metabolite 47.5-fold; rifabutin ↓ unboosted SQV 40%; TPV/r ↑ rifabutin AUC 2.9- fold, ↑ 25-0-desacetyl metabolite 20.7-fold	May consider therapeutic drug monitoring and adjust dose accordingly.
	PIs without RTV		
	FPV	↑ Rifabutin	Rifabutin 150 mg daily or 300 mg 3 times/wk
	IDV	↑ Rifabutin ↓ IDV	Rifabutin 150 mg daily or 300 mg 3 times/wk + IDV 1,000 mg q8h or consider RTV boosting. Levels: rifabutin ↑ 2 times, IDV ↓ 32%
	NFV	↑ Rifabutin 2 times; ↓ NFV 750 mg q8h 32%	Rifabutin 150 mg daily or 300 mg 3 times/wk
Rifampin	All PIs	Approximately >75% ↓ in PI	**Do not coadminister rifampin and PIs.**
Benzodiazepines			
Alprazolam Diazepam	All PIs	May ↑ benzodiazepine levels RTV 200 mg bid × 2 days ↑ Alprazolam half-life 200% and AUC 248%	Consider alternative benzodiazepines such as lorazepam, oxazepam, or temazepam
Lorazepam Oxazepam Temazepam	All PIs	No data	Metabolism of these benzodiazepines via non-CYP450 pathways decreases interaction potential compared with other benzodiazepines.
Midazolam	All PIs	↑ Midazolam SQV/r ↑ midazolam (oral) AUC 1144%, ↑ C_{max} 327%	**Do not coadminister oral midazolam and PIs.** Parenteral midazolam can be used with caution as a single dose and can be given in a monitored situation for procedural sedation.

(continued)

PI DRUG INTERACTIONS TABLE (*continued*)

CONCOMITANT DRUG CLASS/NAME	PROTEASE INHIBITOR (PI)	EFFECT ON PI OR CONCOMITANT DRUG CONCENTRATIONS	DOSING RECOMMENDATIONS AND CLINICAL COMMENTS
Triazolam	All PIs	RTV 200 mg bid: ↑ triazolam AUC by 20 times; Other PIs: no data; may significantly ↑ triazolam concentration	**Do not coadminister triazolam and PIs.**
Calcium Channel Blockers			
Dihydropyridine	ATV + RTV	No data	Caution warranted with ATV. Dose titration should be considered as well as ECG monitoring.
	DRV/r, FPV + RTV, NFV, TPV/r	No data	
	IDV/r	↑ Amlodipine	Monitor closely.
	LPV/r	↑ Dihydropyridine	Caution is warranted and
	SQV/r		clinical monitoring of patients is recommended.
Diltiazem	ATV + RTV	↑ Diltiazem AUC 125%	Decrease diltiazem dose by 50%. ECG monitoring is recommended.
	DRV/r, FPV + RTV, IDV + RTV, LPV/r, NFV, TPV/r	No data	Potential for ↑ diltiazem level.
	SQV/r	↑ Diltiazem	Caution is warranted, and clinical monitoring of patients is recommended.
Herbal Products			
St. John's wort	All PIs	↓ PI	Administration of St. John's wort with PIs is not recommended.
Hormonal Contraceptives			
Hormonal Contraceptives	**RTV-boosted PI** ATV/r	↓ Ethinyl estradiol ↑ Progestin	Oral contraceptive should contain at least 35 μg of ethinyl estradiol. Oral contraceptives containing progestins other than norethindrone or norgestimate have not been studied.

(continued)

PI DRUG INTERACTIONS TABLE (*continued*)

CONCOMITANT DRUG CLASS/NAME	PROTEASE INHIBITOR (PI)	EFFECT ON PI OR CONCOMITANT DRUG CONCENTRATIONS	DOSING RECOMMENDATIONS AND CLINICAL COMMENTS
	DRV/r, IDV/r	No data	Use alternative or additional method because of possible interaction.
	FPV/r	↓ Ethinyl estradiol AUC 37%; ↓ Norethindrone AUC 34%; APV: no change	Use alternative or additional method.
	LPV/r	↓ Ethinyl estradiol 42%	Use alternative or additional method.
	SQV/r	↓ Ethinyl estradiol	Use alternative or additional method.
	TPV/r	↓ Ethinyl estradiol C_{max} and AUC ↓ approximately 50%	Use alternative or additional method. Used as hormone replacement therapy, monitor clinically for signs of estrogen deficiency.
	PIs without RTV		
	ATV	↑ Ethinyl estradiol AUC 48%; ↑ norethindrone AUC 110%	Oral contraceptive should contain no more than 30 μg of ethinyl estradiol, or use alternate method. Oral contraceptives containing less than 25 μg of ethinyl estradiol or progestins other than norethindrone or norgestimate have not been studied.
	FPV	With APV: ↑ ethinyl estradiol, ↑ norethindrone, ↓ APV 20%	Use alternative method.
	IDV	↑ Ethinyl estradiol; ↑ norethindrone	No dose adjustment.
	NFV	Ethinyl estradiol ↓ 47%; norethindrone ↓ 18%	Use alternative or additional method.
HMG-CoA Reductase Inhibitors			
Atorvastatin	All PIs	↑ Atorvastatin; DRV/r + atorvastatin 10 mg similar to atorvastatin 40 mg alone;	Use lowest possible starting dose with careful monitoring, or consider other HMG-CoA reductase

(continued)

PI DRUG INTERACTIONS TABLE (*continued*)

CONCOMITANT DRUG CLASS/NAME	PROTEASE INHIBITOR (PI)	EFFECT ON PI OR CONCOMITANT DRUG CONCENTRATIONS	DOSING RECOMMENDATIONS AND CLINICAL COMMENTS
		FPV ↑ atorvastatin AUC 150%; LPV/r ↑ atorvastatin AUC 5.88-fold; NFV ↑ atorvastatin AUC 74%; SQV/r ↑ atorvastatin levels 450%; TPV/r ↑ atorvastatin AUC 9-fold	inhibitors with less potential for interaction.
Lovastatin	All PIs	Significant ↑ lovastatin level	**Contraindicated—do not coadminister.**
Pravastatin	DRV/r	Mean ↑ in pravastatin AUC 81% and up to 5-fold in some patients	Use lowest possible starting dose with careful monitoring.
	LPV/r	↑ Pravastatin	No dose adjustment necessary.
	NFV, SQV/r	↓ Pravastatin	No dose adjustment necessary.
	TPV/r, ATV, FPV, IDV	No data	
Rosuvastatin	ATV +/− RTV, DRV/r, FPV +/− RTV, IDV +/− RTV, NFV, SQV/r	No data potential for ↑ rosuvastatin level.	Use lowest possible starting dose with careful monitoring, or consider other HMG-CoA reductase inhibitors with less potential for interaction.
	LPV/r	Rosuvastatin AUC ↑ 2.1-fold and C_{max} ↑ 4.7-fold	Use lowest possible starting dose with careful monitoring for rosuvastatin toxicities, or consider other HMG-CoA reductase inhibitors with less potential for interaction.
	TPV/r	Rosuvastatin AUC ↑ 37% and C_{max} ↑ 123%	Use lowest possible starting dose with monitoring for rosuvastatin toxicities, or consider other HMG-CoA reductase inhibitors with less potential for interaction.

(continued)

PI DRUG INTERACTIONS TABLE (*continued*)

CONCOMITANT DRUG CLASS/NAME	PROTEASE INHIBITOR (PI)	EFFECT ON PI OR CONCOMITANT DRUG CONCENTRATIONS	DOSING RECOMMENDATIONS AND CLINICAL COMMENTS
Simvastatin	All PIs	Significant ↑ simvastatin level; NFV ↑ simvastatin AUC 505%	**Contraindicated—do not coadminister.**
Methadone			
Methadone	**RTV-boosted PI** ATV/r, FPV/r, DRV/r, IDV/r, LPV/r, SQV/r, TPV/r	↓ Methadone levels: ATV/r ↓ R-methadone AUC 16%; DRV/r ↓ R-methadone AUC 16%; FPV/r ↓ R-methadone AUC 18%; LPV/r ↓ methadone AUC 26%–53%; SQV/r 1,000/100 mg bid ↓ methadone AUC 19%; TPV/r ↓ R-methadone AUC 48%	Opiate withdrawal unlikely but may occur. No adjustment in methadone usually required but monitor for opiate withdrawal and increase methadone dose as clinically indicated. R-methadone is the active form of methadone.
	PIs without RTV ATV, IDV FPV	No effect No data with FPV; with APV, R-methadone levels ↓ 13%	Monitor and titrate methadone as clinically indicated. The interaction with FPV is presumed to be similar.
	NFV	NFV ↓ methadone AUC 40%	Opiate withdrawal rarely occurs. Monitor and titrate dose as clinically indicated. May require ↑ methadone dose.
Phosphodiesterase Type 5 Inhibitors			
Sildenafil	All PIs	↑ Sildenafil; APV ↑ sildenafil AUC 2- to 11-fold; DRV/r + sildenafil 25 mg similar to sildenafil 100 mg alone; IDV ↑ sildenafil AUC 3-fold; LPV/r ↑ sildenafil 11-fold;	Sildenafil: start with 25 mg every 48 h and monitor for adverse effects of sildenafil.

(*continued*)

PI DRUG INTERACTIONS TABLE (*continued*)

CONCOMITANT DRUG CLASS/NAME	PROTEASE INHIBITOR (PI)	EFFECT ON PI OR CONCOMITANT DRUG CONCENTRATIONS	DOSING RECOMMENDATIONS AND CLINICAL COMMENTS
		NFV ↑ sildenafil 2- to 11-fold; RTV ↑ sildenafil AUC 11-fold	
Tadalafil	All PIs	LPV/r ↑ tadalafil AUC 124%	Tadalafil: start with 5 mg dose and do not exceed a single dose of 10 mg every 72 h. Monitor for adverse effects of tadalafil.
Vardenafil	All PIs	↑ Vardenafil; IDV ↑ vardenafil AUC 16-fold, ↓ IDV AUC 30%; RTV ↑ vardenafil AUC 49-fold, ↓ RTV AUC 20%	Vardenafil: start with 2.5 mg every 72 h and monitor for adverse effects of vardenafil.

From Ref. 38.

PI DRUG-SPECIFIC INTERACTIONS

PROTEASE INHIBITOR (PI)	CONCOMITANT DRUG CLASS/NAME	EFFECT ON PI OR CONCOMITANT DRUG CONCENTRATIONS	DOSING RECOMMENDATIONS AND CLINICAL COMMENTS
DRV/r	**Paroxetine** **Sertraline**	↓ Paroxetine ↓ Sertraline	Monitor closely for antidepressant response. Carefully titrate SSRI dose based on clinical assessment.
IDV	**Grapefruit juice**	↓ IDV	Monitor for virologic responses.
RTV	**Vitamin C >1 g/d** **Desipramine**	↓ IDV RTV ↑ desipramine 145%	Reduce desipramine dose.
	Trazodone	RTV 200 mg bid ↑ trazodone AUC 2.4-fold	Use lowest dose of trazodone, and monitor for CNS and CV adverse effects.
	Theophylline	RTV ↓ theophylline 47%.	Monitor theophylline levels.
SQV	**Grapefruit juice** **Dexamethasone**	↑ SQV ↓ SQV	

From Ref. 38.

■ REFERENCES

1. Elion GB. Acyclovir: discovery, mechanism of action, and selectivity. *J Med Virol*. 1993;(suppl 1):2-6.
2. Whitley RJ, Gnann JW. Acyclovir: a decade later. *N Engl J Med*. 1992;327:782-789.
3. Nikkels AF, Pierard GE. Recognition and treatment of shingles. *Drugs*. 1994;48:528-588.
4. Weller S et al. Pharmacokinetics of the acyclovir pro-drug valaciclovir after escalating single- and multiple-dose administration to normal volunteers. *Clin Pharmacol Ther*. 1993;54:595-605.
5. Soul–Lawton J et al. Absolute bioavailability and metabolic disposition of valaciclovir, the L-valyl ester of acyclovir, following oral administration to humans. *Antimicrob Agents Chemother*. 1995;39:2759-2764.
6. Jacobson MA. Valaciclovir (BW256U87): the L-valyl ester of acyclovir. *J Med Virol*. 1993;(suppl 1):150-153.
7. Laskin OL. Acyclovir, pharmacology and clinical experience. *Arch Intern Med*. 1984;144:1241-1246.
8. Cundy KC et al. Clinical pharmacokinetics of cidofovir in human immunodeficiency virus–infected patients. *Antimicrob Agents Chemother*. 1995;39:1247-1252.
9. Lalezari JP et al. (S)-1-[3-hydroxy-2-(phosphonylmethoxy)propyl]cytosine (cidofovir): results of a phase I/II study of a novel antiviral nucleotide analogue. *J Infect Dis*. 1995;171:788-796.
10. Flaherty JF. Current and experimental therapeutic options for cytomegalovirus disease. *Am J Health Syst Pharm*. 1996;53(suppl 2):S4-S11.
11. Matthews T et al. Enfuvirtide: the first therapy to inhibit the entry of HIV-1 into host CD4 lymphocytes. *Nat Rev Drug Discov*. 2004;3:215-225.
12. Zhang X et al. Population pharmacokinetics of enfuvirtide in HIV-1-infected pediatric patients over 48 weeks of treatment. *J Clin Pharmacol*. 2007;47:510-517.
13. Lalezari J et al. Enfuvirtide, an HIV-1 fusion inhibitor, for drug-resistant HIV infection in North and South America. *N Eng J Med*. 2003;348:2175-2185.
14. Pue MA et al. Linear pharmacokinetics of penciclovir following administration of single oral doses of famciclovir 125, 250, 500 and 750 mg to healthy volunteers. *J Antimicrob Chemother*. 1994;33:119-127.
15. Perry CM, Wagstaff AJ. Famciclovir: a review of its pharmacological properties and therapeutic efficacy in herpesvirus infections. *Drugs*. 1995;50:396-415.
16. Saoka SL, Wilson B, Famciclovir/penciclovir. In: Mills J, ed. *Antiviral Chemotherapy*. Vol 5. New York: Kluwer Academic/Plenum Publishers; 1999:135-147.
17. Minor JR, Baltz JK. Foscarnet sodium. *DICP*. 1991;25:41-47.
18. Wagstaff AJ, Bryson HM. Foscarnet. A reappraisal of its antiviral activity, pharmacokinetic properties and therapeutic use in immunocompromised patients with viral infections. *Drugs*. 1994;48:199-226.
19. Sasadeusz JJ, Sacks SL. Systemic antivirals in herpesvirus infections. *Dermatol Clin*. 1993;11:171-185.
20. Jacobson MA et al. Foscarnet induced hypocalcemia and effects of foscarnet on calcium metabolism. *J Clin Endocrinol Metab*. 1991;72:1130-1135.
21. Crumpacker CS. Ganciclovir. *N Engl J Med*. 1996;335:721-729.
22. Sommadossi J-P et al. Clinical pharmacokinetics of ganciclovir in patients with normal and impaired renal function. *Rev Infect Dis*. 1988;10(suppl 3):S507-S514.
23. Morris DJ. Adverse effects and drug interactions of clinical importance with antiviral drugs. *Drug Saf*. 1994;10:281-291.
24. Erice A et al. Progressive disease due to ganciclovir-resistant cytomegalovirus in immunocompromised patients. *N Engl J Med*. 1989;320:289-293.
25. Dorr P et al. Maraviroc (UK-427,857), a potent, orally bioavailable, and selective small-molecule inhibitor of chemokine receptor ccr5 with broad-spectrum anti human immunodeficiency virus type 1 activity. *Antimicrob Agents Chemother*. 2005;49:4721-4732.
26. Abel S et al. Assessment of the pharmacokinetics, safety and tolerability of maraviroc, a novel CCR5 antagonist, in healthy volunteers. *Br J Clin Pharmacol*. 2008;65:5-18.
27. Abel S et al. Assessment of the absorption, metabolism and absolute bioavailability of maraviroc in healthy male subjects. *Br J Clin Pharmacol*. 2008;65:60-67.
28. Kondru R et al. Molecular interactions of CCR5 with major classes of small-molecule anti-HIV CCR5 antagonists. *Mol Pharmacol*. 2006;73:789-800.
29. Lalezari J et al. Efficacy and safety of maraviroc in antiretroviral treatment-experienced patients infected with CCR5-tropic HIV-1: 48-week results of MOTIVATE 1. Program and abstracts of the 47th Annual Interscience Conference on Antimicrobial Agents and Chemotherapy; September 17-20, 2007; Chicago, Illinois. Abstract H-718a. http://www.abstractsonline.com/viewer/viewAbstractPrintFriendly.asp? Accessed July 26, 2008.
30. Fätkenheuer G et al. Efficacy and Safety of Maraviroc (MVC) Plus Optimized Background Therapy (OBT) in Viremic, Antiretroviral Treatment-Experienced Patients Infected with CCR5-Tropic (R5) HIV-1 in Europe, Australia and North America (MOTIVATE 2): 48-Week Results. Abstract PS3/5. 11th European AIDS Conference/ EACS; 2007; Madrid, Spain. http://www.eacs.eu/conference/madrid07/pdf2.php?pdf=ABS00015. Accessed July 26, 2008.

31. Maraviroc Tablets NDA 22-128. Antiviral Drugs Advistory Committee Briefing Document. April 24, 2007. http://www.fda.gov/OHRMS/DOCKETS/AC/07/briefing/2007-4283b1-01-Pfizer.pdf. Accessed July 24, 2008.

32. Grobler JA et al. HIV-1 reverse transcriptase plus-strand initiation exhibits preferential sensitivity to non-nucleoside reverse transcriptase inhibitors in vitro. *J Biol Chem.* 2007;282:8005-8010.

33. Ruxrungtham K et al. Impact of reverse transcriptase resistance on the efficacy of TMC125 (etravirine) with two nucleoside reverse transcriptase inhibitors in protease inhibitor-naïve, nonnucleoside reverse transcriptase inhibitor-experienced patients: study TMC125-C227. *HIV Med.* 2008;9:883-896.

34. Intelence® [package insert]. Raritan, NJ: Tibotec Therapeutics; January 2008.

35. Rescriptor® [package insert]. New York: Pfizer, Inc.; June 2006.

36. Sustiva® [package insert]. Princeton, NJ: Bristol-Myers Squibb Co; March 2008.

37. Viramune® [package insert]. Ridgefield, CT: Boehringer Ingelheim Pharmaceuticals, Inc.; June 2008.

38. Panel on Antiretroviral Guidelines for Adults and Adolescents. Guidelines for the Use of Antiretroviral Agents in HIV–1–Infected Adults and Adolescents. Department of Health and Human Services. November 3, 2008; 1–139. http://www.aidsinfo.nih.gov/ContentFiles/AdultandAdolescentGL.pdf. Accessed March 18, 2009.

39. Clifford D et al. Impact of efavirenz on neuropsychological performance and symptoms in HIV–infected individuals. *Ann Intern Med.* 2005;143:714-721.

40. Haas DW et al. Pharmacogenetics of efavirenz and central nervous system side effects: an adult AIDS Clinical Trials Group study. *AIDS.* 2004;18:2391-2400.

41. Stern JO et al. A comprehensive hepatic safety analysis of nevirapine in different populations of HIV infected patients. *J Acquir Immune Defic Syndr.* 2003;34(suppl 1):S21-S33.

42. Roder CS et al. Misleading results of screening for illicit drugs during efavirenz treatment. *AIDS.* 2007;21:1390-1391.

43. St Clair MH et al. 3'-Azido-3'deoxythymidine triphosphate as an inhibitor and substrate of purified human immunodeficiency virus reverse transcriptase. *Antimicrob Agents Chemother.* 1987;31:1972-1977.

44. Abacavir® [package insert]. Research Triangle Park, NC: GlaxoSmithKline; July 2008.

45. Yuen GJ et al. A review of the pharmacokinetics of abacavir. *Clin Pharmacokinet.* 2008;47:351-371.

46. Brinkman K et al. Adverse effects of reverse transcriptase inhibitors: mitochondrial toxicity as common pathway. *AIDS.* 1998;12:1735-1744.

47. Birkus G et al. Assessment of mitochondrial toxicity in human cells treated with tenofovir: comparison with other nucleoside reverse transcriptase inhibitors. *Antimicrob Agents Chemother.* 2002;46:716-723.

48. Flexner C. HIV-protease inhibitors. *N Engl J Med.* 1998;338:1281-1292.

49. Hammer SM et al. Antiretroviral treatment of adult HIV infection: recommendations of the international AIDS society USA panel. *JAMA.* 2008;300:555-570.

50. Hirsh MS et al. Antiretroviral drug resistance testing in adults infected with human immunodeficiency virus type 1: 2003 recommendations of an International AIDS Soceity-USA Panel. *Clin Infect Dis.* 2003;37:113-128.

51. Hazuda DJ et al. Inhibitors of strand transfer that prevent integration and inhibit HIV-1 replication in cells. *Science.* 2000;287:646-650.

52. Pommier Y et al. Integrase inhibitors to treat HIV/AIDS. *Nat Rev Drug Discov.* 2005;4:236-248.

53. Markowitz M et al. Antiretroviral activity, pharmacokinetics, and tolerability of KM-0518, a novel inhibitors of HIV-1 integrase, dosed as monotherapy for 10 days in treatment-naïve HIV-1-infected individuals. *J Acquir Immune Defic Syndr.* 2006;43509-43515.

54. Iwamoto M et al. Safety, tolerability, and pharmacokinetics of raltegravir after single and multiple doses in healthy subjects. *Clin Pharmacol Ther.* 2008;83:293-299.

55. Steigbigel RT et al. Raltegravir withoptmized background therapy for resistant HIV-1 infection. *N Engl J Med.* 2008;259:339-354.

56. Isentress® [package insert]. Whitehouse Station, NJ: Merck & Co., Inc.; October 2007.

57. Colman PM. A novel approach to antiviral therapy for influenza. *J Antimicrob Chemother.* 1999;44(suppl B):17-22.

58. Bardsley-Elliot A, Noble S. Oseltamivir. *Drugs.* 1999;58:851-860.

59. Anon. Two neuraminidase inhibitors for treatment of influenza. *Med Lett Drugs Ther.* 1999;41:91-93.

60. Long JK et al. Antiviral agents for treating influenza. *Cleve Clin J Med.* 2000;67:92-95.

61. Rayner CR et al. Population pharmacokinetics of oseltamivir when coadministered with probenecid. *J Clin Pharmacol.* 2008;48:935-947.

62. Dunn CJ, Goa KL. Zanamivir a review of its use in influenza. *Drugs.* 1999;58:761-784.

63. Working Group on Antiretroviral Therapy and Medical Management of HIV-Infected Children. Guidelines for the Use of Antiretroviral Agents in Pediatric HIV Infection. February 23, 2009; 1–139. http://aidsinfo.nih.gov/ContentFiles/PediatricGuidelines.pdf. Accessed March 18, 2009.

β-Lactams

Christopher Betz and Courtney M. Brown

PENICILLINS

Penicillin antibiotics are generally considered bactericidal due to inhibition of cell wall synthesis. The basic structure of penicillin consists of a thiazolidine ring, the β-lactam ring, and a side chain. This side chain is largely responsible for determining the spectrum of activity. Penicillins can be divided into five classes based on antibacterial activity: natural penicillins, penicillinase resistant penicillins, aminopenicillins, carboxypenicillins, and ureidopenicillins.[1] For the purpose of this chapter, carboxypenicillins and ureidopenicillins will be collectively known as extended spectrum penicillins.

AMINOPENICILLINS

AMOXICILLIN · Amoxil, Various

Pharmacology. Amoxicillin differs from ampicillin by the presence of a hydroxyl group on the amino side chain. It has activity essentially identical to ampicillin.[1,2] (*See* Ampicillin and β-Lactams Chart.)

Administration and Adult Dosage. PO—250–500 mg every 8 h OR 500–875 mg twice daily, to a maximum of 4.5 g/d. **PO for endocarditis prophylaxis**—2 g 1 h before dental or upper airway procedures.

Pediatric Dosage. PO—20–40 mg/kg/d in 3 equally divided doses every 8 h. **PO for endocarditis prophylaxis**—50 mg/kg 1 h before dental or upper airway procedures.

Dosage Forms. **Cap** 250, 500 mg; **Chew Tab** 125, 200, 250, 400 mg; **Drp** 50 mg/mL; **Susp** 25, 50 mg/mL; **Tab** 500, 875 mg.

Pharmacokinetics. Amoxicillin is completely absorbed, with approximately 85% bioavailability because of a small first-pass effect. Serum concentrations are greater than those after equal doses of ampicillin; postabsorptive pharmacokinetics are identical to those of ampicillin.

Adverse Reactions. Adverse effects are similar to those of ampicillin, although diarrhea and rashes are much less frequent with amoxicillin.

AMOXICILLIN AND POTASSIUM CLAVULANATE · Augmentin

Pharmacology. Clavulanic acid has weak antibacterial activity but is a potent inhibitor of plasmid-mediated β-lactamases, including those produced by *Haemophilus influenzae*, *Moraxella (Branhamella) catarrhalis*, *Staphylococcus aureus*, *Neisseria gonorrhoeae*, and *Bacteroides fragilis*. Thus, when combined with certain other β-lactam antibiotics, the combination is very active against many bacteria resistant to the β-lactam alone.[3,4]

Administration and Adult Dosage. **PO**—1 250 mg or 500 mg tablet every 8 h or 875 mg tablet every 12 h. (*See* Dosage Forms.)

Pediatric Dosage. **PO**—20–40 mg/kg/d (of the amoxicillin component) in 3 divided doses or 45 mg/kg/d in 2 divided doses. (*See* Dosage Forms.)

Dosage Forms. Do not substitute combinations of lower-dose tablets to make a higher dose because diarrhea is markedly increased. **Tab** (8 h) 250 mg amoxicillin/125 mg clavulanic acid, 500 mg amoxicillin/125 mg clavulanic acid; (12 h) 875 mg amoxicillin/125 mg clavulanic acid; **Chew Tab** (8 h) 125 mg amoxicillin/31.25 mg clavulanic acid, 250 mg amoxicillin/62.5 mg clavulanic acid; (12 h) 200 mg amoxicillin/28.5 mg clavulanic acid, 400 mg amoxicillin/57 mg clavulanic acid; **Susp** (8 h) 25 mg amoxicillin/6.25 mg clavulanic acid/mL, 50 mg amoxicillin/12.5 mg clavulanic acid/mL; (12 h) 40 mg amoxicillin/5.7 mg clavulanic acid/mL, 80 mg amoxicillin/11.4 mg clavulanic acid/mL.

Pharmacokinetics. Peak serum clavulanate concentration is 2.6 mg/L 40–60 min after an oral dose of 250 mg amoxicillin/125 mg clavulanate. Amoxicillin pharmacokinetics are not affected by clavulanic acid. Clavulanic acid half-life is approximately 60 min.

Adverse Reactions. Adverse effects of this preparation include those of amoxicillin; however, diarrhea is more frequent with the combination and depends on the dosage of clavulanate. The 12-h formulations reduce the frequency of diarrhea. Nausea and diarrhea are less frequent when this preparation is administered with food. (*See* β-Lactams Chart.)

AMPICILLIN Various

Pharmacology. Ampicillin has a similar mechanism of action and is comparable in activity to penicillin G against gram-positive bacteria, but is more active than penicillin G against gram-negative bacteria.[1,2] (*See* β-Lactams Chart.)

Administration and Adult Dosage. **PO**—250–500 mg every 6 h. **IM or IV**—500 mg–3 g every 4–6 h to a maximum of 12 g/d. Give the same dose every 12 h with a Cl_{Cr} <20 mL/min. **IV or IM for endocarditis prophylaxis**—2 g within 30 min of procedure.

Pediatric Dosage. **PO**—(<20 kg) 50–100 mg/kg/d in 2–4 divided doses; (>20 kg) 100–400 mg/kg/d in 4–6 divided doses. **IV**—(neonates) 25–100 mg/kg/dose every 6–12 h, higher dosages for meningitis; (<20 kg) 50–100 mg/kg/d in 2–4 divided doses; (>20 kg) 400 mg/kg/d in 4–6 divided doses; **IV or IM for endocarditis prophylaxis**—50 mg/kg within 30 min of procedure.

Dosage Forms. **Cap** 250, 500 mg; **Susp** 25, 50, mg/mL; **Inj** 125, 250, 500 mg, 1, 2, 10 g.

Pharmacokinetics. Oral forms are approximately 50% absorbed in the fasting state; food delays absorption. Plasma protein binding is low, and therapeutic concentrations are attained in most tissues and fluids including CSF (in the presence of inflammation). Approximately 90% is excreted unchanged in urine. Half-life is 1.2 h, 2 h in neonates, increasing to 20 h in anuric patients.

Adverse Reactions. Nausea and diarrhea occur frequently with oral therapy. Other reactions include frequent skin rash (more frequent in patients receiving allopurinol and very frequent in patients with Epstein-Barr virus infection [mononucleosis]). Most of these eruptions probably are not hypersensitivity reactions but immunologically mediated. They are generally dose related (higher frequency at higher dosages), are macular rather than urticarial, and disappear with continued administration of the drug.

AMPICILLIN/SULBACTAM
Unasyn

Pharmacology. Sulbactam is a β-lactamase inhibitor, which when added to ampicillin protects it from hydrolysis by β-lactamase. Although sulbactam lacks significant antimicrobial activity alone, it does offer additional coverage against both *Neisseria* and *Acinetobacter* species. Ampicillin/sulbactam demonstrates high rates of susceptibility toward *Streptococcus pneumoniae, H. influenzae, Moraxella catarrhalis,* and *Bateroides fragillis.* Amid *Enterobacteriaceae* it exhibits moderate activity against *Escherichia coli, Klebsiella pneumoniae, Citrobacter, and Proteus spp.* However, susceptibility rates are less then those of aminoglycosides, carbapenems, third- or fourth-generation cephalosporins, and piperacillin/tazobactam. Additionally, *Enterobacter, Morganella, and Serratia* exhibit high rates of resistance to ampicillin/sulbactam, while *Pseudomonas aeruginosa* and *Enterobacteriaceae* that produce extended-spectrum β-lactamases will not respond at all.[5]

Administration and Adult Dosage. *IM/IV*—1.5–3 g every 6 h, to a maximum of 12 g/d.

Special Populations. *Pediatric Dosage.* (≥1 year) 300 mg/kg/d in equally divided doses every 6 h (300 mg/kg/d = 200 mg ampicillin/100 mg sulbactam/kg/d); (≥ 40 kg) same as adult dosage.

Geriatric Dosage. Same as adult dosage but adjust for age-related reduction in renal function.

Other Conditions. Reduce dosage with renal insufficiency as follows: Cl_{Cr} 15–30 mL/min, give every 12 h; Cl_{Cr} 5–15 mL/min, give every 24 h.

Dosage Forms. *Inj* 1.5 g (1 g ampicillin plus 0.5 g sulbactam), 3 g (2 g ampicillin plus 1 g sulbactam).

Pharmacokinetics. *Fate.* Ampicillin/sulbactam peak concentrations are obtained immediately following a 15-min infusion. Ampicillin serum levels are similar to those produced by the administration of ampicillin alone. Peak ampicillin serum levels ranging from 109 to 150 μg/mL are attained after a 3-g administration of ampicillin/sulbactam and from 40 to 71 μg/mL after a 1.5-g administration. The analogous mean peak serum levels for sulbactam range from 48 to 88 μg/mL and from 21 to 49 μg/mL. Following IM administration of a 1.5-g dose, peak ampicillin serum levels ranging from 8 to 37 μg/mL and peak sulbactam serum levels ranging from 6 to 24 μg/mL are attained. For the first 8 h following administration roughly 75%–85% of ampicillin/sulbactam is expelled from the urine unchanged. Additionally, since ampicillin/sulbactam is primarily eliminated via the kidneys the serum concentration and half-life will be increased in patients with renal impairments. The pharmacokinetics in children and adults do not differ significantly. However, the administration of ampicillin/sulbactam should be avoided in infants <1 week gestation or premature neonates since the half-life can be significantly increased due to the urinary system underdevelopment.[5] **Half-life** (ampicillin) 1 h; (sulbactam) 1 h.

Adverse Reactions. The most prevalent adverse reaction is injection site pain following IM administration (16%). Other common adverse effects include: pain at the IV injection site, thrombophlebitis, diarrhea, and rash.

Precautions. A large percentage of patients who receive ampicillin with concomitant mononucleosis have developed a skin rash. Therefore, ampicillin/sulbactam should not be administered to patients with mononucleosis.

Drug Interactions. Probenecid has been shown to impair renal tubular secretion of ampicillin/sulbactam resulting in extended action and elevated drug concentrations. Allopurinol administered concomitantly with ampicillin has been shown to increase the incidence of rash and should be avoided.

Parameters to Monitor. Obtain renal function tests periodically.

PENICILLINASE RESISTANT PENICILLINS

CLOXACILLIN SODIUM	Cloxapen, Various
DICLOXACILLIN SODIUM	Dynapen, Various
METHICILLIN SODIUM	Staphcillin, Various
NAFCILLIN SODIUM	Nafcil, Various
OXACILLIN SODIUM	Bactocill, Various

Pharmacology. Methicillin, nafcillin, oxacillin, cloxacillin, and dicloxacillin are similar to other penicillins in their mechanism of action. However, these drugs are not hydrolyzed by staphylococcal penicillinases, which is why they are often referred to as antistaphylococcal penicillins. Therefore, nearly all isolates of *S. aureus* and some isolates of coagulase-negative staphylococci are susceptible to these drugs. Methicillin- (actually β-lactam-) resistant staphylococci have altered penicillin-binding proteins (transpeptidases). Although these drugs are used primarily in staphylococcal infection, they retain good activity against most streptococci, except enterococci.[1,6]

Administration and Adult Dosage. Oral administration of nafcillin and oxacillin is not recommended because they are poorly absorbed. (*See* β-Lactams Chart.)

Pediatric Dosage. *See* β-Lactams Chart.

Dosage Forms. *See* β-Lactams Chart.

Pharmacokinetics. Only cloxacillin and dicloxacillin are adequately absorbed from the GI tract. Except for methicillin, these drugs are mostly hepatically eliminated by metabolism and biliary excretion.

Adverse Reactions. Interstitial nephritis is frequent with methicillin but occurs only rarely with the other drugs. Hepatic damage occurs rarely with oxacillin. Nafcillin has a propensity for local irritation at the IV infusion site and causes neutropenia more frequently than other antistaphylococcal penicillins.

NATURAL PENICILLINS

PENICILLIN G AND V SALTS
Various

Pharmacology. Penicillins G and V have activity against most gram-positive organisms and some gram-negative organisms, notably *Neisseria* spp., by interfering with late stages of bacterial cell wall synthesis; resistance is caused primarily by bacterial elaboration of β-lactamases; some organisms have altered penicillin-binding protein targets (e.g., enterococci and pneumococci); others have impermeable outer cell wall layers.[1,2]

Administration and Adult Dosage. PO—(penicillin V) 125–500 mg every 6–8 h for mild to moderate infections; **IV**—(penicillin G) 2–5 million units every 4–6 h to a maximum of 24 million units/day, depending on infection. **IM**—not recommended (very painful); use benzathine or procaine penicillin G as indicated.

Special Populations. *Pediatric Dosage.* PO—(penicillin V) (<12 years) 15–50 mg/kg/d in 3–4 divided doses; (>12 years) same as adult dosage. **IV (preferably) or IM**— (penicillin G) (<1 month) 25,000–50,000 units/kg every 6–12 h; up to 400,000 units/kg/d has been used in meningitis; (>1 month) 100,000–300,000 units/kg/d in 4–6 divided doses.

Geriatric Dosage. Same as adult dosage but adjust for age related reduction in renal function.

Other Conditions. With the usual oral dosage, no dosage adjustment is required in patients with impaired renal function; however, in treating more severe infections with larger IV dosages, careful adjustment is necessary.[7]

Dosage Forms. (Penicillin G) **Inj** (as potassium salt) 1, 5, 10, 20 million units; **Inj** 1, 2, 3 million units/50 mL (frozen); **Inj** (as sodium salt) 5 million units. (Penicillin V) **Susp** 25, 50 mg/mL; **Tab** 125, 250, 500 mg (250 mg = 400,000 units).

Patient Instructions. Take this (oral) drug with a full glass of water on an empty stomach (1 h before or 2 h after meals) for best absorption; refrigerate solution.

Missed Doses. Take this drug at regular intervals. If you miss a dose, take it as soon as you remember. If it is about time for the next dose, take that dose only. Leave at least 4–6 h between doses. Do not double the dose or take an extra dose.

Pharmacokinetics. *Fate.* (Penicillin G) a peak of 20 mg/L is achieved with a dose of 12 million units IV. Widely distributed in body tissues, fluids, and cavities, with biliary levels up to 10 times serum levels; 45%–68% plasma protein bound. Penetration into CSF is poor, even with inflamed meninges; however, large parenteral dosages (>20 million units/d) adequately treat meningitis caused by susceptible organisms. (Penicillin V) oral absorption is 60%–73%, with a peak concentration of 5–6 mg/L after a 500 mg oral dose. It is approximately 80% plasma protein bound and has poor CNS penetration. For both drugs, 80%–85% of the absorbed dose is excreted unchanged in the urine.[1,2] **Half-life** (Penicillins G and V) 30–40 min; 7–10 h in patients with renal failure; 20–30 h in patients with hepatic and renal failure.[7]

Adverse Reactions. Occasionally, nausea or diarrhea occurs after usual oral doses. As with all penicillins, CNS toxicity can occur with massive IV dosages (penicillin G 60–100 million units/d) or excessive dosage in patients with impaired renal function (usually >10–20 million units/d of penicillin G in anuric patients); characterized by confusion, drowsiness, and myoclonus, which can progress to convulsions and result in death. Large dosages of the sodium salt form can result in hypernatremia and fluid overload with pulmonary edema, especially in patients with impaired renal function or heart failure. Large dosages of the potassium salt form can result in hyperkalemia, especially in patients with impaired renal function and with rapid infusions. Occasional positive Coombs' reactions with rare hemolytic anemia have been reported after large IV doses. Interstitial nephritis has been rarely reported after large IV dosages. Hypersensitivity reactions (primarily rashes) occur in 1%–10% of patients. Most serious hypersensitivity reactions follow injection rather than oral administration.[1,8]

Contraindications. History of anaphylactic, accelerated (e.g., hives), or serum sickness reaction to previous penicillin administration. (*See* Notes.)

Precautions. Use caution in patients with a history of penicillin or cephalosporin hypersensitivity reactions, atopic predisposition (e.g., asthma), impaired renal function (hence neonates and geriatric patients), impaired cardiac function, or pre-existing seizure disorder.

Drug Interactions. Physically and/or chemically incompatible with aminoglycosides leading to drug inactivation; never mix them together in the same IV solution or syringe. Probenecid competes with penicillin for renal excretion, resulting in higher and prolonged serum concentrations.[1,2]

Parameters to Monitor. Obtain renal function tests initially when using high dosages. During prolonged high-dose therapy, monitor renal function tests and serum electrolytes periodically.

Notes. Skin testing with **penicilloylpolylysine** (PPL, PrePen) and **minor determinant mixture** (MDM) can help determine the likelihood of serious reactions to penicillin in penicillin-allergic individuals.[1,9] Availability of MDM is limited; it is locally available in small amounts only at larger medical centers. Desensitization is recommended in pregnant women with syphilis and may be attempted (rarely) in patients with life-threatening infections that are likely to be responsive only to penicillin, but this is a dangerous procedure and many alternative antibiotics are available.[1] (*See* β-Lactams Chart.)

EXTENDED SPECTRUM PENICILLINS

PIPERACILLIN/TAZOBACTAM	Zosyn
TICARACILLIN	Ticar
TICARACILLIN/CLAVULANATE	Timentin

Pharmacology. The carboxypenicillin (ticarcillin) and the acylureidopenicillin (piperacillin) have the same mechanisms of action as other penicillins but are more active against enteric gram-negative bacteria and *P. aeruginosa*. Ticarcillin is not active against *Klebsiella* sp., but the acylureido derivatives have activity and are generally more potent against susceptible isolates. The acylureidopenicillins also have activity comparable to those of ampicillin against enterococci. The combination of clavulanic acid plus ticarcillin is active against *Klebsiella* sp. as well as β-lactamase-producing staphylococci, *H. influenzae*, and *Bacteroides* sp. The combination of tazobactam plus piperacillin is similar to clavulanic acid plus ticarcillin. These two combination products are not appreciably more active against *P. aeruginosa* or *Enterobacter cloacae* than ticarcillin or piperacillin alone.[1,2,4,10,11]

Administration and Adult Dosage. *See* β-Lactams Chart.

Pediatric Dosage. *See* β-Lactams Chart.

Dosage Forms. *See* β-Lactams Chart.

Pharmacokinetics. Usual half-life is 1–1.5 h, which is prolonged in anuria, although acylureido derivatives are partially metabolized and accumulate to a lesser extent. The acylureidopenicillins are also subject to capacity-limited elimination (i.e., increasing dosage results in progressive saturation of elimination pathways, resulting in decreased clearance), which allows administration of higher doses at 6- to 8-h intervals.

Adverse Reactions. Adverse effects are similar to those of other penicillins. Sodium content of the usual daily dosage of parenteral ticarcillin approaches the equivalent of 1 L of NS. Prolonged bleeding time can occur as a result of binding to platelets and prevention of platelet aggregation.

CEPHALOSPORINS

Pharmacology. Cephalosporin antibiotics have broad-spectrum activity against many gram-positive and gram-negative pathogens. These agents are generally considered to be bactericidal through binding to various penicillin-binding proteins in bacteria, which results in changes in cell wall structure and function. Members of this class are frequently subdivided into "generations" based on their antimicrobial activity (as well as order of introduction into clinical use).[12–16]

Administration and Adult Dosage. *See* β-Lactams Chart.

Special Populations. *Pediatric Dosage. See* β-Lactams Chart.

Geriatric Dosage. Same as adult dosage but adjust for age-related reduction in renal function.

Other Conditions. Most agents require dosage modification in renal dysfunction; exceptions are ceftriaxone and cefoperazone, which have biliary and renal or primarily biliary elimination, respectively.[15] Dosage reduction of all agents is required in patients with concomitant hepatic and renal dysfunction. (*See* β-Lactams Chart.)

Pharmacokinetics. Some of the greatest differences between agents reside in their pharmacokinetic properties. Of note is the improved CSF penetration of certain later-generation agents over the first-generation agents. Therapeutic CSF concentrations are achieved with cefotaxime, ceftriaxone, and ceftazidime; these agents have proven efficacy in the treatment of meningitis caused by susceptible organisms in adults and children.[12,15,16] Adequate CSF concentrations of ceftizoxime also have been observed, although its use in the treatment of meningitis is less well established. Cefuroxime penetrates adequately into CSF but is less effective for meningitis than third-generation agents.[12,17] No data are available on cefepime concentrations in the CNS, but it does cross the blood–brain barrier.

Adverse Reactions. Most cephalosporins are generally well tolerated, although a few agents have unique adverse reactions. Hypersensitivity reactions can occur in approximately 10% of patients known to be allergic to penicillin; do not administer these agents to patients with histories of an immediate reaction to penicillin.[18] Nausea and diarrhea occur with all agents; however, diarrhea is more common with ceftriaxone and cefoperazone because of high biliary excretion.[12,15,16] Colitis caused by *Clostridium difficile* has been reported with all the cephalosporins but might be more common with ceftriaxone and cefoperazone. Nephrotoxicity is rare, particularly when used without other nephrotoxic agents.[16] All agents with an *N*-methylthiotetrazole (NMTT) moiety in the 3 positions of the cephem nucleus (cefoperazone, cefamandole, cefotetan, and cefmetazole) can produce a disulfiram-like reaction in some patients with ingestion of alcohol-containing beverages. In addition, these agents might be associated to varying degrees with bleeding secondary to hypoprothrombinemia, which is corrected or prevented by vitamin K administration.[12,15,16,19] Although controversial, the mechanism of this reaction appears to involve inhibition of enzymatic reactions requiring vitamin K in the activation of prothrombin precursors by NMTT. However, other factors (e.g., malnutrition, liver disease) might be more important risk factors for bleeding than the NMTT-containing cephalosporins.[19] Thus, cautious use (and perhaps even avoidance) of agents with the NMTT side chain is recommended in patients with poor oral intake and critical illness. Administration of vitamin K and monitoring of the prothrombin time are indicated with these agents, particularly when therapy is prolonged. Positive direct Coombs' tests occur frequently but hemolysis is rare.[12,16] Ceftriaxone has been associated with biliary pseudolithiasis (sludging), which can be asymptomatic or resemble acute cholecystitis.[20] This adverse effect occurs most often with dosages greater than 2 g/d, especially in patients receiving prolonged therapy or those with impaired gallbladder emptying. The mechanism is ceftriaxone-calcium complex formation, and it is usually reversible with drug discontinuation.[20] Neonates given ceftriaxone can develop kernicterus caused by displacement of bilirubin from plasma protein binding sites; its use in this population is best avoided. Development of resistance during treatment of infections caused by *Enterobacter* spp., *Serratia* spp., and *P. aeruginosa* has occurred with all these agents.[12,15,16]

Precautions. Penicillin allergy. Use agents with NMTT side chain with caution in patients with underlying bleeding diathesis, poor oral intake, or critical illness. Use with caution in renal impairment and in those on oral anticoagulants (especially NMTT-containing drugs). Avoid use of ceftriaxone in neonates, particularly premature infants.

Drug Interactions. Avoid concomitant ingestion of alcohol or alcohol-containing products with agents containing the NMTT side chain. Probenecid reduces renal clearance and increases serum levels of most agents, except those that do not undergo renal tubular secretion (e.g., ceftazidime, ceftriaxone).

Parameters to Monitor. Monitor prothrombin time 2–3 times/wk with agents having an NMTT side chain, particularly when using large dosages; monitor bleeding time with high dosages of agents having an NMTT side chain. Obtain antimicrobial susceptibility tests for development of resistance in patients relapsing during therapy. Monitor renal function tests initially and periodically during high-dose regimens or when the drug is used concurrently with nephrotoxic agents. Monitor for diarrhea, particularly with ceftriaxone and cefoperazone; test stool specimen for *Clostridium difficile* toxin if diarrhea persists or is associated with fever or abdominal pain.

FIRST-GENERATION CEPHALOSPORINS

First-generation cephalosporins have activity against gram-positive bacteria (e.g., *Staphylococcus* sp.) and a limited, but important, number of species of aerobic gram-negative bacilli (e.g., *E. coli*, *Klebsiella* spp., *Proteus mirabilis*). *H. influenzae* and most other aerobic gram-negative bacilli often indigenous to hospitals (e.g., *Enterobacter*, *Pseudomonas* spp.) are resistant to these drugs. Anaerobic bacteria isolated in the oropharynx are generally susceptible to these agents; however, anaerobes such as *B. fragilis* are resistant.[12,16]

CEFADROXIL
Duricef

See β-Lactams Chart.

CEFAZOLIN SODIUM
Ancef, Kefzol, Various

Pharmacology. Cefazolin is a first-generation cephalosporin with activity against most gram-positive aerobic organisms except enterococci and some gram-negative bacilli (e.g., *E. coli*, *Klebsiella* sp., *Proteus mirabilis*).[14,16]

Administration and Adult Dosage. IM or IV for treatment—250 mg–2 g every 6–12 h (usually 1–2 g every 8 h), to a maximum of 12 g/d. Decrease dosage in renal impairment. (See β-Lactams Chart.) **IM or IV for surgical prophylaxis**—1 g 30–60 min before surgery. **IM or IV for endocarditis prophylaxis**—1 g within 30 min before a dental or upper airway procedure.

Pediatric Dosage. IM or IV—(≤1 month) 25 mg/kg/dose given every 8–12 h; (>1 month) 50–100 mg/kg/d in 3 divided doses given every 8 h, to a maximum of 6 g/d. **IM or IV for endocarditis prophylaxis**—25 mg/kg within 30 min before a dental or upper airway procedure.

Dosage Forms. Inj 250, 500 mg, 1, 5, 10, 20 g.

Pharmacokinetics. Cefazolin is 75%–85% plasma protein bound and widely distributed throughout the body, with high concentrations in many tissues and cavities but subtherapeutic concentrations in the CSF. Virtually 100% is excreted unchanged in the urine via filtration and secretion; the half-life is about 1.8 h, increasing to 30–40 h in renal impairment.

Adverse Reactions. *See* Cephalosporins.

CEPHALEXIN
Keflex, Various

CEPHRADINE
Velocef, Various

CEPHAPIRIN
Cefadyl

See β-Lactams Chart.

SECOND-GENERATION CEPHALOSPORINS

The second-generation cephalosporins cefamandole, cefonicid, and cefuroxime differ from first-generation agents in their improved activity against *H. influenzae* and some strains of *Enterobacter*, *Providencia*, and *Morganella* spp.[12,16] The oral second-generation cephalosporins cefuroxime axetil, cefprozil, and loracarbef (a carbacephem) have similar but less potent activity.[21–24] Cefoxitin, cefmetazole, and cefotetan (which are actually cephamycins) have increased activity against anaerobes, including *B. fragilis*;[12,25,26] the other second-generation cephalosporins have poor activity against this organism.[12]

CEFACLOR	Ceclor
CEFAMANDOLE	Mandol
CEFONICIDE	Monocid

See β-Lactams Chart.

CEFOTETAN DISODIUM	Cefotan

Pharmacology. Cefotetan is a cephamycin, structurally and pharmacologically similar to the cephalosporins, particularly second-generation agents, and it contains an *N*-methylthiotetrazole side chain. It has greater activity against enteric gram-negative bacteria than first- and second-generation cephalosporins and superior activity against *B. fragilis* and other anaerobic bacteria (comparable to cefoxitin and cefmetazole). Gram-positive activity is less than that of cefazolin.[12,25,27]

Administration and Adult Dosage. **IV or IM for treatment**—500 mg–2 g every 12–24 h (usually 1–2 g every 12 h), to a maximum of 6 g/d. **IV or IM for surgical prophylaxis**—1–2 g 30–60 min before surgery, then 1–2 g 12 h for up to 24 h postoperatively. Reconstitute the drug with 0.5% lidocaine for IM administration because IM injection is painful. Give usual dose every 24 h with a Cl_{Cr} of 10–30 mL/min, and every 48 h in patients with a Cl_{Cr} <10 mL/min.

Pediatric Dosage. Safety and efficacy not established. 40–60 mg/kg/d IV in equally divided doses every 12 h has been used.

Dosage Forms. **Inj** 1, 2, 10 g.

Pharmacokinetics. Cefotetan is excreted primarily unchanged in urine, with an elimination half-life of 3.5 h.

Adverse Reactions. *See* Cephalosporins.

CEFOXITIN	Mefoxin
CEFPROZIL	Cefzil

See β-Lactams Chart.

CEFUROXIME SODIUM	Zinacef
CEFUROXIME AXETIL	Ceftin

Pharmacology. Cefuroxime is a second-generation cephalosporin whose activity is greater than cefazolin but less than cefotaxime, against *H. influenzae*, including β-lactamase–producing strains. The activity of cefuroxime against *S. aureus* is slightly less than that of cefazolin. Its activity against anaerobes is poor, similar to the first-generation cephalosporins.[12,16,17,28]

Administration and Adult Dosage. IM or IV for treatment—750 mg–1.5 g every 8 h (every 6 h in serious infections). **IM or IV for prophylaxis**—1.5 g 1 h before surgery; doses of IM or IV 750 mg may be given every 8 h for up to 24 h postoperatively (1.5 g every 12 h to a total of 6 g for open heart surgery). Reduce parenteral dosage in renal impairment; with a Cl_{Cr} of 10–20 mL/min, give the usual dose every 12 h; with a Cl_{Cr} <10 mL/min, give the usual dose every 24 h. **PO**—125–500 mg every 12 h.

Pediatric Dosage. IM or IV—(newborns) 10–25 mg/kg every 12 h; (older infants and children) 50–100 mg/kg/d, to a maximum of 250 mg/kg/d for meningitis in 3–4 divided doses. **PO**—15–20 mg/kg every 12 h in children (40 mg/kg/d for otitis media); it may be given in applesauce.

Dosage Forms. **Inj** 750 mg, 1.5, 7.5 g; **Susp** 25, 50 mg/mL; **Tab** 125, 250, 500 mg. Do not interchange the tablets and suspension on a mg/kg basis. (*See* β-Lactams Chart.)

Pharmacokinetics. In adults, oral bioavailability appears to be lower with the suspension than with the tablets, and food increases the bioavailability of the tablets. After absorption of oral cefuroxime axetil, it is hydrolyzed in the bloodstream to cefuroxime. Cefuroxime's pharmacokinetics are similar to cefazolin's, but CSF concentrations are adequate for treatment of meningitis caused by certain organisms; however, the third-generation agents ceftriaxone and cefotaxime are superior in *H. influenzae* meningitis. Over 95% of the drug is excreted unchanged in the urine. **Half-life** 1.2 h.

Adverse Reactions. The drug is generally well tolerated. (*See* Cephalosporins.)

LORACARBEF	Lorabid

See β-Lactams Chart.

THIRD-GENERATION CEPHALOSPORINS

Third-generation cephalosporins are noteworthy for their marked potency against common gram-negative organisms (e.g., *E. coli*, *Klebsiella pneumoniae*) and their activity against gram-negative bacilli resistant to older agents (e.g., *Serratia* sp., *P. aeruginosa*). Although grouped together, some agents have better activity against certain organisms (e.g., ceftazidime is better against *P. aeruginosa*), and poorer activity against others (e.g., cefixime and ceftazidime are poorer against *S. aureus*).[12,13,15,16]

CEFDINIR	Omnicef
CEFDITOREN	Spectracef
CEFIXIME	Suprax
CEFOPERAZONE	Cefobid

See β-Lactams Chart.

CEFOTAXIME SODIUM	Claforan

Pharmacology. Cefotaxime is a third-generation cephalosporin with activity against gram-negative organisms resistant to first- and second-generation cephalosporins (e.g., indole-positive *Proteus* sp., *Serratia* spp.). Its desacetyl metabolite (DACM) has good activity and might be synergistic with cefotaxime against certain organisms. The activity of cefotaxime against *P. aeruginosa* is inferior to ceftazidime and against *S. aureus* is inferior to cefazolin. Cefotaxime is more active than other cephalosporins (except ceftriaxone) against *S. pneumoniae* that are intermediately resistant to penicillin G.[12,13,15,16,27]

Administration and Adult Dosage. IM or IV—250 mg–2 g every 6–12 h (usually 1–2 g every 8–12 h), to a maximum of 12 g/d. Reduce dosage by 50% in patients with a Cl_{Cr} <20 mL/min.

Pediatric Dosage. IV—(newborns up to 1 week of age) 50 mg/kg every 12 h; (newborns 1–4 weeks) 50 mg/kg every 8 h; (older infants and children) 50–200 mg/kg/d (200 mg/kg/d for meningitis) given in 3–4 divided doses every 6–8 h.

Dosage Forms. Inj 500 mg, 1, 2, 10 g.

Pharmacokinetics. CSF concentrations range from 0.3 to 0.44 mg/L after a 1-g dose and in higher dosages cefotaxime is effective for treatment of meningitis. Approximately 50% of a dose is excreted unchanged in urine and 50% metabolized to DACM. DACM is metabolized to inactive metabolites and excreted unchanged in urine.

Adverse Reactions. Cefotaxime is well tolerated, with coagulopathies only rarely reported. (*See* Cephalosporins.)

CEFPODOXIME   Vantin

See β-Lactams Chart.

CEFTAZIDIME SODIUM   Ceptaz, Fortaz, Tazicef, Tazidime

Pharmacology. Ceftazidime is a third-generation cephalosporin with activity generally similar to that of cefotaxime, but having superior activity against *P. aeruginosa* and inferior activity against gram-positive (particularly against *S. aureus* and penicillin-resistant pneumococci) and anaerobic bacteria.[12–16,27]

Administration and Adult Dosage. IM or IV—500 mg–2 g every 8–12 h; every 12 h administration appears to be adequate in the elderly. Reduce dosage by 50% with a Cl_{Cr} of 30–50 mL/min; with a Cl_{Cr} of 15–30 mL/min, the maximum dosage is 1 g every 24 h; with a Cl_{Cr} <15 mL/min, the dosage is 500 mg every 24–48 h.

Pediatric Dosage. IV—(newborns) 30 mg/kg every 12 h; (older infants and children) IM or IV—30–50 mg/kg every 8 h, to a maximum of 6 g/d (225 mg/kg/d for treatment of meningitis).

Dosage Forms. Inj 500 mg, 1, 2, 6, 10 g. Conventional formulations of ceftazidime release carbon dioxide during reconstitution; the lysine formulation (e.g., Ceptaz) avoids this problem.

Pharmacokinetics. Ceftazidime is less than 20% plasma protein bound and 80%–90% excreted unchanged in urine by filtration, with a half-life of 1.6 h, which increases to 25–34 h in renal failure.

Adverse Reactions. The drug is generally well tolerated. (*See* Cephalosporins.)

CEFTIBUTEN	Cedax
CEFTRIAXONE	Rocephin
CEFTIZOXIME	Cefizox

See β-Lactams Chart.

FOURTH-GENERATION CEPHALOSPORIN

Fourth-generation cephalosporins have a spectrum similar to that of third-generation drugs, plus activity against some gram-negative strains that are resistant to the third-generation agents, such as *Enterobacter* sp. Their antianaerobic activity is poor. Resistance to cephalosporins is mediated by β-lactamase, reduction in outer cell wall membrane permeability, and alteration of the affinity of these agents for penicillin-binding proteins. Resistance among certain β-lactamase–producing organisms (e.g., *Enterobacter* and *Citrobacter* spp.) to third-generation cephalosporins has increased in recent years such that these agents cannot be relied on to provide effective therapy.[16]

CEFEPIME HYDROCHLORIDE — Maxipime

Pharmacology. Cefepime is a fourth-generation cephalosporin with a broader spectrum of activity than other cephalosporins. Its activity is similar to that of ceftazidime against gram-negative bacteria, including *P. aeruginosa*, but it is also active against some isolates resistant to third-generation cephalosporins (e.g., *Enterobacter* sp.). Cefepime has greater potency against gram-positive organisms (e.g., staphylococci) than ceftazidime and is similar in activity to ceftriaxone. Its anaerobic activity is poor, particularly against *B. fragilis*.[29–31]

Administration and Adult Dosage. IM or IV—500 mg to 2 g every 12 h; moderate to severe infections are treated with IV 1–2 g every 12 h. Higher dosages may be required in pseudomonal infections.

Special Populations. *Pediatric Dosage.* **IM or IV for empiric therapy of febrile neutropenia**— (2 months–16 years) 50 mg/kg every 8 h. **IM or IV for pneumonia, uncomplicated UTI, skin and soft tissue infections**—(2 months–16 years) 50 mg/kg every 12 h.

Geriatric Dosage. Same as adult dosage, adjusting for age-related renal impairment.

Other Conditions. In patients with Cl_{Cr} of 30–60 mL/min, the usual dose is given every 24 h; with a Cl_{Cr} of 10–29 mL/min, 50% of the usual dose is given every 24 h; and with a Cl_{Cr} <10 mL/min, 25% of the dose (but no less than 250 mg) is given every 24 h.

Dosage Forms. **Inj** 500 mg, 1, 2 g.

Pharmacokinetics. *Fate.* After a 30-min IV infusion of 1 g, serum concentrations of 79 mg/L are achieved. It is approximately 20% plasma protein bound. Cefepime penetrates most tissues and fluids well; CSF concentrations are 3.3–6.7 mg/L after 50 mg/kg every 8 h. Approximately 85% of a dose is eliminated renally by glomerular filtration. Elderly patients have a slightly lower total clearance, which parallels Cl_{Cr}. **Half-life** 2.3 h.

Adverse Reactions. The most common adverse reactions are injection-site reactions, rash, positive direct Coombs' test without hemolysis, decreased serum phosphorus, increased hepatic enzymes, eosinophilia, and abnormal PT and PTT. Encephalopathy has been reported in patients with renal impairment given unadjusted dosages. (*See* Cephalosporins.)

Contraindications. Previous immediate hypersensitivity reaction to any β-lactam.

Precautions. Adjust dosage in patients with impaired renal function. Use with caution in patients with GI disease, especially colitis.

Parameters to Monitor. Obtain renal and hepatic function tests, and PT and PTT periodically.

MONOBACTAM

AZTREONAM   Azactam

Pharmacology. Aztreonam is a monobactam with activity similar to that of third-generation cephalosporins against most gram-negative aerobic bacteria (including *P. aeruginosa*) but it is inactive against gram-positive bacteria and anaerobes.[12,32,33] (*See* β-Lactams Chart.)

Administration and Adult Dosage. **IM or IV**—500 mg to 2 g every 6–12 h, to a maximum of 8 g/d, depending on severity and site of infection. Reduce maintenance dosage by 50% with a Cl_{Cr} of 10–30 mL/min and by 75% with a Cl_{Cr} <10 mL/min. Give one-eighth of the initial dose after hemodialysis.

Pediatric Dosage. **IV**—(<1 month) 30 mg/kg every 6–12 h; (1 month–16 years) 30 mg/kg every 6–8 h. Dosages as high as 50 mg/kg every 6 h have been used in children with cystic fibrosis or serious gram-negative infections (e.g., *P. aeruginosa*).

Dosage Forms. **Inj** 500 mg, 1, 2 g.

Pharmacokinetics. Peak serum concentrations of 164 and 255 mg/L occur after 30-min IV infusions of 1 and 2 g, respectively. With inflamed meninges, CSF concentrations are similar to those observed with comparable dosages of third-generation cephalosporins, but experience in treating meningitis is limited. The drug is 60% plasma protein bound and has a V_d of about 0.24 L/kg; 60%–70% is excreted in urine unchanged. **Half-life** 1.5–2 h, increasing to 6 h in renal failure and 3.2 h in alcoholic cirrhosis.

Adverse Reactions. Adverse effects of aztreonam are minimal. Cross-allergenicity between aztreonam and other β-lactams is low, and aztreonam has been used safely in penicillin- or cephalosporin-allergic patients.

CARBAPENEMS

DORIPENEM   Doribax

Pharmacology. Doripenem is a broad-spectrum 1-β-methyl carbapenem indicated in the treatment of serious bacterial infections in adults. The 1-β-methyl segment of doripenem provides protection from renal dehydropeptidases and unlike imipenem does not require the concomitant administration of cilastin. Doripenem exhibits bactericidal activity against various gram-positive and gram-negative bacteria including AmpC producing *Enterobacteriaceae*, extended-spectrum β-lactamase, and anaerobic pathogens. Additionally, it offers the highest level of activity against *P. aeruginosa* in both cystic fibrosis and noncystic fibrosis patients.[34,35]

Administration and Adult Dosage. IV—500 mg every 8 h.

Special Populations. *Pediatric Dosage.* Safety and efficacy not established.

Geriatric Dosage. Same as adult dosage but adjust for age-related reduction in renal function.

Other Conditions. Reduce dosage with renal insufficiency as follows: Cl_{Cr} 30–50 mL/min, give 250 mg IV every 8 h; Cl_{Cr} 10–30 mL/min, give 250 mg every 12 h.

Dosage Forms. Inj 500 mg.

Pharmacokinetics. *Fate.* Doripenem exhibits linear pharmacokinetics at a dose of 500 mg to 1 g infused over 1 h. Plasma protein binding of doripenem is roughly 8.1% independent of drug concentrations, and the median volume of distribution is 16.8 L. Doripenem does not undergo metabolism by hepatic CYP450 isoenzymes, and is primarily eliminated unchanged by the kidneys. Therefore, dosage adjustment is necessary in moderate or severe renal insufficiency. **Half-life** 1 h.

Adverse Reactions. Headache, nausea, diarrhea, rash, and phlebitis are the most common adverse reactions ($\geq 5\%$).

Precautions. Use with caution in any patient who has had a previous hypersensitivity reaction to β-lactam antibiotics to avoid the potential for anaphylaxis or serious skin reactions.

Drug Interactions. Concomitant administration of doripenem with valproic acid has been shown to reduce valproic acid concentrations (63% AUC reduction). Serum valproic acid levels should be drawn if both drugs are coadministered. Probenecid has been shown to impair renal tubular secretion of doripenem resulting in extended action and elevated drug concentrations. Therefore, administration of doripenem with probenecid is not recommended.

Parameters to Monitor. Obtain renal function tests periodically.

ERTAPENEM Invanz

Pharmacology. Ertapenem is a carbapenem that inhibits cell wall synthesis by binding to one or more penicillin binding proteins. Similar to the other carbapenem, ertapenem has activity against both gram-positive and gram-negative organisms, including *Enterobacteriaceae, S. pneumonia,* and most anaerobes. An important difference is the lack of sufficient activity against *P. aeruginosa, Acinetobacter* spp., methicillin-resistant staphylococci and enterococci.[36,37] Like meropenem, ertapenem is not appreciably degraded by renal dehydropeptidase-I and thus does not require concomitant administration of a dehydropeptidase inhibitor.[36–40]

Administration and Adult Dosage. IV and IM—1 g every 24 h.

Special Populations. *Pediatric Dosage.* IV (<3 months) Safety and efficacy not established; (3 months to 12 years) 15 mg/kg twice daily not to exceed 1 g/ d.

Geriatric Dosage. Same as adult dosage but adjust for age-related reduction in renal function.

Other Conditions. **Renal Impairment.** Adults with $Cl_{Cr} \leq 30$ mL/min should receive 500 mg daily.

Dosage Forms. **Inj** 1 g.

Pharmacokinetics. *Fate.* Peak plasma concentrations following a 1-g dose infused over 30 min averages approximately 150 mg/L. Approximately 92% absorption occurs following an intramuscular dosage of ertapenem resulting in modestly lower peak concentrations. However, the AUC is comparable between the two routes of administration. Exhibiting concentration-dependent protein binding, ertapenem is highly protein bound (84%–96%). Nearly 40% of ertapenem is excreted unchanged in the urine.[36,37] **Half-life** 4 h.

Adverse Reactions. Adverse effects are similar to imipenem; the most common are diarrhea, injection-site reactions, nausea, vomiting, and headaches. Similarly with other carbapenems seizures and other CNS reactions have been noted with ertapenem.

Precautions. Use with caution in patients with hypersensitivity to penicillins because ertapenem can cause immediate hypersensitivity reactions in patients allergic to penicillins.[8,36,37]

Drug Interactions. Probenecid can reduce renal clearance of ertapenem and increase its half-life from 4 to 4.8 h and AUC by 25%. Valproic acid plasma levels may be decreased by coadministration.

Parameters to Monitor. Obtain renal function tests periodically.

IMIPENEM AND CILASTATIN SODIUM   Primaxin

Pharmacology. Imipenem is a carbapenem with an extremely broad spectrum of activity against many aerobic and anaerobic gram-positive and gram-negative bacterial pathogens. The commercial preparation contains an equal amount of cilastatin, a renal dehydropeptidase inhibitor that has no antimicrobial activity but prevents imipenem's metabolism by proximal tubular kidney cells, thus increasing urinary imipenem concentrations and possibly decreasing nephrotoxicity.[12,38,41] (*See* Notes.)

Administration and Adult Dosage. **IV**—1–4 g/d in 3 or 4 divided doses (usually 500 mg every 6–8 h). For severe, life-threatening infections, a dose of 1 g every 6 h is recommended (not to exceed 50 mg/kg/d or 4 g/d, whichever is less).[41] Infuse 250–500 mg doses over 20–30 min and 1 g doses over 40–60 min; reduce infusion rate if nausea and/or vomiting develops. **IM**—500–750 mg every 12 h.

Special Populations. *Pediatric Dosage.* (<1 week) 25 mg/kg every 12 h; (1–4 weeks) 25 mg/kg every 8 h; (4 weeks–3 months) 25 mg/kg every 6 h; (3 months–3 years) 25 mg/kg every 6 h; (>3 years) 15 mg/kg every 6 h.[41,42]

Geriatric Dosage. Same as adult dosage but adjust for age-related reduction in renal function.

Other Conditions. **Renal Impairment.** Cl_{Cr} 30–70 mL/min, give 75% of the usual dosage; Cl_{Cr} 20–30 mL/min, give 50% of the usual dosage; Cl_{Cr} <20 mL/min, give 25% of the usual dosage. Give a supplemental dose after hemodialysis.[41]

Dosage Forms. **Inj (IV)**—250 mg imipenem/250 mg cilastatin, 500 mg imipenem/500 mg cilastatin; **Inj (Susp, IM only)**—500 mg imipenem/500 mg cilastatin, 750 mg imipenem/750 mg cilastatin. (*See* Notes.)

Pharmacokinetics. *Fate.* Peak serum imipenem concentrations are 21–58 mg/L after a 30-min infusion of 500 mg and 1–84 mg/L after a 30-min infusion of 1 g; levels are <1 mg/L at 6 h. CSF levels are 0.5–11 mg/L with inflamed meninges and appear to be adequate to treat meningitis, but experience in treating meningitis is limited and seizures can occur in such patients. Imipenem is 20% plasma protein bound; V_d is 0.26 L/kg. Probenecid increases imipenem serum levels and prolongs its half-life. Approximately 70% of imipenem is excreted unchanged in urine when given with cilastatin, with the remainder excreted as metabolite; cilastatin is excreted 90% unchanged in urine.[38,41] **Half-life** (Imipenem) 0.9 ± 0.1 h; 3–4 h in renal failure; (cilastatin) 0.8 ± 0.1 h; 17 h in renal failure.[38,41]

Adverse Reactions. Nausea and vomiting occur in 1%–2% of patients, sometimes associated with hypotension or diaphoresis, particularly with high doses and rapid infusion.[38,41] Rashes occur occasionally, and cross-allergenicity with penicillins has been documented. Convulsions have occurred, primarily in the elderly, in those with underlying CNS disease, with overdosage in patients with renal failure, or with other predisposing factors.[8,38,41,43]

Precautions. Use with caution in elderly patients or those with a history of seizures or who are otherwise predisposed. Adjust dosage carefully in renal impairment. Imipenem can cause immediate hypersensitivity reactions in patients with a history of anaphylaxis to penicillin.[8]

Drug Interactions. Concomitant administration with probenecid produces higher and prolonged serum concentrations of imipenem and cilastatin. Imipenem has been shown in vitro to antagonize the activity of other β-lactams (e.g., acylureidopenicillins, most cephalosporins) presumably via β-lactamase induction; although the clinical relevance is unclear, avoid coadministration.[38] Coadministration of imipenem/cilastatin with ganciclovir has been associated with generalized seizures in a few patients; the mechanism of this interaction is unknown.

Parameters to Monitor. Obtain renal function tests periodically.

Notes. Used alone, emergence of resistance during treatment of *P. aeruginosa* infections occurs frequently; however, cross-resistance to other classes (e.g., aminoglycosides, cephalosporins) does not occur.[38,41] Addition of an aminoglycoside might prevent development of resistance, but in vitro synergism occurs only infrequently.

Vials may be reconstituted into a suspension using 10 mL of the infusion solution and then diluted further by transferring the suspension into the infusion container; alternatively, the powder in the 120-mL vials can be diluted initially with 100 mL of solution. The initial dilution must be shaken well to ensure suspension/solution. Do not inject the suspension. The resulting solution ranges from colorless to yellow. Reconstituted solutions are stable in dextrose-containing solutions for 4 h at room temperature and 24 h under refrigeration, and in normal saline for 10 h at room temperature and 48 h under refrigeration. With IM administration use 2 mL of lidocaine 1% injection to reconstitute a 500-mg vial and give the suspension by deep IM injection into a large muscle mass (e.g., gluteal muscle).[38]

MEROPENEM   Merrem

Pharmacology. Meropenem is a carbapenem with a mechanism of action similar to that of imipenem. Unlike imipenem, meropenem is not appreciably degraded by renal dehydropeptidase-I and thus does not require concomitant administration of a dehydropeptidase inhibitor.[38–40] (*See* Notes.)

Administration and Adult Dosage. **IV for less severe infections**—500 mg–1 g every 8–12 h. **IV for severe or life-threatening infections (e.g., meningitis)**—2 g every 8 h.

Special Populations. *Pediatric Dosage.* IV (<3 months) Safety and efficacy not established, but 20 mg/kg every 12 h has been used; (3 months–12 years) 10–20 mg/kg every 8 h; in meningitis 40 mg/kg every 8 h has been used.[39]

Geriatric Dosage. Same as adult dosage but adjust for age-related reduction in renal function.

Other Conditions. **Renal Impairment.** Cl_{Cr} 26–50 mL/min, give the normal dose every 12 h; with Cl_{Cr} 11–25 mL/min, the dosage is reduced by 50%; Cl_{Cr} <10 mL/min, give one-half the dose once daily.[39,44]

Dosage Forms. Inj 500 mg, 1 g.

Pharmacokinetics. *Fate.* The pharmacokinetics of meropenem are similar to those of imipenem, although meropenem can be given by IV infusion and bolus.[39,43] After IV infusion of 1 g, the peak serum concentration is 39–68 mg/L; the drug distributes well into most tissues and fluids, including the CSF. Plasma protein binding is low and the V_{dss} is 0.32 ± 0.03 L/kg. Meropenem is primarily eliminated renally by glomerular filtration and tubular secretion. Up to 70% of a dose is recovered unchanged in the urine, with a renal metabolite accounting for the remainder of the dose (up to 30%). Meropenem is appreciably removed by hemodialysis, and a supplemental dose is required after dialysis. Children have pharmacokinetics similar to adults; increased clearance and reduced half-life occur in cystic fibrosis.[44] **Half-life** 0.9 ± 0.09 h, increasing to 6.8–13.7 h in end-stage renal disease.[44]

Adverse Reactions. Adverse effects are similar to imipenem; the most common are injection-site reactions, rash, nausea, vomiting, and diarrhea.[38,39] Animal studies suggest that meropenem has a lower epileptogenic potential, which has been supported by a low frequency of seizures in clinical trials, including studies in patients with meningitis.[39]

Precautions. Use with caution in patients with hypersensitivity to penicillins because meropenem can cause immediate hypersensitivity reactions in patients allergic to penicillins.[8] Adjust dosage in renal impairment.

Drug Interactions. Probenecid can reduce renal clearance of meropenem and increase its half-life by 38% and AUC by 56%; avoid the combination.

Parameters to Monitor. Obtain renal function tests periodically.

Notes. Meropenem is more active than imipenem against enteric gram-negative bacilli; the two have equivalent activity against *P. aeruginosa* and *B. fragilis*, and meropenem is slightly less active than imipenem against gram-positive organisms.[38,39]

β-LACTAMS CHART

DRUG CLASS AND DRUG	DOSAGE FORMS	ADULT DOSAGE	PEDIATRIC DOSAGE	ADULT DOSAGE IN RENAL IMPAIRMENT[a]	PEAK SERUM LEVELS (mg/L)[b]	PERCENTAGE PROTEIN BOUND	COMMENTS
CARBAPENEMS							
Doripenem Doribax	Inj 500 mg	IV 500 mg every 8 h.	Not indicated; no data on usage	Cl$_{cr}$ 30–50 mL/min: 250 mg IV every 8 h. Cl$_{cr}$ 10–30 mL/min: 250 mg every 12 h.	23	8.1	Offers the highest level of activity against *P. aeruginosa* in both cystic fibrosis and noncystic fibrosis patients
Ertapenem Invanz	Inj 500 mg	IV 500 mg every 24 h.	IV (<3 mo) safety and efficacy not established; (3 mo–12 y) 5 mg/kg twice daily not to exceed 1 g/d	Cl$_{cr}$ <30 mL/min: 500 mg every 24 h.	150	84–96[c]	Lacks of sufficient activity against *P. aeruginosa*, *Acinetobacter* species, methicillin-resistant staphylococci and entero cocci.
Imipenem and Cilastatin Sodium Primaxin	Inj (IV) 250 plus 250 mg, 500 plus 500 mg; (IM) 500 mg plus 500 mg, 750 plus 750 mg	IV 1–4 g/d (1–2 g/d preferred) in 3 or 4 divided doses; IM 500–750 mg every 12 h	(<3 mo) See monograph; IV (3 mo–3 y) 25 mg/kg every 6 h; (>3 y) 15 mg/kg every 6 h.	Cl$_{cr}$ 31–70 mL/min: 75% of usual dosage. Cl$_{cr}$ <20–30 mL/min: 50% of usual dosage. Cl$_{cr}$ <20 mL/min: 25% of usual dosage.	21–58 (IV 500 mg imipenem)	20	Very broad activity against most aerobic and anaerobic bacteria. Frequent: nausea and dose-related seizure potential.

(continued)

β-LACTAMS CHART (*continued*)

DRUG CLASS AND DRUG	DOSAGE FORMS	ADULT DOSAGE	PEDIATRIC DOSAGE	ADULT DOSAGE IN RENAL IMPAIRMENT[a]	PEAK SERUM LEVELS (mg/L)[b]	PERCENTAGE PROTEIN BOUND	COMMENTS
Meropenem Merrem	Inj 500 mg, 1 g	IV 500 mg–1 g every 8–12 h; 2 g every 8 h in life-threatening infections.	(<3 mo) See monograph; IV (3 mo–12 y) 10–20 mg/kg every 8 h; 40 mg/kg every 8 h in meningitis.	Cl_{Cr} 26–50 mL/min: usual dose every 12 h; Cl_{Cr} 11–25 mL/min: 50% of usual dose every 12 h; Cl_{Cr} <10 mL/min: 50% of usual dose every 24 h.	55	2	Less active than imipenem against Gm+ and more active against most Gm− bacteria; equivalent against *P. aeruginosa* and *B. fragilis.* Less seizure potential than imipenem.
CEPHALOSPORINS, FIRST-GENERATION							
Cefadroxil Duricef Various	Cap 500 mg Susp 25, 50, 100 mg/mL Tab 1 g	PO 1–2 g/d in 1 or 2 divided doses; PO for endocarditis prophylaxis 2 g 1 h prior to dental procedure.	PO 30 mg/kg/d in 1 or 2 divided doses; PO for endocarditis prophylaxis 50 mg/kg 1 h prior to dental procedure.	PO 1 g, then 500 mg at intervals below: Cl_{Cr} 26–50 mL/min: 12 h; Cl_{Cr} 10–25 mL/min: 24 h; Cl_{Cr} >10 mL/min: 36 h.	12–16	20	Spectrum similar to cefazolin.

(continued)

β-LACTAMS CHART (*continued*)

DRUG CLASS AND DRUG	DOSAGE FORMS	ADULT DOSAGE	PEDIATRIC DOSAGE	ADULT DOSAGE IN RENAL IMPAIRMENT[a]	PEAK SERUM LEVELS (mg/L)[b]	PERCENTAGE PROTEIN BOUND	COMMENTS
Cefazolin Sodium Ancef Kefzol Various	Inj 250, 500 mg, 1, 5, 10, 20 g	IM or IV 250 mg–2 g every 6–12 h; (usually every 8 h), to a maximum of 12 g/d. IM or IV for surgical prophylaxis 1 g 30–60 min prior to surgery; IM or IV for endocarditis prophylaxis 1 g within 30 min prior to upper airway procedure.	IM or IV (neonates <1 mo) 25 mg/kg every 8–12 h; (infants >1 mo) 50–100 mg/kg/d in 3 divided doses to a maximum of 6 g/d. IM or IV for endocarditis prophylaxis 25 mg/kg within 30 min of procedure.	Cl_{Cr} 10–30 mL/min: 50% of usual dose every 12 h; Cl_{Cr} >10 mL/min: 50% of usual dose every 24 h.	185	75–85	Good gram + coverage (including S. aureus), plus some gram - activity (E. coli, Klebsiella spp.). Sodium = 2 mEq/g
Cephalexin Keflex Keftab Various	Cap 250, 500 mg Drp 100 mg/mL Susp 25, 50 mg/mL Tab 250, 500 mg, 1 g	PO 250 mg–1 g every 6 h, to a maximum of 4 g/d. PO for endocarditis prophylaxis 2 g 1 h prior to dental procedure.	PO 25–50 mg/kg/d in divided doses every 6 h; severe infections may require 50–100 mg/kg/d, to a maximum of 3 g/d. PO for endocarditis prophylaxis 50 mg/kg 1 h prior to dental procedure.	Cl_{Cr} 10–50 mL/min: 50% of usual dosage; Cl_{Cr} <10 mL/min; 25% of usual dosage.	18–38	6	Oral absorption is almost complete; spectrum similar to cefazolin.

(continued)

β-LACTAMS CHART (continued)

DRUG CLASS AND DRUG	DOSAGE FORMS	ADULT DOSAGE	PEDIATRIC DOSAGE	ADULT DOSAGE IN RENAL IMPAIRMENT[a]	PEAK SERUM LEVELS (mg/L)[b]	PERCENTAGE PROTEIN BOUND	COMMENTS
Cephapirin Sodium Cefadyl Various	Inj 1 g	IM or IV 500 mg–1 g every 4–6 h, to a maximum of 12 g/d.	IM or IV (>3 mo) not well studied; (children) 40–80 mg/kg/d in divided doses every 6 h.	Cl$_{Cr}$ 1C–50 mL/min; usual dose every 6–8 h. Cl$_{Cr}$ >10 mL/min: usual dose every 12 h.	10–20	45–50	Spectrum similar to cefazolin. Sodium = 1.2 mEq/g.
Cephoursadine Velosef Various	Cap 250, 500 mg Susp 25, 50 mg/mL	PO 250 mg–1 g every 6 h to a maximum-of 4 g/d.	PO same as cephalexin.	PO same as cephalexin.	10–20 (PO)	10–20	Oral form comparable to cephalexin; spectrum similar to cefazolin.

CEPHALOSPORINS, SECOND-GENERATION

DRUG CLASS AND DRUG	DOSAGE FORMS	ADULT DOSAGE	PEDIATRIC DOSAGE	ADULT DOSAGE IN RENAL IMPAIRMENT[a]	PEAK SERUM LEVELS (mg/L)[b]	PERCENTAGE PROTEIN BOUND	COMMENTS
Cefaclor Ceclor Various	Cap 250, 500 mg SR Tab 375, 500 mg Susp 25, 37.5, 50, 75 mg/mL	PO 250–500 mg every 8 h SR Tab 375–500 mg every 12 h.	PO 20–40 mg/kg/d in divided doses every 8 h to a maximum of 2 g/d.	Cl$_{Cr}$ 1C–50 mL/min: 50% of usual dosage; Cl$_{Cr}$ >10 mL/min: 25% of usual dosage.	10	25	Spectrum similar to cefazolin, but includes some ampicillin-resistant *H. influenzae.*
Cefamandole Nafate Mandol	Inj 1, 2, g	IM or IV 500 mg–1 g every 4–8 h; life-threatening infections may require 2 g every 4 h.	IM or IV 50–150 mg/kg/d in divided doses every 4–8 h.	Cl$_{Cr}$ 1C–50 mL/min: 50% of usual dose every 8 h; Cl$_{Cr}$ >10 mL/min: 25% of usual dose every 12 h.	80–90	56	NMTT side chain. Spectrum similar to cefuroxime. Sodium = 3.3 mEq/g.

(continued)

β-LACTAMS CHART (*continued*)

DRUG CLASS AND DRUG	DOSAGE FORMS	ADULT DOSAGE	PEDIATRIC DOSAGE	ADULT DOSAGE IN RENAL IMPAIRMENT[a]	PEAK SERUM LEVELS (mg/L)[b]	PERCENTAGE PROTEIN BOUND	COMMENTS
Cefonicid Sodium Monocid	Inj 1 g	IM or IV 500 mg–2 g/d as a single dose.	Not established.	IM or IV 7.5 m2/kg, then 25–50% of usual dose given: Cl_{Cr} 10–50 mL/min: every 24–48 h; Cl_{Cr} >10 mL/min; every 3–5 days.	220 (IV bolus)	83–98[c]	Poor activity against *Staphylococcus* spp. Unbound drug levels low and excreted rapidly because of saturable protein binding. Sodium = 3.7 mEq/g.
Cefotetan Disodium Cefotan	Inj 1, 2, 10 g	IM or IV 500 mg–2 g every 12–24 h.	Not established.	IM or IV give usual dose at intervals below: Cl_{Cr} 10–30 mL/min: 24 h; Cl_{Cr} >10 mL/min: 48 h.	140–180 (IV bolus)	78–91[c]	NMTT side chain. Spectrum similar to cefoxitin Sodium = 3.5 mEq/g. Reconstitute IM with 0.5% lidocaine.
Cefoxitin Sodium Mefoxin	Inj 1, 2, 10 g	IV 1–2 g every 6–8 h.	IV 80–160 mg/kg/d in divided doses every 4–6 h.	Cl_{Cr} 10–50 mL/min: 50% of usual dose every 6–8 h; Cl_{Cr} >10 mL/min: 25% of usual dose every 12 h.	110	75	Gm+ activity less than cefazolin, but better Gm− and anaerobic activity. Sodium = 2.3 mEq/g.

(continued)

β-LACTAMS CHART (continued)

DRUG CLASS AND DRUG	DOSAGE FORMS	ADULT DOSAGE	PEDIATRIC DOSAGE	ADULT DOSAGE IN RENAL IMPAIRMENT[a]	PEAK SERUM LEVELS (mg/L)[b]	PERCENTAGE PROTEIN BOUND	COMMENTS
Cefprozil Cefzil	Tab 250, 500 mg Susp 25, 50 mg/mL	PO 500 mg daily–twice daily.	PO (6 mo–12 y) 15 mg/kg every 12 h.	Cl$_{Cr}$ ≤30 mL/min: 50% of usual dose at same interval.	10.5	36	Spectrum similar to cef-aclor, but more active against *H. influenzae*.
Cefuroxime Sodium Kefurox Zinacef	Inj 750 mg, 1.5, 7.5 g	IM or IV 750 mg–1.5 g 6–8 h; to a maximum of 6 g/d.	IM or IV (neonates) 10–25 mg/kg every 12 h; (children) 50–100 mg/kg/d in divided dose every 6–8 h.	IM or IV: Cl$_{Cr}$ 10–20 mL/min: usual dose every 12 h; Cl$_{Cr}$ <10 mL/min: usual dose every 24 h.	100 (IV 1.5 g)	33–50	Gm+ activity similar to cefazolin, but better Gm– activity, including *H. influenzae*. Sodium = 2.4 mEq/g
Cefuroxime Axetil Ceftin	Susp 25, 50 mg/mL Tab 125, 250, 500 mg	PO 125–500 mg every 12 h.	PO 15–40 mg/kg/d in divided doses every 12 h.	—	3.6 (PO)	33–50	Do not interchange suspension and tablets.
Loracarbef Lorabid	Cap 200, 400 mg Susp 20, 40 mg/mL	PO 200–400 mg every 12–24 h.	PO (6 mo–12 y) 7.5–15 mg every 12 h.	Cl$_{Cr}$ 10–49 mL/min: 50% of Usual dosage; Cl$_{Cr}$ >10 mL/min: Usual dose every 3–5 days.	6.8 (PO 200 mg)	25	Carbacephem analogue of cefaclor with similar spectrum; must be taken on an empty stomach. *(continued)*

208

β-LACTAMS CHART (*continued*)

DRUG CLASS AND DRUG	DOSAGE FORMS	ADULT DOSAGE	PEDIATRIC DOSAGE	ADULT DOSAGE IN RENAL IMPAIRMENT[a]	PEAK SERUM LEVELS (mg/L)[b]	PERCENTAGE PROTEIN BOUND	COMMENTS
CEPHALOSPORINS, THIRD GENERATION							
Cefdinir Omnicef	Cap 300 mg Susp 25 mg/mL	PO 600 mg/d in 1 or 2 doses.	PO 14 mg/kg/d in 1 or 2 doses.	Cl$_{cr}$ >30 mL/min: 300 mg/d.	2.9 (PO 600 mg)	60–70	Spectrum similar to cefixime but better Gm+ activity
Cefditoren Spectracef	Tab 200 mg	PO 200 every 12 h.	PO (>12 y) not established.	Cl$_{cr}$ >50 mL/min: reduce dosage	2.6 (PO 200 mg)	88	Spectrum similar to cefdinir and cefpodoxime but more active.
Cefixime Suprax	Tab 200, 400 mg Susp 20 mg/mL	PO 400 mg/d in 1 or 2 doses. PO for gonorrhea 400 mg once.	PO 8 mg/kg/d in 1 or 2 divided doses.	Cl$_{cr}$ 20–60 mL/min: 75% of usual dosage; Cl$_{cr}$ >20 mL/min: 50% of usual dosage.	4.9	70	More active than cefuroxime or cefaclor against *H. influenzae*, but less Gm+ activity.
Cefoperazone Sodium Cefobid Various	Inj 1, 2, 10 g	IM or IV 2–8 g/d in divided doses every 12 h.	IM or IV (neonates) 50 mg/kg/dose every 12 h; (children) 50–75 mg/kg every 8–12 h.	No change.	125	85–95[c]	Less active than ceftazidime against *P. aeruginosa*. NMTT side chain. Sodium = 1.5 mEq/g.

(continued)

β-LACTAMS CHART (continued)

DRUG CLASS AND DRUG	DOSAGE FORMS	ADULT DOSAGE	PEDIATRIC DOSAGE	ADULT DOSAGE IN RENAL IMPAIRMENT[a]	PEAK SERUM LEVELS (mg/L)[b]	PERCENTAGE PROTEIN BOUND	COMMENTS
Cefotaxime Sodium Claforan	Inj 500 mg, 1, 2, 10 g	IM or IV 1–2 g every 8–12 h; life-threatening infections may require 2 g every 6 h.	IM or IV (neonates ≤1 wk) 50 mg/kg every 12 h; (neonates 1–4 wk) 50 mg/kg every 8 h; (infants >4 wk) 50–200 (200 in meningitis) mg/kg/d in divided doses every 4–6 h.	Cl$_{Cr}$ 10–50 mL/min: usual dose every 8–12 h; <10 mL/min usual dose every 24 h.	40–100	37	Good Gm+ and Gm− activity except for *P. aeruginosa*; modest anti-anaerobic activity. Sodium = 2.2 mEq/g.
Cefpodoxime Proxetil Vantin	Tab 100, 200 mg Susp 10, 20 mg/mL	PO 100–400 mg every 12 h; PO for gonorrhea 200 mg once.	PO 5 mg/kg every 12 h.	Cl$_{Cr}$ <30 mL/min: usual dose given every 24 h.	2.9 (PO 200 mg)	18–30	Spectrum similar to cefixime, but better Gm+ activity.
Ceftazidime Ceptaz Fortaz Tazicef Tazidime	Inj 500 mg, 1, 2, 6 g	IM or IV 500 mg–2 g every 8–12 h.	IM or IV (≤1 mo) 30 mg/kg/dose (every 12 h; (>1 mo) 30–50 mg/kg/dose every 8 h.	Cl$_{Cr}$ 30–50 mL/min: 50% of usual dose every 12–24 h; Cl$_{Cr}$ 15–30 mL/min: 1 g every 24 h; Cl$_{Cr}$ <15 mL/min: 500 mg every 24–48 h.	70–90	17	Best activity against *P. aeruginosa*; poor Gm+ activity. Sodium = 2.3 mEq/g.

(continued)

β-LACTAMS CHART (*continued*)

DRUG CLASS AND DRUG	DOSAGE FORMS	ADULT DOSAGE	PEDIATRIC DOSAGE	ADULT DOSAGE IN RENAL IMPAIRMENT[a]	PEAK SERUM LEVELS (mg/L)[b]	PERCENTAGE PROTEIN BOUND	COMMENTS
Ceftibuten Cedax	Cap 400 mg Susp 18, 36 mg/mL	PO 400 mg every 24 h.	PO 9 mg/kg/d in 1 dose.	Cl_{Cr} 30–49 mL/min: 4.5 mg/kg or 200 mg every 24 h; Cl_{Cr} <30 mL/min: 2.25 mg/kg or 100 mg every 24 h.	11 (PO 200 mg)	60–77	Spectrum similar to cefixime.
Ceftizoxime Sodium Cefizox	Inj 500 mg, 1, 2, 10 g	IM or IV 1–2 g every 8–12 h; life-threatening infections may require up to 4 g every 8 h.	IM or IV (>6 mo) 50 mg/kg/dose every 6–8 h.	Cl_{Cr} 10–50 mL/min: 50% of usual dose every 12–24 h; Cl_{Cr} <10 mL/min: 25%–50% of usual dose every 24–48 h.	60–87	31	Spectrum similar to cefotaxime except slightly more active against anaerobes. Sodium = 2.6 mEq/g.
Ceftriaxone Disodium Rocephin	Inj 250, 500 mg, 1, 2, 10 g	IM or IV 1–2 g/d as a single dose; IV for meningitis 2 g every 12 h; IM for gonorrhea 250 mg once.	IM or IV 50–100 (100 in meningitis) mg/kg/d in 2 divided doses.	No change. (See Comments.)	151	83–96[c]	Spectrum similar to cefotaxime. Reduce dose with concurrent renal and hepatic dysfunction. Sodium = 3.6 mEq/g. *(continued)*

β-LACTAMS CHART (*continued*)

DRUG CLASS AND DRUG	DOSAGE FORMS	ADULT DOSAGE	PEDIATRIC DOSAGE	ADULT DOSAGE IN RENAL IMPAIRMENT[a]	PEAK SERUM LEVELS (mg/L)[b]	PERCENTAGE PROTEIN BOUND	COMMENTS
CEPHALOSPORINS, FOURTH GENERATION							
Cefepime Maxipime	Inj 500 mg, 1, 2 g	IM or IV 500 mg–2 g every 12 h; 2 g every 8 h may be required for pseudomonal infections and febrile neutropenia.	IM or IV (2 mo–16 y) febrile neutropenia 50 mg/kg every 8 h; other infections 50 mg/kg every 12 h.	Cl_{Cr} 30–60 mL/min: usual dose every 24 h; Cl_{Cr} 10–29 mL/min: 50% of usual dose every 24 h; Cl_{Cr} <10 mL/min: 25% of usual dose every 24 h.	79	16–19	Spectrum similar to ceftazidime; more active against Gm+ organisms; also active against resistant *Enterobacter* spp.
MONOBACTAM							
Aztreonam Azactam	Inj 500 mg, 1, 2 g	IM or IV 0.5–2 g every 6–12 h.	Safety and efficacy not established. IV 30 mg/kg every 6–8 h (50 mg/kg every 6–8 h in cystic fibrosis, to a maximum of 200 mg/kg/d).	Cl_{Cr} 10–30 mL/min: 50% of usual dosage; Cl_{Cr} <10 mL/min: 25% of usual dosage.	164	60	Spectrum similar to ceftazidime against aerobic Gm - organisms only. No cross-allergenicity in penicillin-allergic patients.

(continued)

β-LACTAMS CHART (continued)

DRUG CLASS AND DRUG	DOSAGE FORMS	ADULT DOSAGE	PEDIATRIC DOSAGE	ADULT DOSAGE IN RENAL IMPAIRMENT[a]	PEAK SERUM LEVELS (mg/L)[b]	PERCENTAGE PROTEIN BOUND	COMMENTS
PENICILLIN G AND V							
Penicillin G Potassium Various	Inj 1, 5, 10, 20 million units Inj 1, 2, 3 million units/50 mL (frozen)	IV 2–5 million units every 4–6 h.	IV (neonates) 25,000–50,000 units/kg every 6–12 h; (>1 mo) 100,000–300,000 units/kg/d in divided doses every 4–6 h.	Cl$_{Cr}$ 10–50 mL/min: 75% of dosage; Cl$_{Cr}$ <10 mL/min: 25–50% of dosage.	1.5–2.7 (IV 500 mg)	60	Gm+ (except most *Staphylococcus* strains), some Gm– (*Neisseria* spp.), and anaerobes (except *B. fragilis*). Poor oral absorption. Potassium = 1.7 mEq/mill on units.
Penicillin G Benzathine Various	Inj 300,000, 600,000, 1.2 million units/mL	IM for *Strep.* pharyngitis 1.2 million units once; IM for syphilis (early) 2.4 million units once; (late) 2.4 million units/wk for 3 wk.	IM for *Strep.* pharyngitis (<27 kg) 300,000–600,000 units once; (>27 kg) 900,000 units once.	No change.	0.063 (IM 600,000 units)	60	Use limited to syphilis and *Strep.* pharyngitis. For IM use only.

(continued)

213

β-LACTAMS CHART (*continued*)

DRUG CLASS AND DRUG	DOSAGE FORMS	ADULT DOSAGE	PEDIATRIC DOSAGE	ADULT DOSAGE IN RENAL IMPAIRMENT[a]	PEAK SERUM LEVELS (mg/L)[b]	PERCENTAGE PROTEIN BOUND	COMMENTS
Penicillin G Procaine Various	Inj 300,000, 600,000 units/mL	IM 600,000–2.4 million units every 12–24 h (0.6–4.8 million units/d divided every 12–24 h).	IM (neonates) 50,000 units/kg/d in 1–2 divided doses; (>27 kg) 900,000 units once daily.	No change.	0.9 (IM 300,000 units)	60	For IM use only.
Penicillin V Potassium Pen Vee K Veetids Various	Tab 125, 250, 500 mg Susp 25, 50 mg/mL	PO 125–500 mg every 6–8 h.	PO 15–50 mg/kg/d in 3–4 divided doses.	No change.	3–8	78	Spectrum similar to penicillin G. Approximately 60% absorbed; preferred oral form of penicillin.
ANTISTAPHYLOCOCCAL PENICILLINS							
Cloxacillin Sodium Cloxapen Tegopen Various	Cap 250, 500 mg Susp 25 mg/mL	PO 250–500 mg every 6 h.	PO (<20 kg) 50–100 mg/kg/d in divided doses every 6 h; (>20 kg) same as adult dosage.	No change.	7–18	94	Used primarily for *S. aureus* infections. Suspension may be better tolerated than dicloxacillin.

(continued)

214

β-LACTAMS CHART (*continued*)

DRUG CLASS AND DRUG	DOSAGE FORMS	ADULT DOSAGE	PEDIATRIC DOSAGE	ADULT DOSAGE IN RENAL IMPAIRMENT[a]	PEAK SERUM LEVELS (mg/L)[b]	PERCENTAGE PROTEIN BOUND	COMMENTS
Dicloxacillin Sodium Dynapen Pathocil Various	Cap 125, 250, 500 mg Susp 12.5 mg/mL	PO 125–500 mg every 6 h.	PO 12.5–25 mg/kg/d in divided doses every 6 h.	No change.	7–18	98	Comparable to cloxacillin.
Nafcillin Sodium Unipen	Cap 250 mg Inj 500 mg, 1, 2, 4, 10 g	IV 500 mg–2 g every 4–6 h; PO 250 mg–1 g every 4–6 h.	IV (neonates <7 days) 25 mg/kg every 8–12 h; (neonates >7 days) 25 mg/kg every 6–8 h.	No change.	3.4 (PO) 40–57 (IV)	89	Comparable to oxacillin. Reversible neutropenia may be more common with nafcillin. Poorly absorbed orally; cloxacillin or dicloxacillin preferred. IV sodium = 2.9 mEq/g.
Oxacillin Sodium Bactocill Prostaphlin	Cap 250, 500 mg Susp 50 mg/mL Inj 250, 500 mg, 1, 2, 4, 10 g	IV 250 mg–2 g every 4–6 h. PO 500 mg–1 g every 6 h, but not recommended.	IV (≤14 days) 25 mg/kg every 8–12 h; (15–30 days) 25 mg/kg every 6 h (children same as adult dosage. PO 50–100 mg/kg/d in 4–6 divided doses.	No change.	2.5 (PO) 40 (IV)	92	Poorly absorbed orally; cloxacillin or dicloxacillin preferred. Rare hepatic toxicity. IV sodium = 2.9 mEq/g.

(continued)

β-LACTAMS CHART (continued)

DRUG CLASS AND DRUG	DOSAGE FORMS	ADULT DOSAGE	PEDIATRIC DOSAGE	ADULT DOSAGE IN RENAL IMPAIRMENT[a]	PEAK SERUM LEVELS (mg/L)[b]	PERCENTAGE PROTEIN BOUND	COMMENTS
AMPICILLIN DERIVATIVES							
Amoxicillin Amoxil Various	Cap 250, 500 mg Chew Tab 125, 200, 250, 400 mg Drp 50 mg/mL Susp 25, 50 mg/mL Tab 500, 875 mg	PO 250–500 mg 3 times daily, or 500–875 mg twice daily, to a maximum of 4.5 g/d; PO for endocarditis prophylaxis 2 g 1 h before procedure.	PO 20–40 mg/kg/d in 3 divided doses; PO for endocarditis prophylaxis 50 mg/kg 1 h before procedure.	Cl$_{Cr}$ 10–30 mL/min: 250–530 mg twice daily; Cl$_{Cr}$ <10 mL/min: 250–500 mg every 24 h.	9	20	Spectrum similar to ampicillin, but better bioavailability (85%) and less diarrhea.
Ampicillin Sodium Various	Cap 250, 500 mg Susp 25, 50, mg/mL Inj 125, 250, 500 mg, 1, 2, 10 g	PO 250–500 mg 4 times daily; IM or IV 500 mg–3 g every 4–6 h, to a maximum of 12 g/d.	PO (<20 kg) 50–100 mg/kg/d in 2–4 divided doses; PO or IV (>20 kg) 100–400 mg/kg/d in divided doses every 4–6 h.	Cl$_{Cr}$ <20 mL/min: same dose every 12 h.	4 (PO) 58 (IV)	22	Approximately 50% oral bioavailability; GI side effects and rashes are frequent. IV sodium = 3 mEq/g.

(continued)

β-LACTAMS CHART (continued)

DRUG CLASS AND DRUG	DOSAGE FORMS	ADULT DOSAGE	PEDIATRIC DOSAGE	ADULT DOSAGE IN RENAL IMPAIRMENT[a]	PEAK SERUM LEVELS (mg/L)[b]	PERCENTAGE PROTEIN BOUND	COMMENTS
EXTENDED-SPECTRUM PENICILLINS							
Mezlocillin Sodium Mezlin	Inj 1, 2, 3, 4, 20 g	IV 3–4 g every 4–6 h.	IV (<7 days) 50–100 mg/kg every 12 h; (neonates >7 days) 50–100 mg/kg every 6–8 h; (children) 300 mg/kg/d in divided doses every divided doses every of 24 g/d.	Cl$_{Cr}$ 10–30 mL/min: 3 g every 8 h; Cl$_{Cr}$ <10 mL/min: 2 g every 8 h.	263 (IV 4 g)	35	Spectrum similar to ticarcillin, but better enterococcal coverage. Least active drug in this class against *P. aeruginosa.* Sodium = 1.85 mEq/g.
Piperacillin Sodium Pipracil	Inj 2, 3, 4, 40g	IV 3–4 g every 4–6 h, to a maximum of 24g/d.	Not well established. IV (neonates; 100 mg/kg every 12 h; (children) 200–300 (350–500 in cystic fibrosis) mg/kg/d in divided doses every 4–6 h	Cl$_{Cr}$ 20–40 mL/min: 3–4 g every 8 h; Cl$_{Cr}$ <20 mL/min: 3–4 g every 12 h.	244 (IV 4 g)	15–20	Best activity against *P. aeruginosa.* Sodium = 1.85 mEq/g.

(continued)

β-LACTAMS CHART (continued)

DRUG CLASS AND DRUG	DOSAGE FORMS	ADULT DOSAGE	PEDIATRIC DOSAGE	ADULT DOSAGE IN RENAL IMPAIRMENT[a]	PEAK SERUM LEVELS (mg/L)[b]	PERCENTAGE PROTEIN BOUND	COMMENTS
Ticarcillin Disodium Ticar	Inj 1, 3, 6, 20, 30 g	IV 2–4 g every 4–6 h, to a maximum of 24 g/d.	IV (neonates ≤7 days 1 and ≤2 kg) 75 mg/kg every 12 h; (neonates >7 days and <2 kg or ≤7 days and >2kt) 75 mg/kg every 8 h; (neonates ≥7 days and ≥2 kg) 75 mg/kg every 6 h; (children) 200–300 mg/kg/d in divided closes every 6–8 h.	Cl$_{Cr}$ 30–60 mL/min: 2 g every 4 h; Cl$_{Cr}$ 10–30 mL/min: 2 g every 8 h; Cl$_{Cr}$ <10 mL/min: 2 g every 12 h.	260 (IV 3 g)	50–60	Less active than piperacillin against *P. aeruginosa*; no activity against *Klebsiella* spp. More antiplatelet effect than mezlocillin or piperacillin. Sodium = 5.2–6.5 mEq/g.
PENICILLIN AND β-LACTAMASE INHIBITOR COMBINATIONS							
Amoxicillin and Clavuanate Potassium Augmentin	(*See* Monograph.)	PO 250 or 500 every 8 h or 875 tablet every 12 h.	PO 20–40 mg/kg/d (of amoxicillin) in 3 divided doses or 45 mg/kg/d in 2 divided doses.	Cl$_{Cr}$ 10–30 mL/min: 250–500 mg twice daily; Cl$_{Cr}$ <10mL/min 250–500 mg every 24 h.	9 (PO 500 mg amoxicillin) 2.6 (PO 125 mg clavulanate)	20 (amoxicillin) 22 (clavulanate	Active against ampicillin-resistant *S. aureus*, *B. fragilis*, and β-lactamase–producing Enterobacteriaceae. *(continued)*

β-LACTAMS CHART (*continued*)

DRUG CLASS AND DRUG	DOSAGE FORMS	ADULT DOSAGE	PEDIATRIC DOSAGE	ADULT DOSAGE IN RENAL IMPAIRMENT[a]	PEAK SERUM LEVELS (mg/L)[b]	PERCENTAGE PROTEIN BOUND	COMMENTS
							More diarrhea than with amoxicillin. Do not substitute 2 "250" tablets for 1 "500" tablet.
Ampicillin Sodium and Sulbactam Sodium Unasyn	Inj 1 g ampicillin plus 500 mg sulbactam/ vial, 2 g ampicillin plus 1 g sulbactam/ vial, 10 g ampicillin plus 5 g sulbactam/ vial	IM or IV 1.5–3 g of the combination every 6–8 h, to a maximum of 12 g/d.	IM or IV (3 mo–12 y) 150–300 mg of the combination every 6 h, to a maximum of 12 g/d.	Cl_{Cr} 15–30 mL/min: same dose every 12 h; Cl_{Cr} 5–14 mL/min: same dose every 24 h	58 (IV 1 g ampicillin) 30 (IV 500 mg sulbactam)	22 (ampicillin) 38 (sulbactam)	Spectrum similar to Augmentin. Sodium = 5 mEq/1.5 g.
Piperacillin Sodium and Tazobactam Sodium Zosyn	Inj 2.25, 3.375, 4.5, 40.5 g (0.5 g tazobactam/4 g piperacillin)	IV 3.375–4.5 g every 4–6 h; 3.375 g every 4 h or 4.5 g every 6 h for *P. aeruginosa.*	Safety and efficacy not established.	Cl_{Cr} 20–40 mL/min: 2.25 g every 6 h; Cl_{Cr} <20 mL/min: 2.25 g every 8 h.	400 (IV 4 g piperacillin) 34 (IV 0.5 g tazobactam)	15–20 (piperacillin) 1 (tazobactam)	Similar spectrum to Timentin, but better activity against *P. aeruginosa* and enterococcal. Sodium = 2.35 mEq/g of piperacillin. *(continued)*

β-LACTAMS CHART (continued)

DRUG CLASS AND DRUG	DOSAGE FORMS	ADULT DOSAGE	PEDIATRIC DOSAGE	ADULT DOSAGE IN RENAL IMPAIRMENT[a]	PEAK SERUM LEVELS (mg/L)[b]	PERCENTAGE PROTEIN BOUND	COMMENTS
Ticarcillin Disodium and Clavulanate Potassium Timentin	Inj 3.1, 31 (100 mg clavulanate/ 3 g ticarcillin)	IV 3.1 g every 4–6 h.	IV (≥3 mo) <60 kg: 50 mg/kg (of ticarcillin) every 4–6 h; ≥60 kg: same as adult dosage.	Cl$_{Cr}$ 30–60 mL/min: 3.1 g every 6 h; Cl$_{Cr}$ 10–30 mL/min: 3.1 g every 8 h; Cl$_{Cr}$ <10 mL/min: 3.1 g every 12 h.[d]	260 (IV 3 g ticarcillin) 8 (IV 100 mg clavulanate)	50–60 (ticarcillin) 22 (clavulanate)	Improved activity over ticarcillin against, S. aureus, H. influenzae, and anaerobes, but not P. aeruginosa or E. cloacae. Sodium = 4.7 mECl/g of ticarcillin

[a]Usual dose means individual doses given at the specified interval; usual dosage means total daily dosage.
[b]Average peak serum concentrations following administration of a 500-mg oral dose or a 1 g IV infusion over 30 min, except as noted.
[c]Concentration dependent.
[d]With dosages recommended in marked renal impairment, clavulanate concentrations may provide ineffective synergism with ticarcillin.[173]
From Refs. 10, 11, 41, and 45—51 and product information.

■ REFERENCES

1. Chambers HF, Neu HC. Penicillins. In: Mandell GL et al., eds. *Principles and Practice of Infectious Diseases.* 5th ed. New York: Churchill Livingstone; 2000:261-274.
2. Barza M. Antimicrobial spectrum, pharmacology and therapeutic use of antibiotics. Part 2: penicillins. *Am J Hosp Pharm.* 1977;34:57-67.
3. Weber DJ et al. Amoxicillin and potassium clavulanate: an antibiotic combination. *Pharmacotherapy.* 1984;4:12-36.
4. Sutherland R. β-lactam/β-lactamase inhibitor combinations: development, antibacterial activity and clinical applications. *Infection.* 1995;23:191-200.
5. Rafailidia PI et al. Ampicillin/sulbactam current status in severe bacterial infections. *Drugs.* 2007;67:1829-1849.
6. Neu HC. Antistaphylococcal penicillins. *Med Clin North Am.* 1982;66:51-60.
7. Wright AJ. The penicillins. *Mayo Clin Proc.* 1999;74:290-307.
8. Saxon A. Immediate hypersensitivity reactions to beta-lactam antibiotics. *Ann Intern Med.* 1987;107:204-215.
9. Weiss ME, Adkinson NF Jr. β-Lactam allergy. In: Mandell GL et al., eds. *Principles and Practice of Infectious Diseases.* 5th ed. New York: Churchill Livingstone; 2000:299-305.
10. Drusano GL et al. The acylampicillins: mezlocillin, piperacillin, and azlocillin. *Rev Infect Dis.* 1984;6:13-32.
11. Holmes B et al. Piperacillin. A review of its antibacterial activity, pharmacokinetic properties and therapeutic use. *Drugs.* 1984;28:375-425.
12. Donowitz GR, Mandell GL. Beta-lactam antibiotics (2 parts). *N Engl J Med.* 1988;318:419-426 and 490-500.
13. Cunha BA. Third-generation cephalosporins: a review. *Clin Ther.* 1992;14:616-647.
14. Nightingale CH et al. Pharmacokinetics and clinical use of cephalosporin antibiotics. *J Pharm Sci.* 1975;64:1899-1927.
15. Barriere SL, Flaherty JF. Third-generation cephalosporins: a critical evaluation. *Clin Pharm.* 1984;3:351-373.
16. Karchmer AW. Cephalosporins. In: Mandell GL et al., eds. *Principles and Practice of Infectious Diseases.* 5th ed. New York: Churchill Livingstone; 2000:274-291.
17. Schaad UB et al. A comparison of ceftriaxone and cefuroxime for the treatment of bacterial meningitis in children. *N Engl J Med.* 1990;322:141-147.
18. Petz LD. Immunologic cross-reactivity between penicillins and cephalosporins: a review. *J Infect Dis.* 1978;137(suppl):S74-S79.
19. Lipsky JJ. Antibiotic-associated hypoprothrombinemia. *J Antimicrob Chemother.* 1988;21:281-300.
20. Schaad UB et al. Reversible ceftriaxone-associated biliary pseudolithiasis in children. *Lancet.* 1988;2:1411-1413.
21. Rodman DP et al. A critical review of the new oral cephalosporins. *Arch Fam Med.* 1994;3:975-980.
22. Fassbender M et al. Pharmacokinetics of new oral cephalosporins, including a new carbacephem. *Clin Infect Dis.* 1993;16:646-653.
23. Force RW, Nahata MC. Loracarbef: a new orally administered carbacephem antibiotic. *Ann Pharmacother.* 1993;27:121-129.
24. Cooper RDG. The carbacephems: a new beta-lactam antibiotic class. *Am J Med.* 1992;92(suppl 6A):2S-6S.
25. DiPiro JT, May JR. Use of cephalosporins with enhanced anti-anaerobic activity for treatment and prevention of anaerobic and mixed infections. *Clin Pharm.* 1988;7:285-302.
26. Ward A, Richards DM. Cefotetan. A review of its antibacterial activity, pharmacokinetic properties and therapeutic use. *Drugs.* 1985;30:382-426.
27. Friedland IR, McCracken GH Jr. Management of infections caused by antibiotic-resistant *Streptococcus pneumoniae. N Engl J Med.* 1994;331:377-382.
28. Smith BR, LeFrock JL. Cefuroxime: antibacterial activity, pharmacology, and clinical efficacy. *Ther Drug Monit.* 1983;5:149-160.
29. Shiffman ML et al. Pathogenesis of ceftriaxone-associated biliary sludge. *Gastroenterology.* 1990;99:1772-1778.
30. Cunha BA, Gill MV. Cefepime. *Med Clin North Am.* 1995;79:721-732.
31. Barradell LB, Bryson HM. Cefepime. A review of its antibacterial activity, pharmacokinetic properties and therapeutic use. *Drugs.* 1994;47:471-505.
32. Johnson DH, Cunha BA. Aztreonam. *Med Clin North Am.* 1995;79:733-743.
33. Brogden RN, Heel RC. Aztreonam. A review of its antibacterial activity, pharmacokinetic properties and therapeutic uses. *Drugs.* 1986;31:96-130.
34. Keam SJ. Doripenem: a review of its use in the treatment of bacterial infections. *Drugs.* 2008;68:2021-2057.
35. Walsh F. Doripenem: a new carbapenem antibiotic a review of comparative bactericidal activities. *Ther Clin Risk Manag.* 2007;3:789-794.
36. Nix DE et al. Pharmacokinetics and pharmacodynamics of ertapenem: an overview for clinicians. *J Antimicro Chemother.* 2004;53(suppl 2):23-28, ii.
37. Wexler HM. *In vitro* activity of ertapenem: review of recent studies. *J Antimicrob Chemother.* 2004;53(suppl 2):11-21, ii.

38. Norrby SR. Carbapenems. *Med Clin North Am.* 1995;79:745-759.

39. Wiseman LR et al. Meropenem. A review of its antibacterial activity, pharmacokinetic properties and clinical efficacy. *Drugs.* 1995;50:73-101.

40. Pryka RD, Haig GM. Meropenem: a new carbapenem antimicrobial. *Ann Pharmacother.* 1994;28:1045-1054.

41. Clissold SP et al. Imipenem/cilastatin. A review of its antibacterial activity, pharmacokinetic properties and therapeutic efficacy. *Drugs.* 1987;33:183-241.

42. Ahonkhai VI et al. Imipenem-cilastatin in pediatric patients: an overview of safety and efficacy in studies conducted in the United States. *Pediatr Infect Dis J.* 1989;8:740-747.

43. Calandra GB et al. Review of adverse experiences and tolerability in the first 2,516 patients treated with imipenem/cilastatin. *Am J Med.* 1985;78(suppl 6A):73-78.

44. Mouton JW, van den Anker JN. Meropenem clinical pharmacokinetics. *Clin Pharmacokinet.* 1995;28:275-286.

45. Plaisance KI, Nightingale CH. Pharmacology of cephalosporins. In: Queener SF et al., eds. *Beta-Lactam Antibiotics for Clinical Use.* New York: Marcel Dekker; 1986:285-347.

46. Dudley MN, Nightingale CH. Effects of protein binding on the pharmacology of cephalosporins. In: Neu HC, ed. *New Beta-Lactam Antibiotics: A Review from Chemistry to Clinical Efficacy of the New Cephalosporins.* Philadelphia, PA: Francis Clarke Wood Institute for the History of Medicine; 1982:227-239.

47. Carver P et al. Pharmacokinetics and pharmacodynamics of total and unbound cefoxitin and cefotetan in healthy volunteers. *J Antimicro Chemother.* 1989;23:99-106.

48. Wise R. The pharmacokinetics of the oral cephalosporins: a review. *J Antimicrob Chemother.* 1990;26(suppl E):13-20.

49. Melikian DM, Flaherty JF. Antimicrobial agents. In: Schrier RW, Gambertoglio JG, eds. *Handbook of Drug Therapy in Liver and Kidney Disease.* Boston, MA: Little, Brown; 1991:14-45.

50. Klepser ME et al. Clinical pharmacokinetics of newer cephalosporins. *Clin Pharmacokinet.* 1995;28:361-384.

51. Hardin TC et al. Comparison of ampicillin-sulbactam and ticarcillin-clavulanic acid in patients with chronic renal failure: effects of differential pharmacokinetics on serum bactericidal activity. *Pharmacotherapy.* 1994;14:147-152.

Chapter 12

Macrolides

Davey P. Legendre

AZITHROMYCIN Zithromax, Various

Pharmacology. Azithromycin is a macrolide with a 15-membered ring (making it an azalide) that binds to the 50S ribosomal subunit, inhibiting messenger RNA-directed polypeptide and protein synthesis.[1] It is slightly less active than erythromycin against gram-positive bacteria, but it is substantially more active against *Moraxella (Branhamella) catarrhalis, Haemophilus* sp., *Legionella* sp., *Neisseria* sp., *Bordetella* sp., *Mycoplasma* sp., and *Chlamydia trachomatis.* The drug also has activity against aerobic gram-negative bacilli and *Mycobacterium avium* and is comparable to erythromycin in its activity against *Campylobacter* sp. It is the most active macrolide for *Toxoplasma gondii*, including activity against the cyst form.[2-5] The incidence of *Streptococcus pneumoniae* resistant to macrolide antibiotics is increasing[6,7] and this resistance is responsible for clinical failure.[8,9] Mechanisms of resistance to macrolides include alteration of the target site, efflux pumps, decreased permeability, and enzyme inactivation.

Administration and Adult Dosage. **PO for mild to moderate acute bacterial exacerbations of COPD, pharyngitis, or tonsillitis**—500 mg as a single dose on the first day followed by 250 mg/d on days 2–5 OR 500 mg once daily for 3 days for a total dosage of 1.5 g. **PO for community-acquired pneumonia, skin and skin structure infections, and shigellosis**—500 mg as a single dose on the first day followed by 250 mg/d on days 2–5 OR 2 g oral suspension 1 time as a single dose (community-acquired pneumonia only). **PO for sinusitis**—500 mg once daily for 3 days. **PO for gastroenteritis due to *Camphylobacter jejuni***—500 mg once daily for 7–14 days. **PO for nongonococcal urethritis and cervicitis caused by *C. trachomatis* or for chancroid (*Haemophilus ducreyi*), sexually transmitted infectious disease prophylaxis in victims of sexual aggression**—1 g as a single dose.[10] **PO for granuloma inguinale**—1 g once per week for at least 3 weeks OR until all lesions have healed. **PO for disseminated infection due to *Mycobacterium* avium-intracellulare (MAI) group in HIV infection**—500–600 mg daily in combination with ethambutol 15 mg/kg daily ± rifabutin 300 mg daily.[11] **PO for *Mycobacterium* avium complex infection (MAC) in nodular/bronchiectatic lung disease**—500–600 mg 1 times weekly in combination with ethambutol 25 mg/kg 3 times weekly and rifampin 600 mg 3 times weekly. **PO for MAC infection in cavitary lung disease**—250 mg daily in combination with ethambutol 15 mg/kg daily and rifampin 10 mg/kg daily, to a maximum of 600 mg daily. PO for MAC infection in severe lung disease—250–300 mg daily in combination with ethambutol 15 mg/kg daily and rifabutin 150–300 mg daily OR rifampin 10 mg/kg daily, and streptomycin OR amikacin. **PO for prevention of disseminated infection due to (MAI) group in HIV infection**—(primary prevention) 1200 mg once weekly OR 600 mg orally twice weekly;[12] (secondary prevention) 500–600 mg daily in combination with ethambutol 15 mg/kg daily ± rifabutin 300 mg daily. **PO for early localized or early disseminated Lyme disease associated with erythema migrans or borrelial lymphocytoma**—500 mg once daily for 7–10 days. **PO for babesiosis**—500–1000 mg on day 1 followed by 250 mg/d thereafter plus atovaquone 750 mg every 12 h for 7–10 days. **PO for endocarditis prophylaxis**—500 mg 30–60 min before procedure. **IV for pelvic inflammatory disease**—500 mg/d for 1–2 days, followed by PO 250 mg/d to complete 7 days of therapy. **IV for community-acquired pneumonia**—500 mg/d for at least 2 days followed by PO 500 mg/d to complete 7–10 days of therapy; ophthalmic for bacterial conjunctivitis. 1 drop in affected eye(s) twice daily (8–12 h apart) for 2 days, followed by 1 drop in affected eye(s) daily for an additional 5 days.

Special Populations. *Pediatric Dosage.* **PO**—(<6 months) Safety and efficacy not established. **PO for otitis media**—(≥6 months) 10 mg/kg as a single-daily dose on day 1, followed by 5 mg/kg/d as a single dose on days 2–5 OR 10 mg/kg daily for 3 days OR 30 mg/kg as a single dose. **PO for streptococcal pharyngitis/tonsillitis**—(≥2 years) 12 mg/kg/d as a single dose for 5 days.[13–15] **PO for endocarditis prophylaxis**—15 mg/kg 30–60 min before procedure. **PO for *C. trachomatis*—**(≥45 kg and 8-year-old) 1 g as a single dose. **PO for sinusitis**—10 mg/kg once daily for 3 days. **PO for community-acquired pneumonia**—(tablets OR suspension) 30 mg/kg as a single dose OR 10 mg/kg once daily for 3 days OR 10 mg/kg on day 1 followed by 5 mg/kg on day 2–5 (*See* Notes for ER Suspension.). **PO for early localized or early disseminated Lyme disease associated with erythema migrans or borrelial lymphocytoma**—10 mg/kg/d for 7–10 days, to a maximum of 500 mg/d; **PO for *Mycobacterium* avium-intracellulare group**—10–12 mg/kg daily in combination with ethambutol 15–25 mg/kg daily ± rifabutin 10–20 mg/kg daily; **PO for prevention of disseminated infection due to *Mycobacterium* avium-intracellulare group in HIV infection.** (Primary prevention)—20 mg/kg mg once weekly, secondary prevention—5 mg/kg daily in combination with ethambutol 15 mg/kg daily ± rifabutin 5 mg/kg daily. **PO for babesiosis**—10 mg/kg on day 1, to a maximum of 500 mg/dose, followed by 5 mg/kg/d, to a maximum of 250 mg/dose, thereafter and atovaquone 20 mg/kg, to a maximum of 750 mg/dose, every 12 h for 7–10 days. **Opthalmic for bacterial conjunctivitis**—(≥1 year) 1 drop in the affected eye(s) twice daily (8–12 h apart) for 2 days, followed by 1 drop in the affected eye(s) daily for an additional 5 days. **IV** (<16 years) Safety and efficacy not established.

Geriatric Dosage. Same as adult dosage.

Other Conditions. Dosage reduction may be needed in severe hepatic impairment, but specific adjustments are not defined.

Dosage Forms. **Tab** 250, 500, 600 mg; **Susp** 20, 40 mg/mL; **Pwdr for Oral Susp** 1 g/packet, 2 g/60 mL; **Inj** 250 mg, 500 mg; **Ophth Soln** 1%.

Patient Instructions. Take the oral suspension with a full glass of water on an empty stomach (1 h before or 2 h after meals) for best absorption. Tablets may be taken without regard to meals, but food or milk may improve tolerability. Do not take aluminum- or magnesium-containing antacids with azithromycin. If the patient vomits within 5 min of the dose, give another dose. If the patient vomits between 5 and 60 min, consider alternate therapy.

Missed Doses. Take this drug at regular intervals. If you miss a dose, take it as soon as you remember. If it is about time for the next dose, take that dose only. Leave at least 12 h between doses. Do not double the dose or take an extra dose.

Pharmacokinetics. *Fate.* Oral bioavailability is 38%. After a 500-mg oral tablet, a peak serum concentration of 0.41 mg/L (0.55 mol/L) is achieved in approximately 2 h. Plasma protein binding is 7%–51%, primarily to α_1-acid glycoprotein.

Azithromycin penetrates macrophages and polymorphonuclear leukocytes, accounting for intracellular concentrations that are 40-fold extracellular concentrations. Azithromycin is widely distributed throughout the body, and tissue concentrations (including the CNS) range from 10- to 150-fold higher than those in serum. Tissue concentrations peak 48 h after administration, and high concentrations persist for several days after drug discontinuation. Elimination is polyphasic, reflecting rapid initial distribution into tissues, followed by slow elimination. Oral V_d is 23–31 L/kg; clearance is 38 L/h in adults. Azithromycin is metabolized in the liver and eliminated largely through biliary excretion; only 6% is excreted unchanged in urine.[3,5,16,17] **Half-life** Terminal phase—11–68 h.[3,17]

Adverse Reactions. The drug is well tolerated. Frequent adverse effects are mild to moderate diarrhea, nausea, and abdominal pain. Headache and dizziness occur occasionally. Rash, angioedema, hepatomegaly, and cholestatic jaundice are reported rarely.[3] Myasthenia gravis has been reported

Contraindications. Hypersensitivity to any macrolide; fatalities due to allergic reaction have been reported.

Precautions. Pregnancy category B. Use during pregnancy only if clearly needed. Use caution in patients with impaired hepatic function or severely impaired renal function (GFR <10 mL/min).

Drug Interactions. Azithromycin does not interact with hepatic cytochrome P450 enzymes and, unlike erythromycin and clarithromycin, is not associated with these types of interactions.[18]

Parameters to Monitor. Baseline and periodic liver function tests during prolonged therapy.

Notes. The oral extended-release suspension is only approved for community-acquired pneumonia in children older than 6 months of age. If <34 kg, 60 mg/kg as a single dose should be administered; but if ≥34 kg, administer a 2-g single dose. Infuse the IV formulation at 1 mg/mL over 3 h OR 2 mg/mL over 1 h. Do not infuse over less than 60 min.

CLARITHROMYCIN
Biaxin, Various

Pharmacology. Clarithromycin is a semisynthetic macrolide antibiotic that is slightly more active than erythromycin against gram-positive bacteria, *Moraxella (Branhamella) catarrhalis*, and *Legionella* sp. It is very active against *Chlamydia* sp. and superior to other macrolides in its activity against MAC.[3,5,16,19,20] Like azithromycin, resistance to clarithromycin is a growing concern. A recent study comparing resistance patterns of macrolides demonstrated that azithromycin led to resistance in *S. pneumoniae* quicker than clarithromycin (4 vs. 8 days).[21] However, the same study demonstrated that clarithromycin led to a higher level resistance gene (ermB vs. mef).[21] Whether this phenomenon is clinically important, meaning that azithromycin resistance can be treated with clarithromycin, is unknown.

Administration and Adult Dosage. **PO for respiratory, sinusitis, and skin infections**—250–500 mg twice daily for 7–14 days or 1000 mg XL daily for 7–14 days. **PO for pharyngitis or tonsillitis**—250 mg twice daily for 10 days. **PO for endocarditis prophylaxis**—500 mg 30–60 min before procedure. **PO for eradication of *Helicobacter pylori***—500 mg 3 times daily for 10–14 days in combination with other medications based on current recommendations. (*See* Acid-Peptic Therapy.)[22] **PO for early localized or early disseminated Lyme disease associated with erythema migrans or borrelial lymphocytoma**—500 mg twice daily for 14–21 days. **PO for MAC infection in nodular/bronchiectatic lung disease**—1000 mg 3 times weekly in combination with ethambutol 25 mg/kg 3 times weekly and rifampin 600 mg 3 times weekly. **PO for MAC infection in cavitary lung disease**—1000 mg daily OR 500 mg twice daily in combination with ethambutol 15 mg/kg daily and rifampin 10 mg/kg daily, to a maximum of 600 mg daily. **PO MAC infection severe lung disease**—1000 mg daily OR 500 mg twice daily in combination with ethambutol 15 mg/kg daily, rifabutin 150–300 mg daily OR rifampin 10 mg/kg daily, and streptomycin OR amikacin.

Special Populations. *Pediatric Dosage.* **PO for community-acquired pneumonia**—7.5 mg/kg every 12 h for 10 days. **PO for otitis media, sinusitis, pharyngitis, tonsillitis, infection of skin, AND/OR subcutaneous tissue**—7.5 mg/kg twice daily for 10 days, to a maximum of 500 mg twice daily. **PO for prevention of disseminated infection due to (MAI) group in HIV infection**—(Primary prevention) 7.5 mg/kg ORALLY twice daily, to a maxiumum of 500 mg twice daily; (Secondary prevention) 7.5 mg/kg twice daily, to a maximum of 500 mg twice daily, in combination with ethambutol 15–25 mg/kg daily (maximum of 2.5 g/d) ± rifabutin 5 mg/kg daily (maximum of 300 mg/d). **PO for treatment of disseminated infection due to (MAI) group in HIV infection**—7.5–15 mg/kg twice daily, to a maximum of 500 mg twice daily, in combination with ethambutol 15–25 mg/kg once daily (maximum of 2.5 g/d) ± rifabutin 10–20 mg/kg once daily (maximum of 300 mg/d). **PO for early localized or early disseminated Lyme disease associated with erythema migrans, or borrelial lymphocytoma**—7.5 mg/kg twice daily for 14–21 days, to a maximum of 1000 mg/d. **PO for MAC infection in lung disease**—7.5 mg/kg twice daily, to a maximum of 500 mg twice daily, in combination with other antimycobacterial medications. **PO for endocarditis prophylaxis**—15 mg/kg 30–60 min before the procedure.

Geriatric Dosage. Same as adult dosage.

Other Conditions. Reduce dosage by 50% with Cl_{Cr} <30 mL/min.

Dosage Forms. **Tab** 250, 500 mg; **ER Tab** 500 mg; **Susp** 25, 50 mg/mL.

Pharmacokinetics. *Fate.* Clarithromycin is acid-stable and absorbed well with or without food. Bioavailability is 55%, with peak serum concentrations of about 2 mg/L attained after a 400-mg oral dose. The hydroxy metabolite is active and may be synergistic in vitro with the parent drug.[17] **Half-life** (Clarithromycin) 4.5 h; (hydroxy-metabolite) 4–9 h.[17]

Adverse Reactions. Similar to erythromycin, but clarithromycin has better gastrointestinal (GI) tolerance. As with all antibiotics, clarithromycin increases the chance of pseudomembranous colitis.

Contraindications. Hypersensitivity to any macrolide antibiotic; concurrent use with certain other drugs. (*See* Drug Interactions.)

Precautions. Pregnancy category C. Use with caution in severe renal (Cl$_{Cr}$ <25 mL/min) or hepatic function impairment; dosage reduction is advised.

Drug Interactions. Clarithromycin has a lower affinity for CYP3A4 than erythromycin, and therefore has fewer clinically important drug interactions; however, its use is contraindicated with astemizole, pimozide, terfenadine, ergotamine, dihydroergotamine, and cisapride. Serum concentrations of theophylline, sulfonylureas, and carbamazepine also can be increased by clarithromycin. Clarithromycin may induce toxicity of digoxin and rifabutin. Nonnucleoside reverse transcriptase inhibitors (e.g., efavirenz and nevirapine) may reduce clarithromycin concentration, but concomitant use with efavirenz may increase risk of forming a rash. Cardiotoxicity may occur in combination with quinidine. Some protease inhibitors (e.g., darunavir and tipranavir) may increase clarithromycin concentrations.

Notes. Clarithromycin immediate-release formulation indications are not synonymous to the extended-release formulation.

ERYTHROMYCIN AND SALTS   Various

Pharmacology. Erythromycin is a bacteriostatic macrolide antibiotic with a spectrum similar to that of penicillin G; it is also active against *Mycoplasma pneumoniae* and *Legionella pneumophila*.[23–25] It acts by binding to the 50S ribosomal subunit, inhibiting protein synthesis. Gram-positive organisms develop resistance via R-factor mediated alteration of the binding site. Gram-negative organisms are resistant because of cell wall impermeability. Erythromycin is now commonly used for gastroparesis.

Administration and Adult Dosage. *See* Erythromycin Comparison Chart.

ERYTHROMYCIN COMPARISON CHART

DRUG	DOSAGE FORMS	ADULT DOSAGE	PEDIATRIC DOSAGE	COMMENTS
Dirithromycin Dynabac	EC Tab 250 mg	PO 500 mg once daily for 7–14 days	<12 y not recommended	Spectrum similar to erythromycin, but less GI intolerance and little or no P450 inhibition
Erythromycin **Base** E-Mycin Ery-Tab ERYC various	EC Tab 250, 333, 500 mg EC Tab 333, 500 mg SR Cap 250 mg	PO 1 g/d in 2–4 doses, to a maximum of 4 g/d	PO 30–50 mg/kg/d in 4 doses; may double in severe infection[a]	Food interferes with absorption of uncoated products; EC products appear to be among the best tolerated erythromycin formulations[b]
Erythromycin **Estolate** Ilosone Various	Cap 250 mg Susp 25, 50 mg/mL Tab 500 mg	PO 250–500 mg every 6 h, to a maximum of 4 g/d	PO 30–50 mg/kg/d in 3–4 doses[a]	PO well absorbed; unaffected by food and highly resistant to gastric acid hydrolysis; absorbed as propionate ester which predominates in serum (8:1) and might be less active; rare intrahepatic cholestatic jaundice[b]
Erythromycin **Ethylsuccinate** E.E.S. EryPed Various	Drp 40 mg/mL Susp 40, 80 mg/mL Chew Tab 200 mg EC Tab 400 mg	PO 400 mg every 6 h, to a maximum of 4 g/d	PO 30–50 mg/kg/d in 3–4 doses; may double in severe infection[a]	Absorbed better than base; intermediate susceptibility to gastric acid hydrolysis; absorbed as ester, which predominates in serum (3:1) and may be less active; rare intrahepatic cholestatic jaundice[b]
Erythromycin **Gluceptate** Ilotycin	Inj (IV only) 1 g	IV 15–20 mg/kg/d in 3–4 doses, to a maximum of 4 g/d	IV same as adult dosage in 2–4 doses; may double in severe infection[a]	Painful; phlebitis frequent; avoid use if possible; infuse over 20–60 min[b]

(continued)

ERYTHROMYCIN COMPARISON CHART (*continued*)

DRUG	DOSAGE FORMS	ADULT DOSAGE	PEDIATRIC DOSAGE	COMMENTS
Erythromycin Lactobionate Erythrocin Various	Inj (IV only) 500 mg, 1 g	Same as erythromycin gluceptate	Same as erythromycin gluceptate[a]	Same as erythromycin gluceptate[b]
Erythromycin Stearate Various	EC Tab 250, 500 mg	PO 1 g/d in 2 OR 4 doses, to a maximum of 4 g/d	PO 30–50 mg/kg/d in 4 doses; may double in severe infections	Absorption about equal to ethylsuccinate, although food interferes markedly with absorption; hydrolyzed to free base before various absorption[b]
Erythromycin Romycin	Ophth Oint 0.5%	Apply a thin ribbon twice daily for 2 mo for chlamydial conjunctivitis in conjunction with oral therapy	Apply a thin ribbon to conjunctival sac within 1 h after birth to prevent ophthalmia neonatorum	Ribbon should be 0.5–2 cm long; ointment may blur vision

[a]In newborns, data are available for erythromycin estolate only, suggesting an oral dosage of 40 mg/kg•d in 2–4 divided doses.
[b]Despite differences in oral absorption, no clinical studies have shown any salt to be clearly superior in any particular therapeutic use.
From Refs. 33–38 and product information.

229

Special Populations. *Pediatric Dosage. See* Erythromycin Antibiotics Comparison Chart.

Geriatric Dosage. Same as adult dosage.

Other Conditions. Dosage adjustment is probably unnecessary in renal impairment.[13,23]

Dosage Forms. *See* Erythromycin Antibiotics Comparison Chart.

Patient Instructions. Take this drug with a full glass of water on an empty stomach (1 h before or 2 h after meals) for best absorption. Refrigerate the suspension.

Missed Doses. Take this drug at regular intervals. If you miss a dose, take it as soon as you remember. If it is about time for the next dose, take that dose only. Leave at least 4–6 h between doses. Do not double the dose or take an extra dose.

Pharmacokinetics. *Fate.* Oral absorption varies widely with the salt and dosage forms (*see* Erythromycin Antibiotics Comparison Chart), with peak serum concentrations occurring from 30 min (suspension) to 4 h (coated tablet) after administration. However, enteric-coated erythromycin base tablets, stearate tablets, and estolate capsules produce equivalent erythromycin serum levels when administered to fasting subjects. Food or restricted water intake (e.g., <20 mL) with a dose dramatically lowers the absorption of the stearate form. The drug is 83% ± 5% plasma protein-bound and widely distributed into most tissues, cavities, and body fluids except the brain and CSF (even with meningeal inflammation). V_d is 0.6 ± 0.1 L/kg; clearance is 0.55 ± 0.25 L/h/kg. Erythromycin is partially metabolized in the liver by CYP3A3/4 and excreted primarily as unchanged erythromycin with high concentrations in the bile and feces. Only 12%–15% of an IV dose is excreted unchanged in urine.[23] **Half-life** 1.6 ± 0.7 h; unchanged or slightly prolonged in anuric patients, based on minimal data; prolonged in cirrhosis.

Adverse Reactions. Frequent GI distress. IM form is very painful, despite local anesthetic (butamben) in the product, and might produce sterile abscesses. IV administration frequently produces pain, venous irritation, and phlebitis. Mild elevations of serum hepatic enzymes occur frequently. Transient deafness occurs occasionally with high dosages.[23,26] Rare, but potentially serious, reversible intrahepatic cholestatic jaundice occurs primarily with the estolate and ethylsuccinate forms, usually in adults after 10–14 days of therapy, although it can occur after the first dose if there is a history of previous use. Prodrome includes malaise, nausea, vomiting, fever, and abdominal pain (which can be severe and misdiagnosed as acute surgical abdomen). Symptoms resolve in 1–2 weeks, and serum enzymes return to normal over several months.

Contraindications. Concurrent use with astemizole, cisapride, or pimozide; IM form in patients with hypersensitivity to local anesthetics of the para-aminobenzoic acid type (e.g., procaine); hepatic dysfunction (estolate and ethylsuccinate forms).

Precautions. Pregnancy. Use with caution in patients with liver disease because of possibly impaired excretion.

Drug Interactions. Erythromycin inhibits CYP3A4 and can reduce hepatic metabolism of some drugs, including astemizole, carbamazepine, cisapride, cyclosporine, theophylline, triazolam, warfarin, and others.[27] (*See* Contraindications.)

Parameters to Monitor. Liver function tests in patients who experience prodromal symptoms (*see* Adverse Reactions) while receiving the estolate or ethylsuccinate form; check daily for vein irritation and phlebitis in patients receiving IV forms. Closely monitor the effects of other drugs that interact with erythromycin during concurrent use.

Notes. Avoid injectable forms if at all possible, and oral suspension is preferred. Erythromycin is more active in an alkaline environment. Unrelated to its antibacterial effect, erythromycin in low doses binds to motilin receptors in the GI tract to stimulate gastric emptying. Erythromycin is commonly used therapeutically for **gastroparesis** 150–250 mg PO before meals and at bedtime or 200 mg IV of the lactobionate salt, 250 mg of the ethylsuccinate salt or 500 mg of the base 15–120 min before meals and at bedtime.[28–32]

■ REFERENCES

1. Retsema J et al. Spectrum and mode of action of azithromycin (CP-62,993), a new 15-membered-ring macrolide with improved potency against gram-negative organisms. *Antimicrob Agents Chemother.* 1987;31:1939-1947.
2. Bahal N, Nahata MC. The new macrolide antibiotics: azithromycin, clarithromycin, dirithromycin, and roxithromycin. *Ann Pharmacother.* 1992;26:46-55.
3. Schlossberg D. Azithromycin and clarithromycin. *Med Clin North Am.* 1995;79:803-815.
4. Berry A et al. Azithromycin therapy for disseminated *Mycobacterium avium-intracellulare* in AIDS patients. First National Conference on Human Retroviruses. Washington, DC; 1993. Abstract 292.
5. Zuckerman JM. The newer macrolides: azithromycin and clarithromycin. *Infect Dis Clin North Am.* 2000;14:449-462.
6. Waterer GW et al. Decreasing β-lactam resistance in pneumococci from the Memphis region: analysis of 2,152 isolates from 1996 to 2001. *Chest.* 2003;124:519-525.
7. Perez-Trallero E et al. Geographical and ecological analysis of resistance, coresistance, and coupled resistance to antimicrobials in respiratory pathogenic bacteria in Spain. *Antimicrob Agents Chemother.* 2005;49:1965-1972.
8. Musher DM et al. Emergence of macrolide resistance during treatment of pneumococcal pneumonia. *N Engl J Med.* 2002;346:630-631.
9. Lonks JR et al. Failure of macrolide antibiotic treatment in patients with bacteremia due to erythromycin-resistant *Streptococcus pneumoniae*. *Clin Infect Dis.* 2002;35:556-564.
10. Anon. 1993 Sexually transmitted diseases treatment guidelines. *MMWR Morb Mortal Wkly Rep.* 1993; 42(RR-14):1-102.
11. Centers for Disease Control and Prevention. Recommendations on prophylaxis and therapy for disseminated *Mycobacterium avium* complex for adults and adolescents infected with human immunodeficiency virus. *MMWR Morb Mortal Wkly Rep.* 1993;42(RR-9):14-20.
12. Havlir D et al. Prophylaxis against disseminated *Mycobacterium avium* complex with weekly azithromycin, daily rifabutin, or both. *N Engl J Med.* 1996;335:392-398.
13. McLinn S. Double blind and open label studies of azithromycin in the management of acute otitis media in children: a review. *Pediatr Infect Dis J.* 1995;14:S62-S66.
14. Hopkins SJ, Williams D. Clinical tolerability and safety of azithromycin in children. *Pediatr Infect Dis J.* 1995;14:S67-S71.
15. Nahata MC. Pharmacokinetics of azithromycin in pediatric patients: comparison with other agents used for treating otitis media and streptococcal pharyngitis. *Pediatr Infect Dis J.* 1995;14:S39-S44.
16. Piscitelli SQ et al. Clarithromycin and azithromycin: new macrolide antibiotics. *Clin Pharm.* 1992;11:137-152.
17. Rodvold KA, Piscitelli SQ. New oral macrolide and fluoroquinolone antibiotics: an overview of pharmacokinetics, interactions, and safety. *Clin Infect Dis.* 1993;17(suppl 1):S192-S199.
18. Dunn CJ, Barradell LB. Azithromycin: a review of its pharmacological properties and use as 3-day therapy in respiratory tract infections. *Drugs.* 1996;51:483-505.
19. McConnell SA, Amsden GW. Review and comparison of advanced-generation macrolides clarithromycin and dirithromycin. *Pharmacotherapy.* 1999;19:404-415.
20. Matsiota-Bernard P et al. Comparison of clarithromycin-sensitive and clarithromycin-resistant Mycobacterium avium strains isolated from AIDS patients during therapy regimens including clarithromycin. *J Infect.* 2000;40:49-54.

21. Malhotra-Kumar S et al. Effect of azithromycin and clarithromycin therapy on pharyngeal carriage of macrolide-resistant streptococci in healthy volunteers: a randomised, double-blind, placebo-controlled study. *Lancet.* 2007; 369:482-490.

22. Markham A, Mctavish D. Clarithromycin and omeprazole as *Helicobacter pylori* eradication therapy in patients with *H. pylori*-associated gastric disorders. *Drugs.* 1996;51:161-178.

23. Brittain DC. Erythromycin. *Med Clin North Am.* 1987;71:1147-1154.

24. Washington JA, Wilson WR. Erythromycin: a microbial and clinical perspective after 30 years of clinical use. (2 parts). *Mayo Clin Proc.* 1985;60:189-203, 271-278.

25. Smilack JD et al. Tetracyclines, chloramphenicol, erythromycin, clindamycin, and metronidazole. *Mayo Clin Proc.* 1991;66:1270-1280.

26. Eichenwald HF. Adverse reactions to erythromycin. *Pediatr Infect Dis J.* 1986;5:147-150.

27. Amsden GW. Macrolides versus azalides: a drug interaction update. *Ann Pharmacother.* 1995;29:906-917.

29. Peeters TL. Erythromycin and other macrolides as prokinetic agents. *Gastroenterology.* 1993;105:1886-1899.

28. Weber FH et al. Erythromycin: a motilin agonist and gastrointestinal prokinetic agent. *Am J Gastroenterol.* 1993;88:485-490.

30. Lartey PA et al. New developments in macrolides: structures and antibacterial and prokinetic activities. *Adv Pharmacol.* 1994;28:307-343.

31. Kreek MJ, Culpepper-Morgan JA. Constipation syndromes. In: Lewis JH, ed. *A Pharmacologic Approach to Gastrointestinal Disorders.* Baltimore: Williams & Wilkins; 1994:179-208.

32. Dive A et al. Effect of erythromycin on gastric motility in mechanically ventilated critically ill patients: a double-blind, randomized, placebo-controlled study. *Crit Care Med.* 1995;23:1356-1362.

33. Guay DRP. Macrolide antibiotics in paediatric infectious diseases. *Drugs.* 1996;51:515-536.

34. Bloomfield G. A comparison of gastrointestinal tolerance to five different forms of erythromycin. *P&T* 1996;April:209-214.

35. Dajani AS et al. Prevention of bacterial endocarditis. Recommendations by the American Heart Association. *JAMA.* 1990;264:2919-2922.

36. Ginsburg CM. Pharmacology of erythromycin in infants and children. *Pediatr Infect Dis J.* 1986;5:124-129.

37. Brogden RN, Peters DH. Dirithromycin. A review of its antimicrobial activity, pharmacokinetic properties and therapeutic efficacy. *Drugs.* 1994;48:599-616.

38. Anon. Dirithromycin. *Med Lett Drugs Ther.* 1995;37:109-110.

Chapter 13

Quinolones

Mary Gauthier-Lewis and Treavor T. Riley

Fluoroquinolones (FQ) are the only class of antimicrobial agents in clinical use that are direct inhibitors of bacterial DNA synthesis. Thus, FQ are bactericidal agents. While there are 6 available FQ, multiple FQ have been withdrawn from the market for various reasons: sparfloxacin (lack of sales, QT-interval prolongation and increased risk of heart arrhythmias), lomefloxacin (unknown), gatifloxacin (greater variability regarding blood glucose compared to other FQ), trovafloxacin (severe liver toxicity), and enoxacin (unknown).

CIPROFLOXACIN	Ciloxan, Cipro, Proquin XR, Cirpodex

Pharmacology. Ciprofloxacin is a FQ that inhibits bacterial DNA gyrase (an essential enzyme that is involved in the replication, transcription, and repair of bacterial DNA) and topoisomerase IV (an enzyme known to play a key role in the partitioning of the chromosomal DNA during bacterial cell division),[1] enzymes responsible for the unwinding of DNA for transcription and subsequent supercoiling of DNA for packaging into chromosomal subunits. It is highly active against aerobic, gram-negative bacilli, especially *Enterobacteriaceae*, with MICs often <0.1 mg/L. It is also active against some strains of *Pseudomonas aeruginosa* and *Staphylococcus* spp., with an MIC[90] of 0.5–1 mg/L; atypical pneumonias, including *Legionella pneumophila*, *Mycoplasma pneumoniae*, and *Chlamydophila* (formerly *Chlamydia*) *pneumoniae*, and against genital pathogens such as *Chlamydia trachomatis*, *Ureaplasma urealyticum*, and *Mycoplasma hominis*. However, recent reports indicate increasing resistance to this agent in methicillin-resistant *S. aureus* and *P. aeruginosa*.[2,3] The likelihood of developing quinolone resistance is thought to be related to the intensity and duration of therapy. Support for the importance of duration comes from an in vitro model of *Staphylococcus aureus* infection, in which exposure to a quinolone for five days or more was associated with significant drug resistance.[4] Ciprofloxacin has poor activity against streptococci and anaerobes.[5,6]

Administration and Adult Dosage. **PO for uncomplicated UTI**—250 mg every 12 h for 3 days. **PO for moderate to severe systemic infections**—500–750 mg every 12 h for 7–14 days (28 days if bacterial prostatitis). **PO for urethral/cervical gonococcal infections**—250–500 mg once (Centers for Disease Control and Prevention recommend concomitant doxycline or azithromycin due to possible coinfection with *Chlamydia*). **PO for chancroid**—500 mg every 12 h for 3 days.[7] **IV for mild to moderate UTI and systemic infections**—200–400 mg every 12 h. **IV for severe bronchitis, lower respiratory tract, and skin/subcutaneous tissue infections**—750 mg every 12 h for 7–14 days. Ciprofloxacin is also used topically as the hydrochloride salt in eardrops containing the equivalent of 0.2% or 0.3% of ciprofloxacin, usually with a corticosteroid (such as dexamethasone or hydrocortisone) for the treatment of otitis externa and chronic suppurative otitis media caused by susceptible strains of bacteria.

Special Populations. *Pediatric Dosage.* (<18 years) Safety and efficacy not established. Use has been limited because of the potential for arthropathy. Ciprofloxacin has been used in children younger than 18 years in limited situations to treat anthrax and complicated UTI. **IV for** *P. aeruginosa* **infections in cystic fibrosis**—30 mg/kg/d in 2–3 divided doses. **PO for** *P. aeruginosa* **infections in cystic fibrosis**—40 mg/kg/d in 2 divided doses.[8]

Geriatric Dosage. Reduce dosage for age-related reduction in renal function, although dosage reduction is not necessary with only minor age-related renal function changes.[9] The risk of torsades de pointes and tendon inflammation and/or rupture associated with concomitant use of corticosteroids and quinolones is increased in the elderly.

Other Conditions. Reduce dosage to 200–400 mg IV every 18–24 h OR 250–500 mg PO every 18 h (every 24 h if on dialysis) when Cl_{Cr} <30 mL/min; dosage adjustments in patients with cystic fibrosis are not necessary.[10]

Dosage Forms. **Inj** 200, 400 mg; **Susp** 50, 100 mg/mL; **Tab** 100, 250, 500, 750 mg; **Ophth Drp** (Ciloxan) 3.5 mg/mL (equivalent to 3 mg/mL base); **Otic Susp** (CiproHC) 2 mg plus hydrocortisone 10 mg/mL; (Ciprodex) 3 mg plus dexamethasone 1 mg/mL.

Patient Instructions. This drug may be taken with food to minimize stomach upset. Avoid antacid use during treatment; calcium, iron, or zinc supplements can reduce absorption. Avoid excessive exposure to sunlight during ciprofloxacin treatment. Report any tendon pain or inflammation that occurs during therapy.

Missed Doses. Take this drug at regular intervals. If you miss a dose, take it as soon as you remember. If it is about time for the next dose, take that dose only. Leave at least 6–8 h between doses.

Pharmacokinetics. *Fate.* A peak serum level of 4–6 mg/L (12–18 mmol/L) 2 h after an oral 750–1000 mg dose is proposed as evidence of absorption adequate for tuberculosis therapy.[11] Approximately 70%–80% absorbed orally; food decreases the rate but not the extent of absorption. Aluminum-, calcium-, or magnesium-containing antacids or sucralfate markedly decrease the extent of absorption. Peak serum concentrations are 3 ± 0.6 mg/L (9 ± 1.8 mmol/L) after a 750-mg oral dose; a 200-mg IV dose infused over 30 min results in a peak concentration of about 3.2 ± 0.6 mg/L. V_d averages 2 L/kg. Renal clearance averages 0.26 L/h/kg. Less than 30% is plasma protein bound. Ciprofloxacin attains very high concentrations in many body fluids and tissues, most notably urine, prostate, and pulmonary mucosa. CSF concentrations are <1 mg/L; experience with the drug in the treatment of meningitis is very limited. From 45% to 60% of a parenteral dose is recovered unchanged in urine; the remainder is excreted as 4 metabolites with limited activity—oxociprofloxacin appears to be the major urinary metabolite and sulfociprofloxacin the primary fecal metabolite.[9,12–16] **Half-life** 4.2 ± 0.63 h,[15] 6.9 ± 2.9 h in severe renal impairment.[16]

Adverse Reactions. GI intolerance (e.g., nausea, vomiting, diarrhea, and abdominal discomfort) occurs frequently. CNS effects, such as headaches and restlessness, have occurred in 1%–2% of patients. Other CNS effects (e.g., dizziness, insomnia, anxiety, irritability, and seizures) have been reported in less than 1% of patients. Hallucinations, delirium, and seizures are rare. Seizures may have resulted in some, but not all cases, from theophylline accumulation or from the ability of theophylline and NSAIDs to augment quinolone-mediated displacement of GABA from its receptors.[17] Skin rashes and photosensitivity occur occasionally. Anaphylaxis rarely occurs.[12]

Contraindications. Hypersensitivity to ciprofloxacin, any quinolone, or any component of the formulation; concomitant tizanidine use.

Precautions. Pregnancy; lactation; high risk for tendon rupture; excessive sunlight; high risk for seizures.

Drug Interactions. When coadministered by mouth with aluminum-, magnesium-, or, to a lesser extent, calcium-containing antacids, quinolones have markedly reduced oral bioavailability, presumably because of the formation of cation–quinolone complexes, which are poorly absorbed.[14] Although there is some information that spacing administration by ≥2 h might minimize these interactions, it is best not to use ciprofloxacin in patients taking long-term antacid therapy. Iron supplements and zinc-containing multivitamins can reduce absorption. Nutritional supplements given by nasogastric tube may reduce the absorption of quinolones given concurrently by the same route, likely because these supplements also contain multivalent cations, such as iron and zinc. Theophylline clearance and ropinirole metabolism can be reduced in some patients receiving ciprofloxacin (20%–90% increase in theophylline concentrations). Patients receiving FQ and methylxanthines, such as theophylline or caffeine, might be at increased risk of CNS toxicity (e.g., convulsions). Warfarin metabolism can be decreased by ciprofloxacin, although studies with a different fluoroquinolone (enoxacin) indicate that only the metabolism of the less active (R)-warfarin isomer is affected. Use caution when adding ciprofloxacin in a patient taking warfarin. The solubility of ciprofloxacin is reduced at higher pH values; thus, avoid alkalinization of the urine.[14] Ciprofloxacin has demonstrated variable effects on glucose in patients taking antidiabetic medications, including insulin. Monitor blood glucose closely in such patients. FQ can prolong QT interval by inhibiting potassium channels involved in cardiac repolarization.[18] This effect may be augmented if FQ are given together with class III (e.g., sotalol) and class IA antiarrhythmics (e.g., quinidine) or other drugs that prolong QT interval. Because of the increased risk of arrhythmias associated with prolongation of QT interval, in general, FQ should not be given together with other drugs known to prolong QT interval.[19] It is also recommended that gemifloxacin, levofloxacin, moxifloxacin, and ofloxacin be avoided in patients with predisposing factors or who are also receiving other drugs that are known to cause this effect; while norfloxacin should be used with caution in these situations.[20]

Parameters to Monitor. Monitor serum theophylline levels closely in patients receiving theophylline. Monitor prothrombin time and signs of bleeding in patients on warfarin, CBC, renal and hepatic function during prolonged use.

Notes. If infusion is given over less than 30 min OR small veins in the hand are used, there is an increased risk of local site reaction. Preferred is a slow infusion over 60 min. FQ are no longer recommended by the CDC for the treatment of gonorrhea. Most active against *P. aeruginosa*. Do not use against gram-positive organisms, such as *S. aureus*.

OFLOXACIN	Floxin, Ocuflox
LEVOFLOXACIN	Levaquin, Iquix, Quixin

Pharmacology. Ofloxacin is a systemic fluoroquinolone similar to ciprofloxacin. Levofloxacin is the active L-isomer of ofloxacin that allows higher dosages of the active form to be given with fewer side effects. Ofloxacin has greater activity against *Chlamydia trachomatis*, *Ureaplasma urealyticum*, *Mycoplasma pneumoniae*, and *Mycobacterium tuberculosis* than ciprofloxacin, but less activity against *P. aeruginosa*.[5,6,11,12,21] Levofloxacin is the active (S)-enantiomer of ofloxacin and has the same spectrum of activity as ofloxacin but is generally 2-fold more potent.

Administration and Adult Dosage. (Ofloxacin) **IV or PO for community-acquired pneumonia, bronchitis, pelvic inflammatory disease, and skin/subcutaneous tissue infection**—400 mg every 12 h for 10–14 days. **PO for non-gonococcal urethritis, *Chlamydia*, and epididymitis**—300 mg every 12 h for 7–10 days. **PO for Traveler's diarrhea**—300 mg twice daily for 1–3 days. **PO for prostatitis**—300 mg twice daily for 6 weeks. **PO for acute, uncomplicated gonorrhea**—400 mg once. **IV or PO for urinary tract infections and cystitis**—200 mg every 12 h for 7–10 days. **Ophthalmic**—1–2 drops every 30 min while awake and every 4–6 h after retiring for 2 days, then every hour while awake for 4–6 days, then 1–2 drops 4 times daily until cured. **Otic for chronic purulent otitis media**—10 drops twice daily for 14 days. **Otic for otitis externa**—10 drops once daily for 7 days. (Levofloxacin) **PO or IV for chronic bronchitis**—500 mg every 24 h for at least 7 days. **PO or IV for pneumonia, sinusitis, and skin infections**—500 mg every 24 h for 7–14 days OR 750 mg every 24 h for 5 days (7–14 days, if noscomial pneumonia). **PO or IV for UTI**—250 mg once daily for 3–10 days OR 750 mg daily for 5 days. **PO or IV for prostatitis**—500 mg every 24 h for 28 days. **Ophthalmic**—1–2 drops every 2 h while awake up to 8 times/d for 2 days, then every 4 h while awake for 5 days.

Special Populations. *Pediatric Dosage.* **PO, IV**—(<18 years) Safety and efficacy not established. **Ophthalmic**—(<1 year) Safety and efficacy not established, (>1 year) Same as adult dosage. **Otic for otitis externa**—(Ofloxacin) (6 months–13 years) 5 drops once daily for 7 days, (>13 years) Same as adult dosage. **Otic for acute otitis media**—(1–12 years) 5 drops twice daily for 10 days. **Otic for chronic purulent otitis media**—Same as adult dosage.

Renal Impairment. (Levofloxacin) After an initial dose of 750 mg daily and Cl_{Cr} of 20–49 mL/min, subsequent doses are 750 mg every 48 h; Cl_{Cr} up to 19 mL/min (including hemodialysis and continuous peritoneal dialysis patients), subsequent doses are 500 mg every 48 h. After an initial dose of 500 mg daily and Cl_{Cr} of 20–49 mL/min, subsequent doses are 250 mg every 24 h; Cl_{Cr} up to 19 mL/min (including haemodialysis and continuous peritoneal dialysis patients), subsequent doses are 250 mg every 48 h. After an initial dose of 250 mg daily, Cl_{Cr} 10–19 mL/min, subsequent doses are 250 mg every 48 h. (Ofloxacin) after a normal initial dose; Cl_{Cr} 20–50 mL/min, administer usual dose every 24 h; Cl_{Cr} <20 mL/min, administer 50% of the usual dose every 24 h.

Hepatic Impairment. (Ofloxacin) in cirrhosis, the maximum PO dose is 400 mg every 24 h.

Geriatric Dosage. The risk of torsades de pointes and tendon inflammation and/or rupture associated with concomitant use of corticosteroids and quinolones is increased in the elderly.

Other Conditions. The clearance of ofloxacin is reduced in patients with severe hepatic impairment or cirrhosis and lower doses should be used; a maximum dose of 400 mg daily has been recommended.

Dosage Forms. (Ofloxacin) **Inj** 200, 400 mg; **Tab** 200, 300, 400 mg; **Ophth Drp** (Ocuflox) 3 mg/mL; **Otic Drp** 3 mg/mL. (Levofloxacin) **Inj** 5, 25 mg/mL; **Tab** 250, 500 mg; **Ophth Drp** (Quixin) 5 mg/mL.

Pharmacokinetics. *Fate.* Ofloxacin is >95% bioavailable orally. A peak serum concentration of 8–12 mg/L (22–33 mmol/L) 2 h after an oral dose of 600–800 mg is proposed as evidence of absorption adequate for tuberculosis therapy. Ofloxacin is predominantly renally excreted with a half-life of 5–7 h. Levofloxacin is rapidly and completely absorbed after oral administration. Peak plasma concentrations are usually attained 1–2 h after oral dosing. Steady state is reached within 48 h following a 500 or 750 mg once-daily dosage regimen The mean peak and trough concentrations attained following multiple once-daily oral dosage regimens were approximately 5.7 and 0.5 μg/mL after the 500 mg doses, and 8.6 and 1.1 μg/mL after the 750 mg doses, respectively.[22] The mean peak and trough plasma concentrations attained following multiple once-daily IV regimens were approximately 6.4 and 0.6 μg/mL after the 500 mg doses and 12.1 and 1.3 μg/mL after the 750 mg doses, respectively.[22] The mean volume of distribution of levofloxacin generally ranges from 74 to 112 L after single and multiple 500 or 750 mg doses, indicating widespread distribution into body tissues. It reaches peak levels in skin tissues and in blister fluid at ~3 h after dosing.[22] Levofloxacin also penetrates well into the lung tissues. Lung tissue concentrations were generally 2- to 5-fold higher than plasma concentrations. Levofloxacin undergoes limited metabolism and is primarily excreted as unchanged drug in the urine. Less than 4% of the dose was recovered in the feces in 72 h. Less than 5% of an administered dose was recovered in the urine as the desmethyl and N-oxide metabolites. These metabolites have little relevant pharmacological activity. The mean apparent total body clearance and renal clearance range from approximately 144 to 226 mL/min and 96–142 mL/min, respectively.[22] **Half-life** (Levofloxacin) 6.3–7.5 (single dose oral or IV); 7–8.8 (multiple dose oral or IV).[22] (Ofloxacin) biphasic: 5–7.5 h and 20–25 h (accounts for <5%).[10]

Adverse Reactions. *See* Ciprofloxacin.

Drug Interactions. (*See* Ciprofloxacin.) Ofloxacin does not alter hepatic metabolism of methylxanthine compounds (e.g., caffeine or theophylline). However, like other FQ, cations markedly reduce the absorption of this agent.

Special Instructions. Levofloxacin tablets can be administered without regard to food. It is recommended that Levofloxacin oral solution be taken 1 h before or 2 h after eating.

Notes. FQs are no longer recommended by the CDC for the treatment of gonorrhea. Levofloxacin has been used for inhaled anthrax prophylaxis in children older than 6 months with weight-base dosing. Use longer durations of therapy for more complicated infections. Levofloxacin is not appreciably removed from the body during hemodialysis or peritoneal dialysis. Ofloxacin is most active against *Chlamydia* spp.

MOXIFLOXACIN
Avelox, Vigamox

Pharmacology. Moxifloxacin is an 8-methoxyquinolone that has an increased spectrum of activity against gram-negative and gram-positive microorganisms, including *Streptococcus pneumoniae*.[23–25] Levofloxacin and moxifloxacin have gram-negative coverage similar to that of ciprofloxacin but all may be less active particularly against some strains of *P. aeruginosa* and moxifloxacin is less active against some strains of *Providencia spp*, *Proteus spp*, and *Serratia marcescens*. All of the newer quinolones, as well as ciproxacin and ofloxacin, are highly active against *H. influenzae* and *Moraxella catarrhalis*. However, levofloxacin and moxifloxacin exhibit increased potency relative to ciprofloxacin and ofloxacin against *S. pneumoniae* (MIC^{90} values of 1–2 µg/mL for levofloxacin and 0.12–0.25 µg/mL for moxifloxacin.[26,27] Most methicillin-susceptible strains of *S. aureus* are susceptible to levofloxacin (MIC^{90} of 0.5–1 µg/mL),[28] moxifloxacin (MIC^{90} of 0.12 µg/mL),[27] and gemifloxacin (MIC^{90} of 0.03 µg/mL).[29] Activity against enterococci is marginal, with MIC^{90} values of 3.1 µg/mL for levofloxacin and 0.5–8 µg/mL for moxifloxacin.[27]

Administration and Adult Dosage.[30] **IV or PO for acute bacterial sinusitis**— 400 mg every 24 h for 10 days. **PO for acute bacterial exacerbation of COPD**— 400 mg every 24 h for 5 days. **IV or PO for intra-abdominal infections**—400 mg every 24 h for 5–14 days; **IV or PO for community-acquired pneumonia**—400 mg every 24 h for 7–14 days. **IV or PO for skin and skin structure infections**— 400 mg every 24 h for 7–21 days. **Ophthalmic for bacterial conjunctivitis**— 1 drop 3 times daily for 7 days.

Special Populations. *Pediatric Dosage.* **PO, IV**—(<18 years) Safety and efficacy not established. **Ophthalmic for bacterial conjunctivitis**—(≥1 year) Same as adult dosage.

Other Conditions. The pharmacokinetic parameters of moxifloxacin are not significantly altered by mild, moderate, or severe renal impairment. No dosage adjustment is necessary, including patients on hemodialysis or continuous renal replacement therapy. No dosage adjustment is required in mild to moderate hepatic insufficiency or the elderly. Not recommended in patients with severe hepatic insufficiency.

Dosage Forms. (Avelox) **Inj** 400 mg; **Tab** 400 mg; **Ophth Sol** (Vigamox) 0.5%.

Pharmacokinetics. *Fate.* Moxifloxacin oral bioavailability ranges from 86% to 100% (mean 91.8%). Moxifloxacin is well absorbed from the GI tract. Coadministration with a high-fat meal (e.g., 500 calories from fat) does not affect the absorption of moxifloxacin. Consumption of 1 cup of yogurt with moxifloxacin does not significantly affect the extent or rate of systemic absorption (AUC). The C_{max} is attained 1–3 h after oral dosing. The mean trough concentration is approximately 0.95 µg/mL. Plasma concentrations increase proportionally. Steady state is achieved after ≥3 days with a 400 mg once-daily regimen. The volume of distribution ranges from 1.7–2.7 L/kg. Moxifloxacin is widely distributed throughout the body, with tissue concentrations often exceeding plasma concentrations. The rates of elimination of moxifloxacin from tissue generally parallel the elimination from plasma. Moxifloxacin is metabolized via glucuronide and sulfate conjugation. The cytochrome P450 system is not involved and is not affected by moxifloxacin. The sulfate-conjugate (M1) accounts for approximately 38% of the dose and is eliminated primarily in the feces. Approximately 14% of an oral or IV dose are converted to a glucuronide conjugate (M2), which is excreted exclusively in the urine. A total of 95% of an oral dose is excreted as either unchanged drug or known metabolites. The mean apparent total body clearance and renal clearance are approximately 12 L/h and 2.6 L/h, respectively.[31] **Half-life** (PO) 12 h; (IV) 15 h.[30]

Adverse Reactions. (*See* Ciprofloxacin.) Moxifloxacin tends to have fewer CNS effects than some FQ (e.g., norfloxacin) and more than others (e.g., ciprofloxacin, levofloxacin).[31,32]

Drug Interactions. (See Ciprofloxacin.) Concomitant antiarrhythmic agents (e.g., amiodarone, bretylium, disopyramide, procainamide, quinidine, sotalol) increase the risk of life-threatening cardiac arrhythmias, including torsades de pointes. The mechanism is unknown.[33] No effect on theophylline or warfarin metabolism.

Notes. Use longer durations of therapy for more complicated infections. Enhanced activity against common community-acquired pneumonia pathogens.

GEMIFLOXACIN MESYLATE   Factive

Pharmacology. Gemifloxacin is a synthetic, broad-spectrum antibacterial agent that inhibits DNA gyrase and topoisomerase IV, similar to ciprofloxacin. Gemifloxacin is distinctive for its unusually high potency against pneumococci (MIC90 value of 0.03 µg/mL).[34] Gemifloxacin is reported to have greater activity against gram-positive bacteria, including pneumococci, than ciprofloxacin.[35]

Administration and Adult Dosage. **Acute bacterial exacerbation of chronic bronchitis** –(*S. pneumoniae, Haemophilus influenzae, Haemophilus parainfluenzae,* or *Moraxella catarrhalis*) 320 mg daily for 5 days. **Community-acquired pneumonia (mild to moderate)**—(*Haemophilus influenzae, Moraxella catarrhalis, Mycoplasma pneumoniae, Chlamydia pneumoniae, Klebsiella pneumoniae,* or *Streptococcus pneumoniae*) 320 mg daily for 5–7 days.[36–38]

Special Populations. *Pediatric Dosage.* PO, IV—(<18 years) Safety and efficacy not established.

Other Conditions. *Renal Impairment.* (Cl$_{Cr}$ ≤40 mL/min OR patient on hemodialysis) 160 mg once daily and dose should be administered after dialysis. No dose adjustment necessary for hepatic impairment.

Dosage Forms. Tab 320 mg.

Pharmacokinetics. *Fate.* Gemifloxacin is rapidly absorbed from the GI tract with an absolute bioavailability of approximately 71%. Peak plasma concentrations occur 0.5–2 h. Gemifloxacin is widely distributed into body tissues including the bronchial mucosa and lungs and is 55% to 73% bound to plasma proteins.[39] It undergoes limited hepatic metabolism. It is predominately excreted as unchanged drug and metabolites in the feces and urine. **Half-life** 7 h (range 4–12 h).[39]

Adverse Reactions. (*See* Ciprofloxacin.) Almost 14% of women younger than 40 years developed a rash when taking this agent for more than 7 days. This adverse effect is largely avoided by using a 5-day course of treatment. Treatment with gemifloxacin should be stopped if this occurs.

Contraindications. *See* Ciprofloxacin.

Precautions. *See* Ciprofloxacin.

Drug Interactions. *See* Ciprofloxacin.

Notes. Reported to have greater activity against gram-positive bacteria, including pneumococci, than ciprofloxacin.

NORFLOXACIN   Noroxin

Pharmacology. Norfloxacin is a synthetic broad spectrum FQ used in the treatment of prostatitis caused by *Escherichia coli,* and UTI (including cystitis) caused by *Enterococcus faecalis, E. coli, Klebsiella pneumoniae, Protus mirabilis, Pseudomonas aeruginosa, Staphylococcus epidermidis, Staphylococcus saprophyticus, Citrobacter freundii, Enterobacter aerogenes, Enterobacter cloacae, Proteus vulgaris, Staphylococcus aureus* or *Streptococcus agalactiae.* Complicated UTIs caused by *Enterococcus faecalis, E. coli, K. pneumoniae, P. mirabilis, P. aeruginosa,* or *Serratia marcescens.*

Administration and Adult Dosage. **PO for UTI**—400 mg twice daily for 3 days (if uncomplicated AND due to *E. coli, K. pneumoniae* OR *P. mirabilis*) OR 7–21 days (if complicated OR due to other organisms). **PO or IV for prostatitis**—400 mg every 12 h for 28 days. **PO for gonorrhea**—800 mg as a single dose.

Special Populations. *Pediatric Dosage.* (<18 years) Safety and efficacy not established.

Renal impairment. (Cl_{Cr} ≤30 mL/min) 400 mg every 24 h.

Dosage Forms. **Tab** (Noroxin) 400 mg.

Pharmacokinetics. *Fate.* Absorption is rapid following single doses of 200 mg, 400 mg, and 800 mg. At the respective doses, mean peak serum and plasma concentrations of 0.8, 1.5, and 2.4 μg/mL are attained approximately 1 h after dosing. **Half-life** 3–4 h.

Adverse Reactions. *See* Ciprofloxacin.

Contraindications. See Ciprofloxacin.

Monitoring Parameters. *See* Ciprofloxacin.

Precautions. *See* Ciprofloxacin.

Notes. Use longer durations of therapy for complicated infections. Norfloxacin is primarily used for prostatitis, urinary tract, and GI tract infections because of poor oral bioavailability. It has limited activity against streptococci and many anaerobes.

■ REFERENCES

1. Drlica K, Zhao X. DNA gyrase, topisomerase IV, and the 4-quinolones. *Microbiol Mol Biol Rev.* 1997;61:377-392.
2. Coronado VG, et al. Ciprofloxacin resistance among nosocomial Pseudomonas aeruginosa and Staphylococcus aureus in the United States. *Infect Control Hosp Epidemiol.* 1995;16:71-75.
3. Polk RE et al. Predicting hospital rates of fluoroquinolone-resistant Pseudomonas aeruginosa from fluoroquinolone use in US hospitals and their surrounding communities. *Clin Infect Dis.* 2004;39:497-503.
4. Tam VH et al. Impact of drug-exposure intensity and duration of therapy on the emergence of Staphylococcus aureus resistance to a quinolone antimicrobial. *J Infect Dis.* 2007;195:1818-1827.
5. Just PM. Overview of the fluoroquinolone antibiotics. *Pharmacotherapy.* 1993;13:4S-17S.
6. Suh B, Lorber B. Quinolones. *Med Clin North Am.* 1995;79:869-894.

7. Wokowski KA, Berman, SM. Sexually transmitted diseases treatment guidelines. *MMWR Morb Mortal Wkly Rep.* 2006;55:1-94.
8. Schaad UB et al. Use of fluoroquinolones in pediatrics: consensus report of an international society of chemotherapy commission. *Pediatr Infect Dis J.* 1995;14:1-9.
9. Schentag JJ, Gross TF. Quinolone pharmacokinetics in the elderly. *Am J Med.* 1992;92(suppl 4A):33S-37S.
10. Rodvold KA, Neuhauser M. Pharmacokinetics and pharmacodynimics of fluoroquinolones. *Pharmacotherapy.* 2001;21:233S-252S.
11. Peloquin CA. Pharmacology of the antimycobacterial drugs. *Med Clin North Am.* 1993;77:1253-1262.
12. Rodvold KA, Piscitelli SQ. New oral macrolide and fluoroquinolone antibiotics: an overview of pharmacokinetics, interactions, and safety. *Clin Infect Dis.* 1993;17(suppl 1):S192-S199.
13. Nightingale CH. Pharmacokinetic considerations in quinolone therapy. *Pharmacotherapy.* 1993;13:34S-38S.
14. Radandt JM et al. Interactions of fluoroquinolones with other drugs mechanisms, variability, clinical significance, and management. *Clin Infect Dis.* 1992;14:272-284.
15. Dudley MN et al. Effect of dose on the serum pharmacokinetics of intravenous ciprofloxacin with identification and characterization of extravascular compartments using noncompartmental and compartmental pharmacokinetic models. *Antimicrob Agents Chemother.* 1987;31:1782-1786.
16. Forrest A et al. Relationships between renal function and disposition of oral ciprofloxacin. *Antimicrob Agents Chemother.* 1988;32:1537-1540.
17. Halliwell RF et al. Antagonism of GABAA receptors by 4-quinolones. *J Antimicrob Chemother.* 1993;31: 457-462.
18. Owens RC. QT prolongation with antimicrobial agents: understanding the significance. *Drugs.* 2004;64: 1091-1124.
19. Knorr JP et al. Ciprofloxacin-induced Q-T interval prolongation. *Am J Health Syst Pharm.* 2008;65:547-551.
20. Frothingham R. Rates of torsades de pointes associated with ciprofloxacin, ofloxacin, levofloxacin, gatifloxacin, and moxifloxacin. *Pharmacotherapy,* 2001;21:1468-1472.
21. Davis R, Bryson HM. Levofloxacin. *Drugs.* 1994;47:677-700.
22. Anderson VR, Perry CM. Levofloxacin: a review of its use as a high-dose, short-course treatment for bacterial infection. *Drugs.* 2008;68:535-565.
23. Wise R. A review of the clinical pharmacology of moxifloxacin, a new 8-methoxyquinolone, and its potential relation to therapeutic efficacy. *Clin Drug Investig.* 1999;17:365-387.
24. Blondeau JM, Felmingham D. In vitro and in vivo activity of moxifloxacin against community respiratory tract pathogens. *Clin Drug Investig.* 1999;18:57-78.
25. Balfour JA, Lamb HM. Moxifloxacin: a review of its clinical potential in the management of community-acquired respiratory tract infections. *Drugs.* 2000;59:115-139.
26. Thomson KS. Gatifloxacin and moxifloxacin: two new fluoroquinoolones. *Med Lett Drugs Ther.* 2000;42:15-17.
27. Blondeau JM. A review of the comparative in-vitro activities of 12 antimicrobial agents, with a focus on five new respiratory quinolones. *J Antimicrob Chemother.* 1999;43(suppl B):1-11.
28. von Fiff C, Peters G. In-vitro activity of ofloxacin, levofloxacin and D-ofloxacin against staphylocci. *J Antimicrob Chemother.* 1996;38:259-263.
29. Dalhoff A, Schmitz FJ. In vivo antibacterial activity and pharmacodynamics of new quinolones. *Eur J Clin Microbiol Infect Dis.* 2003;22:203-221.
30. Nightingale CH. Moxifloxacin, a new antibiotic designed to treat community-acquired respiratory tract infections: a review of microbiologic and pharmacokinetic-pharmaco-dynamic characteristics. *Pharmacotherapy.* 2000;20:245-256.
31. De Sarro A, De Sarro G. Adverse reactions to fluoroquinolones: an overview on mechanistic aspects. *Curr Med Chem.* 2001;8:371-384.
32. Mandell L, Tillotson G. Safety of fluoroquinolones: an update. *Can J Infect Dis.* 2002;13:54-61.
33. Fish D. Fluoroquinolone adverse effects and drug interactions. *Pharmacotherapy.* 2001;21(10 Pt 2):253S-272S.
34. Zhanel GG et al. Antimicrobial resistance in respiratory tract Streptococcus pneumoniae isolates: results of the Canadian Respiratory Organism Susceptibility Study, 1997 to 2002. *Antimicrob Agents Chemother.* 2003;47:1867-1874.
35. Morrissey I, Tillotson G. Activity of gemifloxacin against Streptococcus pneumoniae and Haemophilus influenzae. *J Antimicrob Chemother.* 2004;53:144-148.
36. Blondeau JM, Tillotson G. Role of gemifloxacin in the management of community-acquired lower respiratory tract infections. *Int J Antimicrob Agents.* 2008;31:299-306.
37. Yoo BK et al. Gemifloxacin: a new fluoroquinolone approved for treatment of respiratory infections. *Ann Pharmacother.* 2004;38:1226-1235.
38. File TM, Tillotson GS. Gemifloxacin: a new, potent fluoroquinolone for the therapy of lower respiratory tract infections. *Expert Rev Anti Infect Ther.* 2004;2:831-843.
39. Bhavnani SM, Andes DR. Gemifloxacin for the treatment of respiratory tract infections: in vitro susceptibility, pharmacokinetics and pharmacodynamics, clinical efficacy, and safety. *Pharmacotherapy.* 2005;25:717-740.

Chapter 14

Sulfonamides

Davey P. Legendre

TRIMETHOPRIM AND SULFAMETHOXAZOLE Bactrim, Septra, Various

Pharmacology. Sulfamethoxazole (SMZ) is a synthetic analogue of para-aminobenzoic acid (PABA), which competitively inhibits the synthesis of dihydropteric acid (an inactive folic acid precursor) from PABA in microorganisms. Mammalian cells do not synthesize folic acid and are not affected. Trimethoprim (TMP) acts at a later step to inhibit the enzymatic reduction of dihydrofolic acid to tetrahydrofolic acid. Mammalian cells require this step, but significantly higher concentrations are needed to inhibit this process in eukaryotes. The most important determinant of efficacy is usually the level of susceptibility to TMP. Resistance to the combination is increasing worldwide, especially in the HIV population receiving the drug for routine prophylaxis.[1] Resistance is likely due to alteration of target enzymes through a plasmid. The combination is active against many bacteria except anaerobes, *Pseudomonas aeruginosa*, and many *Enterococcus* spp. It is active and effective against *Pneumocystis jiroveci, Stenotrophomonas maltophilia*,[2] and *Burkholderia cepacia*.[2] TMP/SMZ has in vitro activity against methicillin-resistant *Staphylococcus aureus* (MRSA), but clinical success has been variable and unpredictable.[3–5]

Administration and Adult Dosage. **PO for cystitis**—160 mg of TMP and 800 mg of SMZ every 12 h for 3 days (uncomplicated) up to 7 days or longer (complicated). **PO for pyelonephritis**—160 mg of TMP and 800 mg of SMZ every 12 h for 10–14 days (uncomplicated) OR for 14–21 days (complicated). **PO for prophylaxis of recurrent UTI**—40 mg TMP and 200 of SMZ at bedtime 3 times a week. **PO for traveler's diarrhea, *Shigella* spp., *Vibrio cholera*, or *Salmonella* spp**—160 mg of TMP and 800 of SMZ every 12 h for 5 days. **IV for moderate to severe infections**—6–10 mg/kg/d of TMP and 30–50 mg/kg/d of SMZ in 2–4 equally divided doses for moderate infection, 15–20 mg/kg/d of TMP and 75–100 mg/kg/d of SMZ in 3–4 equally divided doses for severe infection. **PO OR IV for *P. jiroveci* pneumonia (PCP)**—15–20 mg/kg/d of TMP and 75–100 mg/kg/d of SMZ in 2–4 equally divided doses for 21 days. **PO for PCP infection prophylaxis (also for Toxoplasmosis prophylaxis)**—160 mg of TMP and 800 mg of SMZ once daily; intermittent dosage (e.g., 3 times a week) is also used. (*See* Notes.)

Special Populations. *Pediatric Dosage.* **PO for UTI, otitis media, cystitis, pyelonephritis, or shigellosis**—(2 months–12 years) 8 mg/kg/d of TMP and 40 mg/kg/d of SMZ (suspension 1 mL/kg/d) in 2 equally divided doses; (>12 years) Same as adult mg/kg dosage. **IV for moderate to severe infection**—(>2 months) Same as adult mg/kg dosage. **PO or IV for PCP**—Same as adult mg/kg dosage.

PO for *PCP* infection prophylaxis—150 mg/m²/d of TMP and 750 mg/m²/d of SMZ, in divided doses, given 3 days a week.[6]

Geriatric Dosage. Reduce dosage for age-related reduction in renal function, although dosage reduction is not necessary with only minor age-related renal function changes. (*See* Precautions.)

Other Conditions. For a Cl_{Cr} 10–30 mL/min, reduce dose by 50%. For Cl_{Cr} <10 mL/min, reduce dose by 50%–75%. This drug should be given after dialysis,[7] but less is known about its pharmacokinetics using modern dialysis techniques and filters. Monitoring of serum concentrations may be required for patients on dialysis or for patients requiring higher doses for serious infections.

Dosage Forms. Susp 8 mg/mL of TMP and 40 mg/mL of SMZ; **Tab** 80 mg of TMP and 400 mg of SMZ (single strength), 160 mg of TMP and 800 mg of SMZ (double strength); **Inj** 16 mg/mL of TMP and 80 mg/mL of SMZ.

Patient Instructions. Take this medication with a full 8-fluid oz glass of water on an empty stomach (1 h before or 2 h after meals) for best absorption. Drink several additional glasses of water daily, unless directed otherwise.

Missed Doses. Take this drug at regular intervals. If you miss a dose, take it as soon as you remember. If it is about time for the next dose, take that dose only. If you are taking the drug once a day, leave at least 10–12 h between doses. If you are taking the drug twice a day, leave at least 5–6 h between doses. Do not double the dose or take an extra dose.

Pharmacokinetics. *Serum Levels.* TMP levels >5 mg/L (>17 mol/L) and SMZ peak levels of about 100 mg/L (396 mol/L) may be required in PCP.[8]

Fate. TMP/SMZ is 90%–100% absorbed orally. In normal adults, peak serum concentrations of 0.9–1.9 mg/L (3.1–6.5 mol/L) of TMP and 20–50 mg/L (79–198 mol/L) of SMZ occur about 1–4 h after 160 mg of TMP and 800 mg of SMZ. An additional 10–20 mg/L of SMZ exists in the serum as inactive metabolites. IV infusion of 160 mg of TMP and 800 mg of SMZ over 1 h produces peak serum levels of 3.4 mg/L (11.7 μmol/L) of TMP and 46.3 mg/L (183 μmol/L) of SMZ. TMP/SMZ are widely distributed in the body, although TMP is much more widely distributed because of its greater lipophilicity. TMP is 45% plasma protein bound and has a V_d of 1–2 L/kg; SMZ is 60% plasma protein bound and has a V_d of 0.36 L/kg. TMP concentrations in various tissues and fluids (including the prostate, bile, and sputum) are several times greater than concomitant serum concentrations; CSF concentrations in normal adults are approximately 50% of serum concentrations. Nearly all TMP is excreted in the urine within 24–72 h, 50%–75% as unchanged drug. SMZ undergoes extensive liver metabolism, producing N^4-acetylated and N^4-glucuronidated derivatives; 85% is excreted in the urine within 24–72 h, 10%–30% as unchanged drug. The pharmacokinetics of these drugs are essentially unchanged when given in combination. The pH of the urine influences renal excretion of both drugs but does not markedly alter overall elimination.[9] **Half-life** 11 ± 2.3 h for TMP and 8 ± 0.4 h for SMZ in normal adults.[9] 20–30 h or more for TMP in severe renal failure; 18–24 h for SMZ in anuria.[5]

Adverse Reactions. Gastrointestinal irritation, including nausea, vomiting, and anorexia occur frequently, while both frequency and severity appear to be dose related. Rashes and other hypersensitivity reactions similar to those caused by other sulfonamides occur occasionally. In patients with AIDS, allergic skin reactions with rash (usually diffuse, erythematous or maculopapular, and pruritic) are frequent and might be associated with fever, leukopenia, neutropenia, thrombocytopenia, and increased transaminase levels.[10] Desensitization has been successful. (*See* Notes.) In patients without underlying myelosuppression and treated with conventional dosages, the frequency of megaloblastic anemia and other hematologic disorders is rare but might be higher in folate-deficient patients. Hepatotoxicity and nephrotoxicity are rare; renal dysfunction can occur in patients with preexisting renal disease, but it is reversible.[5,9] Allergic skin reactions, including toxic epidermal necrolysis, exfoliative dermatitis, Stevens-Johnson syndrome, erythema multiforme, and fixed drug eruptions, occur rarely. Other rare adverse effects are cholestatic jaundice, pancreatitis, pseudomembranous colitis, hyperkalemia, myalgia, headache, insomnia, fatigue, ataxia, vertigo, depression, and anaphylaxis.[5]

Contraindications. Pregnancy at term; infants <2 months; history of hypersensitivity reaction to sulfonamide derivatives or trimethoprim; megaloblastic anemia caused by folate deficiency. Lactation is stated by manufacturer to be a contraindication, but risk is probably limited to nursing infants younger than 2 months.

Precautions. G-6-PD deficiency; impaired renal or hepatic function. Adverse reactions can be more frequent in the elderly, especially with impaired hepatic or renal function OR in those taking thiazide diuretics.

Drug Interactions. The effects of methotrexate, sulfonylureas, and warfarin are increased when used with TMP/SMZ. Enhanced bone marrow suppression can occur with the combination of TMP/SMZ and mercaptopurine. A decreased effect of cyclosporine and an increased risk of nephrotoxicity can occur. High-dose TMP/SMZ with didanosine can increase the risk of pancreatitis. Phenytoin clearance can be decreased with concurrent use. Concomitant use with rosiglitazone increases risk of rosiglitazone toxicity and adverse effects. Hyperkalemia and acute renal failure has been reported with TMP/SMZ and ACE inhibitor use.

Parameters to Monitor. Baseline and periodic CBC counts for patients on long-term or high-dose treatment. Monitor SMZ serum levels in patients treated for PCP if absorption is questionable or response is poor. In patients with AIDS, monitor for hypersensitivity skin reactions (e.g., rash and urticaria).

Notes. Protect all dosage forms from light. The efficacy and safety of TMP/SMZ and SMZ have been demonstrated in numerous infectious conditions (e.g., chronic UTI, chronic bronchitis, sepsis, enteric fever, prostatitis, endocarditis, meningitis, and gonorrhea), and the combination is considered an effective alternative to conventional therapy in most cases.[4,9] TMP/SMZ is the treatment of choice for PCP because of high efficacy, efficacy in disseminated disease, low cost, and convenience.[8] Oral desensitization or rechallenge with TMP/SMZ has been successful in permitting continued use in patients with AIDS who experience hypersensitivity reactions.[11] Desensitization can be done outpatient over 9 days. Rapid desensitization consists of giving increasing doses of TMP/SMZ oral suspension once every hour with 6 oz of water (*See* Table 1).[12]

**TABLE 1.   RAPID ORAL DESENSITIZATION METHOD FOR
TRIMETHOPRIM/SULFAMETHOXAZOLE**

HOUR	DOSE TMP/SMZ IN MG
0	0.004/0.02
1	0.04/0.2
2	0.4/2
3	4/20
4	40/200
5	160/800

■ REFERENCES

1. Martin JN et al. Emergence of trimethoprim-sulfamethoxazole resistance in the AIDS era. *J Infect Dis.* 1999;180:1809-1818.

2. Poulos CD et al. In vitro activities of antimicrobial combinations against Stenotrophomonas (Xanthomonas) maltophilia. *Antimicrob Agents Chemother.* 1995;39.2220-2223.

3. Foltzer MA, Reese RE. Trimethoprim-sulfamethoxazole and other sulfonamides. *Med Clin North Am.* 1987;71:1177-1194.

4. Markowitz N et al. Trimethoprim-sulfamethoxazole compared with vancomycin for the treatment of *Staphylococcus aureus* infection. *Ann Intern Med.* 1992;117:390-398.

5. Lundstrom TS, Sobel JD. Vancomycin, trimethoprim-sulfamethoxazole, and rifampin. *Infect Dis Clin North Am.* 1995;9:747-767.

6. Goodwin SD. *Pneumocystis carinii* pneumonia in human immunodeficiency virus–infected infants and children. *Pharmacotherapy.* 1993;13:640-646.

7. Nissenson AR et al. Pharmacokinetics of intravenous trimethoprim-sulfamethoxazole during hemodialysis. *Am J Nephrol.* 1987;7(4):270-274.

8. Davey RT Jr., Masur H. Recent advances in the diagnosis, treatment, and prevention of *Pneumocystis carinii* pneumonia. *Antimicrob Agents Chemother.* 1990;34:499-504.

9. Pratt WB, Fekety R. The antimetabolites. In: Pratt WB, Fekety R, eds. *The Antimicrobial Drugs.* New York: Oxford University Press; 1986:229-251.

10. Masur H. Prevention and treatment of pneumocystis pneumonia. *N Engl J Med.* 1992;327:1853-1860.

11. Absar N et al. Desensitization to trimethoprim/sulfamethoxazole in HIV-infected patients. *J Allergy Clin Immunol.* 1994;93:1001-1005.

12. Gluckstein D, Ruskin J. Rapid oral desensitization to trimethoprim-sulfamethoxazole (TMP-SMZ): use in prophylaxis for pneumocystis carinii pneumonia in patients with AIDS who were previously intolerant to TMP-SMZ. *Clin Infect Dis.* 1995;20:849-853.

Chapter 15

Tetracyclines

Roxie L. Stewart

Tetracyclines are broad-spectrum bacteriostatic compounds that inhibit protein synthesis at the 30S ribosomal subunit. Activity includes gram-positive, gram-negative, aerobic, and anaerobic bacteria, as well as spirochetes, mycoplasmas, *rickettsia*, *chlamydia*, and some protozoa. Many bacteria have developed plasmid-mediated resistance. Most *Enterobacteriaceae* and *Pseudomonas aeruginosa* are resistant.

DOXYCYCLINE AND SALTS
Vibramycin, Adoxa, Oracea

Pharmacology. Doxycycline is somewhat more active than other tetracyclines against anaerobes and facultative gram-negative bacilli.[1,2]

Administration and Adult Dosage. **PO or IV for community-acquired pneumonia or bronchitis**—100 mg every 12 h. **PO for rosacea**—40 mg once daily. **PO or IV for rickettsial disease**—100 mg every 12 h (7–14 days). **PO for nonspecific urethritis**—100 mg every 12 h for seven days. **PO for uncomplicated chlamydial genital infections**—100 mg twice daily for at least 7 days. **PO for primary and secondary syphilis**—100 mg 3 times daily for at least 10 days. **PO for prophylaxis against travelers' diarrhea**—200 mg en route, then 100 mg/d for duration of travel (6 weeks maximum). **PO for brucellosis**—100 mg every 12 h (adjunct with rifampin or streptomycin for 6 weeks). **PO for vibrio cholerae**—300 mg (single dose). **PO for malaria prophylaxis in short-term (<4 months) travelers**—100 mg/d beginning 1–2 days before travel to malarious areas and for 4 weeks after leaving the area. **PO for Lyme disease, tularemia, or Q-fever**—100 mg every 12 h for 2 or 3 weeks. **PO for plague**—100 mg every 12 h for 1 week. **PO for anthrax postexposure prophylaxis or cutaneous anthrax treatment**—100 mg twice daily for 60 days.[3] **IV for treatment of inhalational, gastrointestinal, and oropharyngeal anthrax**—100 mg every 12 h (in combination with 1 or 2 additional antimicrobials). Switch to oral antimicrobial therapy when clinically appropriate. Continue for 60 days (IV and PO combined).[3] **Intrapleural for pleural effusions**—500 mg in 25–30 mL of NS daily; most patients require 2–4 infusions for maximum efficacy.[4] **Not for SQ or IM use.**

Special Populations. *Pediatric Dosage.* Not recommended ≤8 years (exception in anthrax). **PO**—(<45 kg) 2.2 mg/kg every 12 h for 2 doses, then 2.2–4.4 mg/kg/d in 1 or 2 divided doses, depending on the severity of the infection, (>45 kg) Same as adult dosage. **PO for malaria prophylaxis in short-term (<4 months) travelers**—2.2 mg/kg/d to a maximum of 100 mg/d beginning 1–2 days before travel to malarious areas and for 4 weeks after leaving the area. **PO for anthrax postexposure prophylaxis or cutaneous anthrax treatment**—(>45 kg) 100 mg twice daily, (≤45 kg) 2.2 mg/kg twice daily, (≤8 years) 2.2 mg/kg twice daily for 60 days.[3] **IV**—(<45 kg) 4.4 mg/kg in 1 or 2 divided doses for 1 day followed by 2.2–4.4 mg/kg/d in 1 or 2 divided doses, infused at a concentration of 0.1–1 g/L over 1–4 h, (>45 kg) Same as adult dosage. **IV for treatment of inhalational, gastrointestinal, and oropharyngeal anthrax**—Same dose as prophylaxis. Begin IV therapy and switch to oral therapy when clinically appropriate. Continue for 60 days (IV and PO combined).[3]

Geriatric Dosage. Same as adult dosage.

Other Conditions. No dosage adjustment is necessary in renal impairment.

Dosage Forms. **Cap** (as hyclate) 20, 50, 75, 100 mg; **Tab** (as hyclate) 20, 100 mg; **Tab & Cap** (as monohydrate) 50, 75, 100, 150 mg; delayed-release (as hyclate) 75, 100, 150 mg. Variable-release capsule 40 mg (30 mg immediate release, 10 mg delayed release); **Susp** (as monohydrate) 5 mg/mL (reconstituted); **Syrup** (as calcium) 10 mg/mL; **Inj** (as hyclate) 100, 200 mg.

Patient Instructions. Take doxycycline by mouth with a full glass of water on an empty stomach; if stomach upset occurs, the drug may be taken with food or milk but not with antacids or iron products. Avoid prolonged exposure to direct sunlight while taking this drug.

Missed Doses. Take this drug at regular intervals. If you miss a dose, take it as soon as you remember. If it is about time for the next dose, take that dose only. Leave at least 6–8 h between doses. Do not double the dose or take an extra dose.

Pharmacokinetics. *Onset and Duration.* Duration of protection against travelers' diarrhea is about 1 week after drug discontinuation.[5]

Fate. Approximately 93% is orally absorbed, producing a peak of 3 mg/L (6.5 μmol/L) 2–4 h after administration of a 200-mg dose; antacids and iron can markedly impair oral absorption; milk causes about a 30% decrease in bioavailability and food has little effect. Widely distributed in the body, penetrating most cavities including CSF (12%–20% of serum levels). The drug is 88% ± 5% plasma protein bound. V_d is 0.75 ± 0.32 L/kg; Clearance is 0.032 ± 0.01 L/h/kg. Approximately 41% ± 19% is excreted unchanged in the urine in normal adults; the remainder is eliminated in feces via intestinal and biliary secretion.[5,6,7] **Half-life** 16 ± 6 h in normal adults; slightly prolonged in severe renal impairment.[5,6]

Adverse Reactions. IV administration frequently produces phlebitis. Oral doxycycline causes less alteration of intestinal flora than other tetracyclines but can cause nausea and diarrhea with equal frequency. It binds to calcium in teeth and bones, which can cause discoloration of teeth in children, especially during growth; however, doxycycline has a lower potential for this effect than most other tetracyclines. In contrast to other tetracyclines, doxycycline is not very antianabolic and will not further increase azotemia in renal failure. Phototoxic skin reactions occur occasionally.[1,2,5]

Contraindications. Hypersensitivity to any tetracycline.

Precautions. Pregnancy category D. Not recommended in pregnancy or in children younger than 8 years because permanent staining of the child's teeth will occur. Use with caution in severe hepatic dysfunction. The syrup contains sulfites.

Drug Interactions. Antacids containing di- or tri-valent cations, bismuth salts, or zinc salts interfere with absorption of oral tetracyclines. Oral iron salts lower doxycycline serum levels, even of IV doxycycline, by interfering with absorption and enterohepatic circulation. Barbiturates, carbamazepine, and phenytoin can enhance doxycycline hepatic metabolism, possibly decreasing its effect. Tetracyclines can interfere with enterohepatic circulation of contraceptive hormones, causing menstrual irregularities and possibly unplanned pregnancies. Combined use of tetracyclines with the bactericidal agents (e.g., penicillins) can result in decreased activity in some infections.

Parameters to Monitor. Check for signs of phlebitis daily during IV use. Complete blood count along with liver and renal function tests should be monitored periodically. Diarrhea should be assessed at each subsequent contact.

Notes. Doxycycline is the tetracycline of choice because it is better tolerated than other tetracyclines, although tetracyclines are the drugs of choice for very few infections.[1,2] Doxycycline is also used in combined therapy in the treatment of gonococcal urethritis, acute pelvic inflammatory disease, endometritis, salpingitis, peritonitis, and epididymitis when coinfection with *Chlamydia trachomatis*. Each vial for injection contains 480 mg of ascorbic acid per 100 mg of doxycycline hyclate. (*See* Tetracyclines Comparison Chart.)

TETRACYCLINE AND SALTS   Various

Pharmacology. Tetracycline has an antimicrobial spectrum of activity and indications similar to doxycycline. (*See* Doxycycline monograph.) Current uses are for treatment of similar infections treated with doxycycline caused by nearly 40 species, including *Chlamydia* spp., *Mycoplasma* spp., *Brucella* spp., and as a 2nd line agent when penicillin is contraindicated.[1,2] It is also used as a treatment for acne and in some regimens against *Helicobacter pylori*. (*See* Acid-Peptic Therapy.)

Adult Dosage. PO for infection—1–2 g/d in 2–4 divided doses. Reduce dosage, or preferably use another drug, in severe renal or hepatic impairment.

Pediatric Dosage. Not recommended ≤8 years. **PO for infection**—25–50 mg/kg/d in 2–4 divided doses.

Dosage Forms. *See* Tetracyclines Comparison Chart.

Pharmacokinetics. Tetracycline is well absorbed from the gastrointestinal (GI) tract. Multivalent cations chelate tetracyclines and inhibit absorption; warn patients to avoid concurrent antacids, dairy products, iron, or sucralfate. The half-life of tetracycline is about 10 h, increasing to as high as 108 h in anuria.

Fate. Approximately 77% is orally absorbed. The drug is 65% ± 3% plasma protein-bound. V_d is 1.5 ± 0.1 L/kg; clearance is 1.67 ± 0.24 L/h/kg. Approximately 58% ± 8% is excreted in the urine in normal adults.[6]

Adverse Reactions. GI irritation is frequent and can result in esophageal ulceration if the drug is taken at bedtime with insufficient fluid. Disruption of bowel flora occurs frequently and can result in diarrhea, candidiasis, or rarely pseudomembranous colitis. Antianabolic effects produce elevated BUN, hyper phosphatemia, and acidosis in patients with renal failure. Acute fatty infiltration of the liver with pancreatitis occurs rarely with large (>2 g) IV doses, especially in pregnancy; avoid tetracyclines in pregnancy. Do not give tetracyclines to children ≤8 years because of binding of calcium in teeth and resultant discoloration.

Contraindications. (*See* Doxycycline Contraindications.) Late 2nd and 3rd trimester during pregnancy; ≤8 years.

Precautions. *See* Doxycycline Precautions.

Drug Interactions. Oral absorption is markedly inhibited by di- and tri-valent cations (e.g., antacids, iron salts). (*See* Doxycycline Interactions.)

GLYCYLCYCLINES Tygacil

Pharmacology. Tigecycline, a glycylcycline, carries a glycylamido moiety attached to the 9-position of minocycline. Tigecycline inhibits protein translation in bacteria by binding to the 30S ribosomal subunit and blocking entry of aminoacyl tRNA molecules into the A site of the ribosome.[8] Tigecycline is not affected by ribosomal protection and efflux, two major tetracycline resistance mechanisms, thus retaining activity against both tetracycline- and minocycline-resistant bacteria.[8,9] Tigecycline has shown broad spectrum activity against gram positive and gram-negative aerobic and anaerobic bacteria, including resistant strains.

Administration and Adult Dosage. **IV for community-acquired pneumonia, intra-abdominal, and skin/soft tissue infections**—100 mg, followed by 50 mg every 12 h for 5–14 days (7 day minimum if community-acquired pneumonia).

Special Populations. *Pediatric Dosage.* Not recommended ≤8 years; (8–18 years) Safety and efficacy not established

Geriatric Dosage. Same as adult dosage.

Other Conditions. No dosage adjustment is necessary in patients with renal impairment, on hemodialysis, mild to moderate hepatic impairment, or based on race. In patients with severe hepatic impairment, decrease dose to 100 mg followed by a maintenance dose of 25 mg every 12 h.

Dosage Forms. Pwdr for Soln 50 mg.

Pharmacokinetics. Plasma protein binding ranges from 71% to 89%. The steady-state V_d averaged 7–9 L/kg, indicating extensive distribution beyond the plasma volume into the tissues. Tigecycline is not extensively metabolized. The primary route of elimination is biliary excretion (59%). Secondary routes of elimination include renal excretion (22% unchanged through urine) and glucuronidation.[8,10]

Adverse Reactions. GI intolerance is the predominate adverse effect with nausea, vomiting, and diarrhea occurring in >10% of patients. Nearly one-third of patients will have some degree of nausea. Glycylcyclines may have similar adverse effects as tetracyclines such as photosensitivity, pseudomotor cerebri, and antianabolic action (which has led to increased BUN, azotemia, acidosis, and hyperphosphatemia). Pancreatitis has been reported. Anaphylaxis/anaphylactoid reactions have also been reported.

Contraindications. Hypersensitivity.

Precautions. Pregnancy category D. Use during late 2nd and 3rd trimester during pregnancy and ≤8 years may cause permanent discoloration of teeth.

Drug Interactions. Anticoagulation tests should be monitored if tigecycline is administered with warfarin. Concurrent use of antibacterial drugs with oral contraceptives may render oral contraceptives less effective. Tigecycline does not inhibit metabolism mediated by CYP450.

Parameters to Monitor. Abnormalities in total bilirubin concentration, prothrombin time, and transaminases have been seen in patients treated with tigecycline, these should be monitored carefully. Symptoms of diarrhea should be closely monitored and *Clostridium difficile* should be considered as a possible cause.

Notes. Doses should be infused over 30 to 60 min. In clinical studies, tigecycline monotherapy has been shown to be as effective as comparators against a broad spectrum of bacteria, including MRSA.

TETRACYCLINES COMPARISON CHART

DRUG	DOSAGE FORMS	ADULT DOSAGE	PERCENTAGE ORAL ABSORPTION	HALF-LIFE (h) NORMAL	HALF-LIFE (h) ANURIA	PERCENTAGE EXCRETED UNCHANGED IN URINE	COMMENTS
Demeclocycline Hydrochloride Declomycin Various	Tab 150, 300 mg	PO 600 mg/d in 2–4 divided doses PO for SIADH 300 mg 3–4 times daily	66	15	40–60	42	Most phototoxic tetracycline; declomycin PO for SIADH; causes nephrogenic diabetes insipidus rarely
Doxycycline Calcium	(See monograph.)	PO 100 mg every 12 h for 2 doses,	93	16 ± 6	12–22	41	Safest in renal failure because of its lack of accumulation and lack of antianabolic effects; well tolerated when given IV
Doxycyclin Hyclate	(See monograph.)	then 50–100 mg/d in 1–2 divided doses IV 200 mg in 1–2 divided doses on day 1, then 100–200 mg/d					

(continued)

TETRACYCLINES COMPARISON CHART (*continued*)

DRUG	DOSAGE FORMS	ADULT DOSAGE	PERCENTAGE ORAL ABSORPTION	HALF-LIFE (h) NORMAL	HALF-LIFE (h) ANURIA	PERCENTAGE EXCRETED UNCHANGED IN URINE	COMMENTS
Doxycycline Monohydrate Vibramycin Oracea Various	(*See monograph.*)						
Minocycline Hydrochloride Minocin Various	Tab and Cap 50 mg, 75 mg, 100 mg ER Tab 45 mg, 90 mg, 135 mg Cap (pellet-filled) 50 mg, 100 mg Susp 10 mg/mL Inj (IV only) 100 mg	PO or IV 200 mg initially, then 100 mg every 12 h	95–100	16 ± 2	11–23	11	Very frequent transient vestibular toxicity

(continued)

TETRACYCLINES COMPARISON CHART (*continued*)

DRUG	DOSAGE FORMS	ADULT DOSAGE	PERCENTAGE ORAL ABSORPTION	HALF-LIFE (h) NORMAL	HALF-LIFE (h) ANURIA	PERCENTAGE EXCERTED UNCHANGED IN URINE	COMMENTS
Tetracycline Various	Cap 100, 250, 500 mg	PO 1–2 g/d in 2–4 divided doses	77	10.6 ± 5	57–108	60	(*See* monograph)
Tetracycline Hydrochloride Various	Susp 25 mg/mL		N/A				
Tigecycline Tygacil	Inj 50 mg powder for reconstitution	Initial 100 mg as a single dose Maintenance 50 mg every 12 h	N/A				Infuse over 30–60 min

From Ref. 6 and product information.
Abbreviation: SIADH, syndrome of inappropriate antidiuretic hormone hypersecretion

■ REFERENCES

1. Standiford HC. Tetracyclines and chloramphenicol. In: Mandell GL et al., eds. *Principles and Practice of Infectious Diseases*. 5th ed. New York: Churchill Livingstone; 2000:336-348.

2. Chambers HF. Chemotherapy of microbial diseases: protein synthesis inhibitors and miscellaneous antibacterial agents. In: Brunton L et al., eds. *Goodman and Gilman's the Pharmacological Basis of Therapeutics*. 11th ed. New York: McGraw-Hill; 2006:1173-1199.

3. Center for Disease Control and Prevention. Update: investigation of bioterrorism-related anthrax and interim guidelines for exposure management and antimicrobial therapy. *MMWR Morb Mortal Wkly Rep*. 2001;50:909-919.

4. Fingar BL. Sclerosing agents used to control malignant pleural effusions. *Hosp Pharm*. 1992;27:622-628.

5. Francke EL, Neu HC. Chloramphenicol and tetracyclines. *Med Clin North Am*. 1987;71:1155-1168.

6. Thummel KE et al. Design and optimization of dosage regimens; pharmacokinetic data. In: Brunton L et al., eds. *Goodman and Gilman's the Pharmacological Basis of Therapeutics*. 11th ed. New York: McGraw-Hill; 2006:1787-1888.

7. Kasten MJ. Clindamycin, metronidazole, and chloramphenicol. *Mayo Clin Proc*. 1999;74:825-833.

8. Wyeth Pharmaceuticals, Inc. Tygacil (tigecycline) product information. Philadelphia, PA: Wyeth Pharmaceuticals, Inc.; Revised February 2009.

9. Meagher AK et al. The pharmacokinetic and pharmacodynamic profile of tigecycline. *Clin Infect Dis*. 2005;41(suppl 5):S333-S340.

10. Peterson LR. A review of tigecycline—the first glycyclicine. *Int J Antimicrob Agents*. 2008;32(suppl 4):S215-S222.

Chapter 16

Hepatitis Antiviral Drugs

Julianna Chan

ADEFOVIR DIPIVOXIL Hepsera

Pharmacology. Adefovir dipivoxil is an oral acyclic nucleotide monophosphate (9-[2-[[bis[(pivaloyloxy)methoxy]-phosphinyl]-methoxy]ethyl]adenine), a prodrug of adefovir. Adefovir dipivoxil has antiviral activity against the hepatitis B virus (HBV), herpes viruses, and retroviruses with some activity also against the human immunodeficiency virus (HIV). This antiviral agent is phosphorylated to its active form, adefovir. Once adefovir enters the cell, it inhibits HBV replication by competing with the substrate, deoxyadenosine triphosphate, thus inhibiting HBV DNA chain termination.[1]

Administration and Adult Dosage. **PO for treatment of chronic hepatitis B (CHB) or lamivudine-resistant with active HBV replication and either elevated ALT or AST levels or histologically active disease**—10 mg once daily with or without food.

Special Populations. *Pediatric Dosage.* (<12 years) Safety and efficacy not established.

Geriatric dosage. Same as adult dosage.

Other Conditions. Renal Impairment. (Cl_{Cr} 20–49 mL/min) 10 mg every 48h; (Cl_{Cr} 10–19 mL/min) 10 mg every 72h; (hemodialysis) 10 mg every 7d following dialysis.

Dosage Forms. Tab 10 mg.

Patient Instructions. Do not discontinue adefovir dipivoxil without talking to the doctor first. Abrupt discontinuation of this medication may worsen the liver disease. Confirm that the HIV test is negative and if unknown, have the clinician confirm by testing. If you are HIV positive, do not treat with only adefovir because more than one medication is needed to treat the HIV infection. Take adefovir dipivoxil with water on either a full or empty stomach. If a dose is missed, take it later that same day if possible and then resume the regularly scheduled regimen the following day. Do not take 2 doses at once to make up for missing a dose.

Pharmacokinetics. Adefovir dipivoxil is a prodrug of adefovir which has an oral bioavailability of ~59%. C_{max} of adefovir dipivoxil is 18.4 ± 6.26 ng/mL (~67 nmol/L).[2] The plasma protein binding of adefovir is less than 4% and the V_d is 0.35–0.39 L/kg following IV administration of 1 or 3 mg/kg/d, respectively.[2] Adefovir dipivoxil is rapidly converted to the active metabolite adefovir by adefovir diphosphate. The active metabolite is excreted by a combination of glomerular filtration and active tubular secretion. In patients with normal renal function, 45% of the active metabolite is recovered in the urine. **Half-life** ~7 h and is prolonged in patients with renal insufficiencies.

Adverse Reactions. Asthenia is the most common adverse effect, while abdominal pain, diarrhea, dyspepsia, headaches, nausea, and flatulence also occur. In children <12 years of age, similar side effects were observed.[3] Lactic acidosis, pancreatitis, and hepatomegaly have been reported rarely. Adefovir dipivoxil is associated with a dose-related nephrotoxicity, which was most commonly seen in HIV patients receiving doses > 60 mg. The dose of adefovir dipivoxil must be adjusted in patients with renal insufficiency (Cl$_{Cr}$ <50 mL/min). Aminotransferase levels should be monitored more closely when therapy is discontinued, as an increase in ALT concentrations may indicate a flare in disease activity leading to liver failure.

Precautions. Pregnancy category C. Rare cases of lactic acidosis and severe hepatomegaly have been reported during adefovir dipivoxil treatment. ALT levels 10 times the upper limit of normal (ULN) have been observed in approximately 25% of the patients when adefovir dipivoxil was discontinued. These events mostly occur within 12 weeks upon treatment discontinuation and may require reinitiation of adefovir. Confirm patient is HIV negative prior to initiating therapy. There is a risk of developing HIV drug resistance (*see* Patient Instructions).

Drug Interactions. Agents that are nephrotoxic and coadministered with adefovir dipivoxil may increase the risk of renal toxicity. Ribavirin may increase the risk of developing lactic acidosis and pancreatitis while taking nucleosides such as adefovir dipivoxil.

Parameters to Monitor. *See* Parameters to Monitor for Hepatitis B Therapy.

Notes. Adefovir dipivoxil 0.14 mg/kg and 0.3 mg/kg have been evaluated in children aged 2–11 years for CHB infections.[3] Adefovir dipivoxil is effective in suppressing HBV replication, normalizing ALT levels, and improving liver histology.[4,5] Twenty-one percent of the HbeAg-positive CHB patients had a significant loss of serum HBV DNA level compared to 0% of patients receiving placebo at the end of 48 weeks of therapy. Normalizing ALT levels and improvement in histology was observed in ~50% of patients. HBeAg loss was observed in 24%, 46%, and 53% of the subjects at the end of 48, 96, and 144 weeks of treatment, respectively.[6] Even though adefovir dipivoxil has adequate virological, biological, and histological response, this drug is no longer considered first-line therapy for CHB infections due to frequent biochemical and virologic breakthroughs leading to the development of drug resistance.[6,7] Resistance rates up to 30% have been reported at 5 years of treatment.[7] The optimal treatment duration for the treatment of hepatitis B is unknown.

ENTECAVIR	Baraclude

Pharmacology. Entecavir is an oral guanosine nucleoside analogue (2-amino-1,9-dihydro-9-[(1S,3R,4S)-4-hydroxy-3-(hydroxymethyl)-2-methylenecyclopentyl]-6H-purin-6-one) having antiviral activity against the HBV and HIV.[8] Entecavir is phosphorylated to active entecavir-triphosphate, which inhibits the HBV DNA polymerase replication.[1]

Administration and Adult Dosage. PO for treatment-naïve CHB infection with active HBV viral replication and elevated aminotransferases or histologically active disease—0.5 mg once daily without food. **PO for lamivudine-resistant or**

known lamivudine or telbivudine resistance mutations—1 mg once daily without food.

Special Populations. *Pediatric Dosage.* (<16 years) Safety and efficacy not established.

Geriatric dosage. Same as adult dosage. Older individuals have a greater AUC than young healthy subjects with normal renal function.

Other Conditions. **Renal Impairment.** (Treatment-naïve) (Cl_{Cr} 30–49 mL/min) 0.25 mg once daily or 0.5 mg every 48h; (Cl_{Cr} 10–29 mL/min) 0.15 mg once daily or 0.5 mg every 72h; (Cl_{Cr} <10 mL/min, hemodialysis, or continuous ambulatory peritoneal dialysis (CAPD)) 0.5 mg every 7d. (Lamivudine-resistant) (Cl_{Cr} 30–49 mL/min) 0.5 mg once daily or 1 mg every 48h; (Cl_{Cr} 10–29 mL/min) 0.3 mg once daily or 1 mg every 72h; (Cl_{Cr} <10 mL/min, Hemodialysis, or CAPD) 0.1 mg once daily or 1 mg every 7d.

Dosage Forms. **Tab** 0.5 mg, 1 mg. **Soln** 0.05 mg/mL.

Patient Instructions. Do not discontinue entecavir without talking to the doctor first. Abrupt discontinuation may worsen the liver disease. Confirm that the HIV test is negative and if unknown, have the clinician confirm by testing. If you are HIV positive, do not treat with only entecavir because more than one medication is needed to treat the HIV infection. Take entecavir with water on an empty stomach. If a dose is missed, take it later that same day if possible and then resume the regularly scheduled regimen the following day. Do not take 2 doses at once to make up for missing a dose.

Pharmacokinetics. Entecavir is 100% bioavailable after oral administration; both the tablet and oral solution may be used interchangeably. C_{max} of entecavir ranges between 0.6 and 11.8 ng/mL for 0.1–1 mg doses, respectively.[9] Absorption of the drug is delayed with food resulting in a decrease in C_{max} of approximately 45%.[9] The plasma protein binding in vitro of entecavir is ~13%. The apparent V_d is greater than the total body water, thus the drug is distributed into tissue extensively. Entecavir is mostly eliminated by the kidneys, 62%–73%. Entecavir is not metabolized by the cytochrome, CYP P450 enzyme system and has a minimal phase II hepatic metabolism. **Half-life** ~55 h.[9]

Adverse Reactions. Adverse effects include headaches, upper respiratory tract infection, cough, nasopharyngitis, abdominal pain, fatigue, and fever.[9] In rare cases, pancreatitis, hepatomegaly, and potentially fatal lactic acidosis have been reported. ALT levels should be monitored carefully, as mild elevations between 2- and 3-fold increases may be observed. When entecavir is discontinued, aminotransferase levels should be monitored more closely, as increased ALT concentrations may indicate a flare in disease activity leading to liver failure.

Precautions. Pregnancy category C. Rare cases of lactic acidosis and severe hepatomegaly have been reported during entecavir treatment. ALT levels 10 times the ULN and possible exacerbation of hepatitis have been observed in patients when treatment was discontinued. These events mostly occurred within a median time of 23 weeks upon treatment discontinuation. Approximately 2%–8% of patients who are naïve to HBV medications may experience an exacerbation of hepatitis or increased ALT levels. This occurrence increases to ~12% in patients who have lamivudine resistance. Confirm patient is HIV negative prior to initiating therapy. There is a risk of developing HIV drug resistance with entecavir.

Drug Interactions. There is minimal concern with entecavir interacting with medications undergoing CYP P450 metabolism, because the drug is not a substrate of the system. Agents that are nephrotoxic and coadministered with entecavir may increase the risk of renal toxicity thereby increasing serum concentrations of either drug.

Parameters to Monitor. *See* Parameters to Monitor for Hepatitis B Therapy.

Notes. For doses less than 0.5 mg, entecavir oral solution is recommended. Entecavir is highly effective in suppressing HBV replication, normalizing ALT levels, and improving liver histology in patients with HBeAg-positive and HBeAg-negative patients.[6,10,11] Histological improvement is observed in about 70% of those treated with entecavir compared to 60% who are treated with lamivudine after 52 weeks of therapy.[10,11] Entecavir is more effective in achieving undetectable HBV DNA levels (<300 copies/mL) than lamivudine therapy (67% vs. 36%).[10] Sustaining HBeAg seroconversion is more likely to occur in patients with HbeAg-positive CHB who achieved seroconversion at the end of 48 weeks of therapy (70%).[6,12] The relapse rates are unknown for HbeAg-negative patients treated with entecavir. Lamivudine refractory patients may still achieve undetectable HBV DNA levels and improved histology with high dose entecavir, 1 mg daily.[13] Patients with CHB who are naïve to treatment have low resistance rates of 1%–2% when treated with entecavir for up to 5 years. The resistance rate is ~50% at 5 years for patients who were previously treated with lamivudine and switched to entecavir.[6] The optimal treatment duration for the treatment of hepatitis B is unknown. The latest treatment algorithm recommends entecavir, tenofovir, and pegylated interferon α-2a as first-line agents for the treatment of CHB infections.[6]

LAMIVUDINE	Epivir, Epivir-HBV

Pharmacology. Lamivudine is an oral synthetic cytosine nucleoside dideoxy analogue ((-)2′,3′-dideoxy, 3′-thiacytidine) having antiviral effects against HIV and HBV. In the HBV, lamivudine is phosphorylated to 3TC-triphosphate, which inhibits HBV DNA chain termination. 3TC-triphosphate also inhibits RNA and DNA-polymerase viral HIV-1 replication.[1] Lamivudine is approved for the treatment of CHB with active viral replication and liver inflammation. It is also indicated for the treatment of HIV infections when coadministered with other antiretroviral agents.

Administration and Adult Dosage. **PO for the treatment of CHB with active HBV replication and active liver inflammation**—100 mg once daily. **PO for HIV infection**—150 mg twice daily. **For HIV coinfection with CHB**—Use HIV dosage with appropriate combination antiretroviral therapy.

Special Populations. *Pediatric Dosage.* (2–17 years) **PO for the treatment of CHB with active HBV replication and active liver inflammation**—3 mg/kg once daily up to a maximum daily dose of 100 mg/d. **PO for HIV infection** (3 months to 16 years)—4 mg/kg to a maximum of 150 mg twice daily, administered in combination with other antiretrovirals.

Geriatric Dosage. Same as adult dosage.

Other Conditions. **Renal Impairment.** (Cl_{Cr} 30–49 mL/min) 100 mg first dose, then 50 mg once daily; (Cl_{Cr} 15–29 mL/min) 100 mg first dose, then 25 mg once daily; (Cl_{Cr} 5–14 mL/min) 35 mg first dose, then 15 mg once daily; (Cl_{Cr} <5 mL/min) 35 mg first dose, then 10 mg once daily; (hemodialysis) no additional dosing of lamivudine is required after 4 h of hemodialysis or peritoneal dialysis.

Dosage Forms. **Tab** 150 and 300 mg; **Soln** 5 and 10 mg/mL.

Patient Instructions. Confirm HIV test is negative and if unknown, have the clinician confirm by testing. The amount of lamivudine in Epivir-HBV is lower than that needed to treat HIV, therefore Epivir-HBV should not be used as part of an HIV treatment regimen. Do not discontinue lamivudine without talking to the doctor first. Abrupt discontinuation of lamivudine may worsen the liver disease. Take lamivudine with water on either an empty or full stomach. If a dose is missed, take it later that same day if possible and then resume the regularly scheduled regimen the following day. Do not take 2 doses at once to make up for missing a dose.

Pharmacokinetics. Lamivudine is rapidly absorbed after oral administration with absolute bioavailability ranging between 82%–88%.[14] The systemic exposure is similar between the tablet and solution formulations; thus there is no difference in systemic exposure. Lamivudine is poorly bound to plasma protein (<36%). Intravenous lamivudine administered in subjects with HIV resulted in a V_d of 1.3 ± 0.4 L/kg. There is minimal lamivudine metabolism (4.2%); transsulfoxide metabolite is the primary metabolite detected in urine in the first 12 h of administration. Lamivudine is mostly eliminated unchanged in the urine, representing 71% of total clearance of lamivudine. **Half-life** is 5–7 h.

Adverse Reactions. Adverse effects include fatigue, diarrhea, nausea, vomiting, and headaches. In rare cases, pancreatitis, hepatomegaly, lipodystrophy, and potentially fatal lactic acidosis have been reported. ALT levels should be monitored carefully, as mild elevations between 2- and 3-fold increases may be observed. When lamivudine therapy is discontinued, aminotransferase levels should be monitored more closely, as increased ALT concentrations may indicate a flare in disease activity leading to liver failure.

Precautions. Pregnancy category C. Rare cases of lactic acidosis and severe hepatomegaly have been reported during lamivudine treatment. Some of these cases were fatal. Confirm that the HIV test is negative and if unknown, have the clinician confirm by testing. If you are HIV positive, do not treat with only lamivudine because more than one medication is needed to treat the HIV infection. Patients must be monitored after discontinuing lamivudine, as posttreatment exacerbations of the liver disease have been observed, and in some cases were fatal. Reports of pancreatitis have been documented.

Drug Interactions. Hepatic decompensation has been reported in coinfected HIV and hepatitis C virus (HCV) patients treated with ribavirin and interferon-α. Some of these cases have been fatal. Additionally, nucleoside analogues, such as ribavirin, when coadministered with lamivudine may increase the risk of developing lactic acidosis.

Parameters to Monitor. *See* Parameters to Monitor for Hepatitis B Therapy.

Notes. Lamivudine may be considered during the third trimester in pregnant patients with active hepatitis B and HBV DNA levels greater than 10^7 copies/mL along with elevated ALT levels. There is an increased risk for resistance when lamivudine is used long term, thus caution must be taken.[6] Lamivudine is effective in suppressing HBV replication, normalizing ALT levels, and improving liver histology.[15,16] Forty-four percent of the HbeAg-positive CHB patients had a significant loss of serum HBV DNA level compared to 16% receiving placebo. Normalizing ALT levels and improvement in histology was observed in ~50% of patients. HBeAg loss was observed in 18% of the subjects at the end of 52 weeks of treatment.[6,17] Even though lamivudine therapy produces adequate virological, biological, and histological response, the drug is no longer considered first-line therapy for CHB infections due to frequent biochemical and virologic breakthroughs leading to the development of drug resistance.[6,12] The resistance rate is about 20% after 1 year of lamivudine therapy and may increase to 70% by 5 years of treatment.[18] Available in combination with abacavir, zidovudine, and abacavir/zidovudine.

PEGYLATED INTERFERON   Pegasys, PegIntron

Pharmacology. Interferon α-2a and interferon α-2b are proteins with antiviral activity against hepatitis B and C. Interferon's exact mechanism of action is unknown; however, it is thought to exert its immunomodulatory effects by promoting T-cell proliferation (Th1 T-helper cell) and stimulating natural killer cells hence decreasing HCV RNA replication. Synthesis of several proteins which inhibit HCV RNA replication, including $2',5'$-oligoadenylate synthetase and serum neopterin are also stimulated by interferon.[19] Newer formulations attach interferon to a polyethylene glycol moiety to produce either peginterferon α-2a (Pegasys) or peginterferon α-2b (PegIntron). Pegylation prevents rapid drug degradation and renal clearance thus allowing increased systemic exposure and once weekly dosing (versus 3 times weekly dosing for unmodified interferon).

Administration and Adult Dosage. (PegInterferon α-2a) **SQ for the treatment of CHB**—180 μg once weekly; **SQ for the treatment of HCV with or without HIV**—180 μg once weekly with ribavirin 800–1200 mg in 2 divided doses. (Peginterferon α-2b) **SQ for the treatment of HCV**—(Monotherapy) Weight ≤45 kg = 40 μg; 46–56 kg = 50 μg; 57–72 kg = 64 μg; 73–88 kg = 80 μg; 89–106 kg = 96 μg; 107–136 kg = 120 μg; 137–160 kg = 150 μg. (Combination with ribavirin) Weight ≤40 kg = 50 μg; 40–50 kg = 64 μg; 51–60 kg = 80 μg; 61–75 kg = 96 μg; 76–85 kg = 120 μg; >86 kg = 150 μg.

Special Populations. *Pediatric Dosage.* (Pegylated Interferon) (<18 years) Safety and efficacy not established. (Interferon α-2b) **SQ for treatment of CHB** (3–16 years)—3 million International Units/m² 3 times weekly.

Other Conditions. **Renal Impairment.** Dosage adjustment of peginterferon is necessary in patients with renal impairment. It is recommended that peginterferon monotherapy be used cautiously when Cl_{Cr} is <50 mL/min. Combination with ribavirin should be avoided if Cl_{Cr} is <50 mL/min.

Geriatric dosage. Same as adult dosage.

Dosage Forms. (Peginterferon α-2b) **Inj** 50 μg/0.5 mL; 80 μg/0.5 mL; 120 μg/0.5 mL; 150 μg/0.5 mL; (Peginterferon α-2a) **Inj** 180 μg/mL.

Patient Instructions. Do not discontinue without talking to the doctor first. Peginterferon should be used in combination with ribavirin when indicated for the treatment of HCV. Confirm you are not pregnant prior to initiating peginterferon when used in combination with ribavirin and use two forms of birth control during and 6 months after therapy is completed because ribavirin is known to cause birth defects to the fetus. Laboratory monitoring must be completed as ordered by the clinician to assess for any abnormalities during treatment. If symptoms of chest pains, dizziness, shortness of breath, persistent flulike symptoms, depression, and irritability are experienced, contact the health care provider immediately for medical attention. Discard used peginterferon needles and syringes appropriately to minimize the risk of transmitting the hepatitis virus onto others.

Pharmacokinetics. (Peginterferon α-2a) The absolute bioavailability in healthy volunteers is at least 60%. In patients treated for HCV, the C_{max} was 25.6 $\pm$ μg/L. It will take approximately 4–6 weeks after peginterferon discontinuation for serum levels to become undetectable. The drug is metabolized via the liver and eliminated through the kidneys. With interferon attached to a pegylated moiety, the renal clearance of interferon is decreased 100-fold after a single dose of 180 μg peginterferon α-2a. The mean clearance is 0.06 L/h at the end of 48 weeks of peginterferon α-2a treatment. **Half-life** is 70–80 h in patients infected with HCV.[20] (Peginterferon α-2b) The mean absorption is 4.6 h. The V_d is 0.99 L/kg, which is about 30% less than unmodified interferon. It is recommended that peginterferon α-2b be dosed based on weight because of its large volume of distribution. **Half-life** ranges from 22 to 60 h (mean 40 h). The majority of peginterferon α-2b is cleared by the liver and 30% via the kidneys.[21]

Adverse Reactions. Most studies evaluated the combination regimen of interferon or pegylated interferon with ribavirin. The most common adverse effects with peginterferon are flulike symptoms, depression, irritability, rash, headaches, and laboratory abnormalities (neutropenia, thrombocytopenia, and anemia). Suicidal ideation leading to death has been documented. Other rare adverse effects include hypersensitivity reactions, endocrine disorders (hypothyroidism, hyperthyroidism, diabetes), and ophthalmologic disorders (retinopathy). Approximately 10%–30% of patients receiving peginterferon and/or ribavirin require a dosage reduction or treatment discontinuation to minimize side effects.[22] When peginterferon is used with ribavirin, additional adverse effects may be experienced with the most pronounced being hemolytic anemia. Cardiac (fatal and nonfatal myocardial infarction) and pulmonary events (dyspnea, decreased pulmonary function) may develop and requires hemoglobin monitoring to prevent and minimize symptoms. Ribavirin-induced hemolytic anemia is reversible upon discontinuing ribavirin. It is estimated that 10%–25% of patients will require a dosage adjustment or treatment discontinuation and, in rare cases, blood transfusions may be needed if hemoglobin levels fall below 8.5 g/dL (5.27 mmol/L). Erythropoietin or darbepoetin alpha may be used as an adjunctive therapy for ribavirin-induced hemolytic anemia.[23,24]

Contraindications. Peginterferon is contraindicated in patients with hepatic decompensation defined as having a Child-Pugh score greater than 6. It is also contraindicated when administered with ribavirin in pregnant females and patients with hemoglobinopathies including thalassemia major or sickle cell anemia.

Precautions. (Monotherapy) Pregnancy category C. Animal studies using monkeys resulted in an increase in abortion rates. (Combination with ribavirin) Pregnancy Category X. It is undetermined if ribavirin contained in sperm causes teratogenic and embryocidal effects, thus males should take precaution to prevent impregnating their female partners. Ribavirin has a 12-day half-life; all women of childbearing age and men who are able to father a child must use two forms of contraception during and 6 months after treatment. Peginterferon may induce psychiatric adverse effects (irritability, depression, and rarely, suicidal ideation) or worsen psychiatric conditions already present. Patients with suicidal ideations should discontinue treatment immediately.[25] Hematologic abnormalities associated with peginterferon include thrombocytopenia, neutropenia, or anemia. Other lab abnormalities may develop, thus the need to monitor thyroid function tests, glucose concentrations, and creatinine clearance. The patient may experience more pronounced adverse effects when peginterferon is administered with ribavirin for HCV. Careful, frequent monitoring is required if ribavirin is prescribed in patients with a history of sarcoidosis or cardiac or pulmonary disease. Patients must be compliant with monitoring to assess for hemolytic anemia or any other laboratory abnormalities.

Drug Interactions. Peginterferon α-2a inhibits CYP P450 1A2 in healthy volunteers. Theophylline levels should be monitored frequently when coadministered with peginterferon. Peginterferon α-2b induces CYP2C8/9 and CYP2D6 activity, however, its clinical significance is unknown. Caution should be used when peginterferon α-2b is administered with medications that are metabolized via the CYP2C8/9 or 2D6 pathway (e.g., warfarin, phenytoin, or flecainide). Caution should be exercised when didanosine (and other nucleoside analogues) is used along with peginterferon and ribavirin, as this combination may lead to hepatic failure, lactic acidosis, or death. Ribavirin may antagonize and inhibit the phosphorylation of stavudine and zidovudine, thus decreasing their therapeutic effects for the treatment of HIV.

Parameters to Monitor. *See* Parameters to Monitor for Hepatitis C Therapy.

Notes. (Hepatitis B) Pegylated interferon α-2a is approved for the treatment of CHB and is considered a first-line agent because its drug resistance does not develop with utilization. It should not be used in patients with decompensated liver disease because the drug may induce hepatic failure, or in those with significant and unstable medical comorbidities.[6] (Hepatitis C) Peginterferon α-2a and peginterferon α-2b are approved treatments for HCV. Peginterferon therapy alone for 48 weeks achieves a 25%–40% sustained virological response (SVR), and when used in combination with ribavirin, SVR rates increase to 45%–55%.[26,27] Genotype determines the duration of therapy. The recommended treatment duration for individuals with nongenotype 1 is 24 weeks and 48 weeks for genotype 1.[25,28] Patients should not be treated with peginterferon with or without ribavirin if decompensated liver disease is evident. Peginterferon α-2b administered as 1 μg/kg/wk has been evaluated in children between 3 and 16 years of age for chronic hepatitis C infections.[29] Children with HCV between the ages of 5 and 18 years have been evaluated using peginterferon α-2a administered as 180 μg/1.73 m².[30,31]

RIBAVIRIN
Rebetol, Copegus, Ribasphere, Various

Pharmacology. Ribavirin is a nucleoside analogue, (1-β-D-ribofuranosyl-1H-1,2,4-triazole-3-carboxamide) used for the treatment of HCV when administered with interferon. The mechanism of action of ribavirin is still under investigation, however, several mechanisms have been proposed: ceasing HCV RNA viral replication by inhibiting RNA polymerase, inducing "error catastrophe" to promote mutations during the viral replication process; immunomodulation by shifting the balance to stimulate T_H1 to enhance clearance of the virus; and inhibiting IMPDH (inosine-monophosphate-dehydrogenase) to deplete GTP which prevents further HCV RNA replication.[19,32]

Administration and Adult Dosage. PO for the treatment of HCV infection in combination with interferon or pegylated interferon—(Tab) 400–800 mg twice daily with food; genotype 1 and 4—600 mg twice daily for 48 weeks;[28] genotype 2 and 3—400 mg twice daily for 24 weeks.[28] (Cap) Genotype 1 and 4—treat for 48 weeks;[28] genotype 2 and 4—treat for 24 weeks.[28] Weight <40–65 kg—400 mg twice daily; 66–85 kg—400 mg in the morning and 600 mg in the evening; 86–105 kg—600 mg twice daily, >105–600 mg in the morning and 800 mg in the evening.

Special Populations. *Pediatric Dosage.* 15 mg/kg/d in two divided doses with food.[29,33]

Geriatric Dosage. Same as adult dosage.

Other Conditions. **Renal Impairment.** Not recommended when Cl_{Cr} is <50 mL/min.

History of Cardiac Disease. Should be evaluated prior to initiating therapy. A dosage reduction is required if hemoglobin concentrations decrease by 2 g/dL or more in a 4-week period. If patients are symptomatic (severe fatigue, shortness of breath, chest pains), then ribavirin may need to be discontinued.

Dosage Forms. **Tab** 200 mg, 400 mg, 600 mg; **Cap** 200 mg; **Oral Soln** 40 mg/mL; **Inhal Soln** 6 g.

Patient Instructions. Do not discontinue without talking to the doctor first. Treating HCV with only ribavirin is not effective and must include interferon or pegylated interferon. If symptoms of chest pains, dizziness, or shortness of breath are experienced, contact the health care provider immediately for medical attention. Confirm you are not pregnant prior to initiating ribavirin therapy and agree to use two forms of birth control during and 6 months after therapy is completed because the drug is known to cause birth defects to the fetus.

Pharmacokinetics. The pharmacokinetics of ribavirin have been evaluated with interferon and pegylated interferon. The oral bioavailability ranges from 20% to 64% and is increased when ribavirin is administered with a high-fat meal. The mean C_{max} was 2748 ± 818 ng/mL after 12 weeks of ribavirin 600 mg twice daily. Ribavirin accumulates in the body after multiple dosings where the C_{max} was found to be 4 times higher than after a single dose. **Half-life** 120–170 h and as long as 300 h after a single oral dose and is unbound to plasma proteins. Ribavirin was not found to be a substrate of the cytochrome, CYP P450 enzyme system yet it is metabolized through the reversible phosphorylation and degradative pathways.

Patients with renal insufficiencies must have their dose adjusted accordingly because ribavirin is mostly eliminated by the kidneys.

Adverse Reactions. Most studies evaluated the combination regimen of interferon or pegylated interferon with ribavirin. The most common adverse effect is hemolytic anemia. Cardiac (fatal and nonfatal myocardial infarction) and pulmonary events (dyspnea, decreased pulmonary function) may arise and hemoglobin monitoring is required to prevent the occurrence of these symptoms. Ribavirin-induced hemolytic anemia is reversible upon discontinuing ribavirin. It is estimated that 10%–25% of patients will require a dosage adjustment or treatment discontinuation, and in rare cases blood transfusions may be needed if hemoglobin levels fall below 8.5 g/dL (5.27 mmol/L). Erythropoietin or darbepoetin alpha may be used as an adjunctive therapy for ribavirin-induced hemolytic anemia.[23,24] Other adverse effects include headaches, fatigue, dizziness, gastrointestinal disturbances, pruritus, and rash.

Contraindications. Pregnancy category X. Hemoglobinopathies including thalassemia major or sickle cell anemia.

Precautions. Ribavirin is teratogenic and has embryocidal effects. Women must have a negative pregnancy test prior to starting ribavirin. All women of childbearing age and men who are able to father a child must be educated to use two forms of contraception during and 6 months after treatment. Ribavirin monotherapy is not effective for the treatment of HCV and must be administered with pegylated interferon. Patients must be compliant with monitoring to assess for hemolytic anemia or any other laboratory abnormalities. Careful, frequent monitoring is required if ribavirin is prescribed in patients with a history of sarcoidosis or cardiac or pulmonary disease. Avoid use in patients with renal insufficiencies, specifically when Cl_{Cr} is <50 mL/min.

Drug Interactions. Didanosine (and other nucleoside analogues) administered with ribavirin have lead to hepatic failure and lactic acidosis, and in some cases have resulted in death. Ribavirin may antagonize and inhibit the phosphorylation of stavudine and zidovudine, thus decreasing their therapeutic effects for the treatment of HIV.

Parameters to Monitor. *See* Parameters to Monitor for Hepatitis C Therapy.

Notes. Ribavirin monotherapy for the treatment for HCV is not effective and must include pegylated interferon. (*See* Pegylated Interferon monograph.)

TELBIVUDINE	Tyzeka

Pharmacology. Telbivudine is a synthetic thymidine nucleoside analogue (1-((2S,4R,5S)-4-hydroxy-5-hydroxymethyltetrahydrofuran-2-yl)-5-methyl-1*H*-pyrimidine-2,4-dione) that inhibits HBV replication. Telbivudine is phosphorylated to telbivudine 5′-triphosphate, the active form that inhibits HBV DNA reverse transcription, which in turn terminates HBV replication with no HIV activity.[1]

Administration and Adult Dosage. **PO for the treatment of CHB infection with active HBV viral replication and elevated aminotransferases or histologically active disease—600 mg once daily with or without food.**

Special Populations. *Pediatric Dosage.* (<16 years) Safety and efficacy not established.

Geriatric Dosage. Same as adult dosage.

Other Conditions. **Renal Impairment.** (Cl_{Cr} 30–49 mL/min)—600 mg once every 48h; (Cl_{Cr} <30 mL/min)—600 mg once every 72h; (end-stage renal disease)—600 mg once every 96h, administered after hemodialysis.

Dosage Forms. Tab 600 mg.

Patient Instructions. Do not discontinue telbivudine without talking to the doctor first. Abrupt discontinuation may worsen the liver disease. If symptoms of muscle pain, tiredness, difficulty breathing, or palpitations are experienced, seek immediate medical attention as lactic acidosis may have developed. Tell the health care provider if muscle pain, weakness, or tenderness persist and do not resolve. Take telbivudine with water on a full or empty stomach. If a dose is missed, take it later that same day if possible and then resume the regularly scheduled regimen the following day. Do not take 2 doses at once to make up for missing a dose.

Pharmacokinetics. Telbivudine is rapidly absorbed in healthy subjects after oral administration. After 1–4 h, the mean C_{max} is 3.69 ± 1.25 μg/mL. Drug absorption is not affected with a high-fat or high-calorie meal. The plasma protein binding in vitro of telbivudine is about 3%. The apparent V_d is greater than the total body water, thus the drug is distributed into the tissue extensively. Telbivudine is not metabolized by the cytochrome, CYP P450 enzyme system and is mostly eliminated by the kidneys as an unchanged drug. **Half-life** 40–49 h. Patients with renal insufficiencies must have their dose adjusted accordingly.[34]

Adverse Reactions. Adverse effects include fatigue, headaches, nausea, dizziness, diarrhea, and rash. Laboratory abnormalities include elevated creatine kinase (CK), amylase, and lipase.[35] Generalized weakness and myopathy is not uncommon with telbivudine, which may be seen within 2–20 weeks of therapy.[36] In many cases, CK levels were elevated, however, these levels do not correlate with the severity of the myopathy. The muscle discomfort is somewhat reversible upon discontinuing telbivudine, yet in a few instances, symptoms may persist.[34,36] In rare cases, hepatomegaly with steatosis and potentially fatal lactic acidosis have been reported. ALT flare up may occur while on telbivudine during the first 24 weeks of therapy, therefore aminotransferases monitoring is required.[36] When the drug is discontinued, aminotransferase levels should be monitored more closely as increased ALT concentrations may indicate a flare in disease activity leading to liver failure.

Precautions. Pregnancy category B. Rare cases of lactic acidosis and severe hepatomegaly with steatosis have been reported. Possible exacerbation of hepatitis has been observed when treatment was discontinued. Monitor patient's aminotransferase levels and clinically for flare up of liver disease (pale stools, tea color urine, jaundice) several months posttreatment. Patients complaining of muscle weakness and havng elevated creatinine phosphokinase levels should be evaluated for myopathy. If myopathy is confirmed, telbivudine therapy should be discontinued.

Drug Interactions. There is minimal concern with telbivudine interacting with medications undergoing CYP P450 metabolism because the drug is not a substrate of the system. Agents that are nephrotoxic and coadministered with telbivudine may increase the risk of renal toxicity, thereby increasing serum concentrations of either drug.

Parameters to Monitor. *See* Parameters to Monitor for Hepatitis B Therapy.

Notes. Telbivudine is indicated for HBeAg-positive and HBeAg-negative CHB. It is comparable in efficacy in reducing HBV DNA levels and normalizing aminotransferase levels. Its clinical benefits in improving histology, HBeAg seroconversion, and HBeAg loss continues to be confirmed.[35] Telbivudine's place in therapy for the treatment of HBV is still in question due to its intermediate rate of resistance.[6] The resistance rates with telbivudine are lower than lamivudine. Patients with HbeAg-positive hepatitis B have a resistance rate of about 4% at 1 year and 22% at 2 years. These rates are lower in patients with HbeAg-negative CHB (2.7% at year 1 and 8.6% at year 2).[12] The treatment duration for hepatitis B is still under investigation.

TENOFOVIR   Viread

Pharmacology. Tenofovir disoproxil fumarate is an acyclic nucleotide analogue, (9-[(R)-2-[[bis[[(isopropoxycarbonyl)oxy]methoxy]phosphinyl]methoxy] propyl]) adenine fumarate. Tenofovir disoproxil fumarate undergoes diester hydrolysis to tenofovir, which is then phosphorylated to the active form, tenofovir diphosphate. Tenofovir diphosphate inhibits HBV DNA replication and HIV-1 reverse transcriptase.[1]

Administration and Adult Dosage. **PO for the treatment of CHB infection—** 300 mg once daily without food. **PO in combination with other antiretroviral agents for the treatment of HIV-1 infection—**300 mg once daily without food.

Special Populations. *Pediatric Dosage.* (<18 years) Safety and efficacy not established.

Geriatric Dosage. Same as adult dosage.

Other Conditions. **Renal Impairment.** (Cl_{Cr} 30–49 mL/min) 300 mg every 48h; (Cl_{Cr} 10–29 mL/min) 300 mg every 96h; (Hemodialysis) every 7d or after ~12 h of dialysis (assuming 3 hemodialysis sessions a week of about 4 h duration).

Dosage Forms. **Tab** 300 mg.

Patient Instructions. Do not discontinue tenofovir without talking to the doctor first. Abrupt discontinuation of this medication may worsen the liver disease. If symptoms of muscle pain, tiredness, difficulty breathing or palpitations are experienced, seek immediate medical attention as lactic acidosis may have developed. Tell the health care provider if muscle pain, weakness, or tenderness persist and do not resolve. Tenofovir may increase body fat in the upper back, neck, breast, and trunk whereas a decrease in the amount of fat may be seen in the face, arms, and legs. Confirm that the HIV test is negative and if unknown, have the clinician confirm by testing. If you are HIV positive, do not treat with only tenofovir because more than one medication is needed to treat the HIV infection. Take tenofovir with water on an empty stomach. If a dose is missed, take it later that same day if possible and then resume the regularly scheduled regimen the following day. Do not take 2 doses at once to make up for missing a dose.

Pharmacokinetics. Tenofovir is a prodrug with an oral bioavailability of about 25% in fasting patients. After 1 ± 0.4 h, the mean C_{max} is 0.3 ± 0.09 μg/mL. The protein binding of tenofovir is minimal, 7.2%. The mean V_d at steady state is 1.3 ± 0.6 L/kg with a 1 mg/kg intravenous dose of tenofovir. Tenofovir is not metabolized by the cytochrome, CYP P450 enzyme system and is mostly eliminated by the kidney as unchanged drug. **Half-life** 17 h.

Adverse Reactions. The most common adverse effect is a rash that occurs in 18% of patients. Diarrhea, headache, nausea, and dizziness also occur. Laboratory abnormalities include hypophosphatemia, hypercholesterolemia, hypertriglyceridemia, and elevated serum creatinine.[37,38] Decreased bone mineral density and osteomalacia have been observed in patients treated with tenofovir for HIV.[38,39] In a few case reports, patients coinfected with HIV and HBV have developed nephrotoxicity and Fanconi syndrome.[40,41] Lactic acidosis and severe hepatomegaly with steatosis have been seen in patients while on tenofovir, with some cases leading to death.

Precautions. Pregnancy category B. Tenofovir has been shown to cross the placenta in small trials. Risk versus benefit must be weighed when choosing to treat pregnant individuals infected with HBV with tenofovir.[37] Rare cases of lactic acidosis and severe hepatomegaly with steatosis have been reported. Possible exacerbation of hepatitis has been observed when treatment was discontinued. Monitor patient's aminotransferase levels and clinically for flare up of liver disease (pale stools, tea color urine, jaundice) several months posttreatment. Acute renal failure and Fanconi syndrome have been reported; therefore, monitor creatinine clearance and serum phosphorus for potential renal insufficiency.

Drug Interactions. There is minimal concern with tenofovir interacting with medications undergoing CYP P450 metabolism because the drug is not a substrate of the system. Agents that are nephrotoxic and coadministered with tenofovir may increase the risk of renal toxicity, thereby increasing serum concentrations of either drug. Several tenofovir interactions are associated with HIV medications. Didanosine concentrations are increased with tenofovir therapy. This combination should be avoided as it may lead to didanosine toxicity, a syndrome which includes lactic acidosis, neuropathy, pancreatitis, and diarrhea. Atazanavir and lopinavir/ ritonavir increase tenofovir concentrations.

Parameters to Monitor. *See* Parameters to Monitor for Hepatitis B Therapy.

Notes. Tenofovir has a similar structure to adefovir dipivoxil. It is indicated for HBeAg-positive and HBeAg-negative chronic hepatitis B with compensated liver disease as well as HIV. The potency of tenofovir in suppressing hepatitis B viral replication is greater than adefovir dipivoxil; therefore, it is considered as one of the first-line therapies for CHB infections.[6,42,43] Patients with lamivudine, entecavir, or adefovir resistance may benefit from tenofovir.[44–46] Viral suppression, including significant decrease and undetectable HBV DNA levels has been achieved with tenofovir after switching from other anti-HBV agents. The treatment duration is still under investigation. Available in combination with emtricitabine and emtricitabine/efavirenz.

PARAMETERS TO MONITOR FOR HEPATITIS B THERAPY

MONITOR	HOW OFTEN
Liver function tests (ALT)	Every 12 wk
HBV DNA levels	Every 12–24 wk
HBeAg	Every 24 wk
anti-HBe	Every 24 wk
HBsAg	Every 6–12 mo
Serum creatinine[a]	Every 12 wk
Serum creatine phosphokinase[b]	Every 12 wk

[a]Monitor for nephrotoxicity when tenofovir or adefovir used for treatment.
[b]Monitor when telbivudine used for treatment.
From Refs. 6 and 12.

PARAMETERS TO MONITOR FOR HEPATITIS C THERAPY

TIME	BASELINE	24–48 h	2 wk	4 wk	8 wk	12 wk	16/20 wk	24 wk	28/32 wk	36 wk	40/44 wk	48 wk	72 wk (6 mo off therapy)
CBC	X		X	X	X	X	X	X	X	X	X	X	X
LFTs	X		X	X	X	X	X	X	X	X	X	X	X
BMP[a]	X		X	X	X	X	X	X	X	X	X	X	X
TSH	X					X		X		X		X	
HCV RNA[b]	X					X		X		X		X	X
Lipid panel	X					X		X		X		X	
Flulike symptoms		X	X	X	X	X	X	X	X	X	X	X	
Adverse Effects		X	X	X	X	X	X	X	X	X	X	X	

[a]BMP: Basic Metabolic Panel.
[b]HCV RNA: Hepatitis C RNA level.
From Refs. 25 and 28.

■ REFERENCES

1. Férir G et al. Antiviral treatment of chronic hepatitis B virus infections: the past, the present and the future. *Rev Med Virol.* 2008;18:19-34.
2. Dando T, Plosker G. Adefovir Dipivoxil. A review of its use in chronic hepatitis B. *Drugs* 2003;63:2215–34.
3. Sokal EM et al. The pharmacokinetics and safety of adefovir dipivoxil in children and adolescents with chronic hepatitis B virus infection. *J Clin Pharmacol.* 2008;48:512-517.
4. Marcellin P et al. Adefovir dipivoxil for the treatment of hepatitis B e antigen-positive chronic hepatitis B. *N Engl J Med.* 2003;348:808-816.
5. Hadziyannis SJ et al. Adefovir dipivoxil for the treatment of HBeAg-negative chronic hepatitis B. *N Engl J Med.* 2003;348:800-807.
6. Keeffe EB et al. A treatment algorithm for the management of chronic hepatitis B virus infection in the United States: 2008 Update. *Clin Gastroenterol Hepatol.* 2008;6:1315-1341.
7. McMahon MA et al. The HBV Drug Entecavir – Effects on HIV-1 replication and resistance. *N Engl J Med.* 2007;356:2614-2621.
8. Robinson DM et al. Entecavir: a review of its use in chronic hepatitis B. *Drugs.* 2006;66:1605-1622.
9. Chang TT et al. A comparison of entecavir and lamivudine for HBeAg-positive chronic hepatitis B. *N Engl J Med.* 2006;354:1001-1010.
10. Lai CL et al. Entecavir versus lamivudine for patients with HBeAg-negative chronic hepatitis B. *N Engl J Med.* 2006;354:1011-1020.
11. Lok AS, McMahon BJ. Chronic hepatitis B. *Hepatology.* 2007;45:507-539.
12. Sherman M et al. Entecavir is superior to continued lamivudine for the treatment of lamivudine-refractory, HBeAg(+) chronic hepatitis B: results of phase III study ETV-026. *Hepatology.* 2004;40:664A.
13. Jarvis B, Faulds D. Lamivudine. A review of its therapeutic potential in chronic hepatitis B. *Drugs.* 1999;58:101-141.
14. Lai CL et al. A one-year trial of lamivudine for chronic hepatitis B. *N Engl J Med.* 1998;339:61-68.
15. Dienstag JL et al. Histological outcome during long-term lamivudine therapy. *Gastroenterology.* 2003;124:105-117.
16. Lok AS. The maze of treatments for hepatitis B. *N Engl J Med.* 2005;352:2743-2746.
17. Ayoub WS, Keeffe EB. Review article: current antiviral therapy of chronic hepatitis B. *Aliment Pharmacol Ther.* 2008;28:167-177.
18. Feld JJ, Hoofnagle JH. Mechanism of action of interferon and ribavirin in treatment of hepatitis C. *Nature.* 2005;436:967-972.
19. Perry CM, Jarvis B. Peginterferon-alpha-2a (40 kD): a review of its use in the management of chronic hepatitis C. *Drugs.* 2001;61:2263-2288.
20. Zeuzem S, Welsch C, Herrmann F. Pharmacokinetics of peginterferons. *Semin Liver Dis.* 2003;23(suppl 1):23-28.
21. Fried MW. Side effects of therapy of hepatitis C and their management. *Hepatology.* 2002;36:S237-S244.
22. Younossi ZM et al. A phase II dose finding study of darbepoetin alpha and filgrastim for the management of anaemia and neutropenia in chronic hepatitis C treatment. *J Viral Hepat.* 2008;15:370-378.
23. McHutchison JG et al. Strategies for managing anemia in hepatitis C patients undergoing antiviral therapy. *Am J Gastroenterol.* 2007;102:880-889.
24. Ghany MG et al.; American Association for the Study of Liver Diseases. Diagnosis, management, and treatment of hepatitis C: an update. *Hepatology* 2009;49:1335-74.
25. Manns MP et al. Peginterferon alfa-2b plus ribavirin compared with interferon alfa-2b plus ribavirin for initial treatment of chronic hepatitis C: a randomised trial. *Lancet.* 2001;358:958-965.
26. Fried MW et al. Peginterferon alfa-2a plus ribavirin for chronic hepatitis C virus infection. *N Engl J Med.* 2002;347:975-982.
27. Dienstag JL, McHutchison JG. American Gastroenterological Association technical review on the management of hepatitis C. *Gastroenterology.* 2006;130:231-264.
28. Jara P et al. Efficacy and safety of peginterferon-alfa 2b and ribavirin combination therapy in children with chronic hepatitis C infection. *Pediatr Infect Dis J.* 2008;27:142-148.
29. Murray KF et al. Design of the PEDS-C trial: pegylated interferon +/− ribavirin for children with chronic hepatitis C viral infection. *Clin Trials.* 2007;4:661-673.
30. Schwarz KB et al. Safety, efficacy and pharmacokinetics of peginterferon alpha2a (40 kd) in children with chronic hepatitis C. *J Pediatr Gastroenterol Nutr.* 2006;43:499-505.
31. Martin P, Jensen DM. Ribavirin in the treatment of chronic hepatitis C. *J Gastroenterol Hepatol.* 2008;23:844-855.
32. Elisofon SA, Jonas MM. Hepatitis B and C in children: current treatment and future strategies. *Clin Liver Dis.* 2006;10:133-148.
33. Keam SJ. Telbivudine. *Drugs.* 2007;67:1917-1929.
34. Lai CL et al. Telbivudine versus lamivudine in patients with chronic hepatitis B. *N Engl J Med.* 2007;357:2576-2588.

35. Zhang XS et al. Clinical features of adverse reactions associated with telbivudine. *World J Gastroenterol.* 2008;14:3549-3553.

36. Pozniak A. Tenofovir: what have over 1 million years of patient experience taught us? *Int J Clin Pract.* 2008;62:1285-1293.

37. Wong SN, Lok AS. Tenofovir disoproxil fumarate: role in hepatitis B treatment. *Hepatology.* 2006;44:309-313.

38. Parsonage MJ et al. The development of hypophosphataemic osteomalacia with myopathy in two patients with HIV infection receiving tenofovir therapy. *HIV Med.* 2005;6:341-346.

39. Rifkin BS, Perazella MA. Tenofovir-associated nephrotoxicity: Fanconi syndrome and renal failure. *Am J Med.* 2004;117:282-284.

40. Verhelst D et al. Fanconi syndrome and renal failure induced by tenofovir: a first case report. *Am J Kidney Dis.* 2002;40:1331-1333.

41. Heathcote EJ et al. A randomized, double-blind, comparison of tenofovir (TDF) versus adefovir dipivoxil (ADV) for the treatment of HBeAg-positive chronic hepatitis B (CHB): study GS-US-174-0103. *Hepatology.* 2007;46(suppl 1):861A.

42. Marcellin P et al. A randomized, double-blind, comparison of tenofovir (TDF) versus adefovir dipivoxil (ADV) for the treatment of HBeAg-negative chronic hepatitis B (CHB): study GS-US-174-0102. *Hepatology.* 2007;46(suppl 1):290A-291A.

43. Leemans WF et al. Selection of an entecavir-resistant mutant despite prolonged hepatitis B virus DNA suppression, in a chronic hepatitis B patient with preexistent lamivudine resistance: successful rescue therapy with tenofovir. *Eur J Gastroenterol Hepatol.* 2008;20:773-777.

44. Reijnders JG, Janssen HL. Potency of tenofovir in chronic hepatitis B: mono or combination therapy? *J Hepatol.* 2008;48:383-386.

45. Tan J et al. Tenofovir monotherapy is effective in hepatitis B patients with antiviral treatment failure to adefovir in the absence of adefovir-resistant mutations. *J Hepatol.* 2008;48:391-398.

Chapter 17

Miscellaneous Antimicrobials

Mary Gauthier-Lewis and Treavor T. Riley

ATOVAQUONE Mepron

Pharmacology. Atovaquone is a highly lipophilic hydroxynaphthoquinone with activity against *Pneumocystis jiroveci* (formerly *Pneumocystis carinii*), *Toxoplasma gondii*, and *Plasmodium* spp. It is a structural analogue of ubiquinone, a small hydrophobic respiratory chain electron carrier molecule found in mitochondria. The mechanism of antipneumocystis activity by atovaquone is unclear but there might be inhibition of the mitochondrial electron transport chain, which inhibits pyrimidine synthesis and leads to inhibition of nucleic acid and ATP synthesis.[1,2]

Administration and Adult Dosage. **PO for pneumocystis pneumonia (PCP) treatment**—750 mg twice daily for 21 days; **PO for PCP prophylaxis**—1.5 g once daily. (*See* Notes.)

Special Populations. *Pediatric Dosage.* Safety and efficacy not established.

Geriatric Dosage. (>65 years) not evaluated, but dosage adjustment does not appear to be necessary.

Other Conditions. Dosage alteration is not required with renal or hepatic impairment.

Dosage Forms. **Susp** 150 mg/mL; **Tab** 250 mg (with 100 mg of proguanil), 62.5 mg (with 25 mg of proguanil).

Patient Instructions. It is extremely important to take this medication with food to increase absorption; failure to do so might limit response to therapy. Shake the suspension gently before use.

Missed Doses. Take this drug at regular intervals. If you miss a dose, take it as soon as you remember. If it is about time for the next dose, take that dose only. Leave at least 6–8 h between doses. Do not double the dose or take an extra dose.

Pharmacokinetics. *Serum Levels.* Steady-state serum levels >14 mg/L (>38 μmol/L) are correlated with survival in patients with PCP; serum levels <6 mg/L (<16 μmol/L) might be ineffective.[2]

Fate. Atovaquone exhibits slow, irregular absorption, depending on the formulation. A high-fat meal increases absorption of the suspension 2.3-fold compared with the fasting state. A peak concentration of 11.5 mg/L (31 μmol/L) is achieved with a single 750-mg dose of the suspension. Oral administration of 750 mg bid as the suspension produces a steady-state level of 24 mg/L (65 μmol/L). More than 99.9% is protein bound, and the drug does not appear to cross the blood–brain barrier well. It appears to undergo enterohepatic cycling with >94% excreted over 21 days in the feces, with no metabolite identified and <0.6% renally excreted.[2] **Half-life** 67 ± 10 h.[2]

Adverse Effects. Maculopapular rash occurs frequently, but many patients can continue atovaquone therapy; in most instances, the rash resolves without sequelae. Gastrointestinal (GI) disturbances such as abdominal pain, nausea, vomiting, and diarrhea occur in more than 10% of patients. Fever, headaches, and insomnia also have been reported frequently. Elevations of hepatic transaminases and hyponatremia occur frequently (1%–10% of patients) but do not require cessation of therapy.

Contraindications. Life-threatening hypersensitivity.

Precautions. Pregnancy category C; lactation. Consider alternative therapy in patients who cannot take the drug with food or with GI disorders that might decrease oral absorption. Severe diarrhea or malabsorption syndrome because preexisting diarrhea is associated with poor outcome, presumably as a result of decreased absorption and serum levels.

Drug Interactions. Rifampin and rifabutin can decrease atovaquone serum levels.

Parameters to Monitor. Baseline and periodic liver function tests for patients on prolonged treatment.

Notes. Use atovaquone only in the treatment of mild to moderate episodes of PCP. Atovaquone has been used for prevention of PCP in patients who cannot tolerate or who have failed other traditional prevention medication; although the ongoing clinical trials on the safety, efficacy, and optimal dosage for this indication are not well established. **Malarone** tablets contain atovaquone 250 mg and proguanil 100 mg/tablet; **Malarone pediatric** tablets contain atovaquone 62.5 mg and proguanil 25 mg/tablet. Malarone is used for prevention or treatment of chloroquine-resistant malaria.

CHLORAMPHENICOL AND SALTS   Chloromycetin, Various

Pharmacology. Chloramphenicol is a broad-spectrum bacteriostatic antibiotic isolated from *Streptomyces venezuelae* and is particularly useful against ampicillin-resistant *Haemophilus influenzae; Salmonella* spp.; rickettsial infections such as Rocky Mountain spotted fever, typhoid fever; most anaerobic organisms; and many vancomycin-resistant enterococci. It inhibits protein synthesis by binding the 50S ribosomal subunit and might be bactericidal against some bacteria including pneumococci, meningococci, and *H. influenzae*. Resistance occurs because of impermeability of the cell wall or bacterial production of chloramphenicol acetyltransferase, a plasmid-mediated enzyme that acetylates chloramphenicol into a microbiologically inert form.[3–6]

Administration and Adult Dosage. PO or IV—50–100 mg/kg/d in 4 divided doses, depending on severity, location, and organism, to a maximum of 4 g/d. **IM NOT recommended.**

Special Populations. *Pediatric Dosage.* PO or IV—(<7 days or <2 kg) 25 mg/kg once daily; (neonates >7 days and >2 kg) 25 mg/kg every 12 h; (older infants and children) 50–100 mg/kg/d given every 6 h. These regimens produce unpredictable levels, and serum level monitoring is recommended.[7] **IM NOT recommended.**

Geriatric Dosage. Same as adult dosage.

Other Conditions. Reduce dosage with impaired liver and renal function as guided by serum levels.[7]

Dosage Forms. Cap 250 mg; **Inj** (as sodium succinate) 1 g (100 mg/mL when reconstituted); **Ophth Oint** 10 mg/g; **Ophth Pwdr for Soln** 25 mg/vial; **Ophth Soln** 5 mg/mL.

Pharmacokinetics. *Serum Levels.* Therapeutic peak 10–20 mg/L; therapeutic trough 5–10 mg/L. (*See* Adverse Reactions.)

Fate. Well absorbed orally with 75%–90% bioavailability and a peak serum level of 12 mg/L after administration of 1 g to adults. IV 1 g produces levels of 5–12 mg/L (15–37 μmol/L) 1 h after administration to normal adults. In infants and young children, hydrolysis of succinate to the active form can be slow and incomplete. IM administration produces serum levels of active drugs that are 50% lower than the equivalent oral dose. The drug attains therapeutic levels in most body cavities, the eye, and CSF; it is 53% plasma protein bound. V_d is 0.94 ± 0.06 L/kg; Clearance is 0.14 ± 0.01 L/h/kg. Most of the drug is eliminated by glucuronidation in the liver followed by excretion in the urine; the remainder is excreted in the urine unchanged. The rate of glucuronidation and renal elimination is greatly reduced in neonates; 6.5%–80% of succinate can be excreted unhydrolyzed. Urine concentrations can be inadequate to treat UTIs, especially in patients with moderately to severely impaired renal function. A small amount (2%–4%) of a dose appears in the bile and feces, mostly as the glucuronide.[6,8] **Half-life** 4 ± 2 h in healthy adults[8]; extremely prolonged and variable in neonates, infants, and young children. Unpredictable in patients with impaired liver function. Some normal patients and patients with impaired renal function exhibit impaired free drug elimination.

Adverse Reactions. Serum levels >25 mg/L (>77 μmol/L) frequently produce reversible bone marrow depression with reticulocytopenia, decreased hemoglobin, increased serum iron and iron-binding globulin saturation, thrombocytopenia, and mild leukopenia.[7] The drug inhibits iron uptake by bone marrow, and anemic patients do not respond to iron or vitamin B_{12} therapy while receiving chloramphenicol. This anemia most often follows parenteral therapy, large dosages, long duration of therapy, or impaired drug elimination. Complete recovery usually occurs within 1–2 weeks after drug discontinuation. Aplastic anemia occurs rarely (1/12,000 to 1/50,000) and can be fatal. It is not dose related and can occur long after a short course of oral or parenteral therapy[7]; its occurrence after ophthalmic or parenteral use is controversial.[9] Fatal cardiovascular–respiratory collapse (gray syndrome) can develop in neonates given excessive dosages. This syndrome is associated with serum levels of approximately 50–100 mg/L (155–310 μmol/L).[7] A similar syndrome has been reported in children and adults given large overdoses.

Contraindications. Trivial infections; prophylactic use; uses other than those for which it is indicated.

Precautions. Pregnancy; lactation. Use with caution in patients with liver disease (especially cirrhosis, ascites, and jaundice) or preexisting hematologic disorders or patients receiving other bone marrow depressants. It can cause hemolytic episodes in patients with G-6-PD deficiency; observe dosage recommendations closely in neonates and infants.

Drug Interactions. Chloramphenicol inhibits CYP2C9 and increases serum concentrations of phenytoin, warfarin, and sulfonylurea oral hypoglycemic agents. Phenytoin, phenobarbital, and rifampin can decrease serum levels of chloramphenicol.

Parameters to Monitor. CBC with platelet and reticulocyte counts before and frequently during therapy; serum iron and iron-binding globulin saturation also might be useful. Liver and renal function tests before and occasionally during therapy. Monitor serum levels weekly because of variability in pharmacokinetics. More frequent monitoring might be necessary in patient with hepatic dysfunction and during long-term (>2 weeks) therapy.

CLINDAMYCIN SALTS	Cleocin, Various
LINCOMYCIN HYDROCHLORIDE	Lincocin

Pharmacology. Clindamycin is a semisynthetic 7-chloro, 7-deoxylincomycin derivative that is active against most gram-positive organisms except enterococci and *Clostridium difficile*. Gram-negative aerobes are resistant, but most anaerobes are sensitive. It inhibits bacterial protein synthesis by binding to the 50S ribosomal subunit; it is bactericidal or bacteriostatic depending on the concentration, organism, and inoculum.[10,11]

Administration and Adult Dosage. **PO**—150–450 mg every 6–8 h; **PO for prevention of endocarditis in patients at risk undergoing dental, oral, or upper respiratory tract procedures and who are allergic to penicillin**—600 mg 1 h before procedure.[12] **IM or IV**—600 mg to 2.7 g/d in 2–4 divided doses, to a maximum of 4.8 g/d. **IV for endocarditis prophylaxis**—600 mg within 30 min before a dental procedure. Single IM doses > 600 mg are NOT recommended; infuse IV no faster than 30 mg/min.[12] **Topical for acne**—apply twice daily; **vaginal for bacterial vaginosis**—1 applicatorful at bedtime for 7 days.

Special Populations. *Pediatric Dosage.* **PO**—(<10 kg) give no less than 37.5 mg every 8 h; (>10 kg) 8–25 mg/kg/d in 3 or 4 divided doses; **PO for endocarditis prophylaxis**—20 mg/kg 1 h before a dental procedure; **IM or IV**—(<1 month) 15–20 mg/kg/d in 3 or 4 divided doses; the lower dosage may be adequate for premature infants; (>1 month) 15–40 mg/kg/d in 3 or 4 divided doses (not less than 300 mg/d in severe infection, regardless of weight); **IV for endocarditis prophylaxis**—20 mg/kg (up to 600 mg) PO within 30 min before a dental procedure.[12]

Geriatric Dosage. Same as adult dosage.

Other Conditions. Dosage adjustment is unnecessary in renal impairment or cirrhosis, although the effect of acute liver disease is unknown.[7,10,13]

Dosage Forms. (Clindamycin) **Cap** (as hydrochloride) 75, 150, 300 mg; **Soln** (as palmitate) 15 mg/mL (reconstituted); **Inj** (as phosphate) 150 mg/mL; **Top Soln** (as phosphate) 1%; **Top Gel** (as phosphate) 1%; **Vag Crm** 2%. (Lincomycin) **Inj** 300 mg/mL.

Patient Instructions. Report any severe diarrhea or blood in the stools immediately and do not take antidiarrheal medication. Do not refrigerate the reconstituted oral solution because it will thicken.

Missed Doses. Take this drug at regular intervals. If you miss a dose, take it as soon as you remember. If it is about time for the next dose, take that dose only. Leave at least 4–6 h between doses. Do not double the dose or take an extra dose.

Pharmacokinetics. *Fate.* Absorption is nearly 87% and is the same from the capsule or the solution; food can delay, but not decrease, absorption. The palmitate and phosphate esters are absorbed intact and rapidly hydrolyzed to the active base. Unhydrolyzed phosphate ester usually constitutes <20% of the total peak serum level after parenteral clindamycin but can increase to 40% in patients with impaired renal function. A 500-mg oral dose produces a peak serum level of 5–6 mg/L (12–14 μmol/L) in 1 h. A 300-mg IM dose produces a peak level of 5–6 mg/L 1–2 h postinjection. A 600-mg IV dose infused over 30 min produces a peak serum level of 10 mg/L (23 μmol/L). The drug is widely distributed throughout the body except the CSF. It is 94% plasma protein bound; V_d is 1.1 ± 0.3 L/kg; Clearance is 0.28 ± 0.08 L/h/kg. There is hepatic metabolism and excretion of active forms in the bile. From 5% to 10% of the absorbed dose is recovered as unchanged drug and active metabolites in the urine within 24 h. [7,8,10,14] **Half-life** 2.9 ± 0.7 h; increased in premature infants[8]; unchanged or slightly increased in severe renal disease; might be increased or unchanged in liver disease.[11]

Adverse Reactions. After oral administration, anorexia, nausea, vomiting, cramps, and diarrhea occur frequently.[7,10,13] Oral and rarely parenteral clindamycin can cause severe, sometimes fatal, pseudomembranous colitis (PMC), which might be clinically indistinguishable at onset from non-PMC diarrhea.[10] Antibiotic-associated PMC is secondary to the overgrowth of toxin-producing *C. difficile.* Symptoms usually appear 2–9 days after initiation of therapy. PMC has been reported after topical administration.[13] PMC is terminated in many patients by discontinuing the antibiotic immediately; however, if diarrhea is severe or does not improve promptly after discontinuation, treat with oral metronidazole or vancomycin.[10,11] The value of corticosteroids, cholestyramine, and antispasmodics in the management of antibiotic-associated diarrhea and PMC has not been established.[10] Antidiarrheals (e.g., diphenoxylate, loperamide) may worsen PMC and should NOT be used.

Precautions. Pregnancy; lactation. Use with caution in neonates <4 weeks of age and in patients with liver disease. Discontinue immediately if severe diarrhea occurs. Drug accumulation might occur in patients with severe concomitant hepatic and renal dysfunction, but data are lacking.

Drug Interactions. Clindamycin might enhance the action of non–depolarizing neuromuscular blocking agents. Kaolin–pectin mixture delays but does not decrease oral absorption of clindamycin.

Parameters to Monitor. Observe for changes in bowel frequency.

Notes. Oral clindamycin solution is stable for 2 weeks at room temperature after reconstitution. Do NOT refrigerate.

COLISTIMETHATE SODIUM	Coly-Mycin M
POLYMYXIN B	Various

Pharmacology. Colistimethate is a chemically identical compound to polymyxin E, which exhibits bactericidal activity by penetrating and disrupting bacterial cell membranes. It displays selective activity against aerobic gram-negative bacteria, such as *Enterobacter aerogenes*, *Escherichia coli*, *Klebsiella pneumoniae*, and *Pseudomonas aeruginosa*, and is usually inactive against *Proteus* spp. Synergistic activity against strains of gram-negative bacteria is seen when combined with tetracyclines or chloramphenicol, permitting reduced dosage of colistimethate.[15]

Administration and Adult Dosage. May be given intramuscularly at 2.5–5 mg/kg/d in 2–4 divided doses depending upon the severity of the infection. Colistimethate sodium should not be injected intravenously.

Special Populations. *Pediatric Dosage.* 2.5–5 mg/kg/d in 2–4 divided doses.

Other Conditions. Renal Impairment. (serum creatinine 0.7–1.2 mg/dL) 100–150 mg in 2–4 divided doses, to a maximum of 300 mg/d; (serum creatinine 1.3–1.7 mg/dL) 75–115 mg in 2 divided doses, to a maximum of 150–230 mg/d; (serum creatinine 1.6–2.5 mg/dL) 66–150 mg in 1–2 divided doses, to a maximum of 133–150 mg/d; (serum creatinine 2.6–4 mg/dL) 100–150 mg every 36 h, to a maximum of 100 mg/d.

Dosage Forms. (Colistimethate) **Inj** 150 mg colistin base as lyophilized cake; (polymyxin B) **Inj** 500,000 units; **Top Crm** 10,000 units/g with hydrocortisone 0.5% and neomycin 0.35%.

Pharmacokinetics. Blood levels peak between 6 and 12 μg/mL between 2 and 4 h after IM doses of 2–4 mg/kg.

Fate. Not absorbed from the GI tract. Poor topical absorption. Colistimethate does not reach the central nervous system or cerebral spinal fluid unless injected intrathecally. It also does not reach synovial space of joints (unless injected locally), ocular tissues, or penetrate well into cells.[15] Average urinary levels range from approximately 200 μg/mL at 2 h to approximately 25 μg/mL at 8 h after IM administration. **Half-life** 2–3 h.

Adverse Effects. Respiratory arrest; decreased urine output or increased BUN or serum creatinine; paresthesia; tingling of the extremities or the tongue; generalized itching or urticaria; drug fever; GI upset; vertigo; slurring of speech. The subjective symptoms reported by the adult may not be manifested in infants or young children, thus requiring close attention to renal function.

Contraindications. Hypersensitivity to colistimethate; infections due to *Proteus* or *Neisseria* spp.

Precautions. Pregnancy category C. Do not exceed doses of 5 mg/kg/d in patients with normal renal function.

Drug Interactions. Concurrent use with aminoglycosides has been shown to increase concentrations of colistimethate leading to an increased risk of respiratory paralysis and renal dysfunction. Cephalothin also increases colistimethate concentrations leading to an increased risk of renal dysfunction. When used in combination with non–depolarizing muscle relaxants, neuromuscular blockade may be enhanced.

Parameters to Monitor. CBC, renal function, and signs/symptoms of improvement

Notes. Colistimethate sodium crosses the placental barrier, and blood levels of approximately 1 μg/mL are obtained in the fetus following IV administration to the mother. May also be administered via nebulizer in doses ranging from 30 to 150 mg every 12–24 h.[16]

DAPTOMYCIN Cubicin

Pharmacology. Daptomycin is a lipopeptide used for the treatment of gram-positive infections but is intrinsically inactive against gram-negative bacteria. Daptomycin exerts its bactericidal effect by binding to bacterial membranes causing a rapid depolarization of membrane potential, which inhibits synthesis of protein, DNA, and RNA. Daptomycin has shown bactericidal activity against several multidrug-resistant gram-positive organisms, including staphylococcal (methicillin resistant and vancomycin intermediate) and enterococcal (vancomycin resistant) species. Synergy was seen against *Staphylococcus aureus* with the addition of aminoglycosides. In the case of enterococcus, the addition of rifampin, gentamicin, or ampicillin produces synergistic effects.[17,18]

Administration and Adult Dosage. **IV for complicated skin and soft tissue infections**—4 mg/kg IV over 30 min once every 24 h for 7–14 days; **IV for S. aureus bloodstream infections including those with right-sided endocarditis caused by methicillin-susceptible and methicillin-resistant strains**—6 mg/kg IV over 30 min once every 24 h for a minimum of 2–6 weeks.

Special Populations. *Pediatric Dosage.* Safety and efficacy has not been established.

Geriatric Dosage. In clinical trials, lower clinical success rates were seen in patients ≥65 years of age when treated for both complicated skin and soft tissue infections as well as *S. aureus* bacteremia/endocarditis. Adverse reactions were also more common in this population.

Other Conditions. **Renal Impairment.** (Cl$_{Cr}$ <30 mL/min) 4 mg/kg every 48 h in skin and soft tissue infection, 6 mg/kg every 48 h in *S. aureus* bloodstream infection.

Dosage Forms. Inj 500 mg.

Patient Instructions. You should contact your physician as soon as possible if watery and bloody stools (without stomach cramps and fever) develop.

Pharmacokinetics. *Fate.* A peak concentration of 57.8 μg/mL and 93.9 μg/mL is achieved with a single 4 mg/kg and 6 mg/kg IV dose, respectively. In patients with normal renal function, daptomycin is 90%–93% protein bound. Serum protein binding in patients with impaired renal function (Cl$_{Cr}$ <30 mL/min, including all forms of dialysis) ranging from 83% to 87%. In healthy subjects, the volume of distribution is 0.1 L/kg independent of dose. Daptomycin is excreted in the urine (78% unchanged) and the feces (5.7% unchanged). **Half-life** 8 h (28 h with renal impairment).

Adverse Effects. The most common adverse effects are injection site reactions, pruritus, and rash. GI complications, such as nausea, vomiting, constipation, diarrhea, and indigestion, can also occur. In phase 3 clinical trials, there have been reports of increased creatine kinase levels as well as dizziness, insomnia, and limb pain.

Contraindications. Hypersensitivity.

Precautions. Pregnancy category B. PMC leading to diarrhea may occur as with all antibiotics. Persisting or relapsing *S. aureus* infection due to inadequate response may require MIC susceptibility testing.

Drug Interactions. Daptomycin serum concentrations are increased (up to 12.7%) when coadministered with IV tobramycin, while tobramycin concentrations decrease by 10.7%. May require clinical monitoring.

Parameters to Monitor. CBC and signs and symptoms of improvement. Creatinine kinase levels may also require monitoring if administered concurrently with an HMG-CoA reductase inhibitor (statin).

LINEZOLID
Zyvox

Pharmacology. Linezolid belongs to a new class of anti-infective agents known as oxazolidinones. It inhibits protein synthesis by binding to the bacterial 23S ribosomal RNA of the 50S subunit and prevents the formation of a functional 70S initiation complex inhibiting bacterial translation. It has bacteriostatic activity against staphylococci and enterococci, including vancomycin-resistant *Enterococcus faecium* and *Enterococcus faecalis* and bactericidal activity against most streptococcal strains. In vitro the spectrum also includes certain gram-negative and anaerobic organisms. Linezolid is a reversible, nonselective inhibitor of monoamine oxidase.[19]

Administration and Adult Dosage. **PO or IV for pneumonia, skin and soft tissue infections, and endocarditis**—400–600 mg every 12 h.

Special Populations. *Pediatric Dosage.* Safety not established in infants and children. **PO or IV for pneumonia, skin and soft tissue infections, and endocarditis**—10 mg/kg every 12 h has been used.

Geriatric Dosage. Same as adult dosage.

Other Conditions. No dosage adjustment necessary in renal or hepatic insufficiency.

Dosage Forms. **Tab** 400, 600 mg; **Inj** 2 mg/mL; **Susp** 20 mg/mL.

Patient Instructions. This drug may be taken without regard to meals. Avoid concurrent use of diet pills and cough and cold remedies and restrict consumption of aged foods high in tyramine.

Missed Doses. Take this drug at regular intervals. If you miss a dose, take it as soon as you remember. If it is about time for the next dose, take that dose only.

Pharmacokinetics. *Fate.* Rapidly absorbed orally; bioavailability is approximately 100% and not affected by food. A single dose of 600 mg achieves a peak of 12.7 mg/L when administered orally and 12.9 mg/L IV. Plasma protein binding is 31% and linezolid is readily distributed into well-perfused tissues. Linezolid is primarily metabolized by oxidation. Nonrenal clearance accounts for ~65% of the total clearance. Children appear to have a higher average clearance. **Half-life** 4.7–5.4 h in adults.

Adverse Reactions. Adverse reactions are usually mild to moderate and the most commonly reported are diarrhea, headache, and nausea. Occasional reactions are oral and vaginal candidiasis, hypertension, dyspepsia, abdominal pain, pruritus, and tongue discoloration. Treatment periods beyond 28 days have not been evaluated and are not recommended.

Precautions. Pregnancy; lactation. Linezolid can lead to PMC, so it is an important consideration if patients present with diarrhea. Avoid large quantities of food containing tyramine (>100 mg/meal) with linezolid. Use caution with preexisting myelosuppression, other drugs that cause myelosuppression, or chronic infection with previous or concomitant antibiotic therapy. Myelosuppression (including anemia, leukopenia, pancytopenia, and thrombocytopenia) has been reported; consider discontinuing therapy if this occurs or worsens. Myelosuppression is usually reversible after drug discontinuation.

Drug Interactions. Linezolid is not metabolized by cytochrome P450 and does not inhibit or induce the activities of clinically important CYP isoforms. By inhibiting MAO, it can interact with adrenergic and serotonergic agents such as phenyl-propanolamine and pseudoephedrine; reduce initial doses of epinephrine and dopamine and titrate to response.

Parameters to Monitor. CBC with platelet counts before and during weekly therapy.

Notes. Although the drug is effective for many types of infections, it should generally be reserved for treating resistant organisms.

METRONIDAZOLE
Flagyl, MetroGel, Various

Pharmacology. Metronidazole is a synthetic nitroimidazole active against *Trichomonas vaginalis* (trichomoniasis), *Entamoeba histolytica* (amebiasis), and *Giardia lamblia* (giardiasis); it is bactericidal against nearly all obligate anaerobic bacteria including *Bacteroides fragilis.* It is inactive against aerobic bacteria and requires microbial reduction by a nitroreductase enzyme to form highly reactive intermediates that disrupt bacterial DNA and inhibit nucleic acid synthesis, leading to cell death.[20]

Administration and Adult Dosage. PO or IV for anaerobic infections—15 mg/kg (usually 1 g) initially, followed by 7.5 mg/kg (usually 500 mg) every 6–8 h, to a maximum of 4 g/d. Infuse each IV dose over 1 h. PO for antibiotic-associated colitis—250 mg 4 times daily for 7–10 days.[21] (*See* Notes.) PO for trichomoniasis—2 g as a single dose OR in 2 doses on the same day OR 500 mg twice daily for 7 days.[22] PO for giardiasis—250 mg 3 times daily for 5 days.[21] (*See* Notes.) PO for symptomatic intestinal amebiasis (amebic dysentery)—750 mg 3 times daily for 10 days. PO for extraintestinal amebiasis—750 mg 3 times daily for 10 days.[21] Some practitioners include a drug effective against the intestinal cyst form because occasional failures with metronidazole therapy have been reported. PO for bacterial vaginosis—500 mg twice daily for 7 days OR 2 g as a single dose.[22] Vaginal for bacterial vaginosis—1 applicatorful (5 g) twice daily for 5 days. Topical for rosacea—apply twice daily

Special Populations. *Pediatric Dosage.* IV for anaerobic infections—(preterm infants) 15 mg/kg once, then 7.5 mg/kg every 24–48 h; (term infants) 15 mg/kg once, then 7.5 mg/kg every 12–24 h; (infants >1 week old and children) Same as adult mg/kg dosage. PO for giardiasis—15 mg/kg/d in 3 divided doses for 5 days, to a maximum of 750 mg/d. (*See* Notes.) PO for amebic dysentery or extraintestinal amebiasis—35–50 mg/kg/d in 3 divided doses for 10 days, to a maximum of 2.5 g/d.

Geriatric Dosage. (>65 years) decreased clearance can result in accumulation of the drug. Dosage reduction or changing dosage interval to once or twice daily are reasonable modifications to avoid potential adverse reactions.[23]

Other Conditions. No dosage alteration required with renal impairment. Patients with substantial liver dysfunction metabolize metronidazole slowly, with resultant accumulation of metronidazole and its metabolites in the serum. For such patients, it has been suggested that dosage intervals be increased to 12–24 h, although specific guidelines are not available.[23]

Dosage Forms. **Cap** 375 mg; **SR Tab** 750 mg; **Tab** 250, 500 mg; **Inj** 500 mg; **Crm** 1%; **Top Gel** 0.75%; **Vag Gel** 0.75%.

Patient Instructions. This drug may be taken with food to minimize stomach upset. It can cause a harmless dark discoloration of the urine and metallic taste in the mouth. Nausea, vomiting, flushing, and faintness can occur if alcohol is taken during therapy with this drug.

Missed Doses. Take this drug at regular intervals. If you miss a dose, take it as soon as you remember. If it is about time for the next dose, take that dose only. Leave at least 4–6 h between doses. Do not double the dose or take an extra dose.

Pharmacokinetics. *Serum Levels.* Not used clinically.

Fate. IV 500 mg every 12 h over 1 h produces steady-state peak and trough levels of 23.6 mg/L (138 μmol/L) and 6.7 mg/L (39 μmol/L), respectively. IV 500 mg every 8 h over 1 h produces steady-state peak and trough levels of 27.4 mg/L (160 μmol/L) and 15.5 mg/L (91 μmol/L), respectively. Well absorbed orally with levels similar to those after IV infusion; 250- and 500-mg doses produce peak concentrations of 4–6 mg/L (23–35 μmol/L) and 10–13 mg/L (58–76 μmol/L), respectively, at 1–2 h in adults. Bioavailability of vaginal gel is 53%–58%. Less than 20% plasma protein bound; wide distribution with therapeutic levels in many tissues, including abscesses, bile, bone, breast milk, CSF, and saliva. V_d is 0.85 ± 0.25 L/kg; clearance is 0.07 ± 0.02 L/h/kg. Extensively metabolized in the liver by hydroxylation, oxidation, and glucuronide formation; 44%–80% excreted in the urine in 24 h, approximately 6%–18% as unchanged drug.[21,23] **Half-life** 6–10 h in adults; not increased with impaired renal function; prolonged variably with severe hepatic impairment.[8,21,23]

Adverse Effects. Metallic taste in mouth and GI complaints occur frequently with high dosages. Occasional dizziness, vertigo, and paresthesias have been reported with very high dosages. Reversible mild neutropenia reported occasionally.[3,21] Reversible, rare, but severe peripheral neuropathy can occur with high dosages given over prolonged periods. Antibiotic-associated colitis has been reported rarely with oral metronidazole. The IV preparation is occasionally associated with phlebitis at the infusion site. Experimental production of tumors in some rodent species and mutations in bacteria have raised concern regarding potential carcinogenicity; to date, human epidemiologic research has not detected an appreciable risk, although more data are needed.[21]

Contraindications. First trimester of pregnancy, although there is no direct evidence of teratogenicity in humans or animals.[3]

Precautions. Pregnancy; lactation; active CNS disease or neutropenia; and hepatic impairment.

Drug Interactions. Disulfiram-like reactions are reported with concurrent alcohol use but are uncommon. Confusion and psychotic episodes have been reported with concurrent disulfiram; avoid this combination, if possible. Metronidazole inhibits CYP2C9, CYP3A3/4, and CYP3A5-7 and can affect the metabolism of many drugs; the best documented is an enhanced hypoprothrombinemic response to warfarin. Phenytoin metabolism also might be inhibited. It is also a substrate of CYP2C9.

Parameters to Monitor. Before and after the completion of any lengthy or repeated courses of therapy, monitor WBC count. Monitor signs of toxicity in patients with severe liver disease.[23]

Notes. The treatment of asymptomatic trichomoniasis is controversial. Signs of endocervical inflammation or erosion on physical examination are considered an indication for treatment. Also, most practitioners treat asymptomatic male consorts because lack of such treatment might be a cause of treatment failure or recurrent infection of the female partner.[22] Metronidazole has been used in combination regimens to treat *Helicobacter pylori*–infected patients with duodenal or gastric ulcers. (*See* "Drug Treatment Regimens Used to Eradicate *Helicobacter pylori*" in the section "Gastrointestinal Drugs" of Chapter 43.) Although it is slightly less effective than **vancomycin,** metronidazole is considered by some to be the drug of choice for antibiotic-associated PMC because of its lower cost and the emergence of vancomycin-resistant enterococci.[24]

NITROFURANTOIN
Macrodantin, Macrobid, Various

Pharmacology. Nitrofurantoin is a synthetic nitrofuran that is active against most bacteria that cause urinary tract infections (UTI) except *P. aeruginosa*, *Proteus* sp., many *Enterobacter* spp., and *Klebsiella* spp. The drug is used primarily to prevent recurrent UTIs but is also effective in the treatment of uncomplicated UTIs.[25]

Adult Dosage. PO for treatment of UTI—(macrocrystals) 50–100 mg 4 times daily with meals and at bedtime; (Macrobid) 100 mg twice daily for 7 days; **PO for chronic UTI suppression**—50–100 mg at bedtime with food.

Special Population. *Pediatric Dosage.* PO for treatment of UTI—5–7 mg/kg/d in 4 divided doses, to a maximum of 400 mg/d; **PO for chronic UTI suppression**—1 mg/kg/d in 1–2 doses, to a maximum of 100 mg/d.

Dosage Forms. Cap (macrocrystals) 25, 50, 100 mg; Susp 5 mg/mL; Cap 100 mg, containing 25 mg as macrocrystals and 75 mg in an SR form (Macrobid).

Pharmacokinetics. Well absorbed orally; however, serum and extraurinary tissue concentrations are subtherapeutic. Approximately 60% of drug is metabolized to inactive metabolites; 25%–35% is excreted in urine with a urine concentration of approximately 200 mg/L from an average dose.

Adverse Reactions. Adverse effects are primarily nausea, vomiting, and diarrhea and are dose related; use of the macrocrystalline form and administration with food can minimize GI distress. Hypersensitivity reactions such as rash occur only rarely. Acute allergic pneumonitis is reversible with discontinuation of therapy. Chronic interstitial pulmonary fibrosis also occurs occasionally with long-term therapy and might be irreversible. Ascending polyneuropathy associated with prolonged high-dose therapy or use of the drug in renal failure is only slowly reversible. Intravascular hemolysis can occur in patients with severe G-6-PD deficiency. Although the drug is mutagenic in mammalian cells, there is no clinical evidence of carcinogenicity or teratogenicity.

PENTAMIDINE ISETHIONATE
Pentam 300, NebuPent

Pharmacology. Pentamidine is an aromatic diamidine used in the treatment of trypanosomiasis and PCP. Pentamidine inhibits dihydrofolate reductase, interferes with anaerobic glycolysis, inhibits oxidative phosphorylation, and limits nucleic acid and protein synthesis, but the mechanism by which pentamidine kills PCP is unclear.[26]

Administration and Adult Dosage. IV (preferred) or IM—3–4 mg/kg/d as a single dose for 2–3 weeks; infuse IV over 60 min; **inhalation for PCP prophylaxis in high-risk HIV-infected patients**—300 mg every 4 weeks via Respirguard II Nebulizer. (*See* Notes.)

Special Populations. *Pediatric Dosage.* Same as adult dosage.

Geriatric Dosage. Same as adult dosage.

Other Conditions. Dosage adjustment does not appear necessary in renal impairment.[27]

Dosage Forms. **Inj** 300 mg; **Inhal** 300 mg.

Pharmacokinetics. *Serum Levels.* Not used clinically.

Fate. Negligible oral absorption. Peak serum levels of 0.5–3 mg/L (1.5–8.8 μmol/L) occur after 4 mg/kg IV infusion. Serum levels are very low after inhalation (<0.1 mg/L). Approximately 70% plasma protein bound; distributed widely in tissues, with highest concentrations found in spleen, liver, kidneys, and adrenal glands. V_c is 3 L/kg; terminal V_d is 190 ± 70 L/kg; Clearance is 1.08 ± 0.42 L/h/kg. There are no data on the effects of liver impairment. Less than 20% of a dose is excreted unchanged in urine.[8,28] **Half-life** distribution phase 1.2 ± 0.6 h; terminal elimination half-life is 29 ± 25 days, suggesting rapid tissue uptake with slow release and subsequent urinary excretion.[27]

Adverse Reactions. With IV administration, nephrotoxicity occurs in up to 25% of patients, hypoglycemia in up to 27%, and hypotension in up to 10% of patients. Fever, rash, leukopenia, and liver damage occur occasionally. Hyperglycemia, type 1 diabetes mellitus, and pancreatitis have been reported. Pentamidine-induced torsades de points occur rarely. IM injection frequently produces pain and abscess formation at the injection site. With aerosolized pentamidine, reversible bronchoconstriction and unpleasant taste occur frequently. Severe adverse reactions are less frequent, but reports of pancreatitis, hypoglycemia, and cutaneous eruptions have occurred rarely, suggesting some systemic absorption.[26]

Precautions. Use with caution in diabetes mellitus.

Drug Interactions. IV pentamidine can increase the risk of hypocalcemia with foscarnet; avoid this combination, if possible, although inhaled pentamidine does not seem to be a risk factor. Increased risk of QTc prolongation when coadministered with QTc prolonging agents (e.g., quinine, thioridazine, tetrabenzine, ziprasidone, nilotinib).

Parameters to Monitor. Obtain serum glucose, serum creatinine, BUN, liver function tests, electrolytes, and CBC and platelet counts daily. Monitor blood pressure after administration.

Notes. Concomitant therapy with **pentamidine** and TMP/SMZ appears to offer no benefit and might be additively toxic. There is concern about occupational exposure with inhalation therapy. No studies have determined the health effects of exposure to pentamidine itself; however, transmission of tuberculosis to health care workers has been attributed in part to the use of aerosolized pentamidine among clinic patients coinfected with HIV and tuberculosis. Health care workers administering aerosolized pentamidine should wear masks and protective eye wear.[26]

QUINUPRISTIN AND DALFOPRISTIN   Synercid

Pharmacology. Quinupristin and dalfopristin are streptogramin antibiotics that are naturally occurring compounds isolated from *Streptomyces pristinaspiralis*. Quinupristin, a derivative of pristinamycin IA, and dalfopristin, a derivative of pristinamycin IIA, are combined in a fixed ratio of 30:70 (w/w). This combination inhibits protein synthesis by sequential binding to the 50S subunit of bacterial ribosomes; its synergistic activity can be caused by binding of dalfopristin, altering conformation of the ribosome such that its affinity for quinupristin is increased. Individually, pristinamycin I and II are bacteriostatic, but in combination they are bactericidal against gram-positive bacteria, including MRSA. Synergy has been reported with vancomycin against MRSA and multiply-resistant enterococci. It also has activity against anaerobic organisms, but most gram-negative organisms such as the *Enterobacteriaceae*, *Acinetobacter* spp., and *P. aeruginosa* are resistant.[29–31] Although the drug is effective for many types of infections, it should generally be reserved for treating resistant organisms such as vancomycin-resistant *E. faecium*. It has no activity against *E. faecalis*.

Administration and Adult Dosage. IV 7.5 mg/kg (of the combination) every 8–12 h infused in D5W over 60 min. Consider reducing dosage in patients with hepatic impairment who do not tolerate the usual dosage. However, specific guidelines have not been established.

Dosage Forms. Inj 500 mg (quinupristin 150 mg and dalfopristin 350 mg)/10 mL vial.

Pharmacokinetics. The pharmacokinetics are complex and not fully elucidated. Peak concentrations are 2.4–2.8 mg/L (2.3–2.7 μmol/L) for quinupristin and 6.2–7.2 mg/L (9–10.4 μmol/L) for dalfopristin after a 7.5 mg/kg dose in healthy volunteers. Quinupristin is approximately 90% protein bound and dalfopristin is 10%–36% bound in vitro. Clearance of both drugs decreases with repeated doses and in obese patients. Dalfopristin might have an active metabolite. Both drugs are eliminated primarily in feces, with only approximately 15%–20% excreted unchanged in urine. Half-life ~1 h for quinupristin and 0.5–1 h for dalfopristin, both possibly increased in cirrhosis.

Adverse Reactions. Mild to moderate local reactions of itching, pain, and burning at the injection site are frequent and often lead to drug discontinuation. To avoid such side effects, administer the drug through a central venous catheter. Nausea, vomiting, diarrhea, and headache also have been reported frequently. Occasionally, reversible myalgia and arthralgia occur and liver function tests are increased.

Drug Interactions. Quinupristin/dalfopristin inhibits CYP3A4 and markedly impairs cyclosporine clearance, requiring cyclosporine dosage reduction.

SPECTINOMYCIN HYDROCHLORIDE   Trobicin

Pharmacology. Spectinomycin is an aminocyclitol compound that is structurally similar to aminoglycosides, but lacks some of their potential side effects. Spectinomycin exhibits its mechanism of action by acting at the 30S ribosomal subunit inhibiting bacterial protein synthesis. Spectinomycin displays bacteriostatic activity against numerous gram-positive and gram-negative organisms; however, gram-negative susceptibility is unpredictable.[32] Spectinomycin displays bactericidal activity against *Neisseria gonorrhoeae* and is used as a second-line agent for treatment of gonococcal infections in penicillin allergic patients.

Administration and Adult Dosage. **IM for anogenital gonorrhea**—2 g as a single dose. **IM for disseminated gonococcal infection**—2 g every 12 h.

Special Populations. *Pediatric Dosage.* **IM for uncomplicated gonococcal infections**—40 mg/kg, to a maximum dose of 2 g as a single dose.

Geriatric Dosage. Same as adult dosage.

Pharmacokinetics. *Serum Levels.* Not absorbed from the GI tract, but is well absorbed when administered IM, with peak concentrations seen 1–2 h after IM administration. Spectinomycin serum concentrations after administration of 2- and 4-g doses is around 100 μg/mL and 160 μg/mL, respectively. In pediatrics, serum levels after a 40 mg/kg dose ranged from 22 to 87.5 μg/mL. There is insignificant protein binding.

Fate. Excretion—75% excreted in the urine as the unchanged drug. **Half-life** 1.5–2 h.

Adverse Effects. Very limited. Spectinomycin is usually well tolerated due to single-dose regimen and low total dose. Jaundice, rash, dizziness, and insomnia have occurred.

Contraindications. Hypersensitivity.

Precautions. Pregnancy category B. There is conflicting data concerning spectinomycin in renal impairment. The half-life may be prolonged in patients with decreased renal function.[33]

Drug Interactions. None reported.

Parameters to Monitor. Monitor temperature, CBC, and improvement of infection.

TELITHROMYCIN Ketek

Pharmacology. Telithromycin is a ketolide antibiotic, a class similar to macrolides with a similar mechanism of action. It has good activity against gram-positive organisms, especially respiratory pathogens such as *S. aureus, Streptococcus pneumoniae, H. influenzae, Moraxella catarrhalis* and some atypical organisms and anaerobes. It is active against some macrolide-resistant gram-positive cocci.

Administration and Adult Dosage. **PO for community-acquired pneumonia**—800 mg once daily for 7–10 days. No change required in renal or hepatic dysfunction.

Dosage Forms. **Tab** 300 mg, 400 mg.

Pharmacokinetics. Following an 800-mg oral dose, a peak level of 2.3 mg/L occurs in 1 h. It is primarily metabolized in the liver and approximately 18% is excreted unchanged in urine. **Half-life** is ~10 h with a single dose and ~13 h with multiple doses.

Adverse Reactions. The most frequent adverse reactions are nausea, diarrhea, and GI pain similar to the macrolides. Elevated LFTs and hepatotoxicity have been reported.

Drug Interactions. Coadministration with azole antifungals (e.g., ketoconazole, itraconazole) have been shown to increase telithromycin concentrations by

22%–51%. CYP3A4 inducers (e.g., phenytoin, carbamazepine, phenobarbitol, rifampin) may result in subtherapeutic concentrations of telithromycin. Telithromycin should never be administered with rifampin. Avoid coadministration with class IA and class III antiarrhythmic agents because of an increased risk of life-threatening arrhythmias, including torsades de pointes. Coadministration with cisapride should also be avoided due to a 95% increase in cisapride peak plasma concentrations resulting in QTc prolongation. Telithromycin has also been shown to increase peak and trough concentrations of digoxin. Clinical monitoring is recommended. Avoid administration with HMG-CoA reductase inhibitors (statins metabolized by CYP3A4) because of a 5.3- to 8.9-fold increase in C_{max} and AUC.

TRIMETHOPRIM
Proloprim, Trimpex, Various

Pharmacology. Trimethoprim is a synthetic folate-antagonist antibacterial. (*See* Sulfonamides.) Trimethoprim is effective in acute UTI. It has a potential advantage over the sulfa-containing combination in patients with allergy or toxicity attributed to sulfonamides; however, the relative potential for trimethoprim alone to permit the development of resistance is undetermined. As monotherapy, trimethoprim is ineffective against PCP, but in combination with **dapsone** (a sulfone), it is effective in treating mild to moderate PCP.[34,35]

Administration and Adult Dosage. PO for uncomplicated acute UTI— 200 mg/d in 1 or 2 doses for 10 days. **PO for the treatment of mild to moderate** (PaO$_2$ >**60 mm Hg) PCP**—20 mg/kg/d in 3 or 4 divided doses with dapsone 100 mg once daily.

Special Populations. *Other Conditions.* (Cl$_{Cr}$ 15–30 mL/min) decrease dose by 50%; (Cl$_{Cr}$ < 15 mL/min) not recommended.

Dosage Forms. **Tab** 100, 200 mg; **Soln** 10 mg/mL.

Pharmacokinetics. Trimethoprim is rapidly absorbed orally. A 100-mg dose yields a serum concentration of 1 mg/L (3.4 μmol/L) 1–4 h after the dose. It is 40% plasma protein bound and 50%–60% is excreted unchanged in urine. **Half-life** 8–10 h with normal renal function.

Adverse Reactions. Occasional adverse effects are mild thrombocytopenia, nausea, fever, and rash; the frequency appears to be dose related. Methemoglobinemia and dose-related hemolysis have occurred in patients with G-6-PD deficiency receiving dapsone with trimethoprim; it is important to check G-6-PD status before initiating combination therapy.

Drug Interactions. Coadministration with class I and class III antiarrhythmics, tricyclic antidepressants, amantidine, or any drug shown to prolong QTc may lead to life-threatening arrhythmias, including torsades de pointes.[36] Concomitant use for methotrexate can increase effects on folate and induce methotrexate toxicity via protein displacement and decreased clearance. Trimethoprim administered orally has also been shown to decrease the hepatic metabolism of phenytoin, increasing the phenytoin half-life and decreasing the clearance.

VANCOMYCIN HYDROCHLORIDE
Vancocin, Various

Pharmacology. Vancomycin is a glycopeptide that binds irreversibly to the cell wall in a manner slightly different from β-lactams. Many gram-positive cocci and bacilli, including MRSA and *C. difficile*, are inhibited. Most gram-negative bacteria are resistant, and vancomycin-resistant enterococci have been reported in association with overuse of vancomycin.[37] Glycopeptide intermediately resistant *S. aureus* have been reported.

Administration and Adult Dosage. **IV**—20–30 mg/kg/d (usually 2 g/d) in 2–4 divided doses as a dilute infusion over 1–2 h; **PO for staphylococcal enterocolitis**—2 g/d in 2–4 divided doses; **PO for antibiotic-associated colitis**—125–500 mg every 6 h for 7–10 days; retreat with a longer course if relapse occurs. (*See* Notes.) **Not for IM use.**

Special Populations. *Pediatric Dosage.* **IV**—(neonates) 20 mg/kg/d; (older infants and children) 40 mg/kg/d in 2–4 divided doses. **PO**—10–50 mg/kg/d in 4 divided doses. **Not for IM use.**

Geriatric Dosage. Same as adult dosage, but adjust for age-related reduction in renal function.

Other Conditions. Adjust dosage carefully in renal impairment; clearance is directly related to Cl_{Cr}. Anuric patients on hemodialysis have been given the usual dose every 3–7 days. Dosage adjustment is unnecessary in liver disease.

Dosage Forms. **Cap** 125, 250 mg; **Susp** 1, 10 g; **Inj** 500 mg, 1, 5, 10 g.

Patient Instructions. Report pain at infusion site, dizziness, or fullness or ringing in ears with intravenous use; nausea or vomiting with oral use.

Missed Doses. **PO**—if you miss a dose, take it as soon as you remember. If it is about time for the next dose, take that dose only.

Pharmacokinetics. *Serum Levels.* Ototoxicity has been associated with high serum concentrations but has been noted at lower levels.[38,39] Minimum serum trough concentrations should be maintained above 10 mg/L. For pathogens with an MIC of 1 mg/L, the minimum trough concentration would have to be at least 15 mg/L to generate the target AUC–MIC of 400. A target trough range of 15–20 mg/L should be used in complicated infections (e.g., endocarditis, osteomyelitis, meningitis, and hospital-acquired pneumonia caused by MRSA).[40]

Fate. Oral absorption is negligible, although appreciable serum levels can be observed in patients with renal dysfunction receiving oral vancomycin for *C. difficile*–induced antibiotic-associated colitis. Fecal concentrations with PO 500 mg every 6 h reach 3 mg/g. IV 500 mg produces serum levels of 6–10 mg/L (4–7 μmol/L) in 1 h. Plasma protein binding is 30 ± 10%. The drug is widely distributed, except into the CSF, although some success has been reported in the treatment of meningitis, particularly in children. V_c is 0.1–0.15 L/kg; V_d is 0.39 ± 0.06 L/kg; clearance is 0.084 L/h/kg with normal renal function. In renal impairment, clearance (in mL/min) can be estimated as $[0.79 \times Cl_{Cr} \text{ (in mL/min)}] + 3.5$. Metabolism and biliary excretion are negligible; 80%–90% is excreted unchanged in the urine within 48 h.[8,41] **Half-life** 5.6 ± 1.8 h, 6–10 days with renal impairment. No change with hepatic disease.[8]

Adverse Reactions. Chills, fever, nausea, and phlebitis can occur frequently, especially with direct injection of undiluted drug (not recommended). Rapid infusion can cause transient systolic hypotension.[42] The "red man" or "red neck" syndrome of erythema, pruritus, and localized edema is associated with histamine release caused by rapid infusions of doses ≥500 mg; it often does not occur or is less severe with subsequent doses.[43] Extravasation causes local tissue necrosis. Ototoxicity (auditory and vestibular) and possibly nephrotoxicity occur but have not been definitely linked to high serum levels.[38,44] Eosinophilia, neutropenia, and urticarial rashes have been reported frequently. Side effects of vancomycin might not be as prevalent today as in the past, perhaps because of changes in the manufacturing process that eliminated some impurities.[45]

Precautions. Pregnancy. Use with caution in patients with impaired renal function or preexisting hearing loss or in those receiving other ototoxic or nephrotoxic agents.

Drug Interactions. Administration with an aminoglycoside can increase the risk of nephrotoxicity.[45]

Parameters to Monitor. IV—obtain initial renal function tests and repeat twice weekly during therapy. With aggressive dosing (troughs 15–20 mg/L) and in patients with unstable renal function, at least one steady-state trough level (after the fourth dose) should be attained, and repeated when clinically appropriate.[40] Monitoring of peak serum levels is not recommended.[40] Check for signs of phlebitis daily.

Notes. An alternative agent for treatment or prophylaxis of staphylococcal or streptococcal infections when a less toxic agent is inappropriate (e.g., penicillin or cephalosporin allergy, or resistant organisms) or has not produced an adequate therapeutic response. Use of vancomycin in antibiotic-associated colitis is becoming less desirable because of the emergence of vancomycin-resistant *enterococci*. Reserve vancomycin for cases refractory to metronidazole.[24]

■ REFERENCES

1. Haile LG, Flaherty JF. Atovaquone: a review. *Ann Pharmacother*. 1993;27:1488-1494.
2. Spencer CM, Goa KI. Atovaquone. A review of its pharmacological properties and therapeutic efficacy in opportunistic infections. *Drugs*. 1995;50:176-196.
3. Smilack JD et al. Tetracyclines, chloramphenicol, erythromycin, clindamycin, and metronidazole. *Mayo Clin Proc*. 1991;66:1270-1280.
4. Norris AH et al. Chloramphenicol for the treatment of vancomycin-resistant enterococcal infections. *Clin Infect Dis*. 1995;20:1137-1144.
5. Greenfield RA. Symposium on antimicrobial therapy X. Chloramphenicol, clindamycin, and metronidazole. *J Okla State Med Assoc*. 1993;86:336-341.
6. Kapusnik-Uner JE et al. Antimicrobial agents: tetracyclines, chloramphenicol, erythromycin and miscellaneous antibacterial agents. In: Hardman JG et al., eds. *Goodman and Gilman's the Pharmacological Basis of Therapeutics*. 9th ed. New York: McGraw-Hill; 1996:1130-1135.
7. Kasten MJ. Clindamycin, metronidazole, and chloramphenicol. *Mayo Clin Proc*. 1999;74:825-833.
8. Benet LZ et al. Design and optimization of dosage regimens: pharmacokinetic data. In: Hardman JG et al., eds. *Goodman and Gilman's the Pharmacological Basis of Therapeutics*. 9th ed. New York: McGraw-Hill; 1996:1707-1792.
9. Rayner SA, Buckley RJ. Ocular chloramphenicol and aplastic anemia. Is there a link? *Drug Saf*. 1996;14:273-276.
10. Pratt WB, Fekety R. Bacteriostatic inhibitors of protein synthesis. In: Pratt WB, Fekety R, eds. *The Antimicrobial Drugs*. New York: Oxford University Press; 1986:184-228.
11. Dhawan VK, Thadepalli H. Clindamycin: a review of 15 years of clinical experience. *Rev Infect Dis*. 1982;4:1133-1153.
12. Wilson W et al. Prevention of infective endocarditis. Guidelines from the American Heart Association. A guideline from the American Heart Association Rheumatic Fever, Endocarditis, and Kawasaki Disease Committee, Council on Cardiovascular Disease in the Young, and the Council on Clinical Cardiology, Council on Cardiovascular Surgery and Anesthesia, and the Quality of Care and Outcomes Research Interdisciplinary Working Group. *Circulation*. 2007;116:1736-1754.

13. Klainer AS. Clindamycin. *Med Clin North Am.* 1987;71:1169-1176.

14. Van Arsdel PP et al. The value of skin testing for penicillin allergy diagnosis. *West J Med.* 1986;144:311-314.

15. Jawetz E. Polymyxins, colistin, bacitracin, ristocetin and vancomycin. *Pediatr Clin North Am.* 1968;15:85-94.

16. Brochet MS et al. Comparative efficacy of two doses of nebulized colistimethate in the eradication of *Pseudomonas aeruginosa* in children with cystic fibrosis. *Can Respir J.* 2007;14:473-479.

17. Sauermann R et al. Daptomycin: a review 4 years after first approval. *Pharmacology.* 2008;81:79-91.

18. Tedesco KL, Rybak MJ. Daptomycin. *Pharmacotherapy.* 2004;24:41-57.

19. Anon. Linezolid (Zyvox®). *Med Lett Drugs Ther.* 2000;42:45-46.

20. Smilack JD. The tetracyclines. *Mayo Clin Proc.* 1999;74:729-729.

21. Falagas ME, Gorbach SL. Clindamycin and metronidazole. *Med Clin North Am.* 1995;79:845-867.

22. Anon. Sexually transmitted diseases treatment guidelines. *MMWR Morb Mortal Wkly Rep.* 1993;42(RR-14):1-102.

23. Lau AH et al. Clinical pharmacokinetics of metronidazole and other nitroimidazole anti-infectives. *Clin Pharmacokinet.* 1992;23:328-364.

24. Wenisch C et al. Comparison of vancomycin, teicoplanin, metronidazole, and fusidic acid for treatment of *Clostridium difficile*–associated diarrhea. *Clin Infect Dis.* 1996;22:813-818.

25. Black M et al. Antimicrobial agents: sulfonamides, trimethoprim-sulfamethoxazole, quinolones. In: Hardman JG et al., eds. *Goodman and Gilman's the Pharmacological Basis of Therapeutics.* 9th ed. New York: McGraw-Hill; 1996:1069-1070.

26. Wispelwey B, Pearson RD. Pentamidine: a review. *Infect Control Hosp Epidemiol.* 1991;12:375-382.

27. Conte JE Jr. Pharmacokinetics of intravenous pentamidine in patients with normal renal function or receiving hemodialysis. *J Infect Dis.* 1991;163:169-175.

28. Donnelly H et al. Distribution of pentamidine in patients with AIDS. *J Infect Dis.* 1988;157:985-989.

29. Chant C, Rybak MJ. Quinupristin/dalfopristin (RP 59500): a new streptogramin antibiotic. *Ann Pharmacother.* 1995;29:1022-1027.

30. Bryson HM, Spencer CM. Quinupristin-dalfopristin. *Drugs.* 1996;52:406-416.

31. Griswold MW et al. Quinupristin-dalfopristin (RP 59500): an injectable streptogramin combination. *Am J Health Syst Pharm.* 1996;53:2045-2053.

32. Holloway WJ. Spectinomycin. *Med Clin North Am.* 1982;66:169-173.

33. Kusumi R et al. Pharmacokinetics of spectinomycin in volunteers with renal insufficiency. *Chemotherapy.* 1981;27:95-98.

34. Pratt WB, Fekety R. The antimetabolites. In: Pratt WB, Fekety R, eds. *The Antimicrobial Drugs.* New York: Oxford University Press; 1986:229-251.

35. Masur H. Prevention and treatment of pneumocystis pneumonia. *N Engl J Med.* 1992;327:1853-1860.

36. Lopez JA et al. QT prolongation and torsades de pointes after administration of trimethoprim-sulfamethoxazole. *Am J Cardiol.* 1987;59:376-377.

37. Lundstrom TS, Sobel JD. Vancomycin, trimethoprim-sulfamethoxazole, and rifampin. *Infect Dis Clin North Am.* 1995;9:747-767.

38. Lake KD, Peterson CD. A simplified method for initiating vancomycin therapy. *Pharmacotherapy.* 1985;5:340-344.

39. Rybak MJ et al. Nephrotoxicity of vancomycin, alone and with an aminoglycoside. *J Antimicrob Chemother.* 1990;25:679-687.

40. Rybak M et al. Therapeutic monitoring of vancomycin in adult patients: a consensus review of the American Society of Health-System Pharmacists, the Infectious Disease Society of America, and the Society of Infectious Disease Pharmacists. *Am J Health Syst Pharm.* 2009;66:82-98.

41. Matzke GR et al. Clinical pharmacokinetics of vancomycin. *Clin Pharmacokinet.* 1986;11:257-282.

42. Newfield P, Roizen MF. Hazards of rapid administration of vancomycin. *Ann Intern Med.* 1979;91:581.

43. Healy DP et al. Vancomycin-induced histamine release and "red man syndrome": comparison of 1- and 2-hour infusions. *Antimicrob Agents Chemother.* 1990;34:550-554.

44. Edwards DJ, Pancorbo S. Routine monitoring of serum vancomycin concentrations: waiting for proof of its value. *Clin Pharm.* 1987;6:652-654.

45. Farber BF, Mollering RC. Retrospective study of the toxicity of preparations of vancomycin from 1974–1981. *Antimicrob Agents Chemother.* 1983;23:138-141.

Antineoplastics, Chemoprotectants, and Immunosuppressants

3

Nickole N. Henyan

Chapter 18

Antineoplastics

Shirley Hogan

Antineoplastics. The agents included in this section are those having widespread use in cancer chemotherapy. Antineoplastic agents should be administered only under the supervision of a physician experienced in the use of these medications. Agents with therapeutic importance in small patient populations are not included.

Information on the dosage of these drugs has largely been determined empirically, and clinical investigations are continually being performed to find safer and more effective dosage regimens. Thus, **dosages in this section should be considered as only guidelines based on the most widely accepted usage at the time of this writing.** Because space does not permit detailed discussions of the toxicity, dosage regimens, and other aspects of these drugs, the reader should become familiar with specific agents before initiating treatment. References are provided in this section for more detailed information concerning the proper and safe use of these agents. Specific investigational protocols, if available, can also provide information that is unavailable from other sources, especially with regard to dosage and regimens as well as the use of proper procedures for handling and disposal of chemotherapy agents.

Cancer chemotherapeutic agents as a class are the most toxic drugs in use. Adverse reactions listed represent those most likely to occur with the usual doses and methods of use. Infrequent, but serious reactions are also listed; however, the lists of adverse reactions are not all-inclusive. Nausea and vomiting are important side effects of these agents, which can usually be adequately treated by current antiemetics alone or in combination. To tailor antiemetic therapy better to the emetogenic potential of the chemotherapy agents, a standard rating scale is used in these monographs. Several points to remember are that emetogenicity is both dose

289

and patient dependent, that combinations of chemotherapeutic agents result in greater emetogenic potential than the drug(s) used alone, and that emetogenic potentials are best defined in adults and do not necessarily apply to children. The categories of emetogenicity used are as follows:[1]

EMETOGENICITY CATEGORY	PERCENTAGE OF PATIENTS AFFECTED
High	>90
Moderately high	60–90
Moderate	30–60
Moderately low	10–30
Low	<10

Class Instructions. Antineoplastics. This drug is very powerful, and some side effects can be expected to occur with its use. Be sure that you understand the possible benefits and dangers of the drug before you begin to take it.

Cytotoxic Agents. Because this drug can decrease your body's ability to fight infections, report any signs of infection such as fever, shaking chills, or sore throat immediately. Also, report any unusual bruising or bleeding, shortness of breath, or painful or burning urination. Avoid the use of aspirin-containing products, and avoid alcohol or use it in moderation. Nausea, vomiting, or hair loss can sometimes occur with this drug. The severity of these effects depends on the individual, the dosage, and other drugs that might be given at the same time. This drug can cause temporary or sometimes permanent sterility in men and women. It also can cause birth defects if the father is taking the drug at the time of conception or if the mother is taking it any time during pregnancy. If you are breast-feeding, this drug might appear in the milk and cause problems in your baby; therefore, use an alternate method of feeding your baby.

Missed Doses. This drug should be taken at regular intervals exactly as prescribed. If a dose is missed, it should be taken as soon as it is remembered. If it is almost time for the next dose, only that dose should be taken and the regular dosage schedule should be resumed. The dose should never be doubled nor extra doses taken.

■ REFERENCE

1. Lindley CM et al. Incidence and duration of chemotherapy-induced nausea and vomiting in the outpatient oncology population. *J Clin Oncol.* 1989;7:1142-1149.

Chapter 19

Alkylating Agents

Shirley Hogan

ALTRETAMINE	Hexalen

Pharmacology. Altretamine (formerly hexamethylmelamine) structurally resembles an alkylating agent, yet it has not been found to have alkylating activity, in vitro. There is some evidence that it may inhibit DNA and RNA synthesis.

It is used in combination chemotherapy of refractory ovarian cancer and has shown activity in cervical cancers.[1,2]

Adult Dosage. PO is given 260 mg/m^2/d in 4 divided doses (after meals and at bedtime) to be taken for 14 or 21 consecutive days in a 28-day cycle. This is the recommended dosing regimen; however, the effect of food on the bioavailability has not been evaluated.

Dosage Forms. Cap 50 mg.

Pharmacokinetics. Orally the capsules are well absorbed, but bioavailability is variable due to extensive demethylation in the liver. The serum half-life is 4.7–10.2 h, with >50% of a dose renally excreted in 24 h and <1% excreted unchanged.

Adverse Reactions. Nausea, vomiting can be dose limiting in some patients. Both peripheral and central neurotoxicity have been reported including agitation, ataxia, and confusion. These are more frequent with continuous high-dose daily therapy than with moderate-dose intermittent schedules. Anemia, leukopenia, and thrombocytopenia are typically mild.[1,2]

BUSULFAN	Busulfex, Myleran
CHLORAMBUCIL	Leukeran
MELPHALAN	Alkeran

Pharmacology. These are drugs that alkylate DNA, forming a variety of covalent cross-links. The drugs are bifunctional and can form more than one covalent bond to susceptible cell constituents (typically the N^7 position of guanine). They are cell-cycle phase nonspecific and chemically stable enough for oral absorption before appreciable alkylator activation occurs.

Administration and Dosage.

	BUSULFAN	CHLORAMBUCIL	MELPHALAN
Administration	PO; IV	PO	PO; IV
Adult Dosage	1.8 mg/m^2/d (usually 4–8 mg/d); if remission <3 mo, maintenance of 1–3 mg/d	0.1–0.2 mg/kg/d for 3–6 wk; if maintenance dosage is used, do not exceed 0.1 mg/kg/d. CLL: intermittent, bi-weekly, or once-monthly pulse doses begin with initial single dose 0.4 mg/kg and may be increased by 0.1mg/kg	PO several regimens exist but all begin with an initial dose for limited time (5 d to 2wk) and maintenance therapy after a rest period for counts to recover for multiple myeloma
	IV for HSCT conditioning regimen is based on TDM and AUC target		IV 16 mg/m^2 q2wks for 4 doses, then q4wk, after adequate recovery
Pediatric Dosage	Based on ABW ≤12 kg = 1.1 mg/kg >12 kg = 0.8 mg/kg	—	
Geriatric Dosage	Same as adult dosage, but adjust for age-related reduction in renal function.		

Special Populations. *Other Conditions.* Melphalan elimination is significantly cor-related with Cl_{Cr}, yet recommendations for adjustments in patients with reduced renal function vary with most recommending a 25% decrease for oral melphalan and a 50% decrease for IV melphalan in patients with Cl_{Cr}<30 mL/min.[3]

Dosage Forms. (Busulfan) **Tab** 2 mg; **Inj** 60 mg.(6 mg/mL in 10 mL ampule) (store in refrigerator at 2–8°C). (Chlorambucil) **Tab** 2 mg (store in refrigerator 2–8°C). (Melphalan) **Tab** 2 mg (store in refrigerator 2–8°C, protect from light); **Inj** 50 mg (store at controlled room temperature 15–30°C, protect from light).

Patient Instructions. *See* Antineoplastics Class Instructions.

Pharmacokinetics. *Fate.*

	BUSULFAN	CHLORAMBUCIL	MELPHALAN
Absorption	Reported by manufacturer to be well absorbed orally	Oral doses rapidly and completely absorbed	Oral bioavailability is variable and may be due to incom-plete absorption, first pass metabolism, or lipid hydrolysis
Distribution	Homogeneous; good ascites penetration; V_d is 0.64 L/kg; extensively bound to proteins (32%–47%)	99% plasma protein bound	V_d is 0.5 L/kg; 60%–90% plasma protein bound

(continued)

	BUSULFAN	CHLORAMBUCIL	MELPHALAN
Metabolism	Extensively metabolized by enzymatic activity to at least 12 metabolites	Rapid metabolism to a number of inactive metabolites	Not actively metabolized; spontaneous chemical degradation to mono- and dihydroxy products; Cl_{Cr} is 7–9 mL/min/kg
Excretion	<2% excreted unchanged in urine	Less than 1% excreted unchanged in urine over 24 h	Eliminated from plasma by chemical hydrolysis, renal elimination minimal
$t_{1/2}$.	Rapid initial serum clearance: 90% of dose after 3 min; $t_{1/2}$. β is 2.69 ± 0.49 h	1.5 h (parent drug); 1.8 h (major metabolite-phenylacetic acid mustard)	IV: $t_{1/2}$. α 10 min; $t_{1/2}$. β 75 min

Adverse Reactions. Emetogenic potential is low. Nausea and vomiting occur infrequently. Dose-limiting toxicity for this group is typically myelosuppression, with nadirs of 14–21 days for leukopenia and thrombocytopenia after pulse dosage regimens; daily administration results in chronic low indices with cumulative effects. Blood counts commonly continue to drop after drug discontinuation; fatal pancytopenia has been reported. Therefore, hematologic assessments are important with long-term daily regimens. There might be some selectivity for different normal cell lines by these drugs; busulfan, and perhaps chlorambucil, selectively depresses granulocytes, relatively sparing platelets and lymphoid elements. The nadir for melphalan can be prolonged (4–6 weeks); continuous administration frequently leads to severe myelosuppression (especially platelets) that continues after the drug is discontinued. Pulmonary fibrosis can occasionally occur with all these drugs, especially busulfan; symptoms include cough, dyspnea, and fever; histopathologic changes include bilateral fibrosis. High-dose glucocorticoid therapy might help early evolving pulmonary disease caused by melphalan and chlorambucil, but "busulfan lung" is usually fatal (within 6 months of diagnosis). Busulfan frequently causes hyperpigmentation (especially of intertriginous areas) and broad suppression of adrenal functions (occasionally leading to Addisonian crisis). High-dose busulfan used in BMT regimens is associated with increased seizure activity that can be prevented with prophylactic use of phenytoin. Long-term daily administration of these drugs predisposes patients to drug-induced carcinogenesis, often heralded by preleukemic pancytopenia and culminating in acute myelocytic leukemia. Allergic hypersensitivity reported, especially with melphalan. With prolonged use, sterility occurs with all alkylators; women seem more sensitive than men.[4–6]

Contraindications. Documented hypersensitivity; inadequate marrow reserve.

Precautions. *See* Special Populations for melphalan use in renal impairment.

Drug Interactions. Itraconazole may cause reduced busulfan clearance; added myelosuppression when used with other myelosuppressive drugs.

Parameters to Monitor. Weekly CBC with differential while on therapy.

CARBOPLATIN
Paraplatin

Pharmacology. Carboplatin is a more stable cyclobutane carboxylated derivative of cisplatin that is slowly activated to expose two DNA binding sites on the platinum (II) coordinate complex. The drug binds to DNA by both inter- and intrastrand cross-links in a fashion similar to, but more delayed than, that with cisplatin. It is more water soluble and commensurately less nephrotoxic than cisplatin.[7]

Administration and Adult Dosage. IV for refractory ovarian cancer as monotherapy—360 mg/m^2 q4wk. When used in combination with cyclophosphamide 300 mg/m^2 is recommended. (*See* below for doses based on renal function).

Special Populations. *Pediatric Dosage.* Although not specifically labeled for pediatric use, carboplatin has been safely administered to children. Doses should be based on the regimen being used.

Geriatric Dosage. Same as adult dosage but adjust for age-related reduction in renal function.

Other Conditions. Dosage Adjustment in Renal Impairment: Patients with Cl_{Cr} values below 60 mL/min are at increased risk of severe bone marrow suppression. Dosing recommendations for these patients can be made based on their baseline Cl_{Cr} and renal function as follows: 41–59 mL/min; dose on day 1 = 250 mg/m^2 and 16–40 mL/min; 200 mg/m^2. Data for patients with Cl_{Cr} <15 mL/min is too limited to permit recommendations.[7–8]

Another approach for determining initial doses of carboplatin in patients with impaired kidney function is by use of a mathematical formula. There are several formulas available but the most widely accepted is the Calvert Formula, which individualizes dosing and permits targeting an acceptable level of toxicity. The formula is based upon the patient's glomerular filtration rate and carboplatin target AUC. Total Dose (mg) = (target AUC) × (GFR + 25). It is important to note that the Calvert Formula yields the total dose of carboplatin in mg NOT in mg/m^2. A target AUC of 4–6 will generally provide an appropriate dose range.[7,8]

Dosage Forms. Powder for Inj 50, 150, 450 mg. **IV Soln:** 10 mg/mL.

Do not use needles or IV administration sets that contain aluminum parts; they may come into contact with carboplatin and cause precipitate formation and/or reduction in potency.

Patient Instructions. *See* Antineoplastics Class Instructions, particularly regarding infection risk.

Pharmacokinetics. *Fate.* Carboplatin is not bound to plasma proteins, however, platinum from carboplatin becomes irreversibly bound to plasma proteins. The half-life of this protein-bound fraction is >5 days. V_d is 16 L for carboplatin. Urinary elimination accounts for over 65% of drug elimination in patients with normal renal function.

Half-life ($t_{1/2}$.) α phase 1.1–2 h; β phase 2.6–5.9 h.

Adverse Reactions. The Emetogenic potential is moderately high to high but can usually be controlled with antiemetics. Other GI effects include pain, diarrhea, and/or constipation. Myelosuppression is the primary dose-limiting effect of carboplatin. The median nadir for carboplatin as a single agent is approximately 21 days, and patients with preexisting renal dysfunction or poor bone marrow reserve have an increased risk for severe myelosuppression. Anemia is cumulative and may necessitate transfusions in patients receiving prolonged therapy, but the drug is most toxic to the platelet precursors. Nephrotoxicity is much less than that with cisplatin, but concomitant treatment with aminoglycosides has resulted in increased renal and/or audiologic toxicity. Clinically significant hearing loss has occurred in pediatric patients when high doses of carboplatin were administered. Transient decreases of some serum electrolytes may also occur, specifically magnesium, potassium, sodium, and calcium. The risk of peripheral neuropathies increases in patients >65 years or if large dosages of cisplatin have been administered. Occasional reactions are allergic hypersensitivity, alopecia, and various cardiovascular events (eg, embolism, cerebrovascular accident, cardiac failure).[8]

Contraindications. Severe myelosuppression or significant bleeding.

Precautions. Use with caution in patients with hearing impairment or reduced renal function or if extensive prior chemotherapy has been administered. Patients with prior cisplatin therapy are at a higher risk for nephrotoxic and neurotoxic sequelae. Vigorous hydration and diuretics usually are not required with carboplatin.[8]

Drug Interactions. Myelotoxicity of carboplatin is additive with other myelotoxic drugs. Concurrent use of other nephrotoxic drugs (eg, aminoglycosides) can delay carboplatin elimination and enhance toxicity.

Parameters to Monitor. Measure CL_{Cr} before dosage calculation. Monitor platelet and granulocyte counts and Cr_s during therapy.

CISPLATIN
Platinol-AQ

Pharmacology. Cisplatin is a planar coordinate dichlorodiamino compound of platinum in the +II valence state. It is aquated in vivo to a positively charged species that can alkylate nucleophilic sites in DNA such as purine and pyrimidine bases.

Administration and Adult Dosage. IV bolus or continuous infusion— (usually with aggressive hydration) single doses of up to 120 mg/m² have been used, but the manufacturer warns that pharmacists should contact the prescriber to verify doses >100 mg/m² per cycle.

Pretreatment hydration with 1 to 2 L of fluid infused for 8–12 h prior to a cisplatin dose is recommended. The drug is then diluted in 2 L of 5% dextrose in one-half or one-third normal saline containing 37.5 g of mannitol, and infused over a 6- to 8-h period. If diluted solution is not to be used within 6 h, protect solution from light. Do not dilute cisplatin in just 5% dextrose injection. Adequate hydration and urinary output must be maintained during the following 24 h.

Special Populations. *Pediatric Dosage.* Although not specifically labeled for pediatric use, cisplatin has been safely administered to children. Doses should be based on the regimen being used.

Geriatric Dosage. Same as adult dosage but adjust for age-related reduction in renal function.

Other Conditions. Reduce dosage in renal impairment; specific dosage reduction guidelines have not been established.

Dosage Forms. Inj 50, 100, 200 mg.

Do not use needles or IV administration sets that contain aluminum parts; they may come into contact with cisplatin and cause precipitate formation and/or reduction of potency.

Patient Instructions. (*See* Antineoplastics Class Instructions.) Be prepared for severe nausea and vomiting after drug administration.

Pharmacokinetics.

Fate. 90% of platinum is protein bound. Cisplatin has a rapid distribution phase of 25–80 min with a slower elimination half-life of 60–70 h.[8]

Adverse Reactions. Emetogenic potential is high. Nausea and vomiting are severe and often prolonged (days) and are best managed with aggressive prophylaxis using a serotonin 5HT3-antagonist and a high-dose glucocorticoid. Use of aprepitant, an antagonist of human substance P/neurokinin 1 (NK1) receptors may add to the efficacy of the 5HT3 and steroid combination. Primary toxicity is dose-related nephrotoxicity, especially proximal tubular impairment. Ototoxicity occurs frequently and may require a dosage reduction in children; total dose-related hypomagnesemia and severe cumulative peripheral neuropathy occur. Slight leukopenia, thrombocytopenia, and frequent anemia also occur. Rare toxicities include transient cortical dysfunction (blindness) and hypersensitivity (including anaphylaxis).[8]

Contraindications. Renal impairment; myelosuppression; hearing impairment; previous anaphylaxis. However, some patients with prior anaphylaxis have been successfully retreated with cisplatin and concomitant antihistamines, epinephrine, and glucocorticoids.

Precautions. Use with caution in renal impairment and with other nephrotoxic drugs, especially aminoglycosides. Assure adequate hydration (*see* Notes below) before and during administration. Both furosemide and mannitol are used to decrease platinum nephrotoxicity, although each apparently retards free platinum elimination.

Drug Interactions. Cisplatin can enhance nephrotoxicity and ototoxicity when administered with other drugs that cause these adverse events such as, aminoglycosides and Tacrolimus. Cisplatin also may result in decreased plasma concentrations of antiepileptic drugs such as carbamazepine, phenytoin, and valproic acid. Concomitant administration of other myelosuppressive antineoplastics may result in increased myelosuppression.

Parameters to Monitor. Assess renal function before each dose and serum electrolyte levels periodically.

Notes. Pretreatment hydration with 1–2 L of fluid infused for 8–12 h prior to a cisplatin dose is recommended. The cisplatin dosage may be further diluted in dextrose and saline solutions that contain ≥0.2% sodium chloride, therefore do not dilute cisplatin in 5% dextrose injection. Adequate hydration and urinary output must be maintained during the following 24 h.

CYCLOPHOSPHAMIDE   Cytoxan, Various

Pharmacology. Cyclophosphamide is a prodrug which must be enzymatically activated in the liver to active alkylating metabolites. It is widely used in hematologic and solid malignancies and as an immunosuppressant in a variety of autoimmune disorders.[9,10]

Administration and Adult Dosage. When used as monotherapy to nonmyelosuppressed patients—40–50 mg/kg IV in divided doses over 2 to 5 days or 10–15 mg/kg every 7–10 days or 3–5 mg/kg given twice weekly. PO is given in the range of 1–5 mg/kg/d. Many other regimens have been reported and dosages must be adjusted in accordance with evidence of efficacy.

Special Populations. *Pediatric Dosage.* The safety profile of cyclophosphamide in pediatric patients is similar to that of the adult population. **IV, PO for malignancies**—same as adult dosage. **PO for nephrotic syndrome**—2.5–3 mg/kg/d for 60–90 days.

Geriatric Dosage. Insufficient evidence exists for recommending dosage adjustments in patients ≥65 years of age, but published reports from breast cancer trials suggest that elderly patients may be more susceptible to toxicities. In general, dosing in the elderly should be done with caution and started at the low end of dosing ranges with adjustments made based on patient response.

Other Conditions. There is not sufficient evidence to indicate a need for dosage adjustments in patients with renal function impairment.

Dosage Forms. **Tab** 25, 50 mg; **Inj** 200, 500 mg; 1, 2 g

Patient Instructions. (*See* Antineoplastics Class Instructions.) Drink 2–3 quarts of fluids daily (1–2 quarts in smaller children) and urinate frequently; do *not* take oral doses at bedtime. Report any blood in the urine.

Pharmacokinetics. *Fate.* Bioavailability from oral absorption is >75%. Metabolized to active compounds (including the highly toxic nonalkylating aldehyde, acrolein, and the principal alkylator, phosphoramide mustard (within the cell)) primarily by hepatic microsomal mixed-function oxidases. V_d is 40.59 L ± 18.17; renal elimination accounts for <20% of unchanged drug and 30%–60% of metabolites. Children have a more rapid clearance normalized to BSA relative to adults, although the mechanism is unknown.[11]

$t_{1/2}$. (4-hydroxycyclophosphamide) 7.4 ± 4 h.

Cyclophosphamide is a potent inducer of microsomal enzymes and induces its own metabolism when given as repeated doses for consecutive days, which may result in a decrease in the elimination half-life.[10]

Adverse Reactions. Emetogenic potential is moderate to high. Nausea, vomiting, and alopecia are frequent and dose dependent. Dose-limiting toxicity is myelosuppression, with a leukopenic nadir of about 10 days; platelets also are suppressed at higher doses. Transient, reversible blurred vision occurs frequently. The incidence of cyclophosphamide-induced hemorrhagic cystitis is reported to range from 2% to 78%. The causative agent is the metabolite, acrolin. Prophylactic hydration is recommended as well as frequent voiding. To prevent urotoxicity with high-dose regimens, administer **mesna.** (*See* Mesna.) Ovarian and testicular function can be permanently lost after high-dose, long-term therapy. Rare reactions are a high-dose fatal cardiomyopathy, interstitial pneumonitis, and a transient condition similar to SIADH.

Second malignancies have developed in some patients treated with cyclophosphamide used alone or in association with other antineoplastic drugs.

Contraindications. Previous life-threatening hypersensitivity to cyclophosphamide; severe myelosuppression.

Precautions. Pregnancy. Consider dosage reduction or discontinuation of drug in patients who develop infections.

Drug Interactions. Many drug–drug interactions have been reported, with the underlying mechanism involving the induction or inhibition of CYP enzymes. Possible inhibitors of metabolism include: allopurinol, busulfan, chloramphenicol, chlorpromazine, ciprofloxacin, fluconazole, and thiotepa. Possible inducers include: dexamethasone, ondansetron, Phenobarbital, phenytoin, prednisone/prednisolone, and rifampin. The clinical significance of most drug–drug interactions with cyclophosphamide is unclear.[10]

Parameters to Monitor. Assessment of the patient for adequate numbers of WBCs and platelets should occur regularly. With long-term use, assess these counts at least monthly. Monitor closely for hematuria, especially if the patient has received a large cumulative dosage.

DACARBAZINE	DTIC-Dome, Various

Pharmacology. Dacarbazine is a nonclassic alkylating agent. It undergoes demethylation to an active intermediate monomethyl triazeno-imidazole-carboxamide (MTIC) that interrupts DNA replication by causing methylation of guanine.[12]

Adult Dosage. **Malignant Melanoma—2–4.5 mg/kg/d IV × 10 days repeated at 4-week intervals or 250 mg/m^2 IV × 5 days repeated every 3 wk. Hodgkin's Disease** 150 mg/m^2/d × 5 days in combination therapy repeated every 4 wk.

Dosage Forms. **Inj** 100, 200 mg.

Pharmacokinetics. Dacarbazine is extensively metabolized. It is not appreciably protein bound; 40% of a dose excreted, unchanged in the urine. The drug has an α half-life of 19 min and a β half-life of about 5 h, which can be lengthened in patients with renal and hepatic dysfunction to 55 min and 7.2 h.[12]

Adverse Reactions. Nausea and vomiting, which occasionally are severe, occur almost invariably. The dose-limiting toxicity is myelosuppression, with a leukopenic nadir at 7–10 days. Occasionally, a flulike syndrome of myalgia, fever, and malaise occurs within 1 week of drug administration. Use dacarbazine with caution in patients with preexisting bone marrow aplasia and avoid exposure to sunlight because of possible photosensitivity reactions.

IFOSFAMIDE	Ifex

Pharmacology. Ifosfamide is a structural analogue of the alkylating agent cyclophosphamide (CTX). The rate of hepatic conversion of ifosfamide to the active metabolite 4-hydroxyifosfamide is slightly slower than with CTX, although formation of the bladder toxin acrolein is not reduced. The ultimate metabolite ifosforamide mustard cross-links DNA to impair cell division. The drug is always given with mesna to prevent urotoxicity. Ifosfamide is cell-cycle phase nonspecific.

Administration and Adult Dosage. **IV for refractory testicular cancer**—1.2 g/m^2/d for 5 days. The recommended concurrent IV **mesna** dose is 20% of the ifosfamide dose, given 15 min before ifosfamide and again at 4 and 8 h. It can be directly admixed with ifosfamide. The latter two mesna doses can be given orally at twice the dose (ie, each at 40% of the ifosfamide dose) if patient compliance and a lack of emesis can be assured.[13,14]

Special Populations. *Pediatric Dosage.* Although not specifically labeled for pediatric use, ifosfamide has been safely administered to children. Doses should be based on the regimen being used.

Geriatric Dosage. Same as adult dosage but adjust for age-related reduction in renal function.

Other Conditions. Dosage reduction is indicated in patients with reduced renal function, although specific guidelines are not available.

Dosage Forms. Inj 1, 3 g.

Patient Instructions. *See* Antineoplastics Class Instructions.

Pharmacokinetics. *Fate.* Metabolism begins with hydroxylation that produces 4-hydroxyifosfamide, an active alkylator, in equilibrium with its tautomeric form, aldoifosfamide. Aldoifosfamide undergoes spontaneous β elimination, which frees acrolein to form the primary alkylating agent, ifosforamide mustard. Acrolein is a potent urothelial irritant and is the major cause of Ifosfamide-induced hemorrhagic cystitis.[13]

Exhibits dose-dependent pharmacokinetics with biphasic decay at higher doses (3.8–5 gm/m^2) with a mean terminal $t_{1/2}$ of 15 h and at lower doses (1.6–2.3 gm/m^2) monoexponential decay and a terminal $t_{1/2}$ of 7 h.

Adverse Reactions. Emetogenic potential is moderate; nausea and vomiting can generally be managed with antiemetics. Alopecia occurs in most patients treated with ifosfamide. The major dose-limiting effect of ifosfamide is urotoxicity manifested as hemorrhagic cystitis, dysuria, urinary frequency, and other symptoms of bladder irritation. The incidence and severity of hematuria can be reduced with the use of aggressive hydration, use of a fractionated dose schedule, and concomitant administration of a protector such as mesna. Renal tubular toxicity, manifested by elevations in BUN and Cr$_s$, occurs in <10% of patients. Renal tubular acidosis, Fanconi syndrome and acute renal failure have been reported suggesting that close monitoring of serum and urine chemistries is needed. Myelosuppression can be dose limiting mainly consisting of leucopenia and lesser extent thrombocytopenia. Myelosuppression is usually reversible allowing cycles of treatment every 3–4 weeks. CNS side effects include somnolence, confusion, depressive psychosis and hallucinations have occurred in 12% of patients but may occur more frequently in patients with altered renal function. Other rare CNS neurotoxicities are cerebellar toxicity (ataxia), urinary incontinence, and seizures.

Contraindications. Severe preexisting myelosuppression.

Precautions. Withhold repeat therapy until there is resolution of microscopic hematuria (<10 RBCs per high-power field). An adequate state of hydration is critical to reducing urotoxicity.

Drug Interactions. Use with cisplatin can increase nephrotoxicity and potassium and magnesium loss. Nephrotoxicity is also enhanced when ifosfamide is combined with other nephrotoxic drugs.

Parameters to Monitor. Ensure that renal function and WBC counts are normal before administration. During therapy, monitor for hematuria daily.

MECHLORETHAMINE HYDROCHLORIDE   Mustargen

Pharmacology. Mechlorethamine (nitrogen mustard) is a prototype bischloroethylamine, bifunctional alkylating agent, which causes interstrand and intrastrand DNA–DNA cross-links which are responsible for the cytotoxic activity.

Administration and Adult Dosage. The dosage varies with the clinical situation, but generally a total dose of 0.4 mg/kg/course (6 mg/m^2) is given as a single dose or in divided doses of 0.1–0.2 mg/kg/d. Dosage is based on IBW, and the presence of ascites or edema must be considered in this calculation. Solutions decompose on standing; therefore, solutions of the drug should be prepared immediately prior to use.

Special Populations. *Pediatric Dosage.* Although not specifically labeled for pediatric use, mechlorethamine has been safely administered to children. It has been specifically used in the treatment of children with Hodgkin's disease as a component of the MOPP regimen with vincristine, procarbazine, and prednisone. Doses should be based on the regimen being used.

Geriatric Dosage. Same as adult dosage, but usually starting at the low end of the dosing range.

Dosage Forms. **Inj** 10 mg.

Patient Instructions. *See* Antineoplastics Class Instructions.

Pharmacokinetics. *Fate.* Undergoes rapid chemical transformation and combines with water or reactive compounds of cells so that unchanged drug cannot be detected in the blood within minutes of administration. Therefore, the half-life is so short that it has not been characterized.[15]

Adverse Reactions. Emetogenic potential is high; nausea and vomiting can occur within the first 3 h, and the reactions are severe and can last more than 1 day. The major dose-limiting toxicity is myelosuppression, resulting in lymphocytopenia within 24 h and granulocytopenia nadir within 6–8 days. Extravasation causes delayed and protracted (months) ulceration and necrosis (*see* Notes) Primary reproductive failure may be temporary or permanent and both males and females should be warned of the potential risk to their reproductive capacity.

Contraindications. Prior severe hypersensitivity reactions; presence of known infection.

Precautions. Patients with lymphomas (especially "bulky" lymphomas) may require prophylactic allopurinol 2–3 days before and throughout therapy to prevent hyperuricemia and urate nephropathy associated with tumor lysis.

Parameters to Monitor. Pretreatment and at least monthly assessment of bone marrow function, particularly WBC and platelet counts.

Notes. Mechlorethamine is a powerful vesicant and should be prepared with great caution. Due to the drug's toxic properties, use of appropriate safety equipment is recommended for preparation including mask and rubber gloves during preparation. Avoid inhalation of dust and vapors or contact with skin and mucous membranes, especially the eyes.

MITOMYCIN
Mutamycin

Pharmacology. Mitomycin selectively inhibits the synthesis of DNA. The guanine and cytosine content correlates with the degree of mitomycin-induced cross-linking.

Adult Dosage. IV as a single agent—20 mg/m^2 in a single dose and no repeat dosage given until leukocyte count has returned to 4000/mm^3 and platelet count to 100,000/mm^3.

Dosage Forms. Inj 5, 20, 40 mg.

Pharmacokinetics. The drug is eliminated primarily by hepatic clearance, with 10% of the dose recovered unchanged in the urine.

$t_{1/2}$. 17 min.

Adverse Reactions. The dose-limiting toxicitiy, myelosuppression is common (64.4%). Monitor the patient carefully for delayed and prolonged myelosuppression. Acute effects include nausea, vomiting, anorexia, and fever. Severe ulceration can occur if the drug is extravasated. Other more frequent and potentially lethal adverse events include hemolytic uremic syndrome, interstitial pneumonitis, and cardiac failure.[16]

NITROSOUREAS:

CARMUSTINE
BiCNU, Gliadel

LOMUSTINE
CeeNU

Pharmacology. Carmustine (BCNU) and lomustine (CCNU) are lipid-soluble derivatives of bis-chloroethyl nitrosoureas. They form DNA cross-links by chloroethylation of a nucleophilic DNA site.[15]

Administration and Dosage. *See* Notes.

Dosage Forms. (Carmustine) **Inj** 100 mg with alcohol diluent (BiCNU); **Wafer** 7.7 mg (Gliadel). (Lomustine) **Cap** 10, 40, 100 mg individually or a commercial packet, which contains two of each strength for a total of 300 mg.

Patient Instructions. (*See* Antineoplastics Class Instructions). Take lomustine on an empty stomach to reduce nausea and vomiting.

Pharmacokinetics. *Fate.* For BCNU the plasma concentration decay curves are biexponential, with a distribution phase half-life of 6 min and a second-phase half-life of 68 min. Longer elimination half-lives (22–45 min) are seen with higher doses.[17] BCNU CSF concentrations are 30%–97% of the plasma concentrations.[15]

Rapid absorption of CCNU occurs after oral dosing. CCNU is highly lipid soluble and relatively unionized at physiologic pH. CSF concentrations are >50% of the plasma concentrations.[15]

Adverse Reactions. Delayed hematologic toxicity is dose limiting for both of these drugs, with nadirs of greater than 4 weeks.[15] Emetogenic potential is moderately high to high; prophylactic antiemetics are recommended. Carmustine is associated with burning at injection site, although true thrombosis is rare. Both drugs can transiently elevate liver enzymes. Pulmonary fibrosis has been reported as well as nephrotoxicity in patients receiving large cumulative doses over long periods of time. Other occasional toxicities with lomustine are CNS effects (eg, confusion, lethargy, ataxia), stomatitis, and alopecia.

Contraindications. Demonstrated hypersensitivity; marked preexisting myelosuppression.

Precautions. Pregnancy.

Notes. Store carmustine injection in refrigerator; appearance of an oily film in the vial is evidence of decomposition, and such vials should be discarded. Carmustine should only be dispensed in glass containers. Carmustine wafers must be stored at or below −20°C.[16]

Carmustine implant wafers (Gliadel) are indicated for newly diagnosed high-grade glioma patients as an adjunct to surgery and radiation as well as recurrent glioblastoma multiforme patients as an adjunct to surgery. It is recommended that 8 wafers be placed in the resection cavity if the size and shape of the area resected will accommodate the wafers. If all 8 wafers will not fit, the maximum number of wafers (up to 8) that can be accommodated should be used. Slight overlapping of the wafers is acceptable. A wafer broken in two pieces may be used, but if broken into more than two pieces, all pieces should be discarded in a biohazard container. Adverse events specific to the wafer dosage formulation are: seizures, intracranial infections, healing abnormalities, and brain edema.

PROCARBAZINE HYDROCHLORIDE   Matulane

Pharmacology. Procarbazine is a prodrug that is metabolized to active species. It enters the cell by passive diffusion and is rapidly converted to cytotoxic metabolites by several routes.[18] It is cell-cycle phase nonspecific and used in brain tumors and Hodgkin's and non-Hodgkin's lymphomas.

Adult Dosage. PO to minimize the nausea and vomiting—initiate therapy with single or divided doses of 2–4 mg/kg/d for the first week. Increase to 4–6 mg/kg/d until maximum response is obtained or WBC <4000/cmm or platelets <100,000 /cmm. When maximum response is obtained, continue maintenance dose of 1–2 mg/kg/d.

Special Populations. *Pediatric Dosage.* 50 mg/m^2 × 1 week then increased dosing of 100 mg/m^2 until maximum response, then maintenance dosing at 50 mg/m^2. Very close monitoring is necessary in these patients to prevent toxicity.

Dosage Forms. Cap 50 mg.

Pharmacokinetics. The drug is rapidly and completely absorbed after oral administration. The half-life of the parent compound is only minutes and the half-life of the major metabolite is about 1 h.[15] This metabolite crosses the blood–brain barrier and equilibrates between plasma and CSF. Procarbazine is 70% recovered in the urine, primarily as an acid metabolite.

Adverse Reactions. Nausea and vomiting are the most frequently reported, but may be diminished with the step-wise dosing. Myelosuppression occurs frequently and may be dose-limiting. Hemolysis may occur in G6PD-deficient patients. Neurotoxicity manifests as drowsiness, paresthesias of the extremities, and agitation or depression.[15,18]

Drug Interactions. Because procarbazine inhibits monoamine oxidase, it predisposes patients to acute hypertensive reactions if given concomitantly with tricyclic antidepressants or sympathomimetic drug, as well as after ingestion of tyramine-rich foods, such as red wine, bananas, ripe cheese, and yogurt. A disulfiram-like reaction including sweating, facial flushing, and headache may occur in patients who ingest alcohol while taking procarbazine.[18]

STREPTOZOCIN
Zanosar

Pharmacology. Streptozocin is a unique methylnitrosurea that has methylating activity but no carbamylating activity since the molecule autocarbamylates through internal cyclization.[17]

Adult Dosage. IV There are 2 recommended schedules for dosing: **Daily** schedule—500 mg/m^2 × 5 d given q6wk or **Weekly** schedule—1000 mg/m^2 weekly × 2 week, then dosage escalation can occur in patients who have not had significant toxicity, however a single dose should not exceed 1500 mg/ m^2

Dosage Forms. **Inj** 1 g. Store in refrigerator, protected from light.

Pharmacokinetics. Streptozocin is rapidly and extensively metabolized (unchanged drug half-life is 35 min), and <20% is excreted unchanged in the urine.[15]

Adverse Reactions. Nephrotoxicity is dose limiting. It is cumulative and may be irreversible. Nausea and vomiting are severe and may be difficult to control even with appropriate antiemetics. Myelosuppression may occur, but is usually mild to moderate.[15]

TEMOZOLOMIDE
Temodar

Pharmacology. Temozolomide is not directly active but undergoes rapid nonenzymatic conversion at physiologic pH to the reactive compound 3-methyl-(triazen-1-yl) imidazole-4-carboxamide (MTIC). The cytotoxicity of MTIC is thought to be primarily due to alkylation of DNA, which occurs mainly at the O^6 and N^7 positions of guanine.

Adult Dosage. PO for refractory anaplastic astrocytoma—150 mg/m^2 once daily for 5 consecutive days per 28-day cycle. Adjust subsequent dosages according to nadir neutrophil and platelet counts (*see* package insert for specific guidelines). Dosage for newly diagnosed high-grade glioma is 75 mg/m^2 × 42 days concomitantly with focal radiotherapy (*see* package insert for specific dosing guidelines).

Special Populations. *Pediatric Dosage.* PO effectiveness has not been demonstrated, but several studies have been completed at a dose of 160–200 mg/m^2 daily × 5 days q28d.

Dosage Forms. **Cap** 5, 20, 100, 140, 180, 250 mg.

Pharmacokinetics. Temozolomide's oral bioavailability is 100%; food reduces the rate and extent of absorption. Has a mean elimination half-life of 1.8 h and exhibits linear kinetics over the therapeutic dosing range. Mean volume of distribution is 0.4 L/kg. Weakly protein bound (15%). Mean pharmacokinetic parameters are similar in pediatric patients.[19]

Adverse Reactions. The dose-limiting toxicity of temozolomide, myelosuppression, is noncumulative. The most frequent adverse effects are alopecia, nausea, vomiting, anorexia, headache, constipation, and fatigue. Nausea and vomiting are usually moderate and can be controlled by taking the dose on an empty stomach and using prophylactic antiemetics.

Contraindications. Hypersensitivity to any components of temozolomide or dacarbazine.

Notes. Capsules should not be opened or chewed. They should be swallowed whole with a glass of water.

THIOTEPA Thioplex

Pharmacology. Thiotepa is related chemically and pharmacologically to nitrogen mustard. The action of thiotepa occurs through the release of ethylenimine radicals that disrupt the bonds of DNA.

Adult Dosage. IV—0.3–0.4 mg/kg given at 1- to 4-week intervals. **Intracavitary**— 0.6–0.8 mg/kg with administration usually effected through the same tubing used to remove the fluid from the cavity involved. **Intravesical**—60 mg in 30–60 mL of sodium chloride injection.

Dosage Forms. Inj 15 mg.

Pharmacokinetics. Thiotepa is rapidly desulfurated to triethylenephosphoramide (TEPA) and other alkylating species. Thiotepa plasma terminal has a half-life of 1.2–2 h. TEPA appears in the plasma within 5 min of thiotepa administration and has a half-life of 3–21 h. 1.5% of thiotepa is excreted unchanged in the urine after 24 h and 4.2% TEPA. The pharmacokinetic values in children are similar to those in adults.[17]

Adverse Reactions. The dose-limiting toxicity is myelosuppression, which can occur in those patients receiving the drug by the intravesical or intracavitary routes. Nausea and vomiting can generally be prevented by the use of prophylactic antiemetic regimens. At high doses alopecia, mucositis, stomatitis, and erythematous rash have been reported.[15]

■ REFERENCES

1. Keldsen N, Havsteen H, Vergote I, et al. Altretamine (hexamethylmelamine) in the treatment of platinum-resistant ovarian cancer: a phase II study. *Gynecol Oncol*. 2003;88:118-122.
2. Chan JK, Loizzi V, Manetta A, et al. Oral altretamine used as salvage therapy in recurrent ovarian cancer. *Gynecol Oncol*. 2004;92:368-371.
3. Carlson K, Hjorth M, Knudsen LM. Toxicity in standard melphalan-prednisone therapy among myeloma patients with renal failure—a retrospective analysis and recommendations for dose adjustment. *Br J Haematol*. 2005;128:631-635.
4. Booth BP, Rahman A, Dagher R, et al. Population pharmacokinetic-based dosing of intravenous busulfan in pediatric patients. *J Clin Pharmacol*. 2007;47:101-111.
5. Tran HT, Madden T, Petropoulos D, et al. Individualizing high-dose oral busulfan: prospective dose adjustment in a pediatric population undergoing allogenic stem cell transplantation for advanced hematologic malignancies. *Bone Marrow Transplantation*. 2000;26:463-470.
6. Kalaycio M, Pohlman B, Kuczkowski E, et al. High-dose busulfan and the risk of pulmonary mortality after Autologous stem cell transplant. *Clin Transplantation*. 2006;20:783-787.
7. Knox RJ, Friedlos F, Lydall D, et al. Mechanism of cytotoxicity of anticancer platinum drugs: evidence that *cis*-diamminedichloroplatinum(II) and *cis*diammine-(1,1-cyclobutananedicarboxylato) platinum(II) differ only in the kinetics of their interaction with DNA. *Cancer Res*. 1986;46:1972-1979.
8. O'Dwyer PJ, Stevenson JP, Johnson SW. Clinical pharmacokinetics and administration of established platinum drugs. *Drugs*. 2000;59(suppl. 4):19-27.
9. Xie H, Griskevicius L, Stahle L, et al. Pharmacogenetics of cyclophosphamide in patients with hematological malignancies. *Eur J Pharm Sci*. 2006;27:54-61.
10. Jonge M, Huitema A, Rodenhuis S, et al. Clinical pharmacokinetics of cyclophosphamide. *Clin Pharmacokinet*. 2005;44(11):1135-1164.

11. McCune J, Salinger D, Vicini P, et al. Population pharmacokinetics of cyclophosphamide and metabolites in children with neuroblastoma; a report from the Children's Oncology Group. *J Clin Pharmacol*. 2009;49(1):88-102.

12. Medina P, Fausel C. Oncologic Disorders: Cancer Treatment and Chemotherapy. In: Dipiro JT, Talbert RL, Yee GC, Matzke GR, Wells BG, Posey ML, eds. *Pharmacotherapy a pathophysiologic approach*. 7th ed. New York: McGraw-Hill; 2008:2100.

13. Mace JR, Keohan ML, Bernady H, et al. Crossover randomized comparison of intravenous *versus* intravenous/oral mesna in soft tissue sarcoma treated with high-dose Ifosfamide. *Clin Cancer Res*. 2003;9:5829-5834.

14. Goren MP, Epelman S, Bush D. Urine mesna excretion after intravenous and oral dosing in Ifosfamide-treated children. *Cancer Chemother Pharmacol*. 2004; 54(3):237-240.

15. Grochow LB. Covalent DNA-Binding Drugs. In: Perry MC, ed. *Chemotherapy Source Book*. 3rd ed. Philadelphia, PA: Lippincott-Williams & Wilkins; 2001:192-208.

16. Willems EW, Nooter K, Verweij J. Antitumor Antibiotics. In: Chabner BA, Longo DL, eds. *Cancer Chemotherapy and Biotherapy Principles and Practice*. 4th ed. Philadelphilia, PA: Lippincott-Williams & Wilkins; 2006:359-370.

17. Tew KD, Colvin OM, Jones RB. Clinical and High-Dose alkylating Agents. In: Chabner BA, Longo DL, eds. *Cancer Chemotherapy and Biotherapy Principles and Practice*. 4th ed. Philadelphia, PA: Lippincott-Williams & Wilkins; 2006:283-309.

18. Friedman H, Averbuch SD, Kurtzberg J. Nonclassic Agents. In: Chabner BA, Longo DL, eds. *Cancer Chemotherapy and Biotherapy Principles and Practice*. 4th ed. Philadelphia, PA: Lippincott-Williams & Wilkins; 2006:310-331.

19. Horton TM, Thompson PA, Berg S, et al. Phase I Pharmacokinetic and Pharmacodynamic Study of Temozolomide in pediatric patients with refractory or recurrent leukemia: A Children's Oncology Group Study. *J Clin Oncol*. 2007;25:4922-4928.

Chapter 20

Antimetabolites

Shirley Hogan

CLADRIBINE
Leustatin

Pharmacology. Cladribine's mechanism of cytotoxic activity is multifactorial and includes inhibition of DNA synthesis and repair, incorporation in the DNA promoter sequences, causing an imbalance in deoxyribonucleotide triphosphate pools, and triggering apoptosis by activating caspases.[1,2]

Adult Dosage. IV for hairy cell leukemia—a single *course* given as a continous infusion over 7 days, with each day's dose = 0.09 mg/kg.

Dosage Forms. Inj 10 mg (1 mg/mL). Store refrigerated and protect from light during storage.

Pharmacokinetics. Cladribine has a linear biphasic pharmacokinetic profile with an average half-life of 6.7 ± 2.5 h. Volume of distribution 9 L/kg indicates an extensive distribution in body tissues. It penetrates the CSF with concentrations between 12% and 38% of plasma concentrations during continuous infusions. Approximately 20% bound to plasma proteins. An average of 18% of the administered dose is excreted in the urine.[2]

Adverse Reactions. Myelosuppression occurs frequently and may be dose limiting. Patients may experience neutropenia, severe anemia (hemoglobin <8.5 g/dL), and thrombocytopenia as well as suppression of CD4 counts. Serious infections have occurred and deaths have been attributable to infection. Fever occurs frequently with some patients reporting a $T_{max} \geq 104°F$. Nausea, headache, and rash have also been reported frequently.[1,2]

CYTARABINE (Ara-C)
Cytosar-U, Tarabine PFS, Various

CYTARABNE, LIPOSOMAL
DepoCyt

Pharmacology. Cytarabine is sequentially phosphorylated to ara-CTP by the action of deoxycytidine kinases. It inhibits DNA polymerase α, is incorporated into DNA, and terminates DNA chain elongation.[2,3]

Cytarabine is cell-cycle S-phase specific, with activity markedly enhanced by continuous administration over several days.[3]

Administration and Dosage. (**Conventional**) IV—100 mg/m²/d as a continuous infusion for 7 days. Intensification therapy 1–3 g/m² every 12 h for 8–12 doses. **Intrathecal** dosages ranging from 5 to 75 mg/m² have been used. (**Liposomal**) **intrathecal** 50 mg/dose with frequency determined by the stage of treatment. Patients should be started on dexamethasone 4 mg bid PO or IV for 5 days beginning on the day of administration to reduce neurotoxicity.

Special Populations. *Pediatric Dosage.* (Conventional) same as adult dosage. (Liposomal) safety and efficacy not established.

Geriatric Dosage. Same as adult dosage.

Dosage Forms. **Inj** (conventional) 100 mg, 500 mg, 1 g, 2 g; (liposomal) 50 mg.

Pharmacokinetics. *Fate.* (Conventional) biphasic elimination with an α half-life of 15 min (possibly due to initial elimination by the liver) and a β half-life of 2–3 h. Minimal conversion of ara-C to ara-U takes place in the CSF following intrathecal administration because of the low levels of cytidine deaminase present in the brain and CSF providing concentrations above the threshold for cytotoxicity for 24 h.[2,3]

(Liposomal) following intrathecal administration the terminal half-life is of 5.9–82.4 h. Systemic exposure is negligible following administration of the liposomal product intrathecally. The CSF clearance rate is similar to the CSF bulk flow rate of 0.24 mL/min.

Adverse Reactions. (Conventional) leukopenia and thrombocytopenia are common. GI symptoms that include nausea, vomiting, and diarrhea are frequent during the time of drug administration, but generally subside after course is finished. Oral mucositis may be severe and prolonged in patients receiving drug for >5 days. Conjunctivitis is common with high dose regimens and can be reduced by using prophylactic steroid eye drops. Also with high-dose regimens, approximately 10% of patients experience cerebellar toxicity consisting of slurred speech, unsteady gait, dementia, and even coma.[2,3]

Liposomal or conventional when given intrathecally: nausea, vomiting, fever headache, meningeal signs, paresthesia, paraplegia, and seizures, which may be related to the accumulation of ara-CTP in the CNS.[2,3]

Precautions. Patients receiving cytarabine should have frequent hematological monitoring. Periodic checks of liver and kidney function are also recommended. When administered intrathecally (conventional or liposomal formulations), patients should be monitored for signs of chemical arachnoiditis.

Drug Interactions. Digoxin bioavailability from tablets may be decreased after cytarabine containing combination regimens; therefore, monitoring of plasma digoxin levels may be indicated in patients receiving digoxin.

Parameters to Monitor. *See* Precautions.

Notes. (Liposomal) for intrathecal administration only. The liposomal particles are more dense than the diluent and have a tendency to settle with time; therefore, allow the vial to come to room temperature and *gently* agitate or invert the vial to resuspend the particles just prior to withdrawal of the dose. Use within 4 h of withdrawal from vial and discard any unused drug. Do not dilute or mix with any other medications and do not use an in-line filter.

FLUDARABINE PHOSPHATE

Fludara

Pharmacology. Fludarabine is a monophosphate analog of adenosine arabinoside. It is rapidly converted to 2-fluoro-ara-A, which enters the cell through a carrier-mediated transport process. In the cell it is phosphorylated to 2-fluoro-ara-ATP, which inhibits DNA synthesis through the inhibition of ribonucleotide reductase and DNA polymerase.[1,2]

Adult Dosage. IV—25 mg/m^2 over 30 min × 5 consecutive days. Repeat cycle every 28 days.

Special Populations. *Pediatric Dosage.* IV—there is insufficient data to establish efficacy in any childhood malignancy. Clinical trials in pediatric patients have shown adverse events similar to those seen in adults.

Dosage Forms. Inj 50 mg.

Pharmacokinetics. Fludarabine is rapidly converted to the active metabolite, 2-fluoro-ara-A; therefore, pharmacokinetic values are expressed for this metabolite— terminal half-life 20 h. Renal clearance represents 40% of total body clearance, therefore a 20% reduction in dose is recommended for patients with moderate renal inpairment.

Adverse Reactions. The dose-limiting toxicities are myelosuppression and infection. The degree of leukopenia, granulocytopenia, and thrombocytopenia is dose related. Decreases in T-cell subsets increases the risk of opportunistic infections. Nausea and vomiting can usually be prevented with prophylactic antiemetics. Other commonly reported adverse events include malaise, fatigue, anorexia, and weakness.[2]

FLUOROURACIL Various

Pharmacology. Fluorouracil (5-fluorouracil, 5-FU) acts as a false pyrimidine base. Through a carrier-mediated process fluorouracil enters the cell and is converted to fluorouridine triphosphate and monophosphate as well as fluorodeoxyuridine triphosphate. The incorporation of these metabolites into RNA affects synthesis and function and incorporation into DNA affects stability.[2,4]

Administration and Adult Dosage. IV—300–500 mg/m^2 daily × 4 days not to exceed 800 mg/d per manufacturer. The patient's reaction to the previous course will determine the dose in any further courses. Dosage adjustments should be made in accord with toxic manifestations. Base dosage on ideal body weight in obesity or if the patient has excessive fluid retention.

Topical—apply cream or solution twice daily in an amount sufficient to cover the lesions. Apply with a nonmetal applicator or suitable glove. If fingers are used for application, wash immediately afterward. Duration for keratoses is 2–4 weeks and basal cell carcinoma is 3–6 weeks.[2]

Dosage Forms. Inj 500 mg and 5 g (50 mg/mL); **Top Crm** 0.5%, 1%, 1%, 5%; **Top Soln** 2%, 5%.

Patient Instructions. (*See* Antineoplastics Class Instructions.) When using topical application, patients should be forewarned that the treated areas may be unsightly during therapy and usually for several weeks following cessation of therapy. When applied to a lesion, a response occurs in the following sequence: erythema, usually followed by vesiculation, desquamation, erosion, and reepithelialization.

Pharmacokinetics. *Fate.* Approximately 20% of a dose is excreted in urine unchanged and between 22% and 45% is metabolized by the liver. The mean plasma half-life is 16 min, generally follows first-order kinetics and no intact drug can be detected in the plasma after 3 h. 5-FU diffused readily across the blood–brain barrier and distributes into the CSF and brain. Approximately 10% is bound to plasma proteins.[2–4]

Adverse Reactions. Hematologic effects are less pronounced with continuous infusion than with bolus administration, but leukopenia and thrombocytopenia are common. Anorexia, nausea, and vomiting are generally more severe with continuous infusion schedules. Stomatitis is an early sign of impending severe toxicity and necessitates a delay in therapy. Diarrhea can be life-threatening when high doses of 5-FU are administered with leucovorin (see Drug Interactions). Mild alopecia, increased sensitivity to sunlight, and hyperpigmentation of nail beds and skin are common. Palmer-plantar erythrodysesthesia syndrome (hand-foot syndrome) which manifests as pain and tingling in the hands and feet has been reported with continuous infusion. Asymptomatic ST-wave changes on ECG that are suggestive of cardiac ischemia are common. [2,4]

Drug Interactions. Modulation of the cytotoxicity of fluorouracil has been attempted by coadministration with several other agents such as leucovorin and methotrexate as well as interferon and cisplatin. It is not clear whether these combinations are more efficacious than administering equipotent doses of 5-FU alone. The more common approach of these combinations is the administration of leucovorin. The modulation of 5-FU by leucovorin is based on the ability of leucovorin to increase cellular levels of reduced folates and thereby increase the stability of a ternary complex affording greater cytoxicity. [2]

Parameters to Monitor. Assessment of bone marrow function, particularly WBC and platelet counts prior to each course. In the weeks after administration, observe for severe stomatitis, which can herald life-threatening myelosuppression. [4]

GEMCITABINE
Gemzar

Pharmacology. Gemcitabine is metabolized intracellularly by nucleoside kinases into 2 active metabolites, gemcitabine diphosphate and gemcitabine triphosphate. Its cytotoxic effect is attributed to a combination of 2 actions of these metabolites and leads to inhibition of DNA synthesis. The diphosphate moiety inhibits ribonucleotide reductase, which causes a reduction in the concentration of deoxynucleotides. Gemcitabine triphosphate competes with dCTP and enhances the incorporation of gemcitabine triphosphate into DNA and therefore the inhibition of DNA synthesis. DNA polymerase epsilon is unable to remove the gemcitabine triphosphate and repair the DNA strands. [2]

Administration and Adult Dosage. Gemcitabine has shown activity in a variety of tumor types. The dose and dosing schedule varies greatly with the malignancy that is treated. Many clinical trials are in process to determine the most efficacious and best-tolerated regimens. Refer to the full prescribing information for the most current regimen for the type of malignancy being treated. With any of the regimens, prolongation of the infusion time beyond 60 min and more frequent than weekly dosing have been shown to increase toxicity. [2]

Dosage Forms. **Inj** 200 mg, 1 g.

Pharmacokinetics. *Fate.* >65 years old demonstrate a reduced clearance rate. The volume of distribution is increased with increasing infusion time. After short infusions (<70 min) V_d is 50 L/m^2 while after a longer infusion V_d is 370 L/m^2 indicating limited tissue distribution after short infusions and slow equilibration within the tissue compartment with longer infusion times. Gemcitabine is almost entirely excreted in the urine (92%–98%).[2]

Adverse Reactions. Most adverse events associated with gemcitabine are reversible and should be managed by dose reduction rather than discontinuation of therapy. Myelosuppression is dose limiting. Other common adverse events include constipation, diarrhea, fever or flulike symptoms, nausea and vomiting, dyspnea, peripheral edema, hematuria, proteinuria, alopecia, rash, and injection site reactions. Less frequent are bronchospasm, cardiac arrhythmia, and hypertension.[2]

Contraindications. Severe preexisting thrombocytopenia.

Precautions. Use with caution in patients with preexisting renal impairment or hepatic insufficiency.

Parameters to Monitor. Prior to each dose obtain CBC with differential and platelet count.

METHOTREXATE   Rheumatrex, Trexall

Pharmacology. At lower concentrations, methotrexate enters the cell by facilitated transport, but at higher concentrations it can enter by passive diffusion. Once in the cell, it is metabolized to a polyglutamate derivative, which binds to dihydrofolate reductase, leading to a decrease in tetrahydrofolate and subsequent decrease in DNA synthesis.[2,5]

Administration and Dosage. Methotrexate has shown activity in a variety of tumor types in both adults and children. The dose and dosing schedule varies greatly with the malignancy that is treated and the administration route. Methotrexate is also used to treat nonmalignant conditions such as rheumatoid arthritis. Refer to the full prescribing information for the most current regimen for the type of disease being treated.

Other Conditions. Patients with any "third space" fluid (e.g., ascites, pleural effusions) should have fluid removed before drug administration because of drug retention and slow release of drug from these compartments. Reduce dosage in renal impairment. In patients with Cl_{Cr} between 10 mL/min and 50 mL/min dosage reductions of 50 to 70% are recommended and in patients with Cl_{Cr} less than 10 mL/min, dosage reductions of 85% are recommended.

Dosage Forms. **Tab** 2.5, 5, 7.5, 10, 15 mg; **Inj** 25 mg/mL solution for injection, 1 g powder for injection. When administering intrathecally, be certain that the product used is preservative free.

Pharmacokinetics. *Fate.* Methotrexate is rapidly absorbed from the GI tract by a saturable active transport system; therefore, small doses may be completely absorbed, while larger doses may have incomplete absorption. Food also decreases absorption. Plasma level peaks 1 h after an oral dose; wide distribution in the body tissues with approximately 50% plasma protein binding. Elimination begins with a short α half-life of 0.75–2 h followed by a β half-life of 3.5-10 h and a γ half-life of approximately 27 h. Methotrexate has poor CSF penetration at conventional doses, but cytotoxic concentrations can be achieved by direct instillation into the CSF. The majority of the drug is excreted in the urine unchanged within the first 12 h. Clearance approximates creatinine clearance.[2,5]

Adverse Reactions. *Systemic Administration.* The predominant toxicity is neutropenia, but anemia and thrombocytopenia are also reported. Myelotoxicity is increased in the presence of impaired renal function. With high-dose regimens, the use of leucovorin can prevent or diminish the myelotoxicity. Mucositis is common and usually appears 3–5 days after treatment. Diarrhea can be severe, but nausea and vomiting are usually mild at conventional doses. Renal toxicity following high-dose therapy may be due to precipitation of methotrexate and its metabolite (7-OH methotrexate) in the kidney. Vigorous hydration (>100 mL urine/h) and alkalinization of the urine (>7.0 pH) can lessen the chances of this occurring. Brief elevation in liver transaminases commonly occurs after high-dose therapy, but is not generally associated with liver failure, although portal fibrosis and cirrhosis have been reported. Pulmonary infiltrates and fibrosis have been reported and an erythematous rash is seen in 5%–10% of patients that generally resolves without incident.[2,5]

Intrathecal Administration In addition to any of the above side effects that may occur, side effects common to intrathecal administration include headache, fever, meningismus, vomiting, and CSF pleocytosis. More serious side effects include paralysis, cranial nerve palsies, seizures, and coma.[2,5]

Contraindications. Pregnancy; lactation; severe renal or hepatic dysfunction; psoriasis or rheumatoid arthritis patients with alcoholism, alcoholic liver disease or other chronic liver disease; preexisting immunodeficiency syndromes; blood dyscrasias (bone marrow hypoplasia, leukopenia, thrombocytopenia, or anemia) should not receive methotrexate.

Precautions. Renal function must be determined before administration. Alkalinize the urine before high doses to enhance methotrexate solubility and include vigorous hydration to ensure adequate urine output.

Drug Interactions. Concomitant use with NSAIDs may prolong serum methothrexate levels and even at low doses can reduce tubular secretion, but the clinical significance of this interaction in low-dose rheumatoid regimens is unclear. It may cause unexpected toxicity in patients treated for psoriasis. Because of protein binding, toxicity may occur due to displacement by salicylates, phenylbutazone, phenytoin, and sulfonamides. Oral antibiotics such as tetracycline, chloramphenicol, and nonabsorbable broad-spectrum antibiotics may decrease GI absorption of methotrexate.

Parameters to Monitor. Monitor pretreatment and periodic hepatic, renal, and bone marrow functions (including WBCs, platelets, and RBCs). Follow high doses with 24-h and/or 48-h serum methotrexate levels and institution of appropriate leucovorin rescue. Observe for pulmonary symptoms, especially a dry, nonproductive cough and for diarrhea and ulcerative stomatitis.

Notes. Although carboxypeptidase (glucarpidase) is not commercially available in the United States there are clinical trials in progress to allow its use in patients with delayed methotrexate clearance and intrathecal methotrexate overdose (>100 mg). Availability is through Compassionate Use Program of the Cancer Therapy Evaluation Program of the NCI.[6,7]

PENTOSTATIN Nipent

Pharmacology. Pentostatin is an irreversible inhibitor of the enzyme adenosine deaminase, which intracellularly deaminates deoxyadenosine, therefore, controlling the amount of adenosine or deoxyadenosine that is available for phosphorylation.

The inhibition of adenosine deaminase leads to accumulation of dATP pools, which inhibit DNA replication and repair.[1,2]

Adult Dosage. **IV** for hairy cell leukemia refractory to interferon alfa—4 mg/m^2 every other week.

Dosage Forms. **Inj** 10 mg.

Pharmacokinetics. *Fate.* Pentostatin displays a biphasic pharmacokinetic profile with a short α half-life of 10 min followed by a more prolonged terminal half-life averaging 6 h. Renal elimination is the major route of excretion with 50%–90% of the dose excreted unchanged in the urine making dosage adjustment necessary in patients with renal dysfunction. Plasma clearance averages 68 mL/min/m^2 and correlates with creatine clearance.[1,2]

Adverse Reactions. At lower doses (4 mg/m^2), pentostatin is well tolerated with neutropenia and nausea and vomiting as the most common adverse events. Mild to moderate lethargy, rash, and reactivation of herpes zoster have also been reported. Toxicity from higher doses includes immunosuppression, conjunctivitis, hepatic enzyme elevation, and central nervous system disturbances. Pentostatin is also nephrotoxic at higher doses and acute renal failure can be dose limiting, but renal toxicity can be decreased with adequate hydration.[1,2]

PURINE ANALOGUES

MERCAPTOPURINE   Purinethol

THIOGUANINE

Pharmacology. Mercaptopurine (6-MP) and thioguanine (6-TG) are similar to the purine guanine. Their metabolites are incorporated in DNA causing miscoding during DNA replication.[1,2]

Administration and Adult Dosage. (Mercaptopurine) **PO, IV** (investigational)—75–100 mg/m^2/d.[8] (*See* Drug Interactions.) (Thioguanine) **PO, IV** (investigational)—2–3 mg/kg/d.

Special Populations. *Pediatric Dosage.* Same as adult dosage.

Geriatric Dosage. Same as adult dosage.

Dosage Forms. (Mercaptopurine) **Tab** 50 mg; **Inj** (investigational) 500 mg. (Thioguanine) **Tab** 40 mg; **Inj** (investigational) 75 mg.

Patient Instructions. (*See* Antineoplastics Class Instructions.) To maximize absorption, do not take this drug with meals. Nausea and vomiting are uncommon with usual doses.

Pharmacokinetics. *Fate.* Mercaptopurine: Oral absorption is incomplete and highly variable with a mean bioavailability of 5%–37% and food further decreases absorption. The low bioavailability is the result of a large first-pass effect because of drug absorption through the intestinal wall into the portal circulation and metabolized by xanthine oxidase (*see* drug interaction with allopurinol). Plasma half-life is of 0.5–1.5 h. Elimination is through hepatic metabolism with renal excretion as a minor route.[1,2]

Thioguanine: Oral absorption is also incomplete and variable with food decreasing bioavailability. The metabolism differs from that of mercaptopurine in that it is not a substrate of xanthine oxidase and will not be affected by xanthine oxidase inhibitors such as allopurinol. Median drug half-life is 90 min with a range of 0.5–6 h. Hepatic metabolism accounts for the major portion of elimination.[1,2]

Adverse Reactions. The primary toxicity of either drug is myelosuppression. Anorexia and nausea and vomiting are more common with mercaptopurine, but can also occur with thioguanine (more commonly in adults than children). Hepatotoxicity is more common with mercaptopurine and renal toxicity more common with thioguanine.[1,2]

Contraindications. Pregnancy; preexisting severe bone marrow depression.

Drug Interactions. Patients taking allopurinol *must* receive substantially reduced doses of oral mercaptopurine (25%–33% of the normal dose) to avoid life-threatening myelosuppression caused by blocked inactivation. Thioguanine is inactivated primarily by methylation; thus, no dosage reduction is necessary with concomitant allopurinol. Enhanced bone marrow suppression can occur with the combination of trimethoprim/sulfamethoxazole and mercaptopurine.

■ REFERENCES

1. Hande KR. Purine Antimetabolites. In: Chabner BA, Longo DL, eds. *Cancer Chemotherapy and Biotherapy Principles and Practice*. 4th ed. Philadelphia, PA: Lippincott Williams & Wilkins; 2006:549-577.

2. Gutheil JC, Finucane DM. Antimetabolites. In: Perry MC, ed. *Chemotherapy Source Book*. 3rd ed. Philadelphia, PA: Lippincott Williams & Wilkins; 2001:208-226.

3. Ryan DP, Garcia-Carbonero R, Chabner G. Cytidine analogs. In: Chabner BA, Longo DL, eds. *Cancer Chemotherapy and Biotherapy Principles and Practice*. 4th ed. Philadelphia, PA: Lippincott Williams & Wilkins; 2006:183-211.

4. Grem JL. 5-Fluoropyrimidines. In: Chabner BA, Longo DL, eds. *Cancer Chemotherapy and Biotherapy Principles and Practice*. 4th ed. Philadelphia, PA: Lippincott Williams & Wilkins; 2006:125-182.

5. Monahan BP, Allegra CJ. Antifolates. In: Chabner BA, Longo DL, eds. *Cancer Chemotherapy and Biotherapy Principles and Practice*. 4th ed. Philadelphia, PA: Lippincott Williams & Wilkins; 2006:91-124.

6. Widemann B, Balis FM, Shalabi A, et al. Treatment of accidental intrathecal methotrexate overdose with intrathecal carboxypeptidase. Brief communication. *J Natl Cancer Inst*. 2004;96(20):1557-1559.

7. Green MR, Chamberlain MC. Renal dysfunction during and after high-dose methotrexate. *Cancer Chemother Pharmacol*. 2009;63(4):599-604.

8. Wiernik PH, Serpick AA. A randomized clinical trial of daunorubicin and a combination of prednisone, vincristine, 6-mercaptopurine, and methotrexate in adult acute nonlymphocytic leukemia. *Cancer Res*. 1967;32:2023-2026.

Chapter 21

Cytokines

Shirley Hogan

ALDESLEUKIN Proleukin

Pharmacology. Aldesleukin (interleukin-2, IL-2), produced in *Escherichia coli,* is nonglycosylated and differs in 2 amino acid positions from native IL-2, but its biologic activity is essentially similar. Its biologic effects are thought to be due to its role in potentiating the cytotoxic activity of lymphocytes by binding to a specific cell-surface receptor expressed on T cells, but the exact mechanism of aldesleukin's antitumor activity in humans is unknown.[1,2]

Administration and Adult Dosage. Each course of treatment consists of two 5-day treatment cycles separated by a rest period; 600,000 IU/kg administered every 8 h given as a 15-min infusion for a maximum of 14 doses. Nine days of rest follows, then the schedule is repeated for up to another 14 doses, for a maximum of 28 doses/course as tolerated by the patient. Evaluate for response 4 weeks after completion of a course and immediately prior to scheduled start of next treatment course, with only those patients showing some response being considered for retreatment (also *see* Contraindications section for limitations to retreatment).

Special Populations. *Pediatric Dosage.* (<18 years) safety and efficacy not established.

Geriatric Dosage. Same as adult dosage.

Dosage Forms. Inj 22 million IU.

Pharmacokinetics. *Fate.* Aldesleukin's pharmacokinetic profile is characterized by high plasma concentrations following a short IV infusion, with rapid distribution into the extravascular space and elimination from the body by metabolism in the kidneys with minimal bioactive protein excreted in the urine. Distribution half-life is of 13 min and elimination half-life is of 85 min, and average clearance rate is of 268 mL/min.[2]

Adverse Reactions. Emetogenic potential in low. The severity and nature of side effects are related to the dose and schedule. Most patients develop chills, fever, and malaise. A vascular leak syndrome occurs with higher doses and is characterized by weight gain, oliguria, tachycardia, and hypotension. Hematologic effects include anemia, thrombocytopenia, and leukopenia. Hepatic toxicities include increase in serum bilirubin levels and minimal changes in transaminase levels are common. Neurologic and neuropsychiatric effects include agitation and disorientation. Dermatologic complications have also been reported.[1]

Precautions. Patients should have normal cardiac, pulmonary, hepatic, and CNS function at the start of therapy. Capillary leak syndrome (CLS) may begin immediately after aldesleukin treatment and is marked by increased capillary permeability to protein and fluids and reduced vascular tone. Careful monitoring of the patient's fluid and organ perfusion status is accomplished by frequent measurements of blood pressure and pulse and by monitoring mental status and urine output.[1]

Contraindications. Aldesleukin is contraindicated in patients with a history of hypersensitivity to interleukin-2 or any component of the formulation, an abnormal cardiac stress test or abnormal pulmonary function tests, and those with organ allografts. Retreatment with aldesleukin is contraindicated in patients who have experienced the following drug-related toxicities while receiving an earlier course of therapy: sustained ventricular tachycardia (≥ 5 beats), cardiac arrhythmias not controlled or unresponsive to management, chest pain with ECG changes, consistent with angina or myocardial infarction, cardiac tamponade, intubation for >72 h, renal failure requiring dialysis >48 h, repetitive or difficult to control seizures, bowel ischemia/perforation, or GI bleeding requiring surgery.

Drug Interactions. Glucocorticoids block some aldesleukin actions and usually are reserved for treating severe toxicity.

Parameters to Monitor. Daily monitoring of blood pressure, pulse, respiration rate, and temperature as well as weight and fluid intake/output. During treatment, pulmonary function and cardiac function should be assessed on a regular basis.

INTERFERON ALFA	
ALFA-2a	Pegasys, Roferon-A
ALFA-2b	Intron A, PEG-Intron
ALFA-N3	Alferon N

Pharmacology. Interferons bind to specific membrane receptors on the cell surface and through that binding initiate a complex sequence of intracellular events. The exact mechanism used to exert antitumor or antiviral activity is not completely understood, but is thought to involve direct antiproliferative action against tumor cells, inhibition of virus replication, and modulation of the host immune response.[2,3]

Administration and Adult Dosage. There are a number of products available and dosage recommendations for both hairy cell leukemia and various forms of hepatitis. It is recommended that the product information specific to the disease and regimen being utilized be reviewed for the most appropriate regimen. In general, linking the interferon to polyethylene glycol allows once weekly administration and pegylated forms appear to be more effective against hepatitis C than conventional forms. Interferon alfa-N3 is only indicated for condylomata acuminate.

Special Populations. *Pediatric Dosage.* Interferon alpha-2a has safety data for use in pediatric patients with Ph-positive adult-type chronic myelogenous leukemia, showing a safety profile similar to adults, but for all other indications there is no established safety and effectiveness. Interferon alpha-2b had safety data for use in chronic hepatitis B and chronic hepatitis C, with safety profile similar to adults, except some specific adverse events that occur more often in children, such as suicidal ideation, as well as a decrease in the rate of linear growth and a decrease in the rate of weight gain, both of which reversed in the posttreatment period.

Geriatric Dosage. Same as adult dosage, but administer cautiously if decreased hepatic, renal, bone marrow, or cardiac function.

Dosage Forms. Alfa-2a conventional **Inj**—prefilled syringes 3, 6, 9 million IU/syringe (refrigerate and protect from light during storage).

Pegylated **Inj**—single dose vial 180 μg/1mL; prefilled syringe 180 μg/ 0.5mL; Alfa-2b conventional **Inj** powder for Inj—10, 18, 50 million IU/ vial; solution for **Inj**—vials 18, 25 million IU multidose vial; solution for **Inj** multidose pens—6 doses of 3 million IU, 6 doses of 5 million IU, 6 doses of 10 million IU. Pegylated **Inj** powder for Inj—50, 80, 120, 150 μg/vial. (Alfa-N3) **Inj** 5 million IU/mL.

Patient Instructions. (Subcutaneous use) proper method of aseptic preparation of vials and syringes, proper technique for subcutaneous administration, and proper disposal of syringes and needles should be taught for the specific product that the patient will be using.

Pharmacokinetics. *Fate.* Alfa interferons, in general, are totally filtered through the glomeruli and undergo rapid proteolytic degradation during tubular reabsorption, with an insignificant reappearance of intact alfa interferon in the systemic circulation. Liver metabolism and biliary excretion are minor pathways of elimination. Interferon alfa-2a—average elimination half-life of 5.1 h and average volume of distribution 0.4 L/kg. Multiple IM doses results in accumulation and increased serum concentration. Pegylated interferon alfa-2a terminal half-life after SQ dosing is 160 h. Interferon alfa-2b—IM/SQ elimination half-life of 2–3 h. IV elimination half-life of 2 h.

Adverse Reactions. Depression and suicidal behavior including suicidal ideation, suicidal attempts, and suicides have been reported in association with treatment with alfa interferons in patients without previous psychiatric illness. Cardiovascular events include hypotension and arrhythmias. Bone marrow suppression, endocrine disorders, and pulmonary toxicity have been reported. Hepatotoxicity that has been fatal has occurred; therefore, careful monitoring of hepatic function is recommended. Acute self-limiting toxicities such as fever, chills, and flulike symptoms are very common.

Contraindications. Autoimmune hepatitis or hepatic decompensation before or during treatment.

Drug Interactions. Combining with other myelosuppressive drugs may increase the risk of bone marrow toxicity. Concomitant use with theophylline decreases the theophylline clearance, resulting in a 100% increase in serum theophylline concentrations (25% with the pegylated formulations).

Parameters to Monitor. Standard hematologic parameters—hemoglobin, CBC with differential, and platelets. Blood chemistries, including electrolytes, liver function tests, and TSH. ECG prior to and during treatment for patients with pre-existing cardiac abnormalities.

■ REFERENCES

1. Alatrash G, Bukowski RM, Tannenbaum CS, Finke JH. Interleukins. In: Chabner BA, Longo DL, eds. *Cancer Chemotherapy and Biotherapy Principles and Practice*. 4th ed. Philadelphia, PA: Lippincott Williams & Wilkins; 2006:767-808.
2. Beedassy A, Ozer H. Biologic response modifiers: principles of biotherapy. In: Perry MC, ed. *Chemotherapy Source Book*. 3rd ed. Philadelphia, PA: Lippincott Williams & Wilkins; 2001:105-113.
3. Linder DJ, Taylor KL, Reu FJ, Masci PA, Borden EC. Interferons. In: Chabner BA, Longo DL, eds. *Cancer Chemotherapy and Biotherapy Principles and Practice*. 4th ed. Philadelphia, PA: Lippincott Williams & Wilkins; 2006:699-717.

Chapter 22

DNA Intercalating Drugs

Shirley Hogan

ANTHRACYCLINES	Daunorubicin, Doxorubicin, Idarubicin
DAUNORUBICIN HYDROCHLORIDE	Cerubidine
DAUNORUBICIN CITRATE, LIPOSOMAL	DaunoXome

Pharmacology. Daunorubicin has antimitotic and cytotoxic activity by several mechanisms of action including formation of complexes with DNA by intercalation between base pairs. It inhibits topoisomerase II activity by stabilizing the DNA–topoisomerase II complex causing single strand and double strand DNA breaks. It may also inhibit polymerase activity, affect regulation of gene expression, and produce free radical damage to DNA.[1,2] The liposomal preparation is formulated to maximize the selectivity of daunorubicin for solid tumors in situ. It helps to protect the entrapped daunorubicin from chemical and enzymatic degradation, minimizes protein binding, and decreases the uptake by normal tissue.

Administration and Dosage. Daunorubicin is generally given in combination with other cytotoxic agents; therefore, dosages are dependent upon the concomitant agents used. Refer to the specific combination dosage regimen used for specific dosing recommendations. The liposomal product is indicated for use in advanced HIV-associated Kaposi's sarcoma.

Special Populations. *Other Conditions.* Dosage adjustments are recommended in either hepatic or renal impairment.

Dosage Forms. **Inj** conventional—Pwdr for **Inj** 20 mg, Soln for **Inj** 5 mg/mL. Liposomal—Soln for **Inj** 2 mg/mL.

Patient Instructions. Immediately report any change in sensation (e.g., stinging) at the injection site during infusion (this might be an early sign of infiltration). Red-colored urine is expected and does not indicate toxicity.

Pharmacokinetics. *Fate.* Conventional: Initial phase half-life of 45 min and terminal phase half-life of 18.5 h. Extensively metabolized in the liver and other tissues to the major metabolite daunorubicinol, which has cytotoxic activity. Renal excretion contains 25% of unchanged drug and biliary excretion contains 40%.

Liposomal: The plasma pharmacokinetics of the liposomal formulation differ significantly from the conventional formulation. The apparent elimination half-life is 4.4 h, which is much shorter than that of daunorubicin, may actually represent a distribution half-life.

Adverse Reactions. Dose-limiting toxicities include myelosuppression and cardiotoxicity. Reversible alopecia is common. Acute nausea and vomiting occurs, but can usually be controlled with prophylactic antiemetics. Mucositis may occur 3–7 days after administration. Diarrhea and abdominal pain are infrequent. If extravasation occurs during administration, severe local tissue necrosis, severe cellulitis, thrombophlebitis, or painful induration may occur. A triad of back pain, flushing, and chest tightness has been reported in 13.8% of patients treated with the liposomal formulation. This triad usually occurs during the first 5 min of the infusion and subsides if the infusion is stopped. It generally does not recur if the infusion is then resumed at a slower rate. These symptoms appear to be related to the lipid component of the liposomal formulation, as a similar set of symptoms have been observed in patients with other liposomal formulations not containing daunorubicin.

Precautions.   Careful administration technique is mandatory to avoid extravasation and tissue necrosis.

Parameters to Monitor.   Obtain pretreatment and at least biweekly CBC and platelet counts. Monitor general cardiac status and obtain pretreatment echocardiograph. Track doses administered to monitor cardiotoxicity dosage limit.

| **DOXORUBICIN HYDROCHLORIDE** | Adriamycin |
| **DOXORUBICIN, LIPOSOMAL** | Doxil |

Pharmacology.   The cytotoxic effect is thought to be related to nucleotide base intercalation and cell membrane lipid binding. Intercalation inhibits nucleotide replication and action of DNA and RNA polymerases. It interacts with topoisomerase II to form DNA-cleavable complexes. Free radical formation is thought to contribute to the cardiotoxicity.[1,2] The liposomal formulation is encapsulated in long-circulating liposomes formulated with surface-bound methoxypolyethylene glycol (pegylated) to protect the liposomes from detection by the mononuclear phagocyte system and to increase blood circulation time.

Administration and Dosage.   Doxorubicin has shown activity in a variety of tumor types in both adults and children. The dose and dosing schedule varies greatly with the malignancy that is treated and the administration route. Refer to the full prescribing information for the most current regimen for the type disease being treated.

Dosage Forms.   Inj 10-, 20-, 50-mg single dose vials; 150-mg multidose vial. Liposomal—20 mg/10 mL, 50 mg/30 mL single use vials.

Pharmacokinetics.   *Fate.*   Initial distribution phase half-life of 5 min and terminal half-life of 20–48 h suggests rapid tissue uptake and slow tissue elimination. Volume of distribution values exceeding 20–30 L/kg also suggest extensive uptake into tissue. Approximately 40% of the dose undergoes biliary excretion and 5%–12% renal. Enzymatic reduction and cleavage of the daunosamine sugar yields aglycone, which are accompanied by free radical formation that contributes to the cardiotoxicity.[1,2] The pharmacokinetics of the liposomal formulation also displays a 2 phase disposition with a short initial phase of approximately 5 h and a prolonged second phase of approximately 55 h when given at a dose range of 10–20 mg/m^2, but is nonlinear at the 50 mg/m^2 dose with a longer elimination half-life and lower clearance. The small steady-state volume of distribution suggests that it remains in the vascular fluid volume. The plasma clearance is slow when compared to the conventional formulation with the liposomal average clearance value of 0.041 L/h/m^2 in contrast to the conventional product having a clearance value of 24–35 L/h/m.[2]

Adverse Reactions. Irreversible myocardial toxicity, which presents as potentially fatal congestive heart failure, may occur either during therapy or months to years after termination of therapy. The probability of developing impaired myocardial function increases with increasing cumulative doses.

Contraindications. Doxorubicin should not be started in patients with severe myelosuppression that is due to prior treatment with other chemotherapy agents or radiotherapy. Doxorubicin is contraindicated in patients who received prior treatment with maximum cumulative doses of doxorubicin, daunorubicin, idarubicin, and /or other anthracyclines and anthracenes.

Drug Interactions. Phenobarbital increases the elimination of doxorubicin, phenytoin levels may be decreased by doxorubicin, streptozocin may inhibit the hepatic metabolism of doxorubicin, and concomitant use with cyclosporine may induce coma and/or seizures.

Parameters to Monitor. Evaluation of hepatic function (ALT, AST, alkaline phosphatase, and bilirubin) is recommended prior to each dose.

IDARUBICIN HYDROCHLORIDE   Idamycin

Pharmacology. Idarubicin is a DNA-intercalating analog of daunorubicin. It inhibits nucleic acid synthesis and interacts with the enzyme topoisomerase II. Its high lipophilicity allows a greater rate of cellular uptake than other anthracyclines.[1]

Administration and Adult Dosage. Inj 12 mg/m^2/d × 3 days generally in combination with cytarabine.

Special Populations. *Pediatric Dosage.* Safety and efficacy not established.

Geriatric Dosage. Same as adult dosage.

Other Conditions. In patients that experience severe mucositis, the second course should be delayed until recovery and a dose reduction of 25% is recommended. Patients with a bilirubin level that exceeds 5 mg/dL, should not receive idarubicin. Dosage adjustments for hepatic and/or renal impairment should be considered.

Dosage Forms. Inj 5-, 10-, 20-mg vials also available in Cytosafe vials. Refrigerate and protect from light.

Pharmacokinetics. *Fate.* The elimination rate of idarubicin from plasma is slow with an average terminal half-life of 22 h when used as a single agent and 20 h when used in combination with cytarabine. The primary active metabolite is idarubicinol, which has cytotoxic activity and therefore contributes to the overall effects of idarubicin. The elimination of idarubicinol is slower than the parent drug with an average terminal half-life >45 h providing plasma levels for >8 days. Elimination is predominately by biliary excretion and to a lesser extent as idarubicinol by the kidneys.

Adverse Reactions. Severe myelosuppression is the major toxicity, but is viewed as necessary for maximum effect. Nausea, vomiting, mucositis, abdominal pain, and diarrhea occur frequently, but are severe in <5% of patients. Alopecia and dermatologic reactions also occur frequently. Some cardiac effects have been reported, but most were in patients with sepsis and more frequently in patients >60 years of age.

Precautions. Sensitization of soft tissues to radiation damage can occur. To lessen frequency of irreversible cardiomyopathy, track total anthracycline doses and be aware of lifetime limits. Extravasation of idarubicin can cause severe local tissue necrosis and can occur without stinging/burning sensation.

Parameters to Monitor. Frequent CBC with differential and monitoring of hepatic and renal function are recommended.

DACTINOMYCIN   Cosmegen

Pharmacology. Dactinomycin (actinomycin D) exerts its cytotoxic effects by binding DNA and inhibiting RNA synthesis.[1]

Adult Dosage. IV—a wide variety of regimens, both single agent and combination, have been administered; therefore, refer to the full prescribing information for the most current regimen for the type disease being treated. The dose of dactinomycin is calculated in micrograms and the dose intensity per 2-week cycle should not exceed 15 μg/kg/d or 400–600 μg/m^2/d for 5 days. For obese patients, the dose should be calculated on the basis of body surface area.

Dosage Forms. Inj 0.5-mg vial.

Pharmacokinetics. Minimal metabolism occurs and approximately 30% of the drug is recovered from feces and urine in 1 week. The terminal plasma half-life determined by radioactivity is approximately 36 h.

Adverse Reactions. Severe bone marrow suppression occurs, primarily of leukocytes. Nausea, vomiting, alopecia, and mucositis are common. Radiation recall may occur even 2 years after the radiation treatment. Caution should be taken to avoid extravasation injury.[1]

MITOXANTRONE   Novantrone

Pharmacology. Mitoxantrone binds to nucleic acids and inhibits DNA and RNA synthesis. It binds to DNA through intercalation between opposing DNA strands. It also interferes with RNA and is a potent inhibitor of topoisomerase II.[2]

Administration and Adult Dosage. 12 mg/m^2 (in refractory prostate cancer may increase to 14 mg/m^2) given every 21–28 days. In acute myelogenous leukemia, doses may be given days 1–3 in combination with cytarabine. IV for multiple sclerosis 12 mg/m^2 q^3 months to a usual lifetime maximum of 140 mg/m^2.

Special Populations. *Pediatric Dosage.* Although safety and efficacy have not been established, several pediatric regimens exist utilizing mitoxantrone in the treatment of AML.[3]

Geriatric Dosage. Same as adult dosage.

Dosage Forms. Inj 20-mg vial.

Patient Instructions. This drug might turn urine blue-green for 24 h after administration because of its dark blue color. Bluish discoloration of the sclera may also occur.

Pharmacokinetics. *Fate.* Pharmacokinetic profile fits a 3-compartment model with $t_{1/2}$. α phase 6–12 min; β phase 1.1–3.1 h; γ phase 23–215 h with a median of approximately 75 h. Mitoxantrone is 78% protein bound, and this binding is independent of concentration and is not affected by the presence of other highly protein-bound drugs such as phenytoin, heparin, or aspirin. Only 11% of a dose is recovered in the urine, but 65% of this is unchanged drug; 25% of a dose is recovered in the feces.

Adverse Reactions. Primary and dose-limiting side effects are leukopenia and thrombocytopenia. If anemia occurs, it is usually later than these. Nausea, vomiting, and anorexia occur. Stomatitis and/or mucositis are infrequent with lower doses, but may be observed at higher doses often used in leukemia. Hepatic function abnormalities manifest most often as transient increases in transaminases and occasionally increased alkaline phosphatase and bilirubin. Dosage adjustments are needed for hepatic dysfunction, but no specific data-based recommendations exist. Mitoxantrone has less potential for producing cardiotoxicity than doxorubicin, but the reduction in risk is only moderate; therefore, careful monitoring of cardiac function is warranted. Hypotension, urticaria, dyspnea, and rashes have been reported occasionally.[1]

Contraindication. Multiple sclerosis patients with abnormal liver function tests.

Parameters to Monitor. CBC and liver function tests prior to each course. Female multiple sclerosis patients who are biologically capable of becoming pregnant should have a pregnancy test, even those using birth control. The results of the test should be known prior to receiving each dose.

PLICAMYCIN   Mithracin

Pharmacology. The main cytotoxic effect is due to inhibition of DNA-directed RNA synthesis. It was originally studied as a therapy for advanced testicular, bladder, and prostate cancers; it is now used as a treatment of malignant hypercalcemia.[1]

Adult Dosage. IV for hypercalcemia—25 μg/kg/d for 3–4 days. Dosage adjustments are necessary in renal or hepatic impairment. *Note:* Dosage is in μg/kg.

Dosage Forms. Inj 2.5 mg.

Pharmacokinetics. *Fate.* Unknown.

Adverse Reactions. Common toxicities include nausea, vomiting, mucositis, and bone marrow suppression. The platelet count may be most affected and decreased out of proportion to the erythrocytes and leukocytes. Fever, rash, flushing, and local venous irritation or phlebitis have been reported. Acute hypocalcemia can complicate plicamycin therapy in the absence of other signs of renal injury and the need for intravenous calcium replacement is common.[1]

■ REFERENCES

1. Riggs CE, Jr. Antitumor antibiotics and related compounds. In: Perry MC, ed. *Chemotherapy Source Book.* 3rd ed. Philadelphia, PA: Lippincott Williams & Wilkins; 2001:227-251.

2. Doroshow JH. Anthracyclines and anthracenediones. In: Chabner BA, Longo DL, eds. *Cancer Chemotherapy and Biotherapy Principles and Practice.* 4th ed. Philadelphia, PA: Lippincott Williams & Wilkins; 2006:414-450.

3. Wells RJ, Adams MT, Alonzo T, Areci RJ, et al. Mitoxantrone and cytarabine induction, high-dose cytarabine, and etoposide intensification for pediatric patients with relapsed or refractory acute myeloid leukemia: Children's Cancer Group Study 2951. *J Clin Oncol.* 2003;21(15):2940-2947.

Chapter 23

Hormonal Drugs and Antagonists

Shirley Hogan

ANTIANDROGENS	
BICALUTAMIDE	Casodex
FLUTAMIDE	Eulexin
NILUTAMIDE	Nilandron

Pharmacology. These drugs are nonsteroidal antiandrogens that competitively inhibit binding of testosterone at androgen receptors in the testes and prostate gland, reducing androgen-stimulated cell growth. They are used with a luteinizing hormone–releasing hormone (LHRH) analogue (e.g., leuprolide or goserelin). In combination with the LHRH analogues, these agents inhibit the initial surge of testosterone and "flare" reactions associated with LHRH agonists. Discontinuation of the antiandrogen in patients who progress while taking both of these agents induces a clinical antitumor response in approximately 25% of patients.[1]

Administration and Adult Dosage. **PO for prostatic carcinoma** together with an LHRH analogue—(bicalutamide) 50 mg once daily; (flutamide) 250 mg 3 times daily; (nilutamide) 300 mg once daily for 30 days, then 150 mg once daily.

Special Populations. *Geriatric Dosage.* Same as adult dosage.

Other Conditions. If PSA levels rise with clinical disease progression, consider discontinuing the antiandrogen temporarily and continuing the LHRH antagonist to reestablish androgen-receptor sensitivity. Renal or hepatic impairment does not appear to alter elimination.[1]

Dosage Forms. (Bicalutamide) **Tab** 50 mg; (flutamide) **Cap** 125 mg; (nilutamide) **Tab** 150 mg.

Patient Instructions. Take therapy continuously without interruption. Start at the same time as the LHRH agonist. Hot flashes and some feminizing side effects (especially breast enlargement or tenderness) can occur during therapy.

Pharmacokinetics. *Fate.* These agents are well absorbed orally and absorption is unaffected by food. **Bicalutamide** undergoes stereospecific metabolism with the active (R)-enantiomer of bicalutamide oxidized to an inactive metabolite, which, like the inactive (S)-enantiomer, is glucuronidated and cleared rapidly by elimination in the urine and feces.[2] **Flutamide** and its active metabolite, hydroxyflutamide, are highly bound to plasma proteins (86(–94%). The majority of a flutamide dose is excreted in the urine as 2-amino-5-nitro-4-(trifluoromethyl)phenol (inactive) with little parent and active metabolite (4.2% of a dose) excreted in the bile or feces.[3] **Nilutamide** is extensively metabolized and less than 2% of the drug is excreted unchanged in the urine. There is moderate binding to plasma proteins.

$t_{1/2}$. (bicalutamide) 6 days; (flutamide) 6 h; (nilutamide) 41–49 h.

Adverse Reactions. These agents are relatively well tolerated. When the drugs are combined with an LHRH agonist, the following side effects occur: hot flashes, impotence, general pain, back pain, asthenia, pelvic pain, constipation, diarrhea, nausea, nocturia, liver enzyme elevation, abdominal pain, and chest pain. Hepatic injury and jaundice occur rarely with flutamide or bicalutamide. Patients receiving nilutamide have a greater incidence of hepatic injury and interstitial pneumonitis.[1,3]

Contraindications. Nilutamide is contraindicated in patients with severe hepatic impairment or severe respiratory insufficiency.

Drug Interactions. Dosage adjustment of warfarin, based on INR, might be necessary because of possible displacement of warfarin from protein binding sites.

Parameters to Monitor. Monitor PSA levels every 3 months as an index of disease response and/or need to discontinue medication. Obtain serum transaminases every 3–4 months.

AROMATASE INHIBITORS	
AMINOGLUTETHIMIDE	Cytadren
ANASTROZOLE	Arimidex
EXEMESTANE	Aromasin
LETROZOLE	Femara

Pharmacology. These agents inhibit the aromatase-mediated metabolic conversion of androstenedione to estradiol, primarily in peripheral adipose tissues. Aminoglutethimide is less specific and blocks the cholesterol-based biosynthesis of all corticosteroid precursors (e.g., hydrocortisone, aldosterone) in the adrenal gland and at peripheral sites. Anastrozole, exemestane, and letrozole are much more specific inhibitors of estrogen synthesis that do not affect synthesis of other steroids.[1]

Administration and Adult Dosage. Aminoglutethimide: **PO**—250 mg qid. Anastrozole: **PO**—1 mg/d. Exemestane: **PO**—25 mg/d after a meal. Letrozole: **PO**—2.5 mg/d.

Geriatric Dosage. Same as adult dosage.

Other Conditions. (Anastrozole, exemestane) no change required in hepatic or renal impairment. (Letrozole) no dosage adjustment is required with $Cl_{Cr} \geq 10$ mL/min; in patients with cirrhosis and severe hepatic dysfunction is reduced by 50% (2.5 mg every other day).

Dosage Forms. (Aminoglutethimide) **Tab** 250 mg; (anastrozole) **Tab** 1 mg; (exemestane) **Tab** 25 mg; (letrozole) **Tab** 2.5 mg.

Patient Instructions. (Aminoglutethimide) if severe stress or trauma occurs, increased hydrocortisone dosage might be needed. Marked drowsiness can occur during therapy. Skin rashes are common, especially at the start of therapy. (Exemestane) take this drug after a meal. (Letrozole) this drug may be taken without regard to meals.

Pharmacokinetics. *Fate.* (Aminoglutethimide) plasma protein binding is minimal. Approximately 50% is metabolized in liver to a less active **N**-acetyl derivative; this and other metabolites are excreted renally.[3] (Anastrozole) elimination is primarily by hepatic metabolism (85%) with approximately 11% renal excretion. (Exemestane) absorption is increased by 40% when taken with a high-fat meal; extensively metabolized by CYP3A4 and aldo–keto reductases, with unchanged drug accounting for <10% of drug in plasma. Metabolites have less or no inhibitory activity against aromatase. Less than 1% excreted unchanged in urine. (Letrozole) well absorbed. V_d is 1.9 L/kg. The drug is metabolized to a glucuronide metabolite, which is excreted in urine. Only 6% is excreted unchanged in urine.

$t_{1/2}$. (aminoglutethimide) 13.3 h; (anastrozole) 50 h; (exemestane) 24 h; (letrozole) approximately 2 days.

Adverse Reactions. (Aminoglutethimide) adrenal insufficiency and hematologic suppression are the most serious. Lethargy and somnolence, skin rashes, dizziness, nausea, anorexia, fever, and hypotension are also common. (Anastrozole) asthenia, nausea, headache, hot flashes, back pain, emesis, dizziness, rash, constipation, hypertension, lymphoedema, depression, and insomnia. (Exemestane) hot flashes, nausea, fatigue, depression, insomnia, dizziness, and headache. (Letrozole) musculoskeletal pain, nausea, hot flashes, headache, night sweats, weight gain, and edema are frequent.

Contraindications. These drugs should generally not be given to premenopausal women.

Precautions. (Aminoglutethimide) supplemental **hydrocortisone** (50–100 mg/d) and **fludrocortisone** (0.1 mg/d) are required during therapy.

Drug Interactions. (Aminoglutethimide) several drug interactions can occur because of the drug's enhancement of CYP3A metabolism; the effects of dexamethasone, digoxin, medroxyprogesterone, tamoxifen, theophylline, and warfarin might be reduced. Aminoglutethimide also induces its own metabolism, which decreases blood levels and half-lives during long-term therapy.[3] (Anastrozole) although metabolized by CYP3A4, anastrozole had no effect on clearance of antipyrine; therefore, it is unlikely that clinically significant inhibition by CYP450 will occur. (Exemestane) although metabolized by CYP3A4, ketoconazole does not decease its metabolism, so CYP3A4 inhibitor interactions are unlikely. (Letrozole) studies of possible interactions with cimetidine, warfarin, and diazepam showed no clinically significant effect.

ESTRAMUSTINE PHOSPHATE
Emcyt

Pharmacology. Estramustine originally was thought to act as a hormonally directed alkylating agent, but later studies suggest an alternate effect that major cause of cell death is through a direct effect on microtubules. Once bound to tubulin, estramustine inhibits the growth and shortening of microtubules. It also inhibits proliferation by stabilizing microtubules that compromise the mitotic spindle apparatus.[4,5]

Administration and Adult Dosage. PO—14 mg/kg/d in 3–4 divided doses. *Note*: treat for 30–90 days before evaluation efficacy.

Special Populations. *Geriatric Dosage.* Same as adult dosage.

Other Conditions. Closely monitor diabetic and hypertensive patients as they might require increased doses of insulin or antihypertensives because of estrogenic effects.

Dosage Forms. Cap 140 mg.

Patient Instructions. Take this drug on an empty stomach—at least 1 h before or 2 h after a meal; particularly avoid taking with milk, milk products, or calcium-containing foods or drugs (e.g., calcium-containing antacids).

Pharmacokinetics. *Fate.* Most of the absorbed dose is metabolized to estromustine, the principal metabolite detected in the plasma. The elimination half-life of estromustine averages 14 h. Major route of elimination is in the feces with <1% excreted in the urine.[4,5]

Adverse Reactions. Emetogenic potential is low. The major side effects are caused by estrogenic actions such as very frequent gynecomastia and impotence, cardiovascular effects (frequent edema, occasional leg cramps, or thrombophlebitis, and rare pulmonary embolism and infarction), and GI effects (frequent nausea without vomiting, diarrhea, and occasional anorexia). Estramustine may influence the metabolism of calcium and phosphorus.

Contraindications. Thrombophlebitis or thromboembolic conditions (except when tumor is the cause).

Precautions. Use with caution in patients with severe underlying cardiovascular diseases. Poorly controlled CHF can be exacerbated by estrogen-induced fluid retention. Other diseases that may be affected by fluid retention, such as epilepsy, migraine, or renal dysfunction require additional monitoring. Patients with diabetes and patients on antihypertensive medications can have increased medication requirements.

Drug Interactions. Dairy products or calcium salts can reduce estramustine bioavailability.

Parameters to Monitor. Attention to cardiovascular or thromboembolic signs and symptoms is important. Prostate cancer patients with osteoblastic metastases are at risk for hypocalcemia; therefore, monitor calcium levels.

GONADOTROPIN-RELEASING HORMONE ANALOGUES	
GOSERELIN ACETATE	Zoladex
LEUPROLIDE ACETATE	Lupron, Viadur, Eligard
TRIPTORELIN PAMOATE	Trelstar

Pharmacology. These drugs are synthetic peptide analogues of the natural hypothalamic hormone, gonadotropin-releasing hormone (GnRH). This hormone controls the release of pituitary luteinizing hormone (LH) and follicle-stimulating hormone (FSH) to stimulate sex hormone production in the testes (testosterone) and ovaries (estradiol, others). FSH and LH are initially stimulated, followed by suppression or "downregulation" of these hormones and consequent suppression of ovarian and testicular steroidogenesis.[1,6]

Administration and Adult Dosage. **SQ for prostatic carcinoma**—(goserelin) insert 3.6-mg implant into upper abdominal wall every 28 days; (leuprolide aqueous) 1 mg/d. **IM for prostatic carcinoma**—(leuprolide depot) 7.5 mg of 1-month formulation every 28–33 days, 22.5 mg of the 3-month formulation every 3 months or 30 mg of the 4-month formulation every 16 weeks; (triptorelin pamoate depot) 3.75 mg once monthly or 11.25 mg of the 3-month formulation (LA) every 3 months.

SQ for endometriosis—(goserelin) insert 3.6-mg implant into upper abdominal wall every 28 days for 6 months. **IM for endometriosis**—(leuprolide depot) 3.75 mg monthly for 6 months.

Special Populations. *Pediatric Dosage.* **SQ for central precocious puberty (CPP)**—(leuprolide depot-ped). **IM for CPP**—initial dosage is (≤ 25 kg) 7.5 mg monthly; (25–37.5 kg) 11.25 mg monthly; (>37.5 kg) 15 mg monthly. Increase in 3.75 mg/mo increments until total downregulation is achieved, then continue the same as the maintenance dose.

Geriatric Dosage. (Prostatic carcinoma) same as adult dosage.

Dosage Forms. (Goserelin) **Implant** 3.6 mg. (Leuprolide) **Inj (aqueous)** 14-mg vial; **Inj** powder for suspension 3.75, 7.5, 11.25, 22.5, and 30 mg; **Inj** (depot-ped) 7.5 mg, 11.25 mg, and 15 mg. (Triptorelin) **Inj (depot)** 3.75 mg (LA) 11.25 mg.

Patient Instructions. (Prostate cancer) disease symptoms such as bone pain and urinary retention might become worse briefly following initiation of therapy. (Endometriosis) do not become pregnant while on this drug; always use a barrier contraceptive. Notify your physician if regular menstruation continues. Because therapy can cause a loss of bone density, calcium supplementation is recommended. (Pediatric CPP) a slight increase in pubertal signs and symptoms might occur initially. Adherence to therapy is critical; symptoms such as menses or breast or testicular development might indicate inadequate therapy.

Pharmacokinetics. *Fate.* These drugs are inactive orally. The SQ, IM, and IV routes provide comparable bioavailability. The metabolism of these compounds has not been described. (Goserelin) goserelin is slowly absorbed over the first 8 days. Thereafter, absorption is steady for the remaining 28 days, with no evidence of dose-to-dose accumulation. Goserelin serum levels of approximately 2.5 μg/L occur on days 15–16 in males with prostate cancer. (Leuprolide) the absorption profile of leuprolide 3-month formulation is similar to the 7.5 mg 1-month formulation. Leuprolide serum levels after a 7.5 mg depot injection are 20 μg/L at 4 h and 0.36 μg/L at 4 weeks. (Triptorelin) triptorelin peak levels occur within 1 week and persist for 4 weeks.

$t_{1/2}$. (goserelin) 4.2 h; (leuprolide) 3 h; (triptorelin) 3 compartments with half-lives of 6 min, 45 min, and 3 h.

Adverse Reactions. Emetogenic potential is low; nausea occurs in <5% of patients. Prostate cancer symptoms flare initially, causing bone pain or urinary retention. Sexual dysfunction and decreased erections are reported in approximately 20% of males. Hot flashes initially can occur in up to 80% of patients with endometriosis, who also might experience calcium loss and estrogen-deficiency side effects (e.g., decreased libido, vaginal discomfort, dizziness, general malaise, emotional lability, and depression). Mild injection site reactions are rare, except with leuprolide depot for pediatric use, where 5% of patients may experience a site reaction including abscess.

Contraindications. Pregnancy (teratogenic activity has been established in animals). Do not initiate therapy for endometriosis until after negative pregnancy test.

Precautions. Monitor carefully, initially in prostate cancer patients. Those with severe metastatic vertebral lesions are subject to spinal cord compression, and those with severe urinary retention might develop renal impairment.

Parameters to Monitor. (Prostate cancer) monitor serum LH, FSH, estradiol, and testosterone; concentrations should fall to castrate levels with adequate GnRH analogue therapy. Close initial monitoring of disease symptom severity (bone pain, urinary retention) is required. Serum PSA levels should fall and remain low in patients who respond. (Endometriosis) monitor pain and menstrual symptoms.

TAMOXIFEN CITRATE	Various

Pharmacology. Tamoxifen is a synthetic, nonsteroidal antiestrogen. The principal action of antiestrogens is to inhibit estrogen's action at the cellular level. Tamoxifen affects organ systems besides the breast such as endometrium (endometrial cancer and hypertrophy), the coagulation system (thrombosis), bone (modulation of mineral density), and liver (alterations of blood lipid profile). In these systems it acts as an agonist, mimicking the effect of estrogen in contrast to its action on breast epithelial cells, where it acts as an antagonist. Because of these actions in different tissues, tamoxifen is correctly described as a selective estrogen–receptor modulator (SERM) with organ-specific mixed agonist and antagonist effects.[1,6]

Administration and Adult Dosage. PO for breast cancer—usually 20–40 mg/d (doses >20 should be divided bid). PO for reduction of breast cancer risk in high-risk women—20 mg/d for 5 years.

Special Populations. *Geriatric Dosage.* Same as adult dosage.

Dosage Forms. Tab 10, 20 mg.

Patient Instructions. In premenopausal patients, the chance of becoming pregnant is increased and a barrier contraceptive should be used. You should have regular gynecologic examinations after taking this drug and report any menstrual irregularities, abnormal vaginal discharge or bleeding, or pelvic pain or pressure. Lactation can occur while you are taking tamoxifen.

Pharmacokinetics. *Fate.* Metabolism is mediated in the liver by CYP450-dependent oxidases. The metabolites are excreted primarily in the bile as conjugates with only minimal amounts excreted as intact drug. The initial half-life of tamoxifen ranges between 4 and 14 h, with a secondary half-life of approximately 7 days. Steady-state concentrations are not achieved until 4–16 weeks of therapy. The biologic half-life of the metabolite N-desmethyltamoxifen is 14 days with steady state reached in 8 weeks. These long half-lives are due to the high level of plasma protein binding (>99%).

$t_{1/2}$. (tamoxifen) 7 days; (N-desmethyltamoxifen) 14 days.[6]

Adverse Reactions. At standard doses, tamoxifen is usually well tolerated and safe. Serious side effects include pulmonary embolus, deep venous thrombosis, and cerebral vascular accident. Cataract and endometrial cancer have been reported. Other less serious side effects include hot flashes, nausea, and vaginal discharge. Depression is also considered a side effect of tamoxifen, though no clear evidence is available as to this association.[6]

Precautions. Pregnancy. Use with caution in patients with preexisting leukopenia and thrombocytopenia.

Drug Interactions. Drugs that are substrates for CY3A could potentially interfere with tamoxifen metabolism. Tamoxifen lowers plasma levels of letrozole. Aminoglutethimide and medroxyprogesterone can decrease tamoxifen serum levels.

Supratherapeutic effects of warfarin have been reported with tamoxifen use; therefore, it is critical to closely monitor coagulation indices when these are administered together.[6]

Notes. The response rate in breast cancer is approximately 50%–70% in ER-positive patients, whereas the rate in ER-negative patients is only approximately 5%–10%.[7] Tamoxifen has been used in endometrial, stage D prostatic, and renal cell cancers and melanoma. It has been used investigationally to decrease the size and pain of gynecomastia.

TOREMIFENE CITRATE   Fareston

Pharmacology. Toremifene is a chloro derivative of tamoxifen that binds to high-affinity estrogen receptors in hormonally dependent tissues and may exhibit estrogenic, antiestrogenic, or both activities. The antitumor effects in breast cancer are thought to be mainly due to its antiestrogenic effects such as its ability to compete with estrogen for binding sites in the cancer, blocking the growth-stimulating effects of estrogen in the tumor.

Administration and Adult Dosage. **PO for breast cancer**—60 mg/d.

Special Populations. *Geriatric Dosage.* Same as adult dosage.

Dosage Forms. **Tab** 60 mg.

Pharmacokinetics. *Fate.* Well absorbed orally and absorption not affected by food. Extensively metabolized by CYP3A4 to *N*-demethyltoremifene, which has serum concentration 2–4 times higher than toremifene at steady state. Toremifene is eliminated as metabolites primarily in the feces with approximately 10% excreted in the urine during a 1-week period. The average distribution half-life is 4 h and the elimination half-life is approximately 5 days. The elimination is slowed by enterohepatic circulation.

Adverse Reactions. Toremifene is generally well tolerated with most adverse reaction due to the antiestrogenic actions, including hot flashes in 34%, vaginal discharge or bleeding occurs in 13%, dizziness in 9%, and edema in 5% of patients. It causes minimal GI toxicity, consisting of nausea in 14% and vomiting in 4% of patients. Acute tumor flare occurs, marked by transient increases in bone or musculoskeletal pain, cutaneous erythema, and/or hypercalcemia.

Drug Interactions. Drugs that induce CYP3A4 can decrease toremifene levels and those that inhibit CYP3A4 can increase levels. Toremifene can increase prothrombin time in patients taking warfarin. Drugs that decrease renal calcium excretion (thiazide diuretics) may increase the risk of hypercalcemia.

■ REFERENCES

1. DiPaola RS, Reiss M, Aisner J. Hormones. In: Perry MC, ed. *Chemotherapy Source Book.* 3rd ed. Philadelphia, PA: Lippincott Williams & Wilkins; 2001:312-322.
2. Kalaycio M, Pohlman B. Kuczkowski E, et al. High-dose busulfan and the risk of pulmonary mortality after autologous stem cell transplant. *Clin Transplant.* 2006;20:783-787.
3. Dorr RT, Von Hoff DD. Drug monographs. In: Dorr RT, Von Hoff DD, eds. *Cancer Chemotherapy Handbook.* 2nd ed. Norwalk, CT: Appleton and Lange. 1994:518-520.
4. Rowinsky EK. Antimicrotuble agents. In: Chabner BA, Longo DL, eds. *Cancer Chemotherapy and Biotherapy Principles and Practice.* 4th ed. Philadelphia, PA: Lippincott Williams & Wilkins; 2006:237-282.

5. Rowinsky EK, Tolcher AW. Microtubule-targeting drugs. In: Perry MC, ed. *Chemotherapy Source Book*. 3rd ed. Philadelphia, PA: Lippincott Williams & Wilkins; 2001:252-278.
6. Lebowitz PF, Swain S. Hormonal therapy for breast cancer. In: Chabner BA, Longo DL, eds. *Cancer Chemotherapy and Biotherapy Principles and Practice*. 4th ed. Philadelphia, PA: Lippincott Williams & Wilkins; 2006:809-846.
7. Lippman ME, Allegra JC. Receptors in breast cancer: estrogen receptor and endocrine therapy of breast cancer. *N Engl J Med*. 1978;299:930-933.

Chapter 24

Mitotic Inhibitors

Shirley Hogan

DOCETAXEL	Taxotere

Pharmacology. Docetaxel is a semisynthetic derivative of a taxane extracted from the needles of the yew tree, *Taxus baccata*. It acts by disrupting the microtubular network in cells that is essential for mitotic and interphase cellular function. It binds to free tubulin and promotes the assembly of tubulin into stable microtubules while simultaneously inhibiting their disassembly. This leads to the production of microtubule bundles that do not function normally and to the stabilization of microtubules. This results in the inhibition of mitosis in cells.[1,2]

Administration and Adult Dosage. Docetaxel has shown activity in a variety of tumor types. The dose and dosing schedule varies greatly with the malignancy that is treated and the administration route. Refer to the full prescribing information for the most current regimen for the type of disease being treated.

Premedicate all patients with dexamethasone 16 mg/d (8 mg bid) for 3 days, starting 1 day before administering docetaxel, in order to reduce the incidence and severity of fluid retention as well as severity of hypersensitivity reactions.

Special Populations. *Pediatric Dosage.* Safety and efficacy not established.

Geriatric Dosage. Same as adult dosage.

Other Conditions. Patients with bilirubin > Upper limit of normal (ULN) should generally not receive docetaxel or those patients with ALT and/or AST >1.5 × ULN concomitant with alkaline phosphatase >2.5 ULN.

Dosage Forms. **Inj** 20 mg/0.5 mL, 80 mg/2 mL.

Patient Instructions. Immediately report fever or chills occurring 1–2 weeks after drug administration to your provider. This drug can cause swelling of the extremities and tingling sensations.

Pharmacokinetics. *Fate.* Pharmacokinetic profile fits a 3-compartment model with half-lives listed below. The short alpha phase indicates distribution to the peripheral compartments and the terminal phase is due to a slow efflux of the drug from these peripheral compartments. Average steady-state volume of distribution is 113 L. Docetaxel is eliminated mainly in feces (75%) and minimally in urine. Highly protein bound (>80%).[1]

$t_{1/2}$. α phase 4 min; β phase 36 min; γ phase 1.1 h.

Adverse Reactions. Reversible bone marrow suppression is the most common and dose-limiting toxicity. Other common adverse reactions are infections and hypersensitivity reactions. Skin toxicity includes rash and nail disorders characterized by hypo- or hyperpigmentation. Nausea, vomiting, and diarrhea are generally mild to moderate. Severe stomatitis is common. Significant cardiovascular events are rare. Increases in ALT/AST are common.

Contraindications. Docetaxel should not be administered to patients with neutrophil counts of <1500 cells/mm^3.

Precautions. Febrile neutropenia is frequent, necessitating careful follow-up of infectious signs after administration.

Drug Interactions. In vitro metabolism of docetaxel to its hydroxy metabolites is reduced by inhibitors of CYP3A such as cimetidine, erythromycin, ketoconazole, and troleandomycin. The clinical importance of these findings is not known.

Parameters to Monitor. WBC count, peripheral edema, LFTs (ALT, AST, alkaline phosphatase), and signs of infection.

ETOPOSIDE	VePesid
ETOPOSIDE PHOSPHATE	Etopophos

Pharmacology. Etoposide (VP-16) is a semisynthetic derivative of podophyllotoxin. Etoposide phosphate is a water soluble ester of etoposide, which lessens the potential for precipitation following dilution and during infusion. Etoposide phosphate is rapidly and completely converted to etoposide in the plasma. The major cytotoxic activity is the induction of DNA strand breaks by an interaction with DNA–topoisomerase II or the formation of free radicals.[3,4]

Administration and Adult Dosage. IV—50–100 mg/m^2/d × 5 days.

Special Populations. *Pediatric Dosage.* Safety and efficacy are not established. However, etoposide is included in many standard treatment regimens for pediatric malignancies. Dosage calculations are similar to adult dose and are adjusted on the basis of body surface area.

Geriatric Dosage. Same as adult dosage but adjust for age related reduction in renal function.

Other Conditions. Patients with impaired renal function should have the following dosage adjustments: Cl_{Cr} >50 mL/min, 100% of standard dose; Cl_{Cr} 15–50 mL/min, 75% of dose; no data for adjustments in patients with Cl_{Cr} <15 mL/min.

Dosage Forms. **Inj** (etoposide) 100-mg, 500-mg, 1-g vials; (etoposide phosphate) 100-mg vial; **Cap** (etoposide) 50 mg (store in refrigerator).

Pharmacokinetics. *Fate.* Oral bioavailability is 50%. CSF levels are < 10% of serum levels. V_d is 0.36 ± 0.13 L/kg;[5] Cl is 1.1–1.7 L/h/m^2 or 0.04 ± 0.014 L/h/kg.[6,7] Inactive metabolites include the hydroxy acid and *cis*-lactones. Up to 16% of a dose can be eliminated in bile; 30% ± 5% is eliminated in urine, approximately 70% of this is unchanged drug with pharmacokinetic parameters consistently falling into the same range as those for intravenous dose of half the size of the oral dose. On intravenous administration, etoposide exhibits a biphasic distribution with an α half-life of 1.5 h and a terminal elimination half-life ranging from 4 to 11 h. Etoposide binding ratio correlates directly with serum albumin in patients with cancer and in normal volunteers. A significant inverse correlation between albumin concentration and free fraction of etoposide has been reported. Etoposide is cleared through renal processes as well as metabolism and biliary excretion. Patients with impaired renal function have exhibited reduced total body clearance, increased AUC, and a lower volume of distribution at steady state.

Adverse Reactions. Myelosuppression is dose related and dose limiting. Fever and infection have been reported in patients with neutropenia and even death associated with myelosuppression following etoposide administration. Nausea and vomiting are the major gastrointestinal toxicities, but generally can be controlled by standard prophylactic antiemetic therapy. Anaphylactic-type reactions have been reported to occur in all 3 dosage formulations and can occur with the initial infusion. Rash, urticaria, and/or pruritic erythematous maculopapular rash have also been reported. Blood pressure changes (hypotension and hypertension) have been reported. Reversible alopecia occurs commonly.

Precautions. Patients with low serum albumin may be at increased risk for toxicity.

Drug Interactions. High-dose cyclosporine administered with oral etoposide has led to an 80% increase in etoposide exposure with a 38% decrease in total body clearance of etoposide compared to etoposide alone.

Parameters to Monitor. CBC performed prior to each cycle of therapy and at appropriate intervals during and after therapy.

Notes. Concentrated etoposide solutions (>1 mg/mL) can cause cracking of ABS (acrylonitrile butadiene styrene) plastic infusion system components and have short stability times of 2 h. More dilute solutions in NS or D5W of 0.2–0.4 mg/mL have longer stability times of 96 h and 24 h, respectively, at room temperature under normal room fluorescent light in both glass and plastic containers. The phosphate formulation can be diluted to 0.1 mg/mL with either D5W or NS and is stable under refrigeration for 7 days and at controlled room temperature for 24 h.

IRINOTECAN Camptosar

Pharmacology. Irinotecan is a water-soluble camptothecin derivative. It is a prodrug for the lipophilic metabolite SN-38, an inhibitor of topoisomerase I enzymes. Irinotecan and its active metabolite bind to the topoisomerase I–DNA complex and prevent relegation of these single-strand breaks. Newer research also suggests that the cytotoxicity of irinotecan is due to double-strand DNA damage produced during DNA synthesis when replication enzymes interact with the ternary complex formed by topoisomerase I, DNA, and either irinotecan or SN-38.

Adult Dosage. **IV as a single agent or in combination with fluorouracil and leucovorin**—125 mg/m^2 once weekly for 4 consecutive weeks. If severe toxicity occurs, dosage is decreased by 25 mg/m^2 increments. A dose of 180 mg/m^2 every 14 days in combination with fluorouracil and leucovorin is also utilized with dosage adjusted downward in 30 mg/m^2 increments for severe toxicity. **IV as a single agent**—alternatively, 350 mg/m^2 every 3 weeks, with subsequent doses adjusted downward in 50 mg/m^2 increments based on patient tolerability.

Dosage Forms. Inj 40-, 100-mg vials.

Pharmacokinetics. For short IV infusions, the mean terminal elimination half-life for irinotecan is 6.8 h (5.0–9.6 h) but the plasma half-life of the active metabolite,

SN-38, is relatively long compared to other camptothecins at 10.4 h (9.1–11.5). The prolonged half-life is thought to be a function of its sustained production from irinotecan in tissues. Plasma protein binding ranges from 30% to 43% for irinotecan and 92%–96% for SN-38, with serum albumin being the major protein to which they are bound. Urinary excretion is the primary route of disposition of the parent compound, irinotecan, with some biliary excretion (25%) and the conversion to SN-38 also occurring. SN-38 undergoes complex metabolism, but glucuronidation and biliary excretion are the major mechanisms of elimination.

Special Populations. *Pediatric Pharmacokinetics.* The effectiveness of irinotecan in pediatric patients has not been established; however, the results of at least 2 large open-label studies are available and the pharmacokinetic behavior of irinotecan in children appears similar to that in adults. Comparable clearance and dose-normalized AUC values were achieved.

Adverse Reactions. *Diarrhea*: Irinotecan can induce both early and late forms of diarrhea that appear to be mediated by different mechanisms. Early diarrhea is cholinergic in nature. It is usually transient (occurring within first 2 h with a median duration of 30 min) and only infrequently is severe. The diarrhea may be accompanied by other cholinergic symptoms such as rhinitis, increased salivation, miosis, lacrimation, diaphoresis, flushing, and intestinal hyperstalsis that can result in abdominal cramping. Prompt resolution of these symptoms can be obtained by administering atropine 0.5–1 mg subcutaneously or intravenously. Late diarrhea (occurring more than 24 h after administering dose) is pathophysiologically distinct from acute diarrhea. The late diarrhea is common and can be a dose-limiting toxicity. The overall incidence of late diarrhea is approximately 60%–85% with grades 3 and 4 diarrhea occurring in as many as 20%–40%. Treatment of this late diarrhea should begin promptly. Each patient should be instructed to have loperamide readily available and to begin treatment at the first episode of loose stools. The generally accepted regimen (note: this dosage regimen exceeds the usual dosage recommendations for loperamide) is 4 mg at the first onset of late diarrhea and then 2 mg every 2 h until the patient is diarrhea-free for at least 12 h (do not continue at these doses for more than 48 h). The patient may take 4 mg every 4 h overnight to aid sleep. Premedication with loperamide is not recommended. Because of the suspected mechanism of the delayed-onset diarrhea involving the intestinal epithelial damage from direct exposure to SN-38, those patients with abnormalities in SN-38 glucuronidation (Gilbert's syndrome) may be at greater risk for increased GI toxicity.

Other Adverse Reactions: myelosuppression, mainly seen as neutropenia; nausea/vomiting; fatigue, alopecia, and elevated transaminases.[8]

PACLITAXEL
Taxol, Abraxane

Pharmacology. The active ingredient in both products, paclitaxel, is a natural product. Taxol utilizes a semisynthetic process, using product obtained from *T. baccata* and Abraxane product is obtained from *Taxus media*. Paclitaxel promotes the assembly of microtubules from tubulin dimmers and stabilizes microtubules by preventing depolymerization, which results in the inhibition of normal reorganization of the microtubule network.

Administration and Adult Dosage. **Taxol: IV**—135 mg/m^2 over 24 h or 175 mg/m^2 over 3 h every 3 weeks, generally in combination with other chemotherapy agents, commonly cisplatin. Note: Use non-PVC infusion systems. **Abraxane: IV**— 260 mg/m^2 over 30 min every 3 weeks. **Note:** Be sure to follow preparation instructions in order to maintain integrity of the product.

Dosage Forms. **Taxol: Inj** 30 mg/5 mL, 100 mg/16.7 mL, 300 mg/50 mL. **Abraxane: Inj** 100 mg in a single use vial.

Pharmacokinetics. *Fate.* Taxol: Nonlinear pharmacokinetics is more apparent with shorter infusions and result in plasma concentrations that equal or exceed the K_m constants of the saturable elimination or distribution processes. Saturable tissue distribution and drug elimination appear to be responsible for paclitaxel's nonlinear pharmacokinetic process with tissue distribution becoming effectively saturated at relatively lower drug concentrations (175 mg/m^2 over 3 h) compared with elimination processes. These shorter infusions result in higher plasma levels of paclitaxel's polyoxyethylated castor oil vehicle, which may contribute to the apparent nonlinear profile. The nonlinear pharmacokinetic profile yields the following half-lives, which are dose-dependent and infusion-rate dependent: 135 mg/m^2 over 3 h—$t_{1/2}$. 13.1 h; 135 mg/m^2 over 24 h—$t_{1/2}$. 52.7 h; 175 mg/m^2 over 3 h—$t_{1/2}$. 20.2 h; 175 mg/m^2 over 24 h—$t_{1/2}$. 15.7 h. Volume of distribution is much larger than the volume of total body water, indicating extensive protein binding and/or other tissue such as tubulin. Plasma protein binding is greater than 95% and not affected by cimetidine, ranitidine, dexamethasone, or diphenhydramine. The major route of clearance is by hepatic metabolism and excretion of paclitaxel and metabolites into the bile and feces, with renal clearance only accounting for approximately 14%.[1,2]

Abraxane: In contrast to Taxol, Abraxane pharmacokinetic parameters are independent of duration of administration. When administered as the protein-bound product, paclitaxel plasma concentrations decline in a biphasic manner, the initial rapid decline represents a distribution into the peripheral compartment and a slower second phase representing drug elimination. The terminal half-life is approximately 27 h. Abraxane also produces a large volume of distribution, 632 L/m^2, indicating extensive tissue binding and this binding is also unaffected by the presence of cimetidine, ranitidine, dexamethasone, or diphenhydramine. Abraxane utilizes extensive nonrenal clearance with less than 1% excreted unchanged in the urine.

Adverse Reactions. *Hypersensitivity Reactions* Taxol: Anaphylaxis and severe hypersensitivity reactions including dyspnea with bronchospasm, urticaria, and hypotension occur commonly. These reactions may be due to either the paclitaxel itself or its polyoxyethylated castor oil vehicle. The castor oil vehicle is most likely responsible for the hypersensitivity reactions because it induces histamine release. Recommended premedication regimens to reduce the incidence of these reactions include dexamethasone 20 mg orally or IV, 12 and 6 h before treatment; an H1 histamine antagonist (diphenhydramine 50 mg IV) 30 min prior to treatment; and an H2 antagonist (famotidine 20 mg or ranitidine 150 mg IV) 30 min prior to treatment.[1,2]

Abraxane: No premedication to prevent hypersensitivity reactions is recommended prior to administration of Abraxane.

Other Adverse Reactions. With the exception of the hypersensitivity reactions already discussed, the adverse events reported with either agent are similar. These include hematologic toxicity as the major dose-limiting event. Other adverse events of note include hypotension and bradycardia during the infusion, neither of which generally requires treatment, peripheral neuropathy, and elevated hepatic enzymes. Renal toxicity manifested by increases in creatinine was seen more frequently with Abraxane.[1,2]

Contraindications. Neither agent should be used in patients with a baseline neutrophil count <1500 cell/mm[3].

Precautions. *For administration of Taxol*: Contact of the undiluted concentrate with plasticized polyvinyl chloride (PVC) equipment or devices used to prepare solutions for infusion is not recommended. DEHP (Di(2-ethylhexyl) phthalate) may be leached from PVC infusion bags or sets and therefore, to minimize the chance of patient exposure to this plasticizer, diluted Taxol solutions should be stored in bottles or non-PVC–containing bags. It should also be administered via polyethylene-lined administration sets. Use of a 0.22 μm in-line filter is also recommended.[2]

TOPOTECAN   Hycamtin

Pharmacology. Topotecan is a topoisomerase I inhibitor that causes single-strand breaks in DNA. It is a semisynthetic derivative of camptothecin. Topotecan undergoes a reversible pH-dependent hydrolysis of its lactone moiety to form the pharmacologically active moiety.

Adult Dosage. **IV**—for ovarian cancer and small cell lung cancer, the recommended dose is 1.5 mg/m^2/d administered over 30 min daily for 5 days, starting on day 1 of a 21-day course of therapy for at least 4 courses. If patient experiences severe neutropenia or platelet count <25,000 cells/mm^3, reduce the dose for subsequent courses by 0.25 mg/m^2 (to a dose of 1.25 mg/m^2). OR, G-CSF may be administered following subsequent courses starting on day 6 of the course before resorting to dose reduction.

For cervical cancer (in combination with cisplatin), the recommended dose is 0.75 mg/m^2 IV over 30 min on day 1, 2, and 3 of a 21-day course. In the event of febrile neutropenia or platelet count <10,000 cells/mm^3, the dose should be reduced by 20% to 0.6 mg/m^2 for subsequent courses. OR, G-CSF may be administered following the subsequent course starting from day 4 before resorting to dose reduction. If febrile neutropenia occurs despite the use of G-CSF, further dose reduction to 0.45 mg/m^2 should be made.

Dosage Adjustment *Hepatic Impairment:* No dosage adjustment is required for impaired hepatic function. *Renal Impairment:* Dosage adjustments are not necessary until moderate renal impairment occurs (20–39 mL/min) when 0.75 mg/m^2 is recommended. Insufficient data exist for dosage recommendations in severe renal impairment.

Dosage Forms. **Inj** 4-mg single dose vials.

Pharmacokinetics. A linear 2-compartment model is generally used to describe topotecan pharmacokinetics giving an average terminal half-life of 2–3 h, which is relatively short and accounts for lack of accumulation over multiple days of therapy. CNS penetration occurs with a concentration in CNS approximately 29% of plasma concentrations. Renal excretion is the major route of elimination for both parent drug and the hydrolyzed lactone moiety.

Adverse Reactions. The primary dose-limiting side effect of topotecan is bone marrow suppression, primarily neutropenia and thrombocytopenia have also been reported. Therefore, topotecan should only be administered to patients with adequate bone marrow reserves. Baseline measurements should be at least a neutrophil count of 1500 cells/mm^3 and a platelet count of 100,000 cells/mm^3. Frequent monitoring should occur during treatment. GI toxicities include nausea and vomiting that can generally be managed by the use of standard antiemetics; other GI effects are frequent diarrhea, constipation, and abdominal pain. Total alopecia occurs in approximately 31% of patients; headache is the most frequently reported neurologic toxicity.

VINCA ALKALOIDS	
VINBLASTINE SULFATE	Velban
VINCRISTINE SULFATE	Oncovin
VINORELBINE TARTRATE	Navelbine

Pharmacology. The naturally occurring vinca alkaloids, vincristine and vinblastine, are *Vinca rosea* (periwinkle) plant–derived antimitotic agents, and vinorelbine is a semisynthetic derivative. Their cytotoxic activity has been related to the inhibition of microtubule formation in the mitotic spindle, resulting in arrest of dividing cells at the metaphase stage of reproduction.[1,2]

Administration and Dosage. All 3 products require the extra labeling "Fatal if given intrathecally, for IV use only."

Vinblastine **Adults:** Initial dose 3.7 mg/m^2. Additional doses should be administered at a minimum of 7-day intervals and at doses determined by the WBC counts, with second dose of 5.5 mg/m^2, third of 7.4 mg/m^2, fourth of 9.25 mg/m^2 and a maximum of 11.1 mg/m^2. Many patients will not tolerate these increases and their maintenance dose should be 1 dosage increment less than the dose that caused leukopenia. **Pediatrics:** Initial doses of 3–6 mg/m^2 have been utilized with dosage adjustments based on hematologic tolerance.

Vincristine **Adults:** For most malignancies, 1.4 mg/m^2 weekly. **Pediatrics:** ≥10 kg 0.05 mg/kg IV once weekly; >10 kg 1.5–2 mg/m^2 IV once weekly.

Although a maximum single dose of 2 mg is generally recommended, some treatments and protocols allow for doses >2 mg. Any single dose >2 mg should be verified with the specific regimen and an experienced oncologist.

Vinorelbine **Adults:** The initial dose for single-agent is 30 mg/m^2 weekly. Dosage adjustments may be necessary when given in combination chemotherapy regimens.

Special Populations. *Other Conditions.* Vinca alkaloids are eliminated extensively in the bile, and the dosages of vinblastine and vincristine must be reduced by 50% in patients having a direct serum bilirubin value >3mg/dL. Reduce vinorelbine dosages to 50% for a serum total bilirubin of 2.1–3 mg/dL and 25% for a bilirubin >3 mg/dL.

Dosage Forms. (Vinblastine) **Inj** 10 mg/vial. (Vincristine) **Inj** 1 mg/mL 1- and 2-mL preservative-free vials. (Vinorelbine) **Inj** 10 mg/mL 1- and 5-mL vials.

Pharmacokinetics. *Fate.* Pharmacokinetic behavior in plasma fits open 3-compartment models. Pharmacokinetic characteristics include large volumes of distribution, high clearance rates, long terminal half-lives, hepatic metabolism, and biliary/fecal excretion. In comparison, vincristine has the longest terminal half-life and the lowest clearance rate.[1,2]

Adverse Reactions. The neurotoxicity of the vinca alkaloids is most prominent with vincristine, but can occur with any, and is characterized by a peripheral, symmetric mixed sensory motor and autonomic polyneuropathy. These effects manifest as symmetric sensory impairment and paresthesias, which begin in the distal extremities. Neuritic pain and loss of deep tendon reflexes may develop with continued treatment, which can result in foot drop, ataxia, and even paralysis. When the cranial nerves are affected, hoarseness, diplopia, jaw pain, and facial palsies can occur. Neutropenia is the principal dose-limiting toxicity of vinblastine and vinorelbine, but is rare with vincristine unless inadvertent high doses are administered. GI toxicities are rare except for those caused by autonomic dysfunction and manifested as bloating, constipation, and ileus and abdominal pain and are most commonly associated with vincristine. A routine prophylactic regimen to prevent constipation is therefore recommended for all patients receiving vincristine. Various degrees of alopecia can occur with any of these agents.[1,2]

Contraindications. Inadvertent intrathecal administration of any vinca alkaloid is fatal.

Parameters to Monitor. Obtain pretreatment and at least monthly CBC assessments; (vincristine) obtain serial peripheral neurologic assessments; (all drugs) assess biliary function before making dosage adjustments for impaired hepatobiliary status.

Notes. Place individual doses in an overwrap (e.g., plastic bag) that is labeled, "Do not remove covering until the moment of injection. Fatal if given intrathecally; for intravenous use only." The vincas are extremely toxic if inadvertently extravasated; therefore, they should be administered only by appropriately trained health care professionals.[1,7]

■ REFERENCES

1. Rowinsky EK. Antimicrotubule agents. In: Chabner BA, Longo DL, eds. *Cancer Chemotherapy and Biotherapy Principles and Practice.* 4th ed. Philadelphia, PA: Lippincott Williams & Wilkins; 2006:237-282.
2. Rowinsky EK, Tolcher AW. Microtubule-targeting drugs. In: Perry MC, ed. *Chemotherapy Source Book.* 3rd ed. Philadelphia, PA: Lippincott Williams & Wilkins; 2001:252-277.
3. Pommier Y, Goldwasser F. Topoisomerase II inhibitors: the epipodophyllotoxins, acridines, and ellipticines. In: Chabner BA, Longo DL, eds. *Cancer Chemotherapy and Biotherapy Principles and Practice.* 4th ed. Philadelphia, PA: Lippincott Williams & Wilkins; 2006:451-475.
4. Tolcher A, Rowinsky EK. DNA Topoisomerase II inhibitors. In: Perry MC, ed. *Chemotherapy Source Book.* 3rd ed. Philadelphia, PA: Lippincott Williams & Wilkins; 2001:278-288.
5. Benet LZ et al. Design and optimization of dosage regimens: pharmacokinetic data. In: Hardman JG et al., eds. *Goodman and Gilman's the Pharmacological Basis of Therapeutics.* 9th ed. New York: McGraw-Hill; 1996:1707-1792.
6. O'Dwyer PJ et al. Etoposide (VP-16–213): current status of an active anticancer drug. *N Engl J Med.* 1985;312:692-700.
7. Rivera GK et al. Epipodophyllotoxins in the treatment of childhood cancer. *Cancer Chemother Pharmacol.* 1994;34(suppl):S89-S95.

Chapter 25

Monoclonal Antibodies

Amber P. Lawson

ALEMTUZUMAB   Campath

Pharmacology. Alemtuzumab is a DNA-recombinant humanized monoclonal antibody that binds to the CD52 antigen, which exists on the surfaces of T lymphocytes, B lymphocytes, monocytes, macrophages, NK cells, and a subset of granulocytes. The proposed mechanism of action is antibody-dependent cellular cytotoxicity after alemtuzumab binds to leukemic cells.[1] Alemtuzumab is indicated as a single agent for the treatment of B-cell chronic lymphocytic leukemia (B-CLL).

Adult Dosage and Administration. Single-agent alemtuzumab for B-CLL should be dose-escalated to minimize infusion reactions. All alemtuzumab doses should be premedicated with diphenhydramine 50 mg and acetaminophen 500–1000 mg. Dose escalation begins with a dose of 3 mg and increased to 10 mg on the next dose when the infusion reaction is ≤ grade 2 per NCI CTC (National Cancer Institute Common Toxicity Criteria) version 2.0. Final dose escalation to 30 mg when infusion reactions remain ≤ grade 2 per NCI CTC version 2.0. Usually, dose escalation is accomplished within 3–7 days. Alemtuzumab is administered intravenously over 2 h in 100 mL of normal saline or dextrose 5% solutions. Alemtuzumab is given 3 times weekly on alternating days (i.e., Monday, Wednesday, and Friday) for a total of 12 weeks including dose escalation. Individual doses greater than 30 mg or cumulative weekly dosages greater than 90 mg are associated with an increased risk of pancytopenia. Prophylaxis against *Pneumocystis jiroveci* pneumonia and herpes simplex infections is recommended until $CD4^+$ counts ≥ 200/μL or until 2 months after completion of alemtuzumab therapy, whichever occurs later. Administer only irradiated blood products to avoid graft-versus-host disease.

Special Populations. *Pediatric Dosage.* Safety and efficacy not established.

Geriatric Dosage. Same as adult dosage.

Pregnancy Category/Lactation. Pregnancy category C. Although not formally studied, IgG antibodies may pass into breast milk. Use of alemtuzumab during breast-feeding is not recommended.

Dosage Forms. Inj 30 mg.

Patient Instructions. This drug may cause a flulike syndrome including fever, chills, and weakness shortly after you receive it. This drug may make you more likely to get infections because of suppression of the immune system. Ask your physician before receiving live vaccines. Use an effective birth control method during therapy and for 6 months following completion of alemtuzumab therapy.

Pharmacokinetics. *Fate.* Alemtuzumab demonstrates nonlinear elimination kinetics. After the last 30-mg dose, the mean volume of distribution at steady state is 0.18 mL/kg (range 0.1–0.4 mL/kg). Systemic CD52 receptor–mediated clearance decreases with repeated administration. In patients with B-CLL, the AUC is increased 7-fold by the 12th week of therapy. The elimination half-life is approximately 11 h after the first 30-mg dose (range 2–32 h) and increases to 6 days after the last 30-mg dose (range 1–14 days).

Adverse Reactions. Frequent adverse reactions include nausea, emesis, diarrhea, insomnia, and reactivation of cytomegalovirus (CMV) infection. Serious adverse events include cytopenias, immunosuppression/infections, and infusion-related reactions that may result in cardiopulmonary arrest and death in rare cases.

Contraindications. None.

Precautions. Boxed warnings include cytopenias, infusion-related reactions, and prolonged immunosuppression.

Drug Interactions. Infusion-related events may be exacerbated by antihypertensives. The administration of live vaccines is not recommended.

Parameters to Monitor. Obtain complete blood counts (CBC) with differential at weekly intervals during therapy and more frequently when worsening anemia, neutropenia, or thrombocytopenia occurs. Assess $CD4^+$ counts after treatment until recovery to >200 cells/μL. Routine monitoring for CMV reactivation is recommended throughout therapy and for 2 months following discontinuation of alemtuzumab therapy; monitor for signs and symptoms of other bacterial, fungal, viral, or protozoal infections as well. Monitor patient closely for infusion-related events during initiation of therapy.

BEVACIZUMAB Avastin

Pharmacology. Bevacizumab is a recombinant humanized monoclonal antibody that binds to vascular endothelial growth factor (VEGF) and thus prevents VEGF from binding to receptor tyrosine kinases Flt-1 and KDR (kinase insert domain receptor) on the surfaces of endothelial cells. VEGFs play an integral role in new blood vessel formation in a process known as angiogenesis. By interrupting the actions of VEGF, the agent is thought to arrest the further development of tumors by inducing regression of current tumor microvasculature, by normalizing current mature vasculature to facilitate delivery of anticancer therapy, and by inhibiting the formation of new tumor microvasculature.[2]

Adult Dosage and Administration. Bevacizumab should not be administered for at least 28 days following major surgery and should be discontinued when serious adverse events occur. For *metastatic carcinoma of the colon and rectum,* the recommended dose is 5 mg/kg in the IFL (irinotecan, fluorouracil, and leucovorin) regimen[3] and 10 mg/kg when given with the FOLFOX4 regimen[4]; bevacizumab is given once every 14 days in both regimens. For *nonsquamous, non–small cell lung cancer,* the recommended dose is 15 mg/kg given once every 21 days. For *metastatic breast cancer,* the recommended dose is 10 mg/kg given once every 14 days. The dose should be diluted in 100 mL of normal saline; bevacizumab is incompatible with dextrose-containing solutions. The initial bevacizumab is administered intravenously over 90 min. If the first infusion is well tolerated, the second infusion may be administered over 60 min. If the 60-min infusion is well tolerated, all subsequent infusions may be administered over 30 min.

Special Populations. *Pediatric Dosage.* Safety and efficacy not established.

Geriatric Dosage. Same as adult dosage.

Pregnancy Category/Lactation. Pregnancy category C. Although not formally studied, IgG antibodies may pass into breast milk. Use of bevacizumab during breastfeeding is not recommended.

Dosage Forms. **Inj** 100 mg, 400 mg.

Patient Instructions. Seek immediate medical attention if you develop severe stomach/abdominal pain, constipation with vomiting, fever, black/bloody stools, blood in vomit, or coughing up blood. Tell your physician if you have had surgery within the past month or will have surgery in the near future.

Pharmacokinetics. *Fate.* The relationship between bevacizumab exposure and clinical outcomes is unknown. When adjusted for body weight, patients with higher tumor burden demonstrate a higher clearance of the agent and males demonstrate a higher rate of drug clearance than females. The mechanism of metabolism and elimination of bevacizumab is unknown. The elimination half-life is approximately 20 days (range 11–50 days).

Adverse Reactions. The most frequent adverse events seen in patients receiving bevacizumab with other chemotherapy are weakness, pain, abdominal pain, headache, hypertension, diarrhea, nausea, vomiting, loss of appetite, mouth sores, constipation, upper respiratory infection, nosebleeds, difficulty in breathing, skin irritation, and proteinuria. Serious frequent adverse events include gastrointestinal perforation, nongastrointestinal fistula formation, wound healing complications, hemorrhage, arterial thromboembolic events, hypertension, nephritic syndrome, reversible posterior leukoencephalopathy syndrome, neutropenia and infection, and congestive heart failure.

Contraindications. None.

Precautions. Boxed warnings include gastrointestinal perforation, wound healing complications, and hemorrhage. Other precautions include infusion reactions and recent surgery. Warnings include nongastrointestinal fistula formation, arterial thromboembolic events, hypertension, nephritic syndrome, reversible posterior leukoencephalopathy syndrome, neutropenia and infection, and congestive heart failure. Bevacizumab should not be given to patients experiencing these events.

Drug Interactions. No formal drug interaction studies have been conducted.

Parameters to Monitor. Blood pressure monitoring should coincide with bevacizumab administration. Patients with a 2+ or greater urine dipstick reading should undergo further assessment, e.g., a 24-h urine collection. Monitor coagulation parameters and hemoglobin/hematocrit when hemorrhage is suspected. Check vital signs postinfusion and monitor for serious adverse events.

CETUXIMAB Erbitux

Pharmacology. Epidermal growth factor receptors (EGFR, HER-1, c-ErbB-1) are constitutively expressed as glycoprotein transmembrane receptors in both normal epithelial tissues and in many human tumors such as cancers of the head, neck, colon, and rectum. Cetuximab, a chimeric human–mouse monoclonal IgG1 antibody, binds specifically to EGFR on both normal cells and tumor cells that inhibit phosphorylation of membrane-associated kinases. Inhibition of these kinases lead to inhibition of cell growth, induction of apoptosis, decreased matrix metalloproteinase production, and VEGF production.[5]

Adult Dosage and Administration. The initial cetuximab dose should be premedicated with diphenhydramine 50 mg IV (given 30–60 min prior to infusion) to prevent infusion-related reactions; subsequent doses may require premedication based on clinical judgment. Do not dilute.

Initial therapy for squamous cell carcinoma of the head and neck with concurrent radiation. The recommended initial dose is 400 mg/m^2 administered 1 week prior to initiation of a course of radiation therapy as a 120-min intravenous infusion. The recommended subsequent weekly dose (all other infusions) is 250 mg/m^2 infused over 60 min (maximum infusion rate 10 mg/min) for the duration of radiation therapy (6–7 weeks); complete cetuximab administration 1 h prior to radiation therapy.

Monotherapy for recurrent squamous cell carcinoma of the head and neck or failure of platinum-based regimen. Cetuximab 400 mg/m^2 administered as a 120-min intravenous infusion, followed by 250 mg/m^2 over 60 min (maximum infusion rate 10 mg/min) given once weekly until disease progression or unacceptable toxicity.

EGFR-expressing metastatic colorectal cancer as monotherapy after failure of irinotecan- and oxaliplatin-containing regimens; EGFR-expressing metastatic colorectal cancer in combination with irinotecan in patients who are refractory to irinotecan-based therapy. Cetuximab, 400 mg/m^2, administered as a 120-min intravenous infusion, followed by 250 mg/m^2 over 60 min (maximum infusion rate 10 mg/min) given once weekly until disease progression or unacceptable toxicity.

Special Populations. *Pediatric Dosage.* Safety and efficacy not established.

Geriatric Dosage. Same as adult dosage.

Pregnancy Category/Lactation. Pregnancy category C. Although not formally studied, IgG antibodies may pass into breast milk. Use of cetuximab during breastfeeding is not recommended.

Dosage Forms. Inj 100 mg, 200 mg.

Patient Instructions. This medication may cause fever, chills, trouble with breathing, lightheadedness, fainting, or chest pain within a few hours after you receive it; notify nurse or physician when this occurs. You will be monitored by a nurse or a physician for at least 1 h after the dose to make sure this does not happen. If you develop blistering or peeling of the skin, skin lesions, severe acne or skin rash, sores or ulcers on the skin, or fever or chills, contact your physician. Wear sunscreen when outdoors; avoid tanning beds and lamps. Use an effective birth control method during cetuximab therapy and for 6 months after completion of therapy. Avoid breastfeeding during cetuximab therapy and for 2 months after completion of therapy.

Pharmacokinetics. *Onset and Duration.* Intravenous onset occurs within 6 weeks; duration is 4.2–5.7 months for colorectal cancer and 28 months for head and neck cancer.[6,7]

Fate. Cetuximab demonstrates nonlinear pharmacokinetics. Distribution of the agent will approximate plasma volume. The AUC of cetuximab appears to remain constant after dose escalation to >200 mg/m². Steady-state concentrations are achieved after approximately 3 weeks when standard dosing recommendations are followed (*see* **Adult Dosage and Administration**). Female patients with colorectal cancer exhibit an approximate 25% decrease in intrinsic clearance compared to male subjects. Elimination of cetuximab occurs via EGFR binding and subsequent internalization on hepatocytes and skin and is a saturable process. The elimination half-life is estimated to be approximately 112 h (range 63–230 h).

Adverse Reactions. The most frequent adverse reactions (≥25% prevalence) are cutaneous adverse reactions (including rash, pruritus, and nail changes), headache, diarrhea, and infection. Serious frequent adverse events include serious infusion reactions and cardiopulmonary arrest, allergic reactions, skin reactions, serious lung disease, pulmonary embolism, fever, infection, dehydration, renal failure, and diarrhea.

Contraindications. None.

Precautions. Boxed warnings include serious infusion reactions (3%) that may result in fatality and cardiopulmonary arrest/sudden death (2%) in patients receiving concurrent radiation. Pulmonary toxicity and dermatologic toxicity may also occur with the use of cetuximab.

Drug Interactions. Infusion-related events may be exacerbated by antihypertensives.

Parameters to Monitor. *Infusion-related events.* Approximately 90% of severe infusion reactions occurred with the first infusion despite premedication with antihistamines. Monitor patients for at least 1 h following cetuximab infusions in a setting with resuscitation equipment and other agents necessary to treat anaphylaxis; longer monitoring period may be necessary in the event of an infusion reaction. Obtain vital signs before infusion and at least once during infusion and every 15 min for 1 h postinfusion. Reduce the infusion rate by 50% for NCI CTC grade 1 or 2 and nonserious NCI CTC grades 3–4 infusion reactions. Permanently discontinue cetuximab in the event of a severe infusion-related event.

Severe Acneform Rash. After first occurrence, delay treatment by 1–2 weeks; discontinue cetuximab if no improvement occurs. After second and third occurrence, delay treatment by 1–2 weeks with dosage reduction per prescribing information; discontinue cetuximab if no improvement occurs. Permanently discontinue cetuximab after fourth occurrence.

Electrolytes. Monitor for hypomagnesemia, hypocalcemia, and hypokalemia throughout treatment as necessary and for 8 weeks following the completion of therapy.

GEMTUZUMAB   Mylotarg

Pharmacology. Gemtuzumab is a recombinant humanized anti-CD33 monoclonal antibody conjugated to the cytotoxic antibiotic calicheamicin via a Nac-gamma linker molecule. Gemtuzumab selectively binds to CD33 antigen that is expressed on leukemic blasts in more than 80% of patients with AML. Once the antibody binds the CD33 antigen, the complex is internalized by the cell. Once inside the cell, the calicheamicin derivative is released inside cell lysosomes. The derivative binds DNA that ultimately causes DNA double-strand breaks and cell death.

Adult Dosage and Administration. *Treatment of patients with CD33-positive acute myeloid leukemia in first relapse who are 60 years or older and who are not considered candidates for other cytotoxic chemotherapy.* Gemtuzumab 9 mg/m^2 given intravenously over 2 h in 100 mL normal saline for a total of 2 doses given 14 days apart. Prescribers should consider hydroxyurea or leukapheresis to reduce the total WBC to less than 30,000 cells/mm^3 in order to reduce the risk of pulmonary complications and the risk of tumor lysis syndrome prior to the administration of gemtuzumab. Patients should receive the following prophylactic medications 1 h before gemtuzumab administration: diphenhydramine 50 mg PO and acetaminophen 650–1000 mg PO; thereafter, acetaminophen 650–1000 mg PO, one every 4 h as needed for 2 doses.

Special Populations. *Pediatric Dosage.* Safety and efficacy not established.

Geriatric Dosage. Same as adult dosage.

Pregnancy Category/Lactation. Pregnancy category D. Although not formally studied with gemtuzumab, immunoglobulins are excreted into breast milk. Use of gemtuzumab during breast-feeding is not recommended.

Dosage Forms. Inj 5 mg.

Patient Instructions. This medication may cause fever, chills, trouble with breathing, lightheadedness, fainting, or chest pain within a few hours after you receive it; notify nurse or physician when this occurs. Medications will be administered to prevent allergic reaction and you will be monitored for at least 4 h after the dose to make sure this does not happen. You may be more likely to develop an infection or bleeding complication after receiving this medicine. To help with these problems, avoid being near people who are sick. Wash your hands often. Brush and floss your teeth gently. Be careful when using sharp objects, including razors and fingernail clippers. If you have abdominal pain and gain weight, notify your physician.

Pharmacokinetics. *Fate.* After first dose of gemtuzumab at 9 mg/m^2, the elimination half-lives of total and unconjugated calicheamicin are approximately 41 and 143 h, respectively. The elimination half-life of total calicheamicin increases to 64 h following the second dose. The AUC for calicheamicin doubled after the second dose of gemtuzumab as compared to the AUC after the first dose and the AUC of unconjugated calicheamicin increases by 30% following the second dose. The AUC of total calicheamicin has been correlated with an increased risk of hepatic venoocclusive disease (VOD), although dose reduction of gemtuzumab has not been shown to decrease the risk of VOD. In vitro metabolism data has shown that the metabolic products of calicheamicin have been detected in human liver microsomes and cytosol after incubation with the derivative.

Adverse Reactions. The most frequent adverse events ($\geq 20\%$ prevalence) were fever, nausea, chills, vomiting, thrombocytopenia, leukopenia, headache, asthenia, abdominal pain, diarrhea, epistaxis, dyspnea, hypokalemia, sepsis, anorexia, stomatitis, liver function tests abnormal, constipation, anemia, local reaction, herpes simplex, and hypotension. Serious frequent adverse events include myelosuppression, increased opportunistic infection risk, bleeding, anaphylaxis, pulmonary complications including hemorrhage, infusion reactions, hepatotoxicity, VOD, and renal failure secondary to tumor lysis syndrome.

Contraindications. None.

Precautions. Boxed warnings include hepatotoxicity and hypersensitivity reactions including anaphylaxis, infusion reactions, and pulmonary events; other warnings include myelosuppression and risk of tumor lysis syndrome.

Drug Interactions. Infusion-related events may be exacerbated by antihypertensives. No formal studies have evaluated drug interactions with gemtuzumab, but possible interaction via the hepatic cytochrome P450 system cannot be excluded.

Parameters to Monitor. Electrolytes, hepatic function tests, CBC with differential and platelet counts should be monitored periodically as necessary; electrolytes and uric acid should be monitored frequently for 6–72 h after administration of first dose when patients are at risk for tumor lysis syndrome. Vital signs should be monitored during the infusion and for 4 h after the completion of infusion.

IODINE 131 TOSITUMOMAB   Bexxar

Pharmacology. This agent is a mouse-derived monoclonal antibody that binds to the CD20 receptor of normal and malignant B lymphocytes. The β-particle–emitting isotope ^{131}I is coupled to the antibody, forming a selective radioimmuno-conjugate for patients with CD20-positive non-Hodgkin's lymphoma refractory to chemotherapy.[8] Possible mechanisms of action include induction of apoptosis, complement-mediated cytotoxicity, antibody-dependent cellular cytotoxicity, and cell death because of the effect of ionizing radiation from the radioisotope.

Adult Dosage and Administration. Patients should receive one of the following thyroid-protective agents at least 24 h prior to the iodine 131 tositumomab dosimetric dose and for 2 weeks following the iodine 131 tositumomab therapeutic dose: SSKI 4 drops PO tid; potassium iodide tablets 130 mg PO daily; or Lugol's solution 20 drops orally tid.

Treatment of patients with CD20 antigen-expressing relapsed or refractory, low-grade, follicular, or transformed non-Hodgkin's lymphoma. In clinical trials, a 2-stage dosage schedule has been used. First, patients are administered unlabeled antibody IV to suppress nonspecific binding sites. Next, patients are given trace-labeled doses of ^{131}I-labeled antibody (15–20 mg containing 5 mCi IV) to assess antibody distribution. One week later, patients are given a 685-mg dose of unlabeled antibody IV, followed 1 day later by 2 individualized therapeutic (labeled) doses of 135 mg and 685 mg of antibody to deliver up to 75 cGy of whole-body radiation. A total body irradiation dosage of 55 cGy appears to be the maximum tolerated in patients who have undergone bone marrow transplantation. Give diphenhydramine 50 mg and acetaminophen 650 mg before each infusion. Patients who are refractory to rituximab therapy have responded to the Bexxar therapeutic regimen.

Special Populations. *Pediatric Dosage.* Safety and efficacy not established.

Geriatric Dosage. Same as adult dosage.

Pregnancy Category/Lactation. Pregnancy category X. Use during breast-feeding is not recommended.

Dosage Forms. **Inj** 35 mg, 225 mg.

Patient Instructions. This medication may stay in the body for several days after administration. Use effective birth control methods for 12 months after administration of this drug. This medication may cause an endocrine disorder known as hypothyroidism and monitoring and possibly treatment may be required indefinitely. This medication will lower the blood counts for up to 4 months and requires frequent monitoring with blood tests and may require blood or platelet transfusions. The risk of infection will increase after administration of this drug because of low blood counts. In a small number of patients, another cancer may be detected years after the administration of this medication.

Pharmacokinetics. *Fate.* The median blood clearance following administration of 485 mg of tositumomab in 110 patients with non-Hodgkin's lymphoma (NHL) was 68.2 mg/h (range 30.2–260.8 mg/h). Patients with high tumor burden, splenomegaly, or bone marrow involvement were noted to have a faster clearance, shorter terminal half-life, and larger volume of distribution. Approximately 98% of total body clearance occurs by renal excretion of Iodine 131. The median elimination half-life is 67 h.

Adverse Reactions. Nonhematologic toxicities after infusions are mild, with low-grade fever in 31% of patients and chills or rigors in 1%. Mild fatigue and nausea occur in 6%–8% of radiolabeled infusions. The dose-limiting toxicity is hemato logic suppression with grade 3 or 4 leukopenia and thrombocytopenia in 66% of patients who receive a whole-body radiation dose of 85 cGy. All patients develop complete or near-complete depletion of CD19 and CD20-positive B cells from peripheral blood, recovering to normal levels in 3 months. Serum immunoglobulin levels are unchanged. Because of the short, single course of therapy, antimouse antibody (HAMA) reactions are uncommon. However, when they occur, they are usually marked by hypotension that can be treated with fluid hydration and vasopressors. Delayed adverse reactions include hypothyroidism, secondary leukemia or myelodysplastic syndrome (MDS), or development of HAMA.

Contraindications. None.

Precautions. Boxed warnings include hypersensitivity reactions including anaphylaxis and prolonged, severe cytopenias. The regimen should not be administered to patients with >25% lymphoma marrow involvement and/or impaired bone marrow reserve. This regimen is to be administered only by physicians who are in the process of being or have been certified by GlaxoSmithKline in dose calculation and administration of the therapeutic regimen.

Drug Interactions. Infusion-related events may be exacerbated by antihypertensives. No formal studies have evaluated drug interactions with the Bexxar therapeutic regimen. Anticoagulants and medications that interfere with platelet function may increase bleeding risk when administered during periods of severe and prolonged thrombocytopenia.

Parameters to Monitor. Obtain complete blood count with differential prior to therapy and weekly for at least 10 weeks after therapeutic regimen is administered and continue until cytopenias resolve. More frequent monitoring may be necessary when cytopenias are severe. Obtain thyroid stimulating hormone (TSH) prior to treatment and on an annual basis. Obtain baseline serum creatinine measurement before beginning treatment. Obtain HAMA titers before infusion, then 1 month and 6 months after infusion.

IBRITUMOMAB TIUXETAN   Zevalin

Pharmacology. Ibritumomab is a murine IgG1 kappa monoclonal antibody directed against the CD20 antigen. It is covalently linked to tiuxetan, which binds Indium-111 (^{111}In) or Yttrium-90 (^{90}Y). Once ibritumomab binds the CD20 antigen on lymphoid B cells of the bone marrow, lymph nodes, thymus, and other lymphoid tissues, the beta emission from ^{90}Y induces free radical formation and cellular damage in the target B cells and the surrounding cells.[8]

Adult Dosage and Administration. *Treatment of relapsed or refractory, low-grade or follicular B-cell NHL, including patients with rituximab refractory follicular NHL:*

Step 1: Rituximab 250 mg/m^2 given intravenously on day 1 as described in rituximab monograph.

Step 2: 5 mCi ^{111}In Zevalin over 10 min as an intravenous injection within 4 h following completion of the rituximab infusion.

Step 3: Assess the biodistribution of ^{111}In Zevalin by a visual evaluation of whole-body planar view anterior and posterior gamma images obtained at 48–72 h after injection of ^{111}In Zevalin.

Step 4: On day 7,8, or 9, administer rituximab 250 mg/m^2 IV × 1 dose.

Step 5: Within 4 h after completion of rituximab infusion, administer ^{90}Y Zevalin injection through a free-flowing intravenous line. If platelet count is ≥150,000/mm^3, administer 0.4 mCi/kg over 10 min. If platelet count 100,000/mm^3 to 149,000/mm^3, administer 0.3 mCi/kg over 10 min. Doses should be calculated according to actual body weight up to a maximum dose of 32 mCi.

Special Populations. *Pediatric Dosage.* Safety and efficacy not established.

Geriatric Dosage. Same as adult dosage.

Pregnancy Category/Lactation. Pregnancy category D. Although not formally studied, IgG antibodies may pass into breast milk. Use during breast-feeding is not recommended.

Dosage Forms. Inj 3.2 mg.

Patient Instructions. This therapeutic regimen may cause infusion reactions; notify health care personnel when fever, chills, or shortness of breath occur; take premedications as prescribed. When fever, bleeding, bruising, weakness, rash, or other skin changes occurs, contact your physician. Use effective contraception and do not receive live vaccines for 12 months after Zevalin therapy.

Pharmacokinetics. *Fate.* The mean half-life of ^{90}Y activity in the bloodstream is approximately 27–30 h, and approximately 7.2% of the injected activity is excreted in the urine over a 7 days period. No correlation between plasma half-life and severity of hematologic toxicity has been observed.

Contraindications. None.

Warnings/Precautions. Boxed warnings include infusion reactions (rituximab portion); prolonged and severe cytopenias; and severe mucocutaneous and cutaneous reactions. Boxed warning states the importance of avoiding administration in patients with altered distribution and not exceeding 32 mCi of ^{90}Y Zevalin. Do not administer to patients with ≥25% lymphoid marrow involvement in order to avoid severe cytopenias. The use of the agent is rarely associated with the development of MDS or secondary leukemia. Monitor for extravasation and terminate infusion when extravasation occurs.

Adverse Reactions. The most frequent adverse reactions (≥40% prevalence) are neutropenia, thrombocytopenia, anemia, asthenia, and gastrointestinal symptoms. Cytopenias are more likely to occur in patients who have mild baseline thrombocytopenia. Cytopenias may last more than 3 months. Severe cutaneous and mucocutaneous reactions including erythema multiforme, Stevens-Johnson syndrome, toxic epidermal necrolysis, bullous dermatitis, and exfoliative dermatitis may occur up to 4 months following drug administration. MDS and/or AML were reported in 5.2% of patients enrolled in clinical studies and 1.5% of patients included in the expanded-access trial with a median time to onset of 1.9 years after treatment. Because the Zevalin therapeutic regimen contains albumin, a theoretical risk for transmission of Creutzfeldt-Jakob disease (CJD) is possible but is considered extremely rare.

Drug Interactions. Anticoagulants and antiplatelet agents should be used with caution and avoided when possible because of increased bleeding risk in the presence of thrombocytopenia.

Parameters to Monitor. Obtain CBC with differential and platelet count at weekly intervals during therapy and more frequently when worsening anemia, neutropenia, or thrombocytopenia occurs. Monitor blood counts for up to 3 months following therapy or recovery of blood counts. Monitor for extravasation during Zevalin infusion.

PANITUMUMAB Vectibix

Pharmacology. EGFR is a transmembrane glycoprotein that is constitutively expressed in epithelial tissues and is overexpressed in certain human tumors such as colon cancer. EGFR is a member of a subfamily of type I receptor tyrosine kinases, that, upon interaction with its ligand, causes phosphorylation of intracellular proteins and subsequent downstream signaling leads to cell survival, motility, and proliferation.[9] According to in vitro data, panitumumab binds EGFR in normal and tumor cells and thus inhibits phosphorylation of intracellular proteins leading to apoptosis, inhibition of cell growth, and decreases in proinflammatory cytokine and growth factor production.

Adult Dosage and Administration. *For EGFR-expressing, metastatic colorectal carcinoma with disease progression on or following fluoropyrimidine-, oxaliplatin-, and irinotecan-containing chemotherapy regimens.* Panitumumab 6 mg/kg given intravenously in normal saline solution (total volume 100 mL) given every 14 days until disease progression or unacceptable toxicity. The final concentration of the diluted product must not exceed 10 mg/mL. For doses greater than 1000 mg, the dose should be diluted with normal saline to total volume of 150 mL and infused over 90 min. The infusion rate may be decreased by 50% in patients experiencing mild to moderate infusion-related reactions and the infusion should be discontinued for severe infusion-related reactions. Panitumumab should be held for severe or intolerable dermatologic reactions and be resumed at 50% of previous dose upon resolution of toxicity. Panitumumab is not approved for use in combination with chemotherapy.

Special Populations. *Pediatric Dosage.* Safety and efficacy not established. *Geriatric Dosage.* Same as adult dosage.

Pregnancy Category/Lactation. Pregnancy category C. Although not formally studied with panitumumab, immunoglobulins are excreted into breast milk. Use of panitumumab during breast-feeding is not recommended.

Dosage Forms. Inj 100, 200, 400 mg.

Patient Instructions. This medication may cause skin and/or visual changes, coughing, wheezing, dyspnea, or facial swelling; contact your physician when these symptoms occur. Limit sun exposure and wear sunscreen and a hat while outdoors during therapy and for 2 months after therapy is stopped. If fever, chills, or breathing problems occur while receiving the drug, contact the physician or nurse immediately. Blood tests will be monitored periodically to determine if electrolyte replacement is necessary. Use an effective method of birth control during therapy and for 6 months following the last dose of therapy.

Pharmacokinetics. *Fate.* Panitumumab demonstrates nonlinear pharmacokinetics; however, at clinically applicable doses (*see* **Adult Dosage and Administration**), the AUC increased in a dose-proportional manner. Variables such as age, gender, race, mild to moderate renal or hepatic impairment, or degree of EGFR staining intensity have shown no impact on pharmacokinetics. Concentrations may reach steady state by the third infusion. The terminal elimination half-life is approximately 7.5 days (range 3.6–10.9 days).

Adverse Reactions. The most frequent adverse reactions (≥20% prevalence) are skin toxicities (i.e., erythema, dermatitis acneiform, pruritus, exfoliation, rash, and fissures), paronychia, hypomagnesemia, fatigue, abdominal pain, nausea, diarrhea, and constipation. Dermatologic toxicities were reported in 89% of patients and were severe in 12% of patients receiving panitumumab. Severe infusion reactions or pulmonary fibrosis occurred in approximately 1% of patients in clinical trials. Electrolyte depletion requiring electrolyte replacement occurred in 2% of patients receiving panitumumab in clinical trials.

Contraindications. None.

Precautions. Boxed warnings include dermatologic toxicities and severe infusion-related reactions. Other warnings and precautions include hypersensitivity reactions, increased toxicity with combination chemotherapy, pulmonary fibrosis, and electrolyte depletion.

Drug Interactions. No formal studies have evaluated drug interactions with panitumumab. Infusion-related events may be exacerbated by antihypertensives. In clinical studies, the addition of panitumumab to other chemotherapy increased the rate of NCI CTC grade 3–5 adverse reactions.

Parameters to Monitor. Electrolyte screening (magnesium, calcium, potassium) should be performed periodically throughout therapy and until 8 weeks following discontinuation of therapy. Monitor for evidence of severe infusion reactions including hypotension, bronchospasm, anaphylaxis, fever, and/or chills; dermatologic toxicities and subsequent inflammatory or infectious sequelae; and ocular toxicities including conjunctivitis, ocular hyperemia, increased lacrimation, and eye/eyelid irritation.

RITUXIMAB
Rituxan

Pharmacology. Rituximab is a chimeric murine/human monoclonal antibody that binds to the CD20 antigen on the surface of normal and malignant B lymphocytes. This blocks normal CD20-dependent signaling of cell-cycle initiation and differentiation, leading to apoptosis. After binding to CD20, the free Fc portion of the antibody can recruit immune effector functions to cause lysis of B cells of B lymphocytes.[10]

Administration and Adult Dosage. Rituximab may be diluted in normal saline or dextrose 5% solutions to a final concentration of 1 mg/mL to 4 mg/mL. Premedicate the patient with diphenhydramine and acetaminophen and begin the first infusion at a rate of 50 mg/h. Increase the rate by 50 mg/h every 30 min to a maximum of 400 mg/h if no hypotension or hypersensitivity develops. Subsequent infusions are started at a rate of 100 mg/h and increased by 100 mg/h every 30 min to the maximum rate of 400 mg/h, if tolerated. If severe hypersensitivity reactions occur, stop the infusion and treat with diphenhydramine, acetaminophen, and a corticosteroid; for life-threatening reactions, add saline, epinephrine, and bronchodilators. If the reaction is not life-threatening, the infusion may be restarted at one-half of the earlier rate after symptoms subside.

For CD20-positive, B-cell, non-Hodgkin's lymphoma, rituximab is given as an intravenous infusion of 375 mg/m^2 per each schedule according to the indication below.

Relapsed or refractory, low-grade or follicular NHL. Administer once weekly for 4 or 8 doses.

Retreatment for relapsed or refractory, low-grade or follicular NHL. Administer once weekly for 4 doses.

Previously untreated follicular NHL. Administer on day 1 of each cycle of CVP chemotherapy, for up to 8 doses.

Nonprogressing, low-grade NHL, after first line CVP chemotherapy. Following completion of 68 cycles of CVP chemotherapy, administer once weekly for 4 doses at 6-month intervals to a maximum of 16 doses.

Diffuse large B-cell NHL. Administer on day 1 of each cycle of chemotherapy for up to 8 doses.

Recommended dose as a component of Zevalin. Infuse rituximab 250 mg/m^2 within 4 h prior to the administration of ^{111}In Zevalin and within 4 h prior to the administration of ^{90}Y Zevalin. Refer to the Zevalin package insert for full prescribing information regarding the Zevalin therapeutic regimen.

Recommended dose for Rheumatoid Arthritis. Rituximab 1000 mg/m^2 given intravenously every 2 weeks for a total of 2 doses. Methylprednisolone 100 mg given intravenously or its equivalent 30 min prior to each infusion is recommended to reduce the incidence and severity of infusion reactions. In this setting, rituximab is combined with methotrexate. Safety and efficacy of retreatment have not been established.

Special Populations. *Pediatric Dosage.* Safety and efficacy not established.

Geriatric Dosage. Same as adult dosage.

Pregnancy Category/Lactation. Pregnancy category C. Although not formally studied with rituximab, immunoglobulins are excreted into breast milk. Use of rituximab during breast-feeding is not recommended unless treatment of the mother outweighs unknown risks to the infant.

Dosage Forms. Inj 100, 500 mg.

Patient Instructions. This drug may cause a flulike syndrome including fever, chills, and weakness shortly after infusion. Tell your physician if you experience painful sores, blisters, or ulcers on your skin or mouth; if you experience severe stomach pain; or if you experience changes in thinking, walking, strength, or vision over a period of several days.

Pharmacokinetics. *Serum levels.* Peak serum levels are inversely correlated with the number of CD20-positive B cells. Levels average approximately 280 mg/L.

Fate. Major sites of antibody distribution are to lymphoid cells of the thymus gland, white pulp of the spleen, and B lymphocytes in peripheral blood and lymph nodes. Cl averages 0.054 L/h; the antibody is still detectable in serum 3–6 months after the last dose. Half-life is proportional to the dose (range 11–105 h) with an average of 60 h after a dosage of 375 mg/m^2.

Adverse Reactions. Most patients experience an infusion-related symptom complex with fever, chills, and rigors on the first infusion. Other frequent, immediate infusion-related symptoms are nausea (18%), vomiting (10%), angioedema (13%), urticaria or pruritus (10%), and bronchospasm and rhinitis (8%). Hypotension and other immediate effects are moderate or severe in 10% of the first doses. Overall, the frequency and severity of all reactions diminish with subsequent injections. Most first-dose reactions occur within 30 min to 2 h and resolve with slowing of the infusion rate for mild-to-moderate reactions or temporarily halting the infusion and treating with supportive medications for severe reactions. Epinephrine is required only occasionally.

Myelosuppression (neutropenia and thrombocytopenia) is typically mild and occurs in only 10% of patients, although long-term depletion of B cells occurs in 70%–80%; a minority also has decreased serum immunoglobulins. The frequency of grade 3 infections during the 4-week treatment period is 9% and grade 4 infections generally do not occur.

The most serious adverse reactions of rituximab are infusion reactions, tumor lysis syndrome, mucocutaneous toxicities, hepatitis B reactivation with fulminant hepatitis, PML, other viral infections, cardiac arrhythmias, renal toxicity, and bowel obstruction and perforation.

Contraindications. None.

Precautions. Black box warnings include fatal infusion reactions, tumor lysis syndrome with white blood cell count (WBC) $\geq$ 25,000 cells/mm^3, severe mucocutaneous reactions, and progressive multifocal encephalopathy. Other warnings with rituximab use include reactivation of hepatitis B (HBV) infection or other viral infections, cardiovascular or renal complications, and bowel obstruction or perforation. The ability to respond immunologically to a vaccination is compromised after therapy; the safety of live virus vaccination is not known. Consider stopping antihypertensive medications on the day of treatment to reduce hypotensive reactions. Cardiac monitoring is recommended only in patients with preexisting arrhythmias and angina that have worsened during the infusion.

Drug Interactions. Additive hypotension can occur in patients on antihypertensive therapy. No formal studies have evaluated drug interactions with rituximab.

Parameters to Monitor. Monitor vital signs frequently during rituximab infusion. Obtain CBC with differential and platelet count periodically and more frequently in patients developing cytopenias. Obtain HBV infection screening before initiation of rituximab for patients at high risk of HBV infection; cardiac monitoring during rituximab infusion in patients with preexisting arrhythmias, angina, or history of arrhythmias during rituximab infusion. Monitor patient for tumor lysis syndrome when appropriate; patients with large tumor burdens and presumed chemosensitive tumors are at risk for tumor lysis syndrome.

TRASTUZUMAB   Herceptin

Pharmacology. Trastuzumab is a humanized monoclonal antibody that binds to the HER-2 protein found on the surfaces of some normal cells and plays a role in regulating cell growth. It is used only to treat tumors with an overexpression of HER-2 protein. In vitro, trastuzumab has been shown to be a mediator of antibody-dependent cellular cytotoxicity, thus inhibiting the proliferation of tumor cells that exhibit HER-2 expression. Immunohistochemistry (IHC) and fluorescence in situ hybridization (FISH) of fixed tumor blocks are methods used to determine HER-2 protein overexpression.

Administration and Adult Dosage. Trastuzumab should be diluted in 250 mL of normal saline. Do not dilute in dextrose-containing solutions.

   Treatment of HER-2 overexpressing node-positive or node-negative breast cancer (adjuvant therapy or metastatic therapy). Initial dose of 4 mg/kg over 90-min IV infusion, then 2 mg/kg over 30-min IV infusion weekly for 52 weeks. Alternatively, an initial dose of 8 mg/kg over 90-min IV infusion, then 6 mg/kg over 90-min IV infusion every 3 weeks for 52 weeks may be given in the adjuvant setting. Trastuzumab should be permanently discontinued when severe infusion reactions occur or in cases of severe cardiomyopathy. The infusion rate may be decreased in cases of mild-to-moderate infusion-related reactions; the infusion should be interrupted for dyspnea or marked hypotension.

Special Populations. *Pediatric Dosage.* Safety and efficacy not established.

Geriatric Dosage. Same as adult dosage.

Pregnancy Category/Lactation. Pregnancy category C. Although not formally studied with rituximab, immunoglobulins are excreted into breast milk. Use of rituximab during breast-feeding is not recommended unless treatment of the mother outweighs unknown risks to the infant.

Dosage Forms. Inj 440 mg.

Patient Instructions. Contact your physician immediately for any of the following: new onset or worsening shortness of breath, cough, swelling of the ankles/legs, swelling of the face, palpitations, weight gain of more than 5 lb in 24 h, and dizziness or loss of consciousness. Use an effective method of birth control for 6 months following completion of trastuzumab therapy.

Pharmacokinetics. With the recommended dosage regimen, steady-state peak and trough concentrations are 123 and 79 mg/L, respectively. Trough serum levels are 1.5 times higher when given with paclitaxel, possibly because of inhibition of metabolism. The drug is distributed primarily in serum, with a V_d of 0.44 L/kg. Pharmacokinetics appear to be dose related: Cl decreases and half-life increases with increasing dosages. Half-life averages 25 days (range 1–32 days) with the recommended regimen. Renal impairment appears not to affect pharmacokinetics.

Adverse Reactions. Side effects are frequent but usually not severe. Mild-to-moderate chills with or without fever occur in 40% of patients during the infusion and can usually be treated with acetaminophen, diphenhydramine, and/or meperidine. Other frequent side effects are diarrhea, pain, asthenia, nausea, vomiting, flulike symptoms, cough, dyspnea, rash, edema, anemia, and leukopenia. Occasional serious reactions include anaphylaxis, thrombosis, pancytopenia, convulsions, apnea, hypoxia, and renal failure. Cardiac dysfunction and CHF have occurred. Use the drug with caution in preexisting cardiac dysfunction; monitor cardiac function during therapy, and consider discontinuation when clinically important CHF develops. Serious infusion-related reactions including hypersensitivity (including anaphylaxis) and pulmonary events occur in approximately 0.25% of patients.

Contraindications. None.

Precautions. Boxed warnings include cardiomyopathy, infusion-related reactions, and pulmonary toxicity. Trastuzumab can cause left ventricular cardiac dysfunction, arrhythmias, hypertension, disabling cardiac failure, cardiomyopathy, and cardiac death. Trastuzumab may worsen chemotherapy-induced neutropenia and may cause fetal harm when administered to a pregnant female.

Drug Interactions. When administered with paclitaxel, a 1.5-fold increase in trastuzumab serum levels has been observed.

Parameters to Monitor. Left ventricular ejection fraction (LVEF) via MUGA scan or echocardiogram should be obtained at baseline and every 3 months during trastuzumab therapy and every 6 months for 2 years following trastuzumab therapy. More frequent cardiac monitoring is necessary when decreases in left ventricular ejection fraction occur. Patients should also be monitored for infusion-related reactions, which may occur within 24 h following therapy.

■ REFERENCES

1. Ravandi F, O'Brien S. Alemtuzumab in CLL and other lymphoid neoplasms. *Cancer Invest.* 2006;24(7):718-725.
2. Krämer I, Lipp HP. Bevacizumab, a humanized anti-angiogenic monoclonal antibody for the treatment of colorectal cancer. *J Clin Pharm Ther.* 2007;32(1):1-14.
3. Hurwitz H et al. Bevacizumab plus irinotecan, fluorouracil, and leucovorin for metastatic colorectal cancer. *N Engl J Med.* 2004;350:2335.
4. Giantonio BJ et al. Bevacizumab in combination with oxaliplatin, fluorouracil, and leucovorin (FOLFOX4) for previously treated metastatic colorectal cancer: results from the Eastern Cooperative Oncology Group Study E3200. *J Clin Oncol.* 2007;25:1539.
5. Rivera F et al. Cetuximab, its clinical use and future perspectives. *Anticancer Drugs.* 2008;19(2):99-113.
6. Robert F et al. Phase I/IIa study of cetuximab with gemcitabine plus carboplatin in patients with chemotherapy-naive advanced non-small-cell lung cancer. *J Clin Oncol.* 2005;23(36):9089-9096.
7. Robert F et al. Phase I study of anti-epidermal growth factor receptor antibody cetuximab in combination with radiation therapy in patients with advanced head and neck cancer. *J Clin Oncol.* 2001;19:3234-3243.
8. Cheson BD. Radioimmunotherapy of non-Hodgkin lymphomas. *Blood.* 2003;101(2):391-398.
9. Carteni G et al. Panitumumab a novel drug in cancer treatment. *Ann Oncol.* 2007;18(suppl 6):16-21, vi.
10. Smith MR. Rituximab (monoclonal anti-CD20 antibody): mechanisms of action and resistance. *Oncogene.* 200320;22(47):7359-7368.

Chapter 26

Tyrosine Kinase Inhibitors

Amber P. Lawson

DASATINIB   Sprycel

Pharmacology. Dasatinib inhibits the abnormal BCR-ABL tyrosine kinase created by the Philadelphia chromosome abnormality of CML, inhibiting proliferation and inducing apoptosis in leukemic cells displaying this abnormality. Dasatinib binds the ABL kinase in multiple conformations. In addition, dasatinib also has been shown to inhibit c-kit, EPHA2, PDGFR, and the SRC family of tyrosine kinases. Dasatinib lacks activity against the T315I mutation of BCR-ABL tyrosine kinase associated with CML.

Adult Dosage and Administration. *PO for chronic-phase CML*—100 mg once daily. *PO for accelerated-phase CML, lymphoid or myeloid blast phase CML, or Ph+ ALL*—140 mg once daily

Dosage Forms. Tab 20, 50, 70, 100 mg.

Patient Instructions. Dasatinib may be taken with or without food. Take at the same time every day. When a dose is missed, take at the next scheduled time. Do not chew, crush, or break tablets. Do not consume grapefruit juice or grapefruit-containing products while taking dasatinib. Notify health care provider immediately when fever, bleeding, easy bruising, swelling, weight gain, or shortness of breath occurs. Notify your health care provider of all medications you are currently taking. Do not take medications that reduce stomach acid, as these medications may reduce the absorption of dasatinib. Medications that neutralize stomach acid (e.g., Maalox, Tums, Rolaids) may be taken up to 2 h before or 2 h after taking dasatinib. Use effective contraception while receiving dasatinib therapy.

Pharmacokinetics. *Fate.* After oral administration, dasatinib is rapidly absorbed and maximum plasma concentrations have been achieved between 0.5 and 6 h and dose-responsive increases in AUC have been observed. Oral bioavailability in preclinical studies has been estimated at 14%–34%. Although absorption increases by 14% when dasatinib is administered with a high-fat meal, there does not appear to be any important change in clinical effects. Pharmacokinetic studies suggest that dasatinib is extensively protein bound in the extravascular space. Metabolism occurs via cytochrome P450 3A4 pathway and dasatinib exhibits weak, time-dependent CYP3A4 inhibition in human liver microsomes. Major metabolites of dasatinib are not thought to contribute to the pharmacology of the agent. The terminal half-life of dasatinib is between 3 h and 5 h; dasatinib is eliminated almost exclusively via the feces.

Adverse Reactions. The most common adverse reactions include fluid retention events, diarrhea, headache, skin rash, nausea, hemorrhage, fatigue, elevated LFTs, and dyspnea. The most frequently reported serious adverse reactions included pleural effusion, pyrexia, pneumonia, infection, febrile neutropenia, GI bleeding, dyspnea, sepsis, diarrhea, CHF, and pericardial effusion. Myelosuppression may occur more frequently in patients with advanced phase CML and Ph+ ALL than with chronic-phase CML. Occasionally, hemorrhage likely related to thrombocytopenia has occurred. The potential for QTc prolongation exists during dasatinib therapy; monitor patients at risk of QTc prolongation (electrolyte disturbances, coadministration of QTc prolonging medications, or existing QTc prolongation).

Contraindications. None.

Warnings/Precautions. Myelosuppression, bleeding-related events associated with thrombocytopenia, fluid retention, QTc prolongation, and pregnancy.

Drug Interactions. Drugs that inhibit CYP3A4 should be avoided because of increases in dasatinib levels. Drugs that are inducers of CYP3A4 should be avoided when possible. When dasatinib is coadministered with a known inducer of CYP3A4, consider increase in dasatinib dosage. H2 antagonists and proton pump inhibitors should not be administered with dasatinib, because of decreased dasatinib levels. Antacids should be taken at least 2 h before or 2 h after dasatinib.

Monitoring Parameters. Bone marrow assessments should be performed every 1–3 months to assess efficacy. Complete blood counts should be monitored weekly for the first 2 months of therapy then monthly thereafter. Hepatic function tests should be assessed at baseline and as clinically indicated thereafter.

ERLOTINIB   Tarceva

Pharmacology. Although the mechanism of action has not been fully elucidated, erlotinib inhibits the intracellular phosphorylation of tyrosine kinase associated with the epidermal growth factor receptor (EGFR). Specificity of inhibition with regard to other tyrosine kinase receptors has not been fully characterized. EGFR is expressed on the cell surface of normal cells and cancer cells.

Adult Dosage and Administration. *PO for treatment of locally advanced or metastatic non–small cell lung cancer after failure of at least one prior chemotherapy regimen*—150 mg once daily, taken at least 1 h before or 2 h after the ingestion of food. Treatment should continue until disease progression or unacceptable toxicity occurs. *PO for first-line treatment of locally advanced, unresectable, or metastatic pancreatic cancer in combination with gemcitabine*—100 mg once daily, taken at least 1 h before or 2 h after the ingestion of food, in combination with gemcitabine. Treatment should continue until disease progression or unacceptable toxicity occurs.

DOSE MODIFICATIONS

EVENT	DOSE ADJUSTMENT
Diagnosis of interstitial lung disease, hepatic failure, GI perforation, renal failure, exfoliative skin conditions, or acute/worsening ocular disorders	Discontinue Erlotinib.

Concomitant strong CYP3A4 inhibitors	Decrease dose in 50-mg increments when severe adverse reactions occur.
Concomitant strong CYP3A4 inducers	Consider increase in erlotinib dose as tolerated at 2-wk intervals while monitoring the patient's safety.
	The maximum dose of erlotinib studied in combination with rifampicin is 450 mg/d.
	Erlotinib dose will need to be reduced immediately to the indicated starting dose upon discontinuation of rifampin or other inducers.
Cigarette smoking	When a patient continues to smoke, a cautious increase in the erlotinib dose, not exceeding 300 mg/d, may be considered while monitoring the patient's safety.
	Efficacy and long-term safety (>14 d) of a dose higher than the recommended starting doses have not been established in patients who continue to smoke cigarettes.
	When the erlotinib dose is adjusted upward, the dose should be reduced immediately to the indicated starting dose upon cessation of smoking.

Special Populations. *Pediatric Dosage.* Safety and efficacy not established in pediatric patients.

Geriatric Dosage. Safety profiles and clinical effectiveness are similar between younger patients and patients older than 65 years.

Pregnancy Category/Lactation. Pregnancy category D. Use during breast-feeding is not recommended.

Hepatic Impairment. Patients should be closely monitored when total bilirubin is greater than the ULN or has Child-Pugh A, B, or C hepatic insufficiency. Treatment with erlotinib should be used with extreme caution in patients with total bilirubin greater than 3 times the ULN.

Dosage Forms. Tab 25, 100, 150 mg.

Patient Instructions. Take erlotinib on an empty stomach, at least 1 h before or 2 h after meals. Do not consume grapefruit juice or grapefruit-containing products while receiving this medication. Use alcohol-free emollients and sunscreen when going out into the sun to avoid skin toxicity. A rash may develop while taking this medication. Your health care provider will discuss options for treating rash when a rash develops while taking this medication; do not use skin treatments containing alcohol as these agents may aggravate the condition. Women of childbearing age should use effective contraceptive methods while receiving erlotinib. If you smoke, it is highly recommended to stop smoking while receiving erlotinib; talk to your health care provider regarding options to help you quit smoking. Call your health care provider immediately when eye irritation, onset/worsening of shortness of breath and cough, onset/worsening of rash, or severe and persistent nausea, anorexia, vomiting, or diarrhea occurs.

Pharmacokinetics. *Fate.* Erlotinib is almost 60% absorbed after oral administration; the bioavailability approaches 100% when erlotinib is administered with food. The solubility of erlotinib decreases as the pH in the GI tract increases. The AUC of erlotinib is decreased by approximately 50% when administered with proton pump inhibitors. The AUC of erlotinib in cigarette smokers is decreased one-third to one-half compared to nonsmokers. Erlotinib is extensively protein bound. Erlotinib undergoes hepatic metabolism via primarily CYP3A4; CYP1A2 and CYP1A1 are also involved in the metabolism of erlotinib to a lesser extent. The median half-life of erlotinib is estimated to be 36.2 h. Approximately 91% of the dose is recovered in feces, while 8% of the dose is recovered in the urine as metabolites.

Adverse Reactions. The most common adverse reactions of erlotinib include rash, diarrhea, anorexia, nausea, fatigue, dyspnea, cough, infection, stomatitis, pruritis, conjunctivitis, increased LFTs, and abdominal pain. Frequent and serious adverse effects include CVA and MI, bullous and exfoliative skin disorders, GI perforation, and hemorrhage. Occasional and serious adverse effects include pulmonary toxicity, microangiopathic anemia with thrombocytopenia, bullous and exfoliative skin disorders, bleeding, GI perforation, renal failure, liver failure, and hepatorenal syndrome.

Contraindications. None.

Warnings/Precautions. Pulmonary toxicity, renal failure, hepatic failure, GI perforation, bullous and exfoliative skin disorders, MI/ischemia, CVA, microangiopathic hemolytic anemia with thrombocytopenia, ocular disorders, pregnancy, elevated international normalized ratio, and bleeding.

Drug Interactions. Erlotinib is predominately metabolized by CYP3A4; therefore, strong inhibitors and inducers of CYP3A4 are thought to increase and decrease serum concentrations of erlotinib, respectively. Cigarette smoking will decrease the AUC of erlotinib and should be avoided. Medications that alter the pH of the upper GI tract such as histamine-2 receptor blockers and proton pump inhibitors should be avoided because the absorption of erlotinib is decreased when administered with these medications. Erlotinib may increase the international normalized ratio when administered with warfarin. Patients receiving concomitant antiangiogenic agents, corticosteroids, nonsteroidal anti-inflammatory drugs, and/or taxane-based chemotherapy appear to be more at risk for developing GI perforation.

Monitoring Parameters. Baseline and periodic monitoring of serum electrolytes, LFTs, and renal function is indicated. Monitoring of the international normalized ratio in patients receiving warfarin or other anticoagulants should be done at baseline and on a regular basis. Patients should be monitored for skin rash, tumor progression, and signs and symptoms of GI perforation or interstitial lung disease including dyspnea, cough, and fever.

IMATINIB MESYLATE
Gleevec

Pharmacology. Imatinib inhibits the abnormal BCR-ABL tyrosine kinase created by the Philadelphia chromosome (Ph+) abnormality of CML, inhibiting proliferation and inducing apoptosis in leukemic cells with this abnormality. It may also inhibit the tyrosine kinase of platelet-derived growth factor, stem cell factor, and c-kit. In vitro, imatinib inhibits proliferation and induces apoptosis in gastrointestinal stromal tumor (GIST) cells that express an activating c-kit mutation.

Adult Dosage and Administration. All doses of imatinib should be taken orally with food. Doses of 400 or 600 mg should be administered once daily, whereas a dose of 800 mg should be administered as 400 mg twice a day. Imatinib can be dissolved in water or apple juice for patients having difficulty in swallowing. Daily dosing of 800 mg and above should incorporate the use of 400-mg tablets (i.e., 400-mg tablet twice daily) to reduce iron exposure.

DOSAGE BY INDICATION	
INDICATION	STARTING DOSE
Adults with chronic-phase CML	400 mg daily
Adults with accelerated-phase CML or CML in blast crisis	600 mg daily
Pediatrics with CML	340 mg/m^2/d or 260 mg/m^2/d
Adults with Ph+ ALL	600 mg daily
Adult patients with myelodysplastic/myeloproliferative diseases (MDS/MPD) associated with PDGFR (platelet-derived growth factor receptor) gene rearrangements	400 mg daily
Adult patients with aggressive systemic mastocytosis	100 mg daily or 400 mg daily
Adult patients with hypereosinophilic syndrome (HES) and/or chronic eosinophilic leukemia (CEL)	100 mg daily or 400 mg daily
Adult patients with unresectable, recurrent and/or metastatic dermatofibrosarcoma protuberans	800 mg daily
Adults with metastatic and/or unresectable GIST and adjuvant treatment of adults with GIST	400 mg daily

Special Populations. *Pediatric Dosage.* Safety and efficacy have been established in pediatric patients with newly diagnosed chronic-phase CML and recurrent CML after stem cell transplantation or resistance to interferon alfa therapy. There is no data in children younger than 2 years. The recommended doses of 260 mg/m^2/d or 340 mg/m^2/d achieve an AUC comparable to a 400-mg dose in adult patients.

Geriatric Dosage. Safety profiles and clinical effectiveness are similar between younger patients and patients older than 65 years. Edema may be more prevalent in patients older than 65 years.

Pregnancy Category/Lactation. Pregnancy category D. Use during breast-feeding is not recommended.

Hepatic Impairment. Dose reduction of 25% of recommended dose is suggested for severe hepatic impairment.

Renal Impairment. Dose reduction of at least 50% of recommended dose is suggested for moderate or severe renal impairment.

Dosage Forms. **Tab** 100, 400 mg.

Patient Instructions. Imatinib should be taken with food and a full glass of water. Imatinib can be dissolved in water or apple juice. Do not crush, break, or chew tablets. Take dose as prescribed by health care provider; when a dose is missed, take dose as soon as possible unless it is time for the next scheduled dose. Do not double up doses to make up for a missed dose. Notify your health care provider of all the medications you are currently taking. Do not consume grapefruit juice or grapefruit-containing products while taking imatinib. Effective birth control methods should be undertaken in patients of childbearing age while receiving imatinib therapy. Notify your health care provider when side effects occur including fever, shortness of breath, blood in stools, jaundice, sudden weight gain, symptoms of cardiac failure, or if you have a history of heart disease.

Pharmacokinetics. *Fate.* Oral bioavailability is 98% with a peak at 2–4 h after the dose. It is 95% plasma protein bound. Metabolism is primarily by CYP3A4 to the N-desmethyl metabolite that has activity similar to the parent drug. The drug is eliminated in feces, mostly as metabolites. Elimination half-lives are 18 and 40 h for the drug and active metabolite, respectively.

Adverse Reactions. Most adverse reactions are mild to moderate and more frequent during the accelerated phase and especially during blast crisis. The most frequent are nausea, vomiting, and periorbital or lower limb edema. Edema is occasionally severe and can be managed by diuretics, supportive measures, or imatinib dosage reduction. Muscle cramps and pain, hemorrhage, skin rash, headache, fatigue, abdominal pain, arthralgia, and fever are also frequent. Dose-related neutropenia (duration 2–3 weeks) and thrombocytopenia (duration 3–4 weeks) also occur, and respond to dosage reduction or interruption of therapy. Elevated transaminases and bilirubin can occur, sometimes requiring dosage reduction or treatment interruption; one death from hepatotoxicity has been reported.

Contraindications. None.

Warnings/Precautions. Edema, fluid retention, cytopenias, severe CHF, hepatotoxicity, GI perforation, hemorrhage, bullous dermatologic reactions, cardiogenic shock, hypothyroidism, pregnancy.

Drug Interactions. Inhibitors and inducers of CYP3A4 are expected to alter the metabolism of imatinib and should be used with caution. Imatinib decreases the metabolism of simvastatin, apparently through CYP3A4 inhibition. Use other drugs with caution that are metabolized by CYP3A4. Patients requiring anticoagulation should receive heparin or a LMWH rather than warfarin. Systemic exposure to acetaminophen is increased when administered with imatinib.

Monitoring Parameters. Complete blood counts should be performed on a weekly basis for the first month, every 2 weeks for the second month, and every 3 months thereafter. LFTs should be performed at baseline and monthly thereafter. Monitor renal function and electrolytes at baseline and as clinically indicated. Montior TSH levels in patients with a history of thyroidectomy receiving levothyroxine replacement because hypothyroidism in this patient population has been reported. Echocardiograms and determination of serum troponin should be considered prior to initiating imatinib in patients with hypereosinophilic syndrome and cardiac involvement and in patients with myelodysplastic/myeloproliferative disease or systemic mastocytosis associated with high eosinophil levels; concomitant use of prophylactic systemic steroids may be necessary. Patients with a history of cardiac failure or risk factors for cardiac failure should be monitored closely for signs or symptoms of exacerbation. Monitor patient weight for signs of fluid retention and edema.

LAPATINIB   Tykerb

Pharmacology. Lapatinib is a 4-anilinoquinazoline kinase inhibitor of the intracellular tyrosine kinase domains of both the epidermal growth factor receptor (EGFR [ErbB1]) and of human epidermal receptor type 2 (HER-2 [ErbB2]) receptors. On the basis of in vitro data, cross-resistance is not thought to exist between lapatinib and trastuzumab.

Adult Dosage and Administration. *PO for HER-2 positive advanced or metastatic breast cancer after therapy with an anthracycline, a taxane, and trastuzumab*—1250 mg once daily in combination with capecitabine 1000 mg/m^2 orally every 12 h on days 1–14 of a repeating 21-day cycle. Lapatinib should be taken at least 1 h before or 1 h after a meal.

DOSE MODIFICATIONS

EVENT	DOSE ADJUSTMENT
Severe hepatic impairment	Decrease dose to 750 mg once daily.
Concomitant strong CYP3A4 inhibitors	Decrease dose to 500 mg once daily; a washout period of 7 d is recommended when an inhibitor is discontinued before adjusting the lapatinib dose upward.
Concomitant strong CYP3A4 inducers	Dose should be gradually increased from 1250 mg once daily up to 4500 mg once daily based on tolerability.
Left ventricular ejection fraction decrease (NCI Common Toxicity Criteria for Adverse Events ≥ grade 2 and below institutional upper limit of normal)	Hold lapatinib. It may be restarted at a reduced dose of 1000 mg once daily after a minimum of 2 wk when the patient is asymptomatic and the left ventricular ejection fraction recovers to normal.

Special Populations. *Pediatric Dosage.* Safety and efficacy not established in pediatric patients.

Geriatric Dosage. Safety profiles and clinical effectiveness are similar between younger patients and patients older than 65 years when laptinib is used in combination with capecitabine.

Pregnancy Category/Lactation. Pregnancy category D. Use during breast-feeding is not recommended.

Dosage Forms. Tab 250 mg.

Patient Instructions. This medication should be taken on an empty stomach. Do not consume grapefruit juice or grapefruit-containing products while taking lapatinib. This medication is given in combination with another oral chemotherapy agent called capecitabine. Lapatinib should be taken once daily as directed by your health care provider for 21 days of a 28-day cycle. Notify your health care provider if you have a history of heart problems or liver problems before starting lapatinib. If you are pregnant, breast-feeding, or may become pregnant, notify your health care provider before staring lapatinib. Notify your health care provider of all medications and herbal supplements you are taking because many medications may interact with lapatinib. Call your health care provider when you experience severe diarrhea, heart palpitations, or shortness of breath as these symptoms may represent serious side effects of lapatinib.

Pharmacokinetics. *Fate.* Absorption is variable and incomplete after administration of lapatinib. Serum concentrations appear after approximately 0.25–0.5 h (range 0–1.5 h). Peak plasma concentrations are achieved after approximately 4 h. Administering lapatinib in divided doses compared to once daily doses increases the AUC by approximately 2-fold. When lapatinib is administered with food, systemic exposure to the drug increases. The AUC increased by 167% and 325% when lapatinib was administered with a low-fat meal and a high-fat meal, respectively. Lapatinib is highly protein bound and in vitro studies suggest that lapatinib is an inhibitor of P-glycoprotein. Approximately 70% of lapatinib is metabolized through CYP3A4 with minor contributions from CYP3A5, CYP2C19, and CYP2C8.[1] One metabolite (GW690006) remains active against EGFR but not HER-2; no other active metabolites have been identified. The terminal phase half-life is 14.2 h following single doses; with repeated dosing, the half-life may reach 24 h. Approximately 27% of the parent compound is recovered in feces and less than 2% is recovered in urine.

Adverse Reactions. The most common adverse reactions of lapatinib when combined with capecitabine include diarrhea, palmar-plantar erythrodysesthesia, nausea, rash, vomiting, back pain, mucosal inflammation, dyspnea, insomnia, and fatigue. Frequently reported serious adverse effects include palmar-plantar erythrodysesthesia and diarrhea. Occasionally, cardiac toxicity resulting in a decrease in left ventricular ejection fraction of ≥20% has been reported. In the majority of cases, the cardiac toxicity was apparent within the initial 9 weeks of therapy during clinical trials. In an uncontrolled, open-label study, lapatinib was also shown to prolong the QTc interval.

Contraindications. None.

Warnings/Precautions. Decreased left ventricular ejection fraction, diarrhea, and QTc prolongation; use with caution in pregnancy and in patients with hepatic impairment.

Drug Interactions. Lapatinib inhibits CYP3A4, CYP2C8, and P-glycoprotein; this interaction may potentially increase concentrations of drugs metabolized through these pathways. Dose reduction of concomitant substrate drugs should be considered when administered with lapatinib. Lapatinib does not substantially inhibit CYP1A2, CYP2C9, CYP2C19, and CYP2D6 or UGT enzymes in human liver microsomes. Lapatinib is extensively metabolized by CYP3A4, and serum concentrations of lapatinib are markedly altered when administered with these types of medications. Dose adjustment should be considered when lapatinib must be administered with concomitant strong inhibitors or concomitant strong inducers of CYP3A4.

Monitoring Parameters. Hepatic function tests should be obtained at baseline, every 4–6 weeks during therapy, and as clinically indicated. An electrocardiogram (ECG) and assessment of left ventricular ejection fraction should be obtained at baseline and periodically thereafter as clinically indicated. The left ventricular ejection fraction should be assessed periodically (i.e., every 8 weeks) during lapatinib therapy; in clinical trials, the majority of decreases in left ventricular ejection fraction occurred during the initial 9 weeks of therapy. Serum electrolytes should be obtained at baseline and periodically; correcting electrolyte abnormalities such as hypokalemia and hypomagnesemia may potentially decrease risk of QTc prolongation. Monitor for other signs and symptoms of lapatinib toxicity including GI upset, diarrhea, rash, palmar-plantar erythrodysesthesia, and dyspnea.

NILOTINIB Tasigna

Pharmacology. Nilotinib inhibits the abnormal BCR-ABL tyrosine kinase created by the Philadelphia chromosome abnormality of CML, inhibiting proliferation and inducing apoptosis in leukemic cells with this abnormality. Nilotinib binds the inactive, unphosphorylated configuration of the ABL tyrosine kinase. Compared to imatinib, nilotinib may exhibit improved binding to the ABL protein; nilotinib requires 4 hydrogen bonds to bind to the BCR-ABL tyrosine kinase domain while imatinib requires 6 hydrogen bonds.[2] Nilotinib has also been found to inhibit platelet-derived growth factor and c-kit receptor kinase. Nilotinib lacks activity against the T315I mutation of BCR-ABL tyrosine kinase associated with CML.

Administration and Adult Dosage. *PO for chronic or accelerated phase of CML,* **refractory or resistant to imatinib therapy**—400 mg twice daily, approximately 12 h apart. Nilotinib should not be taken with food. No food should be consumed for 2 h before or for 1 h after administration of nilotinib. (*See* tables below for dose adjustments based on QTc prolongation, myelosuppression, and nonhematologic abnormalities.)

DOSE ADJUSTMENTS FOR QTc PROLONGATION

ECG with QTc >480 ms

1. Withhold nilotinib and perform an analysis of serum potassium and magnesium, correcting with supplements when below the lower limit of normal to within normal limits. Concomitant medication usage must be reviewed.
2. Resume within 2 wk at prior dose when QTcF returns to <450 ms and to within 20 ms of baseline.
3. When QTcF is between 450 ms and 480 ms after 2 wk reduce the dose to 400 mg once daily.
4. If, following dose reduction to 400 mg once daily, QTcF returns to >480 ms, nilotinib should be discontinued.
5. An ECG should be repeated approximately 7 d after any dose adjustment.

QTcF = Fridericia's Correction Formula

DOSE ADJUSTMENTS FOR NEUTROPENIA AND THROMBOCYTOPENIA

Chronic- or accelerated-phase CML (400 mg twice daily)	Absolute neutrophil count < 1.0×10^9/L and/or platelet counts < 50×10^9/L	Stop nilotinib and monitor blood counts.
		Resume within 2 wk at prior dose when ANC > 1.0×10^9/L and platelets > 50×10^9/L.
		When blood counts remain low for >2 weeks, reduce the dose to 400 mg once daily.

DOSE ADJUSTMENTS FOR SELECTED NONHEMATOLOGIC LABORATORY ABNORMALITIES

Elevated serum lipase or amylase ≥ grade 3 (≥2 times ULN)	1. Withhold nilotinib and monitor serum lipase or amylase. 2. Resume nilotinib at 400 mg once daily when serum lipase or amylase return to ≤ grade 1 (≤1.5 times ULN).
Elevated bilirubin ≥ grade 3 (>3 times ULN)	1. Withhold nilotinib and monitor bilirubin. 2. Resume nilotinib at 400 mg once daily when bilirubin returns to ≤ grade 1 (≤1.5 times ULN).
Elevated hepatic transaminases ≥ grade 3 (>5 times ULN)	1. Withhold nilotinib and monitor hepatic transaminases. 2. Resume nilotinib at 400 mg once daily when hepatic transaminases return to ≤ grade 1 (≤2.5 times ULN).

Special Populations. *Pediatric Dosage.* Safety and efficacy not established in pediatric patients.

Geriatric Dosage. Safety profiles are similar between younger patients and patients older than 65 years. In accelerated-phase CML patients, the major hematologic response rate is 31% in patients <65 years and 15% in patients ≥65 years.

Pregnancy Category/Lactation. Pregnancy category D. Use during breast-feeding is not recommended.

Dosage Forms. Cap 200 mg.

Patient Instructions. Nilotinib must be taken on an empty stomach. Do not eat 2 h before or 1 h after taking nilotinib. Nilotinib doses should be separated by approximately 12 h. Take at the same time every day. When a dose is missed, take at next scheduled time. Do not chew, crush, or break tablets and take with a full glass of water. Do not consume grapefruit juice or grapefruit-containing products while taking nilotinib. Prior to starting nilotinib therapy, your health care provider will administer a heart test called an electrocardiogram (ECG) to look for irregular heartbeat. If you have a history of an irregular heartbeat, liver problems, heart problems, or a history of pancreatitis, tell your health care provider prior to starting nilotinib. Notify health care provider immediately when fainting or irregular heartbeat occurs as this could represent a serious side effect of nilotinib. Notify health care provider immediately when fever, bleeding, easy bruising, nausea, vomiting, stomach pain, fainting, swelling, weight gain, shortness of breath, or yellowing of the eyes or skin occurs. Notify your health care provider of all medications you are currently taking.

Pharmacokinetics. Age, gender, body weight, or ethnic origin does not appear to affect the pharmacokinetics of nilotinib. *Fate.* Nilotinib reaches peak concentrations approximately 3 h after oral administration. When administered 30 min after a high-fat meal, the systemic exposure (AUC) of nilotinib is increased by 82% compared to the fasted state. Nilotinib is approximately 98% protein bound and no volume of distribution has been reported to date. Nilotinib is metabolized via oxidation and hydroxylation as well as by the CYP3A4 isoenzyme. No metabolites have been suggested to contribute to the pharmacologic activity of nilotinib. The terminal half-life of nilotinib is approximately 17 h and eliminated almost exclusively via feces.

Adverse Reactions. The most common adverse reactions include myelosuppression, rash, nausea, headache, itching, fatigue, diarrhea, or constipation. The most frequently reported serious adverse reactions include QTc prolongation, myelosuppression, febrile neutropenia, electrolyte disturbances, and increased lipase. Occasional and serious adverse effects include hypertensive crisis, pulmonary edema, pleural effusion, pancreatitis, hepatotoxicity, hepatitis, and erectile dysfunction. Occasionally, hemorrhage likely related to thrombocytopenia has occurred. The potential for concentration-dependent QTc prolongation and sudden death exists during nilotinib therapy; monitor patients at risk of QTc prolongation (electrolyte disturbances, coadministration of QTc prolonging medications, or existing QTc prolongation).

Contraindications. Hypokalemia, hypomagnesemia, or long QT syndrome.

Warnings/Precautions. Nilotinib is associated with QTc prolongation and sudden death. An ECG should be performed to assess QTc at baseline, 7 days after initiation, and periodically thereafter as well as following any dosage adjustments. Hypokalemia and hypomagnesemia should be corrected before administering nilotinib. Patients should avoid food with nilotinib for 2 h before and 1 h after nilotinib administration. Medications that are strong inhibitors of CYP3A4 should be avoided. In addition hepatotoxicity, fetal harm, or elevated serum lipase may occur with nilotinib administration.

Drug Interactions. Nilotinib is a competitive inhibitor in vitro of CYP3A4, CYP2B6, CYP2C8, CYP2C9, CYP2D6, and UGT1A1 and may potentially increase concentrations of drugs metabolized through these pathways. Additionally, administering nilotinib with substrates of these enzymes may result in increased nilotinib exposure. Medications known to induce CYP 450 enzymes substantially reduce nilotinib exposure. Patients requiring anticoagulation should receive heparin or a LMWH rather than warfarin. Nilotinib inhibits human P-glycoprotein; caution should be used when administering substrates of human P-glycoprotein with nilotinib because levels of the substrate medication may be increased.

Monitoring Parameters. Bone marrow assessments should be performed every 1–3 months to assess efficacy. Complete blood counts should be monitored every 2 weeks for the first 2 months of therapy then monthly thereafter. Hepatic function tests and serum chemistries (including potassium and magnesium) should be assessed at baseline and as clinically indicated thereafter. ECGs should be obtained at baseline, 7 days after initiation and periodically thereafter as well as following dose adjustments. Serum lipase levels should be monitored periodically in patients with a history of pancreatitis.

SORAFENIB   Nexavar

Pharmacology. Sorafenib is a multikinase inhibitor that decreases tumor cell proliferation in vitro, possibly through interactions with multiple intracellular (CRAF, BRAF and mutant BRAF) and cell surface kinases (KIT, FLT-3, VEGFR-2, VEGFR-3, and PDGFR-β). Several of these kinases are thought to be involved in angiogenesis.

Adult Dosage and Administration. *PO for treatment of advanced renal cell carcinoma*—400 mg twice daily without food. Sorafenib is to be continued until loss of clinical benefit or unacceptable toxicity occurs. *PO for treatment of unresectable hepatocellular carcinoma*[3]—400 mg twice daily without food. Sorafenib is to be continued until loss of clinical benefit or unacceptable toxicity occurs. Dose modifications are suggested for dermatologic toxicities.

SUGGESTED DOSE MODIFICATION FOR SKIN TOXICITIES

SKIN TOXICITY GRADE	OCCURRENCE	SUGGESTED DOSE MODIFICATION
Grade 1: numbness, dysesthesia, tingling, painless swelling, erythema, or discomfort of the hands or feet that does not disrupt the patient's normal activities	Any occurrence	Continue treatment with sorafenib and consider topical therapy for symptomatic relief.

(continued)

SKIN TOXICITY GRADE	OCCURRENCE	SUGGESTED DOSE MODIFICATION
Grade 2: painful erythema and swelling of the hands or feet and/or discomfort affecting the patient's normal activities	First occurrence	Continue treatment with sorafenib and consider topical therapy for symptomatic relief.
		If no improvement in 7 d, *see* below.
	No improvement within 7 d; second or third occurrence	Interrupt sorafenib treatment until toxicity falls to grade 0–1.
		When resuming sorafenib, decrease dose by one dose level (400 mg daily or 400 mg every other day).
	Fourth occurrence	Discontinue sorafenib treatment.
Grade 3: moist desquamation, ulceration, blistering or severe pain of the hands or feet, or severe discomfort that causes the patient to be unable to work or perform activities of daily living	First or second occurrence	Interrupt sorafenib treatment until toxicity falls to grade 0–1.
		When resuming sorafenib, decrease dose by one dose level (400 mg daily or 400 mg every other day)
	Fourth occurrence	Discontinue sorafenib treatment.

Special Populations. *Pediatric Dosage.* Safety and efficacy not established in pediatric patients.

Geriatric Dosage. Safety profiles are similar between younger patients and patients older than 65 years.

Pregnancy Category/Lactation. Pregnancy category D. Use during breast-feeding is not recommended.

Dosage Forms. Tab 200 mg.

Patient Instructions. Sorafenib should be taken without food and at least 1 h before or 2 h following a meal. Take at the same time every day. Do not break, chew, or crush tablets. When a dose is missed, take at the next scheduled time. Do not consume grapefruit juice or grapefruit-containing products while taking sorafenib. Notify your health care provider of all medications you are currently taking. Effective birth control methods should be undertaken during sorafenib therapy and for up to 2 weeks after stopping treatment; birth defects may otherwise occur. Blood pressure may increase during sorafenib therapy and will be monitored by a health care provider. When rash, bleeding, chest pain, or skin reactions on hands and/or feet occur, call health care provider immediately.

Pharmacokinetics. *Fate.* After oral administration, sorafenib reaches peak serum concentrations in approximately 3 h. The bioavailability of sorafenib decreases by 29% when administered with a high-fat meal when compared to administration in the fasted state; therefore, sorafenib should be administered on an empty stomach. The AUC of sorafenib increases at a less than proportionate rate when administered at doses greater than 400 mg twice daily. Limited pharmacokinetic data on sorafenib 400 mg twice daily in a study in Japanese patients showed a 45% lower systemic exposure as compared to pooled phase 1 pharmacokinetic data in Caucasian patients. Sorafenib is extensively protein bound and is metabolized by the liver. Sorafenib undergoes oxidative metabolism involving CYP3A4 and glucuronidation via UGT1A9. Pyridine-N-oxide, the major circulating metabolite of sorafenib in the plasma, demonstrates similar potency compared to sorafenib based on in vitro data. The elimination half-life is estimated to be 25–48 h. The majority of elimination occurs via feces; approximately 19% of the dose is recovered in the urine as glucuronidated metabolites.

Adverse Reactions. The most common adverse reactions include rash, hand-foot skin reaction, nausea, vomiting, diarrhea, fatigue, hypertension, increased amylase and lipase, stomatitis, hoarseness, dysphagia, asthenia, neuropathy, decreased appetite, myelosuppression, hypophosphatemia, increased LFTs, myalgias, and depression. Occasional and serious adverse effects include hypertensive crisis, pancreatitis, myocardial ischemia/infarction, infection, and hemorrhage.

Contraindications. Known hypersensitivity to sorafenib or any other component of sorafenib.

Warnings/Precautions. Pregnancy, hypertension, hemorrhage, cardiac ischemia and/or infarction, wound healing complications, interaction with warfarin resulting in increased PT/INR, potential for decreased drug exposure for persons of Japanese descent.

Drug Interactions. Although sorafenib utilizes the CYP3A4 pathway in its metabolism, studies indicate that CYP3A4 inhibitors do not alter the metabolism of sorafenib. No studies exist regarding coadministration of sorafenib with CYP3A4 inducers, although these medications are thought to increase the metabolism of sorafenib. Sorafenib is a competitive inhibitor of CYP2C19, CYP2D6, and CYP3A4 although no increases in systemic exposure of medications that utilize these pathways have been observed when these medications are coadministered with sorafenib. In vitro data suggests that sorafenib may inhibit CYP2B6 and CYP2C8 and subsequently elevate plasma levels of medications metabolized via these pathways. Sorafenib inhibits glucuronidation via the UGT1A1 and UGT1A9 pathways. Systemic exposure of substrates of UGT1A1 and UGT1A9 may increase when administered with sorafenib. Administration of sorafenib with other neoplastic agents causes a 21% increase in the AUC of doxorubicin and increases of 67%–120% in the AUC of SN-38 (active metabolite of irinotecan) when administered with sorafenib.

Monitoring Parameters. Blood pressure should be monitored weekly throughout the first 6 weeks of therapy and periodically thereafter. Complete blood count and serum chemistries including phosphorus, amylase, and lipase should be obtained periodically as clinically indicated. Monitor PT/INR closely when sorafenib is administered with warfarin. Monitor for dermatologic toxicities such as rash and hand-foot skin reaction. Observe patients for signs and symptoms of unstable angina or MI. Observe progress of wound healing for signs that may indicate the need to hold sorafenib therapy, including the need for major surgery.

SUNITINIB Sutent

Pharmacology. Sunitinib is a small molecule that inhibits multiple receptor tyrosine kinases, some of which are implicated in tumor growth, pathologic angiogenesis, and metastatic progression of cancer. Sunitinib has been identified as an inhibitor of platelet-derived growth factor receptors (PDGFR-α and PDGFR-β), vascular endothelial growth factor receptors (VEGFR-1, VEGFR-2, and VEGFR-3), stem cell factor receptor (KIT), Fms-like tyrosine kinase-3 (FLT-3), colony stimulating factor receptor type 1 (CSF-1R), and the glial cell-line–derived neurotrophic factor receptor (RET).

Adult Dosage and Administration. Note: The manufacturer suggests dose modifications of the recommended dosage for drug interactions. *PO for treatment of advanced renal cell carcinoma*—50 mg once daily taken with or without food. Sunitinib should be taken daily for 4 weeks followed by 2 weeks off the medication. *PO for treatment of GI stromal tumor after disease progression on or intolerance to imatinib mesylate*—50 mg once daily taken with or without food. Sunitinib should be taken daily for 4 weeks followed by 2 weeks off the medication.

SUGGESTED DOSE MODIFICATIONS FOR DRUG INTERACTIONS

ENZYME CLASS/ INTERACTION	SUGGESTED DOSE MODIFICATION
Strong inhibitors of CYP3A4	Consider reducing sunitinib dose to a minimum of 37.5 mg daily.
Strong inducers of CYP3A4	Consider increasing sunitinib dose to a maximum of 87.5 mg daily; monitor closely for toxicities.

Special Populations. *Pediatric Dosage.* Safety and efficacy not established in pediatric patients.

Geriatric Dosage. Safety profiles are similar between younger patients and patients older than 65 years.

Pregnancy Category/Lactation. Pregnancy category D. Use during breast-feeding is not recommended.

Dosage Forms. Cap 12.5, 25, 50 mg.

Patient Instructions. Sunitinib may be taken with or without food. Take at the same time every day. Do not open the capsules. When a dose is missed, take at the next scheduled time. Do not consume grapefruit juice or grapefruit-containing products while taking sunitinib. Notify your health care provider of all medications you are currently taking. Effective birth control methods should be undertaken while receiving sunitinib; birth defects may otherwise occur. Common side effects of sunitinib include stomach upset, diarrhea, rash, lightening of the skin and hair, swelling, taste changes, or blisters on hands or feet. Blood pressure may increase during sunitinib therapy and will be monitored by a health care provider. When rash, swelling, shortness of breath, bleeding, chest pain, or skin reactions on hands and/or feet occur, call health care provider immediately.

Pharmacokinetics. *Fate.* Food does not affect the bioavailability of sutininib. Maximum plasma concentrations of sutininib are observed between 6 and 12 h after oral administration. Sutininib is extensively protein bound. The AUC of sunitinib increases proportionately with dose within the 25–100 mg dosing range. Sunitinib is primarily metabolized hepatically via CYP3A4 to an active metabolite that is also metabolized via CYP3A4. The active metabolite accounts for 23%–37% of the total systemic exposure. The terminal half-life of sunitinib is 40–60 h and the terminal half-life of the metabolite is 80–110 h. Elimination occurs via feces.

Adverse Reactions. The most common adverse reactions include fatigue, asthenia, diarrhea, nausea, mucositis/stomatitis, vomiting, dyspepsia, abdominal pain, constipation, hypertension, rash, hand-foot syndrome, skin discoloration, altered taste, anorexia, and bleeding. Occasional and serious adverse effects include venous thromboembolic events, reversible posterior leukoencephalopathy syndrome, liver failure, pancreatitis, rhabdomyolysis, nephrotic syndrome, QTc prolongation, CHF, adrenal insufficiency, and hypothyroidism.

Contraindications. None.

Warnings/Precautions. Pregnancy, hypertension, left ventricular dysfunction, hemorrhage, QTc prolongation and torsades de pointes, thyroid dysfunction, and adrenal insufficiency.

Drug Interactions. Sunitinib utilizes the CYP3A4 pathway in its metabolism. CYP3A4 inhibitors may increase plasma concentrations of sunitinib; conversely, strong inducers of CYP3A4 may decrease sunitinib plasma concentrations. Dose modifications have been suggested by the manufacturer to account for CYP3A4 drug interactions.

Monitoring Parameters. Complete blood counts with platelet count and serum chemistries including phosphate should be obtained prior to each cycle. Patients with cardiac risk factors such as MI, coronary/peripheral artery bypass graft, symptomatic CHF, CVA, transient ischemic attack, or pulmonary embolism should have baseline and periodic evaluation of left ventricular ejection fraction. Blood pressure should be monitored periodically. Baseline and periodic evaluation of ECG, potassium, and magnesium should be done in patient with a history of QTc prolongation; sunitinib should be used with caution in these patients. Baseline evaluation of thyroid function should be considered and repeated when symptoms of hypothyroidism occur. Adrenocorticotropic stimulation test should be conducted in patients who experience stress while receiving sunitinib because adrenal insufficiency may be present. Monitor for signs and symptoms of bleeding, pancreatitis, hypothyroidism, adrenal insufficiency, and CHF.

■ REFERENCES

1. Medina PJ, Goodin S. Lapatinib: a dual inhibitor of human epidermal growth factor receptor tyrosine kinases. *Clin Ther.* 2008;30(8):1426-1447.
2. DeRemer DL et. al. Nilotinib: a second-generation tyrosine kinase inhibitor for the treatment of chronic myelogenous leukemia. *Clin Ther.* 2008;30(11):1956-1975.
3. Llovet JM et. al. Sorafenib in advanced hepatocellular carcinoma. *N Engl J Med.* 2008;359(4):378-390.

Chapter 27

Miscellaneous Antineoplastics

Shirley Hogan

ASPARAGINASE	Elspar
PEGASPARGASE	Oncaspar

Pharmacology. Asparaginase, isolated from *Escherichia coli*, hydrolyzes L-asparagine to aspartic acid and ammonia. This results in a cellular deficiency of L-asparagine. Normal human cells have high levels of asparagine synthetase, which allows them to synthesize additional L-asparagine, but sensitive tumor cells lack asparagine synthetase and therefore require a source of L-asparagine. Providing tumor cells with L-asparaginase results in rapid inhibition of protein synthesis as well as DNA and RNA synthesis.[1,2]

In an attempt to reduce immunogenicity, the *E. coli* enzyme has been modified by conjugation with monomethoxypolyethylene glycol (PEG). The PEG-asparaginase (pegaspargase) is active and nonimmunogenic in approximately 70% of patients hypersensitive to the nonpegylated product.[1]

Administration and Dosage *Adult Dosage* Elspar: Single induction agent (not recommended) IV—200 IU/kg/d for 28 days. Oncaspar: 2500 IU/m^2 IM or IV no more frequently than every 14 days. Clinical data is not available to support a recommendation for the use of combination regimens in adults. Asparaginase toxicity is reported to be greater in adults than in pediatric patients.

Pediatric Dosage. Elspar: Single induction agent (not recommended) IV—200 IU/kg/d for 28 days. In combination therapy, 2 dosing regimens are approved: 1000 IU/kg/d IV for 10 consecutive days or 6000 IU/m^2 IM every third day for 9 doses. Oncaspar: 2500 IU/m^2 IM or IV no more frequently than every 14 days.

Dosage notes: When administering either product by IM injection, the volume at a single injection site should be limited to 2 mL. If a volume greater than 2 mL is to be administered, 2 injection sites should be used.

Dosage Forms. **Inj** (asparaginase) 10,000 IU vial. (Pegaspargase) 3750 IU/5 mL single-use vial.

Pharmacokinetics. *Fate.* The half-life of IV Elspar (asparaginase) in 8–30 h; the half-life of Oncaspar (pegaspargase) in considerably longer being approximately 3.2 days in patients hypersensitive to asparaginase and 5.7 days in nonsensitive patients. Plasma levels after IM are approximately 10%–50% of those provided by IV administration.[2]

Adverse Reactions. Allergic reactions, including skin rashes, urticaria, arthralgia, respiratory distress, and acute anaphylaxis are common. The addition of the PEG molecule to L-asparaginase (Oncaspar) has shown decreased immunogenicity, though allergic reactions are still reported. Azotemia, usually prerenal, occurs frequently. Pancreatitis, hyperglycemia, hypofibrinogenemia, and depression of various clotting factors are also common events. Liver function abnormalities may also occur, including elevations of AST/ALT.

Contraindications. Elspar: pancreatitis or history of pancreatitis. Oncaspar: history of any of the following with previous L-asparaginase therapy—serious thrombosis, pancreatitis, or serious hemorrhagic events.

Notes. Anaphylaxis can occur with any dose; ensure that emergency resuscitation equipment is available at the time of each dose. Intradermal scratch tests and desensitization procedures are not reliably predictive or preventive for anaphylaxis.[2]

BLEOMYCIN SULFATE   Blenoxane

Pharmacology. Bleomycin is a mixture of glycopeptide antibiotics isolated from a strain of *Streptomyces verticillus*. Antineoplastic effects are generally attributed to the inhibition of DNA synthesis via oxidative cleavage, but other means of exerting deleterious effects on cell growth are also probable.[4]

Administration and Adult Dosage. Patients with lymphoma should receive test doses of 2 units or less for the first 2 doses to observe for anaphylactoid reaction; if no acute reaction occurs with these doses, then regular dosage schedule may be followed.

SQ , IM, or IV—10–20 units/m^2 (0.25–0.5 units/kg) 1–2 times/wk.

Intracavitary for malignant effusion—60 units as a single-dose bolus intrapleural injection.

Pediatric Dosage. Although safety and effectiveness of bleomycin have not been established, it is a well-established agent used in several pediatric malignancies. The pharmacokinetic parameters may vary from adults to children younger than 3 years. Dosages should be determined through the use of established regimens.

Geriatric Dosage. Same as adult dosage but use with caution in patients >70 years and adjust dosage for age-related reduction in renal function.

Other Conditions. Renal insufficiency can reduce bleomycin elimination. The terminal elimination half-life increases exponentially as the creatinine clearance decreases. Established reductions in dose have been proposed for patients with creatinine clearance <50 mL/min as follows: 40–50 mL/min gives 70% of usual dose; 30–40 mL/min, 60%; 20–30 mL/min, 55%; 10–20 mL/min, 45%; 5–10 mL/min, 40%.

Dosage Forms. Inj 15-, 30-unit vials.

Pharmacokinetics. *Fate.* Bleomycin is rapidly absorbed following all routes of administration and reaches a peak plasma concentration in 30–60 min. It is 100% bioavailable following IM and 70% following SQ administration. It is widely distributed with a mean V_d of 17.5 L/m^2 following a 15 units/m^2 IV dose. The primary route of elimination is renal; 45%–70% of a dose is excreted in the urine within 24 h.[4]

Adverse Reactions. Pulmonary toxicities occur in 10% of patients and in approximately 1%, the nonspecific pneumonitis can progress to pulmonary fibrosis and death. This pulmonary toxicity is age (>70 years) and dose (> 400 unit total dose) related, but also unpredictable. Therefore, careful monitoring is necessary. The earliest symptom associated with bleomycin pulmonary toxicity is dyspnea and the earliest sign is fine rales.

Precautions. Use with extreme caution in patients with renal or pulmonary disease, in those with lymphoma, and in those >70 years.

Drug Interactions. Because of the predominant renal excretion, administration of nephrotoxic drugs with bleomycin may affect its elimination. Cisplatin has specifically been reported to cause an increase in terminal half-life of bleomycin, but other nephrotoxic drugs should also be administered with caution when given concomitantly with bleomycin.

Notes. A unit of bleomycin is equal to 1 mg of bleomycin activity.

TRETINOIN	Vesanoid

Pharmacology. Tretinoin (all-*trans*-retinoic acid) is related to retinol (vitamin A). It induces the maturation of acute promyelocytic leukemia (APL) cells. Tretinoin induces cytodifferentiation and decreased proliferation of APL cells, producing an initial maturation of the primitive promyelocytes derived from the leukemic clone. This allows repopulation of the bone marrow and peripheral blood by normal polyclonal hematopoietic cells.[5]

Adult Dosage. PO—45 mg/m^2/d administered as 2 evenly divided doses until remission is documented. Therapy should then be discontinued 30 days after the achievement of complete remission or after 90 days of treatment, whichever occurs first.

Notes. Tretinoin is for the induction of remission only. All patients should receive standard consolidation and/or maintenance chemotherapy regimen after induction therapy with tretinoin, unless otherwise contraindicated.

Dosage Forms. Cap 10 mg.

Pharmacokinetics. Tretinoin activity is primarily due to the parent drug with two-third of orally administered dose excreted in the urine. The terminal elimination half-life following initial dosing is 0.5–2 h in patients with APL, but there is evidence that tretinoin induces its own metabolism with plasma concentrations decreasing during continuous therapy, but increasing the dose to adjust for this change has not shown increased response. Tretinoin is > 95% bound in plasma, predominately to albumin.[5]

Adverse Reactions. Approximately 25%–40% of patients with APL treated with tretinoin will experience retinoic acid–APL syndrome, which is characterized by fever, dyspnea, acute respiratory distress, weight gain, pulmonary infiltrates, as well as pleural or pericardial effusions. Use of high-dose steroids is recommended, beginning with initial symptoms; 40%–50% of patients treated with tretinoin will develop leukocytosis (>20,000/μL). Patients with high WBC at diagnosis have an increased risk of a further rapid increase in WBC.

Dry skin, itching, flaking, nasal stuffiness, xerostomia, and cheilitis are common adverse events. These can usually be managed with topical lubricants and moisturizing agents. Headache that occurs several hours after drug ingestion is also a common adverse event. Sixty percent of the patients experienced elevated cholesterol and/or triglycerides that reversed upon completion of treatment. Elevated liver function test results occur in 50%–60% of patients, necessitating a need for careful monitoring and consideration of at least a temporary withdrawal of the drug if the results reach >5 times ULN. Most of these increases resolve without interruption of drug or after completion of treatment.

Notes. Pregnancy category D: Within 1 week prior to the institution of tretinoin therapy, the patient should have a negative serum or urine pregnancy test with a minimum sensitivity of 50 mIU/mL. Pregnancy testing and contraceptive counseling should be repeated monthly throughout the period of tretinoin treatment. Two reliable forms of contraception should be used simultaneously during therapy and for 1 month following completion of therapy.

■ REFERENCES

1. Chabner BA, Friedmann AM. Asparaginase. In: Chabner BA, Longo DL, eds. *Cancer Chemotherapy and Biotherapy Principles and Practice*. 4th ed. Philadelphia, PA: Lippincott Williams & Wilkins; 2006:476-483.
2. Lyss AP. L-Asparaginase. In: *Chemotherapy Source Book*. 3rd ed. Philadelphia, PA: Lippincott Williams & Wilkins; 2001:323-324.
3. Ohnuma T et al. Biochemical and pharmacological studies with asparaginase in man. *Cancer Res*. 1970;30: 2297–305.
4. Lazo JS, Chabner BA. Bleomycin. In: Chabner BA, Longo DL, eds. *Cancer Chemotherapy and Biotherapy Principles and Practice*. 4th ed. Philadelphia, PA: Lippincott Williams & Wilkins; 2006:344-358.
5. Warrell RP. Differentiation agents. In: *Chemotherapy Source Book*. 3rd ed. Philadelphia, PA: Lippincott Williams & Wilkins; 2001:304-311.

Chapter 28

Chemoprotectants

Shirley Hogan

AMIFOSTINE Ethyol

Pharmacology. Amifostine is an organic thiophosphate cytoprotective agent. It is a prodrug that is dephosphorylated by alkaline phosphatase in tissues to an active free thiol metabolite, which is responsible for the reduction of renal toxicity and toxic effects of radiation on normal oral tissue. The differential protection of normal tissue is attributed to the higher capillary alkaline phosphatase activity, higher pH, and better vascularity of normal tissue relative to tumor tissue, which results in a more rapid generation of the active thiol metabolite as well as a higher rate constant for uptake into cells. Because of this higher concentration of the thiol in normal tissue to bind to, it is able to detoxify reactive metabolites of cisplatin. This thiol metabolite also acts as a scavenger of reactive oxygen species generated by exposure to cisplatin and/or radiation.[1]

Administration and Adult Dosage. **For reduction of cisplatin-induced renal toxicity**—910 mg/m² once daily as a 15-min infusion beginning 30 min before administering cisplatin. The patient should be adequately hydrated prior to infusion and kept in a supine position during the infusion with BP monitored every 5 min during the infusion and as clinically indicated thereafter.

For reduction of xerostomia from radiation—200 mg/m² once daily as a 3-min infusion starting 15–30 min prior to radiation therapy. BP should be monitored at least just prior to and immediately following the infusion and thereafter as clinically indicated.

For either indication, antiemetics are recommended.

Dosage Forms. **Inj** 500 mg/vial lyophilized power in single-use vial.

Pharmacokinetics. *Fate.* Rapidly metabolized to an active free thiol metabolite with an elimination half-life of approximately 8 min.

Adverse Reactions. Hypotension that may necessitate an interruption of the infusion. Serious cutaneous reactions including: erythema multiforme, SJS, toxic epidermal necrolysis, and exfoliative dermatitis. These skin reactions are generally reported more often when amifostine is used for its radioprotective effects. Nausea and vomiting occur frequently and may require additional antiemetic medications. Hypocalcemia may occur, especially in those patients with nephritic syndrome or when multiple doses of amifostine are administered. Serum calcium levels should be monitored in those patients at risk and calcium supplements administered as clinically indicated.

Precautions. Patients must be adequately hydrated prior to infusion. Patients who are hypotensive should not receive amifostine, and patients taking antihypertensive medications should not take a dose 24 h preceding infusion. If interruption of antihypertensive medication for 24 h is not recommended, then the patient should not receive amifostine. There is limited experience in patients with preexisting cardiovascular or cerebrovascular conditions such as ischemic heart disease, arrhythmias, CHF, or history of stroke or TIA, and therefore use in these patients should be with caution.

Parameters to Monitor. Monitor blood pressure frequently during drug administration and immediately after infusion.

DEXRAZOXANE   Zinecard

Pharmacology. Dexrazoxane, a potent intracellular chelating agent, is a derivative of EDTA. Though the mechanism by which dexrazoxane provides cardioprotective activity is not completely understood, it is a cyclic derivative of EDTA that readily penetrates cell membranes. Laboratory studies suggest that dexrazoxane is converted intracellularly to a ring-opened chelating agent that interferes with iron-mediated free radical generation thought to be responsible, at least in part, for anthracycline-induced cardiomyopathy.[2]

Administration and Adult Dosage. **IV as a cardioprotectant**—give in a 10:1 dexrazoxane/doxorubicin (mg/m^2) ratio (e.g., 500 mg/m^2 dexrazoxane and 50 mg/m^2 doxorubicin). May be administered as slow IV push or rapid drip infusion beginning not more than 30 min before an IV push dose of doxorubicin. In patients with Cl_{Cr} <40 mL/min, the dose should be reduced to 5:1. The dexrazoxane dose should be proportionally reduced for any required dosage reductions of doxorubicin, maintaining the appropriate ratio.

Special Populations. *Pediatric Dosage.* Although safety and efficacy are not established in pediatric patients, dexrazoxane had been used in pediatric clinical trials. Recommendations for use and dosages should be determined through the use of established regimens.

Dosage Forms. **Inj** 250, 500 mg/vial lyphilized powder.

Pharmacokinetics. *Fate.* A 2-compartment open model with first-order elimination. The disposition kinetics are dose independent. Elimination half-life is 2.1–2.5 h; primarily excreted in the urine.

Adverse Reactions. It is difficult to determine the adverse effects of dexrazoxane because of its use with chemotherapy regimens, but it does appear to increase the myelosuppressive and emetogenic toxicities of doxorubicin-containing regimens.

MESNA   Mesnex

Pharmacology. Mesna (2-mercaptoethanesulfonate) is a sulfhydryl compound that minimizes urotoxicity from the alkylating agents cyclophosphamide (CTX) and ifosfamide (IFX). Mesna dimerizes to an inactive metabolite in plasma but hydrolyzes in urine to yield the active parent, which reacts chemically with the urotoxic metabolites (acrolein) in the urinary bladder to prevent hemorrhagic cystitis.[2]

Administration and Adult Dosage. **IV** given on a fractionated dosing schedule of 3 bolus doses each equal to 20% of the dose of IFX or CTX. The initial dose is given at the time of the IFX/CTX dose and then repeated at 4 and 8 h afterward. The total daily dose of mesna is 60% of the IFX/CTX dose.

IV/PO combination: IV mesna at a dose of 20% is given with the IFX/CTX dose, then oral doses equal to 40% of the IFX/CTX dose may be given at 2 and 6 h afterward. The total daily dose of mesna for this regimen is 100% of the IFX/CTX dose. Patients who vomit within 2 h of taking oral mesna should repeat the dose or receive IV mesna. The efficacy and safety of this IV/PO ratio has not been established for doses of IFX >2 g/m^2.

Special Populations. *Pediatric Dosage.* Same as adult dosage, though safety and efficacy of the tablets have not been established. Because of the benzyl alcohol content in the multidose vial, its use is not recommended in neonates or infants.

Geriatric Dosage. Same as adult dosage.

Dosage Forms. **Inj** 100 mg/mL. **Tab** 400 mg scored.

Pharmacokinetics. *Fate.* Approximately 48% is orally absorbed.[3] V_d is 0.65 L/kg; Cl is 1.23 L/h/kg. Mesna is oxidized to the inactive dimer, dimesna, which does not inactivate CTX or IFX metabolites in the serum. Approximately 60% of the dimesna is converted back to mesna in the renal tubule and delivered to the bladder in the active sulfhydryl form. Approximately two-thirds of a dose is excreted in the urine, one-half as mesna and one-half as dimesna.[4] $t_{1/2}$ (mesna) 22 min; (dimesna) 1.2 h.[4]

Adverse Reactions. Because mesna is administered in combination with chemotherapy regimens, it is difficult to distinguish the adverse reactions that may be due to mesna from those caused by the cytotoxic agent. However, the most frequently reported side effects are headache, injection site reactions, flushing, dizziness, nausea and vomiting, somnolence, diarrhea, anorexia, fever, pharyngitis, and cough. For patients taking oral doses, flatulence and rhinitis were also reported.[2]

■ REFERENCES

1. Bryer MP. Combined modality therapy. In: *Chemotherapy Source Book.* 3rd ed. Philadelphia, PA: Lippincott Williams & Wilkins; 2001:73-80.
2. Ewer MS, Benjamin RS. Cardiotoxicity of chemotherapeutic drugs. In: *Chemotherapy Source Book.* 3rd ed. Philadelphia, PA: Lippincott Williams & Wilkins; 2001:458-467.
3. Burkert H et al. Bioavailability of orally administered mesna. *Arzneimittelforschung.* 1984;34:1597-1600.
4. Pohl J et al. Toxicology, pharmacology and interactions of sodium 2-mercaptoethanesulfonate (mesna). *Curr Chemother.* 1981;2:1387-1389.

Chapter 29

Immunosuppressants

Timothy M. Clifford

General Precautions for Immunosuppressants. Immunosuppression increases the risk of infectious complications. Serious opportunistic infections can occur during immunosuppressive therapy. Long-term immunosuppression also increases the risk of malignancy or lymphoproliferative disease. Vaccinations might be less effective during immunosuppression. Live or live attenuated vaccines might proliferate excessively in immunosuppressed patients and should be avoided. Immunosuppressants should only be prescribed by physicians experienced in immunosuppressive therapy for the management of transplant recipients.

ANTILYMPHOCYTE IMMUNE GLOBULINS	
ANTITHYMOCYTE GLOBULIN (RABBIT)	Thymoglobulin
LYMPHOCYTE IMMUNE GLOBULIN (EQUINE)	Atgam

Pharmacology. Antilymphocyte immune globulins are polyclonal IgG purified from sera of horses or rabbits immunized with human thymus lymphocytes. These drugs are immunosuppressants that inhibit cell-mediated immunity. The immunosuppressive effects of antilymphocyte immune globulins may be secondary to clearance of alloreactive T lymphocytes from the plasma. However, the exact pharmacologic mechanism of action has not been elucidated.

Administration and Adult Dosage. Antilymphocyte immune globulins are generally used in conjunction with other immunosuppressants. **Intradermal sensitivity testing** to identify patients at risk for anaphylaxis is *strongly* recommended before administration of equine lymphocyte immune globulin. Freshly diluted equine lymphocyte immune globulin (5 μg in 0.1 mL 0.9% NaCl) should be administered intradermally on the anterior aspect of one forearm, with intradermal administration of 0.9% NaCl 0.1 mL on the contralateral forearm as a control. During the hour after administration, the skin test should be observed every 15–20 min for swelling, urticaria, pruritus, and wheel or erythema. A positive skin test is defined as local wheel or erythema formation ≤10 mm in diameter. If the skin test is positive, the risk of serious hypersensitivity or anaphylaxis from drug administration should be weighed carefully against the anticipated benefits of drug administration. A systemic reaction to the skin test generally precludes further administration of equine lymphocyte immune globulin. Administration of equine lymphocyte immune globulin to patients after a positive skin test or systemic reaction to the skin test should be done only in a facility capable of supporting life-threatening allergic reactions. The skin test is not 100% predictive of subsequent hypersensitivity reactions. Allergic reactions and anaphylaxis to equine lymphocyte immune globulin have been reported after a negative skin test. The manufacturer does not recommend a test dose before administration of rabbit antithymocyte globulin. **IV for prevention of renal allograft rejection**—(equine lymphocyte immune globulin) 15 mg/kg/d for 14 doses, followed by the same dose every other day for an additional 14 days. This regimen administers up to 21 doses of equine lymphocyte immune globulin in 28 days. The first dose of equine lymphocyte immune globulin should be administered within 24 h before or after surgery; (rabbit antithymocyte globulin) 1.5 mg/kg/d beginning on the day of surgery, for a total of at least 7 doses, has been used for prevention of renal allograft rejection.[1] **IV for treatment of renal allograft rejection**—(equine lymphocyte immune globulin) same dosage regimen as above, with administration of the first dose at the diagnosis of the initial rejection episode; (rabbit antithymocyte globulin) 1.5 mg/kg/d for 7–14 days. **IV for prevention of rejection after heart transplantation**—(rabbit antithymocyte globulin) 4 mg/kg/d administered as an IV infusion over 6 h on postoperative days 1–5.[2] **IM for prevention of rejection after heart transplantation**—(rabbit antithymocyte globulin) 1.5 mg/kg/d or 200 mg/d for 3–7 days has been administered.[3] **IV for the prevention of rejection after lung transplantation**—(rabbit antithymocyte globulin) 1.5 mg/kg/d for 3 days has been used.[4] **IV for the prevention of rejection after liver transplantation**—(rabbit antithymocyte globulin) 0.5–1 mg/kg/d for up to 5 days has been administered.[5] **IV for the prevention of rejection after simultaneous pancreas–kidney transplantation**—(rabbit antithymocyte globulin) 1.5 mg/kg/d for 4–6 days has been administered.[6] **IV for treatment of aplastic anemia**—(equine lymphocyte immune globulin) 10–30 mg/kg/d for 8–14 days, followed by the same dose every other day for 14 days, has been used. This regimen administers up to 21 doses of equine lymphocyte immune globulin in 28 days. An alternative regimen uses 40 mg/kg every 24–48 h for 3–4 doses; (rabbit antithymocyte globulin) 3.5 mg/kg/d for 5 days has been administered with cyclosporine and filgrastim for treatment of severe aplastic anemia unresponsive to equine lymphocyte immune globulin.[7] **IV for prevention of acute graft-versus-host disease (GVHD) in allogeneic bone marrow transplant recipients**—(equine lymphocyte immune globulin) 7–10 mg/kg every other day for 6 doses; (rabbit antithymocyte globulin) 2, 3.75, or 5 mg/kg/dose for 4–5 doses before unrelated bone marrow transplantation.[8] **IV for treatment of moderate-to-severe steroid-refractory acute GVHD**—(equine lymphocyte immune globulin) 7–15 mg/kg for 6 doses or as indicated by the patient's clinical status. **IV for skin allograft survival in patients with full-thickness burns**—(equine lymphocyte immune globulin) 10–15 mg/kg every other day is generally used; however, doses of 5 mg/kg every other day up to 40 mg/kg/d have been given. The duration of therapy is generally 40–60 days, ending when skin allografts cover <20% of the BSA. **The maximum tolerated cumulative dosage** of antilymphocyte polyclonal immune globulins has not been determined. A total of 50 doses of equine lymphocyte immune globulin have been administered over 4 months, and four 28-day courses of 28 equine lymphocyte immune globulin doses have been administered in renal allograft recipients without changing the frequency, severity, or character of adverse drug reactions. **Intravenous administration**—(equine lymphocyte immune globulin) dilute in 0.45% or 0.9% NaCl to a final concentration >4 mg/mL and infuse slowly over 4–8 h through a high-flow central vein; (rabbit antithymocyte globulin) after reconstitution with the diluent provided, dilute to a final concentration of 0.5 mg/mL in 0.9% NaCl or 5% dextrose injection. Infuse the first dose at 0.25 mg/kg/h (1.5 mg/kg/6 h) through a high-flow vein. In the absence of moderate-to-severe adverse effects, infuse subsequent doses over 4 h. Peripheral administration of rabbit antithymocyte globulin has been described. The total daily dose was admixed with 500 mL of 0.9% NaCl along with 1000 units of heparin and 20 mg of hydrocortisone.[9] Antilymphocyte polyclonal immune globulins should be infused through an inline filter with pore sizes of 0.22–1 μm. Premedication and as-needed administration of a corticosteroid, acetaminophen, and an antihistamine are common practice intended to reduce infusion-related adverse effects.

Special Populations. *Pediatric Dosage.* Same as adult dosage.

Geriatric Dosage. Same as adult dosage.

Dosage Forms. Inj (equine lymphocyte immune globulin) 50 mg/mL; (rabbit antithymocyte globulin) 25 mg.

Patient Instructions. (Equine lymphocyte immune globulin) this medicine can cause serious allergic symptoms, especially in people allergic to horses and horse products. You will receive a skin test to check for allergy to this product. (Rabbit antithymocyte globulin, equine lymphocyte immune globulin) you might experience fever, shaking, and chills when this medication is being given. You may be given additional medications to reduce these side effects.

Pharmacokinetics. *Fate.* (Equine lymphocyte immune globulin) peak concentrations of 727 μg/L occur with repeated doses of 10 mg/kg. Systemic distribution of equine immune globulin is not well defined. In vitro studies predict binding to circulating lymphocytes, granulocytes, and platelets. Binding to bone marrow cells, plus thymus and testis cell membranes, occurs in vitro. (Rabbit antithymocyte globulin) IV infusion of 1.25–1.5 mg/kg/d yields a peak concentration of 10–40 μg/L after the first dose and 23–170 μg/L after repeated doses. V_d is 0.12 L/kg.[10]

$t_{1/2}$. (equine lymphocyte immune globulin) 3–9 days; (rabbit antithymocyte globulin) 14–45 days.[10]

Adverse Reactions. Anaphylaxis can occur anytime during therapy. If signs or symptoms of anaphylaxis occur, the infusion must be stopped immediately and appropriate management must be initiated. Serum sickness occurs frequently. The onset of serum sickness is typically 6–18 days after initiation of therapy with antilymphocyte immune globulins. A morbilliform rash generally starts as a truncal distribution of faint macules, with subsequent progression to the extremities. The macules can become confluent. Erythema can spread to involve palms of the hands and soles of the feet. Antihistamines are helpful for pruritus-associated serum sickness. Although not clearly shown to reduce serum sickness–related adverse effects, corticosteroids have been used. Antilymphocyte immune globulins might bind formed elements in the blood other than T lymphocytes and promote splenic clearance of these blood constituents. Subsequently, patients might experience acute normochromic normocytic anemia, thrombocytopenia, or leukopenia during administration of antilymphocyte immune globulins that is reversible with drug discontinuation. Immunosuppression increases the risk of infectious complications from opportunistic and pathogenic microbes. Rare adverse effects reported with antilymphocyte immune globulins include Epstein-Barr virus infections and lymphoproliferative disorders; (equine lymphocyte immune globulin) periorbital edema, seizures, acute renal failure, headache, hypertension, edema, CHF, bradycardia, adult respiratory distress syndrome, myocarditis, pancytopenia, LFT abnormalities, hyperglycemia, and transient myopia; (rabbit antithymocyte globulin) tachycardia, dyspnea, and dizziness.

Contraindications. (Equine lymphocyte immune globulin) allergy to equine lymphocyte immune globulin, horse serum, or horse products; (rabbit antithymocyte globulin) hypersensitivity or anaphylaxis to rabbit proteins; acute viral illness.

Precautions. Pregnancy; lactation. (*See also* General Precautions for Immunosuppressants.)

Drug Interactions. None identified.

Parameters to Monitor. Observe for anaphylaxis during infusion and serum sickness 6–18 days after initiation of therapy. CBC and platelet count every 1–3 days during therapy.

Notes. Equine lymphocyte immune globulin is also known as ATG, antithymocyte globulin, antithymocyte gamma globulin, antithymocyte immunoglobulin, and horse antihuman thymocyte gamma globulin. Rabbit antithymocyte globulin is also known as r-ATG or RATG. Lot-to-lot variation of immunosuppressive potency and avidity for formed blood elements can occur with these products.

AZATHIOPRINE Imuran, Various

Pharmacology. Azathioprine is a thiopurine prodrug of 6-mercaptopurine (6 MP). Conversion to 6-MP with subsequent phosphoribosylation yields antimetabolites capable of inhibiting DNA and RNA synthesis. The metabolite 6-methylmercaptopurine ribotide is a potent inhibitor of de novo purine synthesis. T lymphocytes are sensitive to inhibition of de novo purine synthesis because these cells lack efficient salvage pathways to maintain adequate intracellular stores.

Administration and Adult Dosage. **PO or IV for immunosuppression after solid organ transplantation**—3–5 mg/kg/d as a single-daily dose beginning the day of, or 1–3 days preceding, transplantation. **Maintenance dosage** is 1–3 mg/kg/d as a single-daily dose. **PO for rheumatoid arthritis**—1 mg/kg/d in 1 or 2 doses. The dosage may be increased after 6–8 weeks if indicated by disease response and patient tolerance. Increase the dosage in increments of 0.5 mg/kg/d q4wk to a maximum of 2.5 mg/kg/d.

Special Populations. *Pediatric Dosage.* **PO or IV for immunosuppression after renal transplantation**—same as adult dosage.

Geriatric Dosage. Same as adult dosage.

Dosage Forms. **Tab** 50 mg; **Inj** 100 mg.

Patient Instructions. This medication may be taken with food to reduce stomach upset. Notify your physician if any of the following symptoms occur: unusual bleeding or bruising, fever, sore throat, mouth sores, abdominal pain, yellowing of the eyes, pale stools, or dark urine, or if nausea, vomiting, diarrhea, skin rash, or joint pains become severe or persistent.

Missed Doses. Take a missed dose as soon as possible. If you take the drug once daily and it is time for the next dose, take it at the regular time. Do not double the dose. If you take 2 or more doses daily and it is time for the next dose, take both doses together. If 2 or more doses are missed, contact your physician.

Pharmacokinetics. *Onset and Duration.* Onset of immunosuppression occurs within days to weeks. Immunosuppression continues for days to weeks after drug discontinuation.

Serum Levels. No correlation between serum concentrations and efficacy or toxicity has been defined.

Fate. After oral absorption, conversion to 6-MP occurs rapidly.[11]

$t_{1/2}$. (azathioprine) ~12 min; (6-MP) 0.7–3 h.[11]

Adverse Reactions. Dose-related bone marrow suppression, which can include leukopenia, thrombocytopenia, and anemia, occurs frequently. Macrocytic anemia, with megaloblastic features, or selective erythrocyte aplasia can occur with long-term azathioprine administration. Skin rash is a common adverse effect. Mouth sores can occur. Dose-related nausea and vomiting are frequent and can be reduced by administration in divided doses. Rare GI hypersensitivity characterized by severe nausea and vomiting, diarrhea, hyperpyrexia, malaise, myalgia, and LFT abnormalities can occur early in the course of therapy. GI hypersensitivity is reversible with discontinuation of azathioprine and can recur with rechallenge. Hepatic venoocclusive disease of the liver, secondary lymphomas, and other malignancies can occur with long-term administration. Azathioprine is teratogenic. Rare adverse effects include pancreatitis, constrictive lung disease, renal failure, alopecia, arthralgia, and retinopathy.

Contraindications. Pregnancy in patients treated for rheumatoid arthritis.

Precautions. Pregnancy; lactation. (*See also* General Precautions for Immunosuppressants.)

Drug Interactions. To reduce the risk of life-threatening myelosuppression, azathioprine dosage must be reduced to 25%–33% of the normal dosage in patients receiving allopurinol. Enhanced bone marrow suppression can occur with concurrent use of drugs that inhibit hematopoiesis. Concurrent corticosteroids used for immunosuppression can mask fever.

Parameters to Monitor. Monitor CBC and platelet count weekly for 1 month after initiation of therapy or any dosage increase. Then, for patients with stable hemograms, the CBC and platelet count may be monitored twice monthly for 2 months and then monthly for the duration of therapy. Monitor serum transaminases, alkaline phosphatase, and total bilirubin periodically. Observe for signs of infection.

Notes. Azathioprine is used in combination with other immunosuppressants as an adjunct in the prevention of renal allograft rejection and for the prevention of solid organ rejection for cardiac and hepatic allografts. It is rarely used for the management of acute or chronic GVHD in allogeneic bone marrow transplant recipients because it markedly increases the risk for infections.[12]

CYCLOSPORINE
Gengraf, Neoral, Sandimmune, Various

Pharmacology. Cyclosporine is a cyclic polypeptide immunosuppressant produced by the fungus *Tolypocladium inflatum* Gams. The intracellular drug–ligand complex formed by cyclosporine and cyclophilin indirectly blocks T lymphocyte activation by inhibiting calcineurin-mediated dephosphorylation of transcription factors necessary for IL-2 transcription.

Administration and Adult Dosage. **PO for prophylaxis of organ rejection or GVHD**—8–12 mg/kg/d in 2 divided doses depending on the type of transplant and the other immunosuppressants being given. To hasten achievement of an immunosuppressant blood level, **an oral loading dose** of cyclosporine 15 mg/kg may be administered. Cyclosporine is usually started 4–12 h before surgery. **Maintenance dosage** is based on cyclosporine blood levels, the risk of organ rejection or GVHD, and patient tolerance. **PO for rheumatoid arthritis**—2.5 mg/kg/d in divided doses bid. As patient tolerance allows, dosage may be increased by 0.5–0.75 mg/kg/d at 8 weeks and again at 12 weeks, to a maximum of 4 mg/kg/d. **PO for psoriasis**—2.5 mg/kg/d in divided doses bid. After 4 weeks of therapy, as patient tolerance allows, the dosage may be increased by 0.5–0.75 mg/kg/d q2wk, to a maximum of 4 mg/kg/d. **An IV loading dose** of 3–4 mg/kg might be useful in patients with low cyclosporine levels during periods of mild-to-moderate diarrhea with oral mainte-nance therapy. **IV for patients unable to take oral medication**—2–6 mg/kg/d in 1–2 divided doses. **IV for prevention of GVHD**—3–4 mg/kg/d in 2 divided doses q12h. Cyclosporine is generally started 1–2 days before bone marrow transplantation. Drug-induced mucositis or diarrhea usually necessitates the use of IV cyclosporine in allogenic bone marrow transplant recipients. Dilute IV cyclosporine in a glass container (it might leach plasticizers from PVC containers) with D5W or NS to a concentration of 50 mg/20–100 mL. Doses may be infused over 2–6 h or given as a continuous infusion. **Conversion from IV to PO administration**—the ratio of IV/PO dosage is typically 1:3 to 1:4 for Sandimmune capsules or 1:1 to 1:3 for microemulsion capsules or solution (Gengraf, Neoral, various). **Conversion from PO Sandimmune to microemulsion capsules or solution**—(Gengraf, Neoral, various) give the same daily dosage or reduce microemulsion dose by 30% with prompt dosage adjustment based on subsequent blood levels. A cyclosporine blood level should be drawn 48 h after dosage form conversion. Because of better bioavailability, maintenance dosages of the microemulsion formulation are usually lower than Sandimmune dosages. **Interchange of various microemulsion capsules or solutions**—(Gengraf, Neoral, various) give the same daily dosage with prompt dosage adjustment based on subsequent blood levels. A cyclosporine blood level should be drawn 48 h after interchange. **Discontinuation**—cyclosporine may eventually be discontinued in certain renal or allogeneic bone marrow transplant recipients. Cyclosporine dosage must be decreased gradually over time to reduce the risk of reactive immune stimulation and graft rejection or GVHD.

Special Populations. *Pediatric Dosage.* Initial dosage same as adult dose. Adjustment based on blood levels. Children may require higher weight-based maintenance dose.

Geriatric Dosage. Same as adult dosage. Age-related loss of renal function and comorbid conditions can predispose geriatric patients to cyclosporine-induced nephrotoxicity or hypertension.

Other Conditions. Use IBW to calculate initial dosage in obese patients.

Dosage Forms. **Cap** (Neoral, various) 25, 100 mg; (Sandimmune) 25, 50, 100 mg; **Oral Soln** 100 mg/mL; **Inj** (Sandimmune) 50 mg/mL.

Patient Instructions. Take this medication on a regular schedule relative to the time of day and meals. Do not discontinue it unless directed to do so. Sandimmune cannot be interchanged with any other brands. The oral solution may taste better if mixed with another liquid. Sandimmune may be mixed with milk, chocolate milk, or orange juice. Neoral may be mixed with orange juice or apple juice. Using a glass container, mix the cyclosporine solution with the milk or juice, stir well, and drink immediately to ensure that the entire cyclosporine dose is swallowed. Do *not* refrigerate the oral solution. Use the oral solution within 2 months after opening. Grapefruit juice can interact with cyclosporine. Talk to the physician or coordinator who monitors your cyclosporine before drinking grapefruit juice and before starting, stopping, or changing the dose of any medication.

Missed Doses. Take a missed dose as soon as possible if you remember within 12 h. If it is within 2 h of the next dose, skip the missed dose and do not double the dose. If you miss 2 or more doses, contact the physician or coordinator who monitors your cyclosporine.

Pharmacokinetics. *Serum Levels.* The serum (blood) concentration–response relationship is not completely defined. Trough blood or serum levels are monitored for toxicity. Therapeutic and toxic concentrations vary with assay, biologic fluid, and time posttransplant. Therapeutic serum or plasma concentrations are radioimmunoassay (RIA) 150–250 μg/L and high-performance liquid chromatography (HPLC) 75–150 μg/L. Therapeutic whole blood concentrations are RIA 375–400 μg/L and HPLC 100–300 μg/L. Peak concentrations 2 h (C_2) post an oral dose can be used for monitoring and dosage adjustment. C_2 concentration range of 1500–2000 μg/L is suggested for the first few months posttransplant. C_2 concentration range of 700–900 μg/L is suggested 6–12 months after transplantation.[11] In routine clinical practice, spurious serum drug levels can result from in vitro drug redistribution. Artifactual serum or whole blood levels can occur when blood is drawn through the same central venous line used for IV cyclosporine administration.[13]

Fate. Oral absorption is formulation dependent (*See* Notes). Sandimmune absorption is incomplete and variable. The mean bioavailability of Sandimmune is 34%; however, the reported range is 5%–90%. Absorption of Sandimmune is improved after a high-fat meal. Peak concentrations occur 2–6 h after ingestion of Sandimmune capsules or oral solution. Absorption of cyclosporine microemulsion formulations is independent of food intake; peak concentrations occur 1.5–2 h after ingestion of microemulsion capsules or solution. Factors that can decrease cyclosporine absorption are diarrhea, gastroenteritis, and short small bowel. Absorption may be reduced in allogeneic bone marrow transplant patients because of residual gut damage from intensive chemotherapy, radiation, or GVHD. Bioavailability of AB therapeutic equivalent cyclosporine capsules and liquid can vary by 20%–30% for a particular patient or when mixed with various juices. Systemic cyclosporine distributes to erythrocytes (45%), leukocytes (15%), and plasma lipoproteins (35%). Marked elevations of plasma lipoproteins can increase measured cyclosporine levels without proportional changes in therapeutic or toxic effects. V_{dss} (whole blood, HPLC) is 4 ± 0.8 L/kg in renal transplant patients and 5.3 ± 2.9 L/kg in bone marrow transplant patients. Cl (whole blood, HPLC) is 0.4 ± 0.2 L/kg/h in renal or liver transplant patients and 0.6 ± 0.4 L/kg/h in allogeneic bone marrow transplant recipients. Cyclosporine is extensively metabolized by CYP3A. At least 25 metabolites, some with immunosuppressant activity, have been identified. Cyclosporine and its metabolites are cleared primarily in the bile. Approximately 6% is excreted in the urine as cyclosporine and metabolites.

$t_{1/2}$. (whole blood, HPLC) 10 ± 3.5 h, possibly prolonged in hepatic failure.

Adverse Reactions. Acute nephrotoxicity, which generally occurs during the first month of treatment, is characterized by Cr_s increasing by ≥ 0.3 mg/dL/24 h or $\geq 30\%/24$ h and usually abates with interruption of drug therapy. Dosage reduction may be required for continuation of therapy. Chronic progressive renal toxicity is characterized by a slow continual increase in Cr_s and BUN, mild proteinuria, and tubular dysfunction. $Cr_s > 2$ mg/dL in adult patients or doubling of Cr_s is an indication for interruption of therapy or dosage reduction. Electrolyte abnormalities, including hypomagnesemia, hypokalemia, hyperkalemia, and renal tubular acidosis, are consequences of cyclosporine-induced nephrotoxicity. Concurrent administration of nephrotoxic drugs increases the likelihood of renal dysfunction. Hypertension occurs frequently. **Calcium channel blockers** and **clonidine** are suitable agents for cyclosporine-induced hypertension because they do not have deleterious effects on renal blood flow. Fine tremors occur frequently and can persist and worsen after drug discontinuation. Neurotoxicity can also present as seizures, cortical blindness, paresthesias, hyperesthesia, headache, or expressive aphasia. Patients with low serum cholesterol may be at increased risk of neurotoxicity. Anaphylactic reactions to cyclosporine or the solubilizing agent, polyoxyethylated castor oil, can occur. Ethanol is a minor constituent in the intravenous and oral formulations. Cyclosporine-induced cholestasis is dose related and transient. Elevated serum transaminases and hypertriglyceridemia can occur. Additional side effects are hemolytic uremic syndrome, pancreatitis, hirsutism, gingival hyperplasia, nausea, vomiting, acne, and gynecomastia. Leukopenia, anemia, and thrombocytopenia occur rarely.

Contraindications. Allergy to cyclosporine or polyoxyethylated castor oil.

Precautions. Pregnancy; lactation. Use cautiously in patients with aldehyde dehydrogenase 2 (ALDH2) deficiency. (*See also* General Precautions for Immunosuppressants.)

Drug Interactions. Numerous important drug interactions have been identified. Additive or synergistic renal toxicity can occur with concomitant administration of nephrotoxic drugs. Sirolimus can potentiate cyclosporine nephrotoxicity. Potassium-sparing diuretics can exacerbate hyperkalemia. Concurrent use of the following drugs frequently increases cyclosporine blood levels: corticosteroids, erythromycin and macrolide antibiotics, azole antifungals, acetazolamide, alcohol, allopurinol, diltiazem, verapamil, cimetidine, colchicine, oral contraceptives, imipenem/cilastatin, metoclopramide, norfloxacin, and sulindac. Grapefruit and grapefruit juice can increase cyclosporine concentrations and therefore should be avoided. Enzyme-inducing drugs such as carbamazepine, phenobarbital, phenytoin, and rifampin reduce cyclosporine blood levels. Octreotide can decrease cyclosporine oral absorption. Additional drugs that can reduce cyclosporine blood levels are St. John's wort, cotrimoxazole, nafcillin, and sulfonamides. Cyclosporine reduces the clearance of HMG-CoA reductase inhibitors, such as lovastatin and atorvastatin, and increases the risk of drug-induced rhabdomyolysis.

Parameters to Monitor. Observe for anaphylaxis with IV administration. Monitor Cr_s every 2–7 days and daily in patients at risk of acute renal dysfunction. Monitor blood pressure regularly. Monitor LFTs weekly and triglycerides and amylase monthly. Monitor blood or serum cyclosporine concentrations every 2–3 days when starting therapy. As the patient's clinical condition and renal function allow, reduce frequency to once or twice weekly and then monthly during the first year of therapy. After the first year of therapy, blood or serum concentration monitoring may be reduced to every 1–2 months in stable patients. Monitor for signs and symptoms of graft rejection or GVHD, especially after dosage reduction.

Notes. Assignment of AB therapeutic equivalency by the FDA requires bioequivalence testing in normal healthy volunteers. Absorption of bioequivalent products can vary in bone marrow or solid organ transplant patients with compromised gut function. Bioequivalence to Neoral in transplant patients has been established for microemulsion Gengraf capsules.

Cyclosporine is generally used in combination with other immunosuppressant drugs for prevention of graft rejection or GVHD. Cyclosporine is used in the management of various immunologic diseases such as aplastic anemia, psoriasis, atopic dermatitis, acute ocular Behçet's syndrome, endogenous uveitis, primary biliary cirrhosis, and acute Crohn's disease.

INTERLEUKIN-2 RECEPTOR ANTAGONISTS

BASILIXIMAB	Simulect
DACLIZUMAB	Zenapax

Pharmacology. Basiliximab and daclizumab (formerly dacliximab) are immunosuppressive, humanized, recombinant IgG1 monoclonal antibodies that bind specifically to the alpha subunit (p55 alpha, CD25, or Tac subunit) of the human high-affinity IL-2 receptor present on the surface of activated lymphocytes. They act as IL-2 receptor antagonists by preventing IL-2 from binding to lymphocytes, subsequently reducing IL-2–mediated immune activation. Both drugs are indicated for prevention of renal allograft rejection in a regimen that includes cyclosporine and a corticosteroid.

Administration and Adult Dosage. IV for prevention of renal allograft rejection—(basiliximab) 20 mg infused over 30 min for 2 doses. The initial dose should be given approximately 2 h before transplantation; the second dose is given 4 days after the transplant. Withhold the second dose if severe hypersensitivity or graft loss occurs. Basiliximab has also been used at this dose for heart, lung, liver, and simultaneous pancreas–kidney transplant.[14–17] (Daclizumab) 1 mg/kg for 5 doses at 14-day intervals. The initial dose should be infused within 24 h preceding surgery. The remaining 4 doses should be administered at 14-day intervals after surgery. This dose has also been used in heart, lung, liver, and simultaneous pancreas–kidney transplant.[11,18–20] Dilute each dose in 50 mL NS and infuse over 15 min through a peripheral or central venous line. **IV for treatment of steroid-refractory GVHD**—(daclizumab) 1 mg/kg on days 1, 4, 8, 15, and 22, with day 1 representing the first day of daclizumab therapy; or 1.5 mg/kg, with repeated administration in 11–48 days for patients with transient improvement.[21,22]

Special Populations. *Pediatric Dosage.* (Basiliximab) in pediatric patients weighing <35 kg, 2 doses of 10 mg each should be used. In those >35 kg, use the adult dosage. (Daclizumab) same as adult dosage. Information about use in pediatric patients is limited.

Geriatric Dosage. Same as adult dosage. Information about use in patients >65 years is limited.

Other Conditions. No dosage adjustment is necessary for patients with severe renal dysfunction.

Dosage Forms. Inj (basiliximab) 10, 20 mg; (daclizumab) 5 mg/mL.

Patient Instructions. This drug is being used as part of combination therapy to prevent rejection of your transplanted kidney.

Pharmacokinetics. *Onset and Duration.* (Basiliximab) receptor saturation is maintained for 36 ± 14 days with the recommended regimen. (Daclizumab) receptor saturation is maintained for approximately 120 days with the recommended regimen.

Serum Levels. (Basiliximab) >200 μg/L maintains complete binding to IL-2 receptor and maintains effective T-lymphocyte suppression. (Daclizumab) 5–10 mg/L inhibits activated T lymphocytes.

Fate. (Basiliximab) peak serum levels of 9.3 ± 4.5 mg/L are attained with the recommended dosage regimen. (Daclizumab) after the first dose of 1 mg/kg, a peak of 21 ± 14 mg/L occurs, and after the fifth dose, a peak of 32 ± 22 mg/L results. The trough is 7.6 ± 4 mg/L after repeated doses of 1 mg/kg in adult renal transplant recipients.

$t_{1/2}$. (basiliximab) approximately 14 days; (daclizumab) 11–38 days.

Adverse Reactions. Both drugs usually are well tolerated. The frequency and type of adverse events were similar between renal transplant patients receiving these drugs or placebo, along with a corticosteroid and cyclosporine. Cases of severe acute hypersensitivity reactions have occurred with basiliximab, usually within 24 h of a dose. Discontinue the drug permanently if this occurs. Hypertension and dehydration with daclizumab might be more frequent in children than in adults.

Precautions. Pregnancy; lactation. Use basiliximab with extreme caution in patients who have had previous courses of therapy. (*See also* General Precautions for Immunosuppressants.)

Drug Interactions. None known.

Parameters to Monitor. Monitor signs and symptoms of infection and graft rejection periodically.

Notes. After preparation, these drugs should be used within 4 h if stored at room temperature or 24 h if refrigerated. Although basiliximab and daclizumab have not been directly compared, their efficacies seem to be similar.

MUROMONAB-CD3   Orthoclone OKT3

Pharmacology. Muromonab-CD3 is a murine monoclonal antibody that recognizes the zeta chain of the CD3 protein complex associated with the T-cell receptor (TCR). CD3 protein complex is an integral component of T-cell receptor signal transduction. Muromonab-CD3 binding to CD3 blocks allograft rejection by inhibition of T-lymphocyte function. Muromonab-CD3 is used to treat acute renal allograft rejection or steroid-resistant heart or liver allograft rejection.

Administration and Adult Dosage. IV for the treatment or prevention of allograft rejection—5 mg/d as an IV push for 10–14 days[11]. Administration of methylprednisolone 8 mg/kg IV 1–4 h before muromonab is strongly recommended by the manufacturer to reduce the frequency and severity of reactions with the first dose. Acetaminophen and diphenhydramine also are often used to control symptoms. The manufacturer recommends that the patient's temperature be <37.8°C (<100°F) before infusion of muromonab-CD3.

Special Populations. *Pediatric Dosage.* Safety and efficacy are not established, but children have received dosages of ≤5 mg/d.

Geriatric Dosage. Same as adult dosage.

Dosage Forms. Inj 1 mg/mL.

Patient Instructions. This medication can cause shortness of breath, fever, and chills during the initial days of treatment.

Pharmacokinetics. *Serum Levels.* Levels ≥ 0.8 mg/L block cytotoxic T-lymphocyte function in vitro and in vivo.

Adverse Reactions. Cytokine release syndrome (CRS) occurs frequently with the initial 2–3 doses; it is related to cytokine release from activated lymphocytes. CRS can present as mild flulike symptoms or as a life-threatening, shocklike reaction. Onset of CRS is usually 30–60 min after drug administration but can be delayed for hours. CRS might last for hours. Pretreatment and symptomatic treatment (*see* Administration and Adult Dosage) can reduce the frequency and severity of reactions with the first dose. Common symptoms are fever, headache, rigors, chills, tremor, nausea, vomiting, abdominal pain, myalgia, arthralgia, and rash. CRS can include CNS and cardiovascular adverse effects. CNS side effects are headache, seizures, encephalopathy, and aseptic meningitis. Cardiovascular side effects are angina, acute MI, CHF, hypertension, hypotension, and arrhythmias. Arterial and venous thromboses of allograft and other vascular beds have occurred. Consider coadministration of prophylactic antithrombotic agents in patients with histories of thrombotic events or underlying vascular disease. Pulmonary edema occurs frequently. Additional respiratory side effects are dyspnea, bronchospasm, wheezing, tachypnea, adult respiratory distress syndrome, and respiratory arrest. Hypersensitivity, including anaphylaxis and Stevens-Johnson syndrome, has been reported. Leukopenia, thrombocytopenia, pancytopenia, and lymphopenia also have occurred. Transient elevations of Cr_s and serum transaminases can occur 1–3 days after initiation of treatment.

Contraindications. Human antimouse antibody titer ≥1:1000.

Precautions. Pregnancy; lactation. Use with caution in patients with volume overload or history of thrombotic events or vascular disease. (*See also* General Precautions for Immunosuppressants.)

Drug Interactions. Concurrent use of indomethacin has been associated with encephalopathy and other CNS side effects.

Parameters to Monitor. A chest X-ray obtained within 24 h before starting muromonab should be free of evidence of volume overload or heart failure. Obtain human antimouse antibody before initiating treatment. (*See* Contraindications.) Obtain Cr_s q2d, AST and ALT q3d, CBC including differential and platelet counts q3d. Monitor one of the following immunologic tests during therapy: serum muromonab concentrations or quantitative T-lymphocyte surface phenotyping (target: $CD3^+$ T lymphocytes <25 cells/μL blood).

Notes. Transfer muromonab into a syringe through a 0.2 μm low protein-binding filter. Do not dilute with IV fluids for administration. Flush IV line with NS before and after injection.

MYCOPHENOLATE MOFETIL	CellCept, Various
MYCOPHENOLATE SODIUM	Myfortic

Pharmacology. Mycophenolate mofetil (MMF) is an ester prodrug of mycophenolic acid. Mycophenolate sodium (MPS-EC) is the sodium salt form of mycophenolic acid in a delayed-release tablet formulation. Mycophenolic acid, which was isolated from the mold *Penicillium glaucum*, inhibits de novo purine synthesis by potent inhibition of inosine monophosphate dehydrogenase. Lymphocyte proliferation and antibody formation are subsequently inhibited by purine deficiency because lymphocytes lack an efficient salvage pathway for biosynthesis of purine bases. MMF is used in combination with cyclosporine and corticosteroids to prevent renal, heart, and liver allograft rejection. MMF can also be used in the prevention of pancreas and lung allograft rejection.[23,24] MPS-EC is used in combination with cyclosporine and corticosteroids to prevent renal allograft rejection. MPS-EC has also been used in pancreas, heart, and liver transplantation.[17,25,26]

Administration and Adult Dosage. **PO or IV for prophylaxis of organ transplant rejection**—(MMF) 1–1.5g bid beginning within 24 h of transplantation. **PO for prophylaxis of renal transplant rejection**—(MPS-EC) 720mg bid within 48 h of transplantation. **PO or IV for treatment of acute or chronic GVHD after allogeneic bone marrow transplantation**—(MMF) 1 g bid as adjunctive therapy for corticosteroid-refractory GVHD or to facilitate use of reduced corticosteroid dosage.[27,28] A dosage of 3 g/d (MMF) does not confer a therapeutic advantage for any condition and is associated with more adverse effects.

Special Populations. *Pediatric Dosage.* **PO for renal transplantation**—(MMF) 600 mg/m² bid, to a maximum of 2 g/d as the suspension. Alternatively, (1.25–1.5 m² BSA) 750 mg bid as capsules; (>1.5 m² BSA) 1 g bid as capsules or tablets. Safety and efficacy of MPS-EC has not been established in pediatric renal transplant recipients.

Geriatric Dosage. Same as adult dosage.

Other Conditions. (MMF) with a chronic Cl_{Cr} <25 mL/min, the dosage should not exceed 1 g bid. This does not apply to the immediate posttransplant period for renal transplant patients.

Dosage Forms. (MMF) **Cap** 250; **Susp** 200 mg/mL; **Tab** 500 mg; **Inj** 500 mg; (MPS-EC) **Tab** 180, 360 mg.

Patient Instructions. Do not stop this medication without consulting your physician.

Missed Doses. Take a missed dose as soon as possible if you remember within 12 h. If it is within 2 h of next dose, skip the missed dose and do not double the next dose. If you miss 2 or more doses, contact your physician.

Pharmacokinetics. *Serum Levels.* Not established; dosage adjustment to a trough concentration of 2.5 mg/L decreased heart transplant rejection rate, but a trough concentration of >3.5 mg/L was associated with greater side effects in liver transplant recipients.[29]

Fate. (MMF) bioavailability is 94% in normal, healthy volunteers. Food decreases the peak serum concentration by 40%, but not bioavailability. Bioavailability is decreased immediately after renal transplantation. Peak serum concentrations after 1 g PO bid are 8.2 ± 4.5 mg/L during the first 40 days posttransplant and 24 ± 12 mg/L 3 months posttransplant (similar to normal volunteers). The mean time to peak is prolonged to 1.3 ± 0.8 h during the first 40 days posttransplant compared with 0.9 ± 0.2 h after 3 months. AUC also is reduced by 42% during the first 40 days posttransplant; AUC is increased approximately 1.5-fold in patients with severe renal impairment. Alcoholic cirrhosis appears not to affect AUC. Mycophenolic acid is 97% bound to albumin. V_d in normal healthy volunteers is 4 ± 1.2 L/kg; Cl is 0.17 ± 0.04 L/h/kg. (MPS-EC) gastrointestinal absorption and absolute bioavailability are 93% and 72%, respectively. Time to peak concentration ranges between 1.5 and 2.75 h. Peak serum concentrations after 720 mg PO bid are 15 ± 10.7 mg/L after 14 days and 26.2 ± 12.7 after 90 days. MMF and MPS-EC are rapidly hydrolyzed to mycophenolic acid, which is subsequently glucuronidated to an inactive metabolite. Enterohepatic recirculation can contribute to the mycophenolic acid AUC. (MMF) less than 1% of the dose is excreted in the urine as mycophenolic acid. (MPS-EC) less than 3% of the dose is excreted in the urine as mycophenolic acid. Equimolar dosing of mycophenolate products is 1g MMF = 720 mg MPS-EC.

$t_{1/2}$. (MMF)16.6 ± 5.8 h; (MPS-EC) 8–16 h.

Adverse Reactions. Hematologic adverse effects are leukopenia, anemia, thrombocytopenia, and pancytopenia. Adverse effects of mycophenolate rarely necessitate discontinuation of therapy, but the drug should be stopped temporarily if neutropenia (ANC <1300/μL) develops during therapy. GI effects, including nausea, vomiting, dyspepsia, abdominal pain, constipation, and diarrhea, occur frequently. GI side effects can be reduced by giving the drug in 3–4 divided doses.

Contraindications. Allergy to mycophenolate.

Precautions. Pregnancy; lactation. Use with caution in patients with renal dysfunction. (*See also* General Precautions for Immunosuppressants.)

Drug Interactions. Concurrent iron or aluminum- or magnesium-containing antacids reduce absorption. Cholestyramine reduces the serum concentration of mycophenolic acid. In vitro, salicylate increases the unbound fraction of mycophenolic acid. (MMF) sevelamer decreases the absorption of MMF. Rifampin decreases the exposure to mycophenolic acid.

Parameters to Monitor. Monitor CBC, including differential and platelet counts, weekly during the first 1–2 months of therapy, q2wk during the 2–4 months of therapy, and monthly thereafter. Monitor for signs and symptoms of infection, graft rejection, and GVHD.

Notes. MMF has been used in the treatment of certain dermatologic and immunologic disorders such as atopic dermatitis, inflammatory bowel disease, lupus nephritis, myasthenia gravis, pemphigus, psoriasis, rheumatoid arthritis, Takayasu's arteritis, uveitis, and Wegener's granulomatosis.

SIROLIMUS   Rapamune

Pharmacology. Sirolimus (formerly known as rapamycin) is a macrocyclic lactone immunosuppressant isolated from *Streptmyces hygroscopicus* that is structurally related to tacrolimus. It binds FK binding protein-12 (FKBP-12) and inhibits the cytosolic enzyme target of rapamycin (TOR). Inhibition of target of rapamycin restricts differentiation and proliferation of T lymphocytes and B lymphocytes subsequent to cytokine stimulation.

Administration and Adult Dosage. PO for prevention of renal allograft rejection ($\geq$ 40 kg)—6 mg on first day of therapy, followed by 2 mg daily. Alternative dosing for patients at high immunologic risk of rejection is 15 mg on first day of therapy, followed by 5 mg daily. Dilute liquid formulation in glass or plastic container with at least 60 mL of water or orange juice. Mix thoroughly and administer immediately. Then fill container with at least 120 mL of liquid, stir vigorously, and administer immediately. Administer with or without food and consistently with respect to meals, oral cyclosporine, and substrates of CYP3A4 or P-glycoprotein.

Special Populations. *Pediatric Dosage.* Same as adult dosage. Safety and efficacy has not been established in patients <13 years of age.

Geriatric Dosage. Same as adult dosage.

Other Conditions. In hepatic failure, reduce maintenance dosage by approximately one-third. In renal dysfunction, no dosage adjustment is necessary.

Dosage Forms. Soln 1 mg/mL; Tab 1, 2 mg.

Patient Instructions. Take this medication on a regular schedule relative to the time of day and meals. Do not discontinue it unless directed to do so. If your sirolimus is in a bottle, use the amber syringe provided by the manufacturer to measure and take each dose out of the container. If your sirolimus is in a packet, squeeze contents to the lower part of the pouch and cut it across the top. Dilute sirolimus in a glass or plastic container with at least 2 fl oz of water or orange juice. Mix thoroughly and swallow immediately. Then fill container with at least 4 fl oz of water or orange juice, stir vigorously, and swallow immediately. Take each dose with or without food but consistently with respect to meals and medications. Refrigerate. Discard bottle 1 month after opening.

Missed Doses. Take a missed dose as soon as possible if you remember within 16 h. If it is within 8 h of the next dose, skip the missed dose and do not double the missed dose. If you miss 2 or more doses, contact the physician or coordinator who monitors your sirolimus.

Pharmacokinetics. *Serum Levels.* Relationship between whole blood levels and therapeutic or toxic effects is not well defined. Whole blood levels are not monitored routinely, although they may be monitored in pediatric patients or patients with markedly impaired hepatic function. Approximate whole blood trough levels (immunoassay) are 9 μg/L and 17 μg/L in patients receiving sirolimus 2 mg/d and 5 mg/d, respectively. The 24 h postdose whole blood concentration correlates with AUC. Marked interpatient variability of whole blood levels occurs. Whole blood therapeutic concentration range by HPLC is 10–15 μg/L in patients also receiving a calcineurin inhibitor or 15–25 μg/L in patients not on a calcineurin inhibitor.[11]

Fate. Oral bioavailability is 14%. Time-to-peak whole blood concentration is 1–2 h; it is delayed and AUC is increased by 35% when sirolimus is taken after a high-fat meal. P-glycoprotein–mediated countertransport affects absorption. The drug is extensively protein bound in plasma, primarily to albumin, α_1-acid glycoprotein, and lipoproteins. There is extensive sequestration in erythrocytes, with a whole blood-to-plasma ratio of 36:1. V_{dss} is 12 ± 7.5 L/kg. Sirolimus is a CYP3A4 substrate. After administration of radiolabeled drug, 2% is recovered in the urine and 91% is recovered in the bile.

$t_{1/2}$. 62 ± 16 h.

Adverse Reactions. Adverse effects related to use of sirolimus include hypercholesterolemia, hypertriglyceridemia, hypertension, anemia, thrombocytopenia, leukopenia, angioedema, delayed wound healing, interstitial lung disease, proteinuria, diarrhea, hypokalemia, arthralgia, rash, and acne. Thrombocytopenia and lipid abnormalities are dose related. Thrombocytopenia generally resolves after drug discontinuation. Additional adverse effects reported in patients taking sirolimus in combination with other immunosuppressants are nausea, emesis, dyspepsia, abdominal pain, diarrhea, constipation; renal and metabolic abnormalities such as increased Cr_s, hypophosphatemia, hyperkalemia, peripheral edema, and weight gain; respiratory system effects are dyspnea, pharyngitis, and upper respiratory tract infection. Fever, headache, asthenia, body pain, arthralgia, insomnia, tremor, and posttransplant lymphoproliferative disorder also have been reported.

Contraindications. Hypersensitivity to sirolimus, derivatives of sirolimus, or any component of the formulation.

Precautions. Pregnancy; lactation. Box warning against use in de novo liver transplant recipients as a result of excessive mortality, graft loss, and hepatic artery thrombosis. Box warning against use in de dovo lung transplant recipients as a result of bronchial anastomotic dehiscence. (*See also* General Precautions for Immunosuppressants.)

Drug Interactions. Concurrent administration of oral cyclosporine microemulsion capsules (Neoral) increases AUC, peak and trough, but administration of oral cyclosporine 4 h after sirolimus has no effect on sirolimus whole blood levels. Sirolimus can potentiate cyclosporine nephrotoxicity. Azole antifungals, macrolide antibiotics, diltiazem, verapamil, bromocriptine, cimetidine, metoclopramide, and HIV protease inhibitors increase sirolimus levels. Grapefruit and grapefruit juice increases sirolimus concentrations. Rifampin, phenytoin, phenobarbital, carbamazepine, and St. John's wort decrease sirolimus levels. AUC is unchanged with concurrent administration of acyclovir, glyburide, digoxin, nifedipine, norgestrel, or ethinyl estradiol. AUC can be affected by substrates, inhibitors, or inducers of CYP3A4 or P-glycoprotein.

Parameters to Monitor. Monitor WBC, erythrocyte, and platelet counts weekly during the first 2–3 months of therapy and monthly thereafter in stable patients. Monitor serum lipids monthly. Monitor for signs and symptoms of graft rejection, especially after dosage reduction.

Notes. Sirolimus has been used in the treatment of psoriasis.

TACROLIMUS
Prograf, Various

Pharmacology. Tacrolimus (formerly FK506) is a macrolide antibiotic produced by *Streptomyces tsukubaensis*. The intracellular drug–ligand complex of tacrolimus and FK506 binding protein (FKBP-12) indirectly blocks T-lymphocyte activation. It inhibits calcineurin-mediated dephosphorylation of factors necessary for IL-2 transcription.

Administration and Adult Dosage. PO for prophylaxis of organ rejection or GVHD—0.075–0.2 mg/kg/d initially, depending on the type of transplant and coadministration of other immunosuppressants. Tacrolimus is usually started no sooner than 6 h after surgery and administered on a bid schedule. **Maintenance dosage** is based on tacrolimus blood concentrations, the magnitude of risk for organ rejection or GVHD, and patient tolerance. **IV for patients unable to take medication orally**—0.01–0.05 mg/kg/d as a continuous infusion diluted in D5W or NS in a glass container (it can leach plasticizers from PVC containers) to a concentration of 2 mg/100–500 mL (final concentration 4–20 mg/L). Mucositis generally necessitates initial use of IV tacrolimus for allogeneic bone marrow transplant recipients. Tacrolimus is generally started 1 or 2 days before bone marrow transplantation. **Conversion from cyclosporine**—the manufacturer recommends at least 24 h between the last **cyclosporine** dose and the first tacrolimus dose. **To convert from IV to PO tacrolimus**—the IV/PO dosage ratio is typically 1:3. A tacrolimus blood level should be drawn 48 h after dosage form conversion. Absorption of oral medications may be reduced in allogeneic bone marrow transplant patients because of residual gut damage from intensive chemotherapy or radiation or GVHD. **Discontinuation**—tacrolimus may be eventually discontinued in certain renal or allogeneic bone marrow transplant recipients. However, it must be decreased gradually to reduce the risk of reactive immune stimulation and consequent graft rejection or GVHD.

Special Populations. *Pediatric Dosage.* Same as adult dosage.

Geriatric Dosage. Same as adult dosage. Age-related reduction in renal function and comorbid conditions may predispose elderly patients to tacrolimus-induced nephrotoxicity and hypertension.

Special Populations. Use IBW to calculate initial dosage in obese patients.

Dosage Forms. Cap 0.5, 1, 5 mg; **Inj** 5 mg/mL.

Patient Instructions. Take this medication on a regular schedule in relation to the time of day and meals. Do not discontinue it unless directed to do so. Grapefruit and grapefruit juice can interact with tacrolimus. Talk to your physician before drinking grapefruit juice and before starting, stopping, or changing the dose of any medication.

Missed Doses. Take a missed dose as soon as possible if you remember within 12 h. If it is within 2 h of next dose, skip the missed dose and do not double the next dose. If you miss 2 or more doses, contact your physician.

Pharmacokinetics. *Serum Levels.* The serum (blood) concentration–response relationship is not completely defined. Trough blood or serum concentrations are monitored to reduce the risk of toxicity. Therapeutic and toxic concentrations vary with assay, biologic fluid, and time posttransplant. Artifactually elevated serum concentrations can occur when blood is drawn through the same central venous line used for IV tacrolimus administration. Whole blood trough levels of 10–20 μg/L are often considered therapeutic.

Fate. The mean absorption of tacrolimus capsules in normal healthy volunteers is $17 \pm 7\%$. In liver transplant patients, absorption is $22 \pm 6\%$. Factors that can decrease absorption are diarrhea, gastroenteritis, and short small bowel. Food does not affect bioavailability but decreases and delays peak serum levels. Whole blood peak concentrations in liver transplant patients after 0.15 mg/kg is 52.4 μg/L fasting and 27.5 μg/L with food. Tacrolimus is extensively bound to erythrocytes and plasma proteins, primarily albumin and α_1-acid glycoprotein. V_d (whole blood) is 0.85 ± 0.3 L/kg in liver transplant patients; Cl (whole blood) is 0.053 ± 0.017 L/h/kg in liver transplant recipients. Tacrolimus is extensively metabolized by CYP3A. At least 10 metabolites, some with immunosuppressant activity, have been identified. Less than 1% is excreted unchanged in the urine.

$t_{1/2}.$ (whole blood) 21.2 ± 8.5 h in normal healthy volunteers; 11.7 ± 3.9 h in liver transplant patients.

Adverse Reactions. Acute nephrotoxicity, which usually occurs within 1 month posttransplant and is characterized by Cr_s increasing ≥ 0.3 mg/mL/24 h, frequently abates with interruption of drug therapy. Dosage reduction might be required for continued administration. Chronic progressive renal toxicity is characterized by a slow, continual increase in Cr_s and BUN, mild proteinuria, and tubular dysfunction. $Cr_s > 2$ mg/dL in adult patients, or doubling of Cr_s, is an indication for interruption of therapy or dosage reduction. Electrolyte abnormalities, including hypomagnesemia, hypokalemia or hyperkalemia, and renal tubular acidosis, are consequences of tacrolimus-induced nephrotoxicity. Concurrent administration of nephrotoxic drugs increases the likelihood of renal dysfunction. Hypertension occurs frequently. **Calcium channel blockers** and **clonidine** are suitable agents for the management of tacrolimus-induced hypertension because these agents do not have deleterious effects on renal blood flow. Fine tremors occur frequently and can persist and worsen after drug discontinuation. Neurotoxicity symptoms are headache, seizures, encephalopathy, confusion, insomnia, cortical blindness, expressive aphasia, paresthesia, hyperesthesia, and myoclonic reactions. Anaphylactoid reactions to tacrolimus or the solubilizing agent, polyoxyethylated castor oil, can occur. After an allergic reaction to IV tacrolimus, patients may receive a trial of oral tacrolimus capsules under close observation. Hyperbilirubinemia, increased γ-glutamyltranspeptidase, serum alkaline phosphatase, and serum transaminases occur frequently. Additional adverse effects are photophobia, rash, hirsutism, pleural effusion, gingival hyperplasia, diarrhea, nausea, vomiting, and hypertriglyceridemia. There is an increased risk of the development of posttransplant diabetes with tacrolimus.

Contraindications. Allergy to tacrolimus or polyoxyethylated castor oil.

Precautions. Pregnancy; lactation. Use with caution in patients at risk for renal dysfunction. (*See also* General Precautions for Immunosuppressants.)

Drug Interactions. Additive or synergistic renal toxicity can occur with concurrent administration of nephrotoxic drugs. Potassium-sparing diuretics can exacerbate hyperkalemia. Because tacrolimus is metabolized by CYP3A, numerous drug interactions are possible with concurrent administration of drugs that affect this enzyme system. The following drugs can increase tacrolimus blood levels: corticosteroids, azole antifungals, macrolide antibiotics, oral contraceptives, calcium channel blockers, cimetidine, danazol, and metoclopramide. Grapefruit and grapefruit juice can increase tacrolimus concentrations. Enzyme-inducing drugs such as carbamazepine, phenobarbital, phenytoin, St. John's wort, rifabutin, and rifampin can decrease tacrolimus blood levels. Tacrolimus can decrease the clearance of HMG-CoA reductase inhibitors and increase the risk of drug-induced rhabdomyolysis.

Parameters to Monitor. Observe for anaphylaxis with IV administration. Monitor Cr_s every 2–7 days and daily in patients at risk for acute renal dysfunction. Monitor LFTs weekly, triglycerides monthly, and blood pressure regularly. Monitor blood or serum concentrations every 2–3 days when starting therapy. As the patient's clinical condition and renal function allow, reduce frequency to 1–2 times weekly and then monthly during the first year of therapy. After the first year of therapy, blood or serum concentration monitoring may be reduced every 1–2 months in stable patients. Monitor for signs and symptoms of graft rejection or GVHD, especially after dosage reduction.

■ REFERENCES

1. Brennan DC et al. A randomized, double-blinded comparison of Thymoglobulin versus Atgam for induction immunosuppression therapy in adult renal transplant recipients. *Transplantation.* 1999;67:1011-1018.
2. Laske A et al. Prophylactic cytolytic therapy in heart transplantation: monoclonal versus polyclonal antibody therapy. *J Heart Lung Transplant.* 1992;11:557-563.
3. Copeland JG et al. Rabbit antithymocyte globulin. A 10-year experience in cardiac transplantation *J Thorac Cardiovasc Surg.* 1990;99:852-860.
4. Palmer SM et al. Rabbit antithymocyte globulin decreases acute rejection after lung transplantation: results of a randomized, prospective study. *Chest.* 1999;116:127-133.
5. Bajjoka I et al. Preserving renal function in liver transplant recipients with rabbit anti-thymocyte globulin and delayed initiation of calcineurin inhibitors. *Liver Transpl.* 2008;14:66-72.
6. Tanchanco R et al. Beneficial outcomes of a steroid-free regimen with Thymoglobulin induction in pancreas-kidney transplantation. *Transplant Proc.* 2008;40:1551-1554.
7. Di Bona E et al. Rabbit antithymocyte globulin (r-ATG) plus cyclosporine and granulocyte colony stimulating factor is an effective treatment for aplastic anaemia patients unresponsive to a first course of intensive immunosuppressive therapy. *Br J Haematol.* 1999;107:330-334.
8. Ringden O et al. Low incidence of acute graft-versus-host disease using unrelated HLA-A-, HLA-B-, and HLA-DR-compatible donors and conditioning, including anti-T-cell antibodies. *Transplantation.* 1998;66:620-625.
9. Wiland AM et al. Peripheral administration of Thymoglobulin for induction therapy in pancreas transplantation. *Transplant Proc.* 2001;33:1910.
10. Bunn D et al. The pharmacokinetics of anti-thymocyte globulin (ATG) following intravenous infusion in man. *Clin Nephrol.* 1996;45:29-32.
11. Schonder KS, Johnson HJ. Solid-organ transplantation. In: Dipiro JT et al, eds. *Pharmacotherapy: A pathophysiologic approach.* New York: McGraw-Hill; 2008:1459-1482.
12. Sullivan KM et al. Prednisone and azathioprine compared with prednisone and placebo for treatment of chronic graft-v-host disease: prognostic influence of prolonged thrombocytopenia after allogenic marrow transplantation. *Blood.* 1988;72:546-554.

13. Brinch L. Fooled by cyclosporin levels. *Bone Marrow Transplant*. 1992;9:77-78.

14. Mattei MF et al. Lower risks of infectious deaths in cardiac transplant patients receiving basiliximab versus anti-thymocyte globulin as induction therapy. *J Heart Lung Transplant*. 2007;26:693-699.

15. Borro JM et al. Comparative study of basiliximab treatment in lung transplantation. *Transplant Proc*. 2005;37:3996-3998.

16. Llado L et al. Immunosuppression without steroids in liver transplantation is safe and reduces infection and metabolic complications: results from a prospective multicenter randomized study. *J Hepatol*. 2006;44:710-716.

17. Zhang R et al. The long-term survival of simultaneous pancreas and kidney transplant with basiliximab induction therapy. *Clin Transplant*. 2007;21:583-589.

18. Ortiz V et al. Induction therapy with daclizumab in heart transplantation—how many doses? *Transplant Proc*. 2006;38:2541-2543.

19. Ailawadi G et al. Effects of induction immunosuppression regimen on acute rejection, bronchiolitis obliterans, and survival after lung transplantation. *J Thorac Cardiovasc Surg*. 2008;135:594-602.

20. Stratta RJ et al. A prospective, randomized, multicenter study evaluating the safety and efficacy of two dosing regimens of daclizumab compared to no antibody induction in simultaneous kidney-pancreas transplantation: results at 3 years. *Transplant Proc*. 2005;37:3531-3534.

21. Przepiorka D et al. Daclizumab, a humanized anti-interleukin-2 receptor alpha chain antibody, for treatment of acute graft-versus-host disease. *Blood*. 2000;95:83-89.

22. Anasetti C et al. Treatment of acute graft-versus-host disease with humanized anti-Tac: an antibody that binds to the interleukin-2 receptor. *Blood*. 1994;84:1320-1327.

23. Singh RP, Stratta RJ. Advances in immunosuppression for pancreas transplantation. *Curr Opin Organ Transplant*. 2008;13:79-84.

24. Snell GI, Westall GP. Immunosuppression for lung transplantation: evidence to date. *Drugs*. 2007;67:1531-1539.

25. Lehmkuhl H et al. Enteric-coated mycophenolate-sodium in heart transplantation: efficacy, safety, and pharmacokinetic compared with mycophenolate mofetil. *Transplant Proc*. 2008;40:953-955.

26. Cantisani GP et al. Enteric-coated mycophenolate sodium experience in liver transplant patients. *Transplant Proc*. 2006;38:932-933.

27. Basara N et al. Mycophenolate mofetil for the treatment of acute and chronic GVHD in bone marrow transplant patients. *Bone Marrow Transplant*. 1998;22:61-65.

28. Mookerjee B et al. Salvage therapy for refractory chronic graft-versus-host disease with mycophenolate mofetil and tacrolimus. *Bone Marrow Transplant*. 1999;24:517-520.

29. Staatz CE, Tett SE. Clinical pharmacokinetics and pharmacodynamics of mycophenolate in solid organ transplant recipients. *Clin Pharmacokinet*. 2007;46:13-58.

Cardiovascular Drugs | 4

Nickole N. Henyan

Chapter 30

Antiarrhythmic Drugs

Kurt Reinhart and C. Michael White

ADENOSINE — Adenocard

Pharmacology. Adenosine is a purinergic agonist that acts on the purine P_1 and P_2 receptors (although P_1 receptors are more sensitive to adenosine). Pharmacologic effects include coronary and peripheral vasodilation, negative inotropic actions, and depression of sinus node and AV nodal conduction. It is used most frequently for supraventricular tachycardia caused by reentry (i.e., AV nodal reentry or AV reentry associated with an extranodal pathway). In these instances, restoration of sinus rhythm occurs in 85%–95% of patients. The drug also can be helpful in diagnosing wide-QRS tachycardias, believed to be supraventricular in origin.[1–3]

Adult Dosage. **IV for supraventricular tachycardia**—administer over 1–2 s through an IV line with minimal dead space, followed by a saline flush; **initial dose** is 6 mg (3 mg if administered through a central line); if this is ineffective, 12 mg can be given 2 min later and repeated once if necessary. An average effective dose of 1 mg has been reported in patients receiving concurrent dipyridamole.[4]

Special Populations. *Pediatric Dosage.* **IV**—0.05–0.1 mg/kg, increased in increments of 0.05–0.1 mg/kg q2min prn, until a maximum of 0.3 mg/kg is reached. Administer the adult dose if body weight $\geq$ 50 kg.

Dosage Forms. Inj 3 mg/mL.

Pharmacokinetics. Adenosine is rapidly metabolized intracellularly to inactive adenosine monophosphate and inosine; elimination half-life is about 1–10 s.

Adverse Reactions. Frequent, but short-lived, subjective complaints include chest discomfort, dyspnea, flushing, and headache. Postconversion arrhythmias also are frequent but transient and include ventricular ectopy, sinus bradycardia, AV block, atrial fibrillation, and rapid reinitiation of supraventricular tachycardia. Adenosine is contraindicated in patients with preexisting sinus node dysfunction or second- or third-degree heart block without a functioning pacemaker because of the risk of prolonged sinus arrest or AV block. Also use adenosine with caution in asthma patients (because it can precipitate bronchospasm) and in patients with atrial fibrillation with an accessory AV pathway (because it can accelerate ventricular response).

Drug Interactions. Dipyridamole blocks the cellular uptake of adenosine, enhancing the pharmacologic effect; methylxanthines inhibit the therapeutic actions of adenosine.

AMIODARONE HYDROCHLORIDE   Cordarone, Pacerone

Pharmacology. Amiodarone is a class III antiarrhythmic that prolongs the effective refractory period of atrial and ventricular tissue by blocking potassium conductance. It decreases sinus rate and slows conduction through the AV node by β-adrenergic blockade. Amiodarone also blocks sodium and calcium channels. The antiarrhythmic actions can be caused by interruption of reentrant substrate or abolition of premature beats that trigger reentry.

Administration and Adult Dosage. PO loading dosage—800–1600 mg/d in divided doses for 1–2 wk. Loading dosages are usually toward the lower end of this range for atrial arrhythmias and toward the upper end of the range for ventricular arrhythmias. PO maintenance dosage—100–600 mg/d (usually 300–400 mg/d for recurrent ventricular tachycardia and 100–200 mg/d for supraventricular tachycardias such as atrial fibrillation). A priming dose of 600–800 mg/d for 1–2 mo after the initial loading period and before maintenance therapy may be used. **IV for treatment or prevention of refractory ventricular tachycardia or fibrillation**—150 mg over 10 min, 360 mg over the next 6 h, and 540 mg over the next 18 h. In one study, amiodarone was administered as a 300 mg IV bolus for cardiac arrest.[5] Initiate amiodarone only during hospitalization for the first several days of the loading phase.

Special Populations. *Pediatric Dosage.* Safety and efficacy not established. PO—10–15 mg/kg/d for 10 d and then 5 mg/kg/d maintenance therapy has been used.[6] IV—5 mg/kg in 1 mg/kg increments over 5–10 min each; an additional 1–5 mg/kg may be given in 30 min if needed.

Geriatric Dosage. Same as adult dosage.

Dosage Forms. Tab 200 mg; Inj 50 mg/mL.

Patient Instructions. Report any shortness of breath, tiredness, abdominal discomfort, or visual abnormalities. Avoid intense sunlight; use sunscreen. Divided doses during loading or maintenance-dose phases can reduce intestinal upset. Do not drink grapefruit juice while taking amiodarone.

Missed Doses. Take this drug at regular intervals. If you miss a dose, do *not* take it. If it is about time for the next dose, take that dose only. Do not double the dose or take extra.

Pharmacokinetics. *Onset and Duration.* Onset is variable, from several days to a month; full effect might not occur for several months.[7]

Serum Levels. 1–2.5 mg/L (1.6–4 μmol/L) proposed but not well established.[8] Desethylamiodarone accumulates to serum levels similar to or greater than the parent drug.

Fate. Oral absorption is erratic and incomplete; bioavailability is 46 ± 22% Peak serum concentrations occur in 3–7 h. The drug is 99.9% plasma protein bound;[7,9] V_d is 66 ± 44 L/kg; Cl is 0.11 ± 0.024 L/h/kg.[7,9,10] Amiodarone is primarily hepatically eliminated with at least one active metabolite, desethylamiodarone. No unchanged amiodarone or desethylamiodarone is found in urine.[7]

Half-life ($t_{1/2}$.). α phase 4–12 h; β phase changes with duration of therapy and study sampling. Reported variously as 25 ± 12 d and 53 ± 23 d.[7,9,10] Similar for desethylamiodarone.[7,10]

Adverse Reactions. Corneal microdeposits occur in virtually all patients and are no reason for stopping treatment; however, visual disturbances are reported in about 5%.[10] Neurologic effects occur frequently and include tremor, ataxia, paresthesias, and nightmares, which can be more common during the loading phase.[10] Anorexia, nausea, vomiting, and/or constipation occur frequently. Transient elevations in hepatic enzymes occur in more than 50% of patients, but clinical hepatitis occurs only occasionally.[11] Photosensitivity occurs frequently, and a blue–gray skin pigmentation (sometimes irreversible) develops in 2%–4% of patients.[10] Hypothyroidism (low T_3 syndrome) or hyperthyroidism occurs frequently.[12] Occasional proximal muscle weakness and myopathy have been reported. Symptomatic pulmonary fibrosis has been reported in 1%–6% of patients; it is probably not immunologic in etiology and seems to occur more often in patients with underlying lung disease.[10,13] Pulmonary symptoms usually improve with drug discontinuation, but up to 10% of cases result in death.[10,13] Aggravation of ventricular tachycardia and drug-induced torsades de pointes can occur.[10,14] Occasional severe sinus bradycardia (requiring a pacemaker) or AV block has been reported.

Contraindications. Sick sinus syndrome or second- or third-degree heart block in the absence of a ventricular pacemaker; patients in whom bradycardia has caused syncope; long-QT syndrome.

Precautions. Electrophysiologic studies may not predict the long-term efficacy of amiodarone.[15] The benzyl alcohol preservative can be hazardous in infants.

Drug Interactions. Amiodarone inhibits a wide array of cytochrome P450 enzymes including CYP1A2, CYP2C9, CYP2D6, and CYP3A4; it also inhibits P-glycoprotein.[16] Amiodarone increases serum levels of cyclosporine, lovastatin, simvastatin, digoxin, flecainide, phenytoin, procainamide, and quinidine. It potentiates the anticoagulant effects of warfarin; reduce the initial dosage of warfarin by one-third to one-half.

Parameters to Monitor. Monitor ECG daily during loading phase for heart rate, PR, QRS, and QT duration. Baseline and periodic thyroid function tests as well as liver enzymes (especially if symptoms present). Obtain baseline pulmonary function tests; repeat chest x-ray and clinical examination every 3–6 months.[10,13]

Notes. Because of the results of the Cardiac Arrhythmia Suppression Trial (CAST),[17] many clinicians use class III antiarrhythmics (e.g., amiodarone, sotalol) as first-line therapy for supraventricular and ventricular arrhythmias. A noniodinated analogue of amiodarone under clinical investigation is **dronedarone.**

DISOPYRAMIDE PHOSPHATE	Norpace, Various

Pharmacology. Disopyramide, a class Ia antiarrhythmic, has qualitatively the same electrophysiologic actions as procainamide and quinidine and is effective for ventricular and (unlabeled) supraventricular tachycardia. It can exert a profound negative inotropic effect and has marked anticholinergic properties systemically and on the heart. The isomers of disopyramide have stereospecific pharmacologic actions.[18,19]

Administration and Adult Dosage. **PO loading dosage**—200–300 mg. **PO maintenance dosage**—400–800 mg/d, to a maximum of 1.6 g/d. Give daily dosage in 4 equally divided doses q6h with non-SR Cap or in 2 equally divided doses q12h with SR Cap. Initiate disopyramide during hospitalization.

Special Populations. *Pediatric Dosage.* PO—(<1 y) 10–30 mg/kg/d; (1–4 y) 10–20 mg/kg/d; (4–12 y) 10–15 mg/kg/d; (12–18 y) 6–15 mg/kg/d. Daily dosage is divided into 4 equal doses q6h.[20] (*See* Notes.)

Geriatric Dosage. Decreased dosage is probably necessary because the elderly might not tolerate the anticholinergic side effects.

Other Conditions. In patients who weigh less than 50 kg or have hepatic disease or moderate renal insufficiency (Cl_{Cr} >40 mL/min), load with 150–200 mg and then give 400 mg/d in 2 or 4 divided doses, depending on the dosage form used. Initial daily dosage in patients with hepatic disease is about 4.4 mg/kg/d.[21,22] In patients with severe renal insufficiency, give 100 mg as follows (non-SR Cap): Cl_{Cr} 30–40 mL/min, q8h; Cl_{Cr} 15–30 mL/min, q12h; Cl_{Cr} <15 mL/min, q24h.

CREATININE CLEARANCE	DISOPYRAMIDE DAILY MAINTENANCE DOSAGE
30–40 mL/min	100 mg tid
15–30 mL/min	100 mg bid
<15 mL/min	100 mg once daily

Dosage Forms. **Cap** 100, 150 mg; **SR Cap** 100, 150 mg. (*See* Notes.)

Patient Instructions. Report any symptoms such as difficulty in urination, constipation, blurred vision, or dry mouth. Also report shortness of breath, weight gain, or edema. Do not crush or chew sustained-release capsules. A sustained-release capsule core in the stool does not indicate lack of absorption.

Missed Doses. Take this drug at regular intervals. If you miss a dose, take it as soon as you remember. If it is about time for the next dose, take that dose only. Leave at least 4 h between regular capsule doses and 6–8 h between sustained-release capsule doses. Do not double the dose or take extra.

Pharmacokinetics. *Onset and Duration.* PO onset is within 1 h. Duration differs with individual differences in drug disposition but is usually 6–12 h.

Serum Levels. Usual range is 2–5 mg/L (6–15 μmol/L),[22,23] with toxicity more likely over 4 mg/L. Therapeutic range of unbound drug is 0.5–2 mg/L (1.5–6 μmol/L).[21] Monitoring unbound concentrations eliminates variability caused by concentration-dependent disposition.[22,24]

Fate. Oral absorption is rapid; systemic availability is $83 \pm 11\%$.[22,23] Unbound drug in serum varies from 19%–46% over a serum concentration range of 2–8 mg/L and is also age dependent.[25] V_d (unbound) is 1.4–1.7 L/kg in normal individuals;[9,22] Cl (unbound) is about 0.25 L/h/kg;[22] Cl is stereospecific.[26] The major metabolite is a mono-N-dealkylated form that has weak antiarrhythmic but potent anticholinergic activity; $55 \pm 6\%$ is excreted unchanged in urine.[9]

$t_{1/2}$. α phase 2–4 min (IV);[23] β phase is concentration dependent, usually 6 ± 1 h;[9] 11–17 h in renal impairment, depending on severity.[25]

Adverse Reactions. Nausea or anorexia occur frequently. Dry mouth, urinary retention, blurred vision, and constipation are dose-related anticholinergic effects that can occur in up to 70% of patients and result in drug discontinuation in about 20%.[27] Through its vagolytic action, disopyramide can cause sinus tachycardia. Severe bradycardia, AV nodal block, or asystole also can occur, especially in patients with SA or AV nodal disease. Exacerbation of CHF is most prevalent (20%–40%) in patients with left ventricular systolic dysfunction.[18] Torsades de pointes, similar to quinidine syncope, has been reported. Rarely rash, hepatic cholestasis, psychosis, or peripheral neuropathy occur. Hypoglycemia also has been reported. Like other class Ia drugs, disopyramide has been associated with torsades de pointes.

Contraindications. History of disopyramide-induced heart block or serious ventricular arrhythmias; second- or third-degree heart block without a ventricular pacemaker; long-QT syndrome; cardiogenic shock or severe CHF.

Precautions. In atrial fibrillation or flutter, give digoxin or drugs that slow AV nodal conduction before giving disopyramide. Use very cautiously, if at all, in patients with CHF because of negative inotropic effects. The drug can worsen sick sinus syndrome or aggravate underlying ventricular arrhythmias. If possible, use other antiarrhythmics in patients with prostatic hypertrophy or preexisting urinary retention. Disopyramide can exacerbate glaucoma or myasthenia gravis.

Drug Interactions. Erythromycin and other CYP3A4 inhibitors inhibit disopyramide metabolism. Phenytoin can decrease disopyramide serum levels and increase its anticholinergic effects. Rifampin, barbiturates, and other enzyme inducers can decrease disopyramide serum levels. Concurrent use of disopyramide and quinidine can increase disopyramide serum levels or decrease quinidine serum levels. Excessive prolongation of the QT interval may occur with other antiarrhythmics.

Parameters to Monitor. Because of concentration-dependent protein binding, total drug levels unreliably reflect active drug concentration, and monitoring unbound drug concentrations is preferable. Monitor serum levels and symptoms or signs of toxicity closely in patients with altered states of drug disposition such as renal dysfunction. When initiating therapy, observe ECG daily for 3–4 d for QT, QRS, or PR prolongation. If QT prolongation of 25% or greater occurs, consider discontinuing disopyramide. Frequently obtain vital signs initially for evidence of adverse hemodynamic effects (e.g., CHF) and less frequently when a maintenance dosage is attained. Question the patient about anticholinergic manifestations such as urinary and visual abnormalities.

Notes. A 1–10 mg/mL suspension, prepared from capsules, in cherry syrup is stable for 1 month with refrigeration in an amber bottle.

DOFETILIDE
Tikosyn

Pharmacology. Dofetilide is a class III antiarrhythmic drug that selectively prolongs atrial and ventricular repolarization by blocking the delayed rectifier (rapid component) potassium current. It is indicated for the termination and prevention of atrial fibrillation and flutter.

Administration and Adult Dosage. PO—125–500 μg bid, adjusted based on response, renal function, and QT-interval prolongation. Initiate therapy during hospitalization and according to the manufacturer's individualized dosing.

Special Populations. *Pediatric Dosage.* Safety and efficacy not established.

Geriatric Dosage. Same as adult dosage.

Other Conditions. Reduce starting dosages for patients with renal dysfunction: 250 μg bid for Cl_{Cr} 40–60 mL/min and 125 μg bid for Cl_{Cr} 20–40 mL/min.[28,29] Avoid the drug in patients with Cl_{Cr} <20 mL/min.

Dosage Forms. Cap 125, 250, 500 μg.

Pharmacokinetics. Oral bioavailability is 96% and peak concentrations occur 2.5 h after oral administration.[28] The V_d is 3 L/kg. About 20% of dofetilide is metabolized hepatically and 80% is eliminated renally as unchanged drug.[28] Elimination half-life is 10 h with normal renal function.

Adverse Reactions. The major side effect is drug-induced torsades de pointes, which occurs in 1%–10% of patients; risk increases with higher dosages.[28] Other risk factors include the female gender and underlying CHF.

Contraindications. Severe renal insufficiency; QT prolongation; hypokalemia; previous history of torsades de pointes; Cl_{Cr} <20 mL/min.

Drug Interactions. Avoid using dofetilide with drugs that interfere with its renal elimination (e.g., cimetidine, ketoconazole, trimethoprim and sulfamethoxazole, prochlorperazine, megestrol).[28,29] Use caution with concurrent use of agents that block CYP3A4 (e.g., verapamil, erythromycin). Do not use with other drugs that can prolong the QT interval.

Parameters to Monitor. Initiate dofetilide during hospitalization with continuous ECG monitoring. Decrease dosage if QT prolongation occurs; discontinue if excessive. Monitor renal function every 3 months.

Notes. When administered properly and monitored closely, dofetilide does not seem to increase mortality in patients with CHF.[30] Prescribers and pharmacies must enroll in a manufacturer-sponsored program in order to prescribe and dispense dofetilide.

DRONEDARONE (Sanofi-Aventis)
Multaq

Pharmacology. Dronedarone is a noniodinated analogue of amiodarone being evaluated for the maintenance of sinus rhythm in patients with atrial fibrillation or flutter. Its nonspecific channel blocking as well as adrenergic blocking properties are similar to those of amiodarone.[31]

Adult Dosage. 400 mg orally twice a day with morning and evening meals.

Dosage Forms. Tab 400 mg.

Pharmacokinetics. Half-life is 24 h and both dronedarone and metabolites are excreted in the feces. Metabolized via CYP3A4.[31]

Adverse Reactions. Because of the lack of an iodine moiety, less lipophilicity, and a much shorter half-life of 24 h, it is hoped that dronedarone will have a better safety profile than amiodarone with similar efficacy. Dronedarone may increase the risk of worsening heart failure and death in patients with severe left heart failure.[32]

FLECAINIDE ACETATE

Tambocor

Pharmacology. Flecainide is a class Ic antiarrhythmic that predominantly slows conduction velocity, with minimal effect on refractoriness. (*See* Electrophysiologic Actions of Antiarrhythmics Comparison Chart.) Compared with class Ia or Ib antiarrhythmics, it binds to and dissociates from the sodium channel very slowly. It can decrease cardiac output by a negative inotropic action.

Administration and Adult Dosage. PO—50 mg q12h initially, increasing in 50-mg increments q12h, q4–7d until desired response. **Usual maintenance dosage** is 100 mg PO q12h to a maximum of 300 mg/d or 400 mg/d for life-threatening ventricular arrhythmias. Initiate flecainide during hospitalization.

Special Populations. *Pediatric Dosage.* Safety and efficacy not established. PO—100–200 mg/m²/d (average 140 mg/m²/d) in 2 divided doses has been used.[33]

Geriatric Dosage. Same as adult dosage.

Other Conditions. Lower maintenance dosage requirements are expected in patients with CHF, liver disease, or renal insufficiency. Start these patients with 50–100 mg q12–24h and cautiously increase dosage as required with the aid of serum levels.[22,34]

Dosage Forms. **Tab** 50, 100, 150 mg.

Patient Instructions. Report any symptoms of dizziness, extra or rapid heartbeats, or visual disturbances. Report symptoms of worsening shortness of breath or exercise intolerance.

Missed Doses. Take this drug at regular intervals. If you miss a dose and it has been less than 4 h since your dose was due, take it as soon as you remember. If it is about time for the next dose, take that dose only. Do not double the dose or take extra.

Pharmacokinetics. *Onset and Duration.* Onset 1–6 h (average 3); duration 12–30 h.[34]

Serum Levels. (Therapeutic trough) 0.2–1 mg/L (0.5–2.5 μmol/L).[34,35]

Fate. Oral bioavailability is $70 \pm 11\%$.[9,35] From 37%–55% is bound to plasma proteins, but the percentage can be higher (61%) post-MI because of increases in $\alpha 1$-acid glycoprotein.[34] V_d is 8–10 L/kg;[34] Cl has been reported as 0.34 ± 0.1 L/h/kg[9] and 0.61 ± 0.23 L/h/kg;[22,34] Cl decreases with CHF, renal failure, and liver disease. Flecainide is about 60% stereoselectively metabolized by the liver through the CYP2D6 isoenzyme[36] and about 30% excreted unchanged in urine.

$t_{1/2}$. α phase 3–8 min; β phase 14 ± 5 h; β phase is 20 ± 4 h in patients with ventricular ectopy and 37.8 ± 39.7 h in those with severe renal dysfunction.[37]

Adverse Reactions. Neurologic side effects, which include dizziness and visual abnormalities, occur frequently. Exacerbation of CHF in patients with underlying left ventricular dysfunction occurs frequently. Nausea, dyspnea, and headache also can occur frequently. Flecainide has proarrhythmic effects that can result in new sustained ventricular tachycardia or aggravation of underlying ventricular arrhythmias. These reactions occur more frequently in patients with left ventricular dysfunction, coronary disease, or ventricular arrhythmias.[17,38] Risk can be sustained over time and not limited to the several days after initiation of therapy. Flecainide-induced ventricular tachycardia may be unresponsive to cardioversion or pacing but responsive to lidocaine therapy or sodium bicarbonate. Aggravation of underlying conduction disturbances also can occur.

Contraindications. Second- or third-degree AV block or bifascicular block without a ventricular pacemaker; severe CHF; history of type Ic–induced arrhythmia.

Precautions. Use with caution in patients with sick sinus syndrome and in combination with other negative inotropic drugs such as calcium channel blockers or β-blockers or after recent therapy with a type Ia antiarrhythmic. Flecainide can increase pacemaker capture threshold.[39] (*See* Notes.)

Drug Interactions. Amiodarone and cimetidine can increase flecainide serum concentrations; flecainide slightly elevates serum digoxin levels.

Parameters to Monitor. Frequent or continuous (preferred) ECG when therapy is initiated and then periodically on an ambulatory basis. Obtain a baseline evaluation of left ventricular function before starting flecainide. Obtain periodic trough serum levels (particularly in those with renal or liver disease and CHF) once an individual's effective level is determined. Observe closely for neurologic toxicities and CHF symptoms when initiating therapy.

Notes. Because the CAST results showed increased mortality in patients with asymptomatic ventricular arrhythmias post-MI who were given flecainide,[17] it should be reserved for individuals with life-threatening ventricular arrhythmias (e.g., sustained ventricular tachycardia) refractory to other drugs.

IBUTILIDE FUMARATE   Corvert

Pharmacology. Ibutilide is a class III antiarrhythmic that selectively prolongs atrial and ventricular repolarizations by increasing sodium influx (the window current) and blocking the rapid component of the delayed rectifier potassium current. It is indicated for the acute termination of atrial fibrillation or atrial flutter of recent onset. In these arrhythmias, sinus rhythm is restored in about 50% of patients.[40,41]

Adult Dosage. **IV for atrial flutter or fibrillation**—(±60 kg) 1 mg over 10 min; (<60 kg) 0.01 mg/kg. If the tachycardia is not terminated 10 min after the end of the initial infusion, the dose can be repeated.

Dosage Forms. **Inj** 0.1 mg/mL.

Pharmacokinetics. Ibutilide is approximately 40% bound to plasma proteins and has a V_d of 11 ± 4 L/kg.[40,41] It is metabolized primarily by the liver. Although many metabolites have been identified, only a hydroxylated form has shown weak class III activity. Less than 10% is excreted unchanged in urine. Elimination half-life is about 6 h (range 2–12 h).[41]

Adverse Reactions. The major side effect is drug-induced proarrhythmia; torsades de pointes (sustained or nonsustained) occurs in 4%–5% of patients. Risk factors are hypokalemia, underlying left ventricular dysfunction, and the female gender.[42] Rapid IV bolus administration can increase the risk of torsades de pointes.[41] Prior administration of IV MgSO$_4$ can prevent torsades de pointes. Heart block and heart failure have occurred rarely.

Contraindications. Preexisting hypokalemia or hypomagnesemia; preexisting long-QT interval; congenital long-QT syndromes; concurrent therapy with other drugs known to delay repolarization.

Precautions. Concurrent use with other medications that prolong the QT interval may increase the risk of arrhythmia.

Parameters to Monitor. Give ibutilide with continuous ECG monitoring. Monitor QT interval before and for at least 4 h after infusion and serum electrolytes before and after administration.

LIDOCAINE HYDROCHLORIDE   Xylocaine, Various

Pharmacology. Lidocaine's electrophysiologic actions differ in healthy and diseased cardiac tissues. (*See* Electrophysiologic Actions of Antiarrhythmics Comparison Chart.) Most of its antiarrhythmic activity is caused by frequency-dependent blockade of the fast sodium channel in Purkinje fibers. In comparison with other antiarrhythmics, lidocaine binds to and dissociates from the sodium channel very quickly. It is used in the acute treatment of ventricular arrhythmias often associated with MI. Effectiveness in the treatment of supraventricular arrhythmia is limited.

Administration and Adult Dosage. **IV loading dose for ventricular tachycardia or fibrillation**—100 mg (1–1.5 mg/kg) over 1 min; if ineffective, repeat with 50–100 mg q5–10 min, to a maximum of 300 mg.[43] **IV maintenance**—2–4 mg/min infusion.[43] **IV for neuropathic pain**—5 mg/kg/h for 60–90 min has been used.[44] (*See* Notes.)

Special Populations. *Pediatric Dosage.* **IV (or intratracheal) loading dose**— 1 mg/kg; can repeat q10–15 min to a maximum of 3–5 mg/kg. **IV maintenance dosage**—20–50 μg/kg/min infusion.[20]

Geriatric Dosage. Same as adult dosage. The elderly can be at increased risk for toxicity because of decreased clearance.

Other Conditions. In CHF, use one-half of IV loading dose and a lower maintenance infusion. In liver disease or CHF, initial maintenance infusion is 1 mg/min, to a maximum of 2–3 mg/min.[43] In MI without CHF, maintenance infusion rate might need to be decreased by 30%–50% in 24 h;[43] however, empiric dosage alterations in MI are not recommended because of increases in α$_1$-acid glycoprotein and lidocaine binding.[45]

Dosage Forms. **Inj** 10, 20, 40, 100, 200 mg/mL. Also available premixed in D5W in concentrations of 2, 4, and 8 mg/mL.

Patient Instructions. Report side effects such as drowsiness, perioral numbness or tingling, dizziness, and nausea during maintenance infusion.

Pharmacokinetics. *Onset and Duration.* IV onset is immediate; duration after initial IV bolus is 10–20 min. IM onset is 10 min; duration is 3 h.[46]

Serum Levels. Therapeutic (total), 1.5–6 mg/L (7–28 μmol/L);[23] unbound, 0.5–1.5 mg/L (2–7 μmol/L).[45] Toxic reactions are more likely at total concentrations >5 mg/L (22 mol/L).[43] (*See* Adverse Reactions.)

Fate. The drug is well absorbed orally, but a large hepatic first-pass effect limits systemic availability to 35 ± 11%.[47] IM absorption half-life is 12–28 min.[48] The drug is 70 ± 5% bound to plasma proteins;[43] V_d is 1.3 ± 0.4 L/kg in normal individuals and 0.9 ± 0.2 L/kg in patients with CHF.[49] Cl is 0.55 ± 0.14 L/h/kg, decreased in CHF, liver disease, and during long-term infusion.[43,49,50] Lidocaine is metabolized primarily in the liver, with 2 ± 1% excreted unchanged in the urine.[49] The major metabolites, monoethylglycinexylidide (MEGX) and glycinexylidide (GX), have neurotoxic[51] and antiarrhythmic[52] actions. Accumulation of these metabolites in renal impairment or during prolonged infusions can contribute to lidocaine toxicity.

$t_{1/2}$. α phase about 8 min;[46,49] β phase 98 ± 24 min.[43,49] The β phases in CHF and liver disease can be prolonged to 4.5 ± 2.4 h and 6.6 ± 1.1 h, respectively.[43,49] Elimination half-life of total lidocaine increases to an average of 3.2 ± 0.5 h 24 h after MI without CHF and up to 10.2 ± 2 h after MI with CHF.[53] In MI, the rise in total lidocaine half-life is greater than that of unbound lidocaine.[54]

Adverse Reactions. Serum level–related neurologic side effects including dizziness, nausea, drowsiness, speech disturbances, perioral numbness, muscle twitching, confusion, vertigo, and tinnitus are frequent at total serum levels >5 mg/L. Serious toxicities including psychosis, seizures, and respiratory depression occur at serum levels >9 mg/L.[43] Sinus arrest or severe bradycardia is associated with sinus node disease, toxic drug levels, or concomitant therapy with other antiarrhythmics. Complete AV block can occur, especially in patients with preexisting bifascicular bundle branch block, AV nodal block, or inferior wall MI.[55,56]

Contraindications. History of hypersensitivity to any amide-type local anesthetic (rare); second- or third-degree heart block unless the site of the block can be localized to the AV node itself[55] or ventricular pacemaker is functional; severe sinus node dysfunction; Stokes-Adams syndrome; atrial fibrillation in association with Wolff–Parkinson–White syndrome.

Precautions. Lidocaine administered to prevent ventricular fibrillation in acute MI is no longer recommended.[56] Toxicity during bronchoscopy caused by tracheal lidocaine absorption has been reported.

Drug Interactions. Propranolol decreases lidocaine clearance, so close monitoring is necessary with concomitant administration of these drugs. Cimetidine can decrease lidocaine clearance, but empiric dosage reduction with concomitant cimetidine is not recommended.[57] Phenytoin can decrease lidocaine serum levels and increase myocardial depression.

Parameters to Monitor. Closely monitor serum levels and signs or symptoms of toxicity in patients with altered drug dispositions such as CHF, hepatic disease, acute MI, or prolonged IV infusion (>24 h). Monitoring unbound levels is preferable post-MI. Minor subjective and objective toxicities are extremely important because they are often subtle and can forecast more serious toxicities (e.g., psychosis or seizures). Continuously observe ECG for therapeutic and/or toxic actions. Frequently monitor vital signs such as blood pressure, heart rate, and respiration.

Notes. IV lidocaine has been used to treat pain of peripheral origin such as neuropathies and burns.[44]

MEXILETINE HYDROCHLORIDE
Mexitil, Various

Pharmacology. Mexiletine has electrophysiologic actions similar to those of lidocaine and tocainide. Depression of conduction is accentuated in ischemic/hypoxic tissue. It is used in the treatment of ventricular arrhythmias; effectiveness in supraventricular tachycardias is limited.

Administration and Adult Dosage. PO loading dose—400 mg once, followed by maintenance dosage in 8 h; **PO maintenance dosage**—200–300 mg q8h, to a maximum of 400 mg q8h. **PO for neuropathic pain**—450 mg/d;[58] dosages as high as 10 mg/kg/d have been used to treat the thalamic pain syndrome.[59] (*See* Notes.) Initiate mexiletine during hospitalization.

Special Populations. *Pediatric Dosage.* Safety and efficacy not established.

Geriatric Dosage. Same as adult dosage.

Other Conditions. Reduce maintenance dosage by 30%–50% in patients with hepatic disease or severe CHF.[22] Dosage also might need to be decreased with Cl_{Cr} <10 mL/min.[60]

Dosage Forms. Cap 150, 200, 250 mg.

Patient Instructions. Report numbness, drowsiness, dizziness, or tingling. Nausea or loss of appetite can occur and may be reduced by taking the drug with food. Report any abnormal bruising.

Missed Doses. Take this drug at regular intervals. If you miss a dose and it has been less than 4 h since your dose was due, take it as soon as you remember. If it is about time for the next dose, take that dose only. Do not double the dose or take extra.

Pharmacokinetics. *Onset and Duration.* PO onset—1–4 h (average 2h); duration 8–16 h.

Serum Levels. Between 0.5 and 2 mg/L (3–11 μmol/L), although not well correlated with therapeutic or toxic effects.[61]

Fate. Oral bioavailability is 87 ± 13%, and, unlike lidocaine, mexiletine undergoes less than 10% first-pass hepatic elimination.[61,62] Absorption can be incomplete in MI patients receiving narcotic analgesics.[61,62] The drug is 63 ± 3% bound to plasma proteins;[9] V_d is large and has been variably reported as 6.6 ± 0.9 L/kg and 10.8 ± 7.2 L/kg.[61,62] Cl is variable, 0.4–0.6 L/h/kg[26] decreased in CHF and liver disease.[61] Mexiletine is metabolized predominantly in the liver, where it undergoes polymorphic metabolism, primarily by the CYP2D6 isozyme;[48] 10%–20% is excreted unchanged in urine, depending on urinary pH.[61,62]

$t_{1/2}$. α phase 3–12 min. β phase 9.2 ± 2.1 hr[63] and 18.5 h in poor metabolizers,[48] 15.7 ± 4.9 h in severe renal dysfunction,[60] and 15 ± 0.6 h in CHF with or without MI;[64,65] half-life can be prolonged in cirrhosis.

Adverse Reactions. Neurologic toxicities are frequent and include tremor, ataxia, drowsiness, confusion, paresthesias, and occasionally psychosis or seizures. Minor CNS side effects can occur in up to 40% of patients.[66] Nausea, vomiting, and anorexia are frequent. Mexiletine can aggravate underlying ventricular arrhythmias or conduction disturbances. Thrombocytopenia has been reported rarely.[66] Mexiletine is an ether analogue of lidocaine, so cross-sensitivity between mexiletine and tocainide or lidocaine is not expected.[67]

Contraindications. Second- or third-degree AV block without a ventricular pacemaker; cardiogenic shock.

Precautions. Sick sinus syndrome can worsen. Mexiletine can increase pacemaker capture threshold and alter the effectiveness of internal defibrillators.[38]

Drug Interactions. Mexiletine increases theophylline concentrations by about 70% by decreasing theophylline metabolism. Phenytoin and rifampin can increase mexiletine metabolism. Quinidine and theophylline occasionally increase serum mexiletine levels.

Parameters to Monitor. ECG for 3–5 d when therapy is initiated and then every 3–6 months on an ambulatory basis. Obtain periodic serum levels once an individual's effective level is determined. Observe closely for neurologic toxicities when initiating therapy.

Notes. The efficacy of mexiletine for ventricular tachycardia can be increased by adding a type Ia antiarrhythmic such as **quinidine.**[68] Mexiletine has been used to treat neuropathic pain such as diabetic neuropathy and for thalamic pain syndrome.[58,59]

PROCAINAMIDE HYDROCHLORIDE   Pronestyl, Various

Pharmacology. Procainamide is a class Ia antiarrhythmic that alters conduction in normal and ischemic tissues by sodium channel blockade in a fashion similar to that of quinidine. It can decrease systemic blood pressure by causing peripheral ganglionic blockade;[69] it also has weak anticholinergic action and a slight negative inotropic action. The active metabolite N-acetylprocainamide (NAPA) has primarily type III antiarrhythmic activity that predominantly delays repolarization by blocking potassium conductance.

Administration and Adult Dosage. **PO loading dose**—(Cap, Tab) 1 g over 2 h in 2 divided doses. **PO maintenance dosage**—(Cap, Tab) 1–6 g/d in 4–6 divided doses, to a maximum of 9 g/d;[70] (SR Tab) can be given q6–8h (Pronestyl-SR), to a maximum of 50 mg/kg/d. **IV loading dose**—1–1.5 g at 20–50 mg/min[69] or 15–20 mg/kg. **IV maintenance dosage**—1.5–5 mg/min (20–80 µg/kg/min) infusion.[69] **Intermittent IV or IM**—1–6 g/d in 4–6 divided doses, to a maximum of 9 g/d. Initiate procainamide during hospitalization.

Special Populations. *Pediatric Dosage.* Safety and efficacy not established. **PO**—15–50 mg/kg/d in 4–8 divided doses, to a maximum of 4 g/d; **IV loading dose**—2–6 mg/kg over 5 min (up to 100 mg/dose); can repeat q5–10 min, to a maximum of 15 mg/kg. **IV maintenance dosage**—20–80 µg/kg/min infusion, to a maximum of 2 g/d. **IM maintenance dosage**—20–30 mg/kg/d in 4–6 divided doses, to a maximum of 4 g/d.[20]

Geriatric Dosage. Same as adult dosage but adjust for age-related decrease in renal function.

Other Conditions. Reduce maintenance dosage in liver disease. In renal insufficiency, procainamide and its active metabolite accumulate, thereby necessitating a lower maintenance dosage.[22] Recent data imply no need for decreasing loading and maintenance dosages in CHF and MI.[71]

Dosage Forms. **Cap, Tab** 250, 375, 500 mg; **SR Tab** (6-h; Pronestyl-SR, various) 250, 500, 750, 1000 mg; **Inj** 100, 500 mg/mL.

Patient Instructions. Report any symptoms such as nausea, vomiting, fever, sore throat, joint pain, rash, chest or abdominal pain, and shortness of breath. Do not chew, split, or crush SR tablets. A sustained-release tablet shell in the stool does not indicate lack of absorption.

Missed Doses. Take this drug at regular intervals. If you miss a dose, take it as soon as you remember. If it is about time for the next dose, take that dose only. Leave at least 2 h between regular capsule or tablet doses and 4–6 h between sustained-release tablet doses. Do not double the dose or take extra.

Pharmacokinetics. *Onset and Duration.* IV onset is immediate; PO and IM onsets occur within 1 h; SR Tab preparations are somewhat slower. Duration is usually 3–6 h.

Serum Levels. Therapeutic range is 4–10 mg/L (17–43 μmol/L);[23] toxicity is more likely at serum levels above 12 mg/L (51 μmol/L). In some arrhythmias (e.g., recurrent ventricular tachycardia), levels of at least 20 mg/L (85 μmol/L) may be required to prevent arrhythmias, with average effective levels of 13 mg/L.[70] Effective serum levels of NAPA are 15–25 mg/L (53–88 μmol/L), with overlap between the toxic and therapeutic ranges.[72]

Fate. Oral bioavailability is $83 \pm 16\%$;[9] about $16 \pm 5\%$ is bound to plasma proteins; V_d is 1.9 ± 0.3 L/kg.[9] The drug is $67 \pm 8\%$ excreted in the urine as unchanged; the remainder is metabolized, mostly to active NAPA by the liver, with smaller amounts excreted as para-aminobenzoic acid. Cl is highly variable depending on acetylator status and renal function. The total quantity of NAPA produced depends on liver function and acetylator phenotype.[9,73]

$t_{1/2}$. (Procainamide) α phase about 6 min; β phase 3 ± 0.6 h in normal individuals, 5.3–20.7 h in patients with renal dysfunction, and 12.5 ± 1.4 h in anephric patients; (NAPA) 7 ± 1 h, 41.5 ± 7.8 h in renal failure.[10,74,75]

Adverse Reactions. About 50%–80% of patients develop a positive ANA, with 30%–50% developing symptoms of SLE; genetically slow acetylators more rapidly develop positive ANA and SLE symptoms.[76] Common SLE symptoms or signs are rash, arthralgias, fever, pericarditis, and pleuritis. Although drug cessation usually reverses these symptoms in about 2 weeks, some patients have prolonged manifestations; for others, the SLE syndrome initially can be life-threatening.[76] Hypotension frequently can occur after rapid IV administration. Severe bradycardia, AV nodal block, or asystole has been reported. Procainamide can aggravate underlying ventricular arrhythmias and cause torsades de pointes.[77] GI symptoms occur frequently and include nausea and vomiting; drug fever and dermatologic reactions occasionally occur.[77] Agranulocytosis has been reported occasionally and can be fatal. Whether the SR product carries a higher risk of neutropenia than the fast-release preparation is controversial.[78] Hepatitis has been reported rarely.

Contraindications. SLE (including that induced by drugs); second- or third-degree heart block without a ventricular pacemaker; long-QT syndrome; severe sinus node dysfunction or torsades de pointes caused by other type Ia antiarrhythmics.

Precautions. In atrial fibrillation or flutter, procainamide paradoxically can increase ventricular rate; administer digoxin or other drugs that slow AV nodal conduction before procainamide. Procainamide can worsen symptoms of sick sinus syndrome and exacerbate myasthenia gravis.

Drug Interactions. Amiodarone, trimethoprim, cimetidine, and, to a lesser extent, ranitidine can increase procainamide levels; alcohol can decrease levels.

Parameters to Monitor. Monitor serum levels and symptoms or signs of toxicity in patients with suspected altered drug dispositions such as hepatic disease or renal dysfunction. Monitor ECG continuously (with IV) or daily initially (with PO) for QRS, QT, and PR prolongation; monitor oral therapy less frequently once maintenance dosage has been established. Monitor blood pressure frequently when therapy is initiated (especially with IV) and less frequently once a maintenance dosage has been established. Periodically monitor WBC count and signs of infection for development of drug-induced agranulocytosis. Observe closely for symptoms of drug-induced SLE.

PROPAFENONE HYDROCHLORIDE   Rythmol

Pharmacology. Propafenone is a sodium channel blocker that slows predominantly atrial and ventricular conduction velocities without appreciably prolonging repolarization. It is therefore classified as a class Ic antiarrhythmic, similar to flecainide. Propafenone is administered as a racemate; the enantiomers and the 5-hydroxy metabolite are equipotent sodium channel blockers. Propafenone, in particular the (S)-enantiomer, and its active 5-hydroxy metabolite also have variable, nonselective β-blocking actions.

Administration and Adult Dosage. **PO**—150 mg q8h initially, increasing q3–4d to desired effect or toxicity. **PO maintenance**—150–200 mg q8h, to a maximum of 1.2 g/d.[79] Initiate propafenone during hospitalization.

Special Populations. *Pediatric Dosage.* Safety and efficacy not established. **PO**—10–20 mg/kg/d in 2–3 divided doses has been used.[80]

Geriatric Dosage. Same as adult dosage. Lower initial dosages and slower titration have been suggested.[81]

Other Conditions. Bioavailability and half-life are increased in patients with hepatic disease, and a dosage reduction of 50% has been suggested[82] and questioned.[79] Lower initial dosages have been suggested for patients with renal dysfunction.[79]

Dosage Forms. Tab 150, 225, 300 mg.

Patient Instructions. Report any symptoms of dizziness, rapid heartbeat, blurred vision, or shortness of breath.

Missed Doses. Take this drug at regular intervals. If you miss a dose, take it as soon as you remember. If it is about time for the next dose, take that dose only. Leave at least 4 h between doses. Do not double the dose or take extra.

Pharmacokinetics. *Onset and Duration.* Onset 2–4 h; peak 2–6 h; duration 4–22 h.[79,81]

Serum Levels. No established therapeutic range. Levels of parent compound and metabolite are highly variable, depending on genetically determined variations in hepatic metabolisms. Mean minimal effective concentration was 0.2 mg/L (6 μmol/L) in one study.[83] Side effects are more frequent when the trough propafenone level exceeds 0.9 mg/L (26 μmol/L).[84]

Fate. Completely absorbed after oral administration, but large hepatic first-pass metabolism limits bioavailability to $12.1 \pm 11\%$. First-pass elimination appears saturable, so bioavailability is highly variable and increases with larger oral doses and long-term therapy.[79,81,84] About 85%–95% is bound to plasma proteins, primarily α_1-acid glycoprotein.[79] V_d is 3.6 ± 2.6 L/kg.[85] The parent drug undergoes polymorphic hepatic metabolism via CYP2D6. Extensive metabolizers (EMs; about 90% of patients) form clinically important quantities of the active metabolite

5-hydroxypropafenone; poor metabolizers (PMs; about 10% of patients) form little of this compound.[81,84] Another active metabolite, *N*-desethylpropafenone, is not subject to genetic polymorphism.[79,84] Cl is 0.96 ± 1.08 L/h/kg in EMs and 0.23 ± 0.042 L/h/kg in PMs.[86] Cl is also stereospecific.

$t_{1/2}$. α phase 5 min; β phase (EMs) 5.5 ± 2 h; (PMs) 17 ± 8 h.[84]

Adverse Reactions. Frequent noncardiac side effects include metallic or bitter taste in 15%–20% of patients, and nausea and CNS toxicity such as dizziness and headache in 10%–15% of patients.[85] Because of the β-blocking activity of propafenone, worsening of asthma or obstructive lung disease can occur.[85] Propafenone has proarrhythmic actions (sometimes life-threatening) that can result in new or worsened ventricular tachycardia. This can occur in 5%–15% of patients, particularly in those with poor left ventricular function caused by structural heart disease or with underlying ventricular tachycardia. Worsening of existing CHF or underlying conduction disturbances, such as AV block or sick sinus syndrome, can occur. Cholestatic jaundice occurs rarely.[87]

Contraindications. Second- or third-degree AV block or bifascicular block without a ventricular pacemaker; history of type Ic-induced arrhythmia; bronchospastic disorders; uncontrolled CHF; cardiogenic shock; marked hypotension; sick sinus syndrome; bradycardia; electrolyte imbalance.

Precautions. Propafenone can increase pacemaker capture threshold and affect the efficacy of internal defibrillators.[38] Because of the CAST results (although not studied in this trial), propafenone is indicated only for arrhythmias where there is a clear benefit to therapy.

Drug Interactions. Inhibitors of CYP2D6, CYP1A2, and CYP3A4 may increase propafenone concentrations. Orlistat may lower the absorption of propafenone. Propafenone inhibits hepatic enzymes (CYP and P-glycoprotein) and reportedly increases serum concentrations of digoxin, theophylline, warfarin, and β-blockers.[81]

Parameters to Monitor. Daily or continuous (preferred) ECG for 3–4 d initially and then every 3–6 months on an ambulatory basis. Observe closely for CNS symptoms such as dizziness.

Notes. Although not a labeled indication, propafenone can be effective for some supraventricular arrhythmias.

QUINIDINE SULFATE	Various
QUINIDINE GLUCONATE	Duraquin, Quinaglute, Quinora, Various

Pharmacology. Quinidine is a class Ia antiarrhythmic that slows conduction velocity, prolongs effective refractory period, and decreases automaticity of normal and diseased fibers. (*See* Electrophysiologic Actions of Antiarrhythmics Comparison Chart.) The cellular mechanism appears to be a frequency-dependent blockade of the fast sodium channel. Quinidine also blocks potassium conductance, particularly at low concentrations. AV nodal conduction can be increased reflexly through vasodilation, attributed to peripheral α-adrenergic blockade or vagolytic action. Slight negative inotropic action might be clinically important in patients with severe CHF.

Administration and Adult Dosage. **IM and PO loading doses**—not recommended. **PO maintenance dosage**—generally 200–400 mg q6–8h; **SR products**—(gluconate) can be given q12h, (polygalacturonate) can be given q8h. **IV loading dose**—(gluconate) 5–8 mg/kg (3.75–6 mg/kg in CHF) at a rate of 0.3 mg/kg/min. (*See* Notes.) Initiate quinidine during hospitalization.

Special Populations. *Pediatric Dosage.* **PO**—(gluconate salt) 15–60 mg/kg/d in 4 divided doses. **IV and IM**—not recommended.

Geriatric Dosage. (>60 y) use lower initial dosages and adjust maintenance dosage based on side effects, therapeutic response, and serum levels.

Other Conditions. In liver disease, CHF, or renal disease, use lower initial dosages and adjust maintenance dosages based on side effects, therapeutic response, and serum levels.[22,88]

Dosage Forms. **Tab**—(sulfate) 200, 300 mg; (polygalacturonate) 275 mg; **SR Tab**—(gluconate) 324, 330 mg; (sulfate) 300 mg; **Inj**—(gluconate) 80 mg/mL. (*See* Notes.)

Patient Instructions. Report any symptoms such as blurred vision, dizziness, tinnitus, diarrhea, abnormal bleeding or bruising, rash, or fainting episodes. Do not crush or chew sustained-release tablets. A sustained-release tablet shell in the stool does not indicate lack of absorption.

Missed Doses. Take this drug at regular intervals. If you miss a dose and it has been less than 2 h since your dose was due, take it as soon as you remember. If it is about time for the next dose, take that dose only. Do not double the dose or take extra.

Pharmacokinetics. *Onset and Duration.* PO onset of sulfate within 1 h; SR gluconate and polygalacturonate salts 2–4 h. IM onset within 1 h; IV is immediate. Duration—(sulfate) 6–8 h,[89] SR (gluconate) 12 h, (polygalacturonate) 8–12 h.

Serum Levels. Therapeutic range about 2–6 mg/L (6–18 μmol/L), depending on assay. Toxicity is more likely with serum levels above 6 mg/L.[22,23]

Fate. Oral sulfate and gluconate are 80 ± 15% and 71 ± 17% bioavailable, respectively, with some first-pass elimination; bioavailability is increased in the elderly; IM absorption is incomplete.[9,89] The drug is 87 ± 3% bound to plasma proteins.[9] V_d is 2.7 ± 1.2 L/kg and 1.8 ± 0.5 L/kg in patients with CHF; Cl is 0.28 ± 0.11 L/h/kg.[9,90] The elderly and patients with liver disease or CHF are likely to have decreased clearance.[9] Quinidine is metabolized primarily in the liver to two active metabolites—3-hydroxyquinidine and 2′-quinidinone, and 18 ± 5% of a dose is excreted unchanged in urine.

$t_{1/2}$. α phase about 7 min; β phase in normal individuals, 6.2 ± 1.8 h.[9] In CHF, Cl and V_d are decreased, so elimination half-life remains about the same.[90] β Half-life in alcoholic cirrhosis is prolonged to 9 ± 1 h.[91]

Adverse Reactions. Diarrhea occurs in up to 30% of patients receiving quinidine and can be treated with **aluminum hydroxide gel** or lessened by using the polygalacturonate salt. Nausea or vomiting occurs frequently. Cinchonism can occur with high levels of quinidine; symptom complex includes tinnitus, blurred vision, headache, and nausea; in severe cases it can progress to delirium and psychosis. Hypotension can occur, especially after IV administration. Quinidine can aggravate underlying ventricular arrhythmias or CHF. Non–dose-related syncope, attributed to drug-induced torsades de pointes, can occur in 1%–8% of patients, usually during the first week of therapy; it can occur in association with hypokalemia.[92] Asystole or AV nodal block has been reported. Rare or occasional idiosyncratic reactions include hepatitis, drug fever, anaphylactoid reactions, SLE, thrombocytopenia, and hemolytic anemia. IM use can cause pain and muscle damage.[89]

Contraindications. History of immunologic reaction to quinidine or quinine; previous occurrence of quinidine syncope; second- or third-degree heart block without a ventricular pacemaker; severe sinus node dysfunction or long-QT syndrome; digitalis intoxication; myasthenia gravis.

Precautions. In atrial fibrillation or flutter, administer digoxin or other drugs that decrease AV nodal conduction before administering quinidine. Chronic quinidine use in patients with atrial fibrillation is associated with increased mortality, which can be caused by torsades de pointes that occurs late in therapy.[92]

Drug Interactions. Quinidine inhibits CYP2D6 and can alter the disposition of many drugs that undergo genetically determined polymorphic metabolism through this pathway. Use care with concurrent digoxin and quinidine therapy because quinidine increases digoxin serum levels approximately two-fold by inhibiting P-glycoprotein.[93] Urinary alkalinization (e.g., with acetazolamide or antacids) can decrease quinidine clearance. Phenytoin can increase quinidine metabolism. Amiodarone and cimetidine can reduce quinidine clearance. Quinidine is a CYP3A4 substrate. Quinidine occasionally increases warfarin response and serum levels of tricyclic antidepressant.

Parameters to Monitor. Monitor serum levels and signs or symptoms of toxicity in patients with altered drug dispositions such as CHF or liver disease. With ECG, monitor daily for QT, QRS, or PR prolongation for the first 2–4 days of therapy and then every 3–6 months on an ambulatory basis. Frequently monitor blood pressure (especially with IV) when therapy is initiated. Monitoring can decrease after a maintenance dosage has been determined. Monitor liver enzymes during the first 4–8 weeks of therapy. Monitor other parameters such as platelet count and hematocrit only if idiosyncratic reactions are suspected.

Notes. Adjust dosage when switching from one salt form to another; sulfate salt contains 83% quinidine, 62% gluconate, and 60% polygalacturonate. The gluconate and polygalacturonate forms are slowly dissociating salts of quinidine.

SOTALOL HYDROCHLORIDE   Betapace, Betapace AF, Various

Pharmacology. Sotalol is a type III antiarrhythmic that is commercially available as a racemate: the L-isomer has nonselective β-blocking actions, and the D- and L-isomers delay repolarization by blockade of potassium channels. (*See* Electrophysiologic Actions of Antiarrhythmics Comparison Chart.) Sotalol is effective for ventricular and (unlabeled) supraventricular arrhythmias.

Administration and Adult Dosage. **PO for ventricular arrhythmias**—(Betapace) 80 mg bid initially, increasing at 2- to 3-d intervals, to a maximum of 640 mg/d in 2 or 3 divided doses. Reserve high dosages (480–640 mg/d) for drug-refractory ventricular arrhythmias. **PO for atrial fibrillation or flutter**—(Betapace AF) 80 mg bid initially, increasing at 3-d intervals, to a maximum of 160 mg bid. Initiate sotalol during hospitalization.

Special Populations. *Pediatric Dosage.* **PO**—Because equal plasma concentrations will have similar potency in pediatrics, the manufacture suggests initiating treatment with 30 mg/m² tid (equivalent to 160 mg daily dose in adults) then slowly titrating to a max of 60 mg/m² (equivalent to 320 mg daily dose in adults). For children younger than 2 years old, this calculated dose should be multiplied by an age factor found in the product labeling for a reduced dosage.

Geriatric Dosage. Same as adult dosage.

Other Conditions. Reduce frequency of administration in patients with renal insufficiency as follows. **Ventricular arrhythmias**—(Betapace) Cl_{Cr} 30–60 mL/min, q24h; Cl_{Cr} 10–29 mL/min, q36–48h. Use with caution, if at all, in patients with Cl_{Cr} <10 mL/min. **Atrial arrhythmias**—(Betapace AF) Cl_{Cr} 40–60 mL/min, q24h; Cl_{Cr} <40 mL/min, contraindicated.

Dosage Forms. **Tab** (Betapace) 80, 120, 160, 240 mg; (Betapace AF) 80, 120, 160 mg.

Patient Instructions. Report any symptoms of fainting, dizziness, shortness of breath, or fatigue.

Missed Doses. Take this drug at regular intervals. If you miss a dose and your next dose is more than 8 h away, take it as soon as you remember. If it is about time for the next dose, take that dose only. Do not double the dose or take extra.

Pharmacokinetics. *Onset and Duration.* PO onset 1–3 h; duration 12–18 h.

Serum Levels. 1–3 mg/L (3.7–11 μmol/L), although not well correlated with therapeutic effect. Concentrations required to achieve delay in repolarization might be greater than those for β-blockade.[94]

Fate. Bioavailability is 90%–100% with negligible first-pass metabolism. AUC is decreased 20% by food. The drug is not bound to plasma proteins. V_d is 1.2–2.4 L/kg; Cl is 0.13 ± 0.04 L/h/kg;[95-97] 80%–90% is excreted unchanged in urine. The disposition of the D-isomer is similar to that of the racemate.[96,97]

$t_{1/2}.$ α phase 3–5 min; β phase variously reported as 7.5 ± 0.8 to 17.5 ± 9.7 h.[97,98] Half-life is highly dependent on renal function: 22.7 ± 6.4 h for Cl_{Cr} 30–80 mL/h; 64 ± 27 h for Cl_{Cr} 10–30 mL/h; and 98 ± 57 h for Cl_{Cr} <10 mL/min.[98]

Adverse Reactions. Fatigue, dyspnea, and bradycardia occur frequently, probably caused by the β-blocking actions of sotalol. Exacerbation of CHF (1.7%) and asthma also can occur. (*See* Propranolol.) Sotalol induces arrhythmias, usually torsades de pointes, in a dose-related fashion. Risk factors for torsades de pointes are the female gender, excessive QT prolongation, CHF, hypokalemia, hypomagnesemia, concurrent diuretic usage, and high sotalol dosages.[99]

Contraindications. (Betapace and Betapace AF) Asthma; second- and third-degree AV blocks without a ventricular pacemaker; sinus bradycardia; cardiogenic shock; long QT-syndrome; uncontrolled CHF. (Betapace AF, additional) sick sinus syndrome; baseline QT interval >450 ms; hypokalemia (<4 mEq/L); Cl_{Cr} <40 mL/min.

Precautions. Use with caution in sinus node dysfunction. Because of its β-blocking actions, use sotalol with caution in patients with diabetes, depressed left ventricular function, obstructive pulmonary disease, or peripheral vascular disease. Do not abruptly discontinue the drug in patients with coronary artery disease. Use with caution with electrolyte disorders, other drugs that prolong QT interval or preexisting QT prolongation. Escalate dosage only after achieving steady state (3 d).

Drug Interactions. Because of its β-blocking actions, observe β-blocker interaction precautions. (*See* Propranolol.)

Parameters to Monitor. Baseline and daily ECG for the first 2–5 d, when therapy is initiated or dosage is adjusted, and then every 3–6 months on an ambulatory basis. QT prolongation to over 550 ms is an indication to discontinue sotalol because of the risk of torsades de pointes.

Notes. Based on the CAST results,[17] many clinicians use type III antiarrhythmics (e.g., amiodarone, sotalol) as first-line therapy in supraventricular and ventricular arrhythmias.

TOCAINIDE Tonocard

Pharmacology. Tocainide has electrophysiologic actions similar to those of lidocaine and mexiletine. Depression of conduction is accentuated in ischemic/hypoxic tissue. Antiarrhythmic actions are somewhat stereospecific. It also has a slight negative inotropic action. It is used in the treatment of ventricular arrhythmias, but it has limited effectiveness in supraventricular tachycardias. There appears to be a concordance of response (and nonresponse) between tocainide and lidocaine.[100]

Administration and Adult Dosage. PO—400 mg q8h initially; **usual maintenance dosage**—1.2–1.8 g/d, to a maximum of 2.4 g/d in 2–3 divided doses. **PO during lidocaine to tocainide conversion**—600 mg q6h for 3 doses, then 600 mg q12h; discontinue lidocaine infusion at the time of the second oral dose of tocainide.[101] Initiate tocainide during hospitalization.

Special Populations. *Pediatric Dosage.* Safety and efficacy not established.

Geriatric Dosage. Same as adult dosage.

Other Conditions. Reduce initial maintenance dosage by 50% in severe liver disease, by 25% in patients with Cl_{Cr} 10–30 mL/min, and by 30% in patients with Cl_{Cr} <10 mL/min.[74] Dosages might have to be reduced slightly in CHF, but more data are needed.[75]

Dosage Forms. Tab 400, 600 mg.

Patient Instructions. Report any symptoms of numbness, drowsiness, dizziness, or tingling. Nausea or loss of appetite can occur and may be reduced by taking the drug with food. Report sore throat, mouth sores, fever, or abnormal bruising.

Missed Doses. Take this drug at regular intervals. If you miss a dose, take it as soon as you remember. If it is about time for the next dose, take that dose only. Leave at least 4–6 h between doses. Do not double the dose or take extra.

Pharmacokinetics. *Onset and Duration.* PO onset 1–2 h (delayed by food); duration 12–24 h.

Serum Levels. 3–10 mg/L (16–52 μmol/L), although not well correlated with therapeutic or toxic effects.[23,102]

Fate. Oral bioavailability is 89 ± 5% with negligible first-pass metabolism.[74,75,102] The drug is 10 ± 15% bound to plasma proteins.[9,103] V_d is 3 ± 0.2 L/kg but slightly lower in CHF;[74,75] Cl is 0.16 ± 0.03 L/h/kg;[9] 38 ± 7% of the drug is excreted unchanged in urine, and 50%–60% is hepatically eliminated.[74,102] Renal clearance depends on urine pH; hepatic metabolism is stereospecific, with the (*S*)-enantiomer eliminated more quickly.[104]

$t_{1/2}$. α phase 5–10 min;[103] β phase 13.5 ± 2.3 h, 14–19 h with ventricular arrhythmia or CHF,[102] and 22 ± 3.1 h in severe renal insufficiency.[105]

Adverse Reactions. Neurologic toxicities, which include dizziness, tremor, ataxia, drowsiness, confusion, and paresthesias, are frequent (30%–50%); psychosis and seizures occur occasionally. The neurologic toxicities of lidocaine and tocainide can be additive. Nausea, vomiting, and anorexia occur frequently. Tocainide can exacerbate underlying ventricular arrhythmias or conduction disturbances. Agranulocytosis and other forms of bone marrow depression have been reported in up to 0.18% of patients.[102] Pulmonary fibrosis or interstitial pneumonitis occurs in 0.03%–0.11% of patients.[101] Rash and fever occur occasionally, and cross-sensitivity between lidocaine and tocainide is possible.[67]

Contraindications. Second- or third-degree AV block without a ventricular pacemaker.

Precautions. Sick sinus syndrome and CHF can worsen.

Drug Interactions. Cimetidine can decrease tocainide serum levels; rifampin can decrease levels.

Parameters to Monitor. Monitor ECG daily for 2–4 d when therapy is initiated and then every 3–6 months on an ambulatory basis. Obtain periodic serum levels once an individual's effective level is determined. Monitor closely for neurologic toxicities when initiating therapy. Monitor WBC counts frequently, particularly during the first 3 months of therapy.[102] Obtain baseline chest x-ray; repeat if pulmonary symptoms arise.

Notes. Because of reports of bone marrow toxicity, pulmonary fibrosis, and hypersensitivity reactions, the indications for tocainide are restricted to patients with life-threatening ventricular arrhythmias.

VERNAKALANT HYDROCHLORIDE
(Investigational, Cardiome, Astellas)

Kynapid

Pharmacology. Vernakalant is a potassium channel blocker, selective for atrial ultrarapid delayed rectifier potassium current (IKur) which prolongs the atrial refractory period with minimal effect of ventricular conduction.[106,107] Vernakalant also blocks sodium channels, slowing conduction in a rate-dependent manner.

Adult Dosage. IV 3 mg/kg over 10 min. Repeat with 2 mg/kg after 15 min if atrial fibrillation persists.[106]

Pediatric Dosage. Not studied.

Pharmacokinetics. IV half life is 2.9–3.3 h; PO sustained-release formulation under development.[106]

Adverse Reactions. Dysgeusia, sneezing, paresthesias occur commonly. Both QT prolongation and torsades de pointes appear uncommon based on two phase II studies of IV vernakalant.[108]

ELECTROPHYSIOLOGIC ACTIONS OF ANTIARRHYTHMICS COMPARISON CHART

CLASS AND DRUG[a,b]	CONDUCTION VELOCITY	REFRACTORY PERIOD	AUTOMATICITY	AV NODAL CONDUCTION
IA (INTERMEDIATE SODIUM CHANNEL BLOCKERS)				
Disopyramide	↓↓	↑↑	↓↓	↑
Procainamide	↓↓	↑↑	↓↓	↑/↓
Quinidine	↓↓	↑↑	↓↓	↑/↓
IB (FAST ON–OFF SODIUM CHANNEL BLOCKERS)				
Lidocaine				
Normal Tissue	0	→	→	0
Ischemic Tissue	↓↓	←	↓↓	0
Mexiletine	0	→	→	0
Phenytoin				
Normal Tissue	0	→	→	←
Ischemic Tissue	↓↓	←	↓↓	←
Tocainide	0	→	→	0
IC (SLOW ON–OFF SODIUM CHANNEL BLOCKERS)				
Flecainide	↓↓↓	0	→	0
Propafenone[c]	↓↓↓	0	→	0
II (β-BLOCKERS)				
Propranolol[d]	→	↓ (acute) ↑ (chronic)	→	↓↓

(continued)

ELECTROPHYSIOLOGIC ACTIONS OF ANTIARRHYTHMICS COMPARISON CHART (*continued*)

CLASS AND DRUG[a,b]	CONDUCTION VELOCITY	REFRACTORY PERIOD	AUTOMATICITY	AV NODAL CONDUCTION
III (POTASSIUM CHANNEL BLOCKERS)				
Amiodarone[c,e]	0/↓	↑↑	0	↓
Dofetilide	0	↑↑	0	0
Ibutilide	0	↑↑	0	0
Sotalol[c,f]	0	↑↑	0	↓
IV (CALCIUM CHANNEL BLOCKERS)				
Diltiazem	0	0	0	↓
Verapamil	0	0	0	↓↓

↑ = increase, ↓ = decrease, 0 = minimal or no effect, ↑/↓ = variable.

[a]Classification system from references 82 and 83.

[b]Type I antiarrhythmics are subdivided into Ia, Ib, and Ic based on their actions on repolarization in normal ventricular tissue and their binding characteristics to the sodium channel: type Ia prolongs repolarization; type Ib shortens repolarization; type Ic causes no change in repolarization.

[c]Amiodarone, propafenone, and sotalol also have type II or β-adrenergic blocking activity.

[d]When caused by sympathetic stimulation.

[e]Amiodarone also has type Ib sodium channel blocking activity.

[f]Most investigational antiarrhythmics are potassium channel blockers, many of which are analogues of sotalol.

■ REFERENCES

1. Parker RB, McCollam PL. Adenosine in the episodic treatment of paroxysmal supraventricular tachycardia. *Clin Pharm.* 1990;9:261-271.

2. DiMarco JP et al. Adenosine for paroxysmal supraventricular tachycardia: dose ranging and comparison with verapamil. *Ann Intern Med.* 1990;113:104-110.

3. McIntosh-Vellin NL et al. Safety and efficacy of central intravenous bolus administration of adenosine for termination of supraventricular tachycardia. *J Am Coll Cardiol.* 1993;22:741-745.

4. Watt AH et al. Intravenous adenosine in the treatment of supraventricular tachycardia: a dose ranging study and interaction with dipyridamole. *Br J Clin Pharmacol.* 1986;21:227-230.

5. 2005 American Heart Association Guidelines for Cardiopulmonary Resuscitations and Emergency Cardiovascular Care. *Circulation.* 2005;112 (suppl 24): IV 1-203. http://circ.ahajournals.org/cgi/content/full/112/24_suppl/IV-58. Accessed October 14, 2008.

6. Gilette PC et al. Amiodarone for children. *Clin Prog Electrophysiol Pacing.* 1986;4:328-330.

7. Roden DM. Pharmacokinetics of amiodarone: implications for drug therapy. *Am J Cardiol.* 1993;72:45F-50F.

8. Rotmensch HH et al. Steady-mate serum amiodarone concentrations: relationship with antiarrhythmic efficacy and toxicity. *Ann Intern Med.* 1984;101:462-469.

9. Benet LZ et al. Design and optimization of dosage regimens; pharmacokinetic data. In: Hardman JG et al., eds. *Goodman and Gilman's The Pharmacological Basis of Therapeutics.* 9th ed. New York: McGraw-Hill; 1996: 1707-1792.

10. Gill J et al. Amiodarone. An overview of its pharmacologic properties, and review of its therapeutic use in cardiac arrhythmias. *Drugs.* 1992;43:69-110.

11. Rigas B et al. Amiodarone hepatotoxicity. A clinicopathologic study of five patients. *Ann Intern Med.* 1986; 104:348-351.

12. Figge HL, Figge J. The effects of amiodarone on thyroid hormone function: a review of the physiology and clinical manifestations. *J Clin Pharmacol.* 1990;30:588-595.

13. Dusman RE et al. Clinical features of amiodarone-induced pulmonary toxicity. *Circulation.* 1990;82:51-59.

14. Hohnloser SH et al. Amiodarone-associated proarrhythmic effects. A review with special reference to torsade de pointes tachycardia. *Ann Intern Med.* 1994;121:529-535.

15. Roberts SA et al. Invasive and noninvasive methods to predict the long-term efficacy of amiodarone: a compilation of clinical observations using meta-analysis. *Pacing Clin Electrophysiol.* 1994;17:1590-1602.

16. Bauman JL et al. Pharmacokinetic and pharmacodynamic drug interactions with antiarrhythmic agents. *Cardiol Rev.* 1997;5:292-304.

17. Echt DS et al. Mortality and morbidity in patients receiving encainide, flecainide, or placebo. The Cardiac Arrhythmia Suppression Trial. *N Engl J Med.* 1991;324:781-788.

18. Podrid PJ et al. Congestive heart failure caused by oral disopyramide. *N Engl J Med.* 1980;302:614-617.

19. Lima JJ et al. Antiarrhythmic activity and unbound concentrations of disopyramide enantiomers in patients. *Ther Drug Monit.* 1990;12:23-28.

20. Siberry GK, Iannone R, eds. *The Harriet Lane Handbook.* 15th ed. St. Louis, MO: Mosby; 2000.

21. Lima JJ. Disopyramide. In: Taylor WJ, Caviness MHD, eds. *A textbook for the clinical application of therapeutic drug monitoring.* Irving, TX: Abbott Diagnostics; 1986:97-108.

22. Bauman JL et al. Practical optimisation of antiarrhythmic drug therapy using pharmacokinetic principles. *Clin Pharmacokinet.* 1991;20:151-166.

23. Latini R et al. Therapeutic drug monitoring of antiarrhythmic drugs: rationale and current status. *Clin Pharmacokinet.* 1990;18:91-103.

24. Piscitelli DA et al. Bioavailability of total and unbound disopyramide: implications for clinical use of the immediate and controlled-release forms. *J Clin Pharmacol.* 1994;34:823-828.

25. Siddoway LA, Woosley RL. Clinical pharmacokinetics of disopyramide. *Clin Pharmacokinet.* 1986;11:214-222.

26. Hasselstrom J et al. Enantioselective steady-state kinetics of unbound disopyramide and its dealkylated metabolite in man. *Eur J Clin Pharmacol.* 1991;41:481-484.

27. Bauman JL et al. Long-term therapy with disopyramide phosphate: side effects and effectiveness. *Am Heart J.* 1986;111:654-660.

28. Lenz TL, Hilleman DE. Dofetilide: a new class III antiarrhythmic agent. *Pharmacotherapy.* 2000;20: 776-786.

29. Kalus JS, Mauro VF. Dofetilide: a class III–specific antiarrhythmic agent. *Ann Pharmacother.* 2000;34:44-56.

30. Torp-Pedersen C et al. Dofetilide in patients with congestive heart failure and left ventricular dysfunction. *N Engl J Med.* 1999;341:857-865.

31. Dale KM, White CM. Dronedarone: an amiodarone analog for the treatment of atrial fibrillation and atrial flutter. *Ann Pharmacother.* 2007;41:599-605.

32. Køber L et al. Increased mortality after dronedarone therapy for severe heart failure. *N Engl J Med.* 2008;358: 2678-2687.

33. Perry JC, Garson A. Flecainide acetate for treatment of tachyarrhythmias in children: review of world literature on efficacy, safety and dosing. *Am Heart J.* 1992;124:1614-1621.

34. Holmes B, Heel RC. Flecainide. A preliminary review of its pharmacodynamic properties and therapeutic efficacy. *Drugs.* 1985;29:1-33.

35. Conrad GJ, Ober RE. Metabolism of flecainide. *Am J Cardiol.* 1984;53:41B-51B.

36. Gross AS et al. Polymorphic flecainide disposition under conditions of uncontrolled urine flow and pH. *Eur J Clin Pharmacol.* 1991;40:155-162.

37. Forland SC et al. Flecainide pharmacokinetics after multiple dosing in patients with impaired renal function. *J Clin Pharmacol.* 1988;28:727-735.

38. McCollam P et al. Proarrhythmia: a paradoxical response to antiarrhythmic drugs. *Pharmacotherapy.* 1989;9:144-153.

39. Tworek DA et al. Interference by antiarrhythmic agents with function of electrical cardiac devices. *Clin Pharm.* 1992;11:48-56.

40. Anonymous. Ibutilide. *Med Lett Drugs Ther.* 1996;38:38.

41. Howard PA. Ibutilide: an antiarrhythmic agent for the treatment of atrial fibrillation or flutter. *Ann Pharmacother.* 1999;33:38-47.

42. Kowey PR et al. Safety and risk/benefit analysis of ibutilide for acute conversion of atrial fibrillation/flutter. *Am J Cardiol.* 1996;78(suppl 8A):46-52.

43. Benowitz NL, Meister W. Clinical pharmacokinetics of lignocaine. *Clin Pharmacokinet.* 1978;3:177-201.

44. Galer BS et al. Response to intravenous lidocaine infusion differs based on clinical diagnosis and site of nervous system injury. *Neurology.* 1993;43:1233-1235.

45. Routledge PA et al. Control of lidocaine therapy: new perspectives. *Ther Drug Monit.* 1982;4:265-270.

46. Rowland M et al. Disposition kinetics of lidocaine in normal subjects. *Ann N Y Acad Sci.* 1971;179:383-398.

47. Boyes RN et al. Pharmacokinetics of lidocaine in man. *Clin Pharmacol Ther.* 1971;12:105-116.

48. Lledo P et al. Influence of debrisoquine hydroxylation phenotype on the pharmacokinetics of mexiletine. *Eur J Clin Pharmacol.* 1993;44:63-67.

49. Thomson PD et al. Lidocaine pharmacokinetics in advanced heart failure, liver disease, and renal failure in humans. *Ann Intern Med.* 1973;78:499-508.

50. Bauer LA et al. Influence of long-term infusions on lidocaine kinetics. *Clin Pharmacol Ther.* 1982;31:433-437.

51. Blumer J et al. The convulsant potency of lidocaine and its N-dealkylated metabolites. *J Pharmacol Exp Ther.* 1973;186:31-36.

52. Burney RG et al. Anti-arrhythmic effects of lidocaine metabolites. *Am Heart J.* 1974;88:765-769.

53. LeLorier J et al. Pharmacokinetics of lidocaine after prolonged intravenous infusions in uncomplicated myocardial infarction. *Ann Intern Med.* 1977;87:700-702.

54. Routledge PA et al. Increased alpha-l-acid glycoprotein and lidocaine disposition in myocardial infarction. *Ann Intern Med.* 1980;93:701-704.

55. Gupta PK et al. Lidocaine-induced heart block in patients with bundle branch block. *Am J Cardiol.* 1974;33:187-192.

56. Singh BN. Routine prophylactic lidocaine administration in acute myocardial infarction, an idea whose time is all but gone? *Circulation.* 1992;86:1033-1035. Editorial.

57. Berk SI et al. The effect of oral cimetidine on total and unbound serum lidocaine concentrations in patients with suspected myocardial infarction. *Int J Cardiol.* 1987;14:91-94.

58. Stracke H et al. Mexiletine in the treatment of diabetic neuropathy. *Diabetes Care.* 1992;15:1550-1555.

59. Awerbuch GI, Sandyk R. Mexiletine for thalamic pain syndrome. *Int J Neurosci.* 1990;55:129-133.

60. Allaf et al. Pharmacokinetics of mexiletine in renal insufficiency. *Br J Clin Pharmacol.* 1982;14:431-435.

61. Schrader BJ, Bauman IL. Mexiletine: a new type I antiarrhythmic agent. *Drug Intell Clin Pharm.* 1986;20:255-260.

62. Woosley RL et al. Pharmacology, electrophysiology, and pharmacokinetics of mexiletine. *Am Heart J.* 1984;107:1058-1065.

63. Campbell NPS et al. The clinical pharmacology of mexiletine. *Br J Clin Pharmacol.* 1978;6:103-108.

64. Leahey EB et al. Effect of ventricular failure on steady state kinetics of mexiletine. *Clin Res.* 1982;31:239A. Abstract.

65. Pentikainen PJ et al. Pharmacokinetics of oral mexiletine in patients with acute myocardial infarction. *Eur J Clin Pharmacol.* 1983;25:773-777.

66. Campbell NPS et al. Long-term oral antiarrhythmic therapy with mexiletine. *Br Heart J.* 1978;40:796-801.

67. Duff HJ et al. Molecular basis for the antigenicity of lidocaine analogs: tocainide and mexiletine. *Am Heart J.* 1984;107:585-589.

68. Duff HJ et al. Mexiletine in the treatment of resistant ventricular arrhythmias: enhancement of efficacy and reduction of dose-related side effects by combination with quinidine. *Circulation.* 1983;67:1124-1128.

69. Hoffman BF et al. Electrophysiology and pharmacology of cardiac arrhythmias. VII. Cardiac effects of quinidine and procainamide. *Am Heart J.* 1975;89:804-808.

70. Greenspan AM et al. Large dose procainamide therapy for ventricular tachyarrhythmia. *Am J Cardiol.* 1980;46:453-462.

71. Kessler KM et al. Procainamide pharmacokinetics in patients with acute myocardial infarction or congestive heart failure. *J Am Coll Cardiol.* 1986;7:1131-1139.

72. Connolly SJ, Kates RE. Clinical pharmacokinetics of *N*-acetylprocainamide. *Clin Pharmacokinet.* 1982;7:206-220.

73. Karlsson E. Clinical pharmacokinetics of procainamide. *Clin Pharmacokinet.* 1978;3:97-107.

74. Routledge PA. Tocainide. In: Taylor WJ, Caviness MHD, eds. *A textbook for the clinical application of therapeutic drug monitoring.* Irving, TX: Abbott Diagnostics; 1986:175-180.

75. Mohiuddin SM et al. Tocainide kinetics in congestive heart failure. *Clin Pharmacol Ther.* 1983;34:596-603.

76. Henningsen NC et al. Effects of long-term treatment with procainamide. A prospective study with special regard to ANF and SLE in fast and slow acetylators. *Acta Med Scand.* 1975;198:475-482.

77. Strasberg B et al. Procainamide-induced polymorphous ventricular tachycardia. *Am J Cardiol.* 1981;47:1309-1314.

78. Meyers DG et al. Severe neutropenia associated with procainamide: comparison of sustained release and conventional preparations. *Am Heart J.* 1985;109:1393-1395.

79. Funck-Brentano C et al. Propafenone. *N Engl J Med.* 1990;322:518-525.

80. Musto et al. Electrophysiological effects and clinical efficacy of propafenone in children with recurrent paroxysmal supraventricular tachycardia. *Circulation.* 1988;78:863-869.

81. Hii JTY et al. Clinical pharmacokinetics of propafenone. *Clin Pharmacokinet.* 1991;21:1-10.

82. Lee JT et al. Influence of hepatic dysfunction on the pharmacokinetics of propafenone. *J Clin Pharmacol.* 1987;27:384-389.

83. Capucci A et al. Minimal effective concentration values of propafenone and 5-hydroxy-propafenone in acute and chronic therapy. *Cardiovasc Drugs Ther.* 1990;4:281-287.

84. Siddoway LA et al. Polymorphism of propafenone metabolism and disposition in man: clinical and pharmacokinetic consequences. *Circulation.* 1987;75:785-791.

85. Parker RB et al. Propafenone: a novel type Ic antiarrhythmic agent. *DICP.* 1989;23:196-202.

86. Bryson HM et al. Propafenone. A reappraisal of its pharmacology, pharmacokinetics and therapeutic use in cardiac arrhythmias. *Drugs.* 1993;45:85-130.

87. Mondardini A et al. Propafenone-induced liver injury: report of a case and review of the literature. *Gastroenterology.* 1993;104:1524-1526.

88. Verme CN et al. Pharmacokinetics of quinidine in male patients. A population analysis. *Clin Pharmacokinet.* 1992;22:468-480.

89. Greenblatt DJ et al. Pharmacokinetics of quinidine in humans after intravenous, intramuscular and oral administration. *J Pharmacol Exp Ther.* 1977;202:365-378.

90. Ueda CT, Dzindzio BS. Quinidine kinetics in congestive heart failure. *Clin Pharmacol Ther.* 1978;23:158-164.

91. Kessler KM et al. Quinidine pharmacokinetics in patients with cirrhosis or receiving propranolol. *Am Heart J.* 1978;96:627-635.

92. Grace AA, Camm AJ. Quinidine. *N Engl J Med.* 1998;338:35-45.

93. Fromm MF et al. Inhibition of P-glycoprotein–mediated drug transport. A unifying mechanism to explain the interaction between digoxin and quinidine. *Circulation.* 1999;99:552-557.

94. Nappi JM, McCollam PL. Sotalol: a breakthrough antiarrhythmic? *Ann Pharmacother.* 1993;27:1359-1368.

95. Hanyok JJ. Clinical pharmacokinetics of sotalol. *Am J Cardiol.* 1993;72:19A-26A.

96. Fiset C et al. Stereoselective disposition of (±)-sotalol at steady-state conditions. *Br J Clin Pharmacol.* 1993;36:75-77.

97. Poirer M et al. The pharmacokinetics of d-sotalol and d,1-sotalol in healthy volunteers. *Br J Clin Pharmacol.* 1990;38:579-582.

98. Dumas M et al. Variations of sotalol kinetics in renal insufficiency. *Int J Clin Pharmacol Ther Toxicol.* 1989;27:486-489.

99. Campbell RW, Furniss SS. Practical considerations in the use of sotalol for ventricular tachycardia and ventricular fibrillation. *Am J Cardiol.* 1993;72:80A-85A.

100. Winkle RA et al. Tocainide for drug-resistant ventricular arrhythmias: efficacy, side effects, and lidocaine responsiveness for predicting tocainide success. *Am Heart J.* 1980;100:1031-1036.

101. Kutalek SP et al. Tocainide: a new oral antiarrhythmic agent. *Ann Intern Med.* 1985;103:387-391.

102. Roden DM, Woosley RL. Tocainide. *N Engl J Med.* 1986;315:41-45.

103. Holmes B et al. Tocainide. A review of its pharmacological properties and therapeutic efficacy. *Drugs.* 1983;26:93-123.

104. Hoffmann K-J et al. Analysis and stereoselective metabolism after separate oral doses of tocainide enantiomers to healthy volunteers. *Biopharm Drug Dispos.* 1990;11:351-363.

105. Braun J et al. Pharmacokinetics of tocainide in patients with severe renal failure. *Eur J Clin Pharmacol.* 1985;28:665-670.

106. Naccarelli GV et al. Vernakalant: pharmacology, electrophysiology, safety and efficacy. *Drugs Today.* 2008;44:325-329.

107. Camm AJ, Savelieva I. New antiarrhythmic drugs for atrial fibrillation: focus on dronedarone and vernakalant. *J Interv Card Electrophysiol.* 2008;23:7-14.

108. Naccarelli GV et al. Vernakalant – a promising therapy for conversion of recent-onset atrial fibrillation. *Expert Opin Investig Drugs.* 2008;17:805-810.

Chapter 31

Antihypertensive Drugs

James J. Nawarskas

Class Instructions. Antihypertensives. This medication can control but not cure hypertension. Long-term treatment is necessary to control hypertension and prevent damage to several body systems. Do not start or stop taking medications or change the dosage without medical supervision, and avoid running out of medications. Some prescription and nonprescription medications can interact with medications for hypertension; make sure that your physician and pharmacist know the names of any other medications that you are taking.

Missed Doses. Take this drug at regular intervals. If you miss a dose, take it as soon as you remember. If it is about time for the next dose, take that dose only. Do not double the dose or take extra.

ALISKIREN	Tekturna

Pharmacology. Aliskiren is a direct renin inhibitor that was approved for use in the United States in March 2007. It decreases plasma renin activity, thereby inhibiting the conversion of angiotensinogen to angiotensin I. This effectively prohibits angiotensin I from being converted to angiotensin II, a substance which increases blood pressure by a variety of mechanisms. Aliskiren therefore reduces blood pressure by ultimately preventing the formation of angiotensin II. In addition, unlike angiotensin-converting enzyme inhibitors and angiotensin II receptor antagonists, which increase plasma renin concentrations via a compensatory feedback loop, aliskiren reduces plasma renin concentrations by about 50%–80%. While in theory this would translate to more effective inhibition of the renin–angiotensin–aldosterone system, the effect of this reduction as it relates to antihypertensive efficacy is currently unknown.

Administration and Adult Dosage. PO for hypertension—150 mg once daily initially, increasing to 300 mg once daily if necessary for additional blood pressure reduction. **Usual maintenance dosage** is 150–300 mg once daily. The majority (85%–90%) of the antihypertensive effect is achieved by 2 weeks after initiation or uptitration of therapy. Additive effects on blood pressure reduction have been seen when either a diuretic or valsartan is added to aliskiren; other combination therapies have not been adequately studied. While aliskiren can be taken with or without food, it is advisable to avoid taking it with high-fat meals as this substantially decreases drug absorption.

Special Populations. *Pediatric Dosage.* Safety and efficacy not established.

Geriatric Dosage. No dosage adjustment necessary.

Other Conditions. No dosage adjustment is necessary for patients with mild-to-severe renal or hepatic insufficiency, although caution should be exercised in these patients because of limited clinical experience.

Dosage Forms. **Tab** (unscored) 150, 300 mg (Tekturna); **Tab** (unscored) 150 or 300 mg with hydrochlorothiazide 12.5 or 25 mg (Tekturna HCT).

Patient Instructions. (*See* Antihypertensives Class Instructions.) As with any medication that lowers blood pressure, dizziness or lightheadedness may occur, which tends to be more noticeable during the first few days of therapy or after a dosage increase. Dehydration may exacerbate these symptoms. Report any loss of consciousness (syncope) to your health care provider. Use potassium supplements or salt substitutes only under medical supervision. Report any of the following to your health care provider, should they occur: angioedema (e.g., swelling of face, eyes, lips, tongue, larynx, extremities, or hoarseness or difficulty in swallowing), skin rash, or persistent, dry cough. If you become pregnant while taking this drug, contact your prescriber immediately. Establish a routing pattern for taking this medication with regards to meals.

Pharmacokinetics. *Onset and Duration.* Significant inhibition of plasma renin activity is seen within 1 h of oral dosing and is sustained beyond 24 h with repeat administration. Sequestration of the drug in the kidneys leads to measurable plasma aliskiren concentrations for 3 weeks after discontinuation of therapy, with inhibition of plasma renin activity and blood pressure reduction being seen for 2–4 weeks after cessation of therapy.[1] The antihypertensive effect of aliskiren extends beyond the 24-h dosing interval, with documented peak-to-trough ratios of up to 0.98 with the 300-mg dose.[1]

Serum Levels. Following a single 300-mg dose of aliskiren, steady-state C_{max} values ranged from 200 to 400 ng/mL (330–660 nmol/L), with trough plasma concentrations of 15–30 ng/mL (25–50 nmol/L). Inhibition of renin by 50% is seen with plasma aliskiren concentrations of 0.6 nmol/L.

Fate. Oral bioavailability is about 2.5%. Peak plasma concentrations are reached within 1–3 h after oral administration. There is much interindividual variability in the pharmacokinetics of aliskiren, with AUC ranging from 40% to 70% and C_{max} ranging from 30% to 50%. This variability is thought to be due to interindividual differences in absorption and hepatobiliary elimination. A high-fat meal has been shown to decrease mean AUC and C_{max} by 71% and 85%, respectively, although this is not believed to have much effect on the inhibition of renin activity. Plasma protein binding is 47%–51%; V_d <2 L/kg; water solubility is modest. CYP3A4 appears to be the major enzyme responsible for the metabolism of aliskiren, although hepatic metabolism is not a major route of drug elimination. Most (>90%; 78% as unchanged drug) of a given dose is eliminated in the feces, with <2% eliminated as oxidized metabolites and <1% eliminated in the urine. The pharmacokinetics of aliskiren is not appreciably affected by race or kidney or liver insufficiency.[1]

Half-life ($t_{1/2}$). The terminal elimination half-life of aliskiren is about 40 h and steady-state blood concentrations are reached in about 7–8 days. The accumulation half-life (based on accumulation of drug at steady-state) is about 24 h. Renal dysfunction does not lead to any significant drug accumulation.

Adverse Reactions. Aliskiren is generally well tolerated. Discontinuation of therapy due to adverse effects in clinical trials was no greater than with placebo. As with ACE inhibitors and angiotensin receptor antagonists, angioedema has been reported in patients taking aliskiren, although the incidence is very low (<1%).

The most common adverse effects seen with aliskiren are gastrointestinal in nature; they are dose-dependent, and usually mild. Diarrhea was reported by 2.3% of patients at 300 mg (1.2% with placebo). Women and the elderly seem more sensitive to this adverse effect, with rates of 2%–3% at 150 mg. Abdominal pain and dyspepsia have also been reported, although at rates distinguishable from placebo only at daily doses of 600 mg. Aliskiren has also been associated with the development of cough (1.1% vs. 0.6% for placebo), although at rates one-third to one-half that seen with ACE inhibitors. Rash (1% vs. 0.3% placebo), elevated uric acid (0.4% vs. 0.1%), gout (0.2% vs. 0.1%), and renal stones (0.2% vs. 0%) have also been associated with aliskiren at rates greater than that of placebo. Tonic–clonic seizures with loss of consciousness were reported in two patients treated with aliskiren in clinical trials. Headache, nasopharyngitis, dizziness, fatigue, upper respiratory tract infection, back pain, and cough were also reported in clinical trials at rates similar or less than that seen with placebo. **Laboratory tests:** As with other drugs that act on the renin–angiotensin system, small decreases in hemoglobin and hematocrit (mean decreases of approximately 0.08 g/dL and 0.16 volume %, respectively) have been seen with aliskiren therapy, which may be due to a reduction in angiotensin II-induced erythropoietin production. This has been linked to slight increases in rates of anemia with aliskiren compared to placebo (0.1% vs. 0%). Increases in serum potassium >5.5 mEq/L have also been seen with aliskiren therapy (0.9% vs. 0.6% with placebo), although this seems to occur less frequently than with ACE inhibitors or angiotensin receptor antagonists. Hyperkalemia has been shown to be more likely when used in combination with an ACE inhibitor in diabetics. Aliskiren may also increase serum uric acid levels (about 6 μmol/L vs. about 30 μmol/L with HCTZ). The combination of aliskiren with HCTZ may lead to an additive (about 40 μmol/L) increase in uric acid concentrations and thereby increases in uric acid-related adverse events.

Contraindications. None.

Precautions. Use aliskiren with caution in patients with greater than moderate renal dysfunction (creatinine 1.7 mg/dL for women and 2.0 mg/dL for men and/or estimated GFR <30 mL/min), a history of dialysis, nephritic syndrome, or renovascular hypertension because of limited clinical experience. Aliskiren may produce hyperkalemia, especially in diabetic patients taking an ACE inhibitor; routine monitoring of electrolytes and renal function is indicated in this population. Use aliskiren cautiously with potassium-sparing diuretics, potassium supplements, salt substitutes containing potassium, or other drugs that increase potassium levels. Also use cautiously in patients with renal artery stenosis because of limited clinical experience.

Drug Interactions. Aliskiren may significantly reduce the blood concentrations of furosemide and dosage adjustments may be necessary. The blood concentrations of aliskiren may significantly increase when taken with cyclosporine; concomitant use of aliskiren with cyclosporine is not recommended. Atorvastatin and ketoconazole have been shown to increase aliskiren levels, while no interactions were seen with the following drugs: allopurinol, amlodipine, atenolol, celecoxib, cimetidine, digoxin, fenofibrate, HCTZ, isosorbide mononitrate, lovastatin, metformin, pioglitazone, valsartan, or warfarin.[1]

Parameters to Monitor. Monitor blood pressure regularly. Obtain baseline serum potassium and then monitor periodically, especially in patients receiving potassium-sparing diuretics, potassium supplements, or salt substitutes. Aliskiren may produce hyperkalemia, especially in diabetic patients taking an ACE inhibitor; routine monitoring of electrolytes and renal function is indicated in this population.

Notes. When corrected for placebo, aliskiren monotherapy reduces systolic blood pressure by 2–11 mm Hg and diastolic blood pressure by 2–8 mm Hg from baseline. Clinical trials have shown aliskiren to be similar to losartan, irbesartan, and valsartan in terms of blood pressure-lowering ability.[2] Additive effects have been seen when aliskiren was added to HCTZ, valsartan, ramipril, and amlodipine. As with ACE inhibitors and angiotensin receptor antagonists, black patients tend to have smaller reductions in blood pressure as compared to Caucasians and Asians.

α_1-ADRENERGIC BLOCKING DRUGS:	
DOXAZOSIN MESYLATE	Cardura, Various
PRAZOSIN HYDROCHLORIDE	Minipress, Various
TERAZOSIN HYDROCHLORIDE	Hytrin, Various

Pharmacology. Doxazosin, prazosin, and terazosin are closely related quinazoline derivatives that selectively block postsynaptic α_1-adrenergic receptors. Total peripheral resistance is reduced through arterial and venous dilatations. Reflex tachycardia that occurs with other vasodilators is infrequent because there is no presynaptic α_2-receptor blockade. The drugs also decrease total cholesterol, increase HDL-C, and may improve glucose tolerance and reduce left ventricular mass during long-term therapy. They increase urine flow in BPH by relaxing smooth muscle tone in the bladder neck and prostate.[3,4]

Administration and Adult Dosage. Give the initial dose and the first dose of all increased dosage regimens at bedtime and observe the patient closely for syncope. **PO for hypertension**—(doxazosin) 1 mg/d initially and then double the dose at 1- to 2-wk intervals to a maximum of 16 mg/d in a single dose, although dosages over 4 mg/d are more likely to cause postural side effects. (Prazosin) 1 mg bid or tid initially, increasing the dosage slowly, based on response, to the usual dosage of 6–15 mg/d; although the maximum effective dosage is usually 20 mg/d, dosages up to 40 mg/d can be effective in some patients who fail to respond to lower dosages. (Terazosin) 1 mg/d initially, increasing to 2, 5, or 10 mg/d in 1–2 doses to a maximum of 20 mg/d. **PO for benign prostatic hypertrophy**—(doxazosin) 1 mg/d initially, doubling the dose at 1- to 2-wk intervals to a maximum of 8 mg/d. (Terazosin) 1 mg/d initially, increasing to 2, 5, and 10 mg once daily.

Special Populations. *Pediatric Dosage.* **PO for hypertension**—(prazosin) 0.05–0.4 mg/kg/d in 2–3 divided doses. Do not exceed single doses of 7 mg and a total daily dosage of 15 mg.[5] (Doxazosin, terazosin) safety and efficacy not established.

Geriatric Dosage. Same as adult dosage.

Dosage Forms. (Doxazosin) **Tab** 1, 2, 4, 8 mg. (Prazosin) **Cap** 1, 2, 5 mg; **Cap** 1, 2, 5 mg with polythiazide 0.5 mg (Minizide). (Terazosin) **Cap** 1, 2, 5, 10 mg.

Patient Instructions. (*See* Antihypertensives Class Instructions.) Take the initial dose of this drug at bedtime. Dizziness or drowsiness can occur with this medication, especially after the first dose or when the dosage is being increased. Do not arise suddenly, stand for long periods, or exercise too vigorously, especially in hot weather. Alcohol can worsen these effects.

Pharmacokinetics. *Onset and Duration.* (Doxazosin) onset 1–2 h, duration 24 h for hypertension; full effect for BPH might not occur for 1–2 wk. (Prazosin) onset 1–2 h, duration about 6–12 h, up to 4–6 wk might be required for full antihypertensive effect. (Terazosin) onset 15 min, duration 24 h, but up to 6–8 wk might be required for full antihypertensive effect. In BPH, at least 4–6 wk might be required to fully evaluate response to a 10-mg/d dosage. (*See* α_1-Adrenergic Blocking Drugs Comparison Chart.)

Serum Levels. No correlation between serum levels and clinical effect has been established.[4,6]

Fate. (Doxazosin) oral bioavailability is 63 ± 14%; absorption is slow, but bioavailability is not affected by food; 98%–99% is bound to plasma proteins. V_d is 1.5 ± 0.3 L/kg; Cl is 0.1 ± 0.024 L/kg/h. Doxazosin is extensively metabolized and excreted primarily in the feces, with only about 9% excreted in urine as unchanged drug and metabolites.[4,6] (Prazosin) bioavailability is 68 ± 17% with 48 ± 16% in the elderly; food can delay but not affect the extent of absorption. About 95% is bound to plasma proteins, decreased in cirrhosis and uremia. V_d is 0.63 ± 0.14 L/kg and Cl is 0.24 ± 0.04 L/h/kg in young patients; V_d is 0.89 ± 0.26 L/kg and Cl is 0.21 ± 0.06 L/h/kg in the elderly; Cl is lower in CHF and pregnancy. Prazosin is metabolized in the liver by demethylation and conjugation; metabolites have about 20% of the activity of the drug. It is excreted renally as metabolites and 3.4% or less as unchanged drug.[7] (Terazosin) pharmacokinetics do not appear to be affected by uremia, CHF, or aging. Oral bioavailability is about 90% with 90%–94% bound to plasma proteins. V_d is 0.8 ± 0.18 L/kg, and Cl is 0.066 ± 0.012 L/h/kg.[6] It is extensively metabolized in the liver, with 18% excreted unchanged in feces, 10% unchanged in urine, and the remainder excreted as metabolites.[8]

$t_{1/2}$. (Doxazosin) 10.5 ± 2.4 h in young adults, 11.9 ± 4.7 h in the elderly. (Prazosin) 2.1 ± 0.3 h in young adults, 3.2 ± 0.6 h in the elderly; also prolonged in CHF and pregnancy. (Terazosin) 13.5 ± 3.5 h in young adults, 16.2 ± 2.2 h in the elderly.[9]

Adverse Reactions. The most important adverse effect is first-dose syncope, which is more likely in patients being treated with other antihypertensive drugs, especially diuretics. During long-term treatment, the most frequent reactions are dizziness, headache, drowsiness, lack of energy or weakness, palpitations, or nausea, all of which occur in 5%–20% of patients. Occasionally reported are rash, vomiting, diarrhea, edema, orthostatic hypotension, syncope, dyspnea, blurred vision, nasal congestion, or urinary frequency. Rarely, allergic reactions, priapism, or impotence occur.[10]

Contraindications. Allergy to a quinazoline derivative.

Precautions. Syncope can occur after the first dose (doxazosin 2–6 h; prazosin 30–90 min; terazosin 1–2 h) and during rapid upward dosage titration or when adding an additional antihypertensive drug. Hold doses of diuretics for 1 day before starting an α_1-blocker. Increase dosage gradually, reduce dosage when adding another antihypertensive, and then retitrate dosage. Use doxazosin with caution in patients with hepatic impairment.

Drug Interactions. β-blockers and verapamil can enhance postural effects of prazosin; NSAIDs can decrease the hypotensive effect of prazosin. The α_1-blockers can decrease the hypotensive effect of clonidine.

Parameters to Monitor. Monitor blood pressure regularly.

Notes. α_1-antagonists can be particularly useful for hypertension (in men with BPH), in hyperlipidemia or renal disease, in diabetics, in physically active young patients (no decrease in cardiac output), and in the elderly.[3,9] However, drugs in this class have not been shown to decrease long-term mortality of hypertension.[4] The doxazosin arm of the ALLHAT study was terminated prematurely because of inferior efficacy in reducing cardiovascular events compared with chlorthalidone.[11] **Tamsulosin** (Flomax) is a selective α_1a-receptor blocker, specific for adrenoreceptors in the prostate. Tamsulosin is not indicated for hypertension but rather for signs and symptoms of BPH. The initial oral dosage is 0.4 mg/d, increasing as needed up to 0.8 mg/d.

CAPTOPRIL
Capoten, Various

Pharmacology. Captopril is an ACE inhibitor pharmacologically similar to enalapril. Captopril's rapid onset and short duration of action are advantageous initially to assess patient tolerance to ACE inhibitors but inconvenient during long-term use. (*See* ACE Inhibitors Comparison Chart.)

Adult Dosage. **PO for hypertension**—12.5–25 mg bid–tid initially, increasing after 1–2 wk to 50 mg bid–tid, to a maximum of 450 mg/d. **PO for CHF**—6.25–25 mg tid initially, increasing over several days based on the patient's tolerance to a dosage of 50 mg tid. Delay further dosage increases, if possible, for at least 2 wk to evaluate response. Most patients respond to 50–100 mg tid. **For hypertension or CHF**—use initial dosages of 6.25–12.5 mg bid–tid and increase slowly in patients on diuretic therapy, with sodium restriction, or with renal impairment. **PO for left ventricular dysfunction post-MI**—6.25 mg once at 3 or more days post-MI and then 12.5 mg tid; increase to 25 mg tid over several days to a target of 50 mg tid over several wk as tolerated. **PO for diabetic nephropathy**—25 mg tid

Pediatric Dosage. **PO for hypertension**—(neonates) 0.01 mg/kg bid–tid initially; (children) up to 0.3 mg/kg tid initially.[5]

Dosage Forms. **Tab** 12.5, 25, 50, and 100 mg, and 25 or 50 mg in combination with hydrochlorothiazide, 15 or 25 mg (Capozide, various).

Pharmacokinetics. Oral bioavailability is about 65%; food decreases absorption, so the drug should be taken on an empty stomach. About 30% is bound to plasma proteins and its V_d is 0.8 ± 0.2 L/kg, higher in CHF; Cl is 0.72 ± 0.08 L/h/kg decreased with renal dysfunction.[6] Approximately 50% of a dose is metabolized, primarily to captopril disulfide, which can be converted back to active captopril in vivo. Urinary excretion of unchanged captopril is 24%–38% over 24 h. Its half-life is 2.2 ± 0.05 h in healthy subjects and is prolonged in renal dysfunction or CHF.[6]

Adverse Reactions. Adverse reactions are similar to those of enalapril, although skin rashes and taste impairment can be more prevalent and cough less prevalent.

CLONIDINE HYDROCHLORIDE	Catapres, Various

Pharmacology. Clonidine stimulates postsynaptic α_2-adrenergic receptors in the CNS by activating inhibitory neurons to decrease sympathetic outflow. Clonidine is not a complete agonist, so some of its effects might result from antagonist actions at presynaptic α-receptors.[12] These actions reduce peripheral vascular resistance, renal vascular resistance, heart rate, and blood pressure.

Administration and Adult Dosage. **PO for hypertension**—0.1 mg bid initially, increasing weekly in increments of 0.1 mg/d until the desired response is achieved. **Maintenance dosage for monotherapy** is usually 0.2–0.6 mg/d, to a maximum of 2.4 mg/d. If rapid lowering of blood pressure is desired (e.g., hypertensive urgency), give 0.1–0.2 mg initially and then 0.1 mg q1h until the desired response is achieved or a total of 0.8 mg has been given. **SR patch for hypertension**—initially apply one #1 (0.1 mg/24 h) patch weekly; dosage can be increased at 1- to 2-wk intervals up to #3 patch that delivers 0.3 mg/24 h. Dosages in excess of two #3 patches/week do not add efficacy. **PO for opiate withdrawal**—1.25–1.5 mg/d in 3–4 divided doses and then decreasing over 14 d by 0.1–0.2 mg/d.[13] **PO for smoking cessation**—0.15–0.675 mg/d in divided doses. **SR patch for smoking cessation**—apply one #1 (0.1 mg/24 h) patch weekly.[14] (*See* Notes.)

Special Populations. *Pediatric Dosage.* **PO for hypertension**—0.05–0.4 mg bid.

Geriatric Dosage. Lower oral dosages might be required, but decreased skin permeability might require higher transdermal dosages.[15]

Other Conditions. In renal impairment, lower oral dosages might be required, but decreased skin permeability might require higher transdermal dosages.[15]

Dosage Forms. **Tab** 0.1, 0.2, 0.3 mg; **Tab** 0.1, 0.2, 0.3 mg with chlorthalidone 15 mg (Combipres, various); **SR Patch** 0.1, 0.2, 0.3 mg/24 h.

Patient Instructions. (*See* Antihypertensives Class Instructions.) Do not abruptly discontinue this drug or interrupt therapy unless under medical supervision. Apply transdermal patches weekly to a clean, hairless area of the upper arm or torso that is free of irritation, abrasions, or scars. Do not touch the adhesive surface. Apply patch to a different location with each application. If the system loosens during the 7 days, apply the adhesive overlay directly over the system. If a generalized rash or moderate-to-severe redness or vesicles appear at the site of application, notify the prescriber. Dispose of the patch by folding the sides together and placing it in a disposal site inaccessible to children.

Missed Doses. Take this drug at regular intervals. If you miss a dose, take it as soon as you remember. If it is about time for your next dose, take that dose only. Do not double the dose or take extra. Contact your physician if you miss two or more doses or if you are late in changing the transdermal system by 3 or more days.

Pharmacokinetics. *Onset and Duration.* (Hypertension) PO onset 30–60 min; peak 2–5 h; duration 6–8 h but can increase to 12–24 h with long-term use.[15] Transdermally, maximal reduction in blood pressure occurs in 2–3 days and persists throughout the 7-day application period. After removal, blood pressure rapidly increases toward baseline, followed by a slower rate of increase, and returns to pretreatment levels over several days.[12]

Serum Levels. (Hypotensive effect) 0.2–2 μg/L (0.9–9 nmol/L); (dry mouth, sedation) 1.5–2 μg/L.[15]

Fate. Oral bioavailability is 75%–95%.[15] Transdermally, maximum serum levels are reached in 3–4 days and remain constant throughout the 7-day application period.[12] Rate of release is a zero-order process and primarily controlled by the delivery system. Serum concentrations remain constant when a patch is removed and another is immediately applied to a different site.[12] Clonidine is 20% bound to plasma proteins; V_d is 2.1 ± 0.4 L/kg; Cl is 0.186 ± 0.072 L/h/kg.[6] It is metabolized in the liver, with drug and metabolites excreted primarily in urine; remaining drug may undergo enterohepatic recycling. About 62% is excreted unchanged in urine.[6]

$t_{1/2}$. (PO) α phase is 10.8 ± 4.7 min; β phase is 12 ± 7 h.[6] (Transdermal) 14 h but can be up to 26 h, reflecting continued absorption from a skin depot.[12]

Adverse Reactions. Frequent adverse reactions include dry mouth (40%), drowsiness (33%), dizziness (16%), constipation (10%), weakness (10%), sedation (10%), nausea or vomiting (5%), nervousness and agitation (3%), orthostatic hypotension (3%), and sexual dysfunction (3%). Occasionally rash, weight gain, anorexia, transient abnormalities in liver function tests, insomnia or vivid dreams, palpitations, tachycardia or bradycardia, or urinary retention occur. Rarely hepatitis, thrombocytopenia, parotitis, elevations of blood glucose or CPK, or cardiac conduction disturbances occur. Allergic contact dermatitis occurs in up to 50% of patients treated with patches.[16] Abrupt withdrawal of oral therapy can result in a withdrawal reaction characterized by rapid reversal of the antihypertensive effect within 24–48 h up to or above pretreatment levels, a rise of blood pressure above 40 mm Hg systolic or 25 mm Hg diastolic, or blood pressure above 225/125 mm Hg. Subjective symptoms of sweating, palpitations, anxiety, and insomnia also can occur, even without marked blood pressure changes. The frequency and severity of symptoms appear to be greater in patients treated with high dosages for more than 3 months and in those with more severe hypertension.[17]

Precautions. Use with caution in patients with severe coronary insufficiency, conduction disturbances, recent MI, cerebrovascular disease, or chronic renal failure. Patients who develop rashes from the transdermal system can develop generalized skin rashes if oral clonidine is substituted.[16] Inadvertent person-to-person transfer of the patches has been reported; check the application site frequently and dispose of the patch by folding adhesive sides together and placing it in a container inaccessible to children.[18]

Drug Interactions. Tricyclic antidepressants can decrease the hypotensive effect of clonidine. Clonidine can inhibit the antiparkinson effect of levodopa. Clonidine use with propranolol can cause hypertension, especially if clonidine is abruptly discontinued. Direct-acting sympathomimetics can have an exaggerated effect during clonidine use. Prazosin can decrease the effects of clonidine. Synergistic hypotension and conduction disturbances can occur with verapamil.

Parameters to Monitor. Monitor blood pressure regularly; check patient compliance.

Notes. Clonidine has been used to suppress symptoms of withdrawal of opiates and to reduce craving and other symptoms in alcohol and tobacco withdrawal.[13,14,19] It also has been used in a variety of psychiatric applications including treatment of mania, anxiety, panic disorders, schizophrenia, and antipsychotic-induced tardive dyskinesia.[19] As an aid in the diagnosis of pheochromocytoma, a single 0.3-mg dose has been administered after determination of baseline catecholamine levels, followed by three subsequent determinations at hourly intervals.[20] Other conditions for which it can be effective include diabetic diarrhea (0.1–0.6 mg q12h), menopausal flushing (0.05–0.15 mg/d in divided doses), and premenstrual syndrome.[21–22]

DIAZOXIDE
Hyperstat I.V., Proglycem

Pharmacology. Diazoxide is a nondiuretic thiazide that reduces total peripheral resistance by direct relaxation of arteriolar smooth muscle. It also increases heart rate, cardiac output, and renal blood flow. Diazoxide increases blood glucose by inhibiting insulin release and peripheral utilization.

Adult Dosage. IV for severe hypertension—1–3 mg/kg, to a maximum single dose of 150 mg administered undiluted over less than 30 sec q5–15 min, until adequate blood pressure reduction is achieved. Repeat q4–24h as needed to maintain blood pressure control to a maximum of 10 d. **PO for hypoglycemia**—3–8 mg/kg/d in 2–3 equal doses q8–12 h, titrated to response.

Pediatric Dosage. IV for severe hypertension—same as adult dosage. **PO for hypoglycemia**—(neonates and infants) 8–15 mg/kg/d in 2–3 divided doses q8–12h, titrated to response; (children) same as adult dosage.

Dosage Forms. **Inj** 15 mg/mL (Hyperstat I.V.); **Cap** 50 mg (Proglycem); **Susp** 50 mg/mL (Proglycem).

Pharmacokinetics. Antihypertensive onset is 1–4 min; peak within 5 min; duration is 3–12 h. Hyperglycemia onset within 1 h; duration 8 h. Oral bioavailability is 86%–96%; 94 ± 14% is bound to plasma proteins at typical concentrations, decreased at higher concentrations and in uremia. V_d is 0.21 ± 0.02 L/kg with normal renal function; Cl is 0.0036 ± 0.0012 L/h/kg. The drug is metabolized by oxidation and sulfate conjugation and excreted slowly in urine as unchanged drug (20%–50%) and metabolites.[6,23] **Half-life.** 48 ± 12 h, prolonged in renal failure in proportion to Cl_{Cr}.[6,23]

Adverse Reactions. (Hypertension) hypotension, nausea and vomiting, dizziness, and weakness are the most frequent reactions. Sodium and water retention and hyperglycemia can occur, especially with repeated administration. (Hypoglycemia) frequent reactions include sodium and fluid retention; hyperglycemia or glycosuria, which might require dosage reduction; hirsutism; tachycardia; palpitations; increases in uric acid; thrombocytopenia with or without purpura, which requires discontinuation of the drug. Rarely, diabetic ketoacidosis or hyperosmolar nonketotic coma can develop rapidly.

Contraindications. Hypersensitivity to thiazides or other sulfonamide derivatives; compensatory hypertension, such as that seen secondary to coarctation of the aorta or arteriovenous shunts; functional hypoglycemia; dissecting aortic aneurysm.

Precautions. Use with caution with impaired cerebral or cardiac circulation. Avoid extravasation of the IV drug. Recent or coadministration of other antihypertensive drugs can produce excessive blood pressure reduction with the IV route.

Drug Interactions. Diazoxide and hydantoins can be mutually antagonistic. Use with a thiazide diuretic can potentiate hyperuricemia and hypotensive effects.

Phenothiazines can potentiate the effects of oral diazoxide and this can antagonize the effects of sulfonylureas.

Parameters to Monitor. (Hypertension) Obtain blood pressure frequently until stable and then hourly; monitor blood glucose and uric acid with repeated doses. Monitor for signs of cerebral or myocardial ischemia. (Hypoglycemia) Obtain frequent blood glucose and urine glucose and ketones initially, when dosage adjustments or dosage form changes are made, and then regularly during stabilization.

ENALAPRIL MALEATE	Vasotec, Various
ENALAPRILAT	Vasotec I.V., Various

Pharmacology. Enalapril is a prodrug that is rapidly converted to its active metabolite, enalaprilat, by ester hydrolysis in the liver. Enalaprilat is a competitive ACE inhibitor. It also reduces serum aldosterone, leading to decreased sodium retention; potentiates the vasodilator kallikrein–kinin system; and can alter prostanoid metabolism, inhibit the sympathetic nervous system, and inhibit the tissue renin–angiotensin system. The net effect is reduction in total peripheral resistance and blood pressure in hypertensive patients, especially those with high pretreatment plasma renin activity and increased renal plasma flow, and reduction of elevated afterload in patients with CHF.[24]

Administration and Adult Dosage. PO for hypertension—5 mg/d initially. **Usual maintenance dosage** is 10–40 mg/d in 1–2 doses. If the patient has recently been receiving a diuretic, discontinue the diuretic for 2–3 d or start with a lower initial enalapril dose of 2.5 mg; bid administration might be necessary in some individuals to achieve adequate 24-h blood pressure control. A diuretic can be added if blood pressure control is inadequate with enalapril monotherapy. **PO for CHF**—2.5 mg daily or bid initially, using the lower dosage for patients taking a diuretic. **Usual maintenance dosage** is 5–20 mg/d, to a maximum of 40 mg; bid administration is preferred. **IV for hypertension**—1.25 mg (0.625 mg initially if patient is taking a diuretic) over 5 min q6h. Dosages as high as 5 mg q6h can be tolerated for up to 36 h, but there is inadequate experience with dosages over 20 mg/d. For patients converting from PO to IV, 5 mg/d PO is equivalent to about 1.25 mg IV q6h.

Special Populations. *Pediatric Dosage.* Safety and efficacy not established.

Geriatric Dosage. No change necessarily required but observe cautions for impaired renal function.

Other Conditions. For patients with $Cl_{Cr} \leq 30$ mL/min, $Cr_s > 3$ mg/dL, or CHF with serum sodium <130 mEq/L, use lower initial doses (2.5 mg PO; 0.625 mg IV). For patients on dialysis, the initial dose should be no greater than 0.625 mg IV q6h or 2.5 mg PO on dialysis days.

Dosage Forms. **Tab** 2.5, 5, 10, 20 mg (Enalapril); **Tab** 5 mg with hydrochlorothiazide 12.5 mg, 10 mg with hydrochlorothiazide 25 mg (Vaseretic); **SR Tab** 5 mg with diltiazem 180 mg (Teczem), 5 mg with 2.5 or 5 mg felodipine (Lexxel); **Inj** 1.25 mg/mL (enalaprilat).

Patient Instructions. (*See* Antihypertensives Class Instructions.) Use potassium supplements or salt substitutes only under medical supervision. Report any signs or symptoms of the following: infection (e.g., sore throat or fever), angioedema (e.g., swelling of face, eyes, lips, tongue, larynx, extremities, or hoarseness or difficulty in swallowing), or excessive fluid loss (e.g., vomiting, diarrhea, or excessive perspiration). Report any skin rash, taste disturbance, or persistent, dry cough. If you become pregnant while taking this drug, contact your prescriber immediately.

Pharmacokinetics. *Onset and Duration.* PO onset is 1 h; peak in 4–6 h; duration is up to 24 h.[25] The onset of action and maximal hemodynamic response correspond to the appearance of enalaprilat in serum.[6] IV onset is 15–30 min; peak is within 1 h; duration is usually 4–6 h with recommended doses but can be as long as 12 h in some patients.[26]

Serum Levels. (Enalaprilat) 5–20 µg/L (13–52 nmol/L) is the EC50 for ACE inhibition; 40 µg/L (104 nmol/L) produces a mean blood pressure reduction of 12 mm Hg.[6,27]

Fate. Oral bioavailability is 41 ± 15%; it is not altered by meals but is decreased in cirrhosis.[6] Peak enalapril and enalaprilat serum levels after a 10-mg oral dose occur at about 1 and 4 h, with ranges of 40–50 µg/L (104–130 nmol/L) and 30–40 µg/L (78–104 nmol/L), respectively.[27] About 60% of a dose is converted to enalaprilat; conversion can be reduced in patients with cirrhosis.[27] Enalapril and enalaprilat levels are increased in renal dysfunction. Less than 50% of enalaprilat is bound to plasma protein.[27] $V_{d\beta}$ is 1.7 ± 0.7 L/kg; Cl is 0.294 ± 0.09 L/h/kg.[28] Cl is decreased in uremia, CHF, the elderly, and neonates.[6] After IV administration, 88% is excreted unchanged in urine;[6] after oral administration, 33% of the dose is recovered in the feces (6% as enalapril, 27% as enalaprilat) and 61% in the urine (18% as enalapril, 43% as enalaprilat).[27,29] Enalapril can be actively secreted into the urine; fecal recovery can indicate unabsorbed drug or biliary excretion.[27]

$t_{1/2}$. (Enalapril) estimated to be 11 h; (enalaprilat) about 30–35 h in normals, increased in CHF, renal dysfunction, cirrhosis, and uremia.[6,27]

Adverse Reactions. ACE inhibitors have a common side effect profile. Most adverse effects are related to dosage and renal function. A dry, nonproductive cough occurs in 1%–3% or more (up to 20% in some surveys) of treated patients, most frequently in women and nonsmokers.[30] The cough is caused by potentiation of tissue kinins or prostaglandins in the lung. It can be more frequent with longer-acting drugs but is usually not resolved by switching to another ACE inhibitor. Taste disturbances occur in 2%–7% but can resolve despite continued therapy.[30,31] Skin rashes occur in 1%–7%, usually within a few days to weeks after starting.[31] Rashes often resolve with continued therapy and do not appear to cross-react among ACE inhibitors.[30] Angioedema is an occasional, serious, potentially fatal reaction, possibly more frequent with longer-acting ACE inhibitors and possibly in blacks.[24,30] Hypotension can occur, especially with the first dose, in vigorously diuresed patients, those who are hyponatremic or hypovolemic, those with severe hypertension, and the elderly. In salt-restricted patients with CHF, receiving ACE inhibitors and continuous diuretic therapy, up to one-third can experience worsening of renal function that can improve when sodium is replenished.[31] Hyperkalemia occurs in 1%–4% of patients, most often in those with diabetes mellitus or renal dysfunction. Proteinuria occurs occasionally with normal renal function and frequently with preexisting renal disease,[24] although patients with progressive renal insufficiency tolerate the drug well and many experience a reduction in proteinuria despite transient reductions in renal function.[32] Neutropenia can occur, usually in the first 3 months of therapy; it is rare in normal patients but more frequent with high doses or in renal impairment.[30] Cholestatic hepatotoxicity is reported rarely and it can cross-react among ACE inhibitors;[30] it is reversible with drug discontinuation, but fatalities have been reported. Serious fetal harm, including renal failure, face or skull abnormalities, and increased risk of miscarriage, occurs with ACE-inhibitor use during the second and third trimesters of pregnancy.[30]

Contraindications. Angioedema caused by any ACE inhibitor.

Precautions. Pregnancy. It is best to avoid ACE inhibitors in women of child-bearing potential who are not actively avoiding pregnancy. Monitor patients on dietary salt restriction, diuretic therapy, or dialysis (salt or volume depletion) for hypotensive episodes after the initial dose. If possible, discontinue these therapies before treatment. Titrate dosage slowly to the minimal effective dosage in patients with impaired renal function or collagen vascular disorders or in patients receiving drugs altering WBC count or immune function.[32,33] Patients with aortic stenosis can develop decreased coronary perfusion when treated with afterload reducers such as ACE inhibitors. Elevations in Cr_s and BUN might require dosage reduction or drug discontinuation. Patients with unilateral or bilateral renal artery stenosis might be more prone to increases in Cr_s and BUN. Hypotension responsive to volume expansion can occur during surgical procedures.

Drug Interactions. Hyperkalemia can develop with concomitant use of potassium-sparing diuretics, potassium supplements, or potassium-containing salt substitutes, particularly with preexisting renal impairment.[30] Sodium and volume depletion because of a loop diuretic can cause postural hypotension when an ACE inhibitor is begun. ACE inhibitors can increase lithium levels. They can potentiate oral hypoglycemic drugs and increase neutropenia caused by azathioprine and hypotensive reactions when used with IV plasma protein solutions. NSAIDs can antagonize the hypotensive effect of ACE inhibitors. Phenothiazines can increase the effects of ACE inhibitors and rifampin can decrease the effects of enalapril. ACE inhibitors can increase serum digoxin concentrations.

Parameters to Monitor. Monitor blood pressure regularly. Obtain baseline Cr_s and BUN to assess the potential for adverse effects and titrate dosages accordingly; then monitor periodically. Obtain WBC count with differential every 2 weeks for the first 3 months and then periodically in renally impaired patients or if signs of infection occur. Obtain baseline serum potassium and then monitor periodically, especially in patients receiving potassium-sparing diuretics, potassium supplements, or salt substitutes. Obtain periodic urinary protein estimates (morning urine) by dipstick in patients with renal impairment.

Notes. ACE inhibitors are considered first-line drugs, along with diuretics, β-blockers, and calcium channel blockers, for the treatment of hypertension.[34] They are also first-line treatments for CHF in combination with digoxin and a diuretic because their use is associated with prolonged survival.[24,35] Regression or attenuation of left ventricular hypertrophy occurs in patients with hypertension and in post-MI patients.[24] Additional advantages of ACE inhibitors are their renal protective effects and improved insulin sensitivity in type 1 diabetics, their lack of adverse effects on serum lipid profile, an improvement in quality of life in hypertensive patients (with one study favoring **captopril** over **enalapril**), and possibly prevention of structural changes in the heart, systemic vasculature, and kidneys.[24,25]

ACE inhibitors with greater tissue ACE inhibition (e.g., **benazepril, quinapril, ramipril**) might be more effective in this latter regard, but studies are lacking.[24] Ramipril and perindopril have been shown to reduce mortality and cardiovascular morbidity in patients without CHF who are at high risk for cardiovascular events, although trandolapril was shown to be neutral in this regard.[36–38] (*See* ACE Inhibitors Comparison Chart.)

FENOLDOPAM   Corlopam

Pharmacology. Fenoldopam is a dopamine D_1-receptor agonist that dilates renal and mesenteric vascular beds, thereby reducing total peripheral resistance and increasing renal blood flow and sodium excretion. Stimulation of postsynaptic D_1-receptors leads to smooth muscle relaxation through activation of adenylate cyclase and a subsequent increase in intracellular cyclic AMP. Unlike dopamine, fenoldopam has no α- or β-adrenergic receptor activity, stimulation of which causes increases in blood pressure or heart rate, respectively.[39]

Administration and Adult Dosage. **IV for the in-hospital, short-term (up to 48 h) management of severe hypertension**—0.03–0.1 µg/kg/min initially, increasing in increments of 0.05–0.1 µg/kg/min at intervals of >20 min to a maximum of 1.7 µg/kg/min.[40] Do not use bolus injections. Lower initial infusion rates and slower titration result in less reflex tachycardia. When the desired effect is achieved, the infusion can be stopped gradually or abruptly because rebound elevation of blood pressure has not been observed.[40]

Special Populations. *Pediatric Dosage.* Safety and efficacy not established.

Geriatric Dosage. Same as adult dosage.

Other Conditions. Dosage adjustments are not necessary for renal or hepatic disease or continuous ambulatory peritoneal dialysis. The effects of hemodialysis have not been evaluated.

Dosage Forms. **Inj** 10 mg/mL.

Pharmacokinetics. *Onset and Duration.* Onset <15 min; peak 2–6 h. Blood pressure returns to baseline 2 h after infusion discontinuation.[41]

Serum Levels. Plasma fenoldopam concentrations of 3.5 µg/L are required for demonstrable reduction in blood pressure. Each 1-µg/L increase in plasma fenoldopam concentration causes a 0.8% decrease in diastolic blood pressure. A concentration of 18 µg/L is required for each 10-mm Hg reduction in diastolic blood pressure.[40]

Fate. Fenoldopam has nonlinear increases in V_d with increases in dosage. V_d is 0.23, 0.66 and 0.67 L/kg at infusion rates of 0.025, 0.25, and 0.5 µg/kg/min, respectively.[40] Cl is dose dependent, increasing from 1.49 L/h/kg at an infusion rate of 0.025 µg/kg/min to 2.29 L/h/kg at a rate of 0.5 µg/kg/min.[42] Fenoldopam is about 88% bound to plasma proteins. Elimination is due primarily to conjugation to inactive metabolites. About 90% is excreted in the urine (4% unchanged), 10% in feces.

$t_{1/2}$. 5–10 min.

Adverse Reactions. Fenoldopam causes dose-related reduction in blood pressure and reflex tachycardia; excessive decreases in blood pressure and vasodilation are responsible for most adverse effects. Frequent adverse effects are headache (11%–36%), flushing (7%–11%), nausea (about 20%), asymptomatic ST-segment abnormalities (6%–33%), and hypotension (>5%).[41] Most adverse events occur during the first 24 h of therapy. Hypokalemia, elevated BUN, serum glucose, transaminase, and LDH have been reported in 0.5%–5% of patients. Fenoldopam can cause reversible, dose-related increases in intraocular pressure.[43]

Contraindications. None known.

Precautions. Use with caution in patients with glaucoma or intraocular hypertension. Fenoldopam causes hypotension and reflex tachycardia, which can lead to increased myocardial oxygen demand and possibly ischemia. Closely monitor patients with low serum potassium concentrations, especially during the first 6 h of fenoldopam therapy.

Drug Interactions. IV allopurinol can attenuate fenoldopam-induced increases in renal blood flow. If possible, avoid concomitant use of β-blockers, which can cause excessive hypotension and inhibition of reflex responses to fenoldopam.

Parameters to Monitor. Monitor blood pressure and heart rate at least q15min because of the rapid onset and termination of effects. Monitor serum potassium frequently during fenoldopam therapy, especially during the first 24 h.

Notes. Fenoldopam reduces blood pressure similar to **nitroprusside**.[44-45] Fenoldopam might be preferred to nitroprusside in patients with renal dysfunction or requiring prolonged therapy due to the accumulation of thiocyanate with nitroprusside.[45,46] Prepare the infusion solution with NS or D5W. It is stable for 24 h under normal light and temperature conditions.

HYDRALAZINE HYDROCHLORIDE   Apresoline, Various

Pharmacology. Hydralazine is a vasodilator that reduces total peripheral resistance by direct action on vascular smooth muscle, with an effect greater on arterioles than on veins. (*See* Notes.)

Administration and Adult Dosage. **PO for hypertension**— 10 mg qid for the first 2–4 d and increase to 25 mg qid for the remainder of the first week; after the first week, the dosage can be increased to 50 mg qid, to a maximum of 300 mg/d; bid administration can be as effective as qid. **PO for CHF**—30–75 mg bid–qid initially. **Usual maintenance dosage** is 200–600 mg/d, but dosages as high as 3 g/d have been used.[47] **IM or IV for hypertension and CHF**—10–40 mg prn.

Special Populations. *Pediatric Dosage.* **PO for hypertension and CHF**— 0.75 mg/kg/d or 25 mg/m^2/d initially in 4 divided doses; the initial dose should not exceed 25 mg. Increase gradually over 3–4 wk, to a maximum of 5 mg/kg/d (infants) to 7.5 mg/kg/d (children) or 200 mg/d. **IM or IV for hypertension and CHF**— 0.1–0.2 mg/kg q4–6h prn; initial parenteral dosage should not exceed 20 mg.

Geriatric Dosage. Lower dosage and slower titration are desirable because of longer half-life in the elderly.

Dosage Forms. **Inj** 20 mg/mL; **Tab** 10, 25, 50, 100 mg; **Cap** 25 mg with hydrochlorothiazide 25 mg, 50 mg with hydrochlorothiazide 50 mg, 100 mg with hydrochlorothiazide 50 mg (Apresazide).

Patient Instructions. (*See* Antihypertensives Class Instructions.) This drug can cause headache, dizziness, or palpitations; report if these symptoms are persistent. Report symptoms of drug-induced SLE such as fever, joint pains, dermatitis, pleuritic chest pain, and generalized malaise.

Pharmacokinetics. *Onset and Duration.* PO onset in 1 h; after 300 mg/d, a minimum of 30 h is required for MAP to return to 50% of baseline value.[48] IV onset is in 10–20 min; peak in 10–80 min; IM onset is in 10–30 min; duration for IV and IM is 3–8 h.

Serum Levels. 100 g/L reduces MAP by 10–20 mm Hg.[6]

Fate. Bioavailability is a function of acetylator phenotype and averages $35 \pm 4\%$ for slow acetylators and $16 \pm 6\%$ for rapid acetylators. Food can enhance the bioavailability; the first-pass effect might be saturable. Plasma protein binding is 87%. V_d is 1.5 ± 1 L/kg; Cl is 3.36 ± 0.78 L/h/kg, reduced in CHF. The drug is metabolized extensively by acetylation to multiple metabolites, principally hydrazones, at a rate that is genetically determined; only 1%–15% of unchanged drug, as well as metabolites, is excreted in the urine.[6]

$t_{1/2}$. β phase 0.96 ± 0.28 h, longer in CHF.[6]

Adverse Reactions. Frequently, headache, anorexia, nausea, vomiting, diarrhea, palpitations, tachycardia, and angina occur. Occasionally, hypotension, edema, peripheral neuritis, dizziness, tremors, muscle cramps, urinary retention, nasal congestion, and flushing occur. A syndrome similar to SLE with joint pain and skin rash (only rarely with cerebritis and nephritis) has been reported at an overall frequency of 6.7% in 281 patients over 51 months; daily dosage affects the frequency, with none at 50 mg/d, 5.4% at 100 mg/d, and 10.4% at 200 mg/d. Women had a higher overall frequency than men (11.6% and 2.8%, respectively), and women taking 200 mg/d had a 19.4% rate; slow acetylator phenotype also can increase the risk; the syndrome is reversible with drug discontinuation, although residual effects can be detected years later.[49] An immune complex glomerulonephritis has been reported in patients with hydralazine-induced SLE.[50]

Contraindications. Coronary artery disease, mitral valvular rheumatic disease.

Precautions. Reflex tachycardia can precipitate anginal attacks or ECG evidence of myocardial ischemia.

Drug Interactions. NSAIDs can antagonize the hypotensive effect of hydralazine.

Parameters to Monitor. Blood pressure and heart rate regularly; baseline and periodic CBC. ANA titers can become positive after several months of therapy; routine monitoring is generally not warranted because the symptoms of hydralazine-induced SLE are characteristic and reversible with drug discontinuation.

Notes. Reflex increases in heart rate, cardiac output, and stroke volume and increases in plasma renin activity and retention of sodium and water can attenuate the antihypertensive action of hydralazine; therefore, long-term regimens for hypertension should include a diuretic and a sympatholytic drug. When hydralazine is used as an afterload-reducing drug in the treatment of CHF in patients on maintenance diuretics, the increase in cardiac output usually prevents the development of reflex tachycardia; likewise, hypotension is usually prevented by the increased cardiac output but can occur if myocardial reserves are inadequate or if the heart cannot respond by increasing output (e.g., severe cardiomyopathy or aortic stenosis).[47]

LABETALOL HYDROCHLORIDE   Normodyne, Trandate, Various

Pharmacology. Labetalol is an adrenergic receptor blocking drug that has selective α1- and nonselective β-adrenergic receptor blocking actions. Although its pharmacologic profile resembles that of other β-blockers and the postsynaptic α1-adrenergic blocking action of prazosin, its β-blocking activity is approximately three times greater than the α-blocking activity after oral administration and 7 times greater after IV administration. During long-term treatment, α-blocking activity is reduced even more.[51,52]

Administration and Adult Dosage. **PO for hypertension**—100 mg bid initially, increasing at 2- to 3-d intervals in 100 mg bid increments until blood pressure is controlled. **Usual maintenance dosage** is 200–400 mg bid, to a maximum of 1.2–2.4 g/d for severe hypertension. **IV for hypertension**—20 mg by slow (2 min) injection, followed by 40–80 mg at 10-min intervals until blood pressure is controlled or to a total of 300 mg. Alternatively, administer a dilute solution by continuous infusion at a rate of 2 mg/min, to a maximum total dosage of 300 mg; the usual effective cumulative dosage is 50–200 mg; the infusion can be repeated q6–8h.[34,51,52]

Special Populations. *Pediatric Dosage.* Safety and efficacy not established, but the following has been used: **IV for hypertension**—0.2–1 (average 0.55) mg/kg initially, followed by a continuous infusion of 0.25–1.5 (average 0.8) mg/kg/h.[53]

Geriatric Dosage. **PO**—Initiate therapy with 50 mg bid.[51]

Other Conditions. Titrate dosage to blood pressure control. No dosage adjustment is required in renal impairment. Patients with hepatic dysfunction might require lower than usual dosages.

Dosage Forms. **Tab** 100, 200, 300 mg; **Inj** 5 mg/mL.

Patient Instructions. (*See* Antihypertensives Class Instructions.) Do not discontinue medication abruptly except under medical supervision. Do not sit up or stand for 3 h after intravenous administration.

Pharmacokinetics. *Onset and Duration.* PO onset is within 2 h, peak in 3 h, and duration of 8–12 h; can be longer with higher dosages. IV injection onset <10 min, peak in 5–15 min, duration 3–6 h.[34,52]

Fate. Almost completely absorbed, but bioavailability is only $18 \pm 5\%$ because of extensive first-pass metabolism, with the higher values reported in the elderly and patients with cirrhosis.[6,54] Peak serum levels occur within 1–2 h after oral administration; food delays the time to peak but can increase bioavailability. Plasma protein binding averages 50%. There is little distribution into the brain because of low lipid solubility. V_d is 9.4 ± 3.4 L/kg; Cl is 1.5 ± 0.6 L/h/kg, lower in young hypertensive patients and the elderly and unchanged in cirrhosis. The drug is metabolized extensively primarily in the liver and possibly gut wall to inactive compounds. Unchanged drug (<5%) and metabolites are excreted in urine and feces.[6,51,52,54]

$t_{1/2}$. β phase 4.9 ± 2 h, independent of route of administration; increased in the elderly.[6,51,54]

Adverse Reactions. These are generally related to α- and β-adrenergic blockade and usually occur during the first few weeks of therapy. Frequently, dizziness, fatigue, headache, scalp tingling, nausea, dyspepsia, and nasal congestion occur. Occasionally, postural hypotension, edema, taste disturbance, impotence, rash, and blurred vision occur. IV administration causes ventricular arrhythmias rarely.

Contraindications. Bronchial asthma; overt cardiac failure; greater than first-degree heart block; cardiogenic shock; bradycardia.

Precautions. Lower dosages might be required in patients with impaired hepatic function.

Drug Interactions. Cimetidine can increase the bioavailability of oral labetalol. Glutethimide can decrease the effect of labetalol by inducing hepatic enzymes. Concurrent use with halothane can produce myocardial depression. Labetalol decreases the reflex tachycardia induced by nitroglycerin and the bronchodilator effects of 2 β2-agonist bronchodilators.

Parameters to Monitor. Monitor blood pressure regularly and hepatic and renal function as indicated.

Notes. Labetalol injection is incompatible with 5% sodium bicarbonate, furosemide, or other alkaline products.

LOSARTAN POTASSIUM   Cozaar

Pharmacology. Losartan is a selective, reversible, nonpeptide, competitive antagonist of the angiotensin II receptor (AT_1), which is responsible for the physiologic effects of angiotensin II including vasoconstriction, aldosterone secretion, sympathetic outflow, and stimulation of renal sodium reabsorption. Losartan and other angiotensin II receptor antagonists are highly selective for the AT_1 receptor over the AT_2 receptor, whose physiologic function is unknown. Angiotensin II receptor antagonists have no inhibitory effects on ACE and therefore decrease blood pressure with no appreciable effect on kinin metabolism.[55]

Administration and Adult Dosage. **PO for hypertension**—50 mg/d initially; 25 mg/d in patients on diuretics or volume depleted. The usual dosage is 25–100 mg/d given once daily without regard to meals; may increase to bid in patients not adequately controlled with once-daily administrations. Most patients respond to 50 mg/d, although further reductions in blood pressure are possible with 100 mg/d.[56] Patients who do not respond to 50 mg/d might benefit more with the addition of hydrochlorothiazide than an increased dosage. Dosages above 100 mg/d offer little added benefit.[55]

Special Populations. *Pediatric Dosage.* Safety and efficacy not established.

Geriatric Dosage. Same as adult dosage.

Other Conditions. No dosage adjustment is necessary in patients with renal impairment or on dialysis. Patients with hepatic insufficiency might require lower doses (e.g., starting dose of 25 mg/d) because of decreased losartan clearance.

Dosage Forms. **Tab** 25, 50, 100 mg (Cozaar); **Tab** 50 mg with 12.5 mg hydrochlorothiazide, 100 mg with 25 mg hydrochlorothiazide (Hyzaar).

Patient Instructions. (*See* Antihypertensives Class Instructions.) This medication can cause dizziness, especially with the first few doses; do not drive or operate dangerous machinery until you know how you will react to this medicine. Do not use this medicine if you are pregnant or planning to become pregnant. If you become pregnant while taking this medicine, contact your prescriber immediately. Report any skin rash or signs or symptoms of angioedema (e.g., swelling of face, eyes, lips, tongue, larynx, extremities, or hoarseness or difficulty in swallowing) immediately to your prescriber.

Pharmacokinetics. *Onset and Duration.* PO onset <2 h; peak 6 h; duration >24 h, can be less with doses (≤25 mg/d.[57] Maximum antihypertensive effect occurs after 1 wk in most patients but can take 3–6 wk.

Serum Levels. Large interindividual variability, with IC50 for AT1 inhibition occurring at losartan concentrations of 1.4–200 nmol/L.[58]

Fate. Oral absorption is rapid, but extensive first-pass metabolism results in a bioavailability of 33%, which might be doubled in hepatic insufficiency. About 14% of an oral dose is converted to an active carboxylic acid metabolite. Peak concentrations of losartan occur in 1 h and those of its metabolite in 3–4 h. The metabolite is approximately 10–40 times more potent than the parent compound and is believed to be responsible for most of the antihypertensive effects of losartan.[59] Losartan and its metabolite are about 99% bound to proteins, mainly to albumin. V_{ds} of losartan and its active metabolite are 34 L and 12 L, respectively. Metabolism of losartan occurs through CYP2C9 and CYP3A4 to the active carboxylic acid metabolite and several inactive metabolites. Cl is about 36 L/h for losartan (12%–15% renal Cl) and 3 L/h for the active metabolite (50% renal Cl). Losartan Cl can be 50% less with hepatic insufficiency.[59] About 4% of an oral losartan dose is excreted unchanged in the urine and 6% of the dose as active metabolite. After oral administration, 60% of a losartan dose is excreted in the feces.

   $t_{1/2}$. (Losartan) 2 h; (metabolite) 6–9 h.

Adverse Reactions. Angiotensin II receptor antagonists are generally well tolerated, with adverse reactions occurring at frequencies similar to those of placebo; adverse events are not related to dose. The most frequent reactions are headache (10%–20%) and upper respiratory tract infection (1%–12%).[60] Nasal congestion, cough, and fatigue occur in fewer than 6% of patients.[60,61] Unlike ACE inhibitors, angiotensin II receptor antagonists induce cough about as frequently as placebo, probably because bradykinin concentrations are not elevated as they are with ACE inhibitors. Angiotensin II receptor antagonists are effective alternatives in patients who experience cough with ACE inhibitors.[62,63] Like ACE inhibitors, angiotensin II receptor antagonists can induce reversible renal dysfunction as a consequence of affecting the renin–angiotensin–aldosterone system. Increases in Cr_s and BUN also can occur in patients with unilateral or bilateral renal artery stenosis. Hypersensitivity reactions (e.g., angioedema, rash) have been reported in patients receiving losartan or **valsartan**. Angiotensin II receptor antagonists can decrease hemoglobin and hematocrit and increase serum bilirubin, but these changes are rarely of clinical importance. Neutropenia has been reported in 1.8% of patients taking valsartan (0.9% for placebo). Hyperkalemia has been reported in 1.5% of losartan-treated patients (1.3% for ACE inhibitor) and 4.4% of valsartan-treated patients (2.9% for placebo).[61]

Contraindications. Hypersensitivity to any product components.

Precautions. Use of drugs affecting the renin–angiotensin–aldosterone system can cause injury and even death to the developing fetus if used in the second or third trimester of pregnancy. Increase dosage slowly in patients with liver dysfunction because of reduced drug clearance (losartan, valsartan) in these patients. Patients taking angiotensin II receptor antagonists whose renal function is dependent on the renin–angiotensin–aldosterone system (e.g., CHF patients) can experience oliguria, progressive azotemia, and (rarely) acute renal failure or death. Reversible increases in Cr_s and/or BUN can occur in patients with unilateral or bilateral renal artery stenosis.

Drug Interactions. Inhibitors of the CYP3A4 or 2C9 isoenzymes (e.g., ketoconazole) can impair the conversion of losartan to the active metabolite. **Telmisartan**

can increase digoxin serum concentrations. No important interactions have been reported with other drugs in this class.

Parameters to Monitor. Monitor for hypersensitivity reactions (e.g., flushing, dyspnea, facial swelling, rash) at the start of therapy. Monitor blood pressure regularly. Monitor patients on dietary salt restriction, diuretic therapy, or dialysis (salt or volume depletion) for hypotensive episodes after the initial dose. Obtain baseline and periodic Cr_s and BUN to assess the potential for adverse effects. Obtain baseline serum potassium, WBC count, hemoglobin, and hematocrit. Monitor periodically for hyperkalemia, neutropenia, and anemia.

Notes. Although the guidelines of the seventh report by the Joint National Committee on Prevention, Detection, Evaluation, and Treatment do not promote this in many situations, many clinicians consider AT_1 antagonists first-line therapy for hypertension because of their efficacy, safety, and ease of administration.[34,60] Losartan is a uricosuric, which can lower plasma uric acid concentration and increase the risk of acute uric acid nephropathy or acute gout.[59] Losartan has been shown to improve cardiac output and reduce peripheral vascular resistance and pulmonary capillary wedge pressure in patients with CHF.[64] The ELITE II study found losartan to be comparable but not superior to captopril in improving survival in elderly patients with CHF, although this study was not designed to test equivalence.[65] **Telmisartan** has been shown to be equivalent to ramipril in preventing major adverse cardiovascular events in patients with vascular disease or high-risk diabetes but without heart failure.[66] (*See* Angiotensin II Receptor Antagonists Comparison Chart.)

METHYLDOPA	Aldomet, Various
METHYLDOPATE HYDROCHLORIDE	Aldomet, Various

Pharmacology. The action of methyldopa is thought to be mediated through stimulation of central α-adrenergic receptors in a manner similar to that of clonidine. Stimulation is caused primarily by the metabolite α-methylnorepinephrine.

Administration and Adult Dosage. **PO for hypertension**—250 mg bid–tid initially, increasing at intervals of no less than 48 h to the usual daily dosage of 500 mg–2 g/d in 2–4 divided doses. **IV for hypertension**—usual dosage is 250–500 mg over 30–60 min in 100 mL D5W q6h, to a maximum of 1 g q6h.

Special Populations. *Pediatric Dosage.* **PO**—10 mg/kg/d in 2–4 doses initially, to a maximum of 65 mg/kg/d or 3 g/d, whichever is less. **IV**—20– 40 mg/kg/d in divided doses q6h, to a maximum of 65 mg/kg/d or 3 g/d, whichever is less.

Geriatric Dosage. Use lower dosages to avoid causing syncope.

Other Conditions. Patients with renal failure might respond to smaller dosages of methyldopa.

Dosage Forms. **Tab** 125, 250, 500 mg; **Tab** 250 mg with chlorothiazide 150 or 250 mg (Aldoclor); **Tab** 250 mg with hydrochlorothiazide 15, 25 mg, 500 mg with hydrochlorothiazide 30, 50 mg (Aldoril, various); **Susp** 50 mg/mL; **IV** 50 mg/mL.

Patient Instructions. (*See* Antihypertensives Class Instructions.) Report changes in mood (depression), loss of appetite, yellowing of eyes or skin, abdominal pain, or unexplained fever or joint pains. This drug can cause your urine to darken if it is exposed to air after voiding.

Pharmacokinetics. *Onset and Duration.* PO onset 2 h; peak within 4–6 h; duration 12–24 h. IV onset 4–6 h; duration 10–16 h.

Serum Levels. No correlation between serum levels and therapeutic effect.

Fate. Oral bioavailability is 42 ± 16%.[6] Peak serum levels occur in 2–4 h but correlate poorly with the hypotensive effect. IV bioavailability is similar to oral, apparently because a large portion of methyldopate ester is not hydrolyzed to methyldopa. From 10% to 15% is bound to plasma proteins. V_d is 0.46 ± 0.15 L/kg; Cl is 0.22 ± 0.06 L/h/kg and is decreased in uremia. The drug is excreted in the urine as metabolites, sulfate conjugate, and unchanged drug. About 49% (IV) and 70% (PO) of a dose are excreted in urine as sulfate conjugate and unchanged drug.[6,67]

$t_{1/2}$. α phase 0.21 h (range 0.16–0.26); β phase 1.8 ± 0.6 h, increased in uremia and in neonates.[6,67]

Adverse Reactions. Frequently, drowsiness, headache, weight gain, nasal stuffiness, postural hypotension, or dry mouth occurs. A positive Coombs' test develops in 10%–20% of patients, usually between 6 and 12 months of therapy; hemolytic anemia is rare. Occasionally, depression, sexual dysfunction, diarrhea, or nightmares occur. Rarely, hepatitis, drug fever, lupuslike syndrome, leukopenia, thrombocytopenia, or granulocytopenia occur.

Contraindications. Active hepatic disease such as acute hepatitis and active cirrhosis or liver dysfunction associated with previous methyldopa therapy; concurrent MAOI therapy.

Precautions. Use with caution in patients with histories of liver disease. A previously positive Coombs' test does not preclude methyldopa use, but early recognition of hemolytic anemia can be more difficult in such patients.

Drug Interactions. Methyldopa can potentiate the effect of tolbutamide and lithium. It can also cause confusion or disorientation when used with haloperidol. An increase in the pressor response of norepinephrine can occur with concurrent use. Iron products reduce methyldopa absorption. Amphetamines and heterocyclic antidepressants can decrease the efficacy of methyldopa. Levodopa and methyldopa can enhance each other's effects.

Parameters to Monitor. Obtain direct Coombs' test initially and at 6 and 12 months. Obtain baseline and periodic CBC and liver function tests to monitor for hemolytic anemia, blood dyscrasias, and hepatic dysfunction.

Notes. Methyldopa is not a first-line drug because of its frequent side effects, but it can be useful in those with ischemic heart disease or diastolic dysfunction because it reduces left ventricular mass.[68] Methyldopa is, however, one of the preferred antihypertensives for use during pregnancy since it is not believed to be harmful to the fetus.[34]

MINOXIDIL   Loniten, Rogaine, Various

Pharmacology. Minoxidil is a potent vasodilator that acts by direct relaxation of arteriolar smooth muscle, thereby reducing total peripheral resistance. The vasodilation and associated reduction in blood pressure lead to reflex sympathetic activation, vagal inhibition, and altered renal homeostatic mechanisms manifested as increases in heart rate and cardiac output, increase in renin secretion, and salt and water retention. Because these responses can attenuate the hypotensive actions, give minoxidil with a sympatholytic drug and a diuretic. Topically, minoxidil stimulates vertex hair growth by an unknown mechanism.

Administration and Adult Dosage. **PO for hypertension**—5 mg/d initially as a single daily dose, increasing to 10, 20, and then 40 mg/d q3d in single or divided doses based on blood pressure response, to a maximum of 100 mg/d; usual dosage is 10–40 mg/d. If a single dose reduces supine diastolic blood pressure by more than 30 mm Hg, divide the total daily dosage into 2 equal doses. **Top for male pattern baldness or female alopecia androgenetica**—1 mL to affected areas bid.

Special Populations. *Pediatric Dosage.* **PO for hypertension**—0.2 mg/kg as a single daily dose, increasing in 50%–100% increments q3d until optimum blood pressure control or a total daily dosage of 50 mg is achieved; usual dosage is 0.25–1 mg/kg/d.

Geriatric Dosage. Same as adult dosage.

Other Conditions. In renal impairment, lower dosages might be required.

Dosage Forms. **Tab** 2.5, 10 mg (Loniten, various); **Top** 20, 50 mg/mL (2.5%) (Rogaine, various).

Patient Instructions. (*See* Antihypertensives Class Instructions.) If a dose is missed, wait until the next regularly scheduled dose and continue with your regular dose; do not double the next dose. Report any of the following: increase in resting heart rate of greater than 20 beats/min, rapid weight gain of more than 5 pounds or the development of edema, increased difficulty in breathing, new or worsening angina, dizziness, lightheadedness, or fainting.

Pharmacokinetics. *Onset and Duration.* PO single dose onset 30 min; peak 2–3 h; duration up to 75 h with a gradual return to baseline at a rate of about 30% per day. Time of maximum effect with repeated administration is a function of dose and averages 7 days at 10 mg/d, 5 days at 20 mg/d, and 3 days at 40 mg/d. Top onset 4 or more months; relapse can occur 3–4 mo after drug discontinuation.

Serum Levels. No correlation between serum levels and effects.

Fate. Oral absorption is at least 90% but bioavailability is probably lower. Protein binding is negligible. V_d is 2.7 ± 0.7 L/kg; Cl is 1.4 ± 0.4 L/h/kg. The drug is primarily metabolized and renally excreted, with about 20% unchanged drug in the urine. The major metabolite, a glucuronide conjugate, is active and might contribute to the drug's effect.[6,68,69]

$t_{1/2}$. 3.1 ± 0.6 h.[6]

Adverse Reactions. Frequently, hypertrichosis (elongation, thickening, and enhanced pigmentation) (80%), transient ECG T-wave changes (60%), temporary edema (7%), or tachycardia occurs. Occasionally, pericardial effusion with or without tamponade (3%), CHF, or angina occurs. Rarely, breast tenderness and rashes (including Stevens-Johnson syndrome) occur. Minor dermatologic reactions occur occasionally after topical application.

Contraindications. (Oral) pheochromocytoma, caused by possible stimulation of catecholamine release from the tumor; acute MI; dissecting aortic aneurysm.

Precautions. For hypertension, minoxidil must usually be administered with a diuretic to prevent fluid retention; a loop diuretic is almost always required. Drugs or regimens that provide around-the-clock sympathetic suppression are usually required to prevent tachycardia, which can precipitate or worsen existing angina. Degenerative myocardial lesions reported in animal studies have yet to be confirmed in humans.

Drug Interactions. Concomitant therapy with guanethidine can result in profound orthostatic hypotension; discontinue guanethidine 1–3 weeks before initiation of oral minoxidil therapy or initiate therapy in the hospital.

Parameters to Monitor. Monitor blood pressure, pulse rate, body weight, cardiac and pulmonary function regularly.

Notes. Minoxidil is reserved for use in severe hypertension in combination with other drugs, usually a diuretic and a sympatholytic drug (e.g., β-blocker).[68]

NITROPRUSSIDE SODIUM   Nitropress, Various

Pharmacology. Nitroprusside is a potent vasodilator that has direct action on vascular smooth muscle to reduce arterial pressure and produce a slight increase in heart rate, a mild decrease in cardiac output, and a moderate reduction in total peripheral resistance. The decrease in total peripheral resistance suggests arteriolar dilation (afterload reduction), whereas the reduction in cardiac output might be caused by peripheral pooling of blood (preload reduction). Nitroprusside is somewhat more active on veins than on arteries. The active component of sodium nitroprusside is the free nitroso (NO^-) group.

Administration and Adult Dosage. IV—0.3 μg/kg/min by continuous infusion initially, increasing to an average rate of 3 μg/kg/min based on blood pressure response with a range of 0.5–10 μg/kg/min. Infusion at the maximum rate should never exceed 10 min. Patients receiving other antihypertensives can usually be controlled with smaller dosages. Control administration rates carefully with a microdrip regulator or an infusion pump; avoid too rapid reduction in blood pressure. Infusion rates greater than 2 μg/kg/min generate more cyanide ion (CN^-) than the body can metabolize or eliminate. Maintain infusions at the lowest possible dosage for the shortest possible duration to avoid toxicity.[70] (*See* Adverse Reactions.)

Special Populations. *Pediatric Dosage.* IV—same as adult dosage.

Geriatric Dosage. Initiate therapy with low infusion rates and carefully titrate the rate and degree of lowering blood pressure to avoid coronary and cerebral hypoperfusion.

Other Conditions. Patients with CHF, stroke, or receiving other antihypertensive drugs might be particularly sensitive to the blood pressure-lowering effects of nitroprusside sodium; initiate therapy with low infusion rates and carefully titrate the rate and degree of lowering blood pressure to avoid coronary and cerebral hypoperfusions. Limit the total dosage in renal failure to avoid accumulation of thiocyanate. Use caution in hepatic insufficiency.

Dosage Forms. **Inj** 50 mg.

Pharmacokinetics. *Onset and Duration.* Onset within 1 min; peak 1–2 min; blood pressure usually returns to pretreatment levels in 2–10 min.[34]

Serum Levels. Therapeutic and toxic levels are not established for nitroprusside because of rapid metabolism to cyanide and thiocyanate. Thiocyanate levels >60 mg/L (1 mμmol/L) are associated with toxicity.

Fate. Nitroprusside is distributed in a volume that approximates the extravascular space, from which it is rapidly metabolized by a reaction with hemoglobin, yielding cyanmethemoglobin and an unstable intermediate that dissociates, releasing cyanide ion. Cyanide is converted to thiocyanate by the enzyme thiosulfate–cyanide sulfurtransferase (rhodanese) in the liver and the kidney. The rate of conversion is determined principally by the availability of sulfur, usually as thiosulfate. Thiocyanate is excreted largely by the kidneys and can accumulate with high infusion rates for prolonged periods of renal dysfunction.

$t_{1/2}$. (Nitroprusside) 2 min; (thiocyanate) 2.7 days, up to 9 days in patients with renal dysfunction.[71]

Adverse Reactions. Most adverse reactions are related to excessive or too rapid reduction of blood pressure and include nausea, retching, diaphoresis, apprehension, restlessness, headache, retrosternal discomfort, palpitations, dizziness, and abdominal pain, all of which resolve when the infusion rate is reduced or the infusion is temporarily discontinued. Thiocyanate is not particularly toxic and usually accumulates to toxic levels only with prolonged (>48 h) or high-dosage (>10 μg/kg/min) infusions, when cyanide elimination is increased by the administration of thiosulfate, or in the presence of renal dysfunction. To limit the risk of thiocyanate toxicity, infuse at <3 μg/kg/min. Manifestations of thiocyanate toxicity include fatigue, anorexia, nausea, disorientation, toxic psychosis, and hallucinations. Cyanide toxicity usually occurs only when large dosages (>10 μg/kg/min) are infused rapidly or for longer than 1 h. An early manifestation of cyanide toxicity can be apparent nitroprusside resistance, so increasing dosage requirements to achieve the same level of blood pressure control is an indication to look for metabolic acidosis, an indicator of cyanide toxicity that might not be evident for more than 1 h after accumulation of dangerous cyanide levels. Other symptoms of cyanide toxicity include dyspnea, vomiting, dizziness, loss of consciousness, weak pulse, distant heart sounds, areflexia, dilated pupils, shallow breathing, convulsions, and the occasional smell of bitter almonds on the breath. **Hydroxocobalamin** (25 mg/h by continuous infusion) can facilitate the conversion of cyanide to cyanocobalamin,[72] but an appropriate hydroxocobalamin dosage form is unavailable. Concurrent **sodium thiosulfate** administration also can prevent cyanide toxicity, but thiocyanate levels can increase.[73] Management of cyanide toxicity includes immediate discontinuation of nitroprusside and the administration of sodium nitrite (0.2 mL/kg of a 3% solution IV over 2–4 min), followed by 12.5 g of sodium thiosulfate infused over 10 min. Methemoglobinemia can develop in patients congenitally unable to convert nitroprusside-induced methemoglobin back to hemoglobin. Management consists of IV administration of **methylene blue** 1–2 mg/kg over several minutes.

Contraindications. Compensatory hypertension (e.g., arteriovenous shunt or coarctation of the aorta); controlled hypotension during surgery in patients with inadequate cerebral circulation; congenital (Leber's) optic atrophy; use of sildenafil. (*See* Drug Interactions.)

Precautions. If an adequate hypotensive response is not achieved after the maximum recommended infusion rate of 10 μg/kg/min for a maximum of 10 min, stop the infusion because these dosages increase the risk of toxicity. Use with caution in renal, hepatic, or thyroid disease, and in vitamin B12 deficiency or elevated intracranial pressure.

Drug Interactions. Use during general anesthesia can impair the capacity to compensate for hypovolemia and anemia and cause abnormal perfusion: ventilation ratio. Use in patients taking sildenafil can result in profound hypotension with serious consequences, including death.

Parameters to Monitor. Monitor blood pressure frequently (i.e., every few minutes) because of the rapid onset and offset of effects. Monitor thiocyanate levels after 24–48 h in patients with normal renal function and daily in patients with impaired renal function or receiving large dosages. However, these levels are of no value in detecting cyanide toxicity. Monitoring of serum cyanide concentrations has been recommended, but the assay is technically difficult and not readily interpretable if fluids other than packed RBCs are analyzed. Frequent monitoring of acid–base balance, particularly in patients with hepatic dysfunction, is considered adequate by most clinicians.

Notes. Protect from light and discard solution after 24 h or if the color changes from the usual faint brownish tint to blue, green, or dark red. Do not administer IV push medications through the same line or use the solution for the simultaneous administration of any other drug.

ACE INHIBITORS COMPARISON CHART

DRUG	DOSAGE FORMS	DAILY ADULT DOSAGE (mg)[a]	INDICATED FOR CHF	PEAK EFFECT (hr)	DURATION (hr)	HALF-LIFE (hr)	ELIMINATION ROUTES
Benazepril Lotensin Various	Tab 5, 10, 20, 40 mg.	20–40	No	2–4	24+	10–11[b]	Renal, Hepatic
Captopril Capoten Various	Tab 12.5, 25, 50, 100 mg.	50–150	Yes	1	6–10	2.2	Renal
Enalapril Vasotec Various	Tab 2.5, 5, 10, 20 mg. Inj 1.25 mg/mL.	PO 10–40; IV 1.25 mg q6h.	Yes	4–6 (PO) 1–4 (IV)	24 (PO) 6 (IV)	11[b]	Renal
Fosinopril Monopril	Tab 10, 20, 40 mg.	20–40	Yes	3–6	24	12–15[b]	Hepatic, Renal
Lisinopril Prinivil Zestril Various	Tab 2.5, 5, 10, 20, 30, 40 mg.	10–40	Yes	6	24	12[b]	Renal
Moexipril Univasc	Tab 7.5, 15 mg.	7.5–30	No	3–8	24	2–9[b]	Hepatic, Renal
Perindopril Aceon	Tab 2, 4, 8 mg.	4–8	No	3–7	24+	3–10[b]	Renal

(continued)

ACE INHIBITORS COMPARISON CHART (*continued*)

DRUG	DOSAGE FORMS	DAILY ADULT DOSAGE (mg)[a]	INDICATED FOR CHF	PEAK EFFECT (hr)	DURATION (hr)	HALF-LIFE (hr)	ELIMINATION ROUTES
Quinapril Accupril	Tab 5, 10, 20, 40 mg.	20–80	Yes	2–4	24+	2–3[b]	Renal
Ramipril Altace	Cap 1.25, 2.5, 5, 10 mg.	2.5–20	Yes[c]	3–8	24+	13–17[b]	Renal Hepatic
Trandolapril Mavik	Tab 1, 2, 4 mg.	2–4	Yes[c]	6–8	24+	10[b]	Hepatic, Renal

[a]Usual maintenance dosage range for hypertension. Initial dosage is often lower, and higher dosages are sometimes effective.
[b]Half-life of active drug.
[c]Indicated for CHF post-MI.
From product information.

ANGIOTENSIN II RECEPTOR ANTAGONISTS COMPARISON CHART

DRUG	DOSAGE FORMS	USUAL DAILY ADULT DOSAGE (mg)	PEAK EFFECT (hr)	DURATION (hr)	HALF-LIFE (hr)	ELIMINATION ROUTES
Candesartan Atacand	Tab 4, 8, 16, 32 mg.	8–32[a]	3–4	24+	9	Hepatic, Renal
Eprosartan Teveten	Tab 400, 600 mg.	400–800[a]	1–3	24+	5–9	Hepatic, Renal
Irbesartan Avapro	Tab 75, 150, 300 mg.	150–300	3–6	24+	11–15	Hepatic, Renal
Losartan Cozaar	Tab 25, 50, 100 mg.	25–100[a]	6	24+	2 6–9[b]	Hepatic Renal, Hepatic[b]
Olmesartan Benicar	Tab 5, 20, 40 mg.	20–40	2	24+	13[b]	Hepatic, Renal
Telmisartan Micardis	Tab 40, 80 mg.	40–80	>3	24+	24	Hepatic
Valsartan Diovan	Cap 80, 160 mg.	80–320	6	24+	6	Hepatic

[a]Occasionally, the daily dosage can be given in 2 divided doses.
[b]For active metabolite, which is responsible for most or all pharmacologic effects.
From product information.

α$_1$-ADRENERGIC BLOCKING DRUGS COMPARISON CHART

DRUG	DOSAGE FORMS	DAILY ADULT DOSAGE (mg)[a]	PEAK EFFECT (hr)	DURATION (hr)	HALF-LIFE (hr)	ELIMINATION ROUTES
Doxazosin Cardura Various	Tab 1, 2, 4, 8 mg.	1–16	2–3	24	10–22	Hepatic
Prazosin Minipress Various	Cap 1, 2, 5 mg.	2–20	1–3	6–12	2–3	Hepatic
Terazosin Hytrin Various	Tab 1, 2, 5, 10 mg.	1–20	1–2	24	9–16	Hepatic, Renal
Tamsulosin Flomax	Cap 0.4 mg.	0.4–0.8[b]	—	—	14–15	Hepatic

[a]Usual maintenance dosage range for hypertension; higher dosages are sometimes effective. Dosage is the same in the elderly.
[b]Not for hypertension; for symptoms of benign prostatic hypertrophy only.
From product information.

447

SECOND-LINE ANTIHYPERTENSIVES COMPARISON CHART

DRUG	DOSAGE FORMS	ADULT DOSAGE	DURATION	ADVERSE EFFECTS	MECHANISM
Guanabenz Acetate Wytensin Various	Tab 4, 8 mg.	PO 4 mg bid, increasing q1–2wk to a maximum of 32 mg bid.	12 h	*See* clonidine monograph.	*See* clonidine monograph.
Guanadrel Sulfate Hylorel Various	Tab 10, 25 mg.	PO 5 mg bid, increasing q1–4wk to 20–75 mg/d. Usual maximum is 150 mg/d in 2 divided doses.	4–14 h	Orthostatic hypotension, diarrhea, drowsiness, sexual dysfunction, peripheral edema, nasal stuffiness, palpitations, shortness of breath, leg cramps, aching limbs.	Postganglionic adrenergic blockade.
Guanethidine Sulfate Ismelin Various	Tab 10, 25 mg.	PO 10 mg/d, increasing q5–7d to 25–50 mg once daily.	1–3 wk	Same as guanadrel, but more frequent.	Postganglionic adrenergic blockade.
Guanfacine Hydrochloride Tenex Various	Tab 1, 2 mg.	PO 1 mg/d, increasing q3–4wk to maximum of 3 mg/d.	2–4 d	*See* clonidine monograph.	*See* clonidine monograph.
Reserpine Various	Tab 0.1, 0.25 mg.	PO 0.5 mg/d for 1–2 wk, then 0.1–0.25 mg/d.	24 h	Drowsiness, weakness, GI disturbances, nasal congestion, sexual dysfunction, bradycardia. Dose-related mental depression occurs.	Depletes norepinephrine from postganglionic adrenergic neurons.

DRUGS FOR HYPERTENSIVE URGENCIES AND EMERGENCIES COMPARISON CHART

DRUG	DOSAGE RANGE	ONSET (min)	DURATION	COMMENTS
ORAL DRUGS FOR HYPERTENSIVE URGENCIES				
Captopril Capoten Various	PO, SL 12.5–25 mg.	10–50	2–6 h	Hypotensive effect is particularly large in patients on a diuretic or in hypertensive crisis. Subsequent doses may be less effective unless given with a diuretic. Acute renal failure can occur.
Clonidine Catapres Various	PO 0.1–0.2 mg initially, then 0.1 mg/h, to a maximum total dosage of 0.8 mg.	30–120	6–8 h	Rate of onset is slower after a meal; drowsiness or dry mouth can occur. Rebound hypertension is possible.
Labetalol Normodyne Trandate Various	PO 200–400 mg, may repeat q2–3h.	30–120	6–12 h	Orthostatic hypotension, bronchoconstriction, and heart block can occur. Avoid in COPD and asthma.
Prazosin Minipress Various	PO 1–2 mg, may repeat q1h.	30–90	1–10 h	Useful in presence of increased circulating catecholamines. First-dose syncope, palpitations, tachycardia, and headache reported.

(continued)

449

DRUGS FOR HYPERTENSIVE URGENCIES AND EMERGENCIES COMPARISON CHART (*continued*)

DRUG	DOSAGE RANGE	ONSET (min)	DURATION	COMMENTS
INTRAVENOUS DRUGS FOR HYPERTENSIVE EMERGENCIES				
Diazoxide Hyperstat I.V. Various	IV 1–3 mg/kg (up to 150 mg) over 30 s; may repeat q5–15min. Alternatively, IV infusion 10–30 mg/min. After 300 mg given, give furosemide IV 40 mg before subsequent doses.	2–4	3–12 h	Now obsolete, but can be useful in hypertensive encephalopathy, malignant hypertension, and eclampsia. Increases cardiac output; requires blood pressure monitoring at hourly intervals. Avoid with ischemic heart disease or intracranial hemorrhage.
Enalaprilat Vasotec I.V. Various	IV 0.625–1.25 mg. (*See monograph.*)	15–30	4–6 h	Useful in CHF and those at risk for cerebral hypotension. Avoid in acute MI or severe renal impairment. Blacks may respond poorly. Hypotension may occur.
Esmolol Brevibloc Various	IV 250–500 mg/kg/min for 1–2 min, Then 50–100 mg/kg/min for 4 min; may repeat sequence.	1–2	10–20 min	Useful in perioperative patients with aortic dissection. Does not cause tachycardia but does decrease heart rate.
Fenoldopam Corlopam	IV 0.1–0.3 mg/kg/min initially by continuous infusion.	<5	30 min	Useful in patients with renal insufficiency who risk cyanide toxicity with nitroprusside. Use with caution in glaucoma.
Hydralazine Apresoline Various	IM or IV 10–40 mg q 3–6 hr.	10–20 (IV) 20–30 (IM)	3–8 h	Limited to treatment of severe pre-eclampsia and eclampsia. Increases cardiac output; many patients sensitive to parenteral doses, resulting in excessive hypotension.

(continued)

DRUGS FOR HYPERTENSIVE URGENCIES AND EMERGENCIES COMPARISON CHART (*continued*)

DRUG	DOSAGE RANGE	ONSET (min)	DURATION	COMMENTS
Labetalol Normodyne Trandate Various	IV push 20 mg initially, then 40–80 mg q 10 min until desired response achieved or a total dose of 300 mg. Alternatively, IV infusion 0.5–2 mg/min.	<10	3–6 h	Hypotensive effect is predictable; contraindicated in CHF, head trauma, and intracranial hemorrhage, often causes marked postural hypotension. Avoid use in patients with COPD, CHF, or bradycardia.
Nicardipine Cardene Various	IV infusion 5–15 mg/hr.	<5–15	1–4 h	Predictable effect. Useful in coronary, cerebral, or peripheral artery disease and in surgical patients. Tachycardia can occur. Use with caution in patients with coronary ischemia.
Nitroglycerin Various	IV 0.3–6 mg/hr by continuous infusion.	1–5	3–5 min	Useful in myocardial ischemia and hypertension associated with MI. Hypotension, headache, tachycardia, and tachyphylaxis occur. Avoid in constrictive pericarditis, pericardial tamponade, or intracranial hypertension.
Nitroprusside Sodium Nipride Various	IV 0.3–10 μg/kg/min by continuous infusion. Infuse at maximal dosage for no more than 10 min. Average dosage is 3 μg/kg/min.	0.5–1	1–2 min	Especially useful in ischemic heart disease. Continuous monitoring required; arterial pressure response adjusted by changing infusion rate; hypotensive effect enhanced by elevating head of patient's bed. Decreases cardiac output; cyanide toxicity with prolonged, high infusion rates.

Adapted From Refs. 34, 57, 74, and 75.

■ REFERENCES

1. Vaidyanathan S, Jarugula V, Dieterich HA, Howard D, Dole WP. Clinical pharmacokinetics and pharmacodynamics of aliskiren. *Clin Pharmacokinet.* 2008;47:515-531.
2. Lam S, Choy M. Aliskiren: an oral renin inhibitor for the treatment of hypertension. *Cardiol Rev.* 2007;15:316-323.
3. Cauffield JS et al. Alpha blockers: a reassessment of their role in therapy. *Am Fam Physician.* 1996; 54:263-270.
4. Fulton B et al. Doxazosin. An update of its clinical pharmacology and therapeutic applications in hypertension and benign prostatic hypertrophy. *Drugs.* 1995;49:295-320.
5. Drug information for the health professional. Vol I. In: *USP DI.* 20th ed. Englewood, CO: Micromedex; 2000.
6. Benet LZ et al. Design and optimization of dosage regimens; pharmacokinetic data. In: Hardman JG et al., eds. *Goodman and Gilman's the pharmacological basis of therapeutics.* 9th ed. New York: McGraw-Hill; 1996:1707-1792.
7. Vincent J et al. Clinical pharmacokinetics of prazosin—1985. *Clin Pharmacokinet.* 1985;10:144-154.
8. Titmarsh S, Monk JP. Terazosin. A review of its pharmacodynamic and pharmacokinetic properties, and therapeutic efficacy in essential hypertension. *Drugs.* 1987;33:461-477.
9. Studer JA, Piepho RW. Antihypertensive therapy in the geriatric patient: II. A review of the alpha₁-adrenergic blocking agents. *J Clin Pharmacol.* 1993;33:2-13.
10. Carruthers SG. Adverse effects of α-adrenergic blocking drugs. *Drug Saf.* 1994;11:12-20.
11. ALLHAT Officers and Coordinators. Major cardiovascular events in hypertensive patients randomized to doxazosin vs chlorthalidone. *JAMA.* 2000;283:1967-1975.
12. Langely MS, Heel RC. Transdermal clonidine: a preliminary review of its pharmacodynamic properties and therapeutic efficacy. *Drugs.* 1988;35:123-142.
13. Guthrie SK. Pharmacologic interventions for the treatment of opioid dependence and withdrawal. *DICP.* 1990;24:721-734.
14. Nunn-Thompson CL, Simon PA. Pharmacotherapy for smoking cessation. *Clin Pharm.* 1989;8:710-720.
15. Lowenthal DT et al. Clinical pharmacokinetics of clonidine. *Clin Pharmacokinet.* 1988;14:287-310.
16. Holdiness MR. A review of contact dermatitis associated with transdermal therapeutic systems. *Contact Dermatitis.* 1989;20:3-9.
17. Reid JL et al. Withdrawal reactions following cessation of central α-adrenergic receptor agonist. *Hypertension.* 1984;6(suppl II):7III-75II.
18. Harris JM. Clonidine patch toxicity. *DICP.* 1990;24:1191-1194.
19. Bond WS. Psychiatric indications for clonidine: the neuropharmacologic and clinical basis. *J Clin Psychopharmacol.* 1986;6:81-87.
20. Bravo EL et al. Clonidine-suppression test: a useful aid in the diagnosis of pheochromocytoma. *N Engl J Med.* 1981;305:623-626.
21. Fedorak RN. Treatment of diabetic diarrhea with clonidine. *Ann Intern Med.* 1985;102:197-199.
22. Nilsson LC et al. Clonidine for the relief of premenstrual syndrome. *Lancet.* 1985;2:549-550.
23. Ogilvie RI et al. Diazoxide concentration-response relation in hypertension. *Hypertension.* 1982;4:167-173.
24. Burris JF. The expanding role of angiotensin converting enzyme inhibitors in the management of hypertension. *J Clin Pharmacol.* 1995;35:337-342.
25. Leonetti G, Cuspidi C. Choosing the right ACE inhibitors. A guide to selection. *Drugs.* 1995;49:516-535.
26. DiPette DJ et al. Enalaprilat, an intravenous angiotensin-converting enzyme inhibitor, in hypertensive crisis. *Clin Pharmacol Ther.* 1985;38:199-204.
27. Todd PA, Heel RC. Enalapril: a review of its pharmacodynamic and pharmacokinetic properties and therapeutic use in hypertension and congestive heart failure. *Drugs.* 1986;31:198-248.
28. Till AE et al. Pharmacokinetics of repeated oral doses of enalapril maleate (MK-421) in normal volunteers. *Biopharm Drug Dispos.* 1984;5:273-280.
29. Ulm EH et al. Enalapril maleate and a lysine analogue (MK-521): disposition in man. *Br J Clin Pharmacol.* 1982;14:357-362.
30. Alderman CP. Adverse effects of the angiotensin-converting enzyme inhibitors. *Ann Pharmacother.* 1996;30:55-61.
31. Brogden RN et al. Captopril. An update of its pharmacodynamic and pharmacokinetic properties, and therapeutic use in hypertension and congestive heart failure. *Drugs.* 1988;36:540-600.
32. Keane WF et al. Angiotensin converting enzyme inhibitors and progressive renal insufficiency; current experience and future directions. *Ann Intern Med.* 1989;111:503-516.
33. Cooper RA. Captopril-associated neutropenia: who is at risk? *Arch Intern Med.* 1983;143:659-660.
34. Chobanian AV, Bakris GL, Black HR, et al. and National High Blood Pressure Education Program Coordinating Committee. The seventh report of the Joint National Committee on Prevention, Detection, Evaluation, and Treatment of High Blood Pressure. Complete report. Bethesda, MD: National Institutes of Health; 2004. http://www.nhlbi.nih.gov/guidelines/hypertension/jnc7full.htm Accessed December 16, 2008.

35. CONSENSUS Trial Study Group. Effects of enalapril on mortality in severe congestive heart failure. *N Engl J Med.* 1987;316:1430-1435.
36. The Heart Outcomes Prevention Evaluation Study Investigators. Effects of an angiotensin-converting enzyme inhibitor, ramipril, on cardiovascular events in high-risk patients. *N Engl J Med.* 2000;342:145-153.
37. EURopean trial on reduction of cardiac events with Perindopril in stable coronary artery disease investigators: efficacy of perindopril in reduction of cardiovascular events among patients with stable coronary artery disease: randomized, double-blind, placebo-controlled, multicentre trial (the EUROPA study). *Lancet.* 2003; 362:782-788.
38. The PEACE Trial Investigators. Angiotensin-converting-enzyme inhibition in stable coronary artery disease. *N Engl J Med.* 2004;351:2058-2068.
39. Murphy MB, Elliott WJ. Dopamine and dopamine receptor agonists in cardiovascular therapy. *Crit Care Med.* 1990;18:S14-S18.
40. Brogden RN, Markham A. Fenoldopam. *Drugs.* 1997;54:634-650.
41. White WB, Halley SE. Comparative renal effects of intravenous administration of fenoldopam mesylate and sodium nitroprusside in patients with severe hypertension. *Arch Intern Med.* 1989;149:870-874.
42. Allison NL et al. The effect of fenoldopam, a dopaminergic agonist, on renal hemodynamics. *Clin Pharmacol Ther.* 1987;41:282-288.
43. Everitt DE et al. Effect of intravenous fenoldopam on intraocular pressure in ocular hypertension. *J Clin Pharmacol.* 1997;37:312-320.
44. Pilmer BL et al. Fenoldopam mesylate versus sodium nitroprusside in the acute management of severe systemic hypertension. *J Clin Pharmacol.* 1993;33:549-553.
45. Bednarczyk EM et al. Comparative acute blood pressure reduction from intravenous fenoldopam mesylate versus sodium nitroprusside in severe systemic hypertension. *Am J Cardiol.* 1989;63:993-996.
46. Reisin E et al. Intravenous fenoldopam versus sodium nitroprusside in patients with severe hypertension. *Hypertension.* 1990;15(suppl I):I-59-I-62.
47. Mulrow JP, Crawford MH. Clinical pharmacokinetics and therapeutic use of hydralazine in congestive heart failure. *Clin Pharmacokinet.* 1989;16.86-99.
48. O'Malley K et al. Duration of hydralazine action in hypertension. *Clin Pharmacol Ther.* 1975;18:581-586.
49. Cameron HA, Ramsay LE. The lupus syndrome induced by hydralazine: a common complication with low-dose treatment. *Br Med J.* 1984;289:410-412.
50. Shapiro KS et al. Immune complex glomerulonephritis in hydralazine-induced SLE. *Am J Kidney Dis.* 1984;3:270-274.
51. Goa KL et al. Labetalol: a reappraisal of its pharmacology, pharmacokinetics and therapeutic use in hypertension and ischaemic heart disease. *Drugs.* 1989;37:583-627.
52. MacCarthy EP, Bloomfield SS. Labetalol: a review of its pharmacology, pharmacokinetics, clinical uses and adverse effects. *Pharmacotherapy.* 1983;3:193-219.
53. Deinchman TE et al. Intravenously administered labetalol for treatment of hypertension in children. *J Pediatr.* 1992;120:140-144.
54. McNeil JJ, Louis WJ. Clinical pharmacokinetics of labetalol. *Clin Pharmacokinet.* 1984;9:157-167.
55. Oliverio MI, Coffman TM. Angiotensin-II receptors: new targets for antihypertensive therapy. *Clin Cardiol.* 1997;20:3-6.
56. Weber MA et al. Blood pressure effects of the angiotensin II receptor blocker, losartan. *Arch Intern Med.* 1995;115:405-411.
57. Abdelwahab W et al. Management of hypertensive urgencies and emergencies. *J Clin Pharmacol.* 1995;35:747-762.
58. Timmermans PBMWM et al. Angiotensin II receptors and angiotensin II receptor antagonists. *Pharmacol Rev.* 1993;45:205-251.
59. Csajka C et al. Pharmacokinetic-pharmacodynamic profile of angiotensin II receptor antagonists. *Clin Pharmacokinet.* 1997;32:1-29.
60. Gavras HP, Salerno CM. The angiotensin II type I receptor blocker losartan in clinical practice: a review. *Clin Ther.* 1996;18:1058-1067.
61. Ellis ML, Patterson JH. A new class of antihypertensive therapy: angiotensin II receptor antagonists. *Pharmacotherapy.* 1996:16:849-860.
62. Benz J et al. Valsartan, a new angiotensin II receptor antagonist: a double-blind study comparing the incidence of cough with lisinopril and hydrochlorothiazide. *J Clin Pharmacol.* 1997;37:101-107.
63. Lacourcière Y et al. Effects of modulators of the renin-angiotensin-aldosterone system on cough. *J Hypertens.* 1994;12:1387-1393.
64. Crozier I et al. Losartan in heart failure. Hemodynamic effects and tolerability. *Circulation.* 1995;91:691-697.
65. Pitt B et al. Effect of losartan compared with captopril on mortality in patients with symptomatic heart failure— the Losartan Heart Failure Survival Study ELITE II. *Lancet.* 2000;355:1582-1587.

66. The ONTARGET Investigators. Telmisartan, ramipril, or both in patients at high risk for vascular events. *N Engl J Med*. 2008;358:1547-1559.

67. Myhre E et al. Clinical pharmacokinetics of methyldopa. *Clin Pharmacokinet*. 1982;7:221-233.

68. Oates JA. Antihypertensive agents and drug therapy of hypertension. In: Hardman JG et al., eds. *Goodman and Gilman's the pharmacological basis of therapeutics*. 9th ed. New York: McGraw-Hill; 1996:780-808.

69. Fleishaker JC et al. The pharmacokinetics of 2.5 to 10 mg oral doses of minoxidil in healthy volunteers. *J Clin Pharmacol*. 1989;29:162-167.

70. Vesey CJ, Cole PV. Blood cyanide and thiocyanate concentrations produced by long-term therapy with sodium nitroprusside. *Br J Anaesth*. 1985;57:148-155.

71. Schultz V et al. Kinetics of elimination of thiocyanate in 7 healthy subjects and in 8 subjects with renal failure. *Klin Wochenschr*. 1979;57:243-247.

72. Cottrell JE et al. Prevention of nitroprusside induced cyanide toxicity with hydroxocobalamin. *N Engl J Med*. 1978;298:809-811.

73. Pasch TH et al. Nitroprusside-induced formation of cyanide and its detoxification with thiosulphate during deliberate hypotension. *J Cardiovasc Pharmacol*. 1983;5:77-82.

74. Stumpf JL. Drug therapy of hypertensive crises. *Clin Pharm*. 1988;7:582-591.

75. Hirschl MM. Guidelines for the drug treatment of hypertensive crisis. *Drugs*. 1995;50:991-1000.

β-Adrenergic Blocking Drugs

Sachin A. Shah

ESMOLOL HYDROCHLORIDE
Brevibloc

Pharmacology. Esmolol is an ultrashort-acting, cardioselective, β1-adrenergic blocking agent. It is effective in controlling ventricular response in patients with atrial fibrillation and other supraventricular tachycardias and in slowing heart rate in patients with sinus tachycardia associated with acute MI or cardiac surgery. Esmolol is useful for treating hypertensive emergencies, particularly in patients with tachycardia, because it has a rapid onset, short duration of action, and reduces heart rate. It also can be effective in perioperative hypertension.[1-4]

Adult Dosage. Dilute injection to a final concentration of 10 mg/mL. IV loading dose is 500 μg/kg/min for 1 min and then 50 μg/kg/min. The IV loading dose can be repeated as often as q5min, with a concomitant increase of infusion rate in 50 μg/kg/min increments, titrated to ventricular response, heart rate, and/or blood pressure. Most patients respond to infusions of 100–200 μg/kg/min. Once the desired endpoint is obtained, the infusion rate can be decreased in 25–50 μg/kg/min increments at 5- to 10-min intervals. Infusions up to 48 h are well tolerated.

Pediatric Dosage. IV 500 μg/kg/min for 1 min and then 25–200 (average 120) μg/kg/min.[4] Weight-adjusted dosages can be higher than in adults because of its more rapid elimination in children; infusion rates as high as 1 mg/kg/min have been required to achieve complete β blockade.[5]

Dosage Forms. Inj 10, 20, 250 mg/mL.

Pharmacokinetics. Effective plasma levels are about 1–1.5 mg/L (3.4–5.1 mol/L). The α half-life is about 2 min; V_d averages 3.5 L/kg (range 2–5). Esmolol is rapidly hydrolyzed by plasma and blood esterases to a metabolite with weak, clinically unimportant β-blocking activity and small amounts of methanol. No unchanged esmolol.[3,4]

Adverse Reactions. The side effect profile is similar to that of other β1-selective β-blockers. Dose-related hypotension is frequent; IV site phlebitis occurs occasionally. Concurrent IV morphine can increase serum levels by 46%.

PROPRANOLOL HYDROCHLORIDE
Inderal, Various

Pharmacology. Propranolol is a nonselective β-adrenergic blocker used in arrhythmias, hypertension, angina pectoris, and CHF. It is also effective in decreasing post-MI mortality. The antiarrhythmic mechanism is caused by decreased AV nodal conduction in supraventricular tachycardias and blockade of catecholamine-induced dysrhythmias. Propranolol and other β-blockers are effective in preventing postoperative atrial fibrillation. The antihypertensive mechanism is unknown, but contributing factors are a CNS mechanism, renin blockade, and decreases in myocardial contractility and cardiac output. Propranolol also lowers myocardial oxygen demand by decreasing contractility and heart rate, which symptomatically alleviates anginal pain and increases exercise tolerance in coronary artery disease. **Metoprolol** and **carvedilol** (and perhaps other β-blockers) are effective in reducing mortality and improving quality of life in patients with CHF by blocking deleterious neurohumoral compensatory factors. β-blockers and diuretics are recommended as first-line drugs for hypertension because of demonstrated reductions in morbidity and mortality.[1] (*See* β-Adrenergic Blocking Drugs Comparison Chart.)

Administration and Adult Dosage. PO—10–20 mg q6h initially, increasing gradually to desired effects. In hypertension, more than 1 g/d has been used; however, consider adding another drug if 480 mg/d is ineffective. In angina pectoris, the dosage is titrated to pain relief and exercise evidence of β-blockade (bradycardia). The endpoint for dosage escalation in acute arrhythmias is the return to sinus rhythm or, in atrial fibrillation or flutter, to a ventricular rate below 100 beats/min with hemodynamic stability. Twice-daily administration is effective in angina pectoris and hypertension. Administer **SR Cap** in the same daily dosage once or twice daily (not indicated post-MI). **PO for post-MI prophylaxis (non-SR)**—180–240 mg/d in 2–3 divided doses. **IV slow push**—1 mg q5min, to a maximum of 0.15 mg/kg; some investigators have recommended that the first dose be given over 2–10 min.

Special Populations. *Pediatric Dosage.* PO for hypertension—0.5–1 mg/kg/d in 2–4 divided doses, increasing to a maximum of 8 mg/kg/d. **IV slow push**—0.01–0.1 mg/kg/dose over 10 min up to 1 mg (infants) or 3 mg (children); may repeat in 6–8 h.[6]

Geriatric Dosage. Bioavailability is increased in the elderly, necessitating lower initial doses.

Other Conditions. Therapeutic endpoints can be achieved with lower dosages in hypothyroidism or liver disease. Begin with lower dosages and titrate to clinical response. Patients with thyrotoxicosis require higher dosages to achieve the desired effect.[7]

Dosage Forms. Soln 4, 8, 80 mg/mL; **Tab** 10, 20, 40, 60, 80, 90 mg; **SR Cap** 60, 80, 120, 160 mg; **Inj** 1 mg/mL.

Patient Instructions. Report any symptoms such as shortness of breath, swelling, wheezing, fatigue, depression, nightmares, or inability to concentrate. Do not stop therapy abruptly. Do not crush or chew SR capsule. A sustained-release capsule core in the stool does not indicate lack of absorption.

Missed Doses. Take this drug at regular intervals. If you miss a dose take it as soon as you remember. If it is about time for the next dose, take that dose only. Leave at least 4 h between regular tablet doses and 6–8 h between extended-release capsule doses. Do not double the dose or take extra.

Pharmacokinetics. *Onset and Duration.* PO onset is variable; the duration varies from 6 to longer than 12 hours.[7]

Serum Levels. No definite relation has been established between serum concentrations and therapeutic effect in the treatment of arrhythmias, angina pectoris, or hypertension. β-blockade is associated with serum concentrations >100 μg/L (340 nmol/L).[8]

Fate. Propranolol is rapidly and completely absorbed after oral administration; however, a large hepatic first-pass effect occurs, limiting systemic availability to $26 \pm 10\%$. First-pass elimination is saturable with an oral dose greater than about 30 mg.[8] The drug is $87 \pm 6\%$ bound to α_1-acid glycoprotein and other plasma proteins.[7,9] V_d is 4.3 ± 0.6 L/kg; Cl is 0.96 ± 0.3 L/h/kg. Unlike most other drugs, displacement from plasma proteins increases elimination half-life and V_d because of high tissue affinity (nonrestrictive elimination). An active metabolite, 4-hydroxypropranolol, is formed after oral, but not IV, administration. Less than 0.5% of a dose is excreted, unchanged in urine.[9]

$t_{1/2}$. About 10 min;[7] β-phase after a single PO dose is 3.9 ± 0.4 h.[9] With long-term oral therapy, β-phase is 4–6 h but can be as long as 10–20 h in patients with liver disease.[10]

Adverse Reactions. Adverse effects often are not related to dose. Depression, nightmares, insomnia, fatigue, and lethargy occur frequently; less often, psychotic changes have been reported. CNS side effects probably occur more often with the lipophilic β-blockers (e.g., propranolol). The drug can cause occasional life-threatening reactions when therapy (especially IV) is initiated, and acute CHF with pulmonary edema and hypotension or symptomatic bradycardia and heart block can occur. Acute drug cessation in patients with coronary artery disease can precipitate unstable angina pectoris or MI. The drug can precipitate hypoglycemia, but probably more important in diabetics is its ability to mask hypoglycemic symptoms (except for sweating). It can exacerbate symptoms of peripheral vascular disease or Raynaud's disease. β-blockers can exacerbate previously stable asthma or chronic airway obstruction by causing bronchospasm or renal dysfunction by further depressing GFR.

Contraindications. Severe obstructive pulmonary disease, asthma or active allergic rhinitis; cardiogenic shock or severe CHF; second- or third-degree heart block; severe sinus node disease.

Precautions. In coronary artery disease, discontinue drug by tapering the dosage over 4–7 days. Use cautiously in patients with Prinzmetal's vasospastic angina to prevent worsening of chest pain. Use caution in peripheral vascular disease or CHF and in patients with brittle diabetes or history of hypoglycemic episodes. Can worsen atrial fibrillation associated with accessory AV pathway.

Drug Interactions. Concurrent digoxin therapy can lessen the β-blocker exacerbation of CHF. When taken with oral hypoglycemics, nonselective β-blockers such as propranolol prolong hypoglycemic episodes and inhibit tachycardia and tremors, which are signs of hypoglycemia (sweating is not inhibited); hypertension can occur during hypoglycemia. Epinephrine can produce hypertensive reactions in patients on propranolol (and probably other nonselective β-blockers); this can occur with other sympathomimetics such as phenylephrine and phenylpropanolamine. Barbiturates and rifampin can increase the metabolism of hepatically eliminated β-blockers such as propranolol. Cimetidine can increase propranolol effects. Combined use of clonidine and propranolol can result in *hyper*tensive reactions, especially if clonidine is abruptly discontinued. β-blockers can increase the first-dose hypotensive effect of prazosin and similar drugs. NSAIDs can blunt the hypotensive response of β-blockers.

Parameters to Monitor. During IV administration, obtain blood pressure and pulse every 5 minutes with constant ECG monitoring for signs of AV nodal block (lengthened PR interval) or bradycardia. Evaluate vital signs routinely for hemodynamic endpoints (e.g., blood pressure in hypertension and heart rate or pressure–rate product in angina pectoris). Question the patient about subjective complaints such as nightmares or fatigue. When a patient at risk for adverse reactions is first given propranolol, evaluate signs and symptoms of toxicity (e.g., CHF, shortness of breath or edema; bronchospasm, wheezing, or shortness of breath; diabetes, bloodglucose; peripheral vascular disease, painful, or cold extremities).

Notes. Propranolol can be beneficial for treatment of symptomatic hypertrophic obstructive cardiomyopathy by increasing end-diastolic volume, producing ventricular relaxation, and relieving ventricular outflow obstruction. Other uses include migraine prophylaxis, pheochromocytoma, essential tremor, prevention of GI bleeding in patients with esophageal varicies, prevention of sudden death in congenital long QT syndromes, and as a cardiac protectant in patients with heart disease undergoing noncardiac surgery. If a β-blocker must be used in lung disease, β_1-selective drugs (e.g., **acebutolol, atenolol,** or **metoprolol**) cause alterations in pulmonary function that are more easily reversed by bronchodilators; these drugs are probably a better choice than propranolol or other nonselective β-blockers. (*See* β-Adrenergic Blocking Drugs Comparison Chart.)

β-ADRENERGIC BLOCKING DRUGS COMPARISON CHART

DRUG	DOSAGE FORMS	CARDIO-SELECTIVITY	β HALF-LIFE (hr)	EXCRETED UNCHANGED IN URINE	PROTEIN BINDING	LABELED USES	STARTING DOSAGE	MAXIMUM DOSAGE
Acebutolol[a] Sectral Various	Cap 200, 400 mg.	+	3–4 (diacetolol) 8–13	30%–40%	25%	Hypertension, arrhythmias.	PO 400 mg/d.	PO 1.2 g/d.
Atenolol Tenormin Various	Tab 25, 50, 100 mg Inj 0.5 mg/mL.	+ (up to 100 mg)	6–7	85%	10%	Hypertension, angina pectoris, acute MI.	PO 50 mg/d, IV 5 mg × 2, then PO 100 mg/d.	PO 200 mg/d.
Betaxolol Kerlone	Tab 10, 20 mg.	+	14–20	15%	50%	Hypertension.	PO 10 mg/d.	PO 40 mg/d.
Bisoprolol Zebeta	Tab 5, 10 mg.	+	9–12	50%	30%	Hypertension.	PO 2.5–5 mg/d.	PO 20 mg/d.
Carteolol[a] Cartrol	Tab 2.5, 5 mg.	0	6–11	15%	30%	Hypertension.	PO 2.5 mg/d.	PO 10 mg/d.
Carvedilol[b] Coreg Coreg CR Various	Tab 3.125, 6.25, 12.5, 25 mg. SR Cap 10, 20, 40, 80 mg.	0	6–8	?%	95%	Hypertension, CHF, post-MI (LVEF ≤40) prophylaxis.	PO 3.125 mg bid. PO 10 mg qd (increasing q2wk) *Refer* to monograph for IR to SR switch.	PO (<85 kg) 50 mg/d; (>85 kg) 100 mg/d. SR PO 80 mg/d.
Esmolol Brevibloc	Inj 10, 20, 250 mg/mL.	+	9 min	0%	55%	Supraventricular tachycardia, intra- and postoperative HTN or tachycardia.	500 µg/kg load, then IV 50 µg/kg/min.	IV 200 µg/kg/min.

(continued)

459

β-ADRENERGIC BLOCKING DRUGS COMPARISON CHART (continued)

DRUG	DOSAGE FORMS	CARDIO-SELECTIVITY	β HALF-LIFE (hr)	EXCRETED UNCHANGED IN URINE	PROTEIN BINDING	LABELED USES	STARTING DOSAGE	MAXIMUM DOSAGE
Labetalol[b] Trandate Normodyne Various	Tab 100, 200, 300 mg Inj 5 mg/mL.	0	4–9	5%	50%	Hypertension.	PO 200 mg/d. IV 20 mg, then 40–80 mg q10min.	PO 2.4 g/d. IV 300 mg.
Metoprolol Lopressor Toprol-XL	Tab 25, 50, 100 mg SR Tab 25, 50, 100, 200 mg Inj 1 mg/mL.	+ (≤100 mg)	3–7	39%	10%	Hypertension, angina pectoris, acute MI, CHF (Toprol-XL).	PO 100 mg/d. PO SR 50–100 mg/d. IV 5 mg × 3, then PO 50 mg q6h × 48 h. PO SR 12.5–25 mg/d.	PO 450 mg/day. PO SR 400 mg/day. PO SR 200 mg/d (CHF)
Nebivolol Bystolic	Tab 2.5, 5, 10 mg	+ (≤10 mg)	10–12	38%	98%	Hypertension.	PO 5 mg/d	PO 40 mg/d
Nadolol Corgard Various	Tab 20, 40, 80, 120, 160 mg.	0	17–24	70%	25%	Hypertension, angina pectoris.	PO 40 mg/d.	PO 320 mg/d.
Penbutolol[a] Levatol	Tab 20 mg.	0	4–8	5%	80%–90%	Hypertension.	PO 20 mg/d.	PO 80 mg/d.
Pindolol[a] Visken	Tab 5, 10 mg.	0	3–4	40%	57%	Hypertension.	PO 10 mg/d.	PO 60 mg/d.

(continued)

β-ADRENERGIC BLOCKING DRUGS COMPARISON CHART (*continued*)

DRUG	DOSAGE FORMS	CARDIO-SELECTIVITY	β HALF-LIFE (hr)	EXCRETED UNCHANGED IN URINE	PROTEIN BINDING	LABELED USES	STARTING DOSAGE	MAXIMUM DOSAGE
Propranolol Inderal Inderal LA Various	(*Refer to* monograph.)	0	4–6	<0.5%	87%	Hypertension, angina pectoris, arrhythmias, post-MI prophylaxis. (*Refer to* monograph)	PO 40–180 mg/d. PO CR 80 mg/d. (*Refer to* monograph)	PO 640 mg/d. (*Refer to* monograph)
Sotalol[c] Betapace Betapace AF	Tab 80, 120, 160, 240 mg	0	7–15	80–90%	0%	Arrhythmias.	PO 160 mg/d.	PO 640 mg/d.
Timolol[b] Blocadren	Tab 5, 10, 20 mg.	0	4–6	20%	<10%	Hypertension, post-MI prophylaxis, migraine prophylaxis.	PO 20 mg/d.	PO 60 mg/d.

[a]Acebutolol, carteolol, penbutolol, and pindolol have intrinsic agonist (sympathomimetic) activity (ISA).
[b]Carvedilol has α₁-blocking actions. Labetalol has potent α₁-blocking actions (ratio of α- to β-blockade 1:3 and 1:7 with PO and IV, respectively).
[c]Sotalol also has type III antiarrhythmic properties.
From Refs. 3 and 11–17 and product information.

■ REFERENCES

1. Joint National Committee on Prevention, Detection, Evaluation, and Treatment of High Blood Pressure. The sixth report of the Joint National Committee on prevention, detection, evaluation, and treatment of high blood pressure. *Arch Intern Med.* 1997;157:2413-2446.

2. Abdelwahab W et al. Management of hypertensive urgencies and emergencies. *J Clin Pharmacol.* 1995;35: 747-762.

3. Angaran DM et al. Esmolol hydrochloride: an ultrashort-acting β-adrenergic blocking agent. *Clin Pharm.* 1986;5:288-303.

4. Cuneo BF et al. Pharmacodynamics and pharmacokinetics of esmolol, a short-acting β-blocking agent, in children. *Pediatr Cardiol.* 1994;15:296-301.

5. Trippel DL et al. Cardiovascular and antiarrhythmic effects of esmolol in children. *J Pediatr.* 1991;119(1, pt 1): 142-147.

6. Siberry GK, Iannone R, eds. *The Harriet Lane Handbook.* 15th ed. St. Louis, MO: Mosby; 2000.

7. Routledge PA, Shand DG. Clinical pharmacokinetics of propranolol. *Clin Pharmacokinet.* 1979;4:73-90.

8. Nies AS, Shand DG. Clinical pharmacology of propranolol. *Circulation.* 1975;52:6-15.

9. Benet LZ et al. Design and optimization of dosage regimens; pharmacokinetic data. In: Hardman JG et al., eds. *Goodman and Gilman's the pharmacological basis of therapeutics.* 9th ed. New York, NY: McGraw-Hill; 1996:1707-1792.

10. Johnsson G, Regardh CG. Clinical pharmacokinetics of β-adrenoreceptor blocking drugs. *Clin Pharmacokinet.* 1976;1:233-263.

11. Nappi JM, McCollam PL. Sotalol: a breakthrough antiarrhythmic? *Ann Pharmacother.* 1993;27:1359-1368.

12. McTavish D et al. Carvedilol. A review of its pharmacodynamic and pharmacokinetic properties, and therapeutic efficacy. *Drugs.* 1993;45:232-258.

13. MacCarthy EP, Bloomfield SS. Labetalol. A review of its pharmacology, pharmacokinetics, clinical uses and adverse effects. *Pharmacotherapy.* 1983;3:193-219.

14. Ryan JR. Clinical pharmacology of acebutolol. *Am Heart J.* 1985;109:1131-1136.

15. Frishman WH, Covey S. Penbutolol and carteolol: two new beta-adrenergic blockers with partial agonism. *J Clin Pharmacol.* 1990;30:412-421.

16. Frishman WH et al. Bevantolol. A preliminary review of its pharmacodynamic and pharmacokinetic properties, and therapeutic efficacy in hypertension and angina pectoris. *Drugs.* 1988;35:1-21.

17. Lancaster SG, Sorkin EM. Bisoprolol. A preliminary review of its pharmacodynamic and pharmacokinetic properties, therapeutic efficacy in hypertension and angina pectoris. *Drugs.* 1988;36:256-285.

Chapter 33

Calcium Channel Blocking Drugs

Sachin A. Shah

DILTIAZEM HYDROCHLORIDE Cardizem, Dilacor XR, Tiazac, Various

Pharmacology. Diltiazem is a calcium channel blocking drug that decreases heart rate, prolongs AV nodal conduction, and decreases arteriolar and coronary vascular tone. It also has negative inotropic properties. Diltiazem is effective in symptomatic angina pectoris, essential hypertension, and supraventricular tachycardias. It also can reduce early reinfarction rates in patients with non–Q-wave MI and normal left ventricular functions. (*See* Calcium Channel Blocking Drugs Comparison Chart.)

Administration and Adult Dosage. **IV loading dose**—0.25 mg/kg (approximately 20 mg) over 2 min; can repeat in 15 min with 0.35 mg/kg (approximately 25 mg). **IV infusion**—5–15 mg/h, titrated to ventricular response. **PO for angina**—30–60 mg q6–8h initially; dosages up to 480 mg/d may be required for symptomatic relief of angina;[1,2] 180–300 mg once daily with Cardizem CD. **PO for hypertension**—120–240 mg/d initially in 2 divided doses using Cardizem SR, or 180–300 mg once daily using Cardizem CD or Dilacor XR, titrated to clinical response; **maintenance dosages**—180–480 mg/d are usually necessary.

Special Populations. *Pediatric Dosage.* Safety and efficacy are not established. **PO**—1.5–2 mg/kg/d in 3–4 divided daily doses up to a maximum of 3.5 mg/kg/d.[3]

Geriatric Dosage. Same as adult dosage but titrate dosage slowly.

Other Conditions. Patients with liver disease may require lower dosages; titrate to clinical response.

Dosage Forms. **Tab** 30, 60, 90, 120 mg; **SR Cap** (12 h; Cardizem SR, various)—60, 90, 120 mg; **SR Cap** (24 h; Cardizem CD)—120, 180, 240, 300 mg; (24 h; Dilacor XR)—120, 180, 240 mg; (24 h; Tiazac)—120, 180, 240, 300, 360 mg; **SR Tab** (Tiamate);—120, 180, 240 mg; **Inj**—5 mg/mL; **SR Tab** (Teczem)—180 mg with enalapril 5 mg.

Patient Instructions. Report dizziness, leg swelling, or shortness of breath. (For angina) maintain a diary to document the number of episodes of chest pain and sublingual (SL) nitroglycerin tablets used.

Missed Doses. Take this drug at regular intervals. If you miss a dose, take it as soon as you remember. If it is about time for the next dose, take that dose only. Do not double the dose or take extra.

Pharmacokinetics. *Onset and Duration.* PO onset 0.5–3 h, duration 6–10 h;[4] 12–24 h with SR cap, depending on the product.

Serum Levels. To cause hemodynamic changes levels >95 μg/L (230 nmol/L) are necessary, but their clinical usefulness is questionable.[5] Levels of desacetyldiltiazem are similar to those of diltiazem.[6]

Fate. Oral bioavailability is 38 ± 11% with the first dose and 90 ± 21% with long-term therapy.[6] The drug is 78 ± 3% bound to plasma proteins; V_d is 5.3 ± 1.7 L/kg;[6] CL is 0.72 ± 0.3 L/h/kg.[7] Enterohepatic recycling occurs. The drug is almost entirely metabolized by the liver, with only 1%–3% excreted unchanged in urine. One metabolite, desacetyldiltiazem, has 40%–50% the activity of diltiazem. Metabolites are excreted primarily in the feces.

$t_{1/2}$. α-phase 2–5 min; β-phase 4.9 ± 0.4 h,[4,6] longer in the elderly.[2] β-phase (desacetyldiltiazem) 6.1 ± 1.2 h.[6]

Adverse Reactions. Frequency of side effects is dose related. Headache, flushing, dizziness, and edema occur frequently. Sinus bradycardia and AV block occur frequently, often in association with concomitant β-blockers.[2] CHF can worsen in patients with underlying left ventricular dysfunction. A variety of skin reactions have been occasionally reported.[2] Hepatitis occurs rarely.

Contraindications. Second- or third-degree block or sick sinus syndrome without a ventricular pacemaker; symptomatic hypotension or severe CHF, acute MI, or pulmonary congestion; atrial fibrillation with accessory AV pathway.

Precautions. Use caution with concomitant use of β-blockers in patients with underlying CHF, especially those with poor left ventricular function.[2]

Drug Interactions. Cimetidine and propranolol increase diltiazem serum levels.[2] Diltiazem inhibits CYP3A4 and the metabolism of many drugs, including carbamazepine, cyclosporine, and theophylline.[2] It also inhibits P-glycoprotein.[8]

Parameters to Monitor. Monitor blood pressure, heart rate, and ECG, especially when initiating therapy. Watch for symptoms of hypotension and CHF. Serial treadmill exercise tests can assess efficacy in angina. Monitor the number of episodes of chest pain and SL nitroglycerin used.

NIFEDIPINE
Adalat, Procardia, Various

Pharmacology. Nifedipine is a dihydropyridine calcium channel blocking drug with potent arterial and coronary vasodilating properties. A reflex increase in sympathetic tone (in response to vasodilation) counteracts the direct depressant effects on SA and AV nodal conduction. This renders nifedipine ineffective in the treatment of supraventricular tachycardias. It is used for vasospastic and chronic stable angina and in the treatment of hypertension. (*See* Calcium Channel Blocking Drugs Comparison Chart.)

Administration and Adult Dosage. **PO for angina** (Cap)—10 mg tid initially, increasing to a usual maximum of 20–30 mg tid or qid; dosages above 180 mg/d are not recommended. **PO for hypertension** (SR Tab only)—30–60 mg/d initially, increasing up to 120 mg/d prn. **PO for severe hypertension** (non-SR)—10 mg, may repeat prn in 20 min. The capsule can be punctured or bitten and swallowed, usually resulting in a more rapid onset than SL administration.[9]

Special Populations. *Pediatric Dosage.* Safety and efficacy not established. **PO for hypertensive crisis**—0.25–0.5 mg/kg q4–6h.[3]

Geriatric Dosage. Same as adult dosage.

Other Conditions. Patients with liver disease might require lower dosages;[10] titrate to clinical response.

Dosage Forms. Cap 10, 20 mg; **SR Tab** 30, 60, 90 mg.

Patient Instructions. Report flushing, edema, dizziness, or increased frequency of chest discomfort. Do not split, chew, or crush sustained-release tablets. A sustained-release tablet core in the stool does not indicate lack of absorption. Maintain a diary to document the number of episodes of chest pain and SL nitroglycerin tablets used.

Missed Doses. Take this drug at regular intervals. If you miss a dose, take it as soon as you remember. If it is about time for the next dose, take that dose only. Do not double the dose or take extra.

Pharmacokinetics. *Onset and Duration.* PO onset 0.5–2 h; duration (Cap) 4–8 h, (SR Tab) 12–24 h. PO (punctured capsule) onset 10–20 min, duration 3–4 h.

Serum Levels. (Therapeutic) >90 μg/L (260 nmol/L), although clinical utility is questionable.[11]

Fate. Bioavailability is 52 ± 37% in normals and 91 ± 26% in cirrhosis because of extensive and variable first-pass hepatic elimination.[10] It is 96 ± 1% bound to plasma proteins; V_d is 0.8 ± 0.2 L/kg;[11,12] Cl is 0.42 ± 0.12 L/h/kg.[7] Nifedipine is almost entirely eliminated by hepatic metabolism via the CYP3A4 isozyme, which is present in variable amounts (but is not a true polymorphism).[13] Only traces of drug are excreted unchanged in urine.[11]

$t_{1/2}$. α-phase 4–7 min; β-phase 2 ± 0.4 h.[11,12]

Adverse Reactions. Most side effects relate to vasodilatory actions and occur frequently; symptoms include dizziness (with or without hypotension), flushing, and headache. These types of side effects seem less frequent with SR dosage forms.[14] Avoid long-term treatment of hypertension with immediate-release products because they can increase mortality.[15,16] Edema occurs frequently and is related to venous pooling and usually not exacerbation of CHF. Nifedipine paradoxically can worsen anginal chest pain, possibly because of a reflex increase in sympathetic tone or redistribution of coronary blood flow away from ischemic areas. Acute, reversible renal failure can occur in patients with chronic renal insufficiency;[17] rare reactions include hepatitis and hyperglycemia.

Contraindications. Symptomatic hypotension.

Precautions. Use with caution in unstable angina pectoris when used alone (i.e., without a β-blocker) and in patients with CHF (caused by systolic dysfunction) because mortality can be increased.[16,18] Do not use immediate-release products to treat hypertension. Nifedipine has an antiplatelet action and can increase bleeding time.[19] Nifedipine can worsen symptoms of obstructive cardiomyopathy.

Drug Interactions. Barbiturates increase nifedipine metabolism. Cimetidine can increase nifedipine serum levels. Nifedipine occasionally increases PT in patients on oral anticoagulants. Nifedipine and IV magnesium sulfate can cause neuromuscular blockade and hypotension.

Parameters to Monitor. Monitor blood pressure and heart rate, especially when initiating therapy. Observe for symptoms of hypotension and edema. Serial treadmill exercise tests can assess efficacy.

Notes. Other potential uses for nifedipine are migraine prophylaxis, achalasia, and Raynaud's phenomenon.

VERAPAMIL HYDROCHLORIDE	Calan, Covera-HS, Isoptin, Verelan, Various

Pharmacology. Verapamil is a calcium channel blocking drug that prolongs AV nodal conduction. It is used to convert reentrant supraventricular tachycardias and slow ventricular rate in atrial fibrillation or flutter. Because it decreases contractility and arteriolar resistance, it is used in angina caused by coronary obstruction or vasospasm. Verapamil also is effective in the treatments of hypertension, hypertrophic obstructive cardiomyopathy, and migraine prophylaxis. (*See* Calcium Channel Blocking Drugs Comparison Chart.)

Administration and Adult Dosage. PO for angina—80–120 mg tid initially, increasing at daily (for unstable angina) or weekly intervals to a maximum of 480 mg/d. **PO for hypertension**—usually 240 mg/d using SR tablet; SR dosages of 120 mg/d to 240 mg bid have been used. Covera-HS is designed to be taken hs. **PO for migraine prophylaxis**—160–320 mg/d. **IV for supraventricular arrhythmias**—5–10 mg (0.075–0.15 mg/kg) over at least 2 min (3 min in elderly); can repeat with 10 mg (0.15 mg/kg) in 30 min if arrhythmia is not terminated or desired endpoint is not achieved. **IV constant infusion**—5–10 mg/h.[20]

Special Populations. *Pediatric Dosage.* PO 4–8 mg/kg/d in 3 divided doses. **IV** (<1 y) 0.1–0.2 mg/kg; (1–15 y) 0.1–0.3 mg/kg, to a maximum of 5 mg over 2–3 min.[3]

Geriatric Dosage. Same as adult dosage but administer over 3 min.

Other Conditions. Dosage might need to be decreased in patients with liver disease; titrate to clinical response.

Dosage Forms. Tab 40, 80, 120 mg; **SR Tab** 120, 180, 240 mg; **SR Cap** 100, 120, 180, 200, 240, 300 mg; **Inj** 2.5 mg/mL; **SR Tab** 180 mg with trandolapril 2 mg, 240 mg with trandolapril 1, 4 mg (Tarka).

Patient Instructions. Report any dizziness, shortness of breath, or edema. Constipation occurs often. Maintain a diary to document the number of episodes of chest pain and SL nitroglycerin tablets used.

Missed Doses. Take this drug at regular intervals. If you miss a dose, take it as soon as you remember. If it is about time for the next dose, take that dose only. Do not double the dose or take extra.

Pharmacokinetics. *Onset and Duration.* IV onset immediate, duration 2–6 h; up to 12 h with long-term use.[21]

Serum Levels. 50–400 μg/L (100–800 nmol/L), although therapeutic range is not well established.

Fate. Although the drug is well absorbed orally, only 22 ± 8% is bioavailable because of extensive first-pass elimination; bioavailability increases in liver disease.[22] Covera-HS provides a 4- to 5-h delay before releasing the drug. Verapamil has stereospecific pharmacology and pharmacokinetics; L-verapamil is a more potent AV nodal blocking drug, but it undergoes greater first-pass metabolism.[23] Norverapamil is an active metabolite. Verapamil is approximately 90 ± 2% bound to plasma proteins, with the more active L-isomer having a greater unbound fraction.[22,24] V_d is 5 ± 2 L/kg and increases in liver disease;[7,22] Cl is 0.9 ± 0.36 L/h/kg. Approximately 1% is excreted unchanged in urine.[7]

$t_{1/2}$. (Verapamil) α-phase 5–30 min; β-phase 4 ± 1.5 h; can increase during long-term use; 13.6 ± 3.9 h in severe liver disease; (norverapamil) 8 ± 1.9 h.[7,22,24]

Adverse Reactions. Constipation occurs frequently (5%–40%), particularly in elderly patients. CHF can occur in patients with left ventricular dysfunction. Serious hemodynamic side effects (e.g., severe hypotension) and conduction abnormalities (e.g., symptomatic bradycardia or asystole) have been reported; these reactions usually occur when the patient is concurrently receiving a β-blocker or has underlying conduction disease.[25] Infants appear to be particularly susceptible to arrhythmias. IV **calcium** (gluconate or chloride salts, 10–20 mL of a 10% solution) and/or **isoproterenol** can, in part, reverse these adverse effects.[25] The administration of IV calcium before verapamil can prevent hypotension without abolishing the antiarrhythmic actions.[26]

Contraindications. Shock or severely hypotensive states; second- or third-degree AV nodal block; sick sinus syndrome, unless functioning ventricular pacemaker is in place; hypotension or CHF unless caused by supraventricular tachyarrhythmias amenable to verapamil therapy; atrial fibrillation and an accessory AV pathway.

Precautions. Use caution with any wide-QRS tachycardia; severe hypotension and shock can ensue if the tachycardia is ventricular in origin. Use with caution in combination with oral β-blockers and poor left ventricular function.

Drug Interactions. Verapamil can increase serum levels of several drugs, including carbamazepine, cyclosporine, digoxin (probably by inhibiting P-glycoprotein[8]), and theophylline. Barbiturates and rifampin can increase verapamil metabolism.

Parameters to Monitor. Monitor blood pressure and ECG continuously during IV administration. Pay particular attention to signs and symptoms of CHF and hypotension. Also, monitor the ECG for PR prolongation and bradycardia.

CALCIUM CHANNEL BLOCKING DRUGS COMPARISON CHART

DRUG	DOSAGE FORMS	ADULT DOSAGE	CONTRACTILITY	HEART RATE	AV NODAL CONDUCTION	VASCULAR RESISTANCE
Amlodipine[a] Norvasc AmVaz	Tab 2.5, 5, 10 mg.	PO for hypertension or angina 5–10 mg/d.	0	0	0	↓↓
Bepridil[b] Vascor	Tab 200, 300, 400 mg.	PO for refractory angina 200–400 mg/d.	0/↓	0/↓	0/↓	→
Clevidipine[c] Cleviprex	Vial 0.5 mg/ml	IV 1–2 mg/h	0/↑	0/↑	0/↑	↓↓
Diltiazem[d] Cardizem Dilacor XR	(See monograph.)	(See monograph.)	→	→	→	→
Felodipine[c] Plendil	SR Tab 2.5, 5, 10 mg.	PO for hypertension 2.5–20 mg once daily.	0/↑	0/↑	0/↑	↓↓
Isradipine[c] DynaCirc DynaCirc CR	Cap 2.5, 5 mg SR Tab 5, 10 mg.	PO for hypertension 2.5–10 mg bid or SR 5–10 mg once daily.	0/↑	0/↑	0/↑	↓↓
Nicardipine[c] Cardene Various	Cap 20, 30 mg SR Cap 30, 45, 60 mg Inj 2.5 mg/mL.	PO for angina or hypertension 20–40 mg tid or SR 30–60 mg q12h. IV for hypertension 5–15 mg/h.	0/↑	0/↑	0/↑	↓↓

(continued)

468 CALCIUM CHANNEL BLOCKING DRUGS COMPARISON CHART (*continued*)

DRUG	DOSAGE FORMS	ADULT DOSAGE	CONTRACTILITY	HEART RATE	AV NODAL CONDUCTION	VASCULAR RESISTANCE
Nifedipine[c] Adalat Procardia	Cap 10, 20 mg SR Tab 30, 60, 90 mg.	(*See* monograph.)	0/↑	0/↑	0/↑	↓↓
Nimodipine[c] Nimotop	Cap 30 mg.	PO postsubarachnoid hemorrhage 60 mg q4h for 21 d.	0/↑	0/↑	0/↑	↓↑
Nisoldipine[c] Sular	SR Tab 10, 20, 30, 40 mg.	PO for hypertension SR 20–40 mg once daily.	0/↑	0/↑	0/↑	↓↓
Verapamil[d] Calan Isoptin Verelan	(*See* monograph.)	(*See* monograph.)	↓↓	↓	↓↓	↓

↑, increase; ↓↓, marked decrease; ↓, decrease; 0, no change.

[a]Selective vascular actions.

[b]Complex pharmacology with probable sodium- and potassium-channel blockade (quinidinelike).

[c]Predominantly vascular actions.

[d]Vascular and electrophysiologic actions.

From Ref. 27 and product information.

■ REFERENCES

1. Petru MA et al. Long-term efficacy of high-dose diltiazem for chronic stable angina pectoris: 16-month serial studies with placebo controls. *Am Heart J.* 1985;109:99-103.

2. Markham A, Brogden RN. Diltiazem. A review of its pharmacology and therapeutic use in older patients. *Drugs Aging.* 1993;3:363-390.

3. Siberry GK, Iannone R, eds. *The Harriet Lane Handbook.* 15th ed. St. Louis, MO: Mosby; 2000.

4. Zelis RF, Kinney EL. The pharmacokinetics of diltiazem in healthy American men. *Am J Cardiol.* 1982;49:529-532.

5. Joyal M et al. Pharmacodynamic aspects of intravenous diltiazem administration. *Am Heart J.* 1986;111:54-60.

6. Smith MS et al. Pharmacokinetic and pharmacodynamic effects of diltiazem. *Am J Cardiol.* 1983;51:1369-1374.

7. Benet LZ et al. Design and optimization of dosage regimens; pharmacokinetic data. In: Hardman JG et al., eds. *Goodman and Gilman's the pharmacological basis of therapeutics.* 9th ed. New York, NY: McGraw-Hill; 1996:1707-1792.

8. Rodriguez I et al. P-glycoprotein in clinical cardiology. *Circulation.* 1999;99:472-474.

9. McAllister RG. Kinetics and dynamics of nifedipine after oral sublingual doses. *Am J Med.* 1986;81(suppl 6A):2-5.

10. Kleinbloesem CH et al. Nifedipine: kinetics and hemodynamic effects in patients with liver cirrhosis after intravenous and oral administration. *Clin Pharmacol Ther.* 1986;40:21-28.

11. Sorkin EM et al. Nifedipine. A review of its pharmacodynamic and pharmacokinetic properties, and therapeutic efficacy, in ischemic heart disease, hypertension and related cardiovascular disorders. *Drugs.* 1985;30:182-274.

12. Kleinbloesem CH et al. Nifedipine: kinetics and dynamics in healthy subjects. *Clin Pharmacol Ther.* 1984;36:742-749.

13. Breimer DD et al. Nifedipine: variability in its kinetics and metabolism in man. *Pharmacol Ther.* 1989;44:445-454.

14. Vetrovec GW et al. Comparative dosing and efficacy of continuous release nifedipine versus standard nifedipine for angina pectoris: clinical response, exercise performance and plasma nifedipine levels. *Am Heart J.* 1988;115:793-798.

15. Joint National Committee on Prevention, Detection, Evaluation, and Treatment of High Blood Pressure. The sixth report of the Joint National Committee on Prevention, Detection, Evaluation, and Treatment of High Blood Pressure. *Arch Intern Med.* 1997;157:2413-2446.

16. Opie LH. Calcium channel blockers for hypertension: dissecting the evidence for adverse effects. *Am J Hypertens.* 1997;10(5, pt 1):565-577.

17. Diamond JR et al. Nifedipine-induced renal dysfunction. Alterations in renal hemodynamics. *Am J Med.* 1984;77:905-909.

18. Elkayam U et al. A prospective, randomized, double-blind, crossover study to compare the efficacy and safety of chronic nifedipine therapy with that of isosorbide dinitrate and their combination in the treatment of chronic congestive heart failure. *Circulation.* 1990;82:1954-1961.

19. Dale J et al. The effects of nifedipine, a calcium antagonist, on platelet function. *Am Heart J.* 1983;105:103-105.

20. Barbarash RA et al. Verapamil infusions in the treatment of atrial tachyarrhythmias. *Crit Care Med.* 1986;14:886-888.

21. Schwartz JB et al. Prolongation of verapamil elimination kinetics during chronic oral administration. *Am Heart J.* 1982;104:198-203.

22. Hamann SR et al. Clinical pharmacokinetics of verapamil. *Clin Pharmacokinet.* 1984;9:26-41.

23. Hoon TJ et al. The pharmacodynamic and pharmacokinetic differences of the D- and L-isomers of verapamil: implications in the treatment of paroxysmal supraventricular tachycardia. *Am Heart J.* 1986;112:396-403.

24. McTavish D, Sorkin EM. Verapamil. An updated review of its pharmacodynamic and pharmacokinetic properties, and therapeutic use in hypertension. *Drugs.* 1989;38:19-76.

25. Singh BN et al. New perspectives in the pharmacologic therapy of cardiac arrhythmias. *Prog Cardiovasc Dis.* 1980;22:243-301.

26. Schoen MD et al. Evaluation of the pharmacokinetics and electrocardiographic effects of intravenous verapamil with intravenous calcium chloride pretreatment in normal subjects. *Am J Cardiol.* 1991;67:300-304.

27. Singh BN et al. Second generation calcium antagonists: search for greater selectivity and versatility. *Am J Cardiol.* 1985;55:214B-221B.

Chapter 34

Hypolipidemic Drugs

Daniel M. Riche and James M. Wooten

Class Instructions. Hypolipidemics. There is a strong relationship between elevated serum cholesterol and death caused by coronary heart disease (CHD). Lowering cholesterol decreases events related to CHD and can slow or even reverse atherosclerosis. These effects are associated with a decrease in CHD mortality. In general, each 1% decrease in low-density lipoprotein cholesterol (LDL-C) results in a 1% decrease in the risk of coronary events. Hypolipidemic medications should be taken daily to achieve these results. Drug therapy does not eliminate the need for appropriate diet, physical activity, and other lifestyle changes, including weight reduction (if appropriate) and smoking cessation. Use of estrogen and progestin in postmenopausal women also has beneficial effects on lipoprotein levels, but the overall risk/benefit assessment of hormone replacement therapy remains controversial. Depending on their overall state of health, elderly patients can benefit from secondary prevention with hypolipidemic therapy.

Missed Doses. Take this drug at regular intervals. If you miss a dose, take it as soon as you remember. If it is about time for the next dose, take that dose only. Do not double the dose or take an extra dose.

CHOLESTYRAMINE Questran, **Questran Light, Prevalite**, Various

Pharmacology. Cholestyramine is a bile acid sequestrant that acts as an anion exchange resin; it releases chloride ions and adsorbs bile acids in the intestine to form a nonabsorbable complex that is excreted in feces. The resulting increase in activity of hepatic LDL-C receptors leads to the oxidation of cholesterol to form new bile acids. Despite a compensatory increase in hepatic cholesterol synthesis, total serum cholesterol, and LDL-C levels are reduced significantly. The increase in cholesterol synthesis sometimes results in an increase in very low-density lipoprotein (VLDL) cholesterol levels, which can correspondingly increase triglyceride levels. [1,2] Cardioprotective HDL-C levels can increase slightly. [2]

Administration and Adult Dosage. PO for hypercholesterolemia; adjunct— 4 g once to twice daily initially, increasing slowly to a maintenance dosage of 8–16 g/d in 1–6 divided doses (typically 2), to a maximum of 24 g/d. Compliance appears to be best in the range of 8–10 g/d in 1–2 divided doses. **PO for treatment of cholestatic pruritus**—Same as for Hypercholesterolemia. The usual dose is 4–8 g/d.

Special Populations. *Pediatric Dosage.* Limited data are available, especially concerning long-term use. Drug therapy is generally reserved for children at least 10 years old, initiated at the lowest possible dosage, and gradually increased until the desired response is achieved. Base initial dosage on serum LDL-C level rather than body weight, and adjust dosage based on response: **PO for hypercholesterolemia—** (LDL-C < 195 mg/dL) 4g/d; (LDL-C-195–235 mg/dL) 8 g/d; (LDL-C-236–280 mg/dL) 12 g/d; (LDL-C > 280 mg/dL) 16 g/d.[3,4] (*See* Precautions.)

Geriatric Dosage. Initiate therapy at lowest possible dosage and slowly titrate to desired effect. Maximum dosage might not be required or tolerated.

Other Conditions. In patients with histories of constipation, start at the low end of the dosage range. In patients with gastrointestinal (GI) intolerance, reduce dosage and increase gradually. (*See* Adverse Reactions.)

Dosage Forms. Pwdr for Susp—4 g resin/9 g pwdr (Questran); 4 g resin/5 g pwdr (Questran Light); 4 g resin/5.5 g pwdr (Prevalite).

Patient Instructions. (*See* Hypolipidemics Class Instructions.) It is preferable to take this drug before meals, but you can adjust the time of the dosages around the scheduling of other oral medications. Take other oral medications at least 1 h before or 4–6 h after taking cholestyramine. Do not take dry; mix each packet or level scoopful with at least 60–180 mL (2–6 fl oz) of water or noncarbonated beverage, highly fluid soup, or pulpy fruit such as applesauce or crushed pineapple. You can experiment with different products and vehicles to determine your preference based on taste, cost, and caloric restrictions. Mixtures can be refrigerated to improve palatability, but do not cook because the drug can be inactivated. This drug frequently causes constipation. If this becomes a problem, contact your physician or pharmacist to discuss measures to minimize constipation. It can cause other gastrointestinal symptoms that usually decrease over time.

Pharmacokinetics. *Onset and Duration.* Reduction in cholesterol begins within the first month.

Fate. It is not absorbed from the GI tract. Resin and complex are excreted in the feces.

Adverse Reactions. Almost 70% of patients experience at least one GI side effect.[5] Constipation frequently occurs, especially with higher dosages, in the elderly and patients with previous constipation; fecal impaction is rare. Nausea, heartburn, abdominal pain, bloating, steatorrhea, and belching also occur frequently but tend to decrease over time. GI side effects tend to be milder in children than in adults. Hemorrhoids can be aggravated or may develop. Rash can occur. Chloride absorption in place of bicarbonate can lead to hyperchloremic acidosis, especially in children, and calcium excretion can increase. Absorption of fat-soluble vitamins (A, D, E, and K) can be impaired, leading to osteomalacia and bleeding. Absorption of folic acid also can be impaired, especially in children. Alimentary cancers in rats are somewhat more prevalent with cholestyramine treatment because of enhancement of other carcinogens, but the importance of this in humans is unknown.[6]

Contraindications. Complete biliary obstruction. Hypersensitivity. Hypertriglyceridemia. Dysbetalipoproteinemia.

Precautions. Possible malabsorption of fat-soluble vitamins. Constipation can be controlled by reducing dosage, slowly titrating dosage, increasing dietary fiber, or using stool softeners/bulk-forming laxatives. Avoid use in the presence of diverticular disease, local intestinal tract lesions, and overt CHD because constipation can be a problem.[7] Discontinue if a clinically important elevation in serum triglycerides occurs. Vitamin supplementation may be needed with high dosage or long-term therapy. Children, in particular, may need a multivitamin with folate and iron.[4] Patients with osteoporosis might need to restrict dietary chloride to limit calcium excretion.[8] Phenylketonurics should avoid Questran Light because it contains aspartame. Pregnancy category C.

Drug Interactions. Absorption of many drugs can be delayed or reduced, including acetaminophen, anticoagulants (including warfarin), cephalosporins, digoxin, ezetimibe, furosemide, oral hypoglycemic drugs,[9] iron, loperamide, methotrexate, NSAIDs, phenobarbital, oral phosphate supplements, pravastatin, thyroid hormones, thiazides, and oral vancomycin. Monitor for concurrent drug therapy effects when initiating and altering sequestrant therapy, particularly for drugs with a narrow therapeutic index.

Parameters to Monitor. Monitor LDL-C and triglycerides 4–6 weeks and 3 months after initiation of therapy. If therapy goals are achieved, monitor every 4 months, unless adverse effects are suspected. Periodically, monitor hemoglobin and serum folic acid during long-term therapy. Monitor efficacy of and appropriate tests for concurrent drug therapy that may be affected by cholestyramine. In children, monitor serum concentrations of fat-soluble vitamins, erythrocyte folate, liver function tests, and CBC annually.[4]

Notes. Bile acid sequestering resins are indicated as an adjunct to diet for primary hypercholesterolemia (types IIa and IIb) in patients for whom hypertriglyceridemia is not a primary concern (triglyceride levels < 400 mg/dL).[8] Bile acid sequestrants moderately lower LDL-C compared with some of the other hypolipidemic drugs, but are considered safer because they are not absorbed. These drugs can be particularly useful with moderately elevated LDL-C in low risk CHD for long-term therapy (e.g., primary prevention and in young men and premenopausal women).[1,10] They can be used in combination with other hypolipidemic drugs for additive effects when a larger decrease in LDL-C is required. Long-term use reduces cardiovascular morbidity and mortality, including the incidence of first heart attacks. Because >1/3 of patients discontinue bile acid sequestrants within the first year, primarily because of adverse effects, conservative dosage titration, education, and support are needed to manage and avoid adverse effects.[5,11] Maximum dosage is rarely needed.[2] Low-dose therapy (8–10 g/d) appears to be best tolerated and the most cost effective, alone or in combination therapy.[1, 12] Increased dosage can increase adverse effects without meaningful decreases in cholesterol. Resins are not effective in patients with homozygous familial hypercholesterolemia.[2] (*See* Recommendations for Initiation of Drug Therapy in Hypercholesterolemia Chart.)

The resins are also used to reduce pruritus caused by dermal deposition of bile acids in patients with partial biliary obstruction. Interference with digoxin absorption suggests a possible role in the management of the mild intoxication caused by these drugs; however, do not rely on cholestyramine alone in cases of severe digoxin toxicity.[9] Questran contains 14 kcal/9 g packet or scoop; Questran Light is flavored with aspartame and contains 1.6 kcal and 16.8 mg of phenylalanine/5 g packet or scoop.

COLESEVELAM HYDROCHLORIDE Welchol

Pharmacology. Colesevelam is a nonabsorbed, polymeric, lipid-lowering agent that binds intestinal bile acids, resulting in the increased clearance of LDL-C and a reduction of total cholesterol. Unlike cholestyramine and colestipol, colesevelam is not an anion exchange resin, but binds bile acids and impedes their reabsorption. Clinical trials have demonstrated modest LDL-C reductions with HDL-C and triglyceride increases compared with placebo.

Administration and Adult Dosage. PO for Primary Hypercholesterolemia—3 tab bid with meals or 6 tab once daily with a meal.[13]

Special Populations. *Pediatric Dosage.* Safety and efficacy not established. *Geriatric Dosage.* Same as adult dosage.

Dosage Forms. **Tab** 625 mg.

Patient Instructions. Take this drug with meals for maximum benefit.

Pharmacokinetics. *Onset and Duration.* Maximum effect occurs after 2 weeks.[13]

Fate. Colesevelam is not absorbed orally. It is excreted unchanged in the feces.

Adverse Reactions. Unlike cholestyramine and colestipol, colesevelam is generally well tolerated. Common adverse effects (>5%) are GI, including constipation and indigestion/dyspepsia, but the frequency is similar to placebo.[13,14]

Contraindications. Bowel obstruction. Hypertriglyceridemia (Triglyceride >500 mg/dL). Triglyceride-induced pancreatitis.

Precautions. Caution in patients with elevated triglyceride levels (>300 mg/dL) or GI disorders (e.g., GI motility disorders, dysphagia, swallowing disorders, or recent GI surgery).

Drug Interactions. Colesevelam does not affect the bioavailability of digoxin, metoprolol, quinidine, valproic acid, or warfarin. The bioavailability of non-dihydropyridine calcium channel blocker, glyburide, levothyroxine, phenytoin, and warfarin can be reduced by colesevelam. Colesevelam does not interfere with the lipid-lowering activity of the HMG–CoA reductase inhibitors. Colesevelam did not appear to affect the bioavailability of vitamin A, D, E, or K during clinical trials of up to 1 year.[13] The manufacturer states that caution should be exercised when treating patients with a susceptibility to vitamin K or fat-soluble vitamin deficiencies.

Parameters to Monitor. Monitor serum total cholesterol, LDL-C, and triglyceride levels initially, 4–6 weeks after initiation and periodically during therapy.

Notes. The tolerability and the relative lack of GI adverse effects make colesevelam the bile acid sequestrant of choice.[13] Colesevelam is also approved as an adjunct for the treatment of type 2 diabetes, the first drug to be approved as both a diabetes and cholesterol therapy.

COLESTIPOL HYDROCHLORIDE Colestid

Pharmacology. Colestipol is a bile acid sequestrant similar to cholestyramine, with equivalent lipid-lowering effects in most patients. Selection of a bile acid sequestrant is generally based on patient preference and cost. The palatability of cholestyramine–vehicle combinations is often preferred over colestipol granules, although colestipol tablets are well tolerated. A 5-g dose of colestipol lowers cholesterol in an amount equivalent to 4 g of cholestyramine; a 4-g dose of colestipol tablets is equivalent to approximately 5 g of the granules.[15–21] (*See* Hypolipidemic Drugs Comparison Chart and Recommendations for Initiation of Drug Therapy in Hypercholesterolemia Chart.)

Adult Dosage. **PO for Primary Hypercholesterolemia**—(Granules) 5 g twice daily initially, increasing in 5 g/d increments at 1–2 month intervals to a maximum of 30 g/d in 1–4 doses; (Tab) 2 g twice daily initially, increasing in 2 g/d increments at 1–2 month intervals to a maximum of 16 g/d. (*See* Adverse Effects.)

Dosage Forms. **Granules** 5 g resin/7.5 g packets and bulk containers; **Tab** 1 g.

Patient Instructions. (*See* Hypolipidemics Class Instructions.) Other medications should be taken at least 1 h before or 4 h after oral administration. Do not crush, cut, or chew the tablet dosage form. Suspension preparation: Do not take in dry form as it may cause esophageal distress; may be mixed with carbonated beverages and slowly stirred; however may be associated with gastrointestinal complaints; mix powder with 3 ounces or more of liquid, soup, cereal, or pulpy fruits; rinse the glass with a small amount of additional beverage to ensure the entire dose is taken; stir until completely mixed.

Adverse Effects. Adverse effects, precautions, monitoring instructions, and drug interactions are similar to those of cholestyramine. Additionally, intestinal impaction may rarely occur. Patients with moderate hypercholesterolemia who cannot tolerate colestipol granules due to GI adverse effects can benefit from one-half of the colestipol dose mixed with 2.5 g of psyllium.

Precautions. May reduce fat-soluble vitamin absorption, increasing bleeding. Also, be careful in patients with preexisting constipation.

| **EZETIMIBE** | Zelia; Vytorin (with simvastatin) |

Pharmacology. Ezetimibe is a cholesterol absorption inhibitor. It reduces the absorption of dietary and biliary cholesterol through selective inhibition of the sterol transporter at the brush border of the small intestine. Reduction in cholesterol absorption results in decreased cholesterol delivery to the liver, reduced stores of hepatic cholesterol, and upregulation of LDL-C receptors causing reduced blood cholesterol. In adults, ezetimibe lowers LDL-C without significant effect on triglycerides or HDL-C. When combined with a statin, synergistic LDL-C reductions can be achieved.

Administration and Adult Dosage. **PO for homozygous familial hypercholesterolemia** (with atorvastatin or simvastatin); **mixed hyperlipidemia** (with fenofibrate); **primary hypercholesterolemia** (monotherapy or combination with a statin); and **homozygous familial sitosterolemia**—10 mg once daily. Maximum ezetimibe dose is 10 mg daily.[22–24]

Special Populations. *Pediatric Dosage.* Not recommended if younger than 10 years old. **PO for homozygous familial hypercholesterolemia** (with atorvastatin or simvastatin) and **homozygous familial sitosterolemia**—10 mg once daily.

Geriatric Dosage. Safety and efficacy have not been established for use in pregnancy

Dosage Forms. Tab 10 mg.

Patient Instructions. (*See* Hypolipidemics Class Instructions.) Take with or without food. Diet and exercise program should be maintained as prescribed. Monitor for signs and symptoms of hepatic, pancreatic, or muscle adverse events (including excessive fatigue, yellowing of skin or eyes, abdominal pain, or muscle pain) and notify provider if present.

Pharmacokinetics. *Onset and Duration.* After oral administration, peak serum concentrations are achieved in 4–12 h. It may take several weeks before ezetimibe achieves its maximum effect.[22–25]

Fate. The oral bioavailability of ezetimibe is variable (35%–65%) and is not influenced by food, although meals high in fat content may somewhat increase absorption. Following absorption, the drug is extensively conjugated to a pharmacologically active phenolic glucuronide (ezetimibe–glucuronide or E–G). The E–G conjugate is highly bound to plasma protein. Oxidative metabolism of the drug and the E–G conjugate is minimal. Ezetimibe and the E–G conjugate are the major drug-derived compounds detected in plasma, accounting for 10%–20% and 80%–90% of the total drug in plasma, respectively. Most of the ezetimibe in the plasma is eliminated in the feces while the E–G conjugate is primarily eliminated in the urine. The half-life of ezetimibe is approximately 22 h. The manufacturer suggests no dosage adjustments for patients with renal impairment, although the elimination rate is reduced for those patients and in the elderly. Hepatic insufficiency may also increase serum concentration and the drug should be avoided in patients with severe hepatic impairment.[22–25]

Adverse Effects. Ezetimibe is fairly well tolerated with common adverse effects occurring in <5% of patients. Diarrhea, myalgia and upper respiratory tract infection are the most common adverse effects. Hepatitis, arthralgia, rhabdomyolysis, and transaminases have also been reported.[22–26]

Contraindications. Ezetimibe is contraindicated as monotherapy or in combination with a statin in patients with active liver disease or unexplained persistent elevations in serum transaminases. The drug should also not be used in patients with a known hypersensitivity to any component of the product.[23]

Precautions. Pregnancy and lactation. Evaluate any reports of muscle pain, tenderness, or weakness for myositis, including a determination of serum creatine phosphokinase, especially when ezetimibe is combined with a statin.[23]

Drug Interactions. Cholestyramine may reduce the absorption of ezetimibe. Cyclosporine and gemfibrozil may increase ezetimibe concentrations and close monitoring is recommended if these agents are used with ezetimibe. When combined with a fibrate, there may be an increased risk of cholelithiasis.[22–25,27]

Parameters to Monitor. Serum lipid panel, initially and 4–6 weeks following initiation, and then approximately every 3 months thereafter.[10] Liver function tests should be monitored according to the statin guidelines, if ezetimibe is used in combination with a statin.[23]

Notes. Although ezetimibe can be used as monotherapy in treating dyslipidemia, it is primarily utilized in combination with a statin to improve LDL-C reduction or in those patients who are being treated with maximum tolerable statin doses. Ezetimibe is available in a single tablet formulation with simvastatin, as Vytorin. Interestingly, Phase II studies indicated that 5 mg/d reduced LDL-C similar to a 10 mg/d, though this dose was not pursued by the manufacturer. To date, ezetimibe used alone or in combination has not been shown to reduce cardiovascular outcomes.

The ENHANCE Study evaluating simvastatin monotherapy or in combination with ezetimibe in 720 patients with heterozygous familial hypercholesterolemia, assessed the effectiveness of ezetimibe by measuring the mean change in the intima media thickness (IMT) at three sites in the carotid arteries over a 2-year period. Ezetimibe provided no additional benefit when added to the statin. Those subjects receiving ezetimibe did achieve a larger reduction in LDL-C compared to the statin alone. Though not powered to detect a difference, there was no difference in cardiovascular events between the two groups. Larger studies are being conducted to further assess cardiovascular safety/benefit of this combination.[22–30]

Another concern occurred in the SEAS (Simvastatin and Ezetimibe in Aortic Stenosis) trial, where the combination of ezetimibe and simvastatin was associated with an increase in the development of cancer as a secondary endpoint. A report combining the data from two large ongoing studies evaluating the effectiveness of the ezetimibe/simvastatin combination [The Study of Heart and Renal Protection (SHARP) trial and the Improved Reduction of Outcomes Vytorin Efficacy International Trial (IMPROVE-IT)]attempted to validate the results of the SEAS trial, but no increased cancer risk was demonstrated in the ezetimibe groups. Further research is necessary to clarify the cancer risk with ezetimibe.[22–30]

FENOFIBRATE	Fenoglide, Lipofen, TriCor, Triglide
FENOFIBRATE, MICRONIZED	Antara, Lofibra
FENOFIBRIC ACID	Trilipix

Pharmacology. Fenofibrate is a fibric acid derivative indicated for the treatment of type IV and V hyperlipidemia. Fenofibrate reduces serum triglycerides and increases HDL. The primary mechanism of action is peroxisome proliferator-activated receptors or PPAR α agonism. There also may be subsequent mechanisms, e.g., enhancing lipoprotein lipase activity, inhibiting VLDL synthesis, and reducing cholesterol synthesis. Fenofibrate can also reduce platelet aggregation and decrease serum uric acid.[31–33]

Adult Dosage. **PO for Primary Hypercholesterolemia or Mixed Dyslipidemia (Fredrickson Type 2a, 2b) Hypercholesterolemia**—130 mg daily (Antara); 120 mg daily (Fenoglide); 200 mg daily (Lofibra); 150 mg daily (Lipofen); 145 mg daily (TriCor); 160 mg daily (Triglide); 135 mg daily (Trilipix). **Fredrickson types 4 and 5 Hyperlipidemia (Hypertriglyceridemia)**—43–130 mg daily (Antara); 40–120 mg daily (Fenoglide); 67–200 mg daily (Lofibra); 50–150 mg daily (Lipofen); 48–145 mg daily (TriCor); 50–160 mg daily (Triglide); 45–135 mg daily (Trilipix). Dose titrations should occur at 4–8 week intervals.

Dosage Forms. **Cap**—*See* Daily Dosing Regimens above.

Pharmacokinetics. After absorption, fenofibrate is hydrolyzed to the active drug, fenofibric acid, which is more than 99% bound to plasma proteins. It is excreted predominantly unchanged in urine with a half-life of 20 h, which is prolonged in renal dysfunction.

Adverse Reactions. Common adverse effects include GI disturbances, skin rash, myalgias, and rhinitis. Elevations in serum transaminases and CPK have occurred, particularly in combination with statins. Rarely, pancreatitis, cholelithiasis, rhabdomyolysis, and hepatotoxicity have been reported. Fenofibrate is precautioned in patients with liver, gallbladder, or kidney disease.

Notes. Trilipix is the most recently approved fenofibrate derivative. Trilipix, the active metabolite of fenofibrate, is the first fenofibrate derivative to be approved for use coadministered with a statin. This approval is for patients with CHD or a CHD risk equivalent.

GEMFIBROZIL	Lopid, Various

Pharmacology. Gemfibrozil is a fibric acid derivative that decreases triglyceride and VLDL concentrations and increases HDL concentrations. Effects on LDL-C are variable. LDL-C can increase in some patients, especially those with type IV hyperlipoproteinemia. Its exact mechanism is unclear, but it appears to act through multiple mechanisms. There is increased secretion of cholesterol into bile, increased affinity of LDL receptors for LDL particles, activation of lipoprotein lipase, inhibition of triglyceride synthesis, suppression of free fatty acid release from adipose tissue, and a change in LDL-C toward a potentially less atherosclerotic form.[2,33]

Administration and Adult Dosage. PO **coronary arteriosclerosis (Fredrickson type 2b)**—600 mg twice daily, 30 min before the morning and evening meal; **Familial hyperlipoproteinemia (Fredrickson type 4)**—600 mg twice daily, 30 min before the morning and evening meal.

Special Populations. *Pediatric Dosage.* Safety and efficacy not established.

Geriatric Dosage. Initiate therapy at lowest possible dosage and slowly titrate to desired effect. Maximum dosage might not be required or tolerated.

Other Conditions. Moderate Renal Impairment—decrease dose by 50%.

Dosage Forms. **Tab** 600 mg.

Patient Instructions. (*See* Hypolipidemics Class Instructions.) Take doses 30 min before morning and evening meals. Gemfibrozil can slightly increase the risk of cancer and is similar to another medication that increases the risk of cancer, gallstones, and pancreatitis. You and your physician might decide that the benefit of reducing the risk of coronary heart disease is worth these other risks. Promptly report any muscle pain, tenderness, or weakness, especially if you also are taking a statin.

Pharmacokinetics. *Onset and Duration.* The maximum decrease in serum triglyceride and total cholesterol occurs within 4–12 weeks; lipids return to pretreatment levels after drug discontinuation.

Fate. The drug is rapidly and completely absorbed after oral administration. Mean peak serum concentrations of 15–25 mg/L (60–100 μmol/L) occur 1–2 h after administration of 600 mg twice daily. Serum concentrations are directly proportional to dose. The drug is 97%–98% bound to albumin. Clearance appears to be independent of renal function. Gemfibrozil is metabolized in the liver to a number of compounds. Approximately 70% of a dose is excreted in the urine, primarily as glucuronide conjugates of the drug and metabolites; less than 2% is excreted renally as unchanged drug. The half-life is reportedly 1.5–2 h, but may be longer.[34,34–36]

Adverse Reactions. The most common adverse effects are dyspepsia, abdominal pain, diarrhea, myalgia, rash, and xerostomia. More serious adverse effects, e.g., acute appendicitis and rhabdomyolysis, may also occur particularly when combined with a statin.[7] Elevations in liver function tests (AST, ALT, LDH, bilirubin, and alkaline phosphatase) can occur and will return to normal with drug discontinuation. Occasional mild decreases in WBC count, hematocrit, and hemoglobin occur, but usually stabilize. However, there have been rare reports of severe blood dyscrasias. Cholelithiasis requiring gallbladder surgery developed in 0.9% of gemfibrozil-treated patients, compared with 0.5% of patients in a placebo group. Routine monitoring of creatine phosphokinase may not detect rhabdomyolysis in a timely manner. Many experts recommend avoiding the combination of gemfibrozil and any HMG–CoA reductase inhibitor, but avoidance of the combination with simvastatin and lovastatin are particularly emphasized.[9]

Contraindications. Hepatic or severe renal dysfunction; primary biliary cirrhosis; preexisting gallbladder disease.

Precautions. Pregnancy and lactation. Evaluate any reports of muscle pain, tenderness, or weakness for myositis, including a determination of serum creatine phosphokinase. Discontinue if an adequate effect does not occur after 3 months, if cholelithiasis is suspected or if liver function tests remain elevated. Not recommended in cholesterol disorders in which an LDL-C elevation predominate.

Drug Interactions. Gemfibrozil can enhance the bleeding risk of oral anticoagulants and hypoglycemia risk of oral antidiabetic agents. Particularly, displacement of glyburide from plasma protein binding sites, an action that produces hypoglycemia, has been reported.[37] Bile acid sequestrants can decrease absorption of gemfibrozil. Gemfibrozil and HMG–CoA reductase inhibitors or colchicine together might increase the risk of myopathy. (*See* Adverse Reactions.) [34,36]

Parameters to Monitor. Serum lipid panel, initially and 4–6 weeks after initiation, and every 3 months thereafter.[10] Liver function tests and CBC every 3–6 months. Monitor serum glucose, if the patient is receiving insulin or an oral hypoglycemic. Monitor prothrombin time, if patient is taking an oral anticoagulant.

Notes. Gemfibrozil is not considered a major treatment for hypercholesterolemia due to the lack of benefit to LDL-C and increased myopathy with statins. However, the improvement to HDL-C and triglycerides make it useful in some patients.[1] The Helsinki Heart Study showed a 34% reduction in the incidence of CHD in middle-aged men (initially without CHD symptoms) treated with gemfibrozil for 5 years, although total death rate was no different between the treated and placebo groups.[38,39] A substudy of the Helsinki Heart Study showed an increase in gallstone and gallbladder surgery in gemfibrozil-treated patients. After a 3.5-year extension of this study, all-cause mortality was slightly higher in the original gemfibrozil group, primarily because of cancer deaths.[39] An ancillary study of the Helsinki Heart Study investigated the use of gemfibrozil in patients with signs or symptoms of CHD.[40] The rate of serious adverse cardiac events and total mortality with gemfibrozil treatment did not significantly differ from that of placebo; however, information on key prognostic indicators and their distribution was not known.[40] Gemfibrozil is chemically and pharmacologically similar to clofibrate. A 44% relative increase in age-adjusted, all-cause mortality occurred in a study of long-term clofibrate use related to a 33% increase in noncardiovascular disease such as malignancy, gallbladder disease, and pancreatitis. Because of the smaller size of the gemfibrozil studies, the increase in mortality in the gemfibrozil group relative to placebo might not be statistically or significantly different from the excess mortality associated with clofibrate use. In the VA-HIT study, gemfibrozil demonstrated significant improvement in major cardiovascular events in patients with CHD when the primary target of therapy was HDL.[41] Though unlikely to occur, further studies would help improve the understanding of gemfibrozil's role in lipid disorders.

| **NIACIN** | Niaspan, Advicor (with lovastatin), Simcor (with simvastatin) |

Pharmacology. Niacin (nicotinic acid), in dosages of ≥ 1 g/d, decreases serum total cholesterol, LDL-C and VLDL, and triglycerides, and increases HDL-C. The mechanism for these effects is not entirely known, but might involve inhibition of lipolysis, reduced LDL and VLDL synthesis, and increased lipoprotein lipase activity.[42,43] Niacin also decreases lipoprotein (a).[1] Niacin is formulated in immediate-release (IR), extended-release (ER), and sustained-release (SR) dosages, as well as in a flush-free formulation. (*See* Notes.)

Administration and Adult Dosage. **PO for Dyslipidemia, Coronary Arteriosclerosis, and in patients with a history of Myocardial Infarction (MI) and Hypercholesterolemia**—(ER) 500 mg at bedtime initially for 4 weeks. May increase dose by 500 mg every 4 weeks to a maximum of 2000 mg/d. **PO for Dyslipidemia**—(IR) 100 mg 3 times daily gradually increasing to 1000 mg three times daily; maximum dose is 4500 mg/d. Risk of hepatotoxicity increases at SR doses >1.5 g/d, and these products are not recommended.[2] **PO for Pellagra**—50–100 mg three times daily to a maximum of 500 mg/d.

Special Populations. *Pediatric Dosage.* **PO for Dyslipidemia**—(IR) 100–250 mg/d in 3 divided doses. May increase by 100 mg/d weekly OR 250 mg/d every 2–3 weeks as tolerated to a maximum of 10 mg/kg/d. **PO for Pellagra**—50–100 mg three times daily to a maximum of 500 mg/d. Although niacin is effective in reducing triglycerides and cholesterol in children and adolescents, adverse effects are common and can be severe. Some investigators have recommended niacin use be avoided in children or be used only under close supervision by a lipid specialist, if diet and bile acid sequestrants have failed.[3,44] In such cases, niacin should generally be used in combination with diet and a bile acid sequestrant, if tolerated.[3] Close monitoring is necessary. (*See* Adverse Reactions and Precautions.)

Geriatric Dosage. Initiate therapy at lowest possible dosage and slowly titrate to desired effect. Maximum dosage may not be required or tolerated.

Patient Instructions. Use only under medical supervision. Effects can differ with different preparations. Many will experience some flushing. Tolerance to flushing generally occurs with time. Taking 325 mg of aspirin or 200 mg of ibuprofen (or an equivalent dose of another NSAID) 30–60 min before each niacin dose may reduce flushing. Taking niacin with meals also might minimize flushing (particularly applesauce) and reduce GI upset. Avoid hot liquids or alcohol after taking a dose. Avoid interruptions in therapy; tolerance can be lost if therapy is interrupted, so slow resumption of the usual dosage is recommended. Avoid sudden changes in posture if you are also taking medicine for high blood pressure. Report any persistent nausea.

Dosage Forms. **ER Tab** 250, 500, 750, 1000 mg; **Elixir** 10 mg/mL; **ER Cap** 250, 500 mg; **IR Tab** 50, 100, 250, 500 mg. (*See* Notes.)

Pharmacokinetics. *Onset and Duration.* The onset of triglyceride and cholesterol reductions usually occurs within several days, although some studies have demonstrated a response after a single dose.[42] Pretreatment lipid levels return 2–6 weeks after drug discontinuation.

Fate. The drug is almost completely absorbed from standard formulations. Peak serum levels 30–60 min after 1 g standard formulations are 15–30 μg/L (120–240 nmol/L). Niacin is largely metabolized in the liver to niacinamide (nicotinamide) and its derivatives (e.g., nicotinuric acid), which can contribute to the lipid-lowering activity, especially after long-term use. The majority is excreted as unchanged drug or metabolites in urine.[42] **Half-life.** 20–48 min.[42]

Adverse Reactions. Dose-related flushing of the neck and face (usually in "blush" areas) occurs in most patients and is related to the rate of rise of serum levels rather than the absolute serum concentrations. Tolerance can develop but dissipate if therapy is interrupted. Administration with food (applesauce), gradual upward dosage titration, use of a non IR formulation, and premedication with 325 mg of aspirin or 200 mg of ibuprofen (or equivalent dose of another NSAID) 30–60 min before each dose can reduce risk of flushing. Postural hypotension can occur, especially when niacin is used with antihypertensive drugs or when it is taken with alcohol or hot liquids. Vasodilatory effects can precipitate or aggravate angina. Rash, pruritus, and stomach discomfort also occur frequently; the latter can occur more commonly with ER preparations. Increases in AST, ALT, bilirubin, and LDH concentrations occur frequently and might be related to increasing the daily dosage by more than 2.5 g/month. Severe hepatotoxicity (hepatic necrosis) is rare and tends to occur with abrupt dosage increases, ER forms substituted for immediate-release products without dosage reduction, or brand interchange. Hepatotoxicity can occur at low dosages (≤3 g/d) of SR products and as soon as 2 d after initiation. Discontinue therapy if liver function tests remain more than 3 times those of pretreatment values.[43]

Contraindications. Arterial hemorrhage; severe hypotension; hepatic dysfunction; unexplained elevations of transaminases, active peptic ulcer disease.

Precautions. Pregnancy; lactation. Use with caution in patients with gallbladder disease or histories of liver disease, unstable angina, gout, gouty arthritis, glaucoma, or diabetes.[2,45] Nausea can be a presenting sign of hepatotoxicity.[2] If the SR form is substituted for the immediate-release form, reduce dosage by approximately one-half. Use with an HMG–CoA reductase inhibitor warrants caution. Some formulations contain tartrazine dye, which can cause allergic reactions in sensitive patients.

Drug Interactions. Concurrent use with HMG–CoA reductase inhibitors can increase the risk of rhabdomyolysis. Concurrent therapy with α-adrenergic blocking antihypertensives can result in hypotension. Diet and/or dosage of oral hypoglycemic drugs or insulin might require adjustment with concurrent niacin use. Hepatotoxic drugs can have additive effects.[1]

Parameters to Monitor. Monitor serum lipids every 4–6 weeks initially and then every 1–3 months. Periodic liver function tests, blood glucose, and serum uric acid levels are recommended, especially at dosages >1.5 g/d.[1] Obtain liver function tests at baseline and every 6–12 weeks for the first year and then semiannually, unless hepatotoxicity is suspected.

Notes. Indicated for type IIa, IIb, III, IV, and V hyperlipoproteinemias. Reductions in sudden cardiac deaths and fatal and nonfatal MI and an 11% decrease in mortality (compared with placebo) occur in patients treated with niacin.[46] The cost of standard niacin formulations can be much lower than alternative drugs; the cost of ER products can be higher. ER products appear to have equal efficacy at lowering LDL-C at one-half the dosage of standard products, but the ER form might be less effective in lowering triglycerides or raising HDL at dosages equal to standard forms.[1,44,47]

Niaspan, the extended-release product, may cause fewer side effects (e.g., flushing) than SR products because of its delayed release. The prescription ER product is available as 500, 750, and 1000 mg tab. Use of >3–4 g/d does not appear to increase efficacy appreciably and is associated with increased side effects.[42]

OMEGA-3 FATTY ACID ESTERS   Lovaza (formerly known as Omacor)

Pharmacology. Various clinical trials have documented the beneficial effects of ingesting fish oil, either through diet or in the form of a pharmaceutical preparation. The active ingredient of fish oil (from coldwater fish) responsible for this effect is omega-3 polyunsaturated fatty acid, which is composed of the essential fatty acids—docosahexaenoic acid (DHA) and eicosapentaenoic acid (EPA).[48–51] Randomized controlled trials have demonstrated that high concentrations of fish oil may reduce serum triglycerides by nearly 50%.[10,50–55] The mechanism of this effect is thought to be due to the ability of the omega-3 fatty acids to inhibit the release of triglycerides from the liver, thus reducing the number of VLDL components and by stimulating lipoprotein lipase, which increases the clearance of triglycerides from the plasma.[50] The benefit of omega-3 fatty acids in reducing cardiovascular events in patients with elevated triglycerides has been impressive.[10,48–55]

Administration and Adult Dosage. **PO for Hypertriglyceridemia as an Adjunct to diet with TG >500 mg/dL**—4 g/d given in 1 or 2 divided doses.

Special Populations. *Pediatric Dosage.* Safety and efficacy not established.

Geriatric Dosage. Same as adult dosage.

Dosage Forms. Cap 1000 mg.

Adverse Effects. Side effects from omega-3 fatty acid therapy include GI upset, including fishy breath and burping. An increase in LDL-C cholesterol (by as much as 40% in some studies), distaste, and diarrhea may also occur.[52] Elevations in liver function tests and bleeding time have also been reported, therefore proper monitoring in patients receiving anticoagulants concomitantly is warranted.

Precautions. Pregnancy Category C. History of sensitivity or allergy to fish. Nonresponders. Concomitant use of medications known to exacerbate hypertriglyceridemia.

Drug Interactions. No significant documented drug interactions.

Parameters to Monitor. Serum lipid panel, initially and 4–6 weeks after initiation, and every 3 months thereafter.[10] Liver function tests every 3–6 months. Monitor serum glucose, if the patient is receiving insulin or an oral hypoglycemic. Monitor prothrombin time, if patient is taking an oral anticoagulant.

Notes. Should be taken with food or milk. If there is not an adequate response following 2 months of therapy, treatment should be withdrawn. Currently, the only approved omega-3 product is Lovaza (formerly known as Omacor). When over-the-counter fish oil is considered, the proposed therapeutic dose is 6–8 g/d. These over-the-counter product contents are not guaranteed by any regulating body. High dose (>10 grams daily) omega-3 fatty acids have also been used to treat psoriasis and rheumatoid arthritis with varying results.[48] Omega-3 fatty acids can be administered with statins (instead of fibric acid derivatives) without an increased risk of rhabdomyolysis. The reduction demonstrated in triglycerides seems to be associated with an increase in LDL-C, occasionally to a significant extent. This triglyceride reduction also seems to display diminished returns (e.g., the higher the triglycerides upon initiation – the larger the percent reduction demonstrated and vice versa).

STATINS (HMG–COA REDUCTASE INHIBITORS)	
ATORVASTATIN	Lipitor; Caduet (with amlodipine)
FLUVASTATIN	Lescol, Lescol XL
LOVASTATIN	Mevacor; Altoprev; Advicor (with niacin), Various
PRAVASTATIN	Pravachol, Various
PITAVASTATIN	Livalo
ROSUVASTATIN	Crestor
SIMVASTATIN	Zocor; Vytorin (with ezetimibe); Simcor (with niacin), Various

Pharmacology. Hydroxymethylglutaryl–CoA (HMG–CoA) reductase inhibitors (or statins) competitively inhibit conversion of HMG–CoA to mevalonate, an early rate-limiting step in cholesterol synthesis. A compensatory increase in LDL receptors, which bind and remove circulating LDL-C, results. Production of LDL-C also can decrease because of decreased production of VLDL or increased VLDL removal by LDL receptors. These medications produce dose-dependent, maximum reductions in LDL of 30%–40% (>50% with atorvastatin and rosuvastatin) and triglycerides of 10%–33% and increases in HDL levels of 5%–10%. (*See* Approximate Dose Equivalence of Statins Based on LDL.) These medications stabilize arterial plaques, which may be an important factor in the reduction of MI risk. They are commonly used in combination with other hypolipidemic medications and are the drug of choice in most cholesterol disorders. (*See* Hypolipidemic Drugs Comparison and Recommendations for Initiation of Drug Therapy in Hypercholesterolemia Charts).

COMBINATION WITH STATIN	CHOLESTEROL ABSORPTION INHIBITOR	BILE ACID SEQUESTRANTS	NIACIN	FISH OIL	FIBRATE
	Ezetimibe	*Colesevelam Cholestyramine Colestipol HCl*	*Niacin ER*	*Omega-3 FA*	*Fenofibrate Gemfibrozil*
LDL	↓ 24%	↓ 8–16%	↓ 10%[a]	↑ 4%	–/↑ 5%
TG	–/↓ 10%	–/↑	↓ 22–24%[a]	↓ 23%[b]	↓ 15–25%
HDL	↑ 2%	–/↑ 7%	↑ 21–24%[a]	↑ 5%	↑ 6–20%

LDL = serum low-density lipoprotein cholesterol, shown to have a graded, positive relationship with coronary heart disease (CHD)
HDL = serum high-density lipoprotein, shown to have a cardioprotective effect against CHD
TG = serum triglycerides, which have a positive relationship to CHD.
[a]At higher doses
[b]TG <500 mg/dL
From Ref. 69–75 and product information

NAME	FREDRICKSON CLASSIFICATION[a]	TC	LDL	TG	HDL	MEDICATION TREATMENT
Hyperlipidemia	IIb	↑	↑	↑	↑	1st Line: Statin 2nd Line: TG = Fibrate, Fish Oil LDL = BAS, CAI
Hypercholesterolemia	IIa	↑	↑↑	–	–	1st Line: Statin 2nd Line: BAS and/or CAI, then Niacin
Atherogenic Dyslipidemia	III	—	—	↑↑	↓↓	1st: Niacin, Fibrate If LDL ↑, then Statin
Mixed Dyslipidemia	IIb	↑	↑	↑	↓	1st Line: Statin 2nd Line: Fibrate, Niacin, CAI, or BAS
Hypertriglyceridemia/ Dysbetalipoproteinemia	III or IV or V	↑	↓	↑↑	–/↓	1st Line: Fibrate, Niacin (if HDL ↓), or Fish Oil (if TG >400 mg/dL)

BAS, Bile Acid Sequestrant; CAI, Cholesterol Absorption Inhibitor.
[a]Fredrickson classifications does not directly account for HDL. Thus, the Fredrickson classifications are approximated into suitable categories

Administration and Adult Dosage. Adjust dosage at no less than 4-week intervals. **PO for Hyperlipidemia**—(Atorvastatin) 10 mg/d initially, increasing to a maximum of 80 mg/d. (Fluvastatin) 20–40 mg at bedtime initially, increasing up to 80 mg/d; a slight increase in fluvastatin LDL-C lowering occurs with a twice daily regimen. (Lovastatin) 10–20 mg with the evening meal initially. Start with 10 mg/d in patients requiring <20% decrease in LDL-C or when concurrent use with CYP3A4 inhibitor is unavoidable. Increase to a maximum of 80 mg/d. Do not exceed a lovastatin dosage of 20 mg/d when used with a CYP3A4 inhibitor (e.g., cyclosporine). (Pravastatin) 40 mg at bedtime initially, increasing to a maximum of 80 mg/d at bedtime. (Rosuvastatin) 5–10 mg/d initially, increasing to a maximum of 40 mg/d. (Simvastatin) 20–40 mg in the evening initially, increasing to maximum of 80 mg/d in the evening.

Special Populations. *Pediatric Dosage.* (Atorvastatin, Fluvastatin, Lovastatin, Rosuvastatin, and Simvastatin)—Safety and efficacy not established for patients younger than 10 years. **PO for Hyperlipidemia**—(Atorvastatin, Lovastatin and Simvastatin) 10–17 years; 10 mg in the evening, increasing to a maximum of 40 mg in the evening (maximum is 20 mg/d for atorvastatin). (Fluvastatin) 10–16 years old, 20 mg at bedtime, increasing to a maximum of 80 mg at bedtime. (Pravastatin) 8–13 years old, 20 mg at bedtime; 14–18 years old, 40 mg at bedtime.

Geriatric Dosage. Same as Adult Dosage. Both initial and maintenance dose reductions should be considered if renal insufficiency is suspected.

Other Conditions. (Atorvastatin) No dosage adjustment necessary in renal impairment. Concomitant cyclosporine: dose limited to 10 mg/d; Concomitant clarithromycin, ritonavir/saquinavir, or lopinavir/ritonavir: lower starting and maintenance doses (≤20 mg/d) should be considered. (Rosuvastatin) Asian patients: 5 mg/d initially; once daily concomitant cyclosporine: maximum dose 5 mg/d; concomitant gemfibrozil OR lopinavir/ritonavir: maximum dose 10 mg/d; severe renal impairment (Cl$_{Cr}$ < 30 mL/min), nondialysis: 5 mg/d initially to a maximum of 10 mg/d. (Lovastatin) Initial dose is 10 mg/d when concurrent use with cyclosporine is unavoidable; maximum dosage is 20 mg/d with concurrent immunosuppressant therapy. Concomitant fibrate, niacin (>1 g/d), amiodarone, or verapamil: maximum dose is 20 mg/d. (Pravastatin) Initial dose is 10 mg/d with renal or hepatic impairment and in patients concurrently on immunosuppressive therapy; do not exceed a dose of 20 mg/d in the latter case. (Simvastatin) Initial dose is 5 mg/d in patients requiring <20% reductions in LDL-C and with severe renal insufficiency or on immunosuppressive therapy. Use dosages >20 mg/d only with extreme caution in patients with Cl$_{Cr}$ < 30 mL/min. Maximum dose is 10 mg/d on gemfibrozil and 20 mg/d on amiodarone or verapamil.

Dosage Forms. *See* Approximate Dose Equivalence of Statins Based on LDL.

Patient Instructions. (*See* Hypolipidemics Class Instructions.) Atorvastatin or rosuvastatin can be taken at any time of day without regard to meals. Take lovastatin with the evening meal to increase its absorption; other drugs can be taken without regard to meals. Take pravastatin 1 h before or 4 h after a dose of a cholesterol-binding resin. Promptly report any unexplained muscle pain or tenderness, especially if accompanied by malaise or fever. Avoid excessive concurrent use of alcohol, but abstinence is not required. Do not take these drugs during pregnancy because of possible harm to the fetus. Inform your physician if you become or intend to become pregnant.

Pharmacokinetics. *Onset and Duration.* Onset is within 2 weeks. Peak effect is within 4–6 weeks. Cholesterol levels return to baseline after drug discontinuation. *Fate.* *See* Fate of Statins Chart.

	LOVASTATIN	SIMVASTATIN	FLUVASTATIN	PRAVASTATIN	ATORVASTATIN	ROSUVASTATIN
Bioavailability	5%	5%	24%	18%	12%	20%
Timing of dose	EVENING - TWICE DAILY	EVENING	AT BEDTIME	AT BEDTIME	DAILY	DAILY
Half-life	3 hr	2 h	1.2 h	1.8 h	14 h	19 h
Renal excretion	10%	10%	6%	20%	<5%	10%
Relative lipophilicity	+ + + + +	+ + + + +	+ + + +	+	+ + + +	+ +
Active metabolites	✓	✓	–	–	✓	±

From product information.

Adverse Reactions. The drugs are generally well tolerated, with discontinuation rates less than other hypolipidemic drugs.[11] The frequency of side effects appears to be similar for all drugs.[46,56–61] GI complaints such as diarrhea, constipation, flatulence, abdominal pain, and nausea occur in approximately 5% of patients. Headache (4%–9%), rash (3%–5%), dizziness (3%–5%), and blurred vision (1%–2%) are other frequent side effects. Myopathy and myositis can occur with single therapy and can be associated with mild elevations of CPK. Rhabdomyolysis leading to acute renal failure is a rare complication but occurs more frequently in combination with gemfibrozil, cyclosporine, or >1 g/d of niacin. Lovastatin and simvastatin have particularly high myopathy risk with a CYP3A4 inhibitor.[56] Increases in liver function tests greater than 3 times the upper limit of normal occur in up to 2% of patients, but most are asymptomatic and reverse with discontinuation.[2] There have been several cases of serious liver disease directly associated with statin use reported to the Food and Drug Administration.[62] Anomalies have been reported with intrauterine exposure. Statins appear to have little to no effect on cancer risk.[63]

Contraindications. Pregnancy; lactation; active liver disease; unexplained persistent elevations of serum transaminases.

Precautions. Administer to women of childbearing age only when possibility of becoming pregnant is unlikely or when utilizing prevention by contraception. Use with caution in patients who consume substantial quantities of alcohol and/or have history of liver disease. Discontinue therapy if liver function tests are greater than 3 times the upper limit of normal. Consider withholding the drug in any patient with risk factors for renal failure secondary to rhabdomyolysis, such as severe acute infection, hypotension, major surgery, trauma, severe electrolyte, endocrine or metabolic abnormalities, and uncontrolled seizures.

Drug Interactions. Myositis and rhabdomyolysis can be more common in combination with cyclosporine (lovastatin levels are quadrupled), erythromycin, gemfibrozil, itraconazole, ketoconazole (and possibly other inhibitors of CYP3A4), or lipid-lowering dosages of niacin (>1 g/d).[56] HMG–CoA reductase inhibitors (other than pravastatin and atorvastatin) may increase the effect of warfarin. Bile acid sequestrants can markedly decrease pravastatin oral bioavailability when taken together; take pravastatin 1 h before or 4 h after resin doses.

Parameters to Monitor. Obtain serum lipid and liver function tests on initiation, 6 and 12 weeks after initiation, after dosage increases, and at least semiannually thereafter. Others have recommended more frequent monitoring.[1,2] Increase the frequency of monitoring if adverse effects are suspected. Routine monitoring of muscle enzymes might not adequately identify patients at risk for rhabdomyolysis but may be warranted in patients with skeletal muscle complaints and risk factors.

Notes. HMG–CoA reductase inhibitors are indicated for the treatment of type IIa and IIb hyperlipoproteinemias. They are the most effective in decreasing LDL-C, and their effect on decreasing coronary morbidity and mortality is proven.[56] The choice of drug depends on cost, amount of cholesterol lowering desired, and risk factors for coronary heart disease. They can have additive effects with many hypolipidemic medications, but may also increase risk of adverse effects. (*See* Adverse Reactions and Drug Interactions.) Cholesterol reduction with these agents can reduce the risk of stroke, MI, and total mortality in both primary and secondary prevention.[64] HMG–CoA reductase inhibitors also exert pleiotropic effect, including anti-inflammatory, antioxidant, and antithrombotic effects. The extent and utility of these pleiotropic effects is not known. HMG–CoA reductase inhibitors can also lower C-reactive protein levels in patients with and without coronary artery disease.[65] C-reactive protein concentrations can be a predictive and sensitive measure of vessel wall inflammation resulting from elevated cholesterol levels.[66]

RECOMMENDATIONS FROM THE THIRD REPORT OF THE NATIONAL CHOLESTEROL EDUCATION PROGRAM (NCEP) EXPERT PANEL ON DETECTION, EVALUATION, AND TREATMENT OF HIGH BLOOD CHOLESTEROL IN ADULTS (ADULT TREATMENT PANEL [ATP] III)

STEP 1. Classification of lipoprotein levels

ATP III CLASSIFICATION OF LDL, TOTAL AND HDL CHOLESTEROL (MG/DL)

LDL CHOLESTEROL—PRIMARY TARGET OF THERAPY		TOTAL CHOLESTEROL		HDL CHOLESTEROL	
<100 mg/dL	Optimal	<200 mg/dL	Desirable	<40 mg/dL	Low
100–129 mg/dL	Near optimal/above optimal	200–239 mg/dL	Borderline high	≥60 mg/dL	Ideal
130–159 mg/dL	Borderline high	≥240 mg/dL	High		
160–189 mg/dL	High				
≥190 mg/dL	Very high				

STEP 2. Identify the presence or absence of clinical atherosclerotic disease that confers a high risk for coronary heart disease (CHD) events. These include clinical CHD, symptomatic carotid artery disease, peripheral arterial disease, or abdominal aortic aneurysm.

STEP 3. Identify major risk factors other than LDL: cigarette smoking, hypertension (BP ≥140/90 mm Hg or on antihypertensive medication, HDL cholesterol <40 mg/dL, family history of premature CHD, age (men ≥45 yr; women ≥55 yr). Diabetes is considered a risk equivalent.

STEP 4. If 2+ risk factors (other than LDL) are present without CHD or CHD risk equivalent, assess 10-yr (short-term) CHD risk (refer to Framingham tables).

STEP 5. Determine Risk Category

RISK CATEGORY	LDL GOAL	LDL LEVEL AT WHICH TO INITIATE THERAPEUTIC LIFESTYLE CHANGES (TLC)	LDL LEVEL AT WHICH TO CONSIDER DRUG THERAPY
CHD or CHD risk equivalents (10-yr risk >20%)	<100 mg/dL	≥100 mg/dL	≥130 mg/dL (100–129 mg/dL: drug therapy optional)
2+ risk factors (10-yr risk ≤20%)	<130 mg/dL	≥130 mg/dL	10-yr risk 10–20%: ≥130 mg/dL; 10-yr risk <10%: ≥160 mg/dL
0–1 risk factor	<160 mg/dL	≥160 mg/dL	≥190 mg/dL (160–189 mg/dL: LDL-lowering drug is optional)

STEP 6. Initiate therapeutic lifestyle changes (TLC); diet (refer to guidelines for precise recommendations), weight management, increased physical activity.

STEP 7. Consider adding drug therapy if LDL exceeds levels shown in Step 5 of table: consider drug simultaneously with TLC for CHD and CHD equivalents; consider adding drug to TLC after 3 mo for other risk categories.

STEP 8. Identify metabolic syndrome and treat, if present, after 3 mo of TLC.

(continued)

RECOMMENDATIONS FROM THE THIRD REPORT OF THE NATIONAL CHOLESTEROL EDUCATION PROGRAM (NCEP) EXPERT PANEL ON DETECTION, EVALUATION, AND TREATMENT OF HIGH BLOOD CHOLESTEROL IN ADULTS (ADULT TREATMENT PANEL [ATP] III) (continued)

CLINICAL IDENTIFICATION OF METABOLIC SYNDROME

Risk Factor	Defined Level
Abdominal obesity	For men: waist circumference >102 cm (40 in.); or women: waist circumference >88 cm (35 in.) ≥150 mg/dL
Triglycerides	≥150 mg/dL
HDL cholesterol	For men: <40 mg/dL; for women: <50 mg/dL
Blood pressure	≥130/≥85 mm Hg
Fasting glucose	≥110 mg/dL

STEP 9. Treat elevated triglycerides

ATP III—CLASSIFICATION OF SERUM TRIGLYCERIDES (TG) (MG/DL)

<150 mg/dL	Normal
150–199 mg/dL	Borderline high
200–499 mg/dL	High
≥500 mg/dL	Very high

- Primary aim of therapy is to reach LDL goal
- Intensify weight management
- Increase physical activity
  If triglycerides are ≥200 mg/dL after LDL goal is reached, set secondary goal for non-HDL cholesterol (total HDL) 33 mg/dL higher than LDL goal.

COMPARISON OF LDL CHOLESTEROL AND NON-HDL CHOLESTEROL GOALS FOR THREE RISK CATEGORIES

Risk Category	LDL Goal	Non-HDL Goal	
CHD and CHD risk equivalent (10-yr risk for CHD >20%)	<100 mg/dL	<130 mg/dL	If TG ≥500 mg/dL: reduce to prevent pancreatitis (low-fat diet, weight management, a fibrate or niacin).
Multiple (2+) risk factors and 10-yr risk ≤20%	<130 mg/dL	<160 mg/dL	Treatment of low HDL: weight management; increased physical activity; if
0–1 risk factor	<160 mg/dL	<190 mg/dL	TG = 200–499 mg/dL, then achieve non-HDL goal; if TG <200 mg/dL in CHD or CHD risk equivalent, consider niacin or a fibrate.

From Ref. 10 and The National Heart Lung and Blood Institute (http://www.nhlbi.nih.gov/).

APPROXIMATE DOSE EQUIVALENCE OF STATINS BASED ON LDL REDUCTION

% LDL REDUCTION	LOVASTATIN MEVACOR ALTOPREV	SIMVASTATIN ZOCOR	FLUVASTATIN LESCOL	PRAVASTATIN PRAVACHOL	ATORVASTATIN LIPITOR	ROSUVASTATIN CRESTOR
17–22%	—	—	20 mg	10 mg	—	—
23–29%	20 mg (M/A)	10 mg	40 mg	20 mg	—	—
30–38%	40 mg[a] (M/A)	20 mg	80 mg[c,d]	40/80 mg[c]	10 mg	—
39–46%	40 mg BID[b] 60 mg (A)	40 mg[a]	—	—	20 mg[b]	5 mg[c]
46–48%	—	80 mg	—	—	40 mg	10 mg[b]
51–52%	—	—	—	—	80 mg	20 mg[b]
55%	—	—	—	—	—	40 mg[b]

[a]Inferior to corresponding dose of atorvastatin
[b]Possible "next level" LDL reduction
[c]Not evaluated (based on product information)
[d]XL daily or IR BID
From Refs. 67 and 68 and product information.

■ REFERENCES

1. Bays HE, Dujovne CA. Drugs for treatment of patients with high cholesterol blood levels and other dyslipidemias. *Prog Drug Res.* 1994;43:9-41.
2. Larsen ML, Illingworth DR. Drug treatment of dyslipoproteinemia. *Med Clin North Am.* 1994;78:225-245.
3. National Cholesterol Education Program. Report of the Expert Panel on Blood Cholesterol Levels in Children and Adolescents. *Pediatrics.* 1992;89: S525-S570.
4. Kwiterovich PO. Diagnosis and management of familial dyslipoproteinemia in children and adolescents. *Pediatr Clin North Am.* 1990;37:1489-1521.
5. Lipid Research Clinics Program. Lipid research clinics coronary primary prevention trial results. I. Reduction in incidence of coronary heart disease. *JAMA.* 1984;251:351-364.
6. Newman TB, Hulley SB. Carcinogenicity of lipid-lowering drugs. *JAMA.* 1996;275:55-60.
7. Smellie WAS, Lorimer AR. Adverse effects of the lipid-lowering drugs. *Adverse Drug React Toxicol Rev.* 1992;11:71-92.
8. Ast M, Frishman WH. Bile acid sequestrants. *J Clin Pharmacol.* 1990;30:99-106.
9. Farmer JA, Gotto AM Jr. Antihyperlipidaemic agents. Drug interactions of clinical significance. *Drug Saf.* 1994;11:301-309.
10. Expert Panel on Detection, Evaluation and Treatment of High Blood Cholesterol in Adults. Executive summary of the third report of the National Cholesterol Education Program (NCEP) Expert Panel on Detection, Evaluation, and Treatment of High Blood Cholesterol in Adults (Adult Treatment Panel III). *JAMA.* 2001;285:2486-2497.
11. Andrade SE et al. Discontinuation rates of antihyperlipidemic drugs—do rates reported in clinical trials reflect rates in primary care settings? *N Engl J Med.* 1995;332:1125-1131.
12. Hilleman DE et al. Comparative cost effectiveness of bile acid sequestering resins, HMG Co-A reductase inhibitors, and their combination in patients with hypercholesterolemia. *J Manag Care Pharm.* 1995;1:188-192.
13. Anonymous. Colesevelam (Welchol) for hypercholesterolemia. *Med Lett Drugs Ther* 2000;42:102 104.
14. Davidson MH et al. Colesevelam hydrochloride (Cholestagel): a new, potent bile acid sequestrant associated with a low incidence of gastrointestinal side effects. *Arch Intern Med.* 1999;159:1893-1900.
15. Jungnickel PW et al. Blind comparison of patient preference for flavored Colestid granules and Questran Light. *Ann Pharmacother.* 1993;27:700-703.
16. Shaefer MS et al. Acceptability of cholestyramine or colestipol combinations with six vehicles. *Clin Pharm.* 1987;6:51-54.
17. Shaefer MS et al. Sensory/mixability preference evaluation of cholestyramine powder formulations. *DICP.* 1990;24:472-474.
18. Ito MK, Morreale AP. Acceptability of cholestyramine and colestipol formulations in three common vehicles. *Clin Pharm.* 1991;10:138-140.
19. Insull W Jr et al. The effects of colestipol tablets compared with colestipol granules on plasma cholesterol and other lipids in moderately hypercholesterolemic patients. *Atherosclerosis.* 1995;112:223-235.
20. Spence JD et al. Combination therapy with colestipol and psyllium mucilloid in patients with hyperlipidemia. *Ann Intern Med.* 1995;123:493-499.
21. Superko HR et al. Effectiveness of low-dose colestipol therapy in patients with moderate hypercholesterolemia. *Am J Cardiol.* 1992;70:135-140.
22. Coleman CI et al. Ezetimibe/simvastatin. *Formulary.* 2004;39:437-444.
23. McEvoy G, ed. Ezetimibe. In: *AHFS Drug Information 2008.* Bethesda, MD: American Society of Health-System Pharmacists; 2008:1711-1714.
24. Caron MF. Ezetimibe. *Formulary.* 2002;37:628-633.
25. Jeu LA, Cheng JWN. Pharmacology and therapeutics of ezetimibe (SCH 58235), a cholesterol-absorption inhibitor. *Clin Ther.* 2003;25:2352-2387.
26. Kashani A et al. Review of side-effect profile of combination ezetimibe and statin therapy in randomized clinical trials. *Am J Cardiol.* 2008;101:1606-1613.
27. Jurado J, Seip R, Thompson PD. Effectiveness of ezetimibe in clinical practice. *Am J Cardiol.* 2004;93:641-643.
28. Peto R et al. Analyses of cancer data from three ezetimibe trials. *N Engl J Med.* 2008;359:1357-1366.
29. Rossebo AB et al. Intensive lipid lowering with simvastatin and ezetimibe in aortic stenosis. *N Engl J Med.* 2008;359:1343-1356.
30. Kastelein JJ et al. Simvastatin with or without ezetimibe in familial hypercholesterolemia. *N Engl J Med.* 2008;358:1431-1433.
31. Balfour JA et al. Fenofibrate. *Drugs.* 1990;40:260-290.
32. Adkins JC, Faulds D. Micronized fenofibrate. *Drugs.* 1997;54:615-633.
33. Shepherd J. Mechanism of action of fibrates. *Postgrad Med J.* 1993;69:S34-S41.

34. Todd PA, Ward A. Gemfibrozil. A review of its pharmacodynamic and pharmacokinetic properties, and therapeutic use in dyslipidemia. *Drugs.* 1988;36:314-339.

35. Evans JR et al. Effect of renal function on the pharmacokinetics of gemfibrozil. *J Clin Pharmacol.* 1987;27:994-1000.

36. Shen D et al. Effect of gemfibrozil treatment in sulfonylurea-treated patients with noninsulin-dependent diabetes mellitus. *J Clin Endocrinol Metab.* 1991;73:503-510.

37. Lozada A, Dujovne CA. Drug interactions with fibric acids. *Pharmacol Ther.* 1994;63:163-176.

38. Frick MH et al. Helsinki heart study: primary prevention trial with gemfibrozil in middle-aged men with dyslipidemia. *N Engl J Med.* 1987;317:1237-1245.

39. Heinonen OP et al. Helsinki heart study: coronary heart disease incidence during an extended follow-up. *J Intern Med.* 1994;235:41-49.

40. Frick MH et al. Efficacy of gemfibrozil in dyslipidaemic subjects with suspected heart disease. An ancillary study in the Helsinki heart study frame population. *Ann Med.* 1993;25:41-45.

41. Rubins HB et al. Gemfibrozil for the secondary prevention of coronary heart disease in men with low levels of high-density lipoprotein cholesterol. Veterans Affairs High-Density Lipoprotein Cholesterol Intervention Trial Study Group. *N Engl J Med.* 1999;341:410-418.

42. Figge HL et al. Nicotinic acid: a review of its clinical use in the treatment of lipid disorders. *Pharmacotherapy.* 1988;8:287-294.

43. American Society of Health System Pharmacists. ASHP Therapeutic Position Statement on the safe use of niacin in the management of dyslipidemias. *Am J Health Syst Pharm.* 1997;54:2815-2819.

44. Colletti RB et al. Niacin treatment of hypercholesterolemia in children. *Pediatrics.* 1993;92:78-82.

45. Hunninghake DB. Diagnosis and treatment of lipid disorders. *Med Clin North Am.* 1994;78:247-257.

46. Canner PL et al. Fifteen year mortality in coronary drug project patients: long-term benefit with niacin. *J Am Coll Cardiol.* 1986;8:1245-1255.

47. McKenney JM et al. A comparison of the efficacy and toxic effects of sustained- vs immediate-release niacin in hypercholesterolemic patients. *JAMA.* 1994;271:672-677.

48. Anonymous. Drugs for lipids. *Med Lett Drugs Ther.* 2008;6:9-16.

49. McEvoy G, ed. Omega-3-acid Ethyl Esters. In: *AHFS Drug Information 2008.* Bethesda, MD: American Society of Health-System Pharmacists; 2008:1761-1762.

50. Holub BJ. Clinical nutrition: 4. Omega-3 fatty acids in cardiovascular care. *CMAJ.* 2002;166:608-615.

51. Bays HE. Safety considerations with omega-3 fatty acid therapy. *Am J Cardiol.* 2007;99(suppl):35C-43C.

52. Nair GM. Should patients with cardiovascular disease take fish oil? *CMAJ.* 2008;178:181-182.

53. Hooper L et al. Omega 3 fatty acids for prevention and treatment of cardiovascular disease. *Cochrane Database Syst Rev.* 2004;CD003177.

54. Oh RC, Lanier JB. Management of hypertriglyceridemia. *Am Fam Physician.* 2007;75:1365-1372.

55. Yokoyama M et al. Effects of eicosapentaenoic acid on major coronary events in hypercholesterolaemic patients (JELIS): a randomized open-label, blinded end point analysis. *Lancet.* 2007;369:1090-1098.

56. Hsu I et al. Comparative evaluation of the safety and efficacy of HMG-CoA reductase inhibitor monotherapy in the treatment of primary hypercholesterolemia. *Ann Pharmacother.* 1995;29:743-759.

57. Henwood JM, Heel RC. Lovastatin. A preliminary review of its pharmacodynamic properties and therapeutic use in hyperlipidaemia. *Drugs.* 1988;36:429-454.

58. McTavish D, Sorkin EM. Pravastatin. A review of its pharmacological properties and therapeutic potential in hypercholesterolemia. *Drugs.* 1991;42:65-89.

59. Todd PA, Goa KL. Simvastatin. A review of its pharmacological properties and therapeutic potential in hypercholesterolemia. *Drugs.* 1990;40:583-607.

60. Mauro VF, MacDonald JL. Simvastatin: a review of its pharmacology and clinical use. *DICP.* 1991;25:257-264.

61. Jungnickel PW et al. Pravastatin: a new drug for the treatment of hypercholesterolemia. *Clin Pharm.* 1992;11:677-689.

62. Anonymous. Statin class labeling should include liver failure as adverse event—OPDRA. *FDC Rep.* 2000; July 24:26-28.

63. Dale KM et al. Statins and cancer risk: a meta-analysis. *JAMA.* 2006;295:74-80.

64. Blauw GJ et al. Stroke, statins, and cholesterol. A meta-analysis of randomized, placebo-controlled, double-blind trials with HMG-CoA reductase inhibitors. *Stroke.* 1997;28:946-950.

65. Ridker PM et al. Long-term effects of pravastatin on plasma concentrations of C-reactive protein. *Circulation.* 1999;100:230-235.

66. Ridker PM et al. C-reactive protein and other markers of inflammation in prediction of cardiovascular disease in women. *N Engl J Med.* 2000;342:836-843.

67. Jones PH et al. Comparative dose efficacy study of atorvastatin versus simvastatin, pravastatin, lovastatin, and fluvastatin in patients with hypercholesterolemia (the CURVES study). *Am J Cardiol.* 1998;81:582-587.

68. Jones PH et al. Comparison of the efficacy and safety of rosuvastatin versus atorvastatin, simvastatin, and pravastatin across doses (STELLAR* Trial). *Am J Cardiol.* 2003;92:152-160.

69. Davidson MH et al. Efficacy and tolerability of adding prescription omega-3 fatty acids 4 g/d to simvastatin 40 mg/d in hypertriglyceridemic patients: an 8-week, randomized, double-blind, placebo-controlled study. *Clin Ther.* 2007;29:1354-1367.

70. Mikhailidis DP et al. Meta-analysis of the cholesterol-lowering effect of ezetimibe added to ongoing statin therapy. *Curr Med Res Opin.* 2007;23:2009-2026.

71. Hunninghake D et al. Coadministration of colesevelam hydrochloride with atorvastatin lowers LDL cholesterol additively. *Atherosclerosis.* 2001;158:407-416.

72. Bays HE et al. Effects of colesevelam hydrochloride on low-density lipoprotein cholesterol and high-sensitivity C-reactive protein when added to statins in patients with hypercholesterolemia. *Am J Cardiol.* 2006;97:1198-1205.

73. Knapp HH et al. Efficacy and safety of combination simvastatin and colesevelam in patients with primary hypercholesterolemia. *Am J Med.* 2001;110:352-360.

74. Derosa G et al. Comparison of fluvastatin + fenofibrate combination therapy and fluvastatin monotherapy in the treatment of combined hyperlipidemia, type 2 diabetes mellitus, and coronary heart disease: a 12-month, randomized, double-blind, controlled trial. *Clin Ther.* 2004;26:1599-1607.

75. Muhlestein JB et al. The reduction of inflammatory biomarkers by statin, fibrate, and combination therapy among diabetic patients with mixed dyslipidemia: the DIACOR (Diabetes and Combined Lipid Therapy Regimen) study. *J Am Coll Cardiol.* 2006;48:396-401.

Chapter 35

Inotropic and Vasopressor Drugs

Robert J. DiDomenico

DOBUTAMINE HYDROCHLORIDE   Dobutrex, Various

Pharmacology. Dobutamine is a synthetic sympathomimetic amine that exists as the racemic mixture of an L-isomer with predominantly α-adrenergic agonist actions and a D-isomer that has β_1- and β_2-adrenergic agonist actions. The net clinical effect is typically that of a potent β_1-agonist with mild vasodilatory properties. At low dosages, it increases myocardial contractility without markedly increasing heart rate; this specificity is dose dependent and is lost at high dosages. Unlike dopamine, dobutamine does not release stored catecholamines and has no effect on dopaminergic receptors.

Administration and Adult Dosage. **IV for inotropic support, by infusion only—** 2.5 μg/kg/min initially, increasing gradually in 2.5 μg/kg/min increments to 20 μg/kg/min, and adjusting dosage to desired response. Maintenance dosages are typically 2–10 μg/kg/min.[1] Although dosages up to 40 μg/kg/min have been used, use dosages above 20 μg/kg/min with caution because of increased risk of tachycardia, arrhythmias, and myocardial ischemia.[1]

Special Populations. *Pediatric Dosage.* Safety and efficacy not established. However, the following dosage is suggested: **IV infusion—**2 μg/kg/min initially, followed by adjustment to desired hemodynamic response, up to 20 μg/kg/min may be used.[2]

Geriatric Dosage. Same as adult dosage. However, use with caution at the lowest effective dose.

Dosage Forms. **Inj** 12.5 mg/mL. Also available prediluted 1, 2, and 4 mg/mL.

Pharmacokinetics. *Onset and Duration.* Onset <2 min; peak within 10 min; duration <10 min.

Fate. Wide interpatient variability exists, especially between adult and pediatric patients. V_d in CHF is 0.2 ± 0.08 L/kg; Cl in CHF is 3.5 ± 1.3 L/h/kg. The drug is eliminated primarily in the liver to inactive glucuronide conjugates and 3-*O*-methyldobutamine.

$t_{1/2}$. 2 min.

Adverse Reactions. Precipitation or exacerbation of ventricular ectopy occurs frequently; atrial and ventricular arrhythmias can occur. Modest increases in heart rate or systolic blood pressure occur frequently; dosage reduction usually reverses these effects rapidly. Occasionally, nausea, headache, angina, nonspecific chest pain, palpitations, and shortness of breath are noted. Patients with atrial fibrillation might be at risk of developing rapid ventricular responses because dobutamine facilitates AV conduction.

Contraindications. Idiopathic hypertrophic subaortic stenosis.

Precautions. Correct hypovolemia before using in patients who are hypotensive. Use with caution in patients with severe aortic stenosis. In the majority of patients hospitalized for acute decompensated heart failure with congestion (not those with a low cardiac output state) there is no rationale for use of IV inotropic drugs.[3] Dobutamine is associated with increased mortality when given chronically as an intermittent infusion, and long-term therapy should only be considered as palliative care in patients with refractory, end-stage heart failure.[4] Outcomes with short-term dobutamine use are poorly studied. Although most cases of extravasation cause no signs of tissue damage, at least one case of dermal necrosis after extravasation has been reported.[5] Dobutamine contains a sulfite preservative that can be problematic in sensitive individuals, especially asthmatics.

Drug Interactions. Heterocyclic antidepressants can potentiate the pressor response to direct-acting vasopressors. Oxytocics used in obstetrics can cause severe, persistent hypertension when used with vasopressors. Halogenated hydrocarbon anesthetics can predispose patients to serious arrhythmias. Use with extreme caution in the presence of monoamine oxidase inhibitors (MAOIs).

Parameters to Monitor. Monitor heart rate, blood pressure, urine output, and ECG for ectopic activity. Invasive hemodynamic monitoring (e.g., cardiac index, pulmonary capillary wedge pressure, systemic vascular resistance) may be necessary in seriously ill patients for adequate dosage titration.

Notes. The drug is physically incompatible with sodium bicarbonate, furosemide, bumetanide, digoxin, magnesium sulfate, and other alkaline solutions. Use the reconstituted solution within 24 h. (*See* Cardiovascular Effects of Inotrope & Vasopressor Drugs Comparison Chart.)

DOPAMINE HYDROCHLORIDE   Dopastat, Intropin, Various

Pharmacology. Dopamine is a catecholamine that acts directly, in a dose-dependent fashion, on postsynaptic dopaminergic (DA_1) receptors to produce renal and mesenteric vasodilation and also acts on postsynaptic α_1-, α_2-, and β_1-adrenergic receptors. It also acts indirectly by releasing norepinephrine from sympathetic nerve storage sites. Clinical response depends on the patient's clinical condition and baseline sympathetic nervous system activity. Approximate ranges: dopaminergic 0.5–2 μg/kg/min; β_1 2–10 μg/kg/min; mixed α and β 10–20 μg/kg/min; predominantly α >20 μg/kg/min.

Administration and Adult Dosage. IV for shock, by infusion only— 2–5 μg/kg/min initially, increasing gradually in 5–10 μg/kg/min increments up to 20–50 μg/kg/min, and adjusting dosage to desired response. If a dosage over 20 μg/kg/min is required, consider other pressors.[1] Use dosages over 50 μg/kg/min only with careful monitoring of hemodynamic parameters and urine output. **IV for chronic refractory CHF**—2–3 μg/kg/min initially and then increasing gradually until desired increases in urine flow, diastolic blood pressure, or heart rate are observed.[6] Dosages over 10 μg/kg/min are rarely used in CHF.[6] (*See* Notes.)

Special Populations. *Pediatric Dosage.* Safety and efficacy not established. However, the following dosage is suggested: **IV for shock**—2–5 μg/kg/min initially, increasing to 10–20 μg/kg/min to improve blood pressure, perfusion, and urine output.[2]

Geriatric Dosage. Same as adult dosage.

Dosage Forms. Inj 40, 80, 160 mg/mL. Also available prediluted 0.8, 1.6, 3.2 mg/mL.

Pharmacokinetics. *Onset and Duration.* Onset within 5 min, duration <10 min.

Fate. There is large interpatient variability. V_d ranges from 19.8–75 L/kg in critically ill patients.[7] Cl varies from 3.9–16.5 L/h/kg.[6] The drug is metabolized by MAO and COMT primarily to homovanillic acid (HVA) and related metabolites; the remainder is hydroxylated to norepinephrine. Most of the drug (>80%) is excreted in urine as HVA and metabolites of both HVA and norepinephrine; very little is excreted as unchanged dopamine.

$t_{1/2}$. 2 min.

Adverse Reactions. Increases in ventricular ectopy, atrial and ventricular arrhythmias can occur, particularly at high dosages; reduce dosage if the number of ventricular ectopic beats increases. Hypertension can occur at high infusion rates. Nausea, vomiting, headache, anxiety, and angina pectoris also have been observed. At high doses, ischemic vasoconstriction of the splanchnic, hepatic, and renal vascular beds may occur.[8] Gangrene of the extremities has occurred in patients given large dosages of dopamine for long periods and in patients with occlusive vascular disease given low dosages.

Contraindications. Pheochromocytoma; presence of uncorrected tachyarrhythmias or ventricular fibrillation.

Precautions. Correct hypovolemia before using in patients with shock. If increased diastolic pressure, decreased pulse pressure, or decreased urine flow occurs, decrease infusion rate and monitor patient for signs of excessive vasoconstriction. Use with caution in patients with occlusive vascular disease and with extreme caution in patients receiving halogenated hydrocarbon anesthesia. Avoid extravasation of solution; however, if it occurs, the area can be infiltrated with 5–10 mg of **phentolamine** diluted in 10–15 mL of NS. Dopamine contains a sulfite preservative that can be problematic in sensitive individuals, especially asthmatics.

Drug Interactions. MAOIs (including furazolidone and linezolid) can dramatically increase the pressor response to dopamine; avoid these combinations or initiate dopamine at 1/10th of the usual dose if given within 3 weeks of MAOIs. Heterocyclic antidepressants can potentiate the pressor response to direct-acting vasopressors. Oxytocics used in obstetrics can cause severe, persistent hypertension when used with vasopressors. IV phenytoin can produce hypotension in severely ill patients receiving dopamine. Halogenated hydrocarbon anesthetics can predispose patients to serious arrhythmias.

Parameters to Monitor. In shock, closely monitor heart rate, ECG, arterial blood pressure, arterial blood gases, acid–base balance, and urine output and watch for signs of vasoconstriction or extravasation (e.g., blanching). Invasive hemodynamic monitoring (e.g., cardiac index, pulmonary capillary wedge pressure, and systemic vascular resistance) may be necessary in seriously ill patients for adequate dosage titration. With low dosages for dopaminergic effects, monitor urine output and ECG.

Notes. The drug is physically incompatible with sodium bicarbonate, furosemide, and other alkaline solutions. A meta-analysis of low-dose dopamine found it was ineffective in preventing renal failure in critically ill patients with signs of early renal dysfunction.[9] (*See* Cardiovascular Effects of Inotrope & Vasopressor Drugs Comparison Chart.)

EPINEPHRINE AND SALTS   Adrenalin, Sus-Phrine, Various

Pharmacology. Epinephrine stimulates α_1-, α_2- (vasoconstriction, pressor effects), β_1- (increased myocardial contractility and conduction), and β_2-adrenergic (bronchodilation and vasodilation) receptors. It is used for reversible bronchospasm, anaphylactic reactions, laryngeal edema (croup), open-angle glaucoma, hemodynamic instability, and cardiac arrest. (*See* Medical Emergencies.)

Administration and Adult Dosage. **SQ for anaphylaxis**—0.2–0.5 mg (0.2–0.5 mL of 1:1000 aqueous soln), may repeat q10–15 min prn. If SQ is ineffective, then **IV** 0.1–0.25 mg (1–2.5 mL of 1:10,000) q5–15min may be given followed by an IV infusion, if necessary. **SQ for asthma**—same dosage as SQ for anaphylaxis; may repeat q20min to 4 h as needed. **IV infusion for hemodynamic support**—(diluted to concentration of 4 μg/mL, range 4–1000 μg/mL)[10] 1 μg/min initially, adjust to hemodynamic response (usually 2–10 μg/min; alternatively, 0.1–2 μg/kg/min).[1,8,11] **IV/IO for cardiac arrest**—1 mg q3–5min.[12] **Endotracheal for cardiac arrest**—2–2.5 mg (diluted in 5–10 mL of NS) q3–5min until IV/IO access is obtained.[12] **Inhal (metered dose) not recommended** because of low efficacy and ultrashort duration of action.

Special Populations. *Pediatric Dosage.* **SQ for anaphylaxis or asthma**— 0.01 mg/kg [0.01 mL/kg of 1:1000 aqueous solution; alternatively, 0.3 mg/m^2 (0.3 mL/m^2)], to a maximum of 0.5 mg (0.5 mL); may repeat q15–20min for 2 doses, then q4h prn. **Inhal for croup**—0.25–0.5 mL of 2.25% racemic aqueous solution diluted in 1.5–4.5 mL of NS q1–2h prn by nebulizer.[13] **IV for hemodynamic support**—0.1 μg/kg/min initially, adjusted to desired hemodynamic response (dosage range 0.1–1 μg/kg/min)[7], doses >0.3 μg/kg/min are associated with greater α mediated vasoconstriction, which may increase the risk of ischemic vasoconstriction.[2] **IV/IO for cardiac arrest**—0.01 mg/kg (0.1 mL/kg of 1:10,000) q3–5min.[2] **Endotracheal for cardiac arrest**—0.1 mg/kg (0.1 mL/kg of 1:1000) q3–5min until IV/IO access is obtained.[2]

Geriatric Dosage. Same as adult dosage. (*See* Precautions.)

Dosage Forms. **Inhal Pwdr** 200 μg/spray; **Inhal Pwdr** (bitartrate) 160 μg/spray; **Inhal Soln** (HCl) 1% (1:100); **Inhal Soln** (racepinephrine) 2.25%; **Inj** (aqueous solution as HCl) 0.01 mg/mL (1:100,000), 0.1 mg/mL (1:10,000), 0.5 mg/mL (1:2000), 1 mg/mL (1:1000).

Patient Instructions. (Autoinjectors) Periodically familiarize yourself with instructions for use so you maintain an adequate comfort level. Obtain new kit by expiration date or sooner if precipitate or color change is noted in solution.

Pharmacokinetics. *Onset and Duration.* Onset SQ 5–10 min (peak effect: 20 min); inhal 1 min (peak effect: 3–5 min). Duration SQ 0.5–2 h; inhal 15–60 min.[14]

Fate. Parenteral action is terminated by uptake into adrenergic neurons. Metabolism is by MAO and COMT primarily to the inactive metabolites, metanephrine and vanillylmandelic acid (VMA). Cl is 2.1–5.3 L/h/kg.[15]

$t_{1/2}$. Approximately 1 min.[16]

Adverse Reactions. Dose-related restlessness, anxiety, tremor, cardiac arrhythmias, palpitations, hypertension, weakness, dizziness, and headache occur. Cerebral hemorrhage can be caused by a sharp rise in blood pressure from overdosage. Angina can be precipitated when coronary insufficiency is present, and elevation of blood glucose has been reported. Local necrosis from repeated injections and tolerance ("epinephrine fastness") with prolonged use also can occur.

Contraindications. Do not use with local anesthetics in fingers or toes or during general anesthesia with halogenated hydrocarbons. Other contraindications include α-adrenergic blocker-induced (including phenothiazines) hypotension, cerebral arteriosclerosis, organic heart disease, narrow-angle glaucoma, shock, difficult labor.

Precautions. Use with caution in patients with cardiovascular disease, hypertension, diabetes, or hyperthyroidism and in psychoneurotic patients. Caution is usually recommended in the elderly because of a higher frequency of cardiovascular intolerance. Intra-arterial administration is not recommended because of marked vasoconstriction. IM injection can produce local tissue necrosis. Epinephrine infusions are administered preferably through a central venous line. Extravasation can cause necrosis; if extravasation occurs, infiltrate the area with **phentolamine** 5–10 mg diluted in 10–15 mL of NS.

Drug Interactions. MAOIs and heterocyclic antidepressants can potentiate the pressor response to epinephrine. Oxytocics used in obstetrics can cause severe, persistent hypertension when used with vasopressors. Halogenated hydrocarbon anesthetics can predispose patients to serious arrhythmias. A hypertensive reaction can occur when epinephrine is given with nonselective β-adrenergic blockers (e.g., propranolol, nadolol).

Parameters to Monitor. Blood pressure, heart rate, ECG; (asthma or allergy) relief of symptoms; (IV infusion): infusion rate and site, signs of excessive vasoconstriction; invasive hemodynamic monitoring (e.g., cardiac index, pulmonary capillary wedge pressure, systemic vascular resistance) may be necessary in seriously ill patients for adequate dosage titration.

Notes. Do not use solution if it is brown or contains a precipitate. Protect solution from light. The solution is incompatible with sodium bicarbonate, furosemide, and other alkaline solutions. Historically, the safety and efficacy of nonprescription epinephrine inhalers has been debated but a 2005 study suggests appropriate doses provide similar symptomatic relief as albuterol with less cardiovascular side effects.[17] Parenteral administration offers no advantage over inhalation for the treatment of acute bronchospasm.[18] (*See* Cardiovascular Effects of Inotrope & Vasopressor Drugs Comparison Chart.)

INAMRINONE LACTATE	Inocor, Various

Pharmacology. Inamrinone (formerly amrinone) increases cyclic AMP and calcium availability through the inhibition of phosphodiesterase (primarily the peak III isoenzyme), which improves cardiac output through vasodilatory and positive inotropic actions.

Administration and Adult Dosage. **IV loading dose**—0.5–1 mg/kg (usually 0.75 mg/kg) over 2–3 min; can repeat in 30 min based on response. **IV maintenance dosage by continuous infusion**—5–10 μg/kg/min.

Special Populations. *Pediatric Dosage.* Safety and efficacy not established, but the following doses are suggested: **IV loading dosage** (neonates and infants)— 0.75–1 mg/kg IV/IO over 5 min (may give up to 2 additional loading doses depending on clinical response), then **IV maintenance dosage by continuous infusion**—2–20 μg/kg/min.[2]

Geriatric Dosage. Same as adult dosage.

Dosage Forms. Inj 5 mg/mL.

Pharmacokinetics. *Onset and Duration.* IV onset 2–5 min after bolus; peak 10 min; duration 0.5–2 h.

Serum Levels. A level of 1.5–4 mg/L (8–21.3 μmol/L) is associated with therapeutic response. Although a correlation exists between inamrinone levels and increased cardiac output, the clinical usefulness of serum level monitoring is not established and pharmacodynamic monitoring is preferred.[19]

Fate. 10%–50% of the drug is bound to plasma proteins; V_d is 1.2 L/kg; Cl is 0.23–0.5 L/h/kg.[20] The drug is eliminated primarily by hepatic metabolism, with 10%–40% excreted unchanged in urine.

$t_{1/2}$. α-phase 4.6 min; β-phase 3.6 h in normal volunteers, 5.8 h in CHF patients.

ISOPROTERENOL HYDROCHLORIDE   Isuprel, isoprenaline

Pharmacology. Isoproterenol is a synthetic, nonselective sympathomimetic agent with potent $β_1$- and $β_2$-adrenergic receptor agonism and low affinity for $α_1$-adrenergic receptors. It has powerful inotropic and chronotropic effects and causes smooth muscle relaxation resulting in both significant vasodilation as well as mild bronchodilation, although tolerance to the latter may occur.[11]

Administration and Adult Dosage. **IV bolus for heart block, Adams-Stokes attacks, and cardiac arrest (including torsades de pointes)**—0.02–0.06 mg [dilute 1 mL (0.2 mg) to 10 mL with NS or D5W, administer 1–3 mL of diluted solution], may give subsequent doses of 0.01 mg (0.5 mL) to 0.2 mg (10 mL). **IV infusion for heart block, Adams-Stokes attacks, and cardiac arrest (including torsades de pointes)**—5 μg/min, titrate to desired response, usual range 2–10 μg/min[11] (alternatively, initiate 0.1 μg/kg/min and titrate up to 1 μg/kg/min) **IM for heart block, Adams-Stokes attacks, and cardiac arrest (including torsades de pointes)**— 0.02 mg (1 mL undiluted solution), may give subsequent doses of 0.02 mg (0.1 mL) to 1 mg (5 mL). **SQ for heart block, Adams-Stokes attacks, and cardiac arrest (including torsades de pointes)**—0.02 mg (1 mL undiluted solution), may give subsequent doses of 0.15 mg (0.75 mL) to 0.2 mg (1 mL). **Intracardiac for heart block, Adams-Stokes attacks, and cardiac arrest (including torsades de pointes)**—0.02 mg (1 mL undiluted solution). **IV infusion for shock and hypoperfusion**—0.5 μg/min, titrate to desired response, usual range 0.5–5 μg/min (doses >30 μg/min have been used in critically ill patients). **IV bolus for bronchospasm during anesthesia**—0.01–0.02 mg [dilute 1 mL (0.2 mg) to 10 mL with NS or D5W, administer 0.5–1 mL of diluted solution], may repeat initial dose as needed.

Special Populations. *Pediatric Dosage.* Safety and efficacy not established, but the following doses have been used: **IV infusion for refractory bradycardia**[2]— 0.05–0.1 μg/kg/min, titrate to desired response, usual range 0.01–5.5 μg/kg/min.[21,22]

Geriatric Dosage. Same as adult dosage.

Dosage Forms. **Inj** 200 µg/mL.

Pharmacokinetics. *Onset and Duration.* Onset (IV) 1–5 min, (IM/SQ) 10–15 min; duration (IV) 15–30 min, (IM) 0.5–2 h, (SQ) 1 h.

Fate. V_d is 0.5 L/kg; Cl is 2.6 L/h/kg.[16] Metabolized primarily in the liver and other tissues by COMT; it is a poor substrate for MAO. The degree to which isoproterenol is taken up by sympathetic neurons is less, compared to epinephrine and norepinephrine.

$t_{1/2}$. 2 min.[16]

Adverse Reactions. Dose-related tachycardia, palpitations, angina, atrial and ventricular tachyarrhythmias, Adams-Stokes attacks, hypotension, hypertension, dyspnea, headache, dizziness, anxiety, nausea, vomiting, flushing of skin, tremors, and diaphoresis. In some patients with impaired AV conduction, isoproterenol may paradoxically worsen heart block.

Contraindications. Tachyarrhythmias, tachycardia or heart block caused by digitalis toxicity, ventricular arrhythmias requiring inotropic support, angina pectoris.

Precautions. Use with caution in patients with known ischemic heart disease, particularly those experiencing acute coronary syndrome as isoproterenol may worsen ischemia by increasing oxygen consumption and reducing coronary perfusion; diabetes, hyperthyroidism; and sensitivity to sympathomimetic drugs. Assure volume status is optimized prior to initiating isoproterenol as hypovolemia may increase the risk of hypotension from isoproterenol. Isoproterenol contains a sulfite preservative that can be problematic in sensitive individuals, especially asthmatics.

Drug Interactions. Avoid concomitant use with epinephrine and other sympathomimetic drugs as these combinations may precipitate serious arrhythmias. Halogenated hydrocarbon anesthetics can predispose patients to serious arrhythmias.

Parameters to Monitor. Arterial blood pressure, arterial blood gases, heart rate, ECG, urine output, and symptoms of angina. Invasive hemodynamic monitoring (e.g., cardiac index, pulmonary capillary wedge pressure, systemic vascular resistance) may be necessary in seriously ill patients for adequate dosage titration.

Notes. If heart rate exceeds 110 beats/min, a reduction in dose or discontinuation is suggested. Do not use solution if it is pinkish, dark yellow, or contains a precipitate. (*See* Cardiovascular Effects of Inotrope & Vasopressor Drugs Comparison Chart.)

MILRINONE LACTATE   Primacor

Pharmacology. Like inamrinone, milrinone is an inhibitor of phosphodiesterase, which increases cyclic AMP and calcium availability leading to positive inotropy and vasodilation. Unlike inamrinone, milrinone is specific to the peak III isoenzyme and it is several times more potent.

Administration and Adult Dosage. **IV loading dose**—50 µg/kg over 10 min and then **IV continuous infusion**—0.375–0.5 µg/kg/min; adjust dosage depending on the patient's response and hemodynamic variables to a maximum of 0.75 µg/kg/min. In renal impairment, reduce dosage as follows: Cl_{Cr} <50 mL/min/m², 0.43 µg/kg/min; <40 mL/min/m², 0.38 µg/kg/min; <30 mL/min/m², 0.33 µg/kg/min; <20 mL/min/m², 0.28 µg/kg/min; <10 mL/min/m², 0.23 µg/kg/min; <5 mL/min/m², 0.2 µg/kg/min.

Special Populations. *Pediatric Dosage.* Safety and efficacy not established, but the following doses are suggested: **IV/IO loading dose**—50–75 μg/kg over 10–60 min and then **IV continuous infusion**—0.5–0.5 μg/kg/min.[2]

Geriatric Dosage. Same as adult dosage.

Dosage Forms. Inj 200 μg/mL (100 mL, 200 mL), 1 mg/mL.

Pharmacokinetics. *Onset and Duration.* Onset 5–15 min; duration 3–6 h.[23]

Fate. 70% bound to plasma proteins; V_d is 0.45 L/kg; Cl is 0.14 L/kg/h. Milrinone is eliminated in the urine (83%) primarily as unchanged drug.

$t_{1/2}$. is 2.3 ± 0.1 h in CHF patients, longer than in normal volunteers.

Adverse Reactions. Thrombocytopenia is less frequent (0.4%) with milrinone than with inamrinone. Ventricular and supraventricular arrhythmias, hypotension, and headaches occur frequently.

Precautions. In the majority of patients hospitalized for acute decompensated heart failure (ADHF) with congestion (not those with a low cardiac output state) there is no rationale for use of IV inotropic drugs.[3] Routine use of milrinone in ADHF has no effect on cumulative days spent in the hospital but does increase the risk of both hypotension and atrial tachyarrhythmias.[24] Because hypotension occurs frequently, the IV loading dose is often avoided when initiating therapy in patients with ADHF and lower initiating doses (0.1 μg/kg/min) and maximum doses (0.2–0.3 μg/kg/min) should be considered.[3] Long-term use of inotropic drugs, including milrinone, has been associated with increased mortality. Chronic infusion therapy should only be considered as palliative care in patients with refractory, end-stage heart failure.[4] Use with caution in patients with severe obstructive aortic or pulmonary disease (e.g., hypertrophic subaortic stenosis).

Drug Interactions. None known.

Parameters to Monitor. Continuous ECG and frequent vital signs. Invasive hemodynamic monitoring (e.g., cardiac index, pulmonary capillary wedge pressure, systemic vascular resistance) may be necessary in seriously ill patients for adequate dosage titration.

Notes. Physically incompatible with IV furosemide. (*See* Cardiovascular Effects of Inotrope & Vasopressor Drugs Comparison Chart.)

NOREPINEPHRINE BITARTRATE	Levophed

Pharmacology. Norepinephrine is a catecholamine that is a potent agonist for α_1- and α_2-adrenergic receptors but only a modest agonist for β_1- and β_2-adrenergic receptors.[11] Therefore, it is a potent vasoconstrictor with less inotropic and minimal chronotropic activity.[11]

Administration and Adult Dosage. **IV for shock, by infusion only** (diluted to a concentration of 16 μg/mL, range 16–128 μg/mL)[10] 8–12 μg/min initially; adjusted to desired hemodynamic response; average maintenance dosage range is 2–4 μg/min. Very large dosages (up to 3 μg/kg/min) may be necessary in patients with refractory hypotension.[11]

Special Populations. *Pediatric Dosage.* Safety and efficacy not established, but the following doses are suggested: **IV for shock, by infusion only**—0.1 μg/kg/min initially, adjusting dosage to desired hemodynamic response to a maximum of 2 μg/kg/min.[2]

Geriatric Dosage. Same as adult dosage. (*See* Precautions.)

Dosage Forms. **Inj** 1 mg/mL.

Pharmacokinetics. *Onset and Duration.* Onset 1–2 min; duration 1–2 min after discontinuing infusion.

Fate. Action is terminated primarily by uptake into adrenergic neurons. Free drug is metabolized primarily by COMT and, to a lesser extent, MAO to inactive metabolites and their conjugates. Epinephrine is an active metabolite of norepinephrine.[16]

$t_{1/2}$. 2 min.[20]

Adverse Reactions. Dose-related hypertension (sometimes indicated by headache), reflex bradycardia, and ischemic vasoconstriction of the renal and splanchnic circulation.[8] Hypovolemia may increase the risk of ischemic vasoconstriction and poor perfusion of extremities and vital organs; therefore, volume resuscitation may be necessary in patients with evidence of volume depletion.[8] Myocardial oxygen consumption is increased, potentially leading to myocardial ischemia and/or infarction.[1] Extravasation can result in tissue necrosis and sloughing of superficial tissues. Arrhythmias can occur in extreme hypoxia or hypercarbia.

Contraindications. Hypotension secondary to uncorrected blood volume deficit; severe visceral or peripheral vasoconstriction; mesenteric or peripheral vascular thrombosis, unless drug is life-saving; halogenated hydrocarbon anesthesia.

Precautions. Use with caution in patients receiving MAOIs or heterocyclic antidepressants. Administer into a large vein (antecubital preferred) to avoid necrosis secondary to vasoconstriction; avoid the leg veins whenever possible, especially in the elderly or in those with occlusive vascular diseases. Avoid extravasation of solution; however, if it occurs, the area can be infiltrated with 5–10 mg of **phentolamine** diluted in 10–15 mL of NS. Norepinephrine contains a sulfite preservative that can be problematic in sensitive individuals, especially asthmatics.

Drug Interactions. MAOIs, methyldopa, and heterocyclic antidepressants can potentiate the pressor response to direct-acting vasopressors. Oxytocics used in obstetrics can cause severe, persistent hypertension when used with vasopressors. Halogenated hydrocarbon anesthetics can predispose patients to serious arrhythmias.

Parameters to Monitor. Arterial blood pressure, heart rate, arterial blood gases, acid–base balance, urine output, and watch for signs of vasoconstriction or extravasation (e.g., blanching). Invasive hemodynamic monitoring (e.g., cardiac index, pulmonary capillary wedge pressure, systemic vascular resistance) may be necessary in seriously ill patients for adequate dosage titration.

Notes. Norepinephrine should be diluted in dextrose-containing solutions to protect against loss of potency due to oxidation. Administration in saline-only solutions is not recommended. Do not mix with alkaline solutions as a precipitate may form, inactivating the drug.[1] Do not use solution if it is brown or contains precipitate. (*See* Cardiovascular Effects of Inotrope & Vasopressor Drugs Comparison Chart.)

PHENYLEPHRINE HYDROCHLORIDE   Neo-Synephrine, Triaminic, others

Pharmacology. Phenylephrine is a synthetic sympathomimetic catecholamine that is a powerful α_1-adrenergic receptor agonist with little, if any, effect on β-adrenergic receptors.[11] It is a potent vasoconstrictor with essentially no inotropic or chronotropic activity.[11]

Administration and Adult Dosage. **IM/SQ for hypotension**—initial dose 2–5 mg, subsequent doses 1–10 mg q10–15min as needed. **IV infusion for shock**—100–180 µg/min initially, adjusting dosage to desired hemodynamic response (alternatively, dosage range 0.4–9.1 µg/kg/min).[11] **IM/SQ for prophylaxis of anesthesia-induced hypotension**—2–3 mg 3–4 min prior to spinal anesthesia, subsequent doses 0.1–0.5 mg q10–15min as needed. **Inj for prolongation of spinal anesthesia**—2–5 mg added to the anesthetic solution. **Inj for vasoconstrictor during regional anesthesia**—1 mg per 20 mL of local anesthetic solution (1:20,000). **IV for paroxysmal supraventricular tachycardia**—0.5 mg over 20–30 s, repeat with 0.5–1 mg q10–15min as needed. **Intranasal for sinus congestion**—1–2 drops/sprays in each nostril q3–4h. **PO for nasal congestion**—10 mg q4h.

Special Populations. *Pediatric Dosage.* Safety and efficacy not established, but the following doses are suggested: **IM/SQ for prophylaxis of anesthesia-induced hypotension**—0.5–1 mg per 25 pounds body weight 3–4 min prior to spinal anesthesia. **Intranasal for nasal congestion**—1–2 drops or sprays in each nostril q3–4h. **PO for nasal congestion**—children (6–12 y) 5 mg q4h; (2–5 y) 2.5 mg q4h.

Geriatric Dosage. Same as adult dosage.

Dosage Forms. **Inj** 10 µg/mL; **Disintegrating filmstrip** 2.5 mg, 10 mg; **Liq** 7.5 mg/5 mL; **Liq drps** 1.25 mg/0.8 mL; **Nasal soln drps** 0.125%, 0.17%, 0.25%, 0.5%, 1%; **Nasal soln spray** 0.25%, 0.5%, 1%; **Susp** 7.5 mg/5 mL; **Chew tab** 10 mg; **Tab** 5 mg, 10 mg; **Dissolving tab** 10 mg.

Pharmacokinetics. Absorption 100%. Bioavailability 38% due to extensive first-pass effect.[25] *Onset and Duration.* Onset (IV) 1–2 min, (IM/SQ/PO) 10–15 min; duration (IV) 15 min, (IM) 0.5–2 h, (SQ) 50 min, (PO) 2–4 h.

Fate. Metabolized by MAO to inactive metabolites. Eliminated in the urine. Cl is 2 L/h. V_d is 340 L.[25]

$t_{1/2}$. 2–3 h.[25]

Adverse Reactions. Headache, reflex bradycardia, and restlessness are common. Ischemic vasoconstriction of the renal and splanchnic circulation.[8] Hypovolemia may increase the risk of ischemic vasoconstriction and poor perfusion of extremities and vital organs; therefore, volume resuscitation may be necessary in patients with evidence of volume depletion.[8] Arrhythmias occur rarely. Extravasation can result in tissue necrosis and sloughing of superficial tissues.

Contraindications. Severe hypertension, ventricular tachycardia.

Precautions. Use with caution in patients receiving MAOIs or heterocyclic antidepressants and during the peripartum period, should oxytocic drugs be given concomitantly as these may cause severe, persistent hypertension. Avoid extravasation of solution; however, if it occurs, the area can be infiltrated with 5–10 mg of **phentolamine** diluted in 10–15 mL of NS. Phenylephrine contains a sulfite preservative that can be problematic in sensitive individuals, especially asthmatics.

Drug Interactions. MAOIs, methyldopa, and heterocyclic antidepressants can dramatically potentiate the pressor response to direct-acting vasopressors. Oxytocics used in obstetrics can cause severe, persistent hypertension when used with vasopressors. Halogenated hydrocarbon anesthetics can predispose patients to serious arrhythmias.

Parameters to Monitor. Arterial blood pressure, heart rate, arterial blood gases, acid–base balance, urine output, and watch for signs of vasoconstriction or extravasation (e.g., blanching). Invasive hemodynamic monitoring (e.g., cardiac index, pulmonary capillary wedge pressure, systemic vascular resistance) may be necessary in seriously ill patients for adequate dosage titration.

Notes. Prolonged topical/intranasal use of phenylephrine can produce rebound congestion;[26] use for >3 days is not recommended. Overdose can cause hypertension and CNS stimulation;[26] therefore, no more than 6 doses of PO phenylephrine should be taken in a 24-h period and self-medication >7 days is not advised without consulting a physician. (*See* Cardiovascular Effects of Inotrope & Vasopressor Drugs Comparison Chart.)

CARDIOVASCULAR EFFECTS OF INOTROPE & VASOPRESSOR DRUGS COMPARISON CHART[a]

Drug	ADRENERGIC RECEPTOR SELECTIVITY				HEMODYNAMIC EFFECTS		
	Inotropic & Chronotropic Activity (β_1)	Vasodilation (β_2)	Vasoconstriction (α)	Other	Cardiac Index	Pulmonary Capillary Wedge Pressure	Systemic Vascular Resistance
Dobutamine Dobutrex Various	+++++	+++	−	—	↑↑	↓	↓
Dopamine Inotropin Various	++++	++	+++	Stimulates dopamine receptors at low doses; releases stored norepinephrine	↑↑	0/↓/↑[b]	0/↑↑[b]
Epinephrine Adrenalin Various	++++	+++	+++++	—	↑↑	↑	0/↑↑[b]
Inamrinone Inocor	0	0	0	PDE inhibitor	↑↑	↓↓	0/↓
Isoproterenol Isuprel Isoprenaline	+++++	+++ − +	+	—	↑↑↑	↓	0/↓

(continued)

CARDIOVASCULAR EFFECTS OF INOTROPE & VASOPRESSOR DRUGS COMPARISON CHART[a] (*continued*)

Drug	ADRENERGIC RECEPTOR SELECTIVITY				HEMODYNAMIC EFFECTS		
	Inotropic & Chronotropic Activity (β₁)	Vasodilation (β₂)	Vasoconstriction (α)	Other	Cardiac Index	Pulmonary Capillary Wedge Pressure	Systemic Vascular Resistance
Milrinone Primacor	0	0	0	PDE inhibitor	⇈	⇊	⇊
Norepinephrine Levophed	+++	++	+++++	—	⇈⇈	0	⇈
Phenylephrine[c] Neo-Synephrine	0	0	+++++	—	0	0	⇈

+ + + + +, Pronounced effect; +, Minimal effect; 0, No effect; ↓, Decreased; ↑, Increased; PDE, = phosphodiesterase.

[a]This table compares only a few of the many factors important in the treatment of hemodynamic instability. Consult references 1–3, 6, 8, and 12 for clinical use. Cross-table comparisons of the adrenergic selectivity properties between this table and the Sympathomimetic Bronchodilators Comparison Chart (Chap 57) cannot be made because: (1) the rating scale of this table reflects a finer degree of differentiation of effects (hence 0–5+ vs 0–4+); (2) the routes of administration are different; and (3) vascular β2-receptors appear to respond slightly differently from bronchiolar β2-receptors.

[b]Dose dependent.

[c]Other pressors are preferred in most shock states because they also have positive inotropic activity. Phenylephrine has no inotropic activity and with its strong α-agonist properties, functions as a pure vasopressor (afterload increaser).

Adapted From Refs. 11, 16.

NITRATES

Class Instructions. **Nitrates.** This drug can cause headache, dizziness, and/or flushing; alcohol can worsen these side effects. Tolerance to side effects of long-acting nitrates such as headache can occur with continued therapy. If necessary, a mild analgesic can be used until tolerance to side effects occurs. During an acute angina attack, discontinue activity, assume a sitting position, and take one dose of sublingual nitroglycerin (tablet or spray) under the tongue. If chest discomfort does not improve within 5 min after one dose of sublingual nitroglycerin (tablet or spray), activate the emergency medical services (EMS) by calling 911; additional sublingual nitroglycerin doses may be taken at 5-min intervals after EMS have been activated (e.g., 911).[27] Keep tablets in the tightly closed original container. If you have been taking this medication for a long time, do not discontinue it abruptly.

ISOSORBIDE DINITRATE
Isordil, Dilatrate, Various

Pharmacology. *See* Nitroglycerin.

Administration and Adult Dosage. **SL tab for acute anginal attack refractory to sublingual nitroglycerin**—2.5–10 mg q5–10min prn, maximum 3 doses in 15–30 min period; **SL tab for prophylaxis of angina prior to angina-provoking activity**—2.5–10 mg 5–10 min prior to activity;[28] **PO for prophylaxis of angina and for CHF**—5–40 mg bid/tid; maintain one dosing interval of >14 h to minimize nitrate tolerance.[24] When used for heart failure, it should be used in combination with hydralazine to achieve optimal benefit.[29] **SR products for prophylaxis of angina**—20–80 mg bid (administered 7 h apart to minimize nitrate tolerance). A daily nitrate-free period of at least 12 h is desirable to minimize tolerance.[28] (*See* Vasodilators in Heart Failure Comparison Chart.)

Special Populations. *Pediatric Dosage.* Safety and efficacy not established.

Geriatric Dosage. Same as adult dosage. However, some clinicians have recommended lower doses due to an increased likelihood of postural hypotension in the elderly.

Dosage Forms. **SL Tab** 2.5, 5 mg; **SR Cap** 40 mg; **ER Tab** 40 mg; **Tab** 5, 10, 20, 30, 40 mg.

Patient Instructions. (*See* Nitrates Class Instructions.) Do not crush or chew sustained-release preparations.

Missed Doses. Take this drug at regular intervals. If you miss a dose, take it as soon as you remember. If it is about time for the next dose, take that dose only. Leave a minimum of 2 h between regular tablet doses and 6 h between sustained-release tablet or capsule doses. Do not double the dose or take extra.

Pharmacokinetics. *Onset and Duration.* Onset is 5 min after SL administration, 7.5 min after PO tab administration, up to 4 h with SR products; peak occurs 15 min after SL administration and 26 min after PO tab administration.[30] Duration is 1 h after SL, 2–6 h after PO tab, and up to 12 h after SR.[28] Long-term, around-the-clock administration is associated with diminished efficacy, probably because of nitrate tolerance.[28]

Fate. Oral bioavailability is 22%–25% for PO, 45% for SL.[30] There is extensive first-pass metabolism by the liver after oral administration to less active isosorbide mononitrate metabolites (2-ISMN, 5-ISMN). The drug is 28% bound to plasma proteins; V_d is 2–4 L/kg; Cl is 2.7 L/h/kg.[30] (*See* Isosorbide Mononitrate *Fate*.)

$t_{1/2}$. (Isosorbide dinitrate) ~1 h; (2-ISMN) ~2 h; (5-ISMN) ~5 h.

Adverse Reactions. *See* Nitroglycerin.

Contraindications. *See* Nitroglycerin.

Precautions. *See* Nitroglycerin.

Drug Interactions. *See* Nitroglycerin.

Parameters to Monitor. Monitor for headache, orthostatic hypotension, and dizziness. In angina, monitor frequency of angina. In CHF, monitor hemodynamic and functional measurements.

Notes. Because of their slower onset of action, reserve SL isosorbide dinitrate (ISDN) for acute anginal attacks only in patients intolerant of or unresponsive to nitroglycerin. Isosorbide dinitrate is efficacious for the treatment of angina and CHF, the eccentric dosing schedule required to maintain at least a 12-h nitrate-free interval may result in worsening or rebound symptoms during the nitrate-free period.

ISOSORBIDE MONONITRATE   Imdur, ISMO, Monoket

Pharmacology. Isosorbide mononitrate (ISMN) is the active 5-mononitrate metabolite of isosorbide dinitrate. (*See* Nitroglycerin.)

Administration and Adult Dosage. PO for prophylaxis of angina—(ISMO, Monoket) 20 mg bid, administered 7 h apart. **SR for prophylaxis of angina**—(Imdur) 30–60 mg once daily in the morning, can increase to 120 mg once daily, to a maximum (rarely) of 240 mg once daily. There can be some attenuation of antianginal efficacy after 6 weeks of therapy with the 30-mg and 60-mg doses, but not with the 120-mg dose.[28]

Special Populations. *Pediatric Dosage.* Safety and efficacy not established.

Geriatric Dosage. Same as adult dosage. However, some clinicians have recommended lower doses due to an increased likelihood of postural hypotension in the elderly.

Other Conditions. For persons of particularly small stature, the manufacturer of Monoket recommends an alternative initial dosage of 5 mg bid, but to increase it to at least 10 mg bid by the second or third day of therapy.

Dosage Forms. SR Tab—(Imdur) 30, 60, 120 mg; **Tab**—(ISMO, Monoket) 10, 20 mg.

Patient Instructions. (*See* Nitrates Class Instructions.) Administer the doses of the twice-daily tablets no more than 7 h apart to minimize the risk of developing nitrate tolerance. Do not crush the sustained-release product.

Missed Doses. Take this drug at regular intervals. If you miss a dose, take it as soon as you remember. If it is about time for the next dose, take that dose only. Leave a minimum of 6 h between regular tablet doses and 12 h between sustained-release tablet doses. Do not double the dose or take extra.

Pharmacokinetics. *Onset and Duration.* Non-SR tablet onset 30–60 min;[31] peak 1–2 h; duration 12–14 h with bid administration.[32] SR Tab onset 4 h; peak 4 h; duration approximately 12 h.[31,32]

Fate. The tablet is rapidly absorbed and essentially 100% bioavailable; The drug is distributed into total body water with negligible plasma protein binding and a V_d of 0.7 L/kg. Cl is 0.11 L/h/kg.[30] It is primarily hepatically metabolized by denitration and glucuronidation to inactive products that are renally eliminated; less than 2% of a dose is excreted unchanged in urine.

$t_{1/2}$. 5 h.

Adverse Reactions. *See* Nitroglycerin.

Contraindications. *See* Nitroglycerin.

Precautions. *See* Nitroglycerin.

Drug Interactions. *See* Nitroglycerin.

Parameters to Monitor. Monitor for headache, orthostatic hypotension, and dizziness; antianginal efficacy; and compliance with 7-h dosage regimen for non-SR tablet.

Notes. ISMN is an effective nitrate with dosage schedules proven to avoid tolerance. Patient compliance is favored with the use of ISMN because the products are administered once (Imdur) or twice (ISMO, Monoket) daily.

NITROGLYCERIN   Various

Pharmacology. Nitroglycerin and other organic nitrates are believed to be converted to nitric oxide (NO) by vascular endothelium. NO activates guanylate cyclase, increasing cyclic GMP that in turn decreases intracellular calcium, resulting in direct relaxation of vascular smooth muscle.[28] The venous (capacitance) system is affected to a greater degree than the arterial (resistance) system. Venous pooling, decreased venous return to the heart (preload), and decreased arterial resistance (afterload) reduce intracardiac pressures and left ventricular size, thereby decreasing myocardial oxygen consumption and ischemia. In myocardial ischemia, nitrates dilate large epicardial vessels, enhance collateral size and flow, and reduce coronary vasoconstriction.[28] The various organic nitrate preparations have the same pharmacologic effects and differ only in bioavailability and pharmacokinetics.

Administration and Adult Dosage. **SL Tab for acute anginal attack**—150–600 μg prn, up to 3 doses in 15 min; **SL aerosol for acute anginal attack**—400–800 μg prn, up to 1200 μg/15 min; **PO SR for prophylaxis of angina**—2.5–26 mg tid/qid; **Top ointment for prophylaxis and treatment of angina pectoris or CHF**— 1.3–5 cm (0.5–2 in.) q6–8h.[28] Start the dosage low and adjust slowly upward over several days to weeks to patient tolerance or to the desired therapeutic effect. Allow at least a 12-h nitrate-free period to minimize the risk of nitrate tolerance.[28] **SR Patch for prophylaxis and treatment of angina pectoris**—0.2–0.8 mg/h, patch applied once daily. Persistent antianginal efficacy for 10–12 h has been noted with patches delivering at least 0.4 mg/h. A daily nitrate-free period of 12 h is desirable to minimize nitrate tolerance.[28] **IV infusion for CHF, post-MI, angina pectoris, perioperative blood pressure control, or hypotensive anesthesia**— 5 μg/min initially, adjusted to the individual patient's response. Increase dosage initially in 5 μg/min increments q3–5min until response is noted. If no response occurs at 20 μg/min, increments of 10 μg/min and then perhaps 20 μg/min can be used. Once partial blood pressure response occurs, decrease incremental increases and increase intervals. (*See* Notes.)

Special Populations. *Pediatric Dosage.* Safety and efficacy not established. **IV**— 0.5–10 μg/kg/min has been suggested.

Geriatric Dosage. Same as adult dosage. However, some clinicians have recommended lower doses due to an increased likelihood of postural hypotension in the elderly.

Dosage Forms. Oint 2%; **SL Aerosol** 400 μg/spray; **SL Tab** 300, 400, 600 μg; **SR Cap** 2.5, 6.5, 9 mg; **SR Patch** 0.1, 0.2, 0.3, 0.4, 0.6, 0.8 mg/h; **Inj** 0.1, 0.2, 0.4, 5 mg/mL.

Patient Instructions. *See* Nitrates Class Instructions.

Pharmacokinetics. *Onset and Duration.* Onset immediate after IV, 2–5 min after SL Tab, 20–45 min after SR Cap, 15–60 min after topical ointment, and 30–60 min after transdermal administration.[33] Peak 4–8 min after SL Tab, 45–120 min after SR Cap, 30–120 min after topical ointment, and 1–3 h after transdermal administration.[33] Duration 10–30 min after IV and SL Tab, 2–6 h after oral, 4–8 h after SR Cap, and 3–8 h after topical administration.[32,33] Although the SR patch can act longer after the first application, long-term continuous therapy limits the duration of action to 4 h or less, probably because of tolerance.[34] With sustained intermittent therapy (removal of patch after 12 h) duration is 8–12 h.[32]

Fate. Bioavailability of SR Cap, SL, and Top are 1%, 38%, and 72%, respectively.[30] The drug is 60% bound to plasma proteins.[30] V_d is 3 L/kg; Cl is 13.8 L/h/kg.[30] Extensive first-pass metabolism occurs after oral administration. It is metabolized in the liver to less active dinitro and inactive mononitro metabolites.

$t\frac{1}{2}$. 2–3 min.[30]

Adverse Reactions. Headache occurs very frequently; dizziness occurs frequently, especially with oral or topical administration. Occasionally, flushing, weakness, nausea, vomiting, palpitations, tachycardia, and postural hypotension occur. Many of these effects are dose related and can be minimized by slowly increasing the dosage. Tolerance and dependence can occur with prolonged use. Contact dermatitis occurs in up to 40% of patients using transdermal patches.[35]

Contraindications. Severe anemia; severe hypotension or uncompensated hypovolemia; increased intracranial pressure; purported hypersensitivity or idiosyncrasy to nitroglycerin, nitrates, or nitrites; use of sildenafil within previous 24 h; use of vardenafil or tadalafil within previous 48 h.[27] (*See* Drug Interactions.) Constrictive or restrictive pericarditis and pericardial tamponade are also contraindications.

Precautions. Some tolerance and cross-tolerance with other nitrates can occur with long-term or excessive use; hemodynamic tolerance to IV nitroglycerin can occur after as little as 3 h of continuous therapy.[36] Use with caution in patients with severe renal or hepatic disease, those with low or normal pulmonary capillary wedge pressure, and those receiving drugs that lower blood pressure. With intermittent therapy, anginal episodes can increase during the nitrate-free interval.[28]

Drug Interactions. Nitrates can produce additive vasodilation and severe postural hypotension when combined with alcohol or hypotensive drugs. Use in patients taking sildenafil, vardenafil, or tadalafil can result in profound hypotension with serious consequences, including death.

Parameters to Monitor. Observe for headache, dizziness, and other side effects. Monitor for orthostatic hypotension, especially with first SL dose in elderly. (Angina) monitor frequency of angina. (CHF) obtain hemodynamic and functional measurements. (IV use) monitor blood pressure and heart rate constantly in all patients; monitoring pulmonary capillary wedge pressure in some patients also can be useful.

Notes. Large and unpredictable amounts of nitroglycerin are lost through polyvinyl chloride (PVC) containers, most IV administration sets and tubing, and certain IV filters. The manufacturers recommend that IV nitroglycerin infusions be prepared and stored in glass bottles and infused through special non-PVC tubing to avoid the use of in-line filters. Some institutions have discontinued use of nitroglycerin tubing to reduce costs and achieved good results clinically when using PVC tubing to infuse nitroglycerin.[37,38] However, because substantial amounts of nitroglycerin are adsorbed onto PVC tubing, special attention to patient response is advisable at the time of IV tubing changes. Stored in glass containers, the diluted injection is stable for 48 h at room temperature and 7 days under refrigeration. When administration sets with large dead spaces are used, flush the line whenever the concentration of solution is changed. (*See* Vasodilators in Heart Failure Comparison Chart.)

DILUTION & CONCENTRATION STANDARDS FOR INOTROPE & VASOPRESSOR INFUSIONS

DRUG	STANDARD DILUTION	STANDARD CONCENTRATION	MAXIMUM CONCENTRATION REPORTED
Dobutamine Dobutrex Various	500 mg/250 mL D5W or NS	2 mg/mL	12.5 mg/mL
Dopamine Inotropin Various	400 mg/250 mL D5W or NS	800 μg/mL	12.8 mg/mL
Epinephrine Adrenalin Various	4 mg/250 mL D5W or NS	16 μg/mL	1 mg/mL
Inamrinone Inocor	250 mg/250 mL NS	1 mg/mL	5 mg/mL
Isoproterenol Isuprel Isoprenaline	1 mg/250 mL D5W or NS	4 μg/mL	100 μg/mL
Milrinone Primacor	50 mg/250 mL D5W or NS	200 μg/mL	400 μg/mL
Norepinephrine Levophed	4 mg/250 mL D5W	16 μg/mL	128 μg/mL
Phenylephrine Neo-Synephrine	5 mg/250 mL D5W or NS	20 μg/mL	6.4 mg/mL

Adapted From Ref. 10.

APPROXIMATE EQUIVALENT DOSAGES OF NITRATES

PRODUCT	LOW DOSAGE	HIGH DOSAGE
Nitroglycerin Ointment	≤1 in. q6h	1–2 in. q6h
Nitroglycerin Patch	0.4 mg/h	0.4–0.8 mg/h
Isosorbide Dinitrate	20 mg tid	20–40 mg tid
Isosorbide Mononitrate		
Immediate-Release	10–20 mg bid	20 mg bid
Sustained-Release	30–60 mg/d	60–120 mg/d

VASODILATORS IN HEART FAILURE COMPARISON CHART

DRUG	DOSAGE[a]	DURATION	SITE OF ACTION[b]	HR	MAP	PCWP	CI	SVR
ACE INHIBITORS								
Captopril Capoten	PO 25–100 mg tid.	hours	A, V	0/↓	→	→	←	→
Enalapril Vasotec	PO 2.5–10 mg bid; IV 0.625–5 mg q6–12h.							
Lisinopril Prinivil Zestril	PO 5–20 mg/d.							
Quinapril Accupril	PO 5–20 mg q12h.							
HYDRALAZINE								
Hydralazine Apresoline Various	PO 50–75 mg q6–8h; usual maintenance 200–600 mg/d	hours	A	0/↑	sl↓	sl↓	←	→

(continued)

VASODILATORS IN HEART FAILURE COMPARISON CHART (*continued*)

DRUG	DOSAGE[a]	DURATION	SITE OF ACTION[b]	HR	MAP	PCWP	CI	SVR
NITRATES								
Isosorbide Dinitrate Isordil Sorbitrate Various	PO 10–60 mg q4–6h.	hours	V, (A)	sl↑/↓	sl↓	↓	↑/↓	sl↓
Nitroglycerin Various	(*See* monograph.)	minutes	V, (A)	sl↑/↓	→	↓	↑/↓	sl↓
NITROPRUSSIDE								
Nitroprusside Sodium Various	IV 0.1–3 mg/kg/min.	minutes	A, V	0	sl↓	↓	↑	→

A, arterial; V, venous; HR, heart rate; MAP, mean arterial pressure; PCWP, pulmonary capillary wedge pressure; CI, cardiac index; SVR, systemic vascular resistance; ↑, increase; ↓, decrease; sl, slight; 0, no change.
[a]Start with low dosages of these drugs and increase gradually with continuous hemodynamic monitoring. To avoid adverse rebound effects, carefully taper the dosages of these drugs if they are to be discontinued. (*See* Nitroglycerin Notes.)
[b]Predominant site of action. Parentheses denote lesser activity.
From Refs. 39–43 and product information.

■ REFERENCES

1. American Heart Association. Part 7.4: Monitoring and medications. *Circulation.* 2005;112:IV-78-IV-83.
2. American Heart Association. 2005 American Heart Association (AHA) guidelines for Cardiopulmonary Resuscitation (CPR) and Emergency Cardiovascular Care (ECC) of pediatric and neonatal patients: pediatric advanced life support. *Pediatrics.* 2006;117:e1005-e1028.
3. Heart Failure Society of America. Section 12: evaluation and management of patients with acute decompensated heart failure. *J Card Fail.* 2006;12:e86-e103.
4. Hunt SA et al. ACC/AHA 2005 guideline update for the diagnosis and management of chronic heart failure in the adult: a report of the American College of Cardiology/American Heart Association Task Force on Practice Guidelines (Writing Committee to Update the 2001 Guidelines for the Evaluation and Management of Heart Failure). American College of Cardiology. http://www.acc.org/qualityandscience/clinical/guidelines/failure/update/index.pdf. Accessed December 7, 2008.
5. Hoff JV, Peatty PA, Wade JL. Dermal necrosis from dobutamine. *N Engl J Med.* 1979;300:1280.
6. McBride BF, White CM. Acute decompensated heart failure: a contemporary approach to pharmacotherapeutic management. *Pharmacotherapy.* 2003;23:997-1020.
7. Karthik S, Lisbon A. Low-dose dopamine in the intensive care unit. *Semin Dial.* 2006;19:465-471.
8. Kellum JA, Pinsky MR. Use of vasopressor agents in critically ill patients. *Curr Opin Crit Care.* 2002;8:236-241.
9. Kellum JA, Decker JM. Use of dopamine in acute renal failure: a meta-analysis. *Crit Care Med.* 2001;29:1526-1531.
10. Sodorff MM et al. Recommended maximum concentrations of common acute care parenteral admixtures. *Hosp Pharm.* 1999;34:937-942.
11. Overgaard CB, Dzavik V. Inotropes and vasopressors: review of physiology and clinical use in cardiovascular disease. *Circulation.* 2008;118:1047-1056.
12. American Heart Association. Part 7.2: Management of Cardiac Arrest. *Circulation.* 2005;112:IV-58-IV-66.
13. Björnson CL, Johnson DW. Croup. *Lancet.* 2008;371:329-339.
14. Tashkin DP, Jenne JW. Alpha and beta adrenergic agonists. In: Weiss EB et al., eds. *Bronchial asthma: mechanisms and therapeutics.* 2nd ed. Boston, MA: Little, Brown; 1985:604-639.
15. Zaritsky AL. Catecholamines, inotropic medications, and vasopressor agents. In: Chernow B et al., eds. *The pharmacologic approach to the critically ill patient.* 3rd ed. Baltimore, MD: Williams & Wilkins; 1994:387-404.
16. Drug information for the health professional, Vol I. In: *USP DI.* 20th ed. Englewood, CO: Micromedex; 2000.
17. Hendeles L et al. Response to nonprescription epinephrine inhaler during nocturnal asthma. *Ann Allergy Asthma Immunol.* 2005;95:530-534.
18. National Asthma Education and Prevention Program Expert Panel Report 3 (EPR3): Guidelines for the Diagnosis and Management of Asthma: Summary Report 2007. National Heart, Lung, and Blood Institute. NIH Publication Number 08-5846: October, 2007. http://www.nhlbi.nih.gov/guidelines/asthma/asthsumm.pdf. Accessed December 7, 2008.
19. Edelson J et al. Relationship between amrinone plasma concentration and cardiac index. *Clin Pharmacol Ther.* 1981;29:723-728.
20. Lehtonen LA et al. Pharmacokinetics and pharmacodynamics of intravenous inotropic agents. *Clin Pharmacokinet.* 2004;43:187-203.
21. Reyes G et al. The pharmacokinetics of isoproterenol in critically ill pediatric patients. *J Clin Pharmacol.* 1993;33:29-34.
22. Zaritsky A. Pharmacology of catecholamines. In: Kacew S, ed. *Drug Toxicity and Metabolism in Pediatrics.* Boca Raton, FL: CRC Press, 1990:49-68.
23. Hilleman DE, Forbes WP. Role of milrinone in the management of congestive heart failure. *Ann Pharmacother.* 1989;23:357-362.
24. Cuffe MS et al. Short-term intravenous milrinone for acute exacerbation of chronic heart failure: a randomized controlled trial. *JAMA.* 2002;287:1541-1547.
25. Hengstmann JH, Goronzy J. Pharmacokinetics of 3H-phenylephrine in man. *Eur J Clin Pharmacol.* 1982;21:335-341.
26. Johnson DA, Hricik JG. The pharmacology of alpha-adrenergic decongestants. *Pharmacotherapy.* 1993;13(suppl):110S-115S.
27. Anderson JL et al. ACC/AHA 2007 guidelines for the management of patients with unstable angina/non-ST-elevation myocardial infarction-executive summary: a report of the American College of Cardiology/American Heart Association Task Force on Practice Guidelines (Writing Committee to Revise the 2002 Guidelines for the management of patients with unstable angina/non-ST-elevation Myocardial Infarction): developed in collaboration with the American College of Emergency Physicians, American College of Physicians, Society for Academic Emergency Medicine, Society for Cardiovascular Angiography and Interventions, and Society of Thoracic Surgeons. *J Am Coll Cardiol.* 2007;50:652-726.
28. Parker JD, Parker JO. Nitrate therapy for stable angina pectoris. *N Engl J Med.* 1998;338:520-531.

29. Cohn JN et al. Effect of vasodilator therapy on mortality in chronic congestive heart failure. Results of a Veterans Administration Cooperative Study. *N Engl J Med*. 1986;314:1547-1552.

30. Kirsten R et al. Clinical pharmacokinetics of vasodilators: Part II. *Clin Pharmacokinet*. 1998;35:9-36.

31. Frishman WH et al. Mononitrates: defining the ideal long-acting nitrate. *Clin Ther*. 1994;16:130-139.

32. Thadani U, Opie LH. Nitrates. In: Opie LH, ed. *Drugs for the heart*. 4th ed. Philadelphia, PA: WB Saunders; 1995:31-48.

33. Abrams J. Nitroglycerin and long-acting nitrates. *N Engl J Med*. 1980;302(22):1234-1237.

34. Anon. Nitroglycerin patches—do they work? *Med Lett Drugs Ther*. 1989;31:65-66.

35. Schrader BJ et al. Acceptance of transcutaneous nitroglycerin patches by patients with angina pectoris. *Pharmacotherapy*. 1986;6:83-86.

36. Elkayam U et al. Comparison of the effects of left ventricular filling pressure of intravenous nesiritide and high-dose nitroglycerin in patients with decompensated heart failure. *Am J Cardiol* 2004;93:237-240.

37. Haas CE et al. Effect of using a standard polyvinyl chloride intravenous infusion set on patient response to nitroglycerin. *Am J Hosp Pharm*. 1992;49:1135-1137.

38. Altavela JL et al. Clinical response to intravenous nitroglycerin infused through polyethylene or polyvinyl chloride tubing. *Am J Hosp Pharm*. 1994;51:490-494.

39. Mulrow CD et al. Relative efficacy of vasodilator therapy in chronic congestive heart failure. Implications of randomized trials. *JAMA*. 1988;259:3422-3426.

40. Chaterjee K et al. Vasodilator therapy in chronic congestive heart failure. *Am J Cardiol*. 1988;62:46A-54A.

41. Cohn JN et al. A comparison of enalapril with hydralazine-isosorbide dinitrate in the treatment of chronic congestive heart failure. *N Engl J Med*. 1991;325:303-310.

42. Parillo JE. Vasodilator therapy. In, Chernow B et al., eds. *The pharmacological approach to the critically ill patient*. 3rd ed. Baltimore: Williams & Wilkins; 1994:470-483.

43. Johnson JA, Lalonde RL. Congestive heart failure. In: DiPiro JT et al., eds. *Pharmacotherapy: a pathophysiologic approach*. 2nd ed. East Norwalk, CT: Appleton & Lange; 1993:160-193.

Central Nervous System 5

Daniel M. Riche

Daniel M. Riche

Chapter 36

Anticonvulsants

April D. Miller

April D. Miller

Class Instructions. *Anticonvulsants.* It is important to take this medication as prescribed to control seizures; stopping it suddenly can increase seizures. This medication can cause drowsiness. Until the extent of this effect is known, use caution when driving, operating machinery, or performing other tasks requiring mental alertness. Avoid concurrent use of alcohol or other drugs that cause drowsiness. Report unusual or bothersome side effects. Always use an effective contraceptive; contact your physician if you plan to become or become pregnant.[1,2]

Alert. The U.S. Food and Drug Administration analyzed reports of suicidality (suicidal behavior or ideation) from placebo-controlled trials of 11 anticonvulsant agents. Patients on therapy with anticonvulsant agents had an almost 2-fold increase in risk of suicidality (0.43%) compared with placebo (0.22%). This risk was observed as early as 1 week following drug initiation and continued through 24 weeks.[3]

All patients who are currently taking or starting therapy with any anticonvulsant agent should be closely monitored for notable changes in behavior that could indicate the emergence or worsening of suicidal thoughts or behavior or depression.[4]

CARBAMAZEPINE
Carbatrol, Tegretol, Various

Pharmacology. Carbamazepine is an iminostilbene compound related structurally to the tricyclic antidepressants. In animals, carbamazepine acts presynaptically to block firing of action potentials, which decreases the release of excitatory neurotransmitters, and postsynaptically by blocking high-frequency repetitive discharge initiated at cell bodies. In bipolar disorder, the mechanism of action is unknown but is believed to be related to effects on sodium and calcium ion channels and receptor-mediated neurotransmission.

Administration and Adult Dosage. **PO for epilepsy**—(tablets/XR) tablets 200 mg twice daily, suspension 100 mg 4 times daily with meals initially, increasing in increments of up to 200 mg/d at weekly intervals to effective dosage. **Usual maintenance**

517

dosage is 800–1200 mg/d in 2–4 divided doses;[5] 3 times daily or 4 times daily administration is recommended when enzyme-inducing antiepileptic drugs are administered concurrently. **XR** product can be given twice daily with concurrent enzyme-inducing antiepileptic drugs. **PO for trigeminal neuralgia**—100 mg twice daily initially, increasing in 200 mg/d using increments of 100 mg every 12 h for tablets or XR tablets, or 50 mg for supension until relief of pain, to a maximum of 1.2 g/d. **Usual maintenance dosage** is 400–800 mg/d in 2–3 divided doses.[5] **PO for bipolar disorder**—200 mg twice daily adjusted in 200 mg daily to achieve optimal clinical response. **Usual maintenance dosage** should not exceed 1600 mg daily.[6] **PO loading dose**—8 mg/kg in a single dose achieves therapeutic levels in 2 h (with suspension) or 5 h (with tablets) and is well tolerated. **Rectal administration** has been reported. (*See* Fate.)

Special Populations. *Pediatric Dosage.* **PO for epilepsy**—(<6 years) 10–20 mg/kg/d in 3–4 divided doses with the chewable tablets or in 4 divided doses with the suspension; (6–12 years) 100 mg twice daily with meals initially, increasing weekly in 100 mg/d increments as needed to achieve optimal clinical response. **Usual maintenance dosage** is 15–35 mg/kg/d or 400–800 mg/d in 3–4 divided doses. (>12 years) Same as adult dosage.[5]

Geriatric Dosage. Clearance of carbamazepine is reduced in some elderly patients, so a lower maintenance dosage might be required.[7]

Other Conditions. During pregnancy, increases in carbamazepine clearance can occur; dosage increases guided by serum levels and patient status might be necessary.[8]

Dosage Forms. **Chew Tab** 100 mg; **Susp** 20 mg/mL; **Tab** 200 mg; **XR Cap** 100, 200, 300 mg (Carbatrol), 100, 200, 300 mg (Equetro); XR Tab 100, 200, 400 mg (Tegretol-XR).

Patient Instructions. (*See* Anticonvulsants, Class Instructions.) Immediately report sore throat, fever, mouth ulcers, or easy bruising, which can be an early sign of a severe, but rare, blood disorder. The Tegretol-XR shell might appear in the stool, but does not indicate a lack of absorption.

Missed Doses. Take this drug at regular intervals. If you miss a dose, take it as soon as you remember. If it is about time for the next dose, take that dose only. Do not double the dose or take an extra dose. If you miss more than one dose in a day, call your physician.

Pharmacokinetics. *Onset and Duration.* Steady-state serum levels are attained within 2–4 days and subsequently can decline because of autoinduction of metabolism.[8] (*See* Fate.)

Serum Levels. (Anticonvulsant) 4–12 mg/L (17–50 mol/L). Variability exists in the relationship between serum levels and central nervous system (CNS) side effects.[5]

Fate. Absorption from tablets is slow and erratic, with a bioavailability of 75%–85%; peak serum levels occur 4–8 h after a dose of immediate-release product and 19 ± 7 h after a dose of XR product.[6] Absorption is rapid with the suspension, with a peak serum level of 7.9 ± 1.9 mg/L at 1.6 ± 1.3 h in the fasting state or 3.4 ± 3.4 h with concomitant enteral tube feeding after a 500 mg oral dose.[9] A peak serum level of 5.1 ± 1.6 mg/L occurs 6.3 ± 1.5 h after rectal administration of 6 mg/kg oral suspension (100 mg/5 mL) diluted with an equal volume of water.[10] The drug is 75%–78% bound to plasma proteins.[5] V_d is 0.88 ± 0.06 L/kg in adults and 1.2 ± 0.2 L/kg in children.[8] Large differences in clearance occur because of autoinduction of liver enzymes; autoinduction is completed within 1–2 weeks of monotherapy; clearance is 0.052 ± 0.04 L/h/kg at the end of week 1, 0.04 ± 0.02 L/h/kg at week 2, and 0.054 ± 0.04 L/h/kg at week 4.[5] Carbamazepine is metabolized to pharmacologically active carbamazepine-10,11-epoxide; the epoxide metabolite (CBZ-E) serum level ratios at steady state are 0.19 ± 0.06 at a carbamazepine level of 6.9 ± 1.5 mg/L and 0.28 ± 1.4 at a carbamazepine level of 10.5 ± 2.6 mg/L.[5] Only approximately 2% of the drug is excreted unchanged in the urine.[5] **Half-life.** There are large interindividual differences because of autoinduction of liver enzymes. (Adults) 31.3 ± 5.9 h after a single dose, 14.5 ± 5.3 h after 2 months; (Children) 29.4 ± 3.6 h after a single dose, 15.2 ± 5.2 h after 5 months.[5,8]

Adverse Reactions. Dizziness, drowsiness, headache, diplopia, nausea, and vomiting occur frequently with initiation of therapy and are minimized by slow titration of dosage. Mild, transient, morbilliform rash and thrombocytopenia also occur frequently. Occasionally, confusion, stomatitis, or rash occur. Hyponatremia and water intoxication occur, and risk factors include carbamazepine monotherapy, elevated serum levels, patient age >25 years, diuretic use, vomiting, or diarrhea.[5] Transient leukopenia has been observed in 10%–20% of patients; persistent leukopenia occurs in 2% of patients.[5] Discontinue drug if leukopenia (absolute neutrophil count < 1500/µL) persists or any evidence of bone marrow depression develops. Rare effects include aplastic anemia, agranulocytosis, hepatitis, lenticular opacities, and arrhythmias. Severe rash including Stevens-Johnson Syndrome (SJS) and toxic epidermal necrolysis (TEN) have been reported.[5] The incidence is increased in patients with a specific allele that is found more commonly in patients of Asian ancestry.

Contraindications. History of bone marrow depression; hypersensitivity to tricyclic antidepressants; concomitant use of an MAOI, or use within 14 days of discontinuing an MAOI; concomitant use of nefazodone.[5]

Precautions. Pregnancy; history of liver disease. Abrupt withdrawal of the drug in patients with epilepsy can precipitate status epilepticus. Exacerbation of atypical absence seizures can occur in children receiving carbamazepine for mixed seizure disorders.[2] Use carbamazepine cautiously in patients with histories of severe hypersensitivity reactions to phenytoin or phenobarbital. In patients of Asian ancestry, testing for the HLA-B*1502 allele should be performed prior to the initiation of therapy because of an increased risk for SJS or TENS. Patients positive for the allele should not receive carbamazepine unless the benefits clearly outweigh the risks.[5]

Drug Interactions. Because of structural similarities to tricyclic antidepressants, discontinue MAOIs for a minimum of 14 days before starting carbamazepine.[5] Carbamazepine can stimulate the metabolism of many drugs metabolized by CYP3A4, including oral anticoagulants, oral contraceptives, corticosteroids, cyclosporine, doxycycline, haloperidol, heterocyclic antidepressants, protease inhibitors, and theophylline. Many drugs inhibit carbamazepine metabolism, including cimetidine, clarithromycin, danazol, erythromycin, fluoxetine, isoniazid, ketoconazole, propoxyphene, quinine, troleandomycin, verapamil, and diltiazem.

Parameters to Monitor. Baseline CBC and platelet counts; monitor more frequently if WBC or platelet counts decrease. Monitor liver function tests periodically during long-term therapy. Monitor serum levels at least weekly during the first month of therapy because of autoinduction. Periodic serum level monitoring is useful in evaluating therapeutic efficacy or potential for adverse effects.[5]

CLONAZEPAM	Klonopin, Various

Pharmacology. Clonazepam is a benzodiazepine anticonvulsant that limits the spread of seizure activity, possibly by enhancing the postsynaptic effect of the inhibitory neurotransmitter, γ-aminobutyric acid (GABA).[11]

Administration and Adult Dosage. **PO for epilepsy**—no more than 0.5 mg 3 times daily initially; increase in 0.5–1 mg/d increments every 3 days to an effective dosage or to a maximum of 20 mg/d. **Usual maintenance dosage** is 4–8 mg/d.[11] **PO for panic disorder**—0.25 mg twice daily initially, increasing to 1 mg/d after 3 days. **Usual maintenance dosage** is 1 mg/d; some patients require up to 4 mg/d. (*See* Notes.) **Rectal administration** has been reported. (*See* Fate.)

Special Populations. *Pediatric Dosage.* **PO for epilepsy**—(≤10 years or ≤30 kg) 0.01–0.03 mg/kg/d initially in 2–3 divided doses, increase in 0.25–0.5 mg/d increments every 3 days to an effective dosage, to a maximum of 0.2 mg/kg/d in 3 divided doses.[11] Rectal administration has been reported. (*See* Fate.)

Geriatric Dosage. No specific clinical trial data exists. Elderly patients should be started at lower doses and observed closely.[11]

Other Conditions. Nursing mothers receiving clonazepam should NOT breast-feed their infants.[11]

Dosage Forms. **Tab** 0.5, 1, 2 mg. **Orally disintegrating Tab** 0.125, 0.25, 0.5, 1, 2 mg (Klonopin Wafer).

Patient Instructions. *See* Anticonvulsants, Class Instructions.

Missed Doses. Take this drug at regular intervals. If you miss a dose, take it as soon as you remember. If it is about time for the next dose, take that dose only. Do not double the dose or take extra.

Pharmacokinetics. *Onset and Duration.* Steady-state serum levels are attained in 4–8 days.[8] (*See* Notes.)

Serum Levels. 13–72 μg/L (40–230 nmol/L); however, some patients controlled with clonazepam can have levels below this range. There is a poor correlation between serum levels and efficacy or adverse effects.[8]

Fate. Rapidly absorbed orally; peak serum levels occur 1–4 h after a dose. Serum levels of 18–40 μg/L occur 20–120 min after rectal administration of a 0.1 mg/kg dose of clonazepam suspension.[12] The drug is 86 ± 0.5% bound to plasma proteins;[8] V_d is 3.1 ± 1.2 L/kg; clearance is 0.059 ± 0.011 L/h/kg.[12] The principal metabolite, 7-aminoclonazepam, is inactive. Less than 0.5% of clonazepam is excreted unchanged in urine.[8] **Half-life.** 30–40 h.[11]

Adverse Reactions. Drowsiness, ataxia, behavior disturbances, and personality changes (hyperactivity, restlessness, and irritability, especially in children) occur frequently and require dosage reduction.[11] Occasionally, hypersalivation and bronchial hypersecretion occur and can cause respiratory difficulties. Rarely, anemia, leukopenia, thrombocytopenia, and respiratory depression occur. Nearly 50% of patients receiving long-term clonazepam can experience transient exacerbations of seizures, dysphoria, restlessness, or autonomic signs during clonazepam withdrawal.[11] An increased seizure frequency and status epilepticus occur rarely, possibly associated with supratherapeutic serum levels.[8]

Contraindications. Severe liver disease; acute narrow-angle glaucoma; hypersensitivity to benzodiazepines.

Precautions. Pregnancy category D; lactation; patients with chronic respiratory disease. Clonazepam can increase frequency of generalized tonic–clonic seizures in patients with mixed seizure types. Abrupt withdrawal of the drug in patients with epilepsy can precipitate status epilepticus. Absence status has been reported in patients receiving valproic acid concurrently. Clonazepam can cause CNS depression. Use caution when operating heavy machinery and operating a motor vehicle.

Drug Interactions. Concurrent use with other CNS depressants can potentiate the sedation caused by clonazepam.

Parameters to Monitor. Periodic serum level monitoring is of limited value. Close attention to changes in patient's seizure frequency is necessary to monitor for the development of tolerance to the therapeutic effect. (*See* Notes.)

Notes. Tolerance to the anticonvulsant effect of clonazepam occurs in approximately one-third of patients within 3–6 months of starting the drug. Taper and discontinue clonazepam if therapeutic benefit cannot be demonstrated. Because of prominent CNS adverse effects and the development of tolerance, it is considered an alternative to **valproic acid** for myoclonic seizures and an alternative to **ethosuximide** or valproic acid for absence seizures.[8] (*See* Anticonvulsants, Comparison Chart.) Clonazepam also has become an alternative to **alprazolam** for treatment of panic disorder. For patients who experience interdose symptom recurrence or morning rebound with alprazolam, clonazepam offers an equally effective alternative with the benefit of a longer duration of effect. When switching a patient from alprazolam to clonazepam, an equivalent dosage of clonazepam is one-half that of alprazolam.[8]

ETHOSUXIMIDE   Zarontin

Pharmacology. Ethosuximide is a succinimide that produces an anticonvulsant effect by blockade of T-type calcium currents in the thalamus. In humans, it suppresses 3 cycles/sec spike-and-wave activity seen in absence seizures.[13] (*See* Notes.)

Administration and Adult Dosage. **PO for absence epilepsy**—250 mg twice daily initially; increase in 250 mg/d increments at 4- to 7-day intervals to an effective dosage, to a maximum of 1.5 g/d. **Usual maintenance dosage**—750–1250 mg/d in 1–2 doses.[13]

Special Populations. *Pediatric Dosage.* **PO for epilepsy**—(3–6 years) 250 mg/d initially; increase in 250 mg/d increments every 4–7 days to effective dosage, to a maximum of 1 g/d. **Usual maintenance dosage**—20 mg/kg/d in 1–2 doses.[1,2] (>6 years) Same as adult dosage.[13]

Geriatric Doses. Same as adult dosage.

Dosage Forms. **Cap** 250 mg; **syrup** 50 mg/mL.

Patient Instructions. (*See* Anticonvulsants, Class Instructions.) This drug can be taken with food or milk to minimize stomach upset.

Missed Doses. Take this drug at regular intervals. If you miss a dose, take it as soon as you remember. If it is about time for the next dose, take that dose only. Do not double the dose or take an extra dose.

Pharmacokinetics. *Onset and Duration.* Steady-state serum levels are attained in 7–12 days.[8]

Serum Levels. 40–100 mg/L (280–710 μmol/L).[13]

Fate. The drug is well absorbed orally, with peak serum level in 3–7 h in adults and children. Plasma protein binding is less than 10%. V_d is 0.69 L/kg; Cl is 0.01 ± 0.04 L/h/kg, greater in children.[8] Ethosuximide is metabolized to 3 inactive metabolites. Approximately 20% of the drug is excreted unchanged in urine.[8]

Half-life. (adults) 52.6 h;[8] (children) 31.6 ± 5.4 h.[8]

Adverse Reactions. Nausea, vomiting, drowsiness, headache, hiccups, and dizziness occur frequently during initiation of therapy and usually are dose related. Occasionally, psychiatric reactions including sleep disturbances, night terrors, inability to concentrate, and aggressiveness occur. Rarely, SLE, leukopenia, aplastic anemia, or SJS occur.[13]

Contraindications. Hypersensitivity to succinimides.

Precautions. Pregnancy; patients with known liver or renal disease. Generalized tonic–clonic seizures can occur in patients with mixed seizure types who are treated with ethosuximide alone. Abrupt withdrawal of the drug can precipitate absence status epilepticus.[13]

Drug Interactions. Ethosuximide can increase phenytoin serum levels and decrease levels of primidone (and its phenobarbital metabolite). Ethosuximide may also increase or decrease valproic acid levels.

Parameters to Monitor. Periodic serum level monitoring, after attaining steady state (7–12 days), is useful in evaluating therapeutic efficacy or potential adverse effects.[8] Periodically monitor CBC, urinalysis, and liver function tests.

Notes. Ethosuximide is indicated only for treatment of absence seizures. Because of the drug's low potential for serious or long-term toxicity and its proven efficacy, it is considered the drug of choice for absence seizures. (*See* Anticonvulsants Comparison Chart.)

FELBAMATE
Felbatol

Pharmacology. Felbamate is a dicarbamate that is structurally related to meprobamate; its mechanism of action is not known but might involve inhibition of *N*-methyl-D-aspartate responses and potentiation of GABA$_A$ receptor chloride currents.[14]

Administration and Adult Dosage. **PO for epilepsy**—1.2 g/d initially in 3–4 divided doses while reducing the dosage of concomitant antiepileptic drugs (phenytoin, carbamazepine, valproic acid, or phenobarbital) by 20%–30%. Increase in 1200 mg/d increments at weekly intervals to a maximum of 3.6 g/d. Further reduction in the dosage of concomitant antiepileptic drugs might be required during felbamate titration.[14]

Special Populations. *Pediatric Dosage.* **PO for epilepsy**—15 mg/kg/d initially in 3–4 divided doses while reducing the dosage of concomitant antiepileptic drugs (phenytoin, carbamazepine, valproic acid, or phenobarbital) by 20%. Increase in 15 mg/kg/d increments at weekly intervals to a maximum of 45 mg/kg/d. Further reduction in the dosage of concomitant antiepileptic drugs may be required during felbamate titration.[14]

Geriatric Dosage. Dosage reduction might be required in patients with reduced hepatic or renal function and should be guided by clinical response.

Renal Impairment. Starting and maintenance doses should be reduced by one-half. Adjunctive therapy with medications, which affect felbamate plasma concentrations, especially antiepileptic drugs, may warrant further reductions in felbamate daily doses in patient with renal dysfunction.[14]

Dosage Forms. **Tab** 400, 600 mg; **Susp** 120 mg/mL.

Patient Instructions. (*See* Anticonvulsants, Class Instructions.) Felbamate has been associated with severe blood and liver disorders that can be fatal. Report signs of infection, bleeding, easy bruising, or signs of anemia (fatigue, weakness) immediately; also report abdominal pain or yellowing of the skin immediately. After an extensive discussion on risks and benefits, informed consent is required for initial prescribing.

Missed Doses. Take this drug at regular intervals. If you miss a dose, take it as soon as you remember. If it is about time for the next dose, take that dose only. Do not double the dose or take extra.

Pharmacokinetics. *Onset and Duration.* Steady-state serum levels are attained in 2–3 days.[14]

Serum Levels. A therapeutic range has not been established. Serum concentrations reported in clinical studies are approximately 20–80 mg/L.[14]

Fate. Rapidly absorbed with over 90% bioavailability; peak serum levels occur 1–4 h after an oral dose.[14] Food and antacids have no appreciable effect on absorption. The drug is 22%–25% bound to plasma proteins, primarily to albumin. V_d is 0.76 ± 0.08 L/kg; Cl is 0.030 ± 0.008 L/h/kg in adults. From 40%–50% is excreted unchanged in urine; 5% is excreted unchanged in feces; the remainder is excreted as inactive metabolites.[14] **Half-life.** 20.2 h in normal volunteers;[14] 14.7 ± 2.8 h in epileptic patients on concomitant enzyme-inducing antiepileptic drugs.

Adverse Reactions. Anorexia, vomiting, insomnia, nausea, headache, weight loss, dizziness, and somnolence occur frequently. Adverse reaction frequency is lower when felbamate is used as monotherapy, and reactions often resolve during long-term therapy. Adverse reactions during adjunctive therapy can be the result of drug interactions. Felbamate is occasionally associated with aplastic anemia and hepatic failure (*see* Precautions), with fatality rates of 20%–30%. It is not known whether the risks of aplastic anemia and hepatic failure are related to the duration of felbamate exposure.[14]

Contraindications. History of any blood dyscrasia or hepatic dysfunction.

Precautions. Do not use felbamate as a first-line antiepileptic drug. Because of the risk of aplastic anemia and hepatic failure, use felbamate only in patients whose seizures cannot be controlled with other antiepileptic drugs or whose epilepsy is so severe that the risks are deemed acceptable. Fully inform patients of the risks of felbamate therapy. (*See* Patient Instructions.)

Drug Interactions. Felbamate increases serum concentrations of phenytoin, CBZ-E (the active metabolite of carbamazepine), and valproate; therefore, reduce the dosage of these antiepileptics by 20%–30% when felbamate is initiated.

Parameters to Monitor. Close monitoring of CBC, platelets, liver function tests, and clinical signs or symptoms of infection, bruising, bleeding, or hepatitis is essential. Monitor liver function tests (i.e., AST, ALT, bilirubin) every 1–2 weeks while treatment continues. The acceptable frequency of hematologic monitoring is not established. Routine monitoring of serum levels is of limited value because of the lack of a well-defined therapeutic range.

Notes. Felbamate is effective for the treatment of partial and secondarily generalized seizures in adults and for partial and generalized seizures associated with the Lennox-Gastaut syndrome in children.

FOSPHENYTOIN   Cerebyx

Pharmacology. Fosphenytoin is a phosphate ester prodrug that is rapidly and completely converted to phenytoin in vivo by phosphatases after parenteral administration. Fosphenytoin has no pharmacologic activity before its conversion to phenytoin. (*See* Phenytoin.)

Administration and Adult Dosage. **IV loading dose**—15–20 mg phenytoin equivalents (PE)/kg at a maximum rate of 150 mg PE/min.[15] **IM loading dose**—10–20 mg PE/kg in 1 or more injection sites. **IV or IM maintenance dosage**—4–6 mg PE/kg/d in 1 or 2 divided doses. Safety and effectiveness have not been established for therapy lasting more than 5 days. **IV or IM substitution for oral phenytoin therapy**—Same total daily dosage in PEs.

Special Populations. *Pediatric Dosage.* Safety and efficacy not established.

Geriatric Dosage. Advanced age has no effect on fosphenytoin pharmacokinetics, but phenytoin clearance and protein binding might be reduced. (*See* Phenytoin.)

Renal or Hepatic Impairment. Fosphenytoin conversion to phenytoin might be increased because of protein binding changes.[15] Because of an increased fraction of unbound phenytoin in patients with renal or hepatic diseases or hypoalbuminemia, dosage adjustments should be guided by patient status and measurement of unbound phenytoin concentrations.

Dosage Forms. **Inj** 50 mg PE/mL.

Patient Instructions. Itching or tingling can occur during intravenous infusion, particularly in the facial and groin areas. These sensations are usually mild and disappear within minutes of stopping the infusion. These symptoms do not indicate an allergic reaction to fosphenytoin or phenytoin.

Pharmacokinetics. *Onset and Duration.* Therapeutic concentrations of unbound phenytoin (>1 µg/mL) are attained within 8–10 min after the start of an IV infusion of fosphenytoin (administered at a rate of 100–150 mg PE/min) and are similar to those attained after an equivalent dose of phenytoin administered at 50 mg/min.[15] Therapeutic concentrations of unbound phenytoin are attained within 30 min after IM injection of fosphenytoin.

Serum Levels. Monitoring fosphenytoin serum concentration is not clinically useful. Phenytoin serum concentrations correlate with efficacy and toxicity. (*See* Phenytoin.)

Fate. Fosphenytoin is completely converted to phenytoin by phosphatases. Peak-free phenytoin concentrations occur 30 min after completion of fosphenytoin infusion administered at the rates of 100–150 mg PE/min and occur 3 h after an IM dose of fosphenytoin.[15] (*See* Onset and Duration.) Fosphenytoin is 95%–99% bound to plasma proteins, primarily albumin. Fosphenytoin binding is saturable and the V_d of fosphenytoin is 4.3–10.8 L depending on plasma concentration. Fosphenytoin displaces phenytoin from protein binding sites. The free (unbound) fraction of phenytoin ranges from 0.30 (in the presence of fosphenytoin) to 0.12 (after complete conversion of fosphenytoin to phenytoin). (*See* Phenytoin.) **Half-life.** (conversion to phenytoin) 15 min.

Adverse Reactions. Fosphenytoin commonly causes burning, itching, or paresthesias during IV infusion, particularly in the groin and facial areas. These symptoms usually disappear within minutes and can be minimized by slowing or stopping the infusion. The frequency and severity of these symptoms increase with fosphenytoin dose and infusion rate and might be related to the phosphate load. Venous irritation including pain, erythema, swelling, tenderness, and cording (hardening of the vessel) occurs less often than with phenytoin.[15] IM fosphenytoin injections are well tolerated and no marked differences in local symptoms were reported when compared with IM saline injections.[15] No appreciable differences between fosphenytoin and phenytoin have been reported with regard to adverse cardiovascular effects with IV infusion. CNS adverse effects are common and likely represent reactions to phenytoin. (*See* Phenytoin.)

Contraindications. Sinus bradycardia; sinoatrial block; second- or third-degree AV block; Adams-Stokes syndrome; hypersensitivity to phenytoin or other hydantoins.

Precautions. Consider the phosphate load of fosphenytoin (0.0037 mmol phosphate/mg PE fosphenytoin) in patients with renal insufficiency and those requiring phosphate restriction. (*See* Phenytoin.)

Drug Interactions. No drugs are known to affect the conversion of fosphenytoin to phenytoin. (*See* Phenytoin.)

Parameters to Monitor. Common immunoassays (e.g., TDx, TDx/FLx) overestimate phenytoin concentrations when fosphenytoin is present. Determine serum phenytoin concentrations no earlier than 2 h after an IV infusion or 4 h after an IM dose of fosphenytoin. Obtain samples in tubes containing ethylenediaminetetraacetic acid to minimize the ex vivo conversion of fosphenytoin to phenytoin. Monitor blood pressure and ECG during and 1–2 h after IV fosphenytoin infusion.

Notes. Unlike parenteral phenytoin, fosphenytoin is not formulated with propylene glycol and is compatible with most common IV solutions including 0.9% saline and 5% dextrose.[15]

GABAPENTIN
Neurontin

Pharmacology. Gabapentin is a cyclohexane compound that is structurally related to GABA; its mechanism of action is not known. Gabapentin does not interact with GABA receptors or alter the formation, release, degradation, or reuptake of GABA.[16]

Administration and Adult Dosage. **PO for epilepsy**—300 mg 3 times daily.[16] Dosage can be increased according to clinical response. **Usual maintenance dosage**—900–1800 mg/d in 3 divided doses. Dosages of 3.6–4.8 g/d have been well tolerated in some patients.[16] Give dosages ≥ 3.6 g/d in 4 divided doses 4 times daily. (*See* Notes.) **PO for postherpetic neuralgia**—300 mg on day 1, 300 mg twice daily on day 2, 300 mg 3 times daily on day 3. **Usual maintenance dosage**—1800–3600 mg/d in divided doses.[16]

Special Populations. *Pediatric Dosage.* (3–12 years) starting dose 10–15 mg/kg/d in 3 divided doses. **Usual maintenance dose**—25–35 mg/kg/d given in 3 divided doses. Maximum dosage 50 mg/kg/d with a maximum time interval of 12 h.[16]

Geriatric Dosage. Lower dosages might be required because of normal age-related decreases in renal function.

Other Conditions. *Renal Impairment.* Reduce dosage in patients with compromised renal function as indicated in the following. (Cl_{Cr} 30–59 mL/min) 400–1400 mg/d in divided doses, (Cl_{Cr} 15–29 mL/min) 200–700 mg/d, (Cl_{Cr} < 15 mL/min) 100–300 mg/d. Use half of this dose for Cl_{Cr} < 7.5 mL/min.

Dosage Forms. **Cap** 100, 300, 400 mg; **Tab** 600 mg, 800 mg; **Oral Soln** 250 mg/5mL.

Patient Instructions. (*See* Anticonvulsants, Class Instructions.) Do not take this drug with antacids, or separate them by at least 2 h. If 600- or 800-mg tablets are broken for administration of a half-tablet, should take the half-tablet at the next dose. Half-tablets not used within several days should be discarded.

Missed Doses. Take this drug at regular intervals. If you miss a dose, take it as soon as you remember. If it is about time for the next dose, take that dose only. Do not double the dose or take an extra dose.

Pharmacokinetics. *Onset and Duration.* Steady-state serum levels are attained in 1–2 days in patients with normal renal function.[8]

Serum Levels. A therapeutic range has not been established. One study found that therapeutic effect correlated with serum concentrations greater than 2 mg/L.

Fate. Rapidly absorbed, and food has no effect on absorption. Absorption occurs via a saturable transport mechanism, so bioavailability decreases with dosages greater than 1.8 g/d; at this dosage it is 60%. At a dosage of 4.8 g/d, bioavailability is 35%.[16] The drug is not bound to plasma proteins. V_d is 58 ± 6 L in adults; Cl is 0.17 ± 0.05 L/kg/h in adults with normal renal function; Cl is linearly related to Cl_{Cr}. Gabapentin is not appreciably metabolized but is eliminated unchanged in urine and normal renal function. **Half-life.** 5–7 h in adults with epilepsy and normal renal function.[16]

Adverse Reactions. Somnolence, dizziness, ataxia, nystagmus, and headache occur frequently. Symptoms are of mild-to-moderate severity and resolve within

2 weeks with continued treatment.[16] Weight gain (mean 4.9% of body weight) and peripheral edema also occur frequently. Occasionally, rash occurs. Rarely, behavioral changes in children occur.[16]

Contraindications. Hypersensitivity to gabapentin or any component of the formulation.[16]

Precautions. Abrupt withdrawal of gabapentin in patients with epilepsy can precipitate status epilepticus. In vivo carcinogenicity studies have demonstrated a high incidence of pancreatic acinar cell tumors in male rats; the relevance of this observation to humans is not known. Gabapentin use in pediatric patients aged 3–12 years is associated with mild-to-moderate central nervous system adverse events such as emotional lability, hostility, thought disorder, and hyperkinesias.[16]

Drug Interactions. Gabapentin does not induce or inhibit hepatic microsomal enzymes and does not affect the metabolism of other antiepileptic drugs or oral contraceptives to a degree considered clinically important. Antacids decrease the oral bioavailability of gabapentin by approximately 20%.[16]

Parameters to Monitor. Serum level monitoring is of limited value because of the lack of a well-defined therapeutic range. Routine monitoring of clinical laboratory parameters during gabapentin therapy is not indicated.[16]

Notes. Gabapentin is indicated as adjunctive treatment for partial and secondarily generalized seizures in adults. Preliminary studies have indicated that the drug can be efficacious as an adjunct in children with refractory partial seizures. Gabapentin might not be effective as monotherapy. Gabapentin is effective for the treatment of postherpetic neuralgia and painful diabetic peripheral neuropathy. Preliminary evidence has suggested efficacy in other painful conditions (e.g., reflex sympathetic dystrophy), bipolar disorder, and other psychiatric conditions.[16]

LAMOTRIGINE	Lamictal, Lamictal ODT, Lamictal XR

Pharmacology. Lamotrigine is a phenyltriazine derivative unrelated to other marketed antiepileptic drugs. Lamotrigine inhibits voltage-dependent sodium channels, thereby stabilizing neuronal membranes and reducing the release of excitatory neurotransmitters such as glutamate and aspartate.[17] Its mechanism in bipolar disorder is unknown. (*See* Notes.)

Administration and Adult Dosage. Adjust starting dosages, titration schedules, and maintenance dosage based on concomitant therapy. Increasing the rate of dosage titration or using higher than recommended initial doses increases the risk of serious rash. **PO for epilepsy in patients receiving enzyme-inducing antiepileptic drugs** (e.g., carbamazepine, phenytoin, phenobarbital, and primidone, but not valproic acid)—50 mg/d for 2 weeks and then increase to 50 mg twice daily for 2 more weeks. Thereafter, increase dosage in 100 mg/d increments at weekly intervals to a maintenance dosage of 300–500 mg/d in 2 divided doses. **PO for epilepsy in patients receiving valproate**—25 mg every other day for 2 weeks and then increase to 25 mg/d for 2 more weeks. Thereafter, increase dosage in 25–50 mg/d increments at 1- to 2-week intervals to a **maintenance dosage** of 100–400 mg/d in 2 divided doses or 200 mg/d with valproate alone. **PO for bipolar disorder in patients receiving enzyme-inducing drugs** (e.g., carbamazepine, phenytoin, phenobarbital, primidone, or rifampin, but not taking valproic acid)—50 mg daily for 2 weeks, then 100 mg/d in divided doses for 2 more weeks. Followed by divided doses in week 5, then 300 mg/d in divided doses in week 6, to a maximum of 400 mg/d in divided doses. **PO for bipolar disorder in patients not taking enzyme-inducing drugs**—25 mg daily for 2 weeks, then 50 mg daily for 2 weeks. In week 5, a maintenance dose of 100 mg daily, then to a maximum of 200 mg daily. **PO for bipolar disorder in patients taking valproic acid**—25 mg every other day for 2 weeks, then 25 mg daily for 2 more weeks. In week 5, a maintenance dose of 50 mg daily, then to a maximum of 100 mg daily.[17]

Special Populations. *Pediatric Dosage.* **PO for epilepsy in patients NOT receiving enzyme-inducing antiepileptic drugs (carbamazepine, phenytoin, phenobarbital, and valproic acid)** (2–12 years old)—0.3 mg/kg/d in 1–2 divided doses for 2 weeks, then 0.6 mg/kg/d in 2 divided doses for 2 weeks, then increase by 0.6 mg/kg/d every 1–2 weeks as needed. **PO for epilepsy in patients receiving enzyme-inducing antiepileptic drugs (carbamazepine, phenytoin, phenobarbital, primidone, but not valproic acid)** (2–12 years old)—0.6 mg/kg/d in 2 divided doses for 2 weeks and then increase to 1.2 mg/kg/d in 2 divided doses for 2 weeks, then increase in 1.2 mg/kg/d every 1–2 weeks. **PO for epilepsy in patients receiving valproate** (2–12 years old)—0.15 mg/kg/d in 1–2 divided doses for 2 weeks and then increase to 0.3 mg/kg/d in 1–2 divided doses. Increase by 0.3 mg/kg/d every 1–2 weeks as needed. All doses should be rounded down to the nearest whole tablet size.[17]

Geriatric Dosage. Dosage reduction might be required in patients with reduced hepatic or renal function and should be guided by clinical response.

Hepatic and Renal Impairment. Patients with chronic renal failure or liver disease might require lower dosages of lamotrigine; specific dosage guidelines are not available.

Dosage Forms. **Chew Tab** 2 mg, 5 mg, 25 mg. **Tab** 25, 100, 150, 200 mg. **Orally Disintegrating Tab** 25 mg, 50 mg, 100 mg, 200 mg. **ER Tab** 25 mg, 50 mg, 100 mg, 200 mg.

Patient Instructions. (*See* Anticonvulsants, Class Instructions.) Only use whole tablets. Inform your physician immediately if a skin rash develops.[17]

Missed Doses. Take this drug at regular intervals. If you miss a dose, take it as soon as you remember. If it is about time for the next dose, take that dose only. Do not double the dose or take extra.

Pharmacokinetics. *Onset and Duration.* Steady-state serum levels are attained in 2–3 days.[8]

Serum Levels. A therapeutic range has not been established. In most clinical trials, trough serum concentrations of lamotrigine were 2–5 mg/L.[17]

Fate. The drug is rapidly absorbed, with a bioavailability of 98 ± 5%; peak serum levels occur 1.4–4.8 h after an oral dose. Food does not affect absorption. Lamotrigine is 55% bound to plasma proteins. V_d is 0.9–1.3 L/kg;[17] 10% is excreted unchanged in urine; 90% is excreted as inactive glucuronide conjugates and minor metabolites. **Half-life.** 25–33 h in normal volunteers taking no other medications;[17] 12–14 h in patients taking enzyme-inducing antiepileptic drugs; 27 h in patients taking enzyme-inducing antiepileptic drugs with valproic acid; 59 h in patients taking valproic acid alone.

Adverse Reactions. Dose-related dizziness, ataxia, somnolence, headache, diplopia, nausea, vomiting, and rash occur frequently.[17] Rash occurs in approximately 10% of patients, usually within 2–6 weeks of treatment initiation. The rash is usually maculopapular and erythematous. Potentially life-threatening rashes (including SJS and TEN) are reported in 1:1000 adults and as many as 1:100 children. Risk factors for rash include concomitant valproic acid therapy, high initial dosage of lamotrigine, and rapid escalation of lamotrigine dosage. Discontinue lamotrigine at the first sign of rash. Acute multiorgan failure has been rarely reported.[17]

Contraindications. Hypersensitivity to lamotrigine or any component of the formulation.

Precautions. Initiate lamotrigine cautiously in patients taking valproic acid because of a higher risk of rash. (*See* Administration and Adult Dosage.)

Drug Interactions. Oral contraceptives decrease plasma levels of lamotrigine, and a rise in lamotrigine levels, by almost 2-fold, has been observed during the hormone-free "pill-free" week of the cycle.[17] Dizziness, diplopia, and ataxia are more common in patients taking carbamazepine concomitantly and appear to be the result of a pharmacodynamic interaction. Lamotrigine has no important effect on blood levels of phenytoin, carbamazepine, or its metabolite CBZ-E. Lamotrigine reduces steady-state valproic acid levels by 25%. Rifampin and valproic acid increase lamotrigine levels by approximately 2-fold, and carbamazepine, phenobarbital, primidone, and phenytoin each decrease lamotrigine serum levels.

Parameters to Monitor. Serum level monitoring is of limited value because of the lack of a well-defined therapeutic range. Routine monitoring of clinical laboratory parameters during lamotrigine therapy is not necessary.

Notes. Lamotrigine is indicated as adjunctive treatment for partial and secondarily generalized seizures in adults and for the treatment of the Lennox-Gastaut syndrome and primarily generalized tonic–clonic seizures in adults and children older than 2 years of age.[17] Lamotrigine can be effective as monotherapy and appears to be better tolerated than carbamazepine monotherapy at dosages that are equally effective for the treatment of partial epilepsy. (*See* Anticonvulsants Comparison Chart.)

LEVETIRACETAM Keppra

Pharmacology. Levetiracetam is a pyrollidine derivative that is structurally unrelated to other antiepileptic drugs.[18] Its mechanism of action is unclear and does not relate to any known mechanisms of neuronal excitation or inhibition. In recordings of epileptiform activity, levetiracetam inhibits burst firing without affecting neuronal excitability, suggesting that it may prevent propagation of seizure activity.

Administration and Adult Dosage. PO for epilepsy—500 mg twice daily initially, increasing in increments of 1 g/d at 2-week intervals as needed.[18] (XR tablets) 1000 mg once daily initially, increasing in 1 g increments every 2 weeks as needed.[19] **Usual maintenance dosage**—2–3 g/d in 2 divided doses. XR tablets may be administered as a single-daily dose. Doses greater than 3 g/d have been used in open-label studies for 6 months or longer. However, there is no evidence that doses greater than 3 g/d confer additional benefit. **Intravenous** Same dose as oral therapy.

Special Populations. *Pediatric Dosage.* (4–16 years) 10 mg/kg twice daily initially, increasing in 2-week intervals to the maximum daily dose of 30 mg/kg twice daily as needed.[18]

Geriatric Dosage. Lower dosages might be required because of age-related decreases in renal function.[8]

Hepatic Impairment. Dosage reduction is not necessary for patients with hepatic impairment.

Renal Impairment. Reduce dosage in patients with compromised renal function as follows, Cl_{Cr} >80 mL/min 500–1500 mg every 12 h; 50–80 mL/min 500–1000 mg every 12 h; 30–50 mL/min 250–750 mg every 12 h; <30 mL/min 250–500 every 24 h, on hemodialysis 500–1000 mg every 24 h.[18]

Dosage Forms. **Tab** 250, 500, 750 1000 mg, **XR Tab** 500 mg, **Oral Soln** 100 mg/mL, **Inj** 100 mg/mL.

Patient Instructions. *See* Anticonvulsants, Class Instructions.

Missed Doses. Take this drug at regular intervals. If you miss a dose, take it as soon as you remember. If it is about time for the next dose, take that dose only. Do not double the dose or take an extra dose.

Pharmacokinetics. *Onset and Duration.* Steady-state serum levels are attained in 2 days.[8]

Serum Levels. Not established.

Fate. Rapidly and completely absorbed within 1 h; food does not affect the extent of absorption but decreases C_{max} by 20% and delays T_{max} by 1.5 h. The drug is largely unbound to plasma proteins (<10% bound). V_d is 0.5–0.7 L/kg in adults; clearance is 0.06 L/h/kg in adults with normal renal function; reduced by 38% in elderly patients with Cl_{Cr} of 30–74 mL/min. Levetiracetam is eliminated primarily as unchanged drug in urine (66% of an administered dose). Metabolism is a minor route of elimination; 3 inactive metabolites have been identified. CYP pathways are not involved.[18] **Half-life.** (adults with normal renal function) 7 ± 1 h.[18]

Adverse Reactions. Somnolence, asthenia, infection, and dizziness occur frequently. Symptoms are of mild-to-moderate severity and usually occur within the first 4 weeks of treatment. Skin rash is rare.[18]

Contraindications. Patients who previously exhibited hypersensitivity to levetiracetam or any of its known components.

Precautions. Minor decreases in RBC and WBC counts, hemoglobin, and hematocrit have been seen. The clinical importance of these findings appears to be minimal.

Drug Interactions. Levetiracetam does not induce or inhibit hepatic microsomal CYP enzymes and does not affect the metabolism of other antiepileptic drugs, oral contraceptives, warfarin, or digoxin. Antacids have no effect on levetiracetam bioavailability.[18]

Parameters to Monitor. Serum level monitoring is not of value because of the lack of a defined therapeutic range. Routine monitoring of clinical laboratory parameters during levetiracetam therapy is not required.

Notes. Levetiracetam is indicated as adjunctive treatment for partial seizures in adults and children >4 years of age, primary generalized tonic–clonic seizures in adults and children >6 years of age, and as an adjunctive treatment of myoclonic seizures in adults and children >12 years of age.[18] There is limited data on its use in status epilepticus.[20]

OXCARBAZEPINE
Trileptal, Various

Pharmacology. Oxcarbazepine is a 10-keto analogue of carbamazepine that exerts its anticonvulsant effect through an active 10-monohydroxy metabolite (MHD).[21] Its mechanism of action is not known but likely involves blockade of voltage-dependent sodium channels and inhibition of repetitive neuronal firing.

Administration and Adult Dosage. **PO for epilepsy**—300 mg twice daily initially, increasing in increments of no more than 600 mg/d at weekly intervals to effective dosage.[21] **Usual maintenance dosage**—1200–2400 mg/d in 2 divided doses.

Special Populations. *Pediatric Dosage.* **PO for epilepsy**—(2–16 years) 8–10 mg/kg/d in 2 divided doses initially, increasing at weekly intervals as needed. **Usual maintenance dosage** in 2 divided doses—(20–29 kg) 900 mg/d; (29.1–39 kg) 1200 mg/d; (>39 kg) 1800 mg/d.

Geriatric Dosage. Clearance of the active MHD is reduced in some elderly patients because of decreased renal function, so lower maintenance dosages might be required.[21]

Hepatic Impairment. No dosage adjustment is required in patients with mild-to-moderate hepatic impairment.

Renal Impairment. Begin oxcarbazepine at one-half the usual starting dosage in patients with $Cl_{Cr} < 30$ mL/min, and reduce the rate of titration.

Dosage Forms. **Tab** 150, 300, 600 mg; **Susp** 60 mg/mL.

Patient Instructions. (*See* Anticonvulsants, Class Instructions.) Report symptoms of nausea, malaise, headache, lethargy, or confusion. This drug may decrease the effect of oral contraceptive; recommend additional form of birth control.

Missed Doses. Take this drug at regular intervals. If you miss a dose, take it as soon as you remember. If it is about time for the next dose, take that dose only. Do not double the dose or take extra.

Pharmacokinetics. *Onset and Duration.* Steady-state serum levels of MHD are attained in 2 days.

Serum Levels. A therapeutic range has not been established.

Fate. Completely absorbed; food has no effect. Oxcarbazepine is converted into MHD, which is primarily responsible for the anticonvulsant activity of oxcarbazepine. MHD is 40% bound to plasma proteins, primarily albumin. V_d (MHD) is 49 L in adults; clearance (MHD) is 2.5 ± 0.1 L/kg/h after a single dose in epilepsy patients taking other antiepileptic drugs. MHD is eliminated primarily by glucuronidation to inactive products (47%) and renal excretion of unchanged MHD (27%). **Half-life.** (oxcarbazepine) 2.4 ± 1.1 h; (MHD) 9.3 ± 1.8 h in healthy adult volunteers.

Adverse Reactions. Dizziness, somnolence, diplopia, fatigue, headache, and nausea occur frequently. Symptoms are more common with rapid dosage titration.

Rash occurs in 2.8% of patients.[21] Among patients with histories of hypersensitivity to carbamazepine, 25%–30% experience hypersensitivity to oxcarbazepine. Hyponatremia (Na <125 mEq/L) occurs in 2.5% of patients.

Contraindications. Patient with known hypersensitivity to oxcarbazepine or to any of its components.

Precautions. Patients with histories of severe hypersensitivity reactions to carbamazepine (e.g., exfoliative dermatitis) appear to be at high risk for similar reactions to oxcarbazepine.[22] Patients should report symptoms of nausea, malaise, headache, lethargy, or confusion, which might indicate hyponatremia.

Drug Interactions. Oxcarbazepine does not induce its own metabolism but does reduce estrogen and progestin levels by 50%. Thus, the efficacy of oral contraceptives might be reduced. Oxcarbamazepine can increase phenytoin levels by up to 40% in adults; no effects on the metabolism of other antiepileptic drugs are reported. Carbamazepine, phenytoin, and phenobarbital increase the metabolism of MHD. Cimetidine, erythromycin, and propoxyphene do not affect MHD levels. Verapamil reduces MHD concentrations by 20%.

Parameters to Monitor. Consider measuring serum sodium levels during oxcarbazepine therapy, particularly in patients taking other drugs known to reduce sodium concentrations or those who develop signs or symptoms of hyponatremia. (*See* Precautions.)

Notes. Oxcarbazepine is indicated as monotherapy and adjunctive therapy for the treatment of partial and secondarily generalized seizures in adults, as adjunctive therapy for the treatment of partial-onset seizures in children (4–16 years), and as adjunctive therapy in children with epilepsy (≥2 years).

PHENOBARBITAL
Luminal, Various

Pharmacology. Phenobarbital is a barbiturate that exerts an anticonvulsant effect by depressing excitatory postsynaptic seizure discharge and increasing the convulsive threshold for electric and chemical stimulation.[23]

Administration and Adult Dosage. **PO or IM for epilepsy**—60–90 mg/d initially, increasing in 30–60 mg/d increments every 7–14 days to an effective dosage. **Usual maintenance dosage**—90–240 mg/d or 1–3 mg/kg/d at bedtime.[23] **IV for status epilepticus**—20 mg/kg at a rate of 100 mg/min. **Rectal administration** has been reported. (*See* Fate, Adverse Reactions and Notes.)

Special Populations. *Pediatric Dosage.* **PO or IM for epilepsy**—0.5 mg/kg/d initially, increasing every 7–14 days to minimize sedation. **Usual maintenance dosage** is 2–5 mg/kg/d or 125 mg/m^2/d given at bedtime.[8] **IV for status epilepticus**—10–20 mg/kg at a rate of 50–100 mg/min.[8] (*See* Adverse Reactions and Notes.)

Geriatric Dosage. Clearance of phenobarbital is reduced in the elderly, so lower maintenance dosages might be required.[8]

Pregnancy Dosage. During pregnancy, phenobarbital clearance can increase. Dosage increases might be necessary and should be guided by serum levels and patient status.

Dosage Forms. **Tab** 15, 16, 30, 60, 90, 100 mg; **Elxr** 3, 4 mg/mL; **Inj** 30, 60, 65, 130 mg/mL.

Patient Instructions. *See* Anticonvulsants, Class Instructions.

Missed Doses. Take this drug at regular intervals. If you miss a dose, take it as soon as you remember. If it is about time for the next dose, take that dose only. Do not double the dose or take an extra dose.

Pharmacokinetics. *Onset and Duration.* Steady-state serum levels are attained in approximately 21 days.[8]

Serum Levels. (Anticonvulsant) 15–35 mg/L (65–150 (mol/L); dysarthria, ataxia, and nystagmus appear as serum level approaches 40 mg/L (172 μmol/L).[23]

Fate. The drug is slowly absorbed orally with 95%–100% bioavailability; peak serum level occurs 2–4 h after a PO or IM dose.[8,23] Rectal bioavailability is 90%, with a peak of 7.2 ± 0.8 mg/L (31 ± 3.4 mol/L) 4.4 ± 0.6 h after rectal administration of a 5 mg/kg dose of parenteral phenobarbital sodium solution. The drug is 45%–60% bound to plasma proteins. V_d is 0.61 ± 0.05 L/kg; Clearance is 0.004 ± 0.0008 L/h/kg in adults, with 50%–80% metabolized in the liver to p-hydroxyphenobarbital (inactive). The drug is 20%–50% excreted unchanged in urine; alkalinization of urine increases renal phenobarbital clearance. **Half-life.** (adults) 100 ± 17 h,[73] (cirrhosis) 130 ± 15 h; (children 1–5 years) 69 ± 3.2 h.

Adverse Reactions. (*See* Serum Levels.) Sedation is frequent and dose related; tolerance usually develops with long-term administration.[8,23] In adults, phenobarbital can impair cognition, reaction time, and motor performance. Loss of concentration, mental dulling, depression, insomnia, and hyperkinetic activity occur frequently with long-term therapy in children and the elderly. Connective tissue disorders associated with barbiturates occur in 6% of patients, usually within the first year of treatment. Occasionally, skin rashes or folate deficiency occur. Rarely, megaloblastic anemia, hepatitis, exfoliative dermatitis, or SJS is reported. Patients can be at risk for similar hypersensitivity reactions if rechallenged with phenytoin or carbamazepine. Neonatal hemorrhage has been reported in newborns whose mothers were taking phenobarbital. SQ or intra-arterial injection can produce tissue necrosis. IV administration, especially when given after IV benzodiazepines, can produce severe respiratory depression and provision for respiratory support should be made.

Contraindications. History of porphyria or severe respiratory disease where dyspnea or obstruction is present; marked hepatic impairment.

Precautions. Pregnancy; lactation; elderly; depression; pulmonary insufficiency. Use with caution in patients with marked liver or renal disease because drug clearance is slowed. Abrupt withdrawal of the drug in patients with epilepsy can precipitate status epilepticus.

Drug Interactions. Concurrent use with other CNS depressants can potentiate the sedation caused by phenobarbital. Numerous drugs can increase phenobarbital serum levels, possibly requiring phenobarbital dosage reduction; phenobarbital can stimulate CYP2D6 and CYP3A and increase the metabolism of many drugs.

Parameters to Monitor. Periodic serum level monitoring (10–40 μg/mL), after attaining steady state (~21 days), is useful in guiding dosage changes or evaluating adverse effects.[8] Monitor CBC and liver function tests periodically during long-term therapy.

Notes. In tonic–clonic status epilepticus, phenobarbital is usually considered a third agent after IV phenytoin plus IV diazepam or lorazepam have failed to control seizures.[8] Considering clinical efficacy and patient tolerance, phenobarbital is a third- or fourth-line choice for single-drug therapy of partial or generalized tonic–clonic seizures compared with the drugs of first choice: carbamazepine, phenytoin, or valproic acid.[23] (*See* Anticonvulsants Comparison Chart.)

PHENYTOIN   Dilantin, Various

Pharmacology. Phenytoin is a hydantoin that suppresses the spread of seizure activity mainly by inhibiting synaptic posttetanic potentiation and blocking the propagation of electric discharge in the motor cortex. Phenytoin might decrease sodium transport and block calcium channels at the cellular level to produce these actions.[24]

Administration and Adult Dosage. **PO maintenance dosage**—300 mg/d in 1–3 doses initially. Using serum levels as a guide, increase in 30–100 mg/d increments every 2–3 weeks to effective dosage.[8] Because of dose-dependent saturable metabolism, small increases in dosage can produce disproportionate increases in serum levels. **Usual maintenance dosage**—300–400 mg/d or 4–8 mg/kg/d in 1 or 2 doses.[8] Only extended-release phenytoin sodium capsules are approved for once-daily administration. **PO loading dosage**—1000 mg in 3 divided doses, administered at 2-h intervals. Using serum levels as a guide, a maintenance dosage can be initiated within 24 h of starting the loading dosage.[24] **IV loading dose**—15–20 mg/kg by direct IV injection, at a rate not greater than 50 mg/min or 0.75 mg/kg/min in adults.[24] Therapeutic serum levels persist for 12–24 h in most patients.[25] Alternatively, dilute the loading dose in 50–150 mL of 0.45% or 0.9% NaCl and infuse through an IV volume control set with an in-line filter at a rate not greater than 50 mg/min.[8] In nonemergency situations, an IV dose of 5 mg/kg every 2 h for 3 doses at a rate of 50 mg/min results in phenytoin serum levels of 10–20 mg/L 12 h after the third dose.[8] (*See* Adverse Reactions and Notes.) **IM administration** is painful and results in slow, but complete, absorption because of deposition of phenytoin crystals in muscle.[8] The IM route is not recommended. The IV route is preferred in patients unable to take phenytoin by mouth.[24] (*See* Fosphenytoin.)

Special Populations. *Pediatric Dosage.* **PO maintenance dosage**—5 mg/kg/d initially in 2–3 divided doses. Increase initial dosage in small increments every 7–10 days to effective dosage.[8,24] Because of dose-dependent metabolism, small increases in dosage can produce disproportionate increases in serum levels. **Usual maintenance dosage**—4–8 mg/kg/d in 2–3 divided doses. **IV loading dose**—(neonates) 15–20 mg/kg given at a rate not exceeding 1–3 mg/kg per min; (older infants and children) Same as adult dosage.[24]

Geriatric Dosage. **PO maintenance dosage**—Advanced age can be associated with a decrease in phenytoin clearance and a reduction in albumin concentration.[24] Dosage adjustment should be guided by phenytoin levels and patient status. (*See* Serum Levels.)

Other Conditions. During pregnancy or febrile illness or after acute traumatic injury, phenytoin clearance can increase; dosage adjustment might be necessary and should be guided by serum levels and patient status.[26–28] Renal disease and hypoalbuminemia can alter phenytoin binding to plasma proteins, resulting in a change in the usual ratio of free to total phenytoin levels; renal disease alters phenytoin protein binding because of decreased affinity of plasma proteins.[8] Increases in fraction unbound are most pronounced in patients with Cl_{Cr} <25 mL/min. Ideally, adjust dosage guided by patient status and actual measurement of unbound and total phenytoin levels. (*See* Serum Levels.)[24]

Dosage Forms. (Phenytoin) **Chew Tab** 50 mg; **Susp** 25 mg/mL. (Phenytoin sodium) **Cap** (extended-release) 30, 100, 200, 300 mg, (prompt) 100mg; **Inj** 50 mg/mL. Phenytoin sodium is 92% phenytoin.[24,29]

Patient Instructions. (*See* Anticonvulsants, Class Instructions.) Good dental hygiene and regular dental visits can minimize gum tenderness, bleeding, or enlargement (especially in children). Shake oral suspension well before each dose and use a calibrated measuring device. (*See* Notes.) Call physician if skin rash develops.[24]

Missed Doses. Take this drug at regular intervals. If you miss a dose, take it as soon as you remember. If it is about time for the next dose, take that dose only. When taking multiple daily doses, leave a minimum of 4–6 h between doses. If you are taking the drug only once daily and you do not remember until the next day, skip the missed dose and return to your normal schedule. Do not double the dose or take extra. If doses are missed for 2 or more days in a row, consult your physician.

Pharmacokinetics. *Onset and Duration.* Time to steady state increases with increasing dosage and serum level. Steady state is usually attained within 7–14 days but can take as long as 28 days.[8]

Serum Levels. 10–20 mg/L (40–80 μmol/L) in patients with normal renal function and serum albumin concentration. Nystagmus, slurred speech, ataxia, or dizziness appear in most patients as serum levels approach 20 mg/L; drowsiness, diplopia, behavioral changes, and cognitive impairment occur with serum levels greater than 30 mg/L (120 μmol/L).[8] The equation $C_{normal} = C_{observed}/([0.2 \times albumin] + 0.1)$ estimates the concentration of phenytoin that would be expected if the albumin concentration were normal (C_{normal}) from the measured total phenytoin concentration in a hypoalbuminemia patient ($C_{observed}$) and the patient's albumin concentration in g/dL (albumin). In patients with end-stage renal disease (Cl_{Cr} <10 mL/min), the equation $C_{normal} = C_{observed}/([0.1 \times albumin] + 0.1)$ is used.[30] (*See* Special Populations, Other Conditions.)

Fate. Oral phenytoin absorption is very slow and incomplete in infants <3 months of age.[8] Bioavailability of the suspension is decreased in patients receiving concomitant enteral feedings. (*See* Precautions.) IM injection is slowly absorbed over several days because of deposition of phenytoin crystals in muscle. Peak serum levels occur 4–12 h after a single dose of an extended-release capsule; after oral loading given in divided doses, the times to reach a serum level of 10 mg/L are 5–7 h for prompt-release capsules and 4–12 h for extended-release capsules.[8,24,29] Time to peak serum level increases with increasing oral dosages. Approximately 90% is bound to plasma proteins. Hypoalbuminemia, chronic liver or renal disease, nephrotic syndrome, AIDS, or acute traumatic injury alter protein binding and increase the fraction of unbound phenytoin. V_d is 0.83 ± 0.2 L/kg in adults with acute seizures[8] and 0.79 ± 0.25 L/kg in critically ill adults after trauma.[26] Hepatic metabolism is capacity limited, exhibiting Michaelis-Menten pharmacokinetics; therefore, clearance decreases as serum level increases. Mean apparent V_{max} is 0.45 mg/L/h; mean apparent K_m is 6.2 mg/L in adults.[8] Approximately 75% of phenytoin is excreted in urine as the inactive metabolite, 5-(p-hydroxyphenyl)-5-phenyl hydantoin. Less than 5% of the parent drug is excreted unchanged in urine.[31] **Half-life.** Phenytoin has no true half-life, but its apparent half-life increases as serum level increases; at phenytoin serum levels of 1, 10, 20, and 40 mg/L, the predicted mean phenytoin half-lives are 13, 26, 40, and 69 h, respectively.[8]

Adverse Reactions. (*See* Serum Levels.) Erythematous morbilliform rash occurs frequently. Do not resume phenytoin if rash is exfoliative, purpuric, bullous, or accompanied by fever. With long-term administration, hirsutism, gingival hypertrophy (especially in children and adolescents), coarsening of facial features, acneiform eruption, osteomalacia, and folate deficiency with mild macrocytosis occur frequently.[8,24] Bradycardia or hypotension caused by rapid IV administration are reported occasionally; slowing the rate of administration can minimize these complications.[8] Severe soft tissue injury after IV phenytoin is more likely in elderly (>70 years) women who receive 2 or more infusions through small (<20 gauge) IV devices. Hepatotoxicity occurs occasionally, usually within the first 6 weeks, and presents with fever, rash, lymphadenopathy, and hepatomegaly.[24] Other idiosyncratic reactions are rare, can occur together within the first 2 months, and include fever, lymphoid hyperplasia, eosinophilia, erythema multiforme, exfoliative dermatitis, SJS, leukopenia, anemia, thrombocytopenia, serum sickness, and SLE.[24] These patients are at risk for similar hypersensitivity reactions if rechallenged with phenobarbital or carbamazepine.[32] Concurrent cranial irradiation predisposes patients to the development of erythema multiforme.[24] A syndrome of anomalies in infants of phenytoin-exposed mothers has been described (fetal hydantoin syndrome).

Contraindications. (Parenteral phenytoin) sinus bradycardia; sinoatrial block; second- and third-degree AV blocks; Adams-Stokes syndrome (intravenous phenytoin only).

Precautions. Pregnancy; lactation. Use with caution in patients with severe liver disease or diabetes or with histories of severe hypersensitivity reactions to carbamazepine or phenobarbital. Abrupt withdrawal of the drug in patients with epilepsy can precipitate status epilepticus. If the patient's nutritional status allows, interrupt tube feeding 2 h before and after the dose and irrigate the feeding tube to improve absorption; nevertheless, the patient might require an increase in phenytoin dosage. If the feedings are discontinued after the phenytoin dosage is increased, the dosage must be adjusted to prevent toxic serum levels from occurring.[24]

Drug Interactions. Chronic alcohol use, barbiturates, rifampin, and some other drugs can stimulate phenytoin metabolism and increase phenytoin dosage requirements. Numerous drugs can increase phenytoin serum levels, possibly requiring phenytoin dosage reduction; phenytoin can stimulate CYP2C8/9/19 and CYP3A4 and increase the metabolism of many drugs. IV phenytoin can produce hypotension in severely ill patients receiving IV dopamine. The antiparkinson effect of levodopa can be inhibited by phenytoin.

Parameters to Monitor. Serum level monitoring, after attaining steady state (10–21 days), is useful in evaluating therapeutic efficacy or potential for adverse effects.[8,24] Monitoring of patient and serum levels are recommended when changing phenytoin dosage form or brand; monitor serum levels 5–7 half-lives (~7–10 days) after treatment initiation to assess trend in concentrations. Monitor CBC and liver function tests periodically with long-term therapy.[29]

Notes. Agitation or shaking is needed to resuspend phenytoin suspension; settling occurs 5 weeks after resuspension. Patients who receive enteral nutrition supplements have had lower than expected phenytoin levels. Phenytoin administration should be separated from enteral nutrition administration.[24] In tonic–clonic status epilepticus, the anticonvulsant effect of phenytoin appears 20–30 min after start of the infusion. Thus, in this situation, concurrent use of phenytoin with a rapidly acting injectable benzodiazepine (**diazepam** or **lorazepam**) is recommended.[8] Phenytoin is recommended, as is **carbamazepine**, as a drug of first choice for single-drug therapy of partial or generalized tonic–clonic seizures.[8] (*See* Anticonvulsants Comparison Chart.)

PREGABALIN   Lyrica

Pharmacology. Pregabalin is a structural derivative of GABA, however, it does not bind directly to GABA receptors or augment the action of GABA. While the exact mechanism of action is unknown, its antiseizure and antinociceptive activity is believed to be related to binding to voltage-gated calcium channels within the central nervous system.[33]

Administration and Adult Dosage. PO for epilepsy—adjunctive therapy 150 mg/d in 2–3 divided doses increasing to a maximum of 600 mg/d in divided doses.[33] **Usual maintenance dosage**—300–600 mg/d in 2–3 divided doses; **PO for diabetic neuropathic pain**—50 mg 3 times daily, increasing to 100 mg 3 times daily in 1 week based on efficacy and tolerability. Doses as high as 600 mg/d have been used, but doses greater than 300 mg/d are not recommended. **Usual maintenance dosage**—100 mg 3 times daily. **PO for postherpetic neuralgia**—150 mg/d in 2–3 divided doses, increasing to 300 mg/d in 1 week. In patients who do not experience adequate pain relief, doses may be increased to 600 mg/d in 2–3 divided doses. **Usual maintenance dosage**—300 mg/d. **PO for fibromyalgia**—150 mg/d in 2–3 divided doses initially, increasing to 300 mg/d in 1 week. **Usual maintenance dosage**—300–450 mg/d in divided doses[33]

Special Populations. *Pediatric Dosage.* Safety and efficacy not established.[33]

Geriatric Dosage. Same as adult dosage.

Renal Impairment. Doses should be adjusted in renal impairment when Cl_{Cr} <60 mL/min.[33]

Dosage Forms. **Cap** 25, 50, 75, 100, 150, 200, 225, 300 mg.

Patient Instructions. (*See* Anticonvulsants, Class Instructions.) Alcohol consumption should be avoided.[33]

Missed Doses. Take this drug at regular intervals. If you miss a dose, take it as soon as you remember. If it is about time for the next dose, take that dose only. Do not double the dose or take an extra dose. If you miss more than one dose in a day, call your physician.[33]

Pharmacokinetics. *Onset and Duration.* Steady-state serum levels are attained within 1–2 days.[33] (*See* Fate.)

Serum Levels. Therapeutic range not established.

Fate. Absorption is rapid, with ≥90% bioavailability; peak serum levels occur within 1.5 h.[33] The drug does not bind to plasma proteins. V_d is 0.5 L/kg in adults. Pregabalin does not undergo metabolism and following administration of single dose 90% was recovered in the urine. Mean renal clearance is approximately 67–81 mL/min.[33] **Half-life.** 6.3 h in adults with normal renal function.[33]

Adverse Reactions. Dizziness, somnolence, dry mouth, edema, blurred vision, weight gain, and difficulties with concentration/attention occur frequently. Angioedema, thrombocytopenia, elevations in creatinine kinase, PR interval prolongation, and hypersensitive skin reactions rarely occur. Animal studies revealed an increased incidence of hemangiosarcoma, but this finding is likely not relevant in humans.[33]

Contraindications. Known hypersensitivity to pregabalin.

Precautions. Pregnancy, peripheral edema has been reported; in patients without clinically evident heart or peripheral vascular disease, this was not associated with cardiovascular complications. Use caution in patients with New York Heart Association (NYHA) class III or IV heart failure or in patients receiving thiazolidinedione antidiabetic agents. Recreational users of sedative/hypnotic drugs reported feelings of euphoria with pregabalin.[33] It is classified as a schedule V controlled substance.

Drug Interactions. Pregabalin does not undergo substantial metabolism and is not subject to interactions with any CYP enzymes. In vivo studies did not demonstrate interactions with gabapentin, oral contraceptives, lorazepam, oxycodone, phenytoin, carbamazepine, valproic acid, and lamotrigine.[33]

Parameters to Monitor. Seizure control; creatinine kinase, with occurrence of myopathy symptoms such as malaise, fever, or muscle pain; symptoms of angioedema, during initial and chronic therapy.

PRIMIDONE   Mysoline, Various

Pharmacology. Primidone (desoxyphenobarbital) is structurally related to the barbiturates. Primidone and its metabolites, phenylethylmalonamide (PEMA) and phenobarbital, exert anticonvulsant activity. The exact mechanism of primidone's antiepileptic action in unknown. In experimental animals, primidone raises electro- or chemishock seizure thresholds or alters seizure patterns; PEMA potentiates the anticonvulsant activity of phenobarbital in animal models.[34] (*See* Phenobarbital.)

Administration and Adult Dosage. **PO for epilepsy**—100–125 mg at bedtime for 1–3 days; increase to 100–125 mg twice daily for days 4–6, increase to 100–125 mg 3 times daily for days 7–9, then to effective dosage, maximum dose 500 mg 4 times daily. **Usual maintenance dosage**—250 mg 3–4 times daily.[34]

Special Populations. *Pediatric Dosage.* **PO for epilepsy**—(<8 years) 50 mg at bedtime for 1–3 days; increase to 50 mg twice daily for days 4–6; increase to 100 mg twice daily for days 7–9, then adjust to effective dosage every 3 days in 50 mg/d increments. **Usual maintenance dosage**—125–250 mg 3 times daily or 10–25 mg/kg/d in divided doses.[34]

Geriatric Dosage. Clearance of primidone is unchanged in elderly patients, but phenobarbital clearance is reduced. Lower maintenance dosages might be required.

Dosage Forms. Tab 50, 250 mg.

Patient Instructions. *See* Anticonvulsants, Class Instructions.

Missed Doses. Take this drug at regular intervals. If you miss a dose, take it as soon as you remember. If it is about time for the next dose, take that dose only. Do not double the dose or take an extra dose.

Pharmacokinetics. *Onset and Duration.* Steady-state serum levels are attained in approximately 3 days.[8]

Serum Levels. (Primidone) 6–12 mg/L (28–55 μmol/L).[8] (*See also* Phenobarbital.) During monotherapy, the serum level ratio of phenobarbital to primidone is approximately 1:1. During polytherapy with enzyme-inducing agents, this ratio increases to 4:1. During monotherapy, the serum level ratio of PEMA to primidone at steady state is 0.74 ± 0.38 for samples drawn before the first morning dose.

Fate. The drug is rapidly absorbed with 90%–100% bioavailability; peak serum levels occur 2–6 h after an oral dose. The drug is up to 20% bound to plasma proteins; V_d is 0.86 ± 0.22 L/kg;[8] clearance with monotherapy is 0.035 ± 0.02 L/h/kg; with concomitant anticonvulsants, it is 0.052 ± 0.02 L/h/kg; in monotherapy with concomitant acute viral hepatitis, it is 0.042 ± 0.14 L/h/kg. Primidone is metabolized in the liver to PEMA and phenobarbital; 76% of the drug is excreted into the urine within 5 days after a single dose as 64% primidone, 7% PEMA, 2% phenobarbital, and 3% unidentified products. **Half-life.** (primidone) 15.2 ± 4.8 h (monotherapy); 8.3 ± 2.9 h (with concomitant enzyme-inducing anticonvulsants); 18 ± 3.1 h (with acute viral hepatitis).[8] (PEMA) 21 ± 3 h (primidone monotherapy); 17 ± 4.3 h (with concomitant anticonvulsants). (*See* Phenobarbital.)

Adverse Reactions. Drowsiness, ataxia, nausea, weakness, and dizziness occur frequently during the first month of therapy and might become tolerable with time. Behavioral disturbances, depression of affect, and cognitive impairment occur frequently with long-term therapy in children and the elderly.[8] Occasionally, skin rashes and, rarely, impotence, leukopenia, thrombocytopenia, megaloblastic anemia, or lymphadenopathy occur.[2,34]

Contraindications. History of porphyria; hypersensitivity to phenobarbital.[34]

Precautions. Pregnancy; lactation. Use with caution in patients with severe liver or renal disease. Abrupt withdrawal of the drug can precipitate status epilepticus. (*See* Phenobarbital.)

Drug Interactions. Concurrent use with other CNS depressants can potentiate the sedation caused by phenobarbital. Primidone levels can be decreased by concurrent carbamazepine, succinimides, phenytoin, rifampin, and other CYP2C19 inducers. Primidone levels can be increased by concurrent hydantoins, isoniazid, niacinamide, and other CYP2C19 inhibitors.

Parameters to Monitor. Periodic serum level monitoring of primidone and phenobarbital, after attaining steady state (primidone, 3 days; phenobarbital, 21 days), is useful in guiding dosage changes, detecting noncompliance, or evaluating adverse effects.[8] Monitor CBC, electrolytes, and liver function tests periodically during long-term therapy.

Notes. Considering comparative efficacy and good patient tolerance of **carbamazepine, phenytoin,** and **valproic acid,** primidone is a fourth- or fifth-line choice for single-drug therapy of generalized tonic–clonic seizures. In a large, multicenter trial comparing carbamazepine, phenytoin, phenobarbital, and primidone, primidone was least successful in controlling seizures with acceptable adverse effects.[35]

TIAGABINE
Gabitril

Pharmacology. Tiagabine is a nipecotic acid derivative unrelated to other marketed antiepileptic drugs. It interacts with the GABA uptake carrier and is thought to enhance the inhibitory effect of GABA by preventing its reuptake into neurons. Tiagabine is indicated in adults and adolescents (>12 years) as adjunctive therapy for patients with partial-onset seizures.[36]

Administration and Adult Dosage. **PO for epilepsy**—in patients taking enzyme-inducing antiepileptic drugs (e.g., carbamazepine, phenytoin, phenobarbital, primidone), initiate at 4 mg/d for 1 week, increasing in increments of 4 mg/d in adolescents and 4–8 mg/d at weekly intervals according to clinical response. **Usual maintenance dosage** is 32–56 mg/d. The daily dosage is given in 2–4 divided doses; with dosages >32 mg/d, 3 or 4 times daily administration might be required. Patients taking only non–enzyme-inducing antiepileptic drugs (e.g., gabapentin, lamotrigine, valproate) might require lower doses or a slower titration schedule. In patients not receiving enzyme-inducing antiepileptic drugs, plasma concentrations are double to those of patients receiving enzyme-inducing agents. Lower initial doses and slower titration schedules should be used.[36]

Special Populations. *Pediatric Dosage.* (<12 years) safety and efficacy not established; (>12 years) Maximum daily dose 32 mg/d in patients on concomitant enzyme inducers.[36]

Geriatric Dosage. Same as adult dosage.

Renal Impairment. No apparent need to adjust tiagabine dosage in renal impairment.

Hepatic Impairment. Patients with liver disease might require lower dosages of tiagabine; however, specific dosage guidelines are not available.

Dosage Forms. **Tab** 2, 4, 12, 16 mg.

Patient Instructions. (*See* Anticonvulsants, Class Instructions.) Take this medication with food.

Missed Doses. Take this drug at regular intervals. If you miss a dose, take it as soon as you remember. If it is about time for the next dose, take that dose only. Do not double the dose or take an extra dose.

Pharmacokinetics. *Onset and Duration.* Steady-state serum levels are attained within 2 days.

Serum Levels. A therapeutic range has not been established.

Fate. Rapidly absorbed with a bioavailability of 90%.[31] Food slows the rate, but not the extent, of tiagabine absorption. Peak serum concentrations of 241 ± 79 g/L occurred 1.3 ± 1 h after a single 12-mg dose was administered in healthy volunteers.[37] Tiagabine is 96% bound to plasma proteins, primarily albumin and α_1-acid glycoprotein. V_d is 1.07 ± 0.22 L/kg and clearance is 6.5 ± 1.5 L/h in healthy volunteers. Clearance is increased in patients taking enzyme-inducing antiepileptic drugs. Tiagabine is metabolized by oxidation (primarily CYP3A) and glucuronidation; approximately 2% is excreted unchanged in urine.[36] **Half-life.** 7–9 h in healthy subjects taking no other medications; reduced by 50%–65% in patients with epilepsy taking enzyme-inducing antiepileptic drugs.[36]

Adverse Reactions. Dizziness, asthenia/lack of energy, somnolence, nausea, nervousness, tremor, abdominal pain, and difficulty with concentration occur frequently. Tremor, difficulty with concentration, and asthenia appear to be dose related. The most common reasons for discontinuation are dizziness, somnolence, depression, confusion, and asthenia. Moderate to severe generalized weakness occurs occasionally. Tiagabine rarely induces absence status and can induce seizures in patients without epilepsy.

Contraindications. Hypersensitivity to tiagabine and any component of the formulation.

Precautions. Dosage reduction might be required in hepatic impairment.

Drug Interactions. Carbamazepine, phenytoin, and phenobarbital reduce tiagabine levels by 60% compared with noninduced patients. Valproate has no important effect on tiagabine levels. Tiagabine has no effect on serum concentrations of phenytoin, carbamazepine, phenobarbital, or primidone. Valproate concentrations decrease approximately 10% during tiagabine therapy. Tiagabine has no effect on the pharmacokinetics of warfarin, theophylline, digoxin, or oral contraceptives.

Parameters to Monitor. Serum level monitoring is of limited value because of the lack of a well-defined therapeutic range. No routine laboratory test monitoring is required during therapy.

TOPIRAMATE   Topamax

Pharmacology. Topiramate, a derivative of the naturally occurring monosaccharide D-fructose, reduces the frequency of action potentials elicited by depolarizing currents in a manner suggestive of sodium channel blocking action. Topiramate also increases GABA-induced chloride flux, although the drug has no direct effect on GABA-binding sites. It also inhibits kainate activation of a subtype of the excitatory glutamate receptor. These properties are believed to contribute to its antiepileptic and antimigraine activity. Topiramate inhibits carbonic anhydrase, but this action might not contribute to the drug's anticonvulsant effect. (*See* Notes.)

Administration and Adult Dosage. PO for epilepsy—50 mg/d in 2 divided doses initially, increasing in 50 mg/d increments at weekly intervals to 200–400 mg/d in 2 divided doses. **Usual maintenance dosage**—400 mg/d. Higher dosages have not been shown to be more effective. **PO for migraine**—25 mg at bedtime for one week, then 25 mg twice daily, increasing in 25 mg/d increments weekly to a target dose of 50 mg twice daily.[38]

Special Populations. *Pediatric Dosage.* PO for epilepsy—(<2 years) safety and efficacy not established; (2–16 years) initiate at 1–3 mg/kg/d, increasing in 1–3 mg/kg/d increments weekly to 5–9 mg/kg in 2 divided doses.[38]

Geriatric Dosage. Same as adult dosage.

Renal Impairment. With Cl_{Cr} <70 mL/min, reduce dosage by 50%. Topiramate clearance increases during hemodialysis to a rate 4–6 times greater than in a normal person. Additional doses of topiramate might be required depending on dialysis method and duration.[38]

Dosage Forms. **Cap** (sprinkle) 15, 25 mg; **Tab** 25, 50, 100, 200 mg. (*See* Notes.)

Patient Instructions. (*See* Anticonvulsants, Class Instructions.) Maintain adequate fluid intake (6–8 glasses of water daily) to minimize the formation of kidney stones. If you are taking oral contraceptives, report any change in menstrual bleeding patterns to your health care provider.

Missed Doses. Take this drug at regular intervals. If you miss a dose, take it as soon as you remember. If it is about time for the next dose, take that dose only. Do not double the dose or take an extra dose.

Pharmacokinetics. *Onset and Duration.* Steady-state serum concentrations are attained in 4 days in patients with normal renal function.[38]

Serum Levels. A therapeutic range has not been established.

Fate. The bioavailability of oral tablets is 80% compared with oral solution and peak concentrations occur 3.5 ± 0.6 h after 400 mg.[8] Administration with food delays absorption (by approximately 2 h) but does not affect the extent of absorption. Topiramate is 15%–41% bound to plasma proteins and binds to a saturable, low-capacity binding site on or in erythrocytes.[38] Less protein binding occurs at higher concentrations. V_d is 0.6–0.8 L/kg in healthy volunteers. Clearance is 20–30 mL/min following oral administration in adults on topiramate monotherapy.[38] Approximately 70% is eliminated unchanged in urine. Six metabolites (each <5% of the administered dose) have been identified. **Half-life.** 23 h after a single 400-mg dose in healthy adults.[8]

Adverse Reactions. Somnolence, dizziness, ataxia, speech problems, psychomotor slowing, nystagmus, and paresthesias occur commonly and are not dose related. Common dose-related adverse effects include fatigue, nervousness, difficulty with concentration or attention, confusion, depression, weight loss, and tremor. These adverse effects are minimized by slow-dose titration. Psychomotor slowing and difficulty with concentration are the most common reasons for topiramate discontinuation. Kidney stones occur in 1.5% of patients and might be related to carbonic anhydrase inhibition.

Contraindications. Hypersensitivity to topiramate or any component of the formulation.[38]

Precautions. Avoid concomitant use of other carbonic anhydrase inhibitors (e.g., acetazolamide) because of the potential increased risk of kidney stones.

Drug Interactions. Concomitant phenytoin and carbamazepine reduce topiramate concentrations by 48% and 40%, respectively.[38] Concomitant valproate reduces topiramate concentrations by 14%.[38] Concomitant lamotrigine reduces topiramate concentrations by 13%. Topiramate variably affects phenytoin concentrations (up to 25% decrease) and has no important effect on other anticonvulsants. Topiramate can reduce the effectiveness of oral contraceptives; consider using products containing ≥35 μg of ethinyl estradiol.[38]

Parameters to Monitor. Serum level monitoring is of limited value because of the lack of a well-defined therapeutic range. Routine monitoring of clinical laboratory parameters during topiramate therapy is not indicated.

Notes. Topiramate is indicated for initial monotherapy epilepsy in adult or pediatric patients ≥10 years and as adjunctive treatment for partial-onset and primary generalized tonic–clonic seizures in pediatric patients ≥2 years.[38] Capsules can be opened and sprinkled on food.

VALPROIC ACID	Depakene, Depacon, Various
DIVALPROEX SODIUM	Depakote

Pharmacology. Valproic acid is a carboxylic acid compound whose anticonvulsant activity might be mediated by an inhibitory neurotransmitter, GABA. Valproic acid might increase GABA levels by inhibiting GABA metabolism or enhancing postsynaptic GABA activity. Valproic acid also limits repetitive neuronal firing through voltage- and usage-dependent sodium channels. Divalproex is comprised of sodium valproate and valproic acid. (*See* Notes.)

Administration and Adult Dosage. PO for epilepsy—(valproic acid) 15 mg/kg/d in 2–3 divided doses initially, increasing in 5–10 mg/kg/d increments at weekly intervals to an effective dosage, to a maximum of 60 mg/kg/d. **Usual maintenance dosage**—15–40 mg/kg/d in 3 divided doses.[39] In patients receiving valproic acid, divalproex extended-release can be substituted at a daily dosage 8%–20% than the immediate-release formulation.[34] **PO for migraine prophylaxis**—(divalproex) 250 mg twice daily or 500 mg once daily of extended-release, to a maximum of 1 g/d. **PO for mania**—(divalproex) 25 mg/kg/d in divided doses, increasing as rapidly as possible to the lowest dosage that produces the desired effect, to a maximum of 60 mg/kg/d. (*See* Serum Levels.) Long-term experience with this use is minimal and characterized by a high dropout rate. **IV for epilepsy**—(valproic acid) same as oral dosage. Administer infusion over 60 min or at a rate of ≤20 mg/min. **Rectal administration** has been reported. (*See* Fate.)

Special Populations. *Pediatric Dosage.* Same as adult dosage.

Geriatric Dosage. Reduce the starting dosage in the elderly. Protein binding and unbound clearance of valproic acid are reduced in the elderly, and the desired clinical response can be achieved with lower dosages than in younger adults. Adjust dosage guided by valproic acid levels (preferably free levels in patients with low serum albumin) and patient status.[8]

Dosage Forms. (Valproic acid) **Cap** 125, 250, 500 mg; **syrup** 50 mg/mL; **Inj** 100 mg/mL; (divalproex) **EC Tab** 125, 250, 500 mg; **Cap** (EC granules) 125 mg; **XR Tab** 250, 500 mg.

Patient Instructions. (*See* Anticonvulsants, Class Instructions). This drug can be taken with food or milk to minimize stomach upset. Do not chew, break, or crush the tablet or capsule because this may irritate your mouth or throat. Sprinkle capsule can be swallowed whole or administered by sprinkling the entire contents on small amount (1 teaspoonful) of soft food such as pudding or applesauce; swallow the drug/food mixture immediately (avoid chewing). Polymer from the sprinkles might appear in the stools, but does not indicate a lack of absorption. Immediately report weakness, tiredness, repeated vomiting, or loss of seizure control, which might be early signs of severe, but rare, liver disorder.

Missed Doses. Take this drug at regular intervals. If you miss a dose, take it as soon as you remember. If it is about time for the next dose, take that dose only. Leave a minimum of 6 h between doses. Do not double the dose or take an extra dose.

Pharmacokinetics. *Onset and Duration.* Steady-state serum levels are attained in 2–4 days.[8,39] Several weeks might be required to attain maximal therapeutic effect. For mania, levels should be above 45 mg/L for efficacy and below 125 mg/L to minimize adverse effects.[39]

Serum Levels. 50–120 mg/L (350–830 μmol/L) for epilepsy and mania. Some patients require and can tolerate serum levels up to 150 mg/L.[8] Tremor, irritability, confusion, and restlessness might be observed with levels >100–150 mg/L.

Fate. The bioavailability of the oral capsule is 90%, with peak levels occurring 1–2 h after the dose. The bioavailability of EC divalproex tablet is 90%, with peak levels in 4 h. V_d is 0.19 ± 0.05 L/kg in adults and 0.26 ± 0.09 L/kg in children.[8] Plasma protein binding is approximately 90%.[40] Increasing serum concentrations, hypoalbuminemia, severe liver disease, renal disease, or pregnancy reportedly increases the unbound fraction and might alter clearance. Clearance is (healthy adults) 0.0066 ± 0.0005 L/h/kg; (epileptic adults) 0.018 ± 0.011 L/h/kg; (children) 0.027 ± 0.015 L/h/kg.[8] Over 96% is metabolized to at least 10 metabolites. Only 1.8%–3.2% of drug is excreted unchanged in urine. **Half-life.** (healthy adults) 13.9 ± 3.4 h; (epileptic adults) 8.5 ± 3.3 h; (children) 7.2 ± 2.3 h.[8]

Adverse Reactions. (*See* Serum Levels.) Nausea, vomiting, diarrhea, and abdominal cramps occur frequently during initiation of therapy and are minimized by slow titration of valproic acid or substitution of EC divalproex for valproic acid. Transient elevations in liver function tests occur frequently. The risk of valproate-exposed women having children with spina bifida is approximately 1%–2%. Drowsiness, ataxia, tremor, behavioral disturbances, transient hair loss, asymptomatic hyperammonemia, or weight gain occurs occasionally. Drowsiness and ataxia are more prominent in patients taking valproic acid with other anticonvulsants.[8] Rarely, thrombocytopenia, acute pancreatitis, abnormal coagulation parameters, or hyperglycinemia occurs. Liver failure occurs rarely; the greatest risk is during the first 6 months of therapy and in children <2 years who receive multiple anticonvulsants.[39] Multiorgan hypersensitivity reactions have also been rarely reported; with cases being reported within 1–40 days of therapy initiation.

Contraindications. Hepatic dysfunction or disease, urea cycle disorders, hypersensitive to valproic acid and its derivatives.

Precautions. Pregnancy; lactation. The drug can alter results of urine ketone tests.

Drug Interactions. Valproate levels can be decreased by concurrent carbamazepine, lamotrigine, phenytoin, or rifampin. Valproate levels can be increased by concurrent aspirin (or other salicylates), chlorpromazine, cimetidine, or felbamate. Lamotrigine and phenobarbital levels can be increased by valproate. Carbapenem antibiotics (e.g., ertapenem, imipenem, meropenem) reduce valproate levels.

Parameters to Monitor. Baseline liver function tests and platelets; repeat liver function tests frequently, especially during the first 6 months. Monitor platelet count and coagulation tests before surgery. Periodic serum level monitoring is useful for guiding dosage changes and evaluating potential adverse effects. Serum levels fluctuate considerably over 24 h, making a single random measurement of limited value. Pre-dose blood sampling at standard times is recommended.[8,39]

Notes. Valproic acid and ethosuximide are equally effective for treating absence seizures, although **ethosuximide** is sometimes preferred as a first-line agent because of its lower risk of serious toxicity. Valproic acid is preferred for patients with absence and generalized tonic–clonic seizures. Many clinicians in the United States use valproic acid as a second-line agent (after **phenytoin** or **carbamazepine**) for the treatment of partial seizures. Valproic acid is as effective as phenytoin and carbamazepine for tonic–clonic seizures and is a drug of choice for atonic and myoclonic seizures.[8] (*See* Anticonvulsants Comparison Chart.) Divalproex plus an antipsychotic is equivalent to **lithium** plus an antipsychotic for manic or mixed episodes in bipolar disorder. Lithium, valproate, or lamotrigine are first-line medications for patients with rapid-cycling bipolar disorder.[41] For migraine prophylaxis, divalproex is effective and well tolerated. It might be more effective in those having frequent migraines than in those characterized as having tension headaches. The sustained-release formulation is approved for migraine prophylaxis only.[39]

ZONISAMIDE   Zonegran

Pharmacology. Zonisamide is a 1,2-benzisoxazole sulfonamide derivative that is chemically unrelated to other antiepileptic drugs. It blocks seizure spread and inhibits epileptic foci in animals. The anticonvulsant effect is likely related to blockade of voltage-sensitive sodium and T-type calcium channels. It is also a weak carbonic anhydrase inhibitor.[42]

Administration and Adult Dosage. PO as adjunctive therapy for partial seizures— 100 mg/d initially, increasing in 100 mg/d increments at intervals of 2 weeks as needed.[42] **Usual maintenance dosage**—200–400 mg/d in 1–2 divided doses. Some patients might require dosages of 600 mg/d; there is little evidence for increased effectiveness above 400 mg/d.[42]

Special Populations. *Pediatric Dosage.* (<16 years) Safety and efficacy not established. Zonisamide is used in Japan for the treatment of epilepsy in children. The recommended dosage is 2–4 mg/kg/d initially, increasing at 2-week intervals to 4–12 mg/kg/d as needed.[43]

Geriatric Dosage. Advanced age has no effect on zonisamide pharmacokinetics. No dosage adjustment is necessary.

Renal Impairment. Zonisamide clearance is reduced in patients with renal disease. These patients might require slower titration because of the prolonged half-life of the drug.

Hepatic Impairment. The effect of liver disease on zonisamide pharmacokinetics is unknown.

Dosage Forms. Cap 25, 50, 100 mg.

Patient Instructions. (*See* Anticonvulsants, Class Instructions). Drink 6–8 glasses of water daily to lessen the likelihood of kidney stone formation.

Missed Doses. Take this drug at regular intervals. If you miss a dose, take it as soon as you remember. If it is about time for the next dose, take that dose only. Do not double the dose or take an extra dose.

Pharmacokinetics. *Onset and Duration.* Steady-state serum levels are attained in 14 days in patients with normal renal function.

Serum Levels. Therapeutic range not established.

Fate. Rapidly absorbed after oral administration with peak serum concentrations occurring 2.8 ± 1.4 h after a dose in healthy volunteers. Food delays the rate but has no effect on the extent of zonisamide absorption. Zonisamide is 40% bound to plasma proteins, mainly albumin. In healthy volunteers, V_d/F is 1.47 ± 0.39 L/kg; Cl/F is 0.019 ± 0.004 L/kg/h. Clearance is increased 30%–40% during concomitant therapy with enzyme-induced antiepileptic drugs. Elimination is mainly by urinary excretion of unchanged drug and glucuronide metabolite. Other metabolic pathways include acetylation and reduction of an acetylated metabolite (via CYP3A4).[8,42] **Half-Life.** (adults with normal renal function) 63 h.

Adverse Reactions. Frequent adverse effects include somnolence, ataxia, anorexia, confusion, abnormal thinking, and nervousness. Kidney stones occur in 2.6% of patients.[2]

Contraindications. Allergy to sulfonamides.

Drug Interactions. Enzyme-inducing antiepileptic drugs (carbamazepine, phenytoin, barbiturates) enhance zonisamide's metabolism and reduce its half-life to 27–36 h. Zonisamide has no apparent effect on the pharmacokinetics of other antiepileptic drugs.[42]

Parameters to Monitor. Seizure control, renal function, serum bicarbonate prior to starting and periodically throughout therapy, signs and symptoms of metabolic acidosis, temperature intolerance (decreased sweating).

Notes. Zonisamide is indicated as adjunctive treatment for partial and secondarily generalized tonic–clonic seizures in adults. It reduces the frequency of seizures by $\geq 50\%$ in 30%–40% of patients as adjunctive therapy. The drug also appears to be effective for generalized and progressive myoclonic epilepsies.[8]

ANTICONVULSANTS COMPARISON CHART

| | CHOICE OF ANTICONVULSANT FOR CLINICAL SEIZURE TYPE[a] | | | | | ANTICONVULSANT DOSAGE RANGE AND SERUM LEVELS | | | |
| | Generalized Seizures | | | | | Dosage Range (mg/kg/d) | | Therapeutic Serum Levels | |
DRUG	Tonic–Clonic	Absence	Myoclonic	Atonic	Partial Seizures[b]	Adult	Pediatric	(mg/L)	(µmol/L)
Carbamazepine	1	W	—	—	1	10–30	15–35	4–12	17–50
Clonazepam	W	3	2	1	—	0.01–0.2	0.01–0.2	13–72 µg/L	40–230 nmol/L
Ethosuximide	—	1	—	—	—	10–30	20–40	40–100	280–710
Gabapentin	—	—	—	—	4	15–35	—	—	—
Lamotrigine	3	—	—	—	3	1.5–7	—	—	—
Levetiracetam	1	—	2	—	1	30–45	—	—	—
Oxcarbazepine	—	—	—	—	1	20–40	30–45	—	—
Phenytoin	1	W	—	—	1	4–8	4–8	10–20	40–80
Pregabalin	—	—	—	—	4	2–8	—	—	—
Tiagabine	—	—	—	—	4	0.5–0.8	—	—	—
Topiramate	3	—	—	—	4	4–8	—	—	—
Valproic acid[c]	1	2	1	1	1	15–60	15–60	50–120	350–830
Zonisamide	—	—	—	—	4	3–6	4–12	—	—

1 = Drug of first choice; initial agent; given as monotherapy.
2 = Drug of second choice; alternative to first choice; given as monotherapy or in combination with agent of first choice.
3 = Drug of third choice; alternative to first or second choice; given as monotherapy or in combination with another agent.
4 = Useful as adjunctive therapy after failure of monotherapy with preferred agents.
W = May worsen clinical seizure type.

[a]Choice of anticonvulsant based on relative and comparative efficacy and potential for adverse effects. Choice of agent should consider individual patient factors. (See Refs. 1 and 2.)
[b]Includes simple-partial, complex-partial, and secondarily generalized tonic–clonic seizures.
[c]Drug of first choice.

■ REFERENCES

1. Glauser T et al. ILAE treatment guidelines: evidence-based analysis of antiepileptic drug efficacy and effectiveness as initial monotherapy for epileptic seizures and syndromes. *Epilepsia.* 2006;47:1094-1120.

2. Azar NJ, Abou-Khalil BW. Considerations in the choice of an antiepileptic drug in the treatment of epilepsy. *Semin Neurol.* 2008;28:305-316.

3. Anon. *Statistical Review and Evaluation. Antiepileptic Drugs and Suicidality.* http://www.fda.gov/ohrms/dockets/ac/08/briefing/2008-4372b1-01-FDA.pdf. Accessed November 6, 2008.

4. Anon. *Suicidality and Antiepileptic Drugs.* http://www.fda.gov/cder/drug/infopage/antiepileptics/default.htm. Accessed October 10, 2008.

5. Product information: Tegretol®, carbamazepine. East Hanover, NJ: Novartis; 2008.

6. Product information: Equetro®, carbamazepine. Wayne, PA: Shire; 2007.

7. Cloyd JC et al. Antiepileptics in the elderly. Pharmacoepidemiology and pharmacokinetics. *Arch Fam Med.* 994;3:589-598.

8. Levy RH et al, eds. *Antiepileptic Drugs.* 5th ed. Philadelphia, PA: Lippincott Williams & Wilkins; 2002.

9. Bass J et al. Effects of enteral tube feeding on the absorption and pharmacokinetic profile of carbamazepine suspension. *Epilepsia.* 1989;30:364-369.

10. Graves NM et al. Relative bioavailability of rectally administered carbamazepine suspension in humans. *Epilepsia.* 1985;26:429-433.

11. Product information: Klonopin®, clonazepam. Nutley, NJ: Roche; 2001.

12. Graves NM, Kriel RL. Rectal administration of antiepileptic drugs in children. *Pediatr Neurol.* 1987;3: 321-326.

13. Product information: Zarontin®, ethosuximide. New York: Parke-Davis; 2007.

14. Product information: Felbatol®, felbamate. Somerset, NJ: MedPointe Pharmaceuticals; 2002.

15. Product information: Cerebyx®, fosphenytoin. Teaneck, NJ: Eisai, Inc.; 2002.

16. Product information: Neurontin®, gabapentin. New York: Pfizer, Inc.; 2007.

17. Product information: Lamictal®, lamotrigine. Research Triangle Park, NC: GlaxoSmithKline; 2007.

18. Product information: Keppra Tablets/Oral Solution®, levetiracetam. Smyrna, GA: UCB Pharma; 2008.

19. Product information: Keppra XR®, levetiracetam. Smyrna, GA: UCB Pharma; 2008.

20. Knake S et al. Intravenous levetiracetam in the treatment of benzodiazepine refractory status epilepticus. *J Neurol Neurosurg Psychiatry.* 2008;79:588-589.

21. Product information: Trileptal®, oxcarbazepine. East Hanover, NJ: Novartis; 2007.

22. Beran RG. Cross-reactive skin eruption with both carbamazepine and oxcarbazepine. *Epilepsia.* 1993;34: 163-165.

23. Kwan P, Brodie MJ. Phenobarbital for the treatment of epilepsy in the 21st century: a critical review. *Epilepsia.* 2004;45:1141-1149.

24. Product information: Dilantin®, phenytoin. New York: Pfizer, Inc.; 2007.

25. Ramsay RE. Pharmacokinetics and clinical use of parenteral phenytoin, phenobarbital, and paraldehyde. *Epilepsia.* 1989;30(suppl 2):S1-S3.

26. Leppik IE et al. Altered phenytoin clearance with febrile illness. *Neurology.* 1986;36:1367-1370.

27. Boucher BA et al. Phenytoin pharmacokinetics in critically ill trauma patients. *Clin Pharmacol Ther.* 1988; 44:675-683.

28. Levy RH, Yerby MS. Effects of pregnancy on antiepileptic drug utilization. *Epilepsia.* 1985;26(suppl 1): S52-S57.

29. Product information: Phenytek®, phenytoin. Research Triangle Park, NC: Bertek Pharmaceuticals, Inc.; 2004.

30. Tozer TN, Winter ME. Phenytoin. In: Evans WE et al., eds. *Applied Pharmacokinetics: Principles of Therapeutic Drug Monitoring.* 3rd ed. Vancouver, BC: Applied Therapeutics; 1992.

31. Yamanaka H et al. Urinary excretion of phenytoin metabolites, 5-(4′-hydroxyphenyl)-5-phenylhydantoin and its o-glucuronide in humans and analysis of genetic polymorphisms of UDP-glucuronoyltransferases. *Drug Metab Pharmacokinet.* 2005;20:135-143.

32. Alldredge BK et al. Anticonvulsant hypersensitivity syndrome: in vitro and clinical observations. *Pediatr Neurol.* 1994;10:169-171.

33. Product information: Lyrica®, pregabalin. New York: Pfizer, Inc.; 2008.

34. Product information: Mysoline®, primidone. Aliso Viejo, CA: Valeant Pharmaceuticals; 2007.

35. Mattson RH et al. Comparison of carbamazepine, phenobarbital, phenytoin, and primidone in partial and secondarily generalized tonic-clonic seizures. *N Engl J Med.* 1985;313:145-151.

36. Product information: Gabitril®, tiagabine. West Chester, PA: Cephalon, Inc.; 2005.

37. Gustavson LE, Mengel HB. Pharmacokinetics of tiagabine, a gamma-aminobutyric acid-uptake inhibitor, in healthy subjects after single and multiple doses. *Epilepsia.* 1995;36:605-611.

38. Product information: Topamax®, topiramate. Titusville, NJ: Ortho-McNeil; 2008.
39. Product information: Depakote ER®, valproic acid. North Chicago, IL: Abbott Laboratories; 2008.
40. Product information: Depakote®, valproic acid. North Chicago, IL: Abbott Laboratories; 2006.
41. Anon. *American Psychiatric Association Practice Guidelines*. http://www.psychiatryonline.com/pracGuide/loadGuidelinePdf.aspx?file=Bipolar2ePG_05-15-06. Accessed October 15, 2008.
42. Product information: Zonegran®, zonisamide. Woodcliff Lake, NJ: Eisai, Inc.; 2007.
43. Hwang H, Kim KJ. New antiepileptic drugs in pediatric epilepsy. *Brain Dev*. 2008;30:549-545.

Chapter 37

Antidepressants

Aaron P. Gibson

Class Instructions. *Antidepressants.* These drugs can cause drowsiness. Until the extent of this effect is known, use caution when driving, operating machinery, or performing other tasks requiring mental alertness. Avoid excessive concurrent use of alcohol or other drugs that cause drowsiness. Patients, their families, and caregivers should be on alert for unusual changes in behavior, worsening of symptoms, or suicidal ideation. These should be reported to their provider immediately, especially if they are severe, abrupt in onset, and not part of the initial presentation of the patient. These symptoms may be associated with an increased risk in suicidal thinking and behavior, indicating a need for very close monitoring and potential changes in therapy. A medication guide detailing the risks and precautions of increased suicidality should be given to patients with every new prescription for these medications. These medications should not be discontinued abruptly because of the risk of rebound symptoms and withdrawal syndrome. Antidepressants should not be administered within 14 days of an MAOI. Caution should also be exercised if multiple antidepressants are used simultaneously because of the increased risk of serotonin syndrome.

BUPROPION	Wellbutrin, Wellbutrin XL, Zyban, Various

Pharmacology. Bupropion is a monocyclic antidepressant, unique as a mild dopamine and norepinephrine uptake inhibitor with no direct effect on serotonin receptors or MAO. It is essentially devoid of anticholinergic, antihistaminic, and peripheral adrenergic effects. In contrast to heterocyclic antidepressants, bupropion produces no clinically important effect on cardiac conduction, no orthostatic hypotension, minimal anticholinergic effects, and it is not associated with weight gain. Compared with selective serotonin reuptake inhibitors (SSRIs), bupropion offers a similar side effect profile without sexual dysfunction. Its lack of sedation and its activating effect can be advantageous for patients with decreased psychomotor activity and lethargy. Disadvantages of bupropion include seizures and the necessity of multiple daily doses.[1-3] (*See* Antidepressants Comparison Chart.)

Administration and Adult Dosage. Small initial doses and gradual dosage escalation is necessary to minimize the risk of seizures. **PO for depression**—(immediate-release) 100 mg twice daily initially, increasing to 100 mg 3 times daily no sooner than 3 days after the start of therapy. The maximum daily dosage is 450 mg, with a maximum single dose of 150 mg; (sustained-release) 150 mg given in the morning initially, increasing to 150 mg twice daily no sooner than 4 days after the start of therapy, to a maximum of 200 mg twice daily; (extended-release) 150 mg given in the morning initially, increasing to 300 mg/d in the morning after 4 days; after several weeks with no response at 300 mg/d, to a maximum of 450 mg/d.

PO for seasonal affective disorder—(Wellbutrin XL only) initial dose of 150 mg/d given in the morning, dose can be increased to the target of 300 mg/d after 4 days.
PO as an aid to smoking cessation—(sustained-release) Same dosage regimen as Wellbutrin SR for depression to a maximum of 300 mg/d for 7–12 weeks.[4]

Special Populations. *Pediatric Dosage.* Safety and efficacy have not been established.

Other Conditions. Hepatic and Renal Impairment: Reduced frequency and/or dose should be considered in patients with mild to moderate hepatic or renal impairment. Extreme caution should be exercised in patients with hepatic cirrhosis and the dose should not exceed 100 mg/d or 150 mg every other day in this population.

Dosage Forms. Tab 75, 100 mg; **SR Tab** 100, 150 mg; **XL Tab** 150, 300 mg.

Patient Instructions. (*See* Class Instructions.) This drug requires at least 2 weeks for a noticeable response in mood and up to 12 weeks for full therapeutic benefit. Taking bupropion close to bedtime can interfere with sleep. Inform your physician of any other medications that you are taking, or if you are pregnant, plan to become pregnant, or are nursing a child during therapy.

Pharmacokinetics. Half-life 11–14 h, but an active hydroxy metabolite has a half-life longer than 24 h. The SR formulation of bupropion has duration of ~12 h, while the duration of the XL formulation is ~24 h.

Contraindications. Seizure disorder; current or previous diagnosis of anorexia nervosa or bulimia (increased risk of seizures) undergoing acute withdrawal from alcohol or sedatives; concomitant use with an MAOI.

Adverse Reactions. Frequent adverse effects include anorexia, rash, sweating, tinnitus, tremor, abdominal pain, dry mouth, myalgia, palpitation, pharyngitis, urinary frequency, anxiety, dizziness, insomnia, agitation, headache, and nausea. There is a dose-dependent risk of seizures when using bupropion. With dosages of ≤450 mg/d, seizures occur in 0.4% of patients, with a 1-year cumulative incidence of 0.5%. Bupropion seems to offer better safety in overdose than heterocyclic antidepressants. Increased risk of suicidal thinking and behavior is a black box warning for bupropion.

Drug Interactions. Bupropion is extensively metabolized by cytochrome (CYP)2B6 and through oxidation, and is also an inhibitor of CYP2D6. Levodopa can increase adverse effects. MAOIs are contraindicated with bupropion because they can increase bupropion levels, leading to toxicity. Lopinavir can decrease bupropion levels due to CYP2B6 induction. Zyban is identical to Wellburtin in SR.

CITALOPRAM   Celexa, Various

Pharmacology. Citalopram has a selective and potent inhibitory effect on serotonergic presynaptic reuptake, similar to fluoxetine. (*See* Antidepressants Comparison Chart.)

Administration and Adult Dosage. (*See* Antidepressants Comparison Chart.) **PO for depression**—20 mg/d initially, administered in the morning. Dose increases should usually occur in 20-mg increments, and at intervals of not less than 1 week. Some patients may require doses up to 60 mg/d.

Special Populations. *Pediatric Dosage.* Safety and efficacy have not been established. Two placebo-controlled trials including 407 pediatric patients with depression did not support a claim for use in this population.[5] Citalopram is frequently used in this population, however, and close monitoring for clinical worsening and an increase in suicidality is warranted. (*See* Class Instructions.)

Geriatric Dosage. The recommended dose for elderly patients is 20 mg/d, with 40 mg/d only for nonresponding patients.

Dosage Forms. **Tab** 10, 20, 40 mg; **Soln** 2 mg/mL.

Patient Instructions. (*See* Class Instructions.) This drug requires at least 2 weeks for a noticeable response in mood and up to 12 weeks for full therapeutic benefit. Take citalopram in the morning or early afternoon. Inform your physician of any other medications that you are taking, or if you are pregnant, plan to become pregnant, or are nursing a child during therapy.

Pharmacokinetics. *Onset and Duration.* Onset of efficacy is delayed 2–4 weeks, which is similar to other antidepressants.

Serum Levels. Not established.

Fate. Oral bioavailability is 80% with all dosage forms. It is 80% bound to plasma proteins, with a V_d of 12 L/kg; clearance is 330 mL/min with ~20% due to renal clearance. Citalopram is metabolized via CYP3A4 and CYP2C19 to the inactive primary metabolites of demethylcitalopram and didemethylcitalopram. **Half-life.** ~35 h.

Adverse Reactions. Frequent adverse events include dry mouth, nausea, insomnia, and somnolence. More serious, life-threatening adverse effects, including serotonin syndrome and/or neuroleptic malignant syndrome (NMS), have been reported with SSRIs including citalopram.

Contraindications. Concomitant use with an MAOI or pimozide.

Precautions. (*See* Class Instructions.) Citalopram may increase the risk of bleeding events. Caution should be exercised when using citalopram with NSAIDs, aspirin, or other drugs that affect coagulation. As with all SSRIs, there is a risk of hyponatremia. This risk is higher in elderly patients and is reversible upon discontinuation of therapy. Abrupt withdrawal may lead to a withdrawal syndrome. There is a risk of switching patients with bipolar disorder into a manic episode.

Drug Interactions. Altered anticoagulant effects including increased bleeding may be seen with concomitant warfarin use. Citalopram plasma levels increase by 39%–43% when coadministered with cimetidine, but the clinical effect of this increase is unknown. Additive QTc intervals were detected when citalopram was administered with pimozide. Because citalopram is metabolized extensively through CYP3A4 and CYP2C19, inhibitors or inducers of these enzymes could potentially interact with citalopram. Coadministration with ketoconazole (a potent inhibitor of CYP3A4) and with carbamazepine (a potent inducer of CYP3A4) showed no differences in citalopram kinetics indicating that inhibition of one metabolic pathway of citalopram is not sufficient to alter metabolism.

CLOMIPRAMINE
Anafranil, Various

Pharmacology. Clomipramine is a 3-chloro analogue of imipramine that is a potent inhibitor of serotonin reuptake and, unlike other tricyclic antidepressants

(TCA), antagonizes dopaminergic neurotransmission. It has a specific indication for treatment of obsessive-compulsive disorder (OCD). Few patients experience complete OCD symptom relief; typically, approximately 40%–50% of patients have marked symptom improvement. Although it is an effective antidepressant, its adverse effect profile makes other antidepressants preferred for this indication.[6–8] (*See* Antidepressants Comparison Chart.)

Administration and Adult Dosage. PO for OCD—25 mg/d initially, increasing to 100 mg/d during the first 2 weeks, and then gradually increasing over several weeks to a maximum of 250 mg/d. Clomipramine can be given safely once daily at bedtime.

Dosage Forms. Cap 25, 50, 75 mg.

Patient Instructions. (*See* Class Instructions.) This drug requires at least 2 weeks for a noticeable response in mood and up to 12 weeks for full therapeutic benefit. Take clomipramine in the evening or at bedtime because of sedation. Inform your physician of any other medications that you are taking, or if you are pregnant, plan to become pregnant, or are nursing a child during therapy.

Pharmacokinetics. Antiobsessional effects are first seen at week 4, with maximum effects between weeks 10 and 18. Clomipramine is a highly lipophilic drug with a large first-pass effect and oral bioavailability of 36%–62%. The major route of elimination is metabolism by demethylation and then hydroxylation and conjugation. **Half-life.** 20–24 h.

Contraindications. Concomitant use of MAOI or use of a MAOI within the past 14 days; during the acute recovery period of a myocardial infarction.

Precautions. (*See* Class Instructions.) There is an increased risk of suicidal ideation or behavior or worsening depression. Abrupt withdrawal can lead to a withdrawal syndrome. There is an increased risk of switching patients with bipolar disorder into mania. Conditions that lower the seizure threshold should be used with caution. Use with caution in patients with cardiovascular disease, liver disease, or glaucoma. NMS has been reported with clomipramine.

Adverse Reactions. Clomipramine's adverse effect profile is similar to that of amitriptyline (e.g., frequent sedation, anticholinergic effects, orthostatic hypotension, tremor, nausea, and sweating), but it has a much higher prevalence of sexual dysfunction and seizures. In controlled studies, 42% of patients experienced ejaculatory failure and 20% were impotent. Frequency of sexual dysfunction increases to >90% of patients when asked directly rather than relying on self-reporting.[9] Seizures occur in 0.5% of patients receiving 250 mg/d or less, and 2% of patients experience seizures with dosages above 250 mg/d. Clomipramine is contraindicated in patients who have received MAOIs within the past 14 days. Use with caution in patients with cardiovascular disease (e.g., arrhythmias, angina, myocardial infarction).

Drug Interactions. Drug interactions are the same as other TCAs. (*See* Heterocyclic Antidepressants.)

DESVENLAFAXINE   Pristiq

Pharmacology. Desvenlafaxine is the major active metabolite of venlafaxine and thus possesses the same mechanism of action, potent reuptake inhibition of serotonin and norepinephrine. Like venlafaxine, it lacks effects on muscarinic, α-adrenergic, or histamine receptors. (*See* Antidepressants Comparison Chart.)

Indications and Adult Dosage. **PO for depression**—50 mg daily, with or without food. Doses up to 400 mg/d were given in clinical trials with no additional efficacy and more frequent adverse events seen than with the 50 mg/d dose.

Special Populations. *Pediatric Dosage.* Safety and efficacy not established.

Geriatric Dosage. No dosage is necessary based on age, but renal clearance should be considered.

Other Conditions. Hepatic Impairment: No dose adjustments are necessary for patients with hepatic impairment; however, doses >100 mg/d are not recommended.

Renal impairment. No dose adjustment is necessary in patients with mild (Cl_{Cr} 50–80 mL/min) or moderate (Cl_{Cr} 30–50 mL/min) renal impairment. The dose should be 50 mg every other day in patients with Cl_{Cr} <30 mL/min.

Dosage Forms. **Tab** 50, 100 mg.

Patient Instructions. (*See* Class Instructions.) This drug requires at least 2 weeks for a noticeable response in mood and up to 12 weeks for full therapeutic benefit. Take desvenlafaxine in the morning or early afternoon. Inform your physician of any other medications that you are taking, or if you are pregnant, plan to become pregnant, or are nursing a child during therapy.

Pharmacokinetics. *Onset and Duration.* Onset of efficacy is delayed 2–4 weeks, which is similar to other antidepressants.

Serum Levels. Not established.

Fate. Oral bioavailability is ~80%. Plasma protein binding is low at 30% and is independent of plasma concentration. Desvenlafaxine has a V_d of 3.4 L/kg following IV administration at steady state. Metabolism occurs through conjugation as well as a minor portion metabolized through oxidation at the CYP3A4 enzyme. The CYP2D6 pathway is not involved. Following oral administration, 45% of the desvenlafaxine dose is excreted unchanged in the urine after 72 h. **Half-life.** ~11 h. Following achievement of steady state, multiple dose accumulation of desvenlafaxine is linear and predictable from the single-dose kinetics.

Adverse Reactions. Similar to venlafaxine, frequent adverse effects include expected serotonin-related effects (e.g., nausea, headache, insomnia or somnolence, and sexual dysfunction). The risk of increasing diastolic blood pressure and cholesterol should be considered.

Contraindications. Concomitant use of MAOIs or use of an MAOI in the previous 14 days.

Precautions. (*See* Class Instructions.) Sustained hypertension was seen with all doses of desvenlafaxine in preliminary trials. Preexisting hypertension should be controlled prior to starting desvenlafaxine, and blood pressure should be monitored frequently during therapy. Desvenlafaxine may increase the risk of bleeding events. Caution should be exercised when using desvenlafaxine with NSAIDs, aspirin, or other drugs that affect coagulation. As with the SSRIs, there is a risk of hyponatremia. This risk is higher in elderly patients, and is reversible upon discontinuation of therapy. Cholesterol and triglyceride elevations have been reported. There is a risk of switching bipolar patients into mania. Abrupt discontinuation can lead to a withdrawal syndrome. Concomitant use with other serotonergic agents increases the risk of developing serotonin syndrome. Patients with narrow-angle glaucoma or increased intraocular pressure can see exacerbations. Interstitial lung disease and eosinophilic pneumonia have been rarely reported.

Drug Interactions. Similar to venlafaxine, desvenlafaxine is not a potent inhibitor of the CYP450 enzyme system, making it different from most of the SSRIs. Avoid it in patients who have received an MAOI within the past 14 days.

Parameters to Monitor. Blood pressure and cholesterol.

DULOXETINE
Cymbalta

Pharmacology. Duloxetine is a potent serotonin and norepinephrine reuptake inhibitor similar to venlafaxine and desvenlafaxine. Unlike venlafaxine, it affects both serotonin and norephinephrine at the lowest available dose and also inhibits dopamine reuptake to a lesser extent than serotonin and norepinephrine. It lacks effects on muscarinic, alpha-adrenergic, or histamine receptors. (*See* Antidepressants Comparison Chart.)

Administration and Adult Dosage. (*See* Antidepressants Comparison Chart.) **PO for depression**—40–60 mg/d given all at once or in divided doses twice daily. Doses up to 120 mg/d have been studied, but there is no evidence that doses >60 mg/d confer any added benefit. **PO for generalized anxiety disorder**—60 mg/d given all at once or as 30 mg twice daily. **PO for diabetic peripheral neuropathic pain**—60 mg/d. Since diabetes is frequently associated with impaired renal function, a lower starting dose may be considered in patients with renal impairment. **PO for fibromyalgia**—30 mg/d for 1 week, followed by 60 mg/d thereafter, if patients do not respond to the initial dose.

Special Populations. *Pediatric Dosage.* Safety and efficacy not established.

Geriatric Dosage. No dosage adjustment is recommended based on age.

Other Conditions. Hepatic and Renal Impairment: Duloxetine should be avoided in patients with any type of hepatic insufficiency or in patients with severe renal insufficiency ($Cl_{Cr} < 30$ mL/min).

Dosage Forms. Cap 20, 30, 60 mg.

Patient Instructions. (*See* Class Instructions.) This drug requires at least 2 weeks for a noticeable response in mood and up to 12 weeks for full therapeutic benefit. Take duloxetine in the morning or early afternoon. Inform your physician of any other medications that you are taking, or if you are pregnant, plan to become pregnant, or are nursing a child during therapy.

Pharmacokinetics. *Onset and Duration.* Onset of efficacy is delayed 2–4 weeks, which is similar to other antidepressants.

Serum Levels. Not established.

Fate. Duloxetine is well absorbed following oral administration. It is highly protein bound (>90%) to albumin and α_1-acid glycoprotein and has a V_d of 1640 L. Trace amounts (<1%) of duloxetine are found unchanged in the urine. Duloxetine is extensively metabolized by CYP1A2 and CYP2D6 and approximately 70% of duloxetine appears in the urine and 20% in the feces as inactive metabolites. **Half-life.** 12 h (range of 8–17 h) and follows linear kinetics over the therapeutic range. Patients with hepatic insufficiency will have a duloxetine half-life that is 3 times longer than normal and will also have an AUC that is 5 times higher than normal. While there is no difference in half-life for patients with severe renal impairment (Cl_{Cr} < 30 mL/min), C_{max} and AUC were ~100% higher. Duloxetine should not be used in either of these patient populations.

Adverse Reactions. Nausea, headache, dry mouth, fatigue, insomnia, dizziness, somnolence, constipation, diarrhea, and decreased appetite were seen in >10% of patients taking duloxetine in controlled trials. Patients taking duloxetine were significantly more likely to have sexual dysfunction than placebo as scored on the Arizona sexual experience scale.

Contraindications. Concomitant use with MAOIs and patients with uncontrolled narrow-angle glaucoma.

Precautions. (*See* Class Instructions.) Patients taking duloxetine may experience increases of up to 2.1 mm Hg in systolic and 2.3 mm Hg in diastolic blood pressure. Preexisting hypertension should be controlled prior to starting duloxetine, and blood pressure should be monitored frequently during therapy. Potentially fatal hepatic toxicity has been seen with duloxetine, and patients who develop jaundice or have other evidence of clinically significant liver dysfunction should discontinue duloxetine and should not be retried unless another definitive cause is identified. Orthostasis and syncope have also been reported on therapeutic doses. Duloxetine may increase the risk of bleeding events. Caution should be exercised when using duloxetine with NSAIDs, aspirin, or other drugs that affect coagulation. As with the SSRIs, there is a risk of hyponatremia. This risk is higher in elderly patients and is reversible upon discontinuation of therapy.

Drug Interactions. CYP1A2 inhibitors (e.g., fluvoxamine) have been shown to greatly increase the half-life, C_{max}, and AUC of duloxetine. Paroxetine, a potent inhibitor of CYP2D6, has been shown to increase the AUC of duloxetine by 60%. Duloxetine does not appear to inhibit or induce any of the CYP450 enzymes to a clinically meaningful degree. Since duloxetine is highly protein bound, coadministration with other highly bound drugs may lead to increased free concentrations of the other drug.

Parameters to Monitor. Blood pressure. No specific laboratory parameters are recommended for monitoring.

ESCITALOPRAM Lexapro

Pharmacology. Escitalopram is the pure (*S*)-enantiomer of citalopram and shares the mechanism of selective serotonin reuptake inhibition.

Administration and Adult Dosage. **PO for depression and generalized anxiety disorder**—10 mg/d initially, administered in the morning or evening. Dose may be increased to 20 mg/d after 1 week.

Special Populations. *Pediatric Dosage.* Safety and efficacy not established. One placebo-controlled trial in 264 pediatric patients with depression had been conducted and was positive, but two positive trials are required in order to receive an indication.[10] Escitalopram is frequently used in this population, however, and close monitoring for clinical worsening and an increase in suicidality is warranted. (*See* Class Instructions.)

Geriatric Dosage. 10 mg/d is the recommended dose for elderly patients.

Other Conditions. Hepatic and Renal Impairment: Dose should be 10 mg/d in patients with hepatic insufficiency. No dosage adjustment is necessary for patients with mild or moderate renal insufficiency. Caution should be used in patients with severe renal insufficiency.

Dosage Forms. **Tab** 5, 10, 20 mg; **Soln** 1 mg/mL.

Patient Instructions. (*See* Class Instructions.) This drug requires at least 2 weeks for a noticeable response in mood and up to 12 weeks for full therapeutic benefit. Take escitalopram in the morning or early afternoon. Inform your physician of any other medications that you are taking or if you are pregnant, plan to become pregnant, or are nursing a child during therapy.

Pharmacokinetics. *Onset and Duration.* Onset of efficacy is delayed 2–4 weeks, which is similar to other antidepressants.

Serum Levels. Not established.

Fate. The bioavailability of escitalopram is approximately 80%. It is 56% bound to human plasma proteins, with a V_d of 12 L/kg; Clearance is ~600 mL/min with 7% of that due to renal clearance. Escitalopram is metabolized by N-demethylation via CYP3A4 and CYP2C19.

Adverse Reactions. *See* Citalopram.

Contraindications. Concomitant use of a MAOI or pimozide.

Precautions. *See* Citalopram.

Drug Interactions. Because escitalopram is metabolized by multiple enzyme systems, inhibition of one enzyme system does not appreciably decrease escitalopram clearance. Altered anticoagulant effects including increased bleeding may be seen with concomitant warfarin use. Escitalopram plasma levels increase by 39%–43% when coadministered with cimetidine, but the clinical effect of this increase is unknown. Additive QTc intervals were detected when citalopram was administered with pimozide.

FLUOXETINE	Prozac, Sarafem, Various

Pharmacology. Fluoxetine is a bicyclic antidepressant that is a selective and potent inhibitor of presynaptic reuptake of serotonin (an SSRI). It does not affect reuptake of norepinephrine or dopamine and has a relative lack of affinity for muscarinic, histamine, α_1- and α_2-adrenergic, and serotonin receptors.[11]

Administration and Adult Dosage. (*See* Antidepressants Comparison Chart.) **PO for depression or OCD**—20 mg/d initially, administered in the morning. Increase dosage no more frequently than every 3–5 weeks. Divide higher dosages, with the last dose given in early afternoon. Although the maximum labeled dosage is 80 mg/d, 20 mg is equal in efficacy for major depression to higher dosages with the benefit of fewer adverse effects.[11,12] For depression maintenance, Prozac Weekly 90 mg once/wk can be started 1 week after the last 20 mg/d dose. **PO for**

bulimia—60 mg/d in the morning. **PO for premenstrual dysphoric disorder**—20 mg/d; higher dosages appear to have no increased efficacy. Administration for the 14 days before menses can be as effective as continuous use.[13]

Special Populations. *Pediatric Dosage.* Fluoxetine is the only antidepressant with an approved indication for the treatment of depression in pediatric patients. The dosage in pediatric patients is not different than adult dosage. Fluoxetine is approved for children/adolescents >8 years of age. The usual starting dose is 10 mg/d.[5] As with all antidepressants used in this population, close monitoring for clinical worsening and an increase in suicidality is warranted. (*See* Class Instructions.)

Geriatric Dosage. Reduce initial dosage and rate of dosage increase in the elderly. Single-dose studies suggest no difference in maintenance dosage in the elderly, but data from multiple-dose studies are needed. (*See* Notes.)

Other Conditions. Reduce initial dosage and rate of dosage increase in patients with hepatic impairment. Dosage adjustment in renal impairment is unnecessary.[11]

Dosage Forms. **Cap** 10, 20, 40 mg; **SR Cap** 90 mg (Prozac Weekly); **Soln** 4 mg/mL; **Tab** 10, 20 mg.

Patient Instructions. This drug requires at least 2 weeks for a noticeable response in mood and up to 4 weeks for full therapeutic benefit. Take fluoxetine in the morning or early afternoon. Inform your physician of any other medications you are taking.

Pharmacokinetics. *Onset and Duration.* Onset is delayed 2–4 weeks, which is similar to other antidepressants.

Serum Levels. Not established.

Fate. Oral bioavailability is 95% with all dosage forms. It is 94% bound to plasma proteins, with a V_d of 35 ± 21 L/kg; Clearance is 0.58 ± 0.41 L/h/kg, decreasing with repeated administration. The primary active metabolite is norfluoxetine; the metabolic rate is possibly under polygenic control. **Half-life.** (fluoxetine) 1–3 days after a single oral dose, increasing with multiple doses to 4–5 days; (norfluoxetine) 7–15 days. Half-lives do not appear to be altered in the elderly or in patients with renal impairment. Patients with alcohol-induced cirrhosis have fluoxetine half-life increased by 100% and norfluoxetine half-life increased by 60% compared with controls.[11,14]

Adverse Reactions. Nausea, anxiety, insomnia, nervousness, diarrhea, anorexia, dry mouth, headache, and tremor occur with a frequency > 10%. Delayed ejaculation and anorgasmia occurs with fluoxetine and all SSRIs in at least 30%–55% of patients.[15,16] Unlike TCAs, which typically cause weight gain, fluoxetine dosages over 40 mg/d cause a weight loss of 1–2 kg within the first 6 weeks of treatment.[17] Fluoxetine rarely causes sedation except at dosages over 40 mg/d and can prolong the QTc interval. Fluoxetine does not appear to have any anticholinergic effects.[18] Initial case reports of patients developing new and intense suicidal preoccupation, agitation, and impulsiveness after several weeks of fluoxetine therapy have been adequately evaluated and found not to be directly related to the drug.[19]

Contraindications. Concurrent use of an MAOI; because of the long half-life, 5 weeks must elapse between discontinuation of fluoxetine and starting an MAOI.[20]

Precautions. (*See* Class Instructions.) Pregnancy category C. Fluoxetine may increase the risk of bleeding events. Caution should be exercised when using fluoxetine with NSAIDs, aspirin, or other drugs that affect coagulation. As with all SSRIs, there is a risk of hyponatremia. This risk is higher in elderly patients, and is reversible upon discontinuation of therapy. Abrupt withdrawal may lead to a withdrawal syndrome. There is a risk of switching patients with bipolar disorder into a manic episode. Episodes of hypoglycemia have been reported with fluoxetine. Use cautiously in the elderly and in patients with hepatic impairment. Use fluoxetine with caution in depressed patients with psychomotor agitation and anxiety or with anorexia and weight loss.

Drug Interactions. Fluoxetine is a potent inhibitor of CYP2D6, causing decreased metabolism and increased serum levels and adverse effects of many drugs, including most other antidepressants, antipsychotics, β-blockers, and class Ic antiarrhythmics. Fluoxetine's effect on other P450 isoenzymes has not been well defined.

Parameters to Monitor. Monitor liver function tests periodically during long-term therapy.

Notes. Fluoxetine is a useful alternative to TCAs because of its greater safety in overdose situations and relative lack of anticholinergic and cardiovascular effects. For severely depressed elderly patients, fluoxetine is less effective than **nortriptyline.**[21] Fluoxetine and other SSRIs have demonstrated efficacy for OCD and panic disorder. (*See* Antidepressants Comparison Chart.)

FLUVOXAMINE	Luvox, Luvox CR, Various

Pharmacology. Fluvoxamine has a selective and potent inhibitory effect on serotonergic presynaptic reuptake, similar to fluoxetine. Although it is also an effective antidepressant, fluvoxamine has been marketed for use in OCD. Fluvoxamine is equal in efficacy to **clomipramine** in OCD and causes fewer anticholinergic effects and sexual dysfunction but more headache and insomnia.[22–24] (*See* Antidepressants Comparison Chart.)

Administration and Adult Dosage. PO for OCD—50 mg/d initially, with a **maintenance dosage** of 100–300 mg/d. Give dosages over 100 mg/d in 2 divided doses. The elderly and those with hepatic impairment might require a lower starting dosage and slower dosage titration. **PO for social phobia**—(extended-release only) 100 mg/d at bedtime, increased by 50 mg to a maximum of 300 mg/d.

Special Populations. *Pediatric Dosage.* Not established for extended-release dosage form OR for children <8 years. **PO for OCD**—(8–17 years) 25 mg at bedtime initially, increasing in 25 mg/d increments every 4–7 days to a **usual maintenance dosage** of 50–200 mg/d. Divide dosages >50 mg/d into 2 doses, either equal or with a greater portion given at bedtime. As with all antidepressants used in this population, close monitoring for clinical worsening and an increase in suicidality is warranted. (*See* Class Instructions.)

Dosage Forms. **Tab** 25, 50, 100 mg. **CR Cap** 100, 150 mg.

Pharmacokinetics. Bioavailability is ~50% and not affected by food. Fluvoxamine is the least protein bound of the SSRIs (77%). On the same dosage, elderly patients have 40% higher serum concentrations than younger patients. Fluvoxamine is metabolized to inactive metabolites. **Half-life.** ~16 h in adults and 26 h in the elderly.

Adverse Reactions. Frequent adverse effects include nausea, somnolence or insomnia, dry mouth, sweating, diarrhea, loss of appetite, xerostomia, dizziness, somnolence, tremor, and sexual dysfunction. Life-threatening adverse events include Stevens-Johnson syndrome and NMS.

Contraindications. Concomitant use with alosetron, pimozide, thioridazine, or tizanidine. Concomitant use with a monoamine oxidase inhibitor (MAOI) or within 14 days following treatment with a MAOI.

Precautions. (*See* Class Instructions.) Fluvoxamine may increase the risk of bleeding events. Caution should be exercised when using fluvoxamine with NSAIDs, aspirin, or other drugs that affect coagulation. As with all SSRIs, there is a risk of hyponatremia. This risk is higher in elderly patients, and is reversible upon discontinuation of therapy. Abrupt withdrawal may lead to a withdrawal syndrome. There is a risk of switching patients with bipolar disorder into a manic episode. Caution should be used in patients with a history of a seizure disorder.

Patient Instructions. (*See* Class Instructions.) This drug requires at least 2 weeks for a noticeable response in mood and up to 12 weeks for full therapeutic benefit. Take fluvoxamine in the evening or before bedtime because it can have a sedating effect. Inform your physician of any other medications that you are taking, or if you are pregnant, plan to become pregnant, or are nursing a child during therapy.

Drug Interactions. Unlike other SSRIs, fluvoxamine is a potent inhibitor of CYP1A2, so increased levels and adverse effects are possible with warfarin, propranolol, metoprolol, caffeine, and theophylline. As with all SSRIs, do not administer fluvoxamine with MAOIs.

HETEROCYCLIC ANTIDEPRESSANTS   Various

Pharmacology. Heterocyclic antidepressants (**TCAs, amoxapine,** and **maprotiline**) have specific effects on neurotransmitters and receptor sensitivity. The primary pharmacologic effect of heterocyclic antidepressants is blockade of presynaptic reuptake of norepinephrine, with subsequent downregulation of adrenergic receptors. Amoxapine, a metabolite of **loxapine**, retains some postsynaptic dopamine reuptake inhibition. Heterocyclic antidepressants have less effect on serotonergic activity than on other neurotransmitters.[25,26]

Administration and Adult Dosage. (*See* Antidepressants Comparison Chart.) **PO for depression**—Initiate dosage at lower limit of range. Administer in divided doses to assess tolerance to side effects and then once daily at bedtime can be used.[25,27] **Maintenance dosage** should be the same as the dosage necessary to treat the acute depressive episode.[28] **Intramuscular** rarely used (e.g., surgical patient NPO for 1–2 days); **PO for chronic pain (amitriptyline** or **imipramine)**—10–25 mg/d initially; most patients respond to a dosage of 25–75 mg/d, although dosages up to 200 mg/d have been used.[29,30] (*See* Notes.)

Special Populations. *Pediatric Dosage.* Not recommended <12 years except for childhood enuresis. **PO for enuresis (imipramine)**—(<12 years) 25–50 mg/d; (≥12 years) up to 75 mg/d.[31] Imipramine maximum dosage in children is 2.5 mg/kg/d; however, use in prepubertal major depression disorder often requires up to 5 mg/kg/d with serum levels over 150 μg/L.[32] As with all antidepressants used in this population, close monitoring for clinical worsening and an increase in suicidality is warranted. (*See* Class Instructions.)

Geriatric Dosage. (>65 years) Reduce initial dosage by at least 50% of adult dosage and increase the dosage slowly.[33]

Other Conditions. Reduce initial dosage and rate of titration in patients with cardiovascular or hepatic disease.[34] During the last trimester of pregnancy, the mean dosage of TCAs required is 1.6 times that of nonpregnant women.[35]

Dosage Forms. *See* Antidepressants Comparison Chart.

Patient Instructions. (*See* Class Instructions.) These drugs usually take 2 weeks for a noticeable response in mood and up to 4 weeks for full therapeutic benefit. If you have small children, be sure to keep this medication in a secure place.

Pharmacokinetics. ***Onset and Duration.*** Physiologic symptoms of depression (e.g., sleep and appetite disturbance, decreased energy) should improve after 1 week, but mood (pessimism, hopelessness, anhedonia) often requires 2–4 weeks for response.

Serum Levels. **Nortriptyline** has a well-established therapeutic range and a curvilinear relationship of serum levels and response ("therapeutic window"). Other antidepressants show a linear response relationship.[36] (*See* Antidepressants Comparison Chart.)

Fate. Bioavailability is variable (30%–70%) because of first-pass metabolism. Major metabolites for TCAs are desmethyl (for tertiary amines) and hydroxy compounds; rate is possibly genetically determined and can result in 30-fold variation in steady-state levels in patients given the same dosage.[37] **Half-life.** (tertiary amine TCAs) 10–25 h; (secondary amine TCAs) 12–44 h.[36]

Adverse Reactions. Sedation, postural hypotension, anticholinergic effects (dry mouth, blurred near vision, constipation, urinary retention, aggravation of narrow-angle glaucoma, and prostatic hypertrophy), weight gain, and cardiac effects (ECG changes and slowed AV conduction) are frequent. **Nortriptyline** is least likely of the TCAs to cause postural hypotension. (*See* Antidepressants Comparison Chart.) Fine hand tremors, seizures, cardiac arrhythmia, or cholestasis can occur, as can hypomanic or manic episodes in bipolar patients. Seizures and blood dyscrasias are rare.[38,39]

Contraindications. Cardiac arrhythmias, especially bundle branch block.

Precautions. Use with caution in the elderly, in pregnancy, or in patients with heart failure and angina pectoris, epilepsy, glaucoma, prostatic hypertrophy, or renal or liver disease. When discontinuing therapy, taper the heterocyclic antidepressant dosage to prevent cholinergic rebound. Cases of sudden cardiac death have been reported in children with attention deficit disorder who received **desipramine** in therapeutic or subtherapeutic dosages.[40] Ingestion of ≥1 g of a heterocyclic antidepressant constitutes a life-threatening medical emergency. Limit the quantities dispensed to depressed patients with suicidal ideation. **Maprotiline** has an increased frequency of seizures at dosages above 225 mg/d. **Amoxapine** has a metabolite with dopamine-blocking activity, resulting in possible extrapyramidal effects, tardive dyskinesia, endocrine effects, and NMS. Neither amoxapine nor maprotiline offers greater efficacy or safety in overdose than TCAs.

Drug Interactions. Many drug interactions occur. Use with caution with MAOIs. The antihypertensive effects of guanethidine, clonidine, and closely related drugs might be reduced. Secondary amines including nortriptyline, desipramine, protriptyline, and amoxapine are all metabolized by CYP2D6. Tertiary amines including amitriptyline, imipramine, clomipramine, and doxepin are all metabolized by CYP2D6 and CYP1A2.

Parameters to Monitor. Monitor hepatic and renal function tests periodically during long-term therapy. Obtain ECG in the elderly, children, and those with preexisting heart disease. With **amoxapine**, monitor carefully for signs of tardive dyskinesia.

Notes. TCAs are commonly used in treating pain associated with diabetic neuropathy and postherpetic neuralgia; **amitriptyline, desipramine,** and **nortriptyline have** proven efficacy, but **SSRIs** are less effective.[29,30] (*See* Antidepressants Comparison Chart.)

MIRTAZAPINE
Remeron, Various

Pharmacology. Mirtazapine is an antidepressant that antagonizes presynaptic α_2-adrenergic auto- and heteroreceptors that are responsible for controlling the release of norepinephrine and serotonin (5-HT). It is also a potent antagonist of postsynaptic $5\text{-}HT_2$ and $5\text{-}HT_3$ receptors. The net outcome of these effects is increased noradrenergic activity and enhanced 5-HT activity, especially at $5\text{-}HT_{1A}$ receptors. This unique mechanism of action preserves antidepressant efficacy but minimizes many of the adverse effects common to heterocyclic antidepressants and SSRIs. Mirtazapine is effective in moderate and severe major depression.[41,42] (*See* Antidepressants Comparison Chart.)

Administration and Adult Dosage. **PO for depression**—15 mg/d at bedtime initially, increasing at 1- to 2-week intervals to a maximum of 45 mg/d.

Dosage Forms. **Tab** (conventional) 7.5, 15, 30, 45 mg; (disintegrating) 15, 30, 45 mg.

Pharmacokinetics. Mirtazapine has an onset of clinical effect in 2–4 weeks, similar to other antidepressants. **Half-life.** 20–40 h, allowing once-daily administration at bedtime.

Contraindications. Hypersensitivity.

Precautions. Abrupt withdrawal may lead to a withdrawal syndrome. There is a risk of switching patients with bipolar disorder into a manic episode. Use cautiously in the elderly and in patients with hepatic or renal impairment. Patients with cardiovascular or cerebrovascular disease or conditions that predispose patients to hypotension should use mirtazapine with caution because of orthostatic hypotension. Orally disintegrating tablets contain phenylalanine. Caution should be used with patients who have a seizure disorder.

Drug Interactions. Mirtazapine is metabolized through CYP2D6, 1A2, and 3A4, and medications that inhibit or induce these enzymes have the potential to interact with mirtazapine. Mirtazapine does not have significant induction or inhibitory effects on these enzymes.

Adverse Reactions. Sedation, increased appetite, and weight gain are the most frequent side effects. Sedation is most frequent at lower doses (15 mg) and decreases in frequency with increasing dosage. Although 2 cases of agranulocytosis occurred in clinical trials, no specific or additional blood count monitoring is required. Mirtazapine has minimal cardiovascular and anticholinergic effects and essentially lacks adverse gastrointestinal effects, insomnia, and sexual dysfunction. Do not use mirtazapine if an MAOI has been administered within the past 14 days. An overdose of up to 975 mg in combination with a benzodiazepine has caused marked sedation but no difficulty with cardiovascular or respiratory effects.

MONOAMINE OXIDASE INHIBITORS   Various

Pharmacology. MAOIs are thought to exert their antidepressant action because of alterations in adrenergic and serotonergic receptor sensitivity. The most consistent findings during long-term MAOI therapy include downregulation of β-adrenergic and adenyl cyclase activities. **Isocarboxazid** and **phenelzine** are hydrazine derivatives; **tranylcypromine** is a nonhydrazine.

Indications and Adult Dosage. PO for depression—(isocarboxazid) 20–30 mg/d; (phenelzine) 45–90 mg/d; (tranylcypromine) 30–60 mg/d. Initiate dosage at the lower limit and titrate upward depending on tolerance to side effects. Dosage schedule should remain divided, usually twice daily or 3 times daily. Avoid bedtime administration because MAOIs can delay onset of sleep.

Special Populations. *Pediatric Dosage.* (<16 years) not recommended.

Geriatric Dosage. Limited information, but decrease initial dosage by 50% because of orthostatic hypotension. Contraindicated in patients >60 years.

Other Conditions. Reduce the initial dosage and rate of upward titration if the patient has taken a heterocyclic antidepressant within 7–10 days.

Dosage Forms. (Isocarboxazid) **Tab** 10 mg; (phenelzine) **Tab** 15 mg; (tranylcypromine) **Tab** 10 mg.

Patient Instructions. (*See* Antidepressants, Class Instructions.) This drug usually takes 2 weeks for noticeable response in mood and up to 4 weeks for full therapeutic benefit to occur. This drug can cause faintness or dizziness, especially after rising suddenly or standing for prolonged periods, or after exertion or alcohol intake. Immediately report nausea, vomiting, sweating, severe occipital headache, and stiff neck, which might be signs of a serious adverse effect. Avoid concurrent use of diet pills and cough and cold remedies and restrict consumption of aged foods high in tyramine. (*See* Foods That Interact with MAO Inhibitors Chart.)

Pharmacokinetics. *Onset and Duration.* Onset 2 weeks; maximum improvement occurs after 3–4 weeks.[43]

Serum Levels. Not used clinically.

Fate. Termination of drug action is dependent on MAO regeneration because the drugs or their active metabolites chemically combine with the MAO enzyme.

Adverse Reactions. Autonomic effects are frequent and not necessarily dose dependent; these include postural hypotension, dry mouth, and constipation. Drowsiness is more frequent with phenelzine, whereas overstimulation and agitation are more likely with tranylcypromine; isocarboxazid is mildly stimulating. Occasionally, delayed ejaculation, edema, skin rash, urinary retention, and blurred vision occur. MAOIs are much less likely than TCAs to cause weight gain, with tranylcypromine being the least likely.[44]

Contraindications. Patients older than 60 years; patients with confirmed or suspected cerebrovascular defect; cardiovascular disease; pheochromocytoma; renal impairment; history of liver disease or abnormal liver function tests; concomitant use with certain drugs. (*See* Drug Interactions.)

Precautions. Always consider the possibility of suicide in depressed patients and take adequate precautions. Like other antidepressant drugs, MAOIs can switch bipolar patients to a hypomanic or manic state.

Drug Interactions. Postural hypotension can increase with coadministration of antipsychotic, heterocyclic antidepressant, or antihypertensive drugs and in patients with heart failure. Concurrent use with buspirone, heterocyclic antidepressants, meperidine, sympathomimetic drugs, SSRIs, and other MAOIs is contraindicated. A 1- to 2-week drug-free interval is necessary when switching from an MAOI to a TCA, but a drug-free interval is not necessary when switching from a TCA to an MAOI.[45] Although uncommon, hypertensive crisis can result from concurrent use of sympathomimetic amines or ingestion of food and drinks high in tyramine or caffeine.[46,47] Avoid diets high in tyramine content. (*See* Foods That Interact with MAO Inhibitors Chart.)

Parameters to Monitor. Monitor blood pressure frequently.

Notes. MAOIs are excellent alternatives to heterocyclic antidepressants in major depressive disorder, are very effective in panic disorder, and are drugs of choice for atypical depression.[46,48]

NEFAZODONE
Serzone, Various

Pharmacology. In 2003, the manufacturer of Serzone discontinued the sale of the drug in the United States and Canada because of cases of potentially fatal hepatotoxicity. Several generic formulations are still available. Nefazodone is a postsynaptic serotonin 5-HT$_{2A}$ antagonist and presynaptic serotonin reuptake inhibitor. These two serotonergic effects make it different from SSRIs and TCAs.[49–52] (*See* Antidepressants Comparison Chart.)

Administration and Adult Dosage. **PO for depression**—100 mg twice daily initially (50 mg twice daily in the elderly), increasing every 4–7 days to the effective dosage range of 150–300 mg twice daily. After initial dosage titration, once-daily bedtime administration is preferred to minimize daytime sedation.[53]

Special Populations. *Pediatric Dosage.* Safety and efficacy not established.

Geriatric Dosage. Starting dose in this population is 50 mg/d, and the total dose is titrated to the adult dose.

Dosage Forms. **Tab** 50, 100, 150, 200, 250 mg.

Pharmacokinetics. Nefazodone has an oral bioavailability of ~20%. Single-dose studies in the elderly have shown a 100% larger AUC; with multiple doses, the AUC differences decreased to 10%–20% above those in younger populations. It is > 99% protein bound and extensively metabolized. **Half-life.** Dose-dependent ~1–2.3 h in young patients, modestly prolonged in the elderly, and 2–3 times longer in hepatic disease. The major active metabolite, hydroxynefazodone, has a half-life of 1.2–1.6 h in young and elderly patients, increasing to 2–4 h with hepatic disease. Renal impairment does not markedly affect nefazodone pharmacokinetics.

Contraindications. Previous withdrawal of nefazodone because of evidence of liver injury. Coadministration of astemizole, carbamazepine, cisapride, pimozide, or terfenadine. Coadministration with full doses of triazolam as it can cause significant increases in triazolam plasma levels.

Precautions. Abrupt withdrawal may lead to a withdrawal syndrome. There is a risk of switching patients with bipolar disorder into a manic episode. Use cautiously in the elderly and in patients with hepatic or renal impairment. Caution should be used in patients with active liver disease as nefazodone may complicate monitoring. Patients with cardiovascular or cerebrovascular disease or conditions that predispose patients to hypotension should use nefazodone with caution because of orthostatic hypotension. Priapism can be a significant complication with nefazodone.

Patient Instructions. (*See* Class Instructions.) This drug requires at least 2 weeks for a noticeable response in mood and up to 12 weeks for full therapeutic benefit. Take nefazodone in the evening or before bedtime because it can be sedating. Inform your physician of any other medications that you are taking, or if you are pregnant, plan to become pregnant, or are nursing a child during therapy.

Adverse Reactions. Although chemically similar to trazodone, it causes less sedation and orthostatic hypotension, and its lower α-adrenergic blockade makes priapism much less likely (no cases reported). Frequent adverse effects include sedation, dry mouth, nausea, and dizziness. Unlike SSRIs, nefazodone's effects on sexual function, agitation, tremor, insomnia, and weight are no different from placebo.

Drug Interactions. Nefazodone is a potent inhibitor of the CYP3A4 isoenzyme and a weak inhibitor of the CYP2D6 isoenzyme. Drug interactions of particular concern include the triazolobenzodiazepines (e.g., alprazolam, triazolam, midazolam). A 1–2 week washout period is recommended when converting a patient to or from an MAOI and nefazodone.

PAROXETINE
Paxil, Paxil CR, Various

Pharmacology. Paroxetine is a highly selective and potent inhibitor of serotonin reuptake (an SSRI) similar to fluoxetine.[22,54–60] (*See* Antidepressants Comparison Chart.)

Administration and Adult Dosage. **PO for depression**—20 mg/d; a few patients require 30–50 mg/d for full efficacy. **PO for generalized anxiety disorder, social phobia, and posttraumatic stress disorder**—20 mg/d in the morning. **PO for panic disorder**—10 mg/d initially; usual maintenance dosage is 20–60 mg/d. **PO for OCD**—20 mg/d initially; maintenance dosage is 40 mg/d to a maximum of 60 mg/d, preferably as a single dose in the morning or evening. **PO for premenstrual dysphoric disorder**—12.5 mg/d in the morning, may increase to 25 mg/d after 1 week.

Special Populations. The starting dosage for all uses in elderly patients and those with marked renal or hepatic impairment is 10 mg/d. For the elderly or those with severe renal or hepatic impairment, the maximum dosage is 40 mg/d.

Dosage Forms. **Tab** 10, 20, 30, 40 mg; **CR Tab** 12.5, 25, 37.5 mg; **Susp** 2 mg/mL.

Pharmacokinetics. Paroxetine is completely orally bioavailable; protein binding is 93%–95%. Unlike fluoxetine, paroxetine is metabolized to inactive metabolites. **Half-life.** 24 h.

Contraindications. Concomitant use of linezolid, pimozide, or thioridazine. Concomitant use of MAOIs.

Precautions. (*See* Class Instructions.) Paroxetine may increase the risk of bleeding events. Caution should be exercised when using paroxetine with NSAIDs, aspirin, or other drugs that affect coagulation. As with all SSRIs, there is a risk of hyponatremia. This risk is higher in elderly patients, and is reversible upon discontinuation of therapy. Abrupt withdrawal may lead to a withdrawal syndrome. There is a risk of switching patients with bipolar disorder into a manic episode.

Patient Instructions. (*See* Class Instructions.) This drug requires at least 2 weeks for a noticeable response in mood and up to 12 weeks for full therapeutic benefit. Take paroxetine in the morning. If excess sedation occurs, switch the dose to bedtime. Inform your physician of any other medications that you are taking, or if you are pregnant, plan to become pregnant, or are nursing a child during therapy.

Adverse Reactions. Paroxetine causes the typical SSRI adverse effects of nausea, sexual dysfunction, and headache but is more likely to cause sedation than insomnia and can cause more delay of orgasm or ejaculation and more impotence than other SSRIs.[61] Like the other SSRIs, it is much safer in overdose than TCAs.

Drug Interactions. Paroxetine is a potent inhibitor of CYP2D6, so most other antidepressants, antipsychotics, β-blockers, and class Ic antiarrhythmics can have increased serum levels and adverse effects when paroxetine is combined with these drugs. Do not use paroxetine within 14 days of using an MAOI.

SERTRALINE
Zoloft, Various

Pharmacology. Sertraline is an SSRI similar to fluoxetine, which indirectly results in a downregulation of β-adrenergic receptors. It has no clinically important effect on noradrenergic or histamine receptors and no effect on MAO. It lacks stimulant, cardiovascular, anticholinergic, and convulsant effects. Sertraline has antidepressant effects equal to TCAs and fluoxetine and might have anorectic effects and efficacy in OCD.[26,62–64] (*See* Antidepressants Comparison Chart.)

Administration and Adult Dosage. **PO for depression, panic disorder, OCD, and posttraumatic stress disorder**—50 mg/d initially, increasing if necessary at weekly intervals to a maximum of 200 mg/d in a single dose in the morning or evening.

Special Populations. *Pediatric Dosage.* Safety and efficacy not established. Sertraline is frequently used in this population. Close monitoring for clinical worsening and an increase in suicidality is warranted. Initial dose for children aged 6–12 years is 25 mg/d, and for adolescents aged 13–17 years, the initial dosage is 50 mg/d. (*See* Class Instructions.)

Geriatric Dosage. No specific dosage adjustment is recommended for geriatric patients.

Other Conditions. Hepatic Impairment: The dose should be decreased or interval increased in patients with liver impairment.

Dosage Forms. **Tab** 25, 50, 100 mg; **Soln** 20 mg/mL.

Pharmacokinetics. Sertraline has an oral bioavailability of 36%, and, when it is taken with food, peak serum concentrations and bioavailability increase by 30%–40%. Peak serum concentrations are reached in 6–8 h. Sertraline concentrations in breast milk are the lowest of the SSRIs and produce minimal serum levels in the breast-fed infant.[65] The primary metabolite is N-desmethylsertraline, which has 5–10 times less activity than sertraline as an SSRI and has no demonstrated antidepressant activity. Clearance is decreased by up to 40% in the elderly. **Half-life.** 27 h.

Contraindications. Concomitant use of MAOIs or pimozide.

Precautions. (*See* Class Instructions.) Paroxetine may increase the risk of bleeding events. Caution should be exercised when using paroxetine with NSAIDs, aspirin, or other drugs that affect coagulation. As with all SSRIs, there is a risk of hyponatremia. This risk is higher in elderly patients, and is reversible upon discontinuation of therapy. Abrupt withdrawal may lead to a withdrawal syndrome. There is a risk of switching patients with bipolar disorder into a manic episode.

Drug Interactions. Sertraline undergoes significant first-pass metabolism via N-demethylation, and is highly protein bound. Coadministration with another highly protein-bound medication (e.g., warfarin, digitoxin) may lead to a shift in plasma concentrations.

Adverse Reactions. Frequent adverse effects include nausea, diarrhea, ejaculatory delay, tremor, and increased sweating. It causes less agitation, anxiety, and insomnia than fluoxetine and is a less potent inhibitor of the CYP2D6 isoenzyme at a dosage of 50 mg/d. Use with caution in patients with renal or hepatic impairment and do not use it within 14 days of using an MAOI. SIADH has been reported.[66]

VENLAFAXINE
Effexor, Effexor XR, Various

Pharmacology. Venlafaxine is a potent reuptake inhibitor of serotonin and norepinephrine, like many TCAs, but lacks effects on muscarinic, α-adrenergic, or histamine receptors.[67–70] (*See* Antidepressants Comparison Chart.)

Administration and Adult Dosage. **PO for depression**—(immediate-release) 75 mg twice daily or 3 times daily initially, increasing every 4–7 days to an effective antidepressant dosage of 225–375 mg/d in 2 or 3 divided doses; (sustained-release) 75 mg once daily initially, increasing in increments of up to 75 mg/d at intervals of 4 or more days to a maximum of 225 mg/d. The sustained-release preparation does not reduce side effects but allows once-daily administration; **PO for generalized anxiety disorder**—75–225 mg/d in 2–3 divided doses. Patients with renal impairment or on hemodialysis require a 25%–50% dosage reduction; **PO for panic disorder**—(sustained-release) 37.5–225 mg; **PO for social phobia**—75 mg/d and can be titrated up to 225 mg/d.

Dosage Forms. **Tab** 25, 37.5, 50, 75, 100 mg; **SR Cap** 37.5, 75, 150 mg (Effexor XR).

Pharmacokinetics. Venlafaxine is well absorbed orally; food has no effect on absorption. Serum concentrations in elderly patients are no different from those in younger patients. Unlike SSRIs, venlafaxine has minimal protein binding (27%–30%). It undergoes extensive hepatic metabolism. **Half-life.** 5 h, and one major active metabolite has an 11 h half-life. Venlafaxine exhibits linear pharmaco-kinetics over the recommended dosage range, and steady state is reached in 3 days.

Contraindications. Concomitant administration with MAOIs.

Precautions. (*See* Class Instructions.) Patients taking venlafaxine may experience increases in systolic and diastolic blood pressure while taking venlafaxine. Preex-isting hypertension should be controlled prior to starting venlafaxine, and blood pressure should be monitored frequently during therapy. Orthostasis and syncope have also been reported on therapeutic doses. Venlafaxine may increase the risk of bleeding events. Caution should be exercised when using venlafaxine with NSAIDs, aspirin, or other drugs that affect coagulation. As with the SSRIs, there is a risk of hyponatremia. This risk is higher in elderly patients and is reversible upon discontinuation of therapy.

Patient Instructions. (*See* Class Instructions.) This drug requires at least 2 weeks for a noticeable response in mood and up to 12 weeks for full therapeutic benefit. Take venlafaxine in the morning or early afternoon. Inform your physician of any other medications that you are taking, or if you are pregnant, plan to become preg-nant, or are nursing a child during therapy.

Adverse Reactions. Frequent adverse effects include nausea, headache, insomnia or somnolence, dizziness, dry mouth, and sexual dysfunction. At higher dosages (375 mg/d), venlafaxine is unique in causing a consistent but mild elevation in diastolic blood pressure (6 mm Hg). Regular blood pressure monitoring is required for all patients.

Drug Interactions. Venlafaxine is not a potent inhibitor of the CYP450 enzyme system, making it different from most of the SSRIs. Use is contraindicated within 14 days of an MAOI.

ANTIDEPRESSANTS COMPARISON CHART[a]

CLASS AND DRUG	DOSAGE FORMS	USUAL DAILY ADULT DOSAGE RANGE (mg)	THERAPEUTIC SERUM LEVELS (μg/L)	RELATIVE FREQUENCY OF SIDE EFFECTS		
				Sedation	Anticholinergic	Orthostatic Hypotension
α-ADRENERGIC BLOCKERS						
Mirtazapine Remeron Various	Tab (conventional and rapidly dissolving) 15, 30, 45 mg	15–45	[b]	Moderate	None	None
CHLOROPROPIOPHENONES						
Bupropion Wellbutrin Zyban Various	Tab 75, 100 mg SR Tab 100, 150 mg	300–450	[b]	None	None	None
DIBENZOXAZEPINES[c]						
Amoxapine Asendin Various	Tab 25, 50, 100, 150 mg	300–600	[b]	Low	Low	Low
MONOAMINE OXIDASE INHIBITORS (MAOIs)						
Phenelzine Nardil	Tab 15 mg	45–90	[b]	Moderate	Low	Very high
Tranylcypromine Parnate	Tab 10 mg	30–60	[b]	Low	Low	Very high

(continued)

569

ANTIDEPRESSANTS COMPARISON CHART[a] (*continued*)

CLASS AND DRUG	DOSAGE FORMS	USUAL DAILY ADULT DOSAGE RANGE (mg)	THERAPEUTIC SERUM LEVELS (μg/L)	RELATIVE FREQUENCY OF SIDE EFFECTS		
				Sedation	Anticholinergic	Orthostatic Hypotension
SELECTIVE SEROTONIN REUPTAKE INHIBITORS (SSRIs)						
Citalopram Celexa Various	Tab 20, 40 mg Soln 2 mg/mL	20–60	b	Very low	Very low	None
Escitalopram Lexapro	5, 10, 20 mg 1 mg/mL	10–20	b	Very low	Very low	None
Fluoxetine Prozac Various	Cap, Tab 10, 20, 40 mg SR Cap 90 mg Soln 4 mg/mL Tab 10 mg	10–80	b	None	Very low	None
Fluvoxamine Luvox	Tab 25, 50, 100 mg	100–300[d]	b	None	None	None
Paroxetine Paxil Various	Tab 10, 20, 30, 40 mg SR Tab 12.5, 25 mg Susp 2 mg/mL	20–50	b	Low	Low	Very low
Sertraline Zoloft Various	Tab 25, 50, 100 mg Soln 20 mg/mL	50–200	b	None	None	None

(continued)

ANTIDEPRESSANTS COMPARISON CHART[a] (continued)

CLASS AND DRUG	DOSAGE FORMS	USUAL DAILY ADULT DOSAGE RANGE (mg)	THERAPEUTIC SERUM LEVELS (μg/L)	RELATIVE FREQUENCY OF SIDE EFFECTS		
				Sedation	Anticholinergic	Orthostatic Hypotension
SEROTONIN NOREPINEPHRINE REUPTAKE INHIBITORS (SNRIs)						
Desvenlafaxine Pristiq	Tab 50, 100 mg	50	[b]	Very low	Very low	Very low
Duloxetine Cymbalta	Cap 20, 30, 60 mg	40–60	[b]	Very low	Very low	Very low
Venlafaxine Effexor Effexor XR Various	Tab 25, 37.5, 50, 75, 100 mg SR Cap 37.5, 75, 150 mg	225–375	[b]	Very low	Very low	Very low
TETRACYCLICS[c]						
Maprotiline Ludiomil Various	Tab 25, 50, 75 mg	150–225	200–300[b]	Moderate	Moderate	Moderate
TRIAZOLOPYRIDINES						
Trazodone Desyrel Various	Tab 50, 100, 150, 300 mg	50–100 (hypnotic) 200–400 (antidepressant)	[b]	High	Very low	High
Nefazodone Serzone Various	Tab 50, 100, 150, 200, 250 mg	300–600	[b]	Moderate	Very low	Moderate

(continued)

ANTIDEPRESSANTS COMPARISON CHART[a] (continued)

CLASS AND DRUG	DOSAGE FORMS	USUAL DAILY ADULT DOSAGE RANGE (mg)	THERAPEUTIC SERUM LEVELS (µg/L)	RELATIVE FREQUENCY OF SIDE EFFECTS		
				Sedation	Anticholinergic	Orthostatic Hypotension
TRICYCLICS (TCAs)[d]						
Amitriptyline Elavil Various	Tab 10, 25, 50, 75, 100, 150 mg Inj 10 mg/mL	150–300	75–175[e]	High	High	High
Clomipramine Anafranil Various	Cap 25, 50, 75 mg	100–250[d] 100–150[f]	b	High	High	High
Desipramine Norpramin Various	Tab 10, 25, 50, 75, 100, 150 mg	150–300	100–160	Low	Low	Moderate
Doxepin Adapin Sinequan Various	Cap 10, 25, 50, 75, 100, 150 mg Soln 10 mg/mL	150–300	110–250[e]	High	Moderate	High
Imipramine Tofranil Janimine Various	Tab 10, 25, 50 mg Cap (as pamoate) 75, 100, 125, 150 mg	150–300	>200[e]	Moderate	Moderate	High

(continued)

ANTIDEPRESSANTS COMPARISON CHART[a] (*continued*)

CLASS AND DRUG	DOSAGE FORMS	USUAL DAILY ADULT DOSAGE RANGE (mg)	THERAPEUTIC SERUM LEVELS (μg/L)	RELATIVE FREQUENCY OF SIDE EFFECTS		
				Sedation	Anticholinergic	Orthostatic Hypotension
Nortriptyline Aventyl Pamelor Various	Cap 10, 25, 50, 75 mg Soln 2 mg/mL	100–200	50–150	Moderate	Moderate	Low
Protriptyline Vivactil Various	Tab 5, 10 mg	30–60	70–260[b]	Very low	Moderate	Moderate
Trimipramine Surmontil	Cap 25, 50, 100 mg	150–300	[b]	Moderate	Moderate	High

[a]Antidepressants with serotonergic activity (SSRIs, nefazodone, venlafaxine, and mirtazapine) have established efficacy for many indications other than depression. Some have received approval for generalized anxiety disorder, bulimia nervosa, obsessive-compulsive disorder, social phobia, panic disorder, posttraumatic stress disorder, and premenstrual dysphoric disorder. Effective doses for major depression for most patients are in the low to moderate ranges listed which is also true for generalized anxiety disorder, social phobia, panic disorder, and premenstrual dysphoric disorder. The middle to high end of the listed dosage ranges is usually necessary for efficacy when treating bulimia nervosa, obsessive-compulsive disorder, and posttraumatic stress disorder.[71]

[b]Not well established.

[c]Amoxapine, maprotiline, and the tricyclic antidepressants are categorized together as heterocyclic antidepressants because their therapeutic and side effect profiles are similar.

[d]For obsessive-compulsive disorder.

[e]Includes active metabolites.

[f]For major depression.

From Refs. 1, 7, 18, 22, 23, 36, 37, 41, 42, 44, 49, 55, 56, 69, and 71–72.

FOODS THAT INTERACT WITH MAO INHIBITORS CHART

Many fermented foods contain tyramine as a byproduct formed by the bacterial breakdown of the amino acid tyrosine; it also can be formed by parahydroxylation of phenylethylamine or dehydroxylation of dihydroxyphenylalanine (DOPA) and dopamine. Tyramine and some other amines found in food can cause hypertensive reactions in patients taking MAO inhibitors. MAO found in the GI tract inactivates tyramine; when drugs prevent this, exogenous tyramine and other monoamines are absorbed and norepinephrine from sympathetic nerve endings and epinephrine from the adrenal gland are released. If sufficient quantities of these pressor compounds are released, palpitations, severe headache, and hypertensive crisis can result.

FOODS THAT CONTAIN TYRAMINE

Avocados	Particularly if overripe.
Bananas	Reactions can occur if eaten in large amounts; tyramine levels are high in peel.
Bean curd	Fermented bean curd, fermented soya bean, soya bean pastes, soy sauces, and miso soup, prepared from fermented bean curd, contain tyramine in large amounts; miso soup has caused reactions.
Beer and ale	Major domestic brands do not contain appreciable amounts; some imported brands have had high levels. Nonalcoholic beer might contain tyramine and should be avoided.
Caviar	Safe if vacuum packed and eaten fresh or refrigerated only briefly.
Cheese	Reactions possible with most, except unfermented varieties such as cottage cheese. In others, tyramine concentration is higher near the rind and close to fermentation holes.
Figs	Particularly if overripe.
Fish	Safe if fresh; avoid dried products. Caution required in restaurants. Vacuum-packed products are safe if eaten promptly or refrigerated only briefly.
Liver	Safe if very fresh, but rapidly accumulates tyramine; caution required in restaurants.
Meat	Safe if known to be fresh; caution required in restaurants.
Milk products	Milk and yogurt appear to be safe.
Protein extracts	See also soups; avoid liquid and powdered protein dietary supplements.
Sausage	Fermented varieties such as bologna, pepperoni, and salami have a high tyramine content.
Shrimp paste	Contains large amounts of tyramine.
Soups	Might contain protein extracts and should be avoided.
Soy sauce	Contains large amounts of tyramine; reactions have occurred with teriyaki.
Wines	Generally do not contain tyramine, but many reactions have been reported with Chianti, champagne, and other wines.
Yeast extracts	Dietary supplements (e.g., marmite) contain large amounts; yeast in baked goods, is safe.

FOODS THAT DO NOT CONTAIN TYRAMINE

Caffeine	A weak pressor agent; large amounts can cause reactions.
Chocolate	Contains phenylethylamine, a pressor agent that can cause reactions in large amounts.
Fava beans	(Broad beans, "Italian" green beans) contain dopamine, a pressor amine, particularly when overripe.
Ginseng	Some preparations have caused headache, tremulousness, and manic-like symptoms.
Liqueurs	Reactions reported with some (e.g., Chartreuse, Drambuie); cause unknown.
New Zealand prickly spinach	Single case report; patient ate large amounts.
Whiskey	Reactions have occurred; cause unknown.

For more information, consult Refs. 75 and 76.
From Ref. 77, reproduced with permission.

■ REFERENCES

1. Davidson JR, Connor KM. Bupropion sustained release: a therapeutic overview. *J Clin Psychiatry.* 1998; 59(suppl 4):25-31.
2. Cooper BR et al. Evidence that the acute behavioral and electrophysiological effects of bupropion (Wellbutrin) are mediated by a noradrenergic mechanism. *Neuropsychopharmacology.* 1994;11:133-141.
3. Walker PW et al. Improvement in fluoxetine-associated sexual dysfunction in patients switched to bupropion. *J Clin Psychiatry.* 1993;54:459-465.
4. Goldstein MG. Bupropion sustained release and smoking cessation. *J Clin Psychiatry.* 1998;59(suppl 4):66-72.
5. Cheung AH et al. Review of the efficacy and safety of antidepressants in youth depression. *J Child Psychol Psychiatry.* 2005,46.735-754.
6. Jermain DM et al. Pharmacotherapy of obsessive-compulsive disorder. *Pharmacotherapy.* 1990;10:175 198.
7. Peters MD et al. Clomipramine: an antiobsessional tricyclic antidepressant. *Clin Pharm.* 1990;9:165-178.
8. Stokes PE. Fluoxetine: a five-year review. *Clin Ther.* 1993;15:216-243.
9. Monteiro WO et al. Anorgasmia from clomipramine in obsessive-compulsive disorder: a controlled trial. *Br J Psychiatry.* 1987;151:107-112.
10. Wagner KD et al. A double-blind, randomized, placebo-controlled trial of escitalopram in the treatment of pediatric depression. *J Am Acad Child Adolesc Psychiatry.* 2006;45:280-288.
11. Sommi RW et al. Fluoxetine: a serotonin-specific second-generation antidepressant. *Pharmacotherapy.* 1987;7:1-15.
12. Schweizer E et al. What constitutes an adequate antidepressant trial for fluoxetine? *J Clin Psychiatry.* 1990;51:8-11.
13. Steiner M et al. Intermittent fluoxetine dosing in the treatment of women with premenstrual dysphoric disorder. *Psychopharmacol Bull.* 1997;33:771-774.
14. Benet LZ et al. Design and optimization of dosage regimens: pharmacokinetic data. In: Hardman JG et al., eds. *Goodman and Gilman's the Pharmacological Basis of Therapeutics.* 9th ed. New York: McGraw-Hill; 1996: 1707-1792.
15. Gutierrez MA, Stimmel GL. Management of and counseling for psychotropic drug-induced sexual dysfunction. *Pharmacotherapy.* 1999;19:823-831.
16. Rothschild AJ. Sexual side effects of antidepressants. *J Clin Psychiatry.* 2000;61(suppl 11):28-36.
17. Kinney-Parker JL et al. Fluoxetine and weight: something lost and something gained? *Clin Pharm.* 1989;8:727-733.
18. Jefferson JW. Cardiovascular effects and toxicity of anxiolytics and antidepressants. *J Clin Psychiatry.* 1989;50:368-378.
19. Tollefson GD et al. Absence of a relationship between adverse events and suicidality during pharmacotherapy for depression. *J Clin Psychopharmacol.* 1994;14:163-169.
20. Feighner JP et al. Adverse consequences of fluoxetine-MAOI combination therapy. *J Clin Psychiatry.* 1990;51: 222-225.

21. Roose SP et al. Comparative efficacy of selective serotonin reuptake inhibitors and tricyclics in the treatment of melancholia. *Am J Psychiatry.* 1994;151:1735-1739.

22. Grimsley SR, Jann MW. Paroxetine, sertraline, and fluvoxamine: new selective serotonin reuptake inhibitors. *Clin Pharm.* 1992;11:930-957.

23. Wilde MI et al. Fluvoxamine: an updated review of its pharmacology and therapeutic use in depressive illness. *Drugs.* 1993;46:895-924.

24. Freeman CPL et al. Fluvoxamine versus clomipramine in the treatment of obsessive-compulsive disorder: a multi-center, randomized, double-blind, parallel group comparison. *J Clin Psychiatry.* 1994;55:301-305.

25. Potter WZ et al. The pharmacologic treatment of depression. *N Engl J Med.* 1991;325:633-642.

26. Preskorn SH. Recent pharmacologic advances in antidepressant therapy for the elderly. *Am J Med.* 1993;94(suppl 5A):2S-12S.

27. Baldessarini RJ. Current status of antidepressants: clinical pharmacology and therapy. *J Clin Psychiatry.* 1989;50:117-126.

28. Frank E et al. Comparison of full-dose versus half-dose pharmacotherapy in the maintenance treatment of recurrent depression. *J Affect Disord.* 1993;27:139-145.

29. Wright JM. Review of the symptomatic treatment of diabetic neuropathy. *Pharmacotherapy.* 1994;14:689-697.

30. Max MB. Treatment of post-herpetic neuralgia: antidepressants. *Ann Neurol.* 1994;35:S50-S53.

31. Rappoport JL et al. Childhood enuresis II. Psychopathology, tricyclic concentration in plasma, and antienuretic effect. *Arch Gen Psychiatry.* 1980;37:1146-1152.

32. Puig-Antich J et al. Imipramine in prepubertal major depressive disorders. *Arch Gen Psychiatry.* 1987;44:81-89.

33. Salzman C. Pharmacologic treatment of depression in the elderly. *J Clin Psychiatry.* 1993;54(suppl 2):23-28.

34. Salzman C. Practical considerations in the pharmacologic treatment of depression and anxiety in the elderly. *J Clin Psychiatry.* 1990;51(suppl 1):40-43.

35. Wisner KL et al. Tricyclic dose requirements across pregnancy. *Am J Psychiatry.* 1993;150:1541-1542.

36. Preskorn SH. Pharmacokinetics of antidepressants. *J Clin Psychiatry.* 1993;54(suppl 9):14-34.

37. DeVane CL. *Fundamentals of Monitoring Psychoactive Drug Therapy.* Baltimore, MD: Williams & Wilkins; 1990.

38. Cole JO, Bodkin A. Antidepressant drug side effects. *J Clin Psychiatry.* 1990;51(suppl 1):21-26.

39. Rosenstein DL et al. Seizures associated with antidepressants: a review. *J Clin Psychiatry.* 1993;54:289-299.

40. Anonymous. Sudden death in children treated with a tricyclic antidepressant. *Med Lett Drugs Ther.* 1990;32:53.

41. Stimmel GL et al. Mirtazapine: an antidepressant with noradrenergic and specific serotonergic effects. *Pharmacotherapy.* 1997;17:10-21.

42. Stimmel GL et al. Mirtazapine safety and tolerability: analysis of the clinical trials database. *Prim Psychiatry.* 1997;4:82-96.

43. Goodman WK, Charney DS. Therapeutic applications and mechanisms of action of monoamine oxidase inhibitors and heterocyclic antidepressant drugs. *J Clin Psychiatry.* 1985;46(10, sec 2):6-22.

44. Cantú TG, Korek JS. Monoamine oxidase inhibitors and weight gain. *Drug Intell Clin Pharm.* 1988;22:755-759.

45. Kahn D et al. The safety of switching rapidly from tricyclic antidepressants to monoamine oxidase inhibitors. *J Clin Psychopharmacol.* 1989;9:198-202.

46. Brown CS, Bryant SG. Monoamine oxidase inhibitors: safety and efficacy issues. *Drug Intell Clin Pharm.* 1988;22:232-235.

47. Shulman KI et al. Dietary restriction, tyramine, and the use of monoamine oxidase inhibitors. *J Clin Psychopharmacol.* 1989;9:397-402.

48. Nierenberg AA, Amsterdam JD. Treatment-resistant depression: definition and treatment approaches. *J Clin Psychiatry.* 1990;51(suppl 6):39-47.

49. Dopheide JA et al. Focus on nefazodone: a serotonergic drug for major depression. *Hosp Formul.* 1995;30:205-212.

50. Fontaine R et al. A double-blind comparison of nefazodone, imipramine, and placebo in major depression. *J Clin Psychiatry.* 1994;55:234-241.

51. Barbhaiya RH et al. Single-dose pharmacokinetics of nefazodone in healthy young and elderly subjects and in subjects with renal or hepatic impairment. *Eur J Clin Pharmacol.* 1995;49:221-228.

52. Barbhaiya RH et al. Steady-state pharmacokinetics of nefazodone in subjects with normal and impaired renal function. *Eur J Clin Pharmacol.* 1995;49:229-235.

53. Voris JC et al. Nefazodone: single versus twice daily dose. *Pharmacotherapy.* 1998;18:379-380.

54. DeWilde J et al. A double-blind, comparative, multicentre study comparing paroxetine with fluoxetine in depressed patients. *Acta Psychiatr Scand.* 1993;87:141-145.

55. Dechant KL, Clissold SPP. Paroxetine. *Drugs.* 1991;41:225-253.

56. DeVane CL. Pharmacokinetics of the selective serotonin reuptake inhibitors. *J Clin Psychiatry.* 1992;53(suppl 2):13-20.

57. Tollefson GD et al. A multicenter investigation of fixed dose fluoxetine in the treatment of obsessive-compulsive disorder. *Arch Gen Psychiatry.* 1994;51:559-567.

58. Greist J et al. Double blind parallel comparison of three dosages of sertraline and placebo in outpatients with obsessive-compulsive disorder. *Arch Gen Psychiatry*. 1995;52:289-295.

59. Johnson MR et al. Panic disorder: pathophysiology and drug treatment. *Drugs*. 1995;49:328-344.

60. Sheehan DV, Harnett-Sheehan K. The role of SSRIs in panic disorder. *J Clin Psychiatry*. 1996;57(suppl 10):51-58.

61. Montejo-Gonzalez AL et al. SSRI-induced sexual dysfunction: fluoxetine, paroxetine, sertraline, and fluvoxamine in a prospective, multicenter, and descriptive clinical study of 344 patients. *J Sex Marital Ther*. 1997;23:176-194.

62. Heym J, Koe BK. Pharmacology of sertraline: a review. *J Clin Psychiatry*. 1988;49(suppl 8):40-45.

63. Doogan DP, Caillard V. Sertraline: a new antidepressant. *J Clin Psychiatry*. 1988;49(suppl 8):46-51.

64. Aguglia E et al. Double-blind study of the efficacy and safety of sertraline versus fluoxetine in major depression. *Int Clin Psychopharmacol*. 1993;8:197-202.

65. Wisner KL et al. Serum sertraline and *N*-desmethylsertraline levels in breast-feeding mother-infant pairs. *Am J Psychiatry*. 1998;155:690-692.

66. Bradley ME et al. Sertraline-associated syndrome of inappropriate antidiuretic hormone: case report and review of the literature. *Pharmacotherapy*. 1996;16:680-683.

67. Cunningham LA. Once-daily venlafaxine extended release (XR) and venlafaxine immediate release (IR) in outpatients with major depression. *Ann Clin Psychiatry*. 1997;9:157-164.

68. Schweizer E et al. Placebo-controlled trial of venlafaxine for the treatment of major depression. *J Clin Psychopharmacol*. 1991;11:233 236.

69. Montgomery SA. Venlafaxine: a new dimension in antidepressant pharmacotherapy. *J Clin Psychiatry*. 1993;54:119-126.

70. Cunningham LA et al. A comparison of venlafaxine, trazodone, and placebo in major depression. *J Clin Psychopharmacol*. 1994;14:99-106.

71. Bryant SG, Freshefsky L. Antidepressant properties of trazodone. *Clin Pharm*. 1982;1:406-417.

72. Milne RJ, Goa KL. Citalopram. *Drugs*. 1991;41:450-477.

73. Montgomery SA et al. The optimal dosing regimen for citalopram—a meta-analysis of nine placebo-controlled studies. *Int Clin Psychopharmacol*. 1994;9(suppl 1):35-40.

74. Schatzberg AF. New indications for antidepressants. *J Clin Psychiatry*. 2000;61(suppl 11):9-17.

75. Lippman SB, Nash K. Monoamine oxidase inhibitor update. Potential adverse food and drug interactions. *Drug Saf*. 1990;5:195-204.

76. Shulman KI, Walker SE. Redefining the MAOI diet: tyramine content of pizzas and soy products. *J Clin Psychiatry*. 1999;60:191-213.

77. Anonymous. Foods interacting with MAO inhibitors. *Med Lett Drugs Ther*. 1989;31:11-12.

Chapter 38

Antipsychotic Drugs

Aaron P. Gibson

Class Instructions. *Antipsychotics.* These drugs can cause drowsiness. Until the extent of this effect is known, use caution when driving, operating machinery, or performing other tasks requiring mental alertness. Avoid excessive concurrent use of alcohol or other drugs that cause drowsiness. Both conventional and atypical antipsychotics have a black box warning for increased risk of mortality in elderly patients treated for dementia-related psychosis.

Missed Doses. If you miss a dose, take it as soon as you remember. If it is almost time for your next dose, skip it and resume your normal schedule. Do not double doses.

ANTIPSYCHOTIC (TYPICAL) CLASS OVERVIEW

Pharmacology. Antipsychotic efficacy is most likely related to blockade of post-synaptic dopaminergic receptors in the mesolimbic and prefrontal cortexes of the brain, although other neurotransmitter systems also are involved.[1]

Administration and Adult Dosage. (*See* Antipsychotic Drugs Comparison Chart.) Initiate therapy with divided doses until therapeutic dosage is found; then, for most patients, once-daily administration at bedtime is preferred. For maintenance, decrease acute dosage by 25% every 3 months, with a target maintenance dosage being 50%–67% of the acute treatment dosage.[2] Recent concern has focused on the need to establish a minimum effective dosage for antipsychotic drugs, and treatment regimens at the low end of the dosage range are preferred. Oral dosages of high-potency antipsychotics (e.g., **fluphenazine, haloperidol**) in the range of 5–20 mg/d are better tolerated and equal in efficacy to dosages >20 mg/d.[3] Most patients can be given a maintenance dosage of 50% of the acute dosage by the end of 1 year, although 10%–15% of chronically ill patients require a maintenance dosage >15 mg/d of **haloperidol** or its equivalent.[4,5] For manic episodes, no additional benefit is achieved with dosages >10 mg/d of haloperidol.[6] **Mesoridazine** and **thioridazine** are indicated only in patients who fail with other drugs because of inefficacy or intolerable side effects.

Special Populations. *Pediatric Dosage.* As with adults, dosage is determined primarily by titration to individual response. No precise dosage range exists, but in general the initial dosage is lower and increased more gradually in children.

Geriatric Dosage. Initial dosage is 20%–25% of the dosage used in younger adults. Typical starting dosages in the elderly are **haloperidol** 0.5–2 mg/d. Dosage adjustments also must be done more slowly than in younger adults.[7] Dosages in the lower range are sufficient for most elderly patients, and the rate of dosage titration is slower.

Dosage Forms. *See* Antipsychotic Drugs Comparison Chart.

Patient Instructions. (*See* Antipsychotics, Class Instructions.) These drugs usually take several weeks for clinical response and up to 8 weeks for full therapeutic response.

Pharmacokinetics. *Onset and Duration.* Onset of antipsychotic activity is variable with noticeable response requiring days to weeks.

Serum Levels. Correlation of serum levels with clinical response is not consistently established. The best evidence exists for **haloperidol**, with serum concentrations of 5–15 µg/L (13–40 nmol/L) correlating well with therapeutic effects in adult psychotic patients, and an increasing risk of adverse effects and decreased efficacy when steady-state concentrations exceed 15 µg/L.[8,9]

Fate. **Haloperidol** is well absorbed; peak serum levels are achieved 2–6 h after liquid or tablets are administered and within 30 min after IM. Oral bioavailability of haloperidol is 60%–70%. Haloperidol is extensively metabolized, with one active hydroxy metabolite. **Chlorpromazine** and other phenothiazines are well absorbed but undergo extensive and variable presystemic metabolism in the gut wall and liver; more than 20 chlorpromazine metabolites with different activities have been identified in human plasma. Sustained-release formulations result in a greater first-pass effect *Half-life.* Serum half-lives have no clinical correlation with biologic half-lives for antipsychotic drugs; **chlorpromazine** 30 h, **thioridazine** 4–10 h, **thiothixene** 34 h, and **haloperidol** 12–24 h. Of more clinical importance is that steady-state central nervous system (CNS) levels and tissue saturation which allow once-daily administration of all antipsychotic drugs.[10]

Adverse Reactions. (*See* Antipsychotic Drugs Comparison Chart for relative frequency of common adverse reactions.) Frequently, sedation, extrapyramidal effects (e.g., parkinsonism, dystonic reactions, akathisia), tardive dyskinesia (TD), anticholinergic effects (e.g., dry mouth, blurred vision, constipation, urinary retention), photosensitivity, and postural hypotension occur. Occasionally, weight gain, amenorrhea, galactorrhea, ejaculatory disturbance, neuroleptic malignant syndrome (NMS), agranulocytosis, skin rash, cholestatic jaundice, and skin or eye pigmentation occur. Rarely, seizures, thermoregulatory impairment, and slowed AV conduction occur. **Mesoridazine** and **thioridazine** can prolong QTc interval, leading to torsades de pointes and sudden death. Low-potency drugs are more likely to cause sedation, anticholinergic effects, and orthostatic hypotension, whereas high-potency drugs cause more extrapyramidal effects. TD is a long-term adverse effect, untreatable, and sometimes irreversible. TD occurs at a 4% yearly incidence for at least the first 5–6 years of treatment. NMS (e.g., fever, extrapyramidal rigidity, autonomic instability, alterations in consciousness) occurs more frequently with high-potency antipsychotics, with a prevalence of 1.4% and a fatality rate of 4%.[3,11,12]

Contraindications. Coma; circulatory collapse or severe hypotension; bone marrow depression; history of blood dyscrasia. (Mesoridazine and thioridazine) concurrent use with drugs that prolong QTc interval; baseline QTc>450 ms.

Precautions. Use cautiously in patients with myasthenia gravis, Parkinson's disease, seizure disorders, or hepatic disease.

Drug Interactions. Barbiturates can enhance phenothiazine metabolism; carbamazepine can enhance haloperidol metabolism. Phenothiazines can decrease efficacy of guanethidine or guanadrel or have additive hypotensive effects with hypotensive drugs. Phenothiazines can inhibit the antiparkinson activity of levodopa. Haloperidol can increase the CNS toxicity of lithium. Combined use of haloperidol and methyldopa can result in dementia.

Parameters to Monitor. (Mesoridazine and thioridazine) obtain baseline and periodic ECGs and serum potassium. Complete blood count (CBC) and absolute neutrophil count (ANC) must be monitored with clozapine therapy.

ARIPIPRAZOLE
Abilify

Pharmacology. Aripiprazole is considered an atypical antipsychotic but has a very unique mechanism of action. It combines partial agonism at D_2 and 5-HT_{1A} with antagonism at 5-HT_{2A}.

Administration and Adult Dosage. **PO for schizophrenia**—10 or 15 mg/d. Doses up to 30 mg/d were studied but did not show a benefit over the 10 or 15 mg/d groups.[13] **PO for acute bipolar disorder**—15 mg/d as monotherapy or as adjunct therapy to lithium or valproic acid. The dose can be increased to 30 mg/d based on response and tolerability. **PO for adjunctive treatment of depression**—2–5 mg/d. Doses up to 15 mg/d were studied. Dose increases should be in 5 mg/d increments and should not occur more frequently than every 7 days. **IM for agitation associated with schizophrenia or bipolar mania**—9.75 mg. Cumulative doses up to 30 mg/d may be given, but doses should not be administered more frequently than every 2 h. Conversion from the oral solution to oral tablets is a 1:1 conversion up to 25 mg. If the patient is taking 30-mg tablets, 25 mg of oral solution should be used.

Special Populations. *Pediatric Dosage.* **PO for schizophrenia**—(13–17 years) 10 mg/d. Doses up to 30 mg/d have been studied, but not found to be more efficacious than the 10 mg/d dose. **PO for bipolar disorder**—(10–17 years) 10 mg/d, but doses up to 30 mg/d have been studied.

Other Conditions. No dosage adjustments are necessary for elderly patients, renal or hepatic impairment.

Dosage Forms. **Tab** 2, 5, 10, 15, 20, 30 mg; **Orally Disintegrating Tab** 10, 15 mg; **Oral Soln** 1 mg/mL; **IM Soln** 9.75 mg/1.3 mL.

Patient Instructions. *See* Class Instructions.

Pharmacokinetics. *Onset and Duration.* Onset of antipsychotic activity is variable, with noticeable response requiring days to weeks.

Serum Levels. Not established.

Fate. Aripiprazole is well absorbed following oral administration with an absolute bioavailability of 87%. It is >99% plasma protein bound (primarily to albumin); the V_d is 4.9 L/kg. Aripiprazole is extensively metabolized by CYP3A4 and CYP2D6 with 1% and 18% unchanged aripiprazole found in urine and feces, respectively. **Half-life.** In extensive metabolizers, the half-life of aripiprazole and its major active metabolite is 75 and 94 h, respectively. In poor metabolizers (~8% of Caucasians), the half life of the parent compound increases to 146 h.

Adverse Reactions. Frequent adverse reactions include akathisia, nausea, constipation, vomiting, headache, dizziness, agitation, insomnia, anxiety, somnolence, extrapyramidal disorder, and fatigue. Adverse reactions that were increased with higher doses include somnolence, extrapyramidal disorder, tremor, and akathisia. Unlike most of the other atypical antipsychotics, aripiprazole appears to be fairly benign with regard to metabolic changes.[13]

Precautions. There has been a documented increase in mortality specifically due to cerebrovascular events in elderly patients treated with antipsychotics for dementia-related psychosis. In patients with depression who take antidepressants, there is also a risk of clinical worsening and increased suicide risk. Rare cases of NMS have been reported with aripiprazole. There is also the risk of the development of the movement disorder TD with all antipsychotics. Aripiprazole may also cause orthostatic hypotension secondary to its blockade of α_1-adrenoreceptors, and aripiprazole also has the potential to lower the seizure threshold, but this effect is less than with other antipsychotics like clozapine.

Drug Interactions. The dose of aripiprazole should be reduced by half when it is administered with potent CYP3A4 inhibitors like ketoconazole. Additionally, the aripiprazole dose should be reduced by half when it is given with potent CYP2D6 inhibitors (e.g, quinidine, fluoxetine, or paroxetine). When aripiprazole is given concomitantly with potent CYP3A4 inducers like carbamazepine, the aripiprazole dose should be doubled.

Parameters to Monitor. ECG should be monitored at baseline. Weight, lipid panel, and fasting glucose should be checked at baseline and then at 3 and 6 months followed by annual evaluation.

CLOZAPINE
Clozaril, Various

Pharmacology. Clozapine is an atypical antipsychotic drug that is chemically similar to loxapine and has unique pharmacologic effects and indications as well as very serious adverse effects. Whereas typical antipsychotic drugs exert their effects primarily with a blockade of dopamine D_2 receptors, clozapine affects several dopamine and serotonin receptors. Its high 5-HT$_2$ to dopamine D_2 ratio is the likely explanation for its unique efficacy. Compared with traditional antipsychotic drugs, clozapine is more effective for negative symptoms of schizophrenia, is more effective in treatment-resistant patients, and rarely causes extrapyramidal effects.[14–17]

Administration and Adult Dosage. **PO for schizophrenia**—100–200 mg 3 times daily is effective for most patients, but some might require up to 900 mg/d. A therapeutic trial of 12–24 weeks is required for the full therapeutic effect to become apparent. Initial dosing recommendation is 12.5 mg once or twice daily. On the basis of patient tolerance, daily dose increases of 25–50 mg may be added to achieve an initial target dose of 300–450 mg at the end of 2 weeks. Any subsequent increases should not occur more frequently than 1–2 times per week and should not exceed 100 mg. Twice-daily dosing is recommended if the patient is able to tolerate it in order to minimize the risk of hypotension, sedation, and seizures.

Dosage Forms. **Tab** 25, 100 mg; **orally disintegrating Tab** (FazaClo) 12.5, 25, 100 mg.

Pharmacokinetics. Clozapine is nearly completely absorbed after oral administration, with approximately 30% oral bioavailability because of extensive first-pass metabolism. Clozapine is 95% bound to plasma proteins with multiple doses. **Half-life.** 12 h.[18]

Adverse Reactions. Frequent adverse effects include sedation, orthostatic hypotension, anticholinergic effects, fever, and excessive salivation. Seizures are dose related, with a frequency up to 5% in the therapeutic dosage range and a 1-year cumulative incidence of 10%. Agranulocytosis is the major adverse effect of concern, occurring in 0.8% of patients after 1 year.[19] Most cases of agranulocytosis occur within the first 3 months of therapy. Substantial weight gain has been reported in most patients receiving clozapine.[20] (*See* Antipsychotic Drugs Comparison Chart.)

Contraindications. Agranulocytosis or severe granulocytopenia; concomitant use with medications known to cause agranulocytosis or suppress bone marrow function; preexisting myeloproliferative or paralytic ileus; uncontrolled epilepsy.

Precautions. Blood counts should be monitored as agranulocytosis can develop. There is an increased risk of cardiovascular or pulmonary adverse events including orthostasis, cardiomyopathy, deep vein thrombosis, and myocarditis. Worsening of narrow angle glaucoma may occur secondary to anticholinergic properties. Metabolic parameters including diabetes mellitus, hyperlipidemia, and hyperglycemia may occur or worsen secondary to treatment with clozapine. NMS and TD have been reported with clozapine use, but are much less of a concern than with other antipsychotics.

Patient Instructions. (*See* Class Instructions.) Tell your doctor if you are pregnant or breast-feeding while taking this medication. Common adverse events you might experience include drowsiness, dizziness, seizures, and increased salivation. Clozapine may also cause an increase in weight. You should notify your doctor if you start to notice weight gain. You should also contact your doctor if you start to experience any uncontrolled movements such as lip smacking or puckering, puffing of the cheeks, rapid or worm-like movements of the tongue, uncontrolled chewing movements, or uncontrolled movements of the arms and legs.

Parameters to Monitor. Patients must have a baseline white blood cell (WBC) count and differential before initiating therapy, mandatory weekly WBC monitoring for the first 6 months, and then every 2 weeks throughout treatment and for 4 weeks after discontinuation. If mild leukopenia or granulocytopenia develops (defined as a WBC $\geq$3000 mm^3 but <3500 mm^3 OR an ANC is $\geq$1500 μL but <2000 μL), the CBC should be repeated. If the results fall into the same range, twice weekly CBC monitoring is required until the WBC is >3500 mm^3 and ANC >1500 μL. Regular weekly monitoring can be resumed after those thresholds are reached. If moderate leukopenia or granulocytopenia develops (defined as a WBC $\geq$2000 mm^3 but <3000 mm^3 OR an ANC is $\geq$1000 μL but <1500 μL), therapy should be interrupted and daily CBCs should be done until WBC >3000 mm^3 and ANC >1500 μL. Once those levels are reached, twice weekly CBCs must be done until the WBC >3500 mm^3 and ANC >2000 μL. Clozapine may be rechallenged once those levels have been reached with normal weekly monitoring resuming.

If severe leukopenia or granulocytopenia develops (defined as a WBC <2000 mm^3 OR an ANC is <1000 mm^3), clozapine must be discontinued and is not eligible for rechallenge. Additionally, CBC monitoring parameters described in moderate leukopenia or granulocytopenia must be followed.

HALOPERIDOL AND HALOPERIDOL DECANOATE

Haldol, Haldol Decanoate, Various

Pharmacology. Haloperidol is a high potency dopamine receptor antagonist typical antipsychotic. Haloperidol decanoate (HD) is the preferred long-acting depot antipsychotic drug. Depot antipsychotics are indicated only for patients who demonstrate good response but are consistently drug-noncompliant with resultant frequent psychotic relapses. Depot antipsychotics provide fewer relapses and hospitalizations, stable serum drug levels, and side effects equal to oral antipsychotic drugs. HD can be given every 4 weeks; **fluphenazine decanoate** (FD) is similar in efficacy and adverse effects, but it must be administered every 2 weeks. Do not use HD or FD to treat acute psychotic symptoms; rather, use the drug only after a patient has been stabilized on an oral antipsychotic drug.[21-24] *See* Antipsychotic (Typical) Class Overview.

Administration and Adult Dosage. **PO for psychotic disorders, schizophrenia, or Tourette's syndrome**—(moderate symptoms) 0.5–2 mg 2–3 times daily, (severe symptoms) 3–5 mg 2–3 times daily. **IM for acute psychosis, schizophrenia, or Tourette's syndrome**—2–5 mg every 4–8 h; may increase to every hour if necessary. **IM decanoate for chronic schizophrenia**—Do not exceed an initial HD dosage of 100 mg, with the first month's dose being 10–15 times the oral haloperidol daily dosage if the PO dose was 10 mg/d or less and 20 times the oral dose if it was greater than 10 mg/d. An IM loading dose technique has been described that gives 20 times the daily oral dosage, using 100–200 mg of depot every 3–7 days to reach the calculated amount, with a maximum of 450 mg.[25] In geriatric or hepatically impaired patients, use a monthly HD dose 10 times the oral haloperidol dosage. Experience with HD doses greater than 500 mg is limited; divide injections >5 mL into 2 equal portions given at 2 sites. PO haloperidol supplementation might be necessary between monthly injections to treat reemergence of psychotic symptoms until steady-state concentrations are reached.

Dosage Forms. **Tab** 0.5, 1, 2, 5, 10, 20 mg; **Inj** (lactate) 5 mg/mL; **Oral Soln** 2 mg/mL; **Inj** (decanoate) 50, 100 mg/mL.

Pharmacokinetics. After IM administration of HD, esterases cleave the decanoate chain to release the active drug. Peak serum concentrations of haloperidol occur in 3–9 days. **Half-life.** 3 weeks. Steady-state levels are reached after 12–16 weeks.

Adverse Reactions. Because of its tight D_2 binding profile, haloperidol is frequently associated with extrapyramidal symptoms (EPS) including Parkinson-like symptoms, akathisia, and dystonias. Cardiovascular side effects include QTc prolongation, tachycardia, and arrhythmias. Withdrawal dyskinesias may present upon abrupt withdrawal. Like all antipsychotics, Haldol has been linked as a causative agent of TD as well as NMS. Endocrine side effects include gynecomastia, lactation, prolactin elevations, menstrual irregularities, and hyperglycemia. Anorexia, dyspepsia, nausea, vomiting, and constipation have all been reported with haloperidol. Xerostomia, blurred vision, and urinary retention have also been reported. There is no evidence that HD causes adverse effects with a frequency different from that of oral haloperidol.

Contraindications. Severe toxic CNS depression or comatose secondary to any cause; Parkinson's disease.

Precautions. Caution should be exercised when using haloperidol in patients with severe cardiovascular disorders because of hypotension and/or ECG changes. Patients with a history of seizures or EEG abnormalities should be closely monitored as haloperidol might lower the convulsive threshold. Patients taking other CNS depressants are at risk of potentiating that effect while taking haloperidol.

Patient Instructions. (*See* Class Instructions.) Tell your doctor if you are pregnant or breast-feeding while taking this medication. Common adverse events you might experience include drowsiness, dizziness, and muscle stiffness. Haloperidol may also cause an increase in weight. You should notify your doctor if you start to notice weight gain. You should also contact your doctor if you start to experience any uncontrolled movements such as lip smacking or puckering, puffing of the cheeks, rapid or worm-like movements of the tongue, uncontrolled chewing movements, or uncontrolled movements of the arms and legs.

Drug Interactions. Haloperidol is a substrate of CYP2D6 and is susceptible to any medications that induce or inhibit this enzyme such as paroxetine or fluvoxamine. Carbamazepine can reduce the effectiveness of haloperidol secondary to inducing its metabolism through CYP2D6 and 3A4. Any medication that increases the QTc interval (e.g., amiodarone, amoxapine, and fluoxetine) should not be used concomitantly with haloperidol. The effects of levodopa may be minimized or alleviated when given concomitantly with haloperidol.

OLANZAPINE
Zyprexa, Various

Pharmacology. Olanzapine is an atypical antipsychotic agent that is a potent serotonin 5-HT_2 and dopamine D_2 antagonist. It also has anticholinergic and histamine H1 receptor antagonistic effects that might account for some of its side effects.[26,27] (*See* Antipsychotic Drugs Comparison Chart.)

Administration and Adult Dosage. **PO for schizophrenia**—5–10 mg/d initially (5 mg/d in patients >65 years, debilitated patients, or those with a predisposition to hypotensive reactions). Increase in 5 mg/d increments at ≥7-day intervals. **Usual maintenance dosage**—10–15 mg/d, to a maximum of 20 mg/d, although dosages ≥10 mg/d are generally no more effective than 10 mg/d. **IM for acute psychosis**—2.5–10 mg/dose. **PO for bipolar disorder**—10-15 mg/d with dose increases of 5 mg/d occurring not more frequently than every 24 h. Doses up to 20 mg/d have been studied.

Dosage Forms. **Tab** 2.5, 5, 7.5, 10, 15, 20 mg; **Orally Disintegrating Tab** 5, 10, 15, 20 mg (Zyprexa Zydis); **Inj** 10 mg. Also available in combination with fluoxetine (Symbyax)

Pharmacokinetics. Olanzapine is well absorbed orally; food has no effect, but bioavailability is approximately 60% because of a first-pass effect. It is 93% bound to plasma proteins and has a V_d of ~1000 L. The drug is hepatically metabolized, probably by CYP1A2 and CYP2D6. Only 7% is excreted unchanged in urine. **Half-life.** 30 h.

Adverse Reactions. Frequent adverse effects include drowsiness, agitation, nervousness, orthostatic hypotension, dizziness, tachycardia, headache, rhinitis, constipation, akathisia, and weight gain. As with other atypical antipsychotic drugs, weight gain is the most troublesome long-term adverse effect, often affecting compliance.

Drug Interactions. Inducers of CYP2D6 may decrease olanzapine serum levels. Olanzapine does not appear to affect CYP450 enzymes.

PALIPERIDONE   Invega Sustenna

Pharmacology. Paliperidone is the major active metabolite of the atypical antipsychotic risperidone. The proposed antipsychotic mechanism for paliperidone is exactly like that of risperidone, which is through D_2 blockade and 5-HT$_{2A}$ antagonism.

Administration and Adult Dosage. PO for schizophrenia—6 mg/d. May increase by 3 mg/d every 5 days. Doses up to 12 mg/d have been studied but did not show any additional benefit. **IM for Schizophrenia**—234 mg IM on day 1 and 156 mg IM one week later. **Usual maintenance dose**—117 mg IM monthly.

Special Populations. Pediatric Dosage. Safety and efficacy not established.

Other Conditions. Renal impairment—(Cl$_{Cr}$ 50–80 mL/min) maximum dose is 6 mg/d, (Cl$_{Cr}$ 10–50 mL/min) maximum dose is 3 mg/d.

Dosage Forms. ER Tab 3, 6, 9 mg. Inj (Invega Sustenna) 39 mg, 78 mg, 117 mg, 156 mg, 234 mg.

Patient Instructions. (See Class Instructions.) Tablets should be swallowed whole, not chewed, cut, or crushed prior to administration.

Pharmacokinetics. Onset and Duration. Onset of antipsychotic activity is variable, with noticeable response requiring days to weeks.

Serum Levels. Not established.

Fate. Oral bioavailability of paliperidone is 28%; plasma protein binding is 74% and the V_d is 487 L. Following oral administration, 56% of the initial dose is found unchanged in the urine. Unlike the parent compound risperidone, CYP2D6 or CYP3A4 do not play a prominent role in the metabolism of the drug. **Half-life.** 23 h in patients with normal renal function (Cl$_{Cr}$ >80 mL/min); the half-life increases to 24, 40, and 51 h in patients with mild, moderate, and severe renal dysfunction, respectively.

Adverse Reactions. See Risperidone, Adverse Reactions.

Precautions. There has been a documented increase in mortality, specifically due to cerebrovascular events in elderly patients treated with antipsychotics for dementia-related psychosis. Rare cases of NMS have been reported. There is also the risk of the development of TD with all antipsychotics. Paliperidone may also cause orthostatic hypotension and syncope secondary to its blockade of α_1-adrenoreceptors and has the potential to lower the seizure threshold (less than with other antipsychotics, like clozapine). Cases of priapism and prolongation of the QTc interval have been reported.

Drug Interactions. Because paliperidone is not extensively metabolized and is primarily cleared by the kidneys, there is little potential for drug interactions through the CYP450 enzyme system.

Parameters to Monitor. ECG should be monitored at baseline. Weight, lipid panel, and fasting glucose should be checked at baseline and then at 3 and 6 months followed by annual evaluation. Renal function should be assessed prior to initiating paliperidone.

PIMOZIDE
Orap

Pharmacology. Pimozide is indicated for the treatment of Tourette's disorder. Although structurally different from other antipsychotic drugs, pimozide shares their ability to block dopaminergic receptors. Its lack of effect on norepinephrine receptors insinuated that pimozide would have a more favorable adverse effect profile than other antipsychotic drugs. **Haloperidol** is the drug of choice for Tourette's disorder.[28,29]

Administration and Adult Dosage. PO for Tourette's syndrome—1–2 mg/d in divided doses initially, with dosage increased every other day, to a maximum of 20 mg/d. Most patients who respond require ≤10 mg/d. Periodically decrease the dosage and attempt to withdraw treatment.

Special Populations. *Pediatric Dosage.* PO for Tourette's syndrome—0.05 mg/kg/d initially (preferably at bedtime), increasing every 3 days to a maximum of 0.2 mg/kg OR 10 mg daily.

Dosage Forms. Tab 1, 2 mg.

Pharmacokinetics. Pimozide is approximately 50% absorbed orally. It undergoes extensive first-pass metabolism in the liver to 2 metabolites with unknown activity. **Half-life.** 55 h.

Adverse Reactions. (*See* Adverse Reactions for Haloperidol). The relative frequencies of adverse effects of pimozide and haloperidol are similar, and pimozide remains an alternative to haloperidol for treating Tourette's disorder.

Contraindications. Aggressive schizophrenia patients when sedation is required; concurrent administration of pemoline, methylphenidate, or amphetamines that may cause motor and phonic tics; concurrent administration with dofetilide, sotalol, quinidine, other Class Ia and III antiarrhythmics, mesoridazine, thioridazine, chlorpromazine, and droperidol; concurrent administration with moxifloxacin, halofantrine, mefloquine, pentamidine, arsenic trioxide, levomethadyl acetate, dolasetron mesylate, probucol, tacrolimus, ziprasidone, sertraline, and macrolide antibiotics; concurrent administration with drugs that have demonstrated QT prolongation as one of their pharmacodynamic effects, and less potent inhibitors of CYP3A4 (e.g., zileuton, fluvoxamine); congenital or drug-induced long QT syndrome; doses >10 mg/d; history of cardiac arrhythmias; Parkinson's disease; hypokalemia; hypomagnesemia; severe CNS depression.

Precautions. Pregnancy category C. Cardiac problems including hypotension, QTc prolongation, and sudden cardiac death are associated with pimozide administration. Metabolic effects (e.g., hyperprolactinemia, weight gain, and hyponatremia) have been reported with pimozide. Significant weight loss has also been reported in chronic schizophrenic patients, which makes pimozide somewhat different than other antipsychotics. EPS, NMS, drowsiness, sedation, and seizures have been reported as well.

Drug Interactions. (*See* Haloperidol, Drug Interactions and Contraindications.) Pimozide is metabolized extensively via CYP3A4, therefore any medications that inhibit this enzyme (e.g., macrolide antibiotics, azole antifungals, and protease inhibitors) may lead to adverse events secondary to increased plasma levels. Conversely, medications that induce CYP3A4 metabolism could potentially decrease pimozide plasma levels.

QUETIAPINE
Seroquel, Seroquel XR, Various

Pharmacology. Quetiapine displays very loose D_2 antagonism in addition to $5\text{-}HT_{2A}$ antagonism. Additionally, it also has antihistaminic properties at the H1 receptor and adrenergic effects at the α_1-receptor. Quetiapine is frequently used without approval for insomnia because of its sedative effects thought to be mediated by histamine antagonism.[30-32]

Administration and Adult Dosage. **PO for schizophrenia**—25 mg twice daily with dose increases of 25–50 mg on the second and third day of therapy to a target dose of 300–400 mg/d in divided doses by the fourth day. Further dose increases should occur no sooner than every 2 days and should be 25–50 mg. **PO for bipolar depression**—similar to schizophrenia dosage except it should be given once daily at bedtime to reach 300 mg/d by day 4. **PO for bipolar mania**—initial dose is 100 mg/d in divided doses titrated up by 100 mg/d in divided doses up to 400 mg/d by day 4. Further dosage titration up to 800 mg/d by day 6 should not be in increments exceeding 200 mg/d. **Usual maintenance dosage**—Same dose as during the stabilization phase.

Dosage Forms. **Tab** 25, 50, 100, 200, 300, 400 mg. **ER Tab** 50, 150, 200, 300, 400 mg.

Pharmacokinetics. Quetiapine is rapidly absorbed following oral administration and reaches peak plasma levels in 1.5 h. The bioavailability is marginally affected by administration with food, but not clinically significant. Apparent volume of distribution for quetiapine is approximately 10 L/kg and it is 83% bound to plasma proteins at therapeutic doses. Metabolism of quetiapine occurs primarily through CYP3A4. **Half-life.** 6 h.

Adverse Reactions. Frequent adverse effects include drowsiness, agitation, nervousness, orthostatic hypotension, dizziness, tachycardia, headache, rhinitis, constipation, akathisia, and weight gain. As with other atypical antipsychotic drugs, weight gain is the most troublesome long-term adverse effect, often affecting compliance. Sedation is often seen with quetiapine, and it is frequently used in low doses to treat insomnia.

Contraindications. Hypersensitivity.

Precautions. (*See* Class Instructions.) Pregnancy category C. Elderly patients with dementia-related psychosis treated with antipsychotic medications are at increased risk of death. Patients with depression may experience worsening of depression and increased suicidal thinking or behavior. Metabolic effects including weight gain, hyperlipidemia, hyperglycemia, and diabetes mellitus have been seen with quetiapine treatment. Like other antipsychotics, NMS and TD are risks of quetiapine therapy. Orthostatic hypotension is also a concern when using quetiapine. Blood dyscrasias including leukopenia, neutropenia, and agranulocytosis have been reported with quetiapine. Chronic dosing of quetiapine in dog studies led to the development of cataracts. While not as severe as other antipsychotics, quetiapine can lower the seizure threshold and should be used with caution in patients with epilepsy or history of seizures. Transient increases in transaminases have been reported, but where asymptomatic and reversible. Because of activity on alpha receptors, quetiapine has the potential to cause priapism. Quetiapine can cause dysphagia and should be used cautiously in patients at risk for aspiration pneumonia. Patients should also be closely monitored for suicide risk.

Drug Interactions. Medications or substances like alcohol that can cause CNS depression should be used cautiously in combination with risperidone because of the risk of additive CNS depression. Because of the potential to cause orthostatic hypotension, patients taking antihypertensive medication along with risperidone should be monitored closely. Like other antipsychotics, quetiapine can minimize or alleviate the effects of levodopa, but because of its loose binding profile at the D_2 receptors it is often used in patients with Parkinson's disease. Inducers of CYP3A4 (e.g., phenytoin, carbamazepine, rifampin) can increase the clearance of quetiapine and thus would require higher doses of to maintain effects. Thioridazine increased plasma clearance of quetiapine by 65%. Inhibitors at CYP3A4 including ketoconazole, erythromycin, and protease inhibitors increased quetiapine plasma concentrations by 335%, therefore caution and dosage decreases of quetiapine should be done when coadministering it with these medications.

RISPERIDONE
Risperdal, Various

Pharmacology. Risperidone is a potent 5-HT_2 antagonist with D_2 antagonism. Whereas typical antipsychotics are dopamine antagonists, the additional serotonin antagonism increases efficacy for negative symptoms of schizophrenia and reduces the likelihood of EPS. Initial evidence also suggests that risperidone is more effective than traditional antipsychotic drugs for treatment-resistant schizophrenic patients.[33–36] (*See* Antipsychotic Drugs Comparison Chart.)

Administration and Adult Dosage. **PO for schizophrenia and bipolar disorder**— 1 mg twice daily initially, increasing by 1 mg/d every 24 h to the usual effective dosage of 4–6 mg/d in 1 or 2 doses. Occasionally, dosages above 6 mg/d might be necessary, but adverse effects increase and efficacy can be less. The solution can be mixed with water, coffee, orange juice, or low-fat milk; do not mix with cola or tea. **PO for irritability associated with autistic disorder**— 0.25 mg for patients <20 kg and 0.5 mg for patients >20 kg. Dose can be increased by 0.25 or 0.5 mg at 2-week intervals to a target dose of 0.5–3 mg/d. **IM long-acting injection for schizophrenia**—25 mg given every 2 weeks, but doses up to 50 mg/d have been studied. Oral overlap therapy with PO risperidone is necessary for the first 3 weeks of therapy due to delayed release of the injectable formulation.

Special Populations. *Geriatric Dosage.* Initial dose is 0.5 mg twice daily.

Other Conditions. Hepatic or Renal Impairment—initial dose is 0.5 mg twice daily.

Dosage Forms. **Tab** 0.25, 0.5, 1, 2, 3, 4 mg; **Soln** 1 mg/mL; **Oral Disintegrating Tab** 0.5, 1, 2, 3, 4 mg; **Inj** 12.5, 25, 37.5, 50 mg.

Pharmacokinetics. Risperidone is well absorbed orally. The free fraction of risperidone in serum increases in hepatic disease, necessitating lower dosages. It is metabolized by CYP2D6 to an active metabolite. **Half-life.** 3 h; its active metabolite has a half-life of 24 h. The half-lives of one or both are prolonged in patients with renal disease.[37] The half-life for the long-acting injection is 3–6 days because of the microsphere formulation.

Adverse Reactions. Frequent dose-related adverse effects are extrapyramidal effects, orthostatic hypotension, headache, rhinitis, and insomnia.

Contraindications. Hypersensitivity.

Precautions. Elderly patients with dementia-related psychosis treated with antipsychotic medications are at increased risk of death. Similar to other antipsychotics, NMS and TD have been reported with risperidone. Metabolic effects (e.g., weight gain, hyperlipidemia, hyperglycemia, and diabetes mellitus) have been seen with risperidone treatment. Even at low doses, risperidone has been shown to increase prolactin levels. Orthostatic hypotension is also a concern when using risperidone. While not as severe as other antipsychotics, risperidone can lower the seizure threshold and should be used with caution in patients with epilepsy or history of seizures. Risperidone can cause dysphagia and should be used cautiously in patients at risk for aspiration pneumonia. Rare cases of priapism have been documented. Patients should also be closely monitored for suicide risk.

Patient Instructions. (*See* Class Instructions.) Tell your doctor if you are pregnant or breast-feeding while taking this medication. Common adverse events you might experience include drowsiness, dizziness, and muscle stiffness. Risperidone may also cause an increase in weight. You should also notify your doctor if you start to notice weight gain. You should also contact your doctor if you start to experience any uncontrolled movements such as lip smacking or puckering, puffing of the cheeks, rapid or worm-like movements of the tongue, uncontrolled chewing movements, or uncontrolled movements of the arms and legs.

Drug Interactions. Inhibitors of CYP2D6 can increase risperidone levels and have adverse effects. Medications or substances like alcohol that can cause CNS depression should be used cautiously in combination with risperidone because of the risk of additive CNS depression. Because of the potential to cause orthostatic hypotension, patients taking antihypertensive medication along with risperidone should be monitored closely. Like other D_2 antagonists, risperidone can minimize or alleviate the effects of levodopa. Cimetidine, fluoxetine, paroxetine, and ranitidine can increase the bioavailability of risperidone. Carbamazepine can decrease risperidone plasma levels by up to 50%.

ZIPRASIDONE   Geodon

Pharmacology. Ziprasidone is an atypical antipsychotic drug with a very high ratio of 5-HT_{2A} to dopamine-2 blockade, suggesting a very low risk of extrapyramidal effects. In addition, it is a 5-HT_{1A} agonist like buspirone, and inhibits reuptake of both serotonin and norepinephrine like antidepressants. The clinical value of the latter two effects is not established.[38]

Administration and Adult Dosage. **PO for schizophrenia**—20 mg twice daily with food initially, increasing as necessary at intervals of at least 2 days to a maximum of 80 mg twice daily. **Maintenance dosage** may be as low as 40 mg/d. **PO for bipolar disorder**—40 mg twice daily on day 1, 60–80 mg twice daily on day 2, maintain with 40–80 mg twice daily. **IM injection for acute agitation in a psychotic patient**—10 mg every 2 h OR 20 mg every 4 h, to a maximum of 40 mg/d for up to 3 days. Switch to PO therapy as soon as possible. Caution should be exercised in patients with renal impairment.[38]

Dosage Forms. Cap 20, 40, 60, 80 mg; **Inj** 20 mg/mL.

Patient Instructions. (*See* Class Instructions.) Take this medication with food.

Pharmacokinetics. Oral bioavailability is 60% when taken with food. With oral twice-daily administration, peak blood levels occur at 6–8 h. Ziprasidone is metabolized by aldehyde oxidase and to a lesser extent by CYP3A4 to inactive metabolites. **Half-life.** 5–10 h (range 3–18 h) for oral ziprasidone and 3 h for IM ziprasidone. The pharmacokinetics are unaffected by sex, age, or moderate renal or hepatic disease.

Adverse Reactions. EPS are minimal, but comparative data with other atypical antipsychotic drugs are not available. A major potential advantage of ziprasidone is that it is the least likely atypical antipsychotic drug to cause weight gain.[39] Compared to placebo, the only side effect greater with ziprasidone is sedation. Ziprasidone increases the QTc interval by up to 14 ms. Ziprasidone should be avoided in patients with preexisting QTc prolongation, after acute MI, in severe heart failure, and in patients taking other drugs that prolong the QTc interval. The drug should be discontinued if the QTc interval is persistently >500 ms.

ANTIPSYCHOTIC DRUGS COMPARISON CHART

DRUG AND CLASS	DOSAGE FORMS	ADULT ORAL DOSAGE RANGE (mg/d)	ORAL EQUIVALENT ANTIPSYCHOTIC DOSE (mg)	USUAL SINGLE IM DOSE (mg)	RELATIVE FREQUENCY OF SIDE EFFECTS			
					Sedation	Anticholinergic	Extrapyramidal	Orthostatic H₂potension

DRUG AND CLASS	DOSAGE FORMS	ADULT ORAL DOSAGE RANGE (mg/d)	ORAL EQUIVALENT ANTIPSYCHOTIC DOSE (mg)	USUAL SINGLE IM DOSE (mg)	Sedation	Anticholinergic	Extrapyramidal	Orthostatic H₂potension
LOW POTENCY								
Chlorpromazine Thorazine Various	Soln 30, 100 mg/mL Syrup 2 mg/mL Tab 10, 25, 50, 100, 200 mg Inj 25 mg/mL Supp 25, 100 mg ER Cap not recommended	50–1200	100	25–50	High	Moderate	Moderate	High
Thioridazine Mellaril Various	Soln 30, 100 mg/mL Susp 5, 20 mg/mL Tab 10, 15, 25, 50, 100, 150 , 200 mg	50–800	100	—	High	High	Low	High
INTERMEDIATE POTENCY								
Loxapine Loxitane Various	Cap 5, 10, 25, 50 mg Soln 25 mg/mL Inj 50 mg/mL	20–250	10	12.5–50	Low	Low	Moderate	Low
Molindone Moban	Tab 5, 10, 25, 50, 100 mg Soln 20 mg/mL	25–225	10	—	Very low	Low	Moderate	Low

(continued)

ANTIPSYCHOTIC DRUGS COMPARISON CHART (continued)

DRUG AND CLASS	DOSAGE FORMS	ADULT ORAL DOSAGE RANGE (mg/d)	ORAL EQUIVALENT ANTIPSYCHOTIC DOSE (mg)	USUAL SINGLE IM DOSE (mg)	RELATIVE FREQUENCY OF SIDE EFFECTS			
					Sedation	Anticholinergic	Extrapyramidal	Orthostatic Hypotension
ATYPICAL								
Aripiprazole Abilify	Tab 2, 5, 10, 15, 20, 30 mg Tab (disintegrating) 10, 15 mg Soln (PO) 1 mg/mL Soln (IM) 9.75 mg/ 1.3 mL	10–30	—	—	Low	Moderate	Low	Low
Clozapine Clozaril FazaClo Various	Tab 25, 100 mg Tab (disintegrating) 12.5, 25, 100 mg	300–900	50	—	High	High	Very low	High
Olanzapine Zyprexa Various	Tab 2.5, 5, 7.5, 10, 15 mg Tab (disintegrating) 5, 10, 15, 20 mg Inj 10 mg	10–15	—	2.5–10	Low	Low	Very low	Low
Paliperidone Invega	ER Tab 3, 6, 9 mg		—	—	Very low	Very low	Low	Moderate

(continued)

ANTIPSYCHOTIC DRUGS COMPARISON CHART (*continued*)

DRUG AND CLASS	DOSAGE FORMS	ADULT ORAL DOSAGE RANGE (mg/d)	ORAL EQUIVALENT ANTIPSYCHOTIC DOSE (mg)	USUAL SINGLE IM DOSE (mg)	RELATIVE FREQUENCY OF SIDE EFFECTS			
					Sedation	Anticholinergic	Extrapyramidal	Orthostatic Hypotension
Quetiapine Seroquel Seroquel XR Various	Tab 25, 100, 200, 300 mg, 400 mg ER Tab 50, 150, 200, 300, 400 mg	150–500	—	—	Moderate	Low	Very low	Low
Risperidone Risperdal Various	Tab 0.25, 0.5, 1, 2, 3, 4 mg Soln 1 mg/mL	4–6[a]	—	—	Very low	Very low	Low[a]	Moderate
Ziprasidone Geodon	Cap 20, 40, 60, 80 mg Inj 20 mg/mL	40–160	—	10	Moderate	Very low	Very low	Low
HIGH POTENCY								
Fluphenazine Permitil Prolixin Various	Elxr 0.5 mg/mL Soln 5 mg/mL Tab 1, 2.5, 5, 10 mg Inj 2.5 mg/mL	2–40	2	2–5	Low	Low	Very high	Low
Fluphenazine Decanoate Prolixin Various	Inj 25 mg/mL	—	—	12.5–75 q 2 weeks	Low	Low	Very high	Low

(continued)

ANTIPSYCHOTIC DRUGS COMPARISON CHART (continued)

DRUG AND CLASS	DOSAGE FORMS	ADULT ORAL DOSAGE RANGE (mg/d)	ORAL EQUIVALENT ANTIPSYCHOTIC DOSE (mg)	USUAL SINGLE IM DOSE (mg)	RELATIVE FREQUENCY OF SIDE EFFECTS			
					Sedation	Anticholinergic	Extrapyramidal	Orthostatic Hypotension
Haloperidol Haldol Various	Soln 2 mg/mL Tab 0.5, 1, 2, 5, 10, 20 mg Inj 5 mg/mL	2–100	2	2–5	Very low	Very low	Very high	Very low
Haloperidol Decanoate Haldol Decanoate Various	Inj 50, 100 mg/mL	—	—	50–450 (monthly)	Very low	Very low	Very high	Very low
Perphenazine Trilafon Various	Soln 3.2 mg/mL Tab 2, 4, 8, 16 mg Inj 5 mg/mL	12–64	8	5–10	Low	Low	High	Low
Trifluoperazine Stelazine Various	Soln 10 mg/mL Tab 1, 2, 5, 10 mg Inj 2 mg/mL	5–40	5	1–2	Low	Low	High	Low
Thiothixene Navane Various	Cap 1, 2, 5, 10, 20 mg Soln 5 mg/mL Inj 5 mg/mL	5–60	4	2–4	Low	Low	High	Low

[a]At dosages over 6 mg/d, nausea and insomnia are limiting side effects; extrapyramidal symptoms markedly increase at dosages over 6 mg/d.
From Refs. 1–3, 13, 14, 20, 22, 26, 30–32, 34, 40, and 41 and from product information.

■ REFERENCES

1. Ereshefsky L et al. Pathophysiologic basis for schizophrenia and the efficacy of antipsychotics. *Clin Pharm.* 1990;9:682-707.
2. Coyle JT. The clinical use of antipsychotic medications. *Med Clin North Am.* 1982;66:993-1009.
3. Kane JM. The current status of neuroleptic therapy. *J Clin Psychiatry.* 1989;50:322-328.
4. Heresco-Levy U et al. Trial of maintenance neuroleptic dose reduction in schizophrenic outpatients: two year outcome. *J Clin Psychiatry.* 1993;54:59-62.
5. Brotman AW et al. A role for high-dose antipsychotics. *J Clin Psychiatry.* 1990;51:164-166.
6. Rifkin A et al. Dosage of haloperidol for mania. *Br J Psychiatry.* 1994;165:113-116.
7. Zaleon CR, Guthrie SK. Antipsychotic drug use in older adults. *Am J Hosp Pharm.* 1994;51:2917-2943.
8. Coryell W et al. Haloperidol plasma levels and dose optimization. *Am J Psychiatry.* 1998;155:48-53.
9. Khot V et al. The assessment and clinical implications of haloperidol acute-dose, steady-state, and withdrawal pharmacokinetics. *J Clin Psychopharmacol.* 1993;13:120-127.
10. DeVane CL. *Fundamentals of Monitoring Psychoactive Drug Therapy.* Baltimore, MD: Williams & Wilkins; 1990.
11. Pearlman CA. Neuroleptic malignant syndrome: a review of the literature. *J Clin Psychopharmacol.* 1986;6:257-273.
12. Gardos G et al. Ten year outcome of tardive dyskinesia. *Am J Psychiatry.* 1994;151:836-841.
13. Harrison TS et al. Aripiprazole: A review of its use in schizophrenia and schizoaffective disorder. *Drugs.* 2004;64:1715-1736.
14. Ereshefsky L et al. Clozapine: an atypical antipsychotic agent. *Clin Pharm.* 1989;8:691-709.
15. Lieberman JA et al. Clozapine: guidelines for clinical management. *J Clin Psychiatry.* 1989;50:329-338.
16. Meltzer HY. An overview of the mechanism of action of clozapine. *J Clin Psychiatry.* 1994;55(suppl 9):47-52.
17. Lieberman JA et al. Clinical effects of clozapine in chronic schizophrenia: response to treatment and predictors of outcome. *Am J Psychiatry.* 1994;151:1744-1752.
18. Jann MW et al. Pharmacokinetics and pharmacodynamics of clozapine. *Clin Pharmacokinet.* 1993;24:161-176.
19. Alvir JM, Lieberman JA. Agranulocytosis: incidence and risk factors. *J Clin Psychiatry.* 1994;55(suppl 9).137-138.
20. Miller DD. Review and management of clozapine side effects. *J Clin Psychiatry.* 2000;61(suppl 8):14-17.
21. Chouinard G et al. A randomized clinical trial of haloperidol decanoate and fluphenazine decanoate in the outpatient treatment of schizophrenia. *J Clin Psychopharmacol.* 1989;9:247-253.
22. Hemstrom CA et al. Haloperidol decanoate: a depot antipsychotic. *Drug Intell Clin Pharm.* 1988;22:290-295.
23. Gerlach J. Oral versus depot administration of neuroleptics in relapse prevention. *Acta Psychiatr Scand.* 1994;89(suppl 382):28-32.
24. Inderbitzin LB et al. A double-blind dose-reduction trial of fluphenazine decanoate for chronic, unstable schizophrenic patients. *Am J Psychiatry.* 1994;151:1753-1759.
25. Ereshefsky L et al. A loading dose strategy for converting from oral to depot haloperidol. *Hosp Community Psychiatry.* 1993;44:1155-1161.
26. Foster RH, Goa KL. Olanzapine. *Pharmacoeconomics.* 1999;15:611-640.
27. Bever KA, Perry PJ. Olanzapine: a serotonin-dopamine receptor antagonist for antipsychotic therapy. *Am J Health Syst Pharm.* 1998;55:1003-1016.
28. Colvin CL, Tankanow RM. Pimozide: use in Tourette's syndrome. *Drug Intell Clin Pharm.* 1985;19:421-424.
29. Tueth MJ, Cheong JA. Clinical uses of pimozide. *South Med J.* 1993;86:344-349.
30. Small JG et al. Quetiapine in patients with schizophrenia. *Arch Gen Psychiatry.* 1997;54:549-557.
31. Anonymous. Quetiapine for schizophrenia. *Med Lett Drugs Ther.* 1997;39:117-118.
32. Arvanitis LA et al. Multiple fixed doses of Seroquel (quetiapine) in patients with acute exacerbation of schizophrenia: a comparison with haloperidol and placebo. *Biol Psychiatry.* 1997;42:233-246.
33. Ereshefsky L, Lacomb S. Pharmacological profile of risperidone. *Can J Psychiatry.* 1993;38(suppl 3):S80-S88.
34. Cohen LJ. Risperidone. *Pharmacotherapy.* 1994;14:253-265.
35. Livingston MG. Risperidone. *Lancet.* 1994;343:457-460.
36. Marder SR, Meibach RC. Risperidone in the treatment of schizophrenia. *Am J Psychiatry.* 1994;151:825-835.
37. Heykants J et al. The pharmacokinetics of risperidone in humans: a summary. *J Clin Psychiatry.* 1994;55(suppl 5): 13-17.
38. Chou JCY, Serper MR. Ziprasidone—a new highly atypical antipsychotic. *Essent Psychopharmacol.* 1998;2: 463-485.
39. Allison DB et al. Antipsychotic-induced weight gain: a comprehensive research synthesis. *Am J Psychiatry.* 1999;156:1686-1696.
40. American Psychiatric Association. Practice guideline for the treatment of patients with schizophrenia. *Am J Psychiatry.* 1997;154(suppl 4):1-63.
41. Beasley CM et al. Safety of olanzapine. *J Clin Psychiatry.* 1997;58(suppl 10):13-17.

Chapter 39

Anxiolytics, Sedatives, and Hypnotics

Aaron P. Gibson

Class Instructions. *Sedatives and Hypnotics.* This drug causes drowsiness and can produce sleep. Do not exceed the prescribed dosage, and use caution when driving, operating machinery, or performing other tasks requiring mental alertness. Avoid concurrent use of alcohol or other drugs that cause drowsiness or sleep. Do not abruptly stop taking this medication; the dosage must be decreased slowly. Complex behaviors such as "sleep driving", preparing and eating meals, engaging in sexual activity, and making phone calls with no memory of the event have been reported in association with hypnotic use. Concomitant alcohol or other CNS depressants may increase the risk of these behaviors.

Missed Doses. If you miss a dose, take it as soon as you remember. If it is almost time for your next dose, skip it and resume your normal schedule. Do not double doses.

ALPRAZOLAM
Xanax, Various

Pharmacology. Alprazolam is a triazolobenzodiazepine that is equal in efficacy to other benzodiazepines for generalized anxiety disorder but more effective in the treatment of panic disorder. Although alprazolam has some efficacy in major depression, it is less effective than heterocyclic antidepressants.[1,2] (*See* Benzodiazepines and Related Drugs Comparison Chart.)

Administration and Adult Dosage. **PO for generalized anxiety disorder**— 0.25 mg 3 times daily initially, increasing gradually to 4 mg/d. **PO for panic disorder**—0.5 mg 3 times daily is recommended initially; most patients require 5–6 mg/d, and occasionally 10 mg/d can be needed for full response. **Sublingual** formulation can be administered with no difference from oral administration in onset, peak, or pharmacokinetics.[3] **Discontinuation**—Decrease the daily dosage by no more than 0.5 mg/d every 3 days until the daily dosage reaches 2 mg and then decrease dosage in 0.25 mg/d increments every 3 days.

Dosage Forms. **Tab** 0.25, 0.5, 1, 2 mg; **ER Tab** 0.5, 1, 2, 3 mg. **Orally Disintegrating Tab** 0.25, 0.5, 1, 2 mg; **Soln** 1 mg/mL.

Pharmacokinetics. Similar to diazepam, alprazolam has a rapid onset of effect after oral administration, but its shorter half-life requires 3 times daily administration. **Half-life.** 11 h in adults; the elderly might have decreased clearance and an increased half-life of 21 h.[2–4]

Adverse Reactions. (*See* Benzodiazepines.) Patients do not show complete cross-tolerance between triazolobenzodiazepines and other benzodiazepines, but **clonazepam** has been shown to be an effective long half-life substitute drug for use in alprazolam withdrawal.[5]

Contraindications. Patients with acute narrow angle glaucoma. Concomitant use of ketoconazole or itraconazole.

Precautions. Precautions should be taken in patients who are severely depressed or in patients who are experiencing suicidal ideation or plans. Caution should be exercised by limiting the administration of the medication to nonlethal quantities. Episodes of mania or hypomania have been reported. As with all benzodiazepines, caution should be exercised when using this medication in the elderly population. Severe pulmonary disease and untreated open angle glaucoma are also precautions for the use of alprazolam. While alprazolam has a weak uricosuric effect, there have been no reports of acute renal failure secondary to the medication.

Patient Instructions. Generally, alcohol should be avoided when taking alprazolam. Inform your physician of alcohol use or other medications that you are taking. Inform your physician if you are pregnant, nursing, become pregnant, or are planning to become pregnant, as alprazolam should be avoided in pregnancy. Operating a vehicle or other heavy machinery should be avoided until you know how this medication will affect you. This medication should not be abruptly stopped.

Drug Interactions. Alprazolam can cause CNS depression, and other medications that also cause CNS depression can potentiate this effect. Plasma levels of imipramine and desipramine have been reported to increase while administered with alprazolam, but the clinical significance of these increases is unknown. Drugs that inhibit CYP3A4 can significantly decrease the clearance of alprazolam. Examples of this interaction include fluoxetine, propoxyphene, and oral contraceptives. Conversely, drugs like carbamazepine that induce CYP3A4 can increase the clearance of alprazolam.

BENZODIAZEPINES

Pharmacology. Benzodiazepines have a more specific anxiolytic effect than other sedatives. Benzodiazepines facilitate the inhibitory effect of GABA on neuronal excitability by increasing membrane permeability to chloride ions.[6]

Administration and Adult Dosage. (*See* Benzodiazepines and Related Drugs Comparison Chart.) Optimal oral use requires individual dosage titration to clinical response. The long-acting drugs can be administered once daily at bedtime; the short-acting drugs require multiple daily doses. (*See* Benzodiazepines and Related Drugs Comparison Chart.) Determine the dosage schedule by the individual patient's relative degree of dysfunction from daytime anxiety compared with insomnia. Despite physiologic dependence, benzodiazepines might need to be used for months and sometimes years for treatment of panic disorder and generalized anxiety disorder; situational anxiety, adjustment disorders, and anxiety secondary to other causes require only days to weeks of drug treatment.[7] **PO for alcohol withdrawal**—Evidence suggests no superiority of any benzodiazepine in alcohol withdrawal, although **chlordiazepoxide** has been most adequately studied; **(chlordiazepoxide)** 25–100 mg for agitation, anxiety, and tremor; on the first day, up to 400 mg can be given in divided doses, with gradual dosage reductions over 4 days; **(diazepam)** 5–20 mg for agitation, anxiety, and tremor; alternatively, it can be given in 20-mg doses every 2 h until complete suppression of signs and symptoms is achieved. After this loading dose, further administration is unnecessary;[8] **(oxazepam)** 15–60 mg every 4–6 h for agitation, anxiety, and tremor. Oxazepam is preferred in patients with severe liver disease. **IM chlordiazepoxide** is not recommended because of slow, erratic absorption; however, **lorazepam** is suitable for intramuscular administration.[8,9] Diazepam injectable solution (Valium, Various) can be administered **IM or IV;** the injectable emulsion (Dizac) is for **IV use only** (do not administer IM or SQ); neither the solution nor the emulsion should be administered faster than 5 mg/min into a peripheral vein, and small veins should be avoided; neither product is recommended to be added to other drugs or solutions. (*See* Fate.) **Rectal diazepam for seizures**—0.2 mg/kg of Diastat rectal gel, rounded up to the next dosage size (2.5, 5, 10, 15, 20 mg); an additional dose can be given 4–12 h after the first dose. Treat no more than 1 episode every 5 days OR 5 episodes/month with Diastat.

Special Populations. *Pediatric Dosage.* PO—(diazepam, >6 months) 1–2.5 mg 3 times daily or 4 times daily. Most benzodiazepines are not recommended in children because of insufficient clinical experience and concern about the stimulating and paradoxical effects that occur because of disinhibition. **Midazolam** is commonly used in children for preanesthetic sedation. (*See* Midazolam.) **Rectal diazepam for seizures**—(2–5 years) 0.5 mg/kg of Diastat rectal gel, rounded up to the next dosage size (2.5, 5, 10, 15, 20 mg); (6–11 years) 0.3 mg/kg of Diastat rectal gel, rounded up to the next dosage size. An additional dose may be given 4–12 h after the first dose. Treat no more than 1 episode every 5 days OR 5 episodes/mo with Diastat.

Geriatric Dosage. The elderly might have reduced clearance and enhanced CNS sensitivity, which requires initial dosage to be reduced by 33%–50%.[10]

Other Conditions. Higher dosages might be needed in heavy smokers. Patients with liver disease might have reduced clearance and/or enhanced CNS sensitivity, which requires reduction of initial and subsequent doses. Alcoholic patients with reduced plasma proteins might require a lower dosage because of decreased protein binding.

Dosage Forms. *See* Benzodiazepines and Related Drugs Comparison Chart.

Patient Instructions. *See* Sedatives and Hypnotics, Class Instructions.

Pharmacokinetics. *Serum Levels.* Not used clinically.

Fate. Diazepam and chlordiazepoxide are absorbed faster and more completely orally than intramuscularly. Lorazepam and midazolam have rapid and reliable IM absorption.[9,11] (*See* Benzodiazepines and Related Drugs Comparison Chart.)

Adverse Reactions. Frequent effects include drowsiness, dizziness, ataxia, and disorientation; these effects rarely require drug discontinuation and are easily managed by dosage reduction. Anterograde amnesia is frequent.[9] Occasionally, agitation and excitement occur.[12] With parenteral therapy, hypotension and respiratory depression occur occasionally. Rarely, hepatotoxicity or blood dyscrasias occur. Diazepam emulsion is associated with less venous thrombosis and phlebitis than the solution, which can be very irritating to veins.

Contraindications. Acute narrow-angle glaucoma; (diazepam emulsion injection) hypersensitivity to soy protein.

Precautions. Pregnancy; impaired hepatic function. Abrupt drug withdrawal can result in rebound insomnia, abstinence syndrome similar to barbiturate withdrawal, seizures, or, rarely, psychosis. Patients do not show complete cross-tolerance between triazolobenzodiazepines and other benzodiazepines. History of substance abuse can indicate increased likelihood of benzodiazepine misuse.[6]

Drug Interactions. Concurrent use with other CNS depressants can potentiate the sedation caused by benzodiazepines. Nefazodone inhibits alprazolam and triazolam metabolism; fluoxetine and fluvoxamine increase levels of alprazolam and diazepam; omeprazole increases serum diazepam levels. Most medications in this class are metabolized through CYP3A4 and are susceptible to inducers and inhibitors of this enzyme.

Parameters to Monitor. Periodically reassess the need for therapy during long-term use.

BUSPIRONE HYDROCHLORIDE   BuSpar, Various

Pharmacology. Buspirone is the first of a class of selective serotonin 5-HT$_{1A}$ receptor partial agonists. It also has some effect on dopamine D$_2$ autoreceptors and, like antidepressants, can downregulate β-adrenergic receptors. Unlike benzodiazepines, it lacks amnestic, anticonvulsant, muscle relaxant, and hypnotic effects. Its exact anxiolytic mechanism of action is complex and not clearly defined.[13,14]

Administration and Adult Dosage. PO for anxiety—5 mg 3 times daily OR 7.5 mg twice daily for 1 week, increasing in 5 mg/d increments every 2–3 days to a maximum of 60 mg/d in 2 or 3 divided doses. Most patients require 20–30 mg/d in divided doses.

Special Populations. *Pediatric Dosage.* Safety and efficacy not established.

Geriatric Dosage. Same as adult dosage.

Other Conditions. Decrease the initial dose to 5 mg twice daily in patients with hepatic or renal impairment.[13,15]

Dosage Forms. Tab 5, 7.5, 10, 15, 30 mg.

Patient Instructions. This drug requires several weeks of continuous use for therapeutic effect and is not effective when used intermittently. Common adverse events include dizziness, headache, nausea, nervousness, lightheadedness, and insomnia. You should avoid drinking large amounts of grapefruit juice while taking buspirone.

Pharmacokinetics. *Onset and Duration.* Onset of anxiolytic effect can take several weeks.

Fate. The drug is well absorbed; oral bioavailability is 3.9 ± 4.3%. Administration after meals increases bioavailability by 80%. It is extensively metabolized by oxidative dealkylation pathways.[16] **Half-life.** 2.1 ± 1.2 h.[16]

Adverse Reactions. Dosages >60 mg/d can cause dysphoria.[6] Frequent nausea, dizziness, headache, and insomnia occur. Unlike benzodiazepines, buspirone does not cause dependence or withdrawal effects.[13,17]

Contraindications. None known.

Precautions. Buspirone has no cross-tolerance with benzodiazepines, so patients being switched from a benzodiazepine should have their dosages of the benzodiazepine decreased slowly.

Drug Interactions. Unlike benzodiazepines, buspirone does not interact with alcohol.[13,17] Buspirone can increase haloperidol serum levels. Avoid concurrent buspirone and an MAOI because the combination can cause hypertension. Because buspirone is primarily metabolized through CYP3A4, it is susceptible to inducers or inhibitors of that enzyme.

Parameters to Monitor. Monitor renal and hepatic function initially and periodically during long-term therapy.

Notes. Buspirone is indicated only for the treatment of generalized anxiety disorder and is not effective as an "as-needed" medication or hypnotic. Buspirone's anxiolytic effect without sedation or respiratory depression has led to its use in agitation and anxiety, dementia, mental retardation, and spinal cord injury. Its unique effect on the 5-HT$_{1A}$ receptor has led to uncontrolled studies and clinical use for premenstrual tension syndrome and to decrease craving in smoking cessation.[18]

ESZOPICLONE   Lunesta

Pharmacology. Eszopiclone is a nonbenzodiazepine hypnotic that, like zolpidem, selectively binds only to the GABA$_1$ receptor. This selectivity suggests a sedative effect with less potential for memory impairment, interaction with alcohol, and psychomotor effects than with benzodiazepines.

Administration and Adult Dosage. **PO for insomnia**—2 mg immediately before bedtime; initial dose that can be increased to 3 mg/d if clinically necessary as it has been shown to be a more effective dose. For patients whose primary complaint is difficulty falling asleep, the initial recommended dose is 1 mg/d and can be increased to 2 mg/d if necessary.

Special Populations. *Pediatric Dosage.* Safety and efficacy not established.

Geriatric Dosage. Initial dose should be 1 mg/d and should not exceed 2 mg/d.

Other Conditions. No dosage adjustment is necessary for patients with mild-to-moderate hepatic impairment. Initial dose should be 1 mg/d in severe hepatic impairment and patients taking potent CYP3A4 inhibitors and should not exceed 2 mg/d. No dosage adjustment is necessary for patients with renal impairment.

Dosage Forms. **Tab** 1, 2, 3 mg.

Patient Instructions. This medication should be taken immediately prior to going to bed, and only if there are 8 full hours to dedicate to sleep. Sleep onset may be delayed if medication is taken with high-fat meal. Alcohol and other sedating medications should not be taken with this medication. "Sleep driving" and other abnormal behaviors while sleeping should be reported immediately to your physician.

Pharmacokinetics. *Onset and Duration.* Decreased sleep latency and improved sleep maintenance should be seen with the first dose of medication.

Serum Levels. Not established.

Fate. Eszopiclone is rapidly absorbed and achieves C_{max} approximately 1 h after administration. Plasma protein binding ranges from 52% to 59% and the drug is extensively metabolized by oxidation and demethylation at CYP3A4 and CYP2E1. **Half-life.** 6 h; if administered with food it may increase the T_{max} to 2 h.

Adverse Reactions. Headache, somnolence, and unpleasant taste were the most common adverse events seen with eszopiclone. Neither dependence nor withdrawal syndrome has been reported.

Precautions. Taking dose earlier than just prior to bedtime might lead to short-termed memory impairment, hallucinations, impaired coordination, dizziness and lightheadedness. Patients with depression should be closely monitored as this population is more likely to intentionally overdose. The least amount of drug that is feasible should be prescribed at one time.

Drug Interactions. When administered concomitantly with alcohol, additive effects on worsening of psychomotor performance were noted for up to 4 h after administration. The eszopiclone dose should be decreased to 1 mg/d when administered with potent CYP3A4 inhibitors like ketoconazole. The dose may be increased to 2 mg/d if necessary.

FLUMAZENIL
Romazicon, Various

Pharmacology. Flumazenil is a selective inhibitor of the CNS effects of benzodiazepine sedatives. It competitively blocks the effect of benzodiazepines and zolpidem on GABA-mediated inhibitory pathways within the CNS. Flumazenil finds its greatest use in the reversal of benzodiazepine sedation after medical and surgical procedures and occasionally in the management of benzodiazepine overdose.[19–21]

Administration and Adult Dosage. **IV for reversal of conscious sedation**—0.2 mg over 15 sec; this dose can be repeated after 45 s and every minute thereafter as needed, to a total dosage of 1 mg. **IV for benzodiazepine overdose**—0.2 mg over 30 s, followed, if necessary, by 0.3 mg after 30 s. Further doses of 0.5 mg over 30 s can be given at 1-min intervals to a cumulative dosage of 3 mg. Rarely, patients who respond partially to 3 mg, respond more completely to a dosage of 5 mg. If resedation occurs after either use, additional doses of up to 1 mg can be given at 20-min intervals to a maximum of 3 mg/h. Flumazenil does not consistently reverse benzodiazepine amnesia, so give patients written instructions to avoid operation of motor vehicles or hazardous equipment, or ingestion of alcohol or nonprescription medications for 18–24 h or longer if benzodiazepine effects persist. **IV for reversal of conscious sedation in pediatric patients**—0.01 mg/kg (up to 0.2 mg) given over 15 s; this dose can be repeated after 45 s and every minute thereafter as needed, to a total dosage of 0.05 mg/kg or 1 mg, whichever is lower.

Special Populations. *Pediatric Dosage.* **IV for reversal of conscious sedation**—(>1 year) 0.01 mg/kg (up to 0.2 mg) over 15 s; this dose can be repeated after 45 s and every minute thereafter as needed, to a total dosage of 1 mg.

Other Conditions. *Hepatic impairment:* The initial dose is the same, but subsequent doses should be reduced in size or frequency to account for reduced clearance.

Dosage Forms. **Inj** 0.1 mg/mL.

Pharmacokinetics. Reversal of benzodiazepine coma can occur within 1–2 min and last 1–5 h, depending on the dosages of the benzodiazepine and flumazenil.

First-pass hepatic metabolism limits the bioavailability of oral flumazenil, so the drug is administered by IV injection. It is rapidly hydroxylated in the liver to inactive metabolites. V_d is 0.6–1.6 L/kg. **Half-life.** 0.7–1.3 h. Flumazenil has a black box warning regarding the increased risk of seizures. Practitioners should individualize the dose and be prepared to manage seizures.

Contraindications. Patients showing signs of serious overdose of cyclic antidepressants; patients given a benzodiazepine for a control of a life-threatening condition such as control of intracranial pressure or status epilepticus.

Precautions. Pregnancy category C. Flumazenil does not alleviate the risks associated with large benzodiazepine doses for sedation. Adequate postprocedure monitoring should be conducted. Patients who are dependent on benzodiazepines or alcohol may experience seizures if given flumazenil. Flumazenil is meant to be used as an adjunct to proper airway management and support. Patients with head injury receiving benzodiazepines who are given flumazenil might experience altered cerebral blood flow or convulsions. Panic attacks have been reported in patients with a history of panic disorder.

Patient Instructions. Following a procedure you may feel alert, but you should be aware that confusion and sedation secondary to benzodiazepines might return. For this reason, you should not operate a motor vehicle or hazardous machinery for 24 h following the procedure. You should also avoid alcohol and nonprescription medications for 24 h following flumazenil administration.

Adverse Reactions. Frequent side effects have been minimal and are usually limited to nausea and vomiting, anxiety, and agitation. However, seizures have occurred, most often in patients on long-term benzodiazepine therapy or after overdose with heterocyclic antidepressants or other potentially convulsant drugs (e.g., bupropion, cocaine, cyclosporine, isoniazid, lithium, methylxanthines, MAOIs, propoxyphene). Be prepared to manage seizures before giving flumazenil.[22]

MIDAZOLAM HYDROCHLORIDE   Versed, Various

Pharmacology. Midazolam is a short-acting triazolobenzodiazepine for use in anesthesia. It is unique in its physicochemical properties; at a pH less than 4, the drug exists as a highly water-soluble, stable compound, but at physiologic pH, it becomes lipophilic. This allows IV administration of a water-soluble, rapidly acting drug with a very low frequency of venous irritation. Midazolam is given intramuscularly for preoperative sedation and intravenously for induction of anesthesia or for conscious sedation for endoscopy and other procedures.[23–25]

Administration and Adult Dosage. **IM for preoperative sedation**—0.07–0.08 mg/kg (approximately 5 mg) 1 h before surgery. **IV for endoscopy and other conscious sedation procedures**—dosage must be individualized and not administered by rapid bolus. Titrate slowly to desired effect; some patients might respond to as little as 1 mg. Give no more than 2.5 mg over at least 2 min as the 1 mg/mL (or more dilute) solution; in elderly, debilitated, or chronically ill patients, limit the initial dose to 1.5 mg. Further small doses can be given after waiting for at least 2 min. Do not give the drug intravenously without oxygen and resuscitation equipment immediately available.

Special Populations. *Pediatric Dosage.* **PO for sedation** (6 months–16 years) 0.25–1 mg/kg (usually 0.5 mg/kg), to a maximum of 20 mg. **PR for preanesthetic sedation**—0.3 mg/kg as a solution diluted in 5 mL of saline is a safe and effective alternative to IM administration.[26]

Dosage Forms. **Inj** 1, 5 mg/mL; **Syrup** 2 mg/mL.

Pharmacokinetics. Midazolam is >90% absorbed after IM injection; peak serum levels occur within 30 min. Peak levels after IM administration are approximately 50% of IV levels. PO onset is 10–20 min; IM onset is approximately 15 min. The drug is 97% bound to plasma proteins and has a V_d of 1–3 L/kg; Clearance is 0.25–0.54 L/h/kg. Midazolam is hepatically metabolized via CYP3A4 to the 1-hydroxy and 4-hydroxy metabolites; the 1-hydroxy metabolite is at least as active as midazolam. **Half-life.** 1.8–6.4 h.

Contraindications. Acute narrow-angle glaucoma.

Precautions. Pregnancy category D. IV doses of midazolam should be decreased for elderly and debilitated patients. Midazolam does not protect against the rise in intracranial pressure or against pulse and blood pressure increases secondary to endotracheal intubation under light general anesthesia.

Patient Instructions. Inform your physician about alcohol consumption and any medications that you are taking, especially blood pressure medications, antibiotics, and over-the-counter medications. You should also inform your doctor if you are pregnant or nursing. Sedation and amnesia are common adverse events that you can expect to experience following midazolam administration.

Drug Interactions. Any medication that can cause CNS depression can interact with midazolam and lead to additive CNS depression. Midazolam is predominantly metabolized by CYP3A4 so inhibitors of that enzyme including cimetidine, erythromycin, diltiazem, verapamil, and ketoconazole can lead to decreased clearance of midazolam resulting in prolonged sedation. Midazolam decreases the minimum alveolar concentration of halothane required for general anesthesia in a dose-dependent fashion.

Adverse Reactions. Respiratory depression and respiratory arrest occur frequently. Impairment of psychomotor skills continues after acute sedation has passed; patients should not drive or operate machinery until it is clear that they have recovered fully.

RAMELTEON	Rozerem

Pharmacology. Ramelteon is a melatonin receptor agonist with selectivity for the M_1 and M_2 receptors. These receptors when acted upon by endogenous mechanisms are responsible for normal circadian rhythm. Ramelteon has no appreciable affinity for the GABA receptor complex.[27]

Administration and Adult Dosage. **PO for insomnia characterized by difficulty with sleep onset**—8 mg within 30 min of bedtime.

Special Populations. *Pediatric Dosage.* Safety and efficacy not established.

Geriatric Dosage. No dosage adjustment is necessary based on age.

Other Conditions. Hepatic Impairment, (severe) Not recommended.

Dosage Forms. **Tab** 8 mg.

Patient Instructions. This medication should be taken immediately prior to going to bed. Alcohol and other sedating medications should not be taken with this medication. "Sleep driving" and other abnormal behaviors while sleeping should be reported immediately to the prescribing physician.

Pharmacokinetics. *Onset and Duration.* This medication has been shown to improve the time to fall asleep by ~12 min.[28]

Serum Levels. Not established.

Fate. Absolute bioavailability is only 1.8% due to extensive first-pass metabolism. The drug is ~82% protein bound, with albumin accounting for ~70% of binding; V_d is 73.6 L. Metabolism is extensive by oxidation primarily via CYP1A2 and to a lesser extent CYP2C subfamily and CYP3A4. **Half-life.** 1–2.6 h in normal healthy subjects. Patients with mild-to-moderate hepatic impairment experienced 4- to 10-fold increases in half-life.

Adverse Reactions. Somnolence, dizziness, fatigue, and nausea were the most common adverse events reported and were only seen in 3%–4% of patients taking ramelteon. Worsening of depression in patients with mood disorders has been reported with the use of hypnotics and may occur with ramelteon. Additionally, there is a risk of activation into mania in patients with bipolar disorder.

Contraindications. Patients who develop angioedema while taking ramelteon should not be rechallenged; concomitant fluvoxamine use.

Precautions. Use with caution in moderate hepatic impairment. Cases of angioedema involving the tongue, glottis, or larynx have been reported with the first and subsequent doses of ramelteon. Sleep disturbances may be the manifestation of a primary psychiatric disorder. If sleep problems do not resolve within 7–10 days of therapy, follow-up is recommended. Abnormal sleep behaviors including "sleep driving" have been reported. Decreases in reproductive hormones including testosterone and elevated prolactin levels have been reported.

Drug Interactions. Fluvoxamine, a potent CYP1A2 inhibitor increased the AUC for ramelteon by approximately 190-fold. The use of fluvoxamine is contraindicated with ramelteon. Drugs with less potent inhibition of CYP1A2 have not been adequately studied, but should be given concomitantly with ramelteon cautiously. Strong CYP450 inducers like rifampin, ketoconazole, and fluconazole should be used with caution when taking ramelteon as they may increase plasma levels.

TRIAZOLAM
Halcion, Various

Pharmacology. Triazolam is a triazolobenzodiazepine hypnotic whose effect is likely related to its facilitation of GABA-mediated neurotransmission, but its exact mechanism is unknown.

Administration and Adult Dosage. (*See* Benzodiazepines and Related Drugs Comparison Chart.) **PO as a hypnotic**—0.25 mg at bedtime initially; do not exceed 0.5 mg/d.

Special Populations. *Pediatric Dosage.* (<18 years) safety and efficacy not established.

Geriatric Dosage. **PO** decrease initial dose to 0.125 mg, increase if necessary to 0.25 mg at bedtime.[28,29]

Other Conditions. **PO**—0.125 mg initially in debilitated patients and those with low body weights or with hepatic impairment.

Dosage Forms. **Tab** 0.125, 0.25 mg.

Patient Instructions. *See* Sedatives and Hypnotics, Class Instructions.

Pharmacokinetics. *Onset and Duration.* Onset of hypnotic effect is 0.5–1 h, with peak serum levels achieved within 2 h.

Fate. Oral bioavailability 44%, SL 53%, because of nonhepatic presystemic metabolism. V_d is 1.2 ± 0.5 L/kg; clearance is 0.34 ± 0.2 L/h/kg. Clearance decreases with advancing age (attributed to reduced hepatic oxidizing capacity in the elderly). Triazolam undergoes hydroxylation and rapid conjugation. Smoking does not affect elimination.[30,31] Accumulation does not occur with multiple doses.

Half-life. 2.6 ± 1 h. Half-life is not affected by end-stage renal disease or liver disease.[30–32]

Adverse Reactions. Frequently, anterograde amnesia,[33] daytime anxiety, and ataxia occur. Occasionally, agitation, confusion, or mood disturbance occur. Rarely, respiratory depression, depersonalization, and derealization, or psychosis occurs. Unlike other benzodiazepines, several fatalities have been reported in elderly patients who overdosed on triazolam.[34,35]

Contraindications. Pregnancy.

Precautions. Impaired hepatic function. Abrupt drug withdrawal can result in rebound insomnia, abstinence syndrome similar to barbiturate withdrawal, seizures, or, rarely, psychosis. Patients do not show complete cross-tolerance between triazolam and other benzodiazepines. History of substance abuse can indicate an increased likelihood of triazolam misuse.[6] Do not prescribe the drug for more than 7–10 days of consecutive therapy or in quantities larger than a 30-day supply.

Drug Interactions. Concurrent use with other CNS depressants can potentiate the sedation caused by benzodiazepines. Nefazodone inhibits triazolam metabolism. Triazolam is extensively metabolized by CYP3A4. Medications that inhibit this enzyme including azithromycin, cimetidine, clarithromycin, diltiazem, erythromycin, and birth control medications can decrease clearance of the drug and lead to adverse events.

Notes. Compared with other benzodiazepine hypnotics, triazolam is equally effective in reducing sleep latency and less likely to cause daytime sedation; however, it is less likely to prevent early morning awakening and more likely to cause rebound insomnia. Hypnotic drugs are most effective when used to treat transient situational insomnia (1–3 days) and short-term insomnia (1–3 weeks maximum).[35,36]

ZALEPLON
Sonata, Various

Pharmacology. Zaleplon is a nonbenzodiazepine hypnotic that, like zolpidem, selectively binds only to the $GABA_1$ receptor. This selectivity suggests a sedative effect with less potential for memory impairment, interaction with alcohol, and psychomotor effects than with benzodiazepines.[37]

Administration and Adult Dosage. **PO as a hypnotic**—10 mg at bedtime initially (5 mg in the elderly), up to 20 mg. Because of its very rapid onset and offset, zaleplon can be given during the night after the patient experiences difficulty falling asleep rather than being given before bedtime in anticipation of sleep difficulty. Zaleplon can be given during the night without morning hangover as long as there are 4 h remaining in bed after administration.

Special Populations. *Pediatric Dosage.* (<18 years) Safety and efficacy not established.

Geriatric Dosage. Initial dose is 5 mg/d with 10 mg/d being the maximum dose.

Other Conditions. Hepatic Impairment, Dose in patients with mild-to-moderate impairment is 5 mg/d.

Dosage Forms. **Cap** 5, 10 mg.

Pharmacokinetics. After oral administration, zaleplon reaches peak serum concentrations in 1.1 h. Zaleplon is metabolized by CYP3A4 but has no active metabolites. **Half-life.** 0.8–1.4 h (average 1 h).[38]

Adverse Reactions. Dose-related side effects include dizziness, headache, and somnolence. Symptoms begin to appear approximately 30 min after a dose, peak at 1–2 h, and are no longer evident at 4 h. After a 10-mg dose, zaleplon has no residual effects on performance and memory tests after 2 h; in contrast, residual effects persist for up to 5 h with zolpidem.[39]

Precautions. (*See* Sedatives and Hypnotics, Class Instructions.) Complex sleep behaviors are possible. Anaphylaxis and angioedema have been seen even with the first dose of the medication. Patients with aspirin sensitivity have increased risk of tartrazine sensitivity and allergic reactions. There is a risk of depression of respiratory drive in patients with compromised respiratory function. Potentiation of CNS depression is possible in patients taking medications that can cause CNS depression. Sedative hypnotics have been linked to worsening depression and zaleplon may have this effect.

Patient Instructions. This medication should be taken just before going to bed and only when you have at least 4 h to devote to sleep. Avoid high-fat meals prior to taking this medication. You should carefully read the medication guide that was given to you when this medication was dispensed. Make sure that your doctor knows if you are pregnant, breast-feeding, or planning to become pregnant.

Drug Interactions. Zaleplon is partially metabolized through CYP3A4 and is thus susceptible to medications that induce or inhibit this enzyme. Inducers like rifampin and carbamazepine can reduce plasma concentrations of zaleplon by up to 80%. Concomitant use of cimetidine with zaleplon leads to an 85% increase in C_{max} for zaleplon.

ZOLPIDEM TARTRATE Ambien, Ambien CR, Zolpimist, Edluar, Various

Pharmacology. Zolpidem is a short-acting non-benzodiazepine hypnotic indicated for the short-term treatment of insomnia. Most benzodiazepines bind to all

GABA–benzodiazepine (ω) receptor complexes, but zolpidem selectively binds only to the ω_1 receptor. This difference suggests a more selective sedative–hypnotic effect without anxiolytic, anticonvulsant, or muscle relaxant effects.[40–42] (*See* Benzodiazepines and Related Drugs Comparison Chart.)

Administration and Adult Dosage. **PO as a hypnotic**—(immediate-release, sublingual tablet, or oral spray) 10 mg or (extended-release) 12.5 mg immediately before bedtime.

Special Populations. *Pediatric Dosage.* (<18 years) safety and efficacy not established.

Geriatric Dosage. (immediate-release) 5 mg/d. (extended-release) 6.25 mg/d.

Other Conditions. *Hepatic Impairment,* (immediate-release, sublingual tablet, or oral spray) 5 mg/d. (extended-release) 6.25 mg/d.

Dosage Forms. **Tab (immediate-release)** 5, 10 mg. **ER Tab** 6.25, 12.5 mg. **Oral Spray** (Zolpimist) 5, 10 mg. **Sublingual Tab** (Edluar) 5, 10 mg.

Pharmacokinetics. After oral administration, zolpidem reaches peak serum concentrations in 1.6 h, is 93% bound to plasma proteins, and has no active metabolites. **Half-life.** 1.5–4 h (average 2.5 h). Half-life is slightly increased in the elderly and greatly increased in patients with hepatic impairment (9.9 h). Onset of action for the immediate-release tablets is 1.5 h and with the extended-release tablets is 1.6 h.

Precautions. (*See* Sedatives and Hypnotics, Class Instructions.) Complex sleep behaviors are possible. Anaphylaxis and angioedema have been seen even with the first dose of the medication. There is a risk of depression of respiratory drive in patients with compromised respiratory function. Potentiation of CNS depression is possible in patients taking medications that can cause CNS depression. Sedative hypnotics have been linked to worsening depression and zolpidem may have this effect.

Patient Instructions. This medication should be taken just before going to bed and only when you have at least 8 h to devote to sleep. It is best to take this medication on an empty stomach. You should carefully read the medication guide that was given to you when this medication was dispensed. Make sure that your doctor knows if you are pregnant, breast-feeding, or planning to become pregnant.

Drug Interactions. An increased risk of hallucinations has been reported when zolpidem is administered with bupropion, fluoxetine, sertraline, venlafaxine, and desipramine. It does not appear that kinetic changes of the medications are responsible for this event. Zolpidem is metabolized by CYP3A4. Increased plasma concentrations and pharmacodynamic effects were seen when ketoconazole was administered with zolpidem and ritonavir. Conversely, rifampin decreased the plasma concentrations and pharmacodynamic effects of zolpidem.

Adverse Reactions. Dose-related side effects include daytime drowsiness, dizziness, and diarrhea. Clinical trials with 20-mg doses have reported headache, nausea, memory problems, and CNS stimulation. Tolerance has not been reported, nor has rebound insomnia after therapeutic doses. Psychomotor performance is impaired when zolpidem is combined with alcohol. Efficacy has been demonstrated for 35 nights at doses of 10 mg without affecting sleep stages or psychomotor performance.

BENZODIAZEPINES AND RELATED DRUGS COMPARISON CHART

DRUG AND SCHEDULE[a]	DOSAGE FORMS	ADULT ORAL DOSAGE RANGE	PEAK ORAL SERUM LEVELS (h)	HALF-LIFE (h)[b]
SHORT-ACTING ANXIOLYTICS				
Alprazolam (C-IV) Xanax Various	Tab 0.25, 0.5, 1, 2 mg Soln 0.1, 1 mg/mL	0.75–4 mg/d[c] 5–10 mg/d[d]	0.7–1.6	11–21
Lorazepam[e] (C-IV) Ativan Various	Tab 0.5, 1, 2 mg Soln 2 mg/mL Inj 2, 4 mg/mL	2–10 mg/d	2	10–20
Oxazepam (C-IV) Serax Various	Cap 10, 15, 30 mg Tab 15 mg	30–120 mg/d	1–2	5–15
LONG-ACTING ANXIOLYTICS				
Chlordiazepoxide (C-IV) Librium Libritabs Various	Cap 5, 10, 25 mg Tab 10, 25 mg Inj 100 mg	15–100 mg/d	2–4	>24
Clorazepate (C-IV) Tranxene Various	Cap 3.75, 7.5, 15 mg Tab 3.75, 7.5, 15 mg SR Tab 11.25, 22.5 mg	15–60 mg/d	1–2[f]	>24
Diazepam (C-IV) Dizac Valium Various	Tab 2, 5, 10 mg Soln 1, 5 mg/mL Inj 5 mg/mL	6–40 mg/d	1–2	>24
Halazepam (C-IV) Paxipam	Tab 20, 40 mg	60–160 mg/d	1–3	>24
SHORT-ACTING HYPNOTICS				
Midazolam[e] (C-IV) Versed Various	Inj 1, 5 mg/mL Syrup 2 mg/mL	—	—	1.5–3
Triazolam (C-IV) Halcion Various	Tab 0.125, 0.25 mg	0.125–0.25 mg	0.5–2	1.5–3.6
Zaleplon[g] (C-IV) Sonata Various	Cap 5, 10 mg	10 mg	1.1	0.8–1.4
Zolpidem[g] (C-IV) Ambien Ambien CR Edluar Zolpimist Various	Tab 5, 10 mg ER Tab 6.25, 12.5 mg Oral Spray 5, 10 mg Sublingual Tab 5, 10 mg	5–20 mg	2	1.5–4

(continued)

BENZODIAZEPINES AND RELATED DRUGS COMPARISON CHART (*continued*)

DRUG AND SCHEDULE[a]	DOSAGE FORMS	ADULT ORAL DOSAGE RANGE	PEAK ORAL SERUM LEVELS (h)	HALF-LIFE (H)[b]
INTERMEDIATE-ACTING HYPNOTICS				
Estazolam (C-IV) ProSom Various	Tab 1, 2 mg	1–2 mg	1–2	12–15
Temazepam (C-IV) Restoril Various	Cap 7.5, 15, 30 mg	7.5–30 mg	2–3	10–15
LONG-ACTING HYPNOTICS				
Flurazepam (C-IV) Dalmane Various	Cap 15, 30 mg	15–30 mg	h	>24[b]
Quazepam (C-IV) Doral	Tab 7.5, 15 mg	7.5–15 mg	1 2	>24[b]

[a]Controlled substance schedule designated after each drug (in parentheses).
[b]Parent drug plus active metabolites.
[c]For generalized anxiety disorder.
[d]For panic disorder.
[e]Also used as an IV anesthetic; well absorbed IM.
[f]Hydrolyzed to nordazepam (desmethyldiazepam) before absorption.
[g]Not a benzodiazepine chemically, but an imidazopyridine, which is a selective benzodiazepine-1 receptor agonist.
[h]Rapidly and completely metabolized to desalkylflurazepam.
From Refs. 2, 3, 6, 11, 23, 31, 33, and 42–46

■ REFERENCES

1. Jonas JM, Cohon MS. A comparison of the safety and efficacy of alprazolam versus other agents in the treatment of anxiety, panic, and depression: a review of the literature. *J Clin Psychiatry.* 1993;54(suppl 10):25-45.
2. Fawcett JA, Kravitz HM. Alprazolam: pharmacokinetics, clinical efficacy, and mechanism of action. *Pharmacotherapy.* 1982;2:243-254.
3. Scavone JM et al. Alprazolam kinetics following sublingual and oral administration. *J Clin Psychopharmacol.* 1987;7:332-334.
4. Kroboth et al. Alprazolam in the elderly: pharmacokinetics and pharmacodynamics during multiple dosing. *Psychopharmacology.* 1990;100:477-484.
5. Patterson JF. Alprazolam dependency: use of clonazepam for withdrawal. *South Med J.* 1988;81:830-832.
6. Dubovsky SL. Generalized anxiety disorder: new concepts and psychopharmacologic therapies. *J Clin Psychiatry.* 1990;51(suppl 1):3-10.
7. Gorman JM, Papp LA. Chronic anxiety: deciding the length of treatment. *J Clin Psychiatry.* 1990;51(suppl 1):11-15.
8. Kranzler HR, Orrok B. The pharmacotherapy of alcoholism. In: Tasman A et al., eds. *Review of Psychiatry.* Vol 8. Washington, DC: American Psychiatric Press; 1989:359-380.
9. DeVane CL. Fundamentals of Monitoring Psychoactive Drug Therapy. Baltimore, MD: Williams & Wilkins; 1990.
10. Roy-Byrne PP, Cowley DS. *Benzodiazepines in Clinical Practice: Risks and Benefits.* Washington, DC: American Psychiatric Press; 1991:213-227.
11. Greenblatt DJ et al. Benzodiazepines: a summary of pharmacokinetic properties. *Br J Clin Pharmacol.* 1981;11:11S-16S.

12. Dietch JT, Jennings RK. Aggressive dyscontrol in patients treated with benzodiazepines. *J Clin Psychiatry.* 1988;49:184-188.

13. Jann MW. Buspirone: an update on a unique anxiolytic agent. *Pharmacotherapy.* 1988;8:100-116.

14. Sussman N. The uses of buspirone in psychiatry. *J Clin Psychiatry Monogr.* 1994;12:3-19.

15. Gammans RE et al. Pharmacokinetics of buspirone in elderly subjects. *J Clin Pharmacol.* 1989;29:72-78.

16. Gammans RE et al. Metabolism and disposition of buspirone. *Am J Med.* 1986;80(suppl 3B):41-51.

17. Newton RE et al. Review of the side-effect profile of buspirone. *Am J Med.* 1986;80(suppl 3B):17-21.

18. Schweizer E, Rickels K. New and emerging clinical uses for buspirone. *J Clin Psychiatry Monogr.* 1994;12:46-54.

19. Brogden RN, Goa KL. Flumazenil. A preliminary review of its benzodiazepine antagonist properties, intrinsic activity and therapeutic use. *Drugs.* 1988;35:448-467.

20. Longmire AW, Seger DL. Topics in clinical pharmacology: flumazenil, a benzodiazepine antagonist. *Am J Med Sci.* 1993;306:49-52.

21. Hoffman EJ, Warren EW. Flumazenil: a benzodiazepine antagonist. *Clin Pharm.* 1993;12:641-656.

22. Spivey WH. Flumazenil and seizures: analysis of 43 cases. *Clin Ther.* 1992;14:292-305.

23. Kanto JH. Midazolam: the first water-soluble benzodiazepine. *Pharmacotherapy.* 1985;5:138-155.

24. Bell GD et al. Intravenous midazolam for upper gastrointestinal endoscopy: a study of 800 consecutive cases relating dose to age and sex of patient. *Br J Clin Pharmacol.* 1987;23:241-243.

25. Daneshmend TK, Logan RFA. Midazolam. *Lancet.* 1988;1:389.

26. Saint-Maurice C et al. The pharmacokinetics of rectal midazolam for premedication in children. *Anesthesiology.* 1986;65:536-538.

27. Simpson D et al. Ramelteon: A review of its use in insomnia. *Drugs.* 2008;68:1901-1919.

28. Yakabowich MR. Hypnotics in the elderly: appropriate usage guidelines. *J Geriatr Drug Ther.* 1992;6:5-21.

29. Weiss KJ. Management of anxiety and depression syndromes in the elderly. *J Clin Psychiatry.* 1994;55(suppl 2):5-12.

30. Benet LZ et al. Design and optimization of dosage regimens: pharmacokinetic data. In: Hardman JG et al., eds. Goodman and Gilman's the Pharmacological Basis of Therapeutics. 9th ed. New York: McGraw-Hill; 1996:1707-1792.

31. Garzone PD, Kroboth PD. Pharmacokinetics of the newer benzodiazepines. *Clin Pharmacokinet.* 1989;16:337-364.

32. Robin DW et al. Triazolam in cirrhosis: pharmacokinetics and pharmacodynamics. *Clin Pharmacol Ther.* 1993;54:630-637.

33. Scharf MB et al. Comparative amnestic effects of benzodiazepine hypnotic agents. *J Clin Psychiatry.* 1988;49:134-137.

34. Roth T et al. Pharmacology and hypnotic efficacy of triazolam. *Pharmacotherapy.* 1983;3:137-148.

35. Gillin JC, Byerley W. The diagnosis and management of insomnia. *N Engl J Med.* 1990;322:239-248.

36. National Institutes of Health. The treatment of sleep disorders of older people. *NIH Consens Statement.* 1990;8:1-22.

37. Stimmel GL, Dopheide JA. Sleep disorders: focus on insomnia. *US Pharm.* 2000;25:69-80.

38. Greenblatt DJ et al. Comparative kinetics and dynamics of zaleplon, zolpidem, and placebo. *Clin Pharmacol Ther.* 1998;64:553-561.

39. Danjou P et al. A comparison of the residual effects of zaleplon and zolpidem following administration 5 to 2 h before awakening. *Br J Clin Pharmacol.* 1999;48:367-374.

40. Scharf MB et al. A multi-center placebo-controlled study evaluating zolpidem in the treatment of chronic insomnia. *J Clin Psychiatry.* 1994;55:192-199.

41. Jonas JM et al. Comparative clinical profiles of triazolam versus other shorter-acting hypnotics. *J Clin Psychiatry.* 1992;53(suppl 12):19-31.

42. Langtry HD, Benfield P. Zolpidem: a review of its pharmacodynamic and pharmacokinetic properties and therapeutic potential. *Drugs.* 1990;40:291-313.

43. Mitler MM. Evaluation of temazepam as a hypnotic. *Pharmacotherapy.* 1981;1:3-13.

44. Kales A. Quazepam: hypnotic efficacy and side effects. *Pharmacotherapy.* 1990;10:1-12.

45. Scherf MB et al. Estazolam and flurazepam: a multicenter, placebo-controlled comparative study in outpatients with insomnia. *J Clin Pharmacol.* 1990;30:461-467.

46. Anonymous. Hypnotic drugs. *Med Lett Drugs Ther.* 2000;42:71-72.

Chapter 40

Lithium

Aaron P. Gibson

LITHIUM CARBONATE	Various
LITHIUM CITRATE	Cibalith-S, Lithonate-S

Pharmacology. Lithium's mechanism of antimanic effect is unknown; it alters the actions of several second-messenger systems (e.g., adenylate cyclase and phosphoinositol).[1,2]

Indications and Adult Dosage. Individualize dosage according to serum levels and clinical response. **PO for bipolar disorder**—(carbonate) **Acute** manic episodes typically requires 1.2–2.4 g/d; **Maintenance therapy** typically requires 900 mg–1.5 g/d. A **loading dose** of 30 mg/kg, in 3 divided doses, can be given to achieve the desired serum level within 12 h.[3] A number of predictive dosage techniques have been developed based on estimated steady state after one serum level.[4,5] The syrup is a citrate salt that contains 300 mg/5 mL. Dosing is the same as with oral tablet formulations.

Special Populations. *Pediatric Dosage.* **PO**—(<12 years) 15–20 mg/kg/d (or 0.4–0.5 mEq/kg/d) in 2–3 divided doses; (12–18 years) same as adult dosage.[6]

Geriatric Dosage. (>65 years) decrease adult dosage by 33%–50%.[7]

Other Conditions. Adjust the dosage more carefully in patients with decreased renal function.

Dosage Forms. **Cap** 150, 300, 600 mg; **Tab** 300 mg; **Tab** SR 300, 450 mg; **Syrup** 1.6 mEq/mL (as citrate).

Patient Instructions. This drug can be taken with food, milk, or antacid to minimize stomach upset. Report immediately if signs of toxicity occur, such as persistent diarrhea, vomiting, coarse hand tremor, drowsiness, or slurred speech, or before beginning any diet. In hot weather, ensure adequate water and salt intake.

Pharmacokinetics. *Onset and Duration.* Onset—7–10 days for therapeutic effect.[8]

Serum Levels. (Acute mania or hypomania) 0.8–1.5 mEq/L; (prophylaxis) 0.6–1.2 mEq/L, although concern about long-term renal effects suggests most patients should be maintained at <0.9 mEq/L. Levels >1.5 mEq/L are regularly associated with signs of toxicity, and levels <2 mEq/L result in serious toxicity.[9] (*See* Adverse Reactions.)

Fate. Absorption is virtually complete 8 h after oral administration, with peak levels occurring in 2–4 h. Distribution is throughout total body water, but tissue uptake is not uniform. The drug is not protein bound or metabolized, but freely filtered through the glomerulus, with approximately 80% being reabsorbed. **Half-life.** >18–20 h; up to 36 h in the elderly.[8]

Adverse Reactions. Frequent, dose-related adverse effects with therapeutic serum levels include nausea, diarrhea, polyuria, polydipsia, fine hand tremor, and muscle weakness. GI adverse effects can be worse with extended-release forms of lithium as these disturbances are directly tied to the time lithium spends in the gut lumen. Signs of toxicity include coarse hand tremor, persistent GI effects, muscle hyperirritability, slurred speech, confusion, stupor, seizures, increased deep tendon reflexes, irregular pulse, and coma. Frequent, non–dose-related effects include nontoxic goiter, hypothyroidism, nephrogenic diabetes insipidus-like syndrome, folliculitis, aggravation of acne or psoriasis, leukocytosis, hypercalcemia, and weight gain.[10–12]

Contraindications. Pregnancy; fluctuating renal function; severe renal or cardiovascular disease.

Precautions. Use with caution in patients with cardiac disease, dehydration, sodium depletion, diuretic therapy, or dementia; in nursing mothers; and in the elderly. (*See* Special Populations.)

Drug Interactions. ACE inhibitors can increase serum lithium concentrations. Theophylline or excess sodium enhances renal lithium clearance; sodium deficiency can promote lithium retention and increase risk of toxicity. Long-term diuretic or NSAID use can result in decreased lithium elimination. Haloperidol can increase the CNS toxicity of lithium. With methyldopa or phenytoin, signs of lithium toxicity can occur without increased serum lithium levels.

Parameters to Monitor. Pre-lithium workup should include thyroid function tests, serum creatinine, BUN, CBC (for baseline WBC count), urinalysis (for baseline specific gravity), electrolytes, and ECG (if patient is <40 years). During therapy, obtain serum lithium levels (drawn 12 h after last dose) weekly during initiation and monthly during maintenance.[12,13]

Notes. **Divalproex sodium** is equivalent in efficacy to lithium for bipolar disorder and more effective than lithium for rapid-cycling bipolar illness.[14–16]

■ REFERENCES

1. Post RM et al. Mechanisms of action of anticonvulsants in affective disorders: comparisons with lithium. *J Clin Psychopharmacol.* 1992;12:23S-35S.
2. Bowden CL. Efficacy of lithium in mania and maintenance therapy of bipolar disorder. *J Clin Psychiatry.* 2000;61(suppl 9):35-40.
3. Kook KA et al. Accuracy and safety of a priori lithium loading. *J Clin Psychiatry.* 1985;46:49-51.
4. Lobeck F. A review of lithium dosing methods. *Pharmacotherapy.* 1988;8:248-255.
5. Gutierrez MA et al. Evaluation of a new steady-state lithium prediction method. *Lithium.* 1991;2:57-59.
6. The United States Pharmacopeial Convention. *USP-DI.* vol I. Rockville, MD: The United States Pharmacopeial Convention; 1996.
7. Hardy BG et al. Pharmacokinetics of lithium in the elderly. *J Clin Psychopharmacol.* 1987;7:153-158.
8. DeVane CL. *Fundamentals of Monitoring Psychoactive Drug Therapy.* Baltimore, MD: Williams & Wilkins; 1990.
9. Jefferson JW. Lithium: a therapeutic magic wand. *J Clin Psychiatry.* 1989;50:81-86.
10. Jefferson JW. Lithium: the present and the future. *J Clin Psychiatry.* 1990;51(suppl 8):4-8.
11. Gitlin MJ et al. Maintenance lithium treatment: side effects and compliance. *J Clin Psychiatry.* 1989;50:127-131.
12. Kilts CD. The ups and downs of lithium dosing. *J Clin Psychiatry.* 1998;59(suppl 6):21-26.
13. Gitlin MJ. Lithium-induced renal insufficiency. *J Clin Psychopharmacol.* 1993;13:276-279.
14. American Psychiatric Association. Practice guideline for the treatment of patients with bipolar disorder. *Am J Psychiatry.* 1994;151(suppl 12):1-36.
15. Guay DRP. The emerging role of valproate in bipolar disorder and other psychiatric disorders. *Pharmacotherapy.* 1995;15:631-647.
16. Bowden CL et al. Relation of serum valproate concentrations to response in mania. *Am J Psychiatry.* 1996;153:765-770.

Chapter 41

Neurodegenerative Disease Drugs

Toy S. Biederman

AMANTADINE Symmetrel, Various

Pharmacology. Amantadine is an antiviral compound that prevents the release of viral nucleic acid into the host cell. In Parkinson's disease, the drug increases presynaptic dopamine release, blocks the reuptake of dopamine into the presynaptic neurons, and exerts anticholinergic effects. Amantadine also can reduce levodopa-induced dyskinesias in patients with Parkinson's disease, possibly by acting as an *N*-methyl-D-aspartate receptor antagonist.[1,2]

Administration and Adult Dosage. PO for parkinsonism—100 mg/d initially, increasing in 100 mg/d increments every 7–14 days to effective dosage. **Usual maintenance dosage**—100 mg twice daily. Occasional patients may benefit from titration up to 400 mg daily in divided doses, under close physician supervision. **PO for extrapyramidal reactions**—100 mg twice daily, to a maximum of 300 mg/d in 3 divided doses. **PO for prophylaxis of influenza A (consult the Centers for Disease Control and Prevention each year for recommendations on effectiveness)**—200 mg/d in 1–2 divided doses continuing for at least 10 days after known exposure, for 2–3 weeks after giving influenza A vaccine, or for up to 90 days when vaccine is unavailable or contraindicated. **PO for treatment of influenza A**—200 mg/d in 1–2 divided doses starting within 24–48 h after onset of illness and continuing for 24–48 h after symptoms disappear.

Special Populations. *Pediatric Dosage.* **PO for prophylaxis or treatment of influenza A**—(<1 year) Safety and efficacy not established; (1–9 years) 4.4–8.8 mg/kg/d in 2 divided doses, to a maximum of 150 mg/d; (9–12 years) 100 mg twice daily. **For prophylaxis**, continue therapy for at least 10 days after exposure, for 2–3 days after giving influenza A vaccine, or for up to 90 days when vaccine is unavailable or contraindicated. **For treatment**, continue for 24–48 h after symptoms disappear.

Geriatric Dosage. **PO for influenza prophylaxis or treatment**—(>65 years) 100 mg/d. **PO for parkinsonism**—Same as adult dosage, adjusting for renal impairment.

Other Conditions. Renal Impairment: Cl_{Cr} of 30–50 mL/min, give 200 mg first day and then 100 mg/d; Cl_{Cr} of 15–29 mL/min, give 200 mg first day and then 100 mg every other day; Cl_{Cr} <15 mL/min or for patients on hemodialysis, give 200 mg every 7 days.[1]

Dosage Forms. Cap, Tab 100 mg; **Soln, Syrup** 10 mg/mL.

Patient Instructions. This medication can cause dizziness, confusion, or difficulty in concentrating. Until the extent of these effects is known, use caution when driving, operating machinery, or performing other tasks requiring mental alertness.

Avoid excessive concurrent use of alcohol. **Parkinson's disease**—stopping this medication suddenly can cause your Parkinson's disease to worsen.

Missed Doses. Take this drug at regular intervals. If you miss a dose, take it as soon as you remember. If it is about time for the next dose, take that dose only. Do not double the dose or take extra.

Pharmacokinetics. *Onset and Duration.* Onset is usually within 48 h. Benefit may fall off after a few months. It may be regained by increasing the dose or temporarily discontinuing and then reinitiating the drug.

Serum Levels. Maximum plasma concentration after 100 mg is 0.22 ± 0.03 mg/L.[1]

Fate. Peak serum levels occur in 1–4 h in young adults, 4.5–7 h in older adults. V_d is 6.6 ± 1.5 L/kg; clearance is 0.39 ± 0.13 L/h/kg with normal renal function; from 78% to 88% is excreted unchanged in the urine.[1] **Half-life.** 11.8 ± 2.1 h,[3] elderly adults—31 ± 7.2 h,[4] during chronic hemodialysis—8.3 ± 1.5 days.[3]

Adverse Reactions. Nausea, dizziness, insomnia, confusion, hallucinations, anxiety, restlessness, depression, irritability, peripheral edema, orthostatic hypotension, and livedo reticularis (purplish mottling of the skin) occur frequently. Occasionally, heart failure, psychosis, urinary retention, or reversible elevation of liver enzymes can occur. Seizures, corneal opacities, or leukopenia rarely occur.

Drug Interactions. Amantadine can potentiate the CNS effects of anticholinergic agents.

Precautions. Pregnancy; lactation. Use with caution in patients with heart failure, seizures, renal or hepatic disease, peripheral edema, orthostatic hypotension, psychosis, or history of eczematoid rash or in those receiving CNS stimulants. Abrupt drug discontinuation in patients with Parkinson's disease can result in rapid clinical deterioration. Observe patients carefully when dosages of amantadine are reduced abruptly or discontinued, especially if patients are receiving neuroleptics. Sporadic cases of neuroleptic malignant syndrome have been reported in association with amantadine withdrawal or dosage reduction. Suicide attempts have been reported in patients treated with amantadine, including short influenza treatment, and in patients with and without psychiatric histories. Amantadine can exacerbate mental problems in patients with psychiatric disorders. Patients with Parkinson's disease are at increased risk for melanoma; monitoring is recommended for all indications. Orthostatic hypotension is a risk; use caution in rising from supine or sitting position.

Parameters to Monitor. Monitor renal function and disease symptoms periodically in parkinsonian patients.

BENZTROPINE MESYLATE Cogentin

Pharmacology. Benztropine is a synthetic competitive antagonist of acetylcholine. In Parkinson's disease, the drug reduces the relative excess of cholinergic activity in the basal ganglia that develops because of absolute dopamine deficiency in this area. Benztropine also possesses antihistaminic effects.[5,6] It is a tertiary amine developed by the union of the tropine segment of atropine and the benzhydryl segment of diphenhydramine hydrochloride.[7]

Administration and Adult Dosage. **PO, IM, or IV for adjunctive use in parkin-sonism**—0.5–1 mg/d initially, increasing in 0.5 mg/d increments every 5–6 days to effective dosage, to a maximum of 6 mg/d. **Usual maintenance dosage**—1–2 mg/d in 2–3 divided doses. When used concurrently with levodopa, the dosages of both drugs might require reduction. **PO, IM, or IV for drug-induced extrapyramidal disorders**—1–4 mg/d in 1–2 doses.

Special Populations. *Pediatric Dosage.* **IM or IV for medication-induced extrapyramidal disorders.** (<3 years) Contraindicated ≥ 0.02–0.05 mg/kg/dose 1 or 2 times daily, to a maximum of 2 mg/d.

Geriatric Dosage. Same as adult dosage, although older patients often can be controlled with 1–2 mg/d. Because of anticholinergic effects, the drug should be used with caution in elderly patients.

Dosage Forms. **Tab** 0.5, 1, 2 mg; **Inj** 1 mg/mL.

Patient Instructions. This drug can cause constipation, difficult or painful urination, dry mouth, blurred vision, or drowsiness. Use caution when driving, operating machinery, or performing other tasks requiring mental alertness. Avoid excessive concurrent use of alcohol and other drugs that cause drowsiness.

Missed Doses. Take this drug at regular intervals. If you miss a dose, take it as soon as you remember. If it is about time for the next dose, take that dose only. Do not double the dose or take extra.

Pharmacokinetics. *Onset and Duration.* Onset of resolution of drug-induced extrapyramidal symptoms is within 15 min after IV or IM administration and 1–2 h after oral administration. Benztropine is a long-acting drug and may be dosed daily or twice daily.[5,7]

Fate. Benztropine pharmacokinetics have not been well studied. Small increases in dose variable increases in anticholinergic activity.[7]

Adverse Reactions. Frequent adverse effects are dose related and include dry mouth, blurred vision, nausea, dizziness, constipation, nervousness, and urinary retention. Confusional states, impairment of recent memory, and hallucinations occur with use of high doses and in patients with advanced age and underlying dementia. Rarely, paralytic ileus, parotitis, hyperthermia, or skin rash occurs.

Contraindications. Children <3 years; angle-closure glaucoma; pyloric or duodenal obstruction; stenosing peptic ulcers; achalasia; bladder-neck obstructions; myasthenia gravis; cognitive disturbances.[5,6]

Precautions. Pregnancy; elderly patients; children >3 years. Use with caution in hot weather or during exercise. May cause anhidrosis and hyperthermia; increased risk in alcoholics. Use with caution in patients with tachycardia, prostatic hypertrophy, glaucoma, or obstructive diseases of the gastrointestinal (GI) tract.[5,6]

Drug Interactions. Carefully observe patients given concomitant phenothiazines and/or heterocyclic antidepressants because intensification of mental symptoms, paralytic ileus, or hyperthermia can occur. Anticholinergics can decrease the effectiveness of phenothiazines. Use with amantadine can result in increased CNS anticholinergic effects. Anticholinergics can decrease digoxin absorption from digoxin tablets.

Parameters to Monitor. Intraocular pressure monitoring and gonioscope evaluation periodically. Monitor for Parkinson's disease symptoms periodically.

CARBIDOPA AND LEVODOPA   Sinemet, Parcopa

Pharmacology. Levodopa is centrally converted to dopamine by DOPA decarboxylase and replenishes dopamine, which is deficient in the basal ganglia of patients with Parkinson's disease. Carbidopa, which does not cross the blood–brain barrier, inhibits peripheral DOPA decarboxylase, thereby increasing the amount of levodopa available to the brain for conversion to dopamine and limiting peripheral side effects. Addition of carbidopa decreases levodopa-induced nausea and vomiting but does not decrease adverse reactions caused by the central effects of levodopa.[8]

Administration and Adult Dosage. **PO for Parkinson's disease in patients not receiving levodopa (standard formulation)**—25 mg carbidopa/100 mg levodopa 3 times daily initially, increasing in 1 tablet/d increments every 1–2 days to effective dosage, to usual maximum of 8 tablets/d. Alternatively, 10 mg carbidopa/100 mg levodopa 3 or 4 times daily initially, to a maximum of 8 tablets/d. Initial use of 10 mg carbidopa/100 mg levodopa can result in more nausea and vomiting because 70–100 mg/d of carbidopa is needed to saturate peripheral DOPA decarboxylase. If initial dosage maximum is reached with 10/100 tablets and further titration is necessary, substitute 25 mg carbidopa/250 mg levodopa 3 or 4 times daily, increasing in increments of 0.5–1 tablet/d every 1–2 days to effective dosage, to a maximum of 8 tablets/d.[8] Some long-term users with advanced disease might need > 2 g/d. **SR Tablet**—(patients already taking non-SR tablets) start with a dosage that provides 10% more levodopa daily. Initially, divide dosage 2 or 3 times daily with an interval of 4–8 h between doses while awake. Ultimately, dosages up to 30% greater might be needed, depending on patient response; (patients not receiving carbidopa/levodopa) 1 tablet twice daily initially, at least 6 h apart, and allow 3 days between dosage adjustments.[8] **Usual maintenance dosage**—2–8 tablets/d. If given in combination with a dopamine agonist or selegiline, lower dosages may be effective.

Special Populations. *Pediatric Dosage.* (<18 years) Safety and efficacy not established.

Geriatric Dosage. Same as adult dosage.

Dosage Forms. **Tab and Orally Disintegrating Tab** (Parcopa) 10 mg carbidopa/100 mg levodopa, 25 mg carbidopa/100 mg levodopa, 25 mg carbidopa/250 mg levodopa;[8,9] **SR Tab** 25 mg carbidopa/100 mg levodopa, 50 mg carbidopa/200 mg levodopa.[8] (*See* Notes.)

Patient Instructions. Stopping this medication suddenly can cause Parkinson's disease to worsen quickly. Report bothersome or unexpected side effects. Unless prescribed, do not take levodopa in addition to this drug. Avoid pyridoxine (vitamin B_6) if you are taking levodopa alone, although it can be taken with carbidopa/levodopa. Avoid high-protein meals for maximum absorption. If you are taking the sustained-release tablet, swallow a whole or one-half tablet without chewing or crushing it. Onset of effect of the first morning dose of the sustained-release product could be delayed up to 1 h compared with the quick-release product. A dark color (red, brown, or black) might appear in saliva, urine, or sweat and can stain clothing.

Missed Doses. Take this drug at regular intervals. If you miss a dose, take it as soon as you remember. If it is about time for the next dose, take that dose only. Do not double the dose or take an extra dose.

Pharmacokinetics. ***Onset and Duration.*** Patients experience a reduction in efficacy, with a narrowing of the therapeutic window and the occurrence of "off episodes," with advanced disease.[8] (*See* Notes.)

Fate. Carbidopa's inhibition of peripheral levodopa decarboxylation doubles the oral bioavailability of levodopa and decreases its clearance by one-half.[8,9] Dietary proteins compete with levodopa for intestinal absorption and decrease its effectiveness. A levodopa peak of $3.2 < 1.1$ mg/L occurs in $0.7 < 0.3$ h.[10] (SR 50 mg carbidopa/200 mg levodopa) levodopa bioavailability is $71 < 24\%$ and increases with food. A peak of $1.14 < 0.42$ mg/L occurs in $2.4 < 1.2$ h.[10] Levodopa V_d is $1.09 < 0.59$ L/kg; clearance is $0.28 < 0.06$ L/h/kg; 90% of clearance is nonrenal.[11] **Half-life.** (carbidopa) $2.1 < 0.6$ h,[10] (levodopa alone) $1.4 < 0.3$ h, (levodopa with carbidopa) 2 ± 1.3 h.[11]

Adverse Reactions. Anorexia, nausea, vomiting, and involuntary muscle movements (dyskinesias) occur frequently and are generally reversible with dosage reduction. Occasionally, mental changes, depression, dementia, palpitations, or orthostatic hypotensive episodes, increased libido, and bullous lesions occur. Rarely, psychosis, hemolytic anemia, leukopenia, or agranulocytosis is reported. Compared with levodopa alone, carbidopa/levodopa has markedly reduced GI and cardiovascular side effects. However, mental disturbances are not eliminated and dyskinesias can appear earlier in therapy. These dyskinesias might require a decrease in dosage or dosage interval. Side effects can be more pronounced in patients receiving selegiline or a dopamine agonist as adjunctive therapy.

Contraindications. Lactation; nonselective MAO inhibitors concurrently or 2 weeks before carbidopa/levodopa; narrow-angle glaucoma; undiagnosed skin lesions; history of melanoma.

Precautions. ***Pregnancy.*** Use with caution in patients with histories of myocardial infarction (MI) complicated by arrhythmias; peptic ulcer disease; severe cardiovascular, pulmonary, renal, hepatic, or endocrine disease; open-angle glaucoma; bronchial asthma; urinary retention; or underlying depression or psychosis. Also, use caution in patients receiving antihypertensives. Symptoms resembling neuroleptic malignant syndrome can occur when carbidopa/levodopa in combination with other antiparkinson agents is reduced abruptly or discontinued.

Drug Interactions. Iron salts, including low doses in multivitamins, can decrease levodopa absorption. Other agents for Parkinson's disease, such as dopamine agonists, COMT inhibitors, and selegiline, can increase levodopa side effects when added to carbidopa/levodopa. Dosage of the levodopa product might need to be reduced by 10%–30%. Metoclopramide and older neuroleptics (e.g., chlorpromazine, haloperidol) have antidopaminergic effects and oppose the action of levodopa. Atypical neuroleptics have less antidopaminergic effect (clozapine has the least) but still can reduce the effectiveness of Parkinson's disease therapy. Cholinergic agents such as donepezil and rivastigmine can worsen Parkinson's symptoms by changing the dopamine–acetylcholine balance in the brain. However, they may also improve symptoms of Lewy body dementia associated with Parkinson's disease. Bupropion elicits a higher frequency of side effects in patients taking levodopa. Administer bupropion with caution, using small initial doses and small, gradual increases. There are rare reports of adverse reactions, including hypertension and dyskinesias, resulting from the concomitant use of TCAs and levodopa. Isoniazid, phenytoin, and papaverine can decrease the therapeutic effects of levodopa. Antihypertensive drugs may increase the risk of postural hypotension when given with carbidopa/levodopa.[8]

Parameters to Monitor. Monitor CBC, renal, cardiovascular, and liver functions periodically during long-term therapy. Monitor symptoms of Parkinson's disease periodically. In patients with open-angle glaucoma, monitor intraocular pressure. May increase risk of GI bleed in patients with history of peptic ulcer disease. Monitor for signs and symptoms of GI bleed.

Notes. Levodopa produces sustained improvement in rigidity and bradykinesia in most patients. Tremor is variably affected, and postural stability is unresponsive. Loss of therapeutic effect is manifested by fluctuations in motor performance. Patients can experience periods of lack of drug effect ("off" periods) alternating with periods of therapeutic efficacy ("on" periods). Response can be predictable, where the effect fades before the next dose ("wearing-off" or "end-of-dose"), or unpredictable ("yo-yo"), where there is no relation to the time of dose. SR carbidopa/levodopa reduces "off" time, an average of 30–40 min/d, and allows a mean 33% reduction in the frequency of administration; the lower bioavailability of the SR product may require a higher daily dosage of levodopa compared with non-SR carbidopa/levodopa.[8] With disease progression, adjunctive therapy with an MAO-B inhibitor, a dopamine agonist, or a COMT inhibitor (e.g., tolcapone, entacapone) might be required to decrease the frequency of fluctuations caused by dyskinesia or dystonia.[8,9]

Notes. Stalevo incorporates carbidopa, levodopa, and entacapone with 200 mg of entacapone in each dose and carbidopa and levodopa in a 1:4 ratio. Doses with amounts of carbidopa, levodopa, and entacapone, respectively are as follows: Stalevo 50 (12.5, 50, 200 mg), Stalevo 75 (18.75, 75, 200 mg), Stalevo 100 (25, 100, 200 mg), Stalevo 125 (31.25, 125, 200 mg), Stalevo 150 (37.25, 150, 200 mg), and Stalevo 200 (50, 200, 200 mg).[12]

DONEPEZIL   Aricept

Pharmacology. Donepezil enhances the action of acetylcholine by reversibly inhibiting acetylcholinesterase (AChE), the enzyme responsible for its hydrolysis. It has a high degree of selectivity for AChE in the CNS, which might explain the relative lack of peripheral side effects. Donepezil is indicated for the treatment of mild to severe dementia of the Alzheimer's type. No evidence suggests that donepezil alters the course of the disease.[13,14]

Administration and Adult Dosage. **PO for mild-to-moderate Alzheimer's disease**—5 mg once daily, with or without food. The 10-mg dose is associated with a higher frequency of side effects but may provide extra benefit in some individuals. If a 10-mg dose is desired, first allow 4–6 weeks at 5 mg/d. **PO for**

severe Alzheimer's disease—5 mg daily for 1 week, then increase to 10 mg daily.[13]

Special Populations. *Geriatric Dosage.* Same as adult dosage.

Other Conditions. No dosage adjustment is necessary in patients with renal or hepatic disease.

Dosage Forms. **Tab** 5, 10 mg; **Orally Disintegrating Tab** 5, 10 mg.

Patient Instructions. This drug can be taken with or without food. Side effects can occur when you first start taking donepezil, but these frequently subside after 1–2 weeks. The maximum benefits of the drug might not occur until 4–8 weeks after starting the drug. Because there is variability in the way patients respond to donepezil, decide with your doctor how long to take donepezil. Do not abruptly discontinue donepezil on your own.

Missed Doses. Take this drug at regular intervals. If you miss a dose, take it as soon as you remember. If it is about time for the next dose, take that dose only. Do not double the dose or take an extra dose.

Pharmacokinetics. *Onset and Duration.* Onset is in approximately 3 weeks, with maximum benefits occurring in 4–8 weeks,[13]

Fate. Donepezil is completely absorbed and is 96% protein bound. C_{max} occurs in 3–4 h. V_{dss} is 12 L/kg; clearance is 0.13 L/h/kg. Approximately 60% is eliminated as hepatic metabolites including products of CYP2D6 and CYP3A4 and glucuronides. Approximately 17% is excreted unchanged in urine.[13] **Half-life.** >70 h.

Adverse Reactions. Occasionally, nausea, vomiting, diarrhea, muscle cramps, fatigue, anorexia, asthenia, flu syndrome, hypotension, bradycardia, headache, ecchymosis, and headache occur.[13]

Contraindications. Hypersensitivity to donepezil or piperidine derivatives (e.g., biperiden, bupivacaine, methylphenidate, paroxetine, rifabutin, trihexyphenidyl).

Precautions. Use with caution in peptic ulcer disease, syncope, sick sinus syndrome, bradycardia, altered supraventricular cardiac conduction, asthma, seizures, or COPD. Donepezil is likely to increase muscle relaxation when used with succinylcholine-type neuromuscular blockers. Use with caution in patients at increased risk of GI bleed, such as those taking NSAIDs.

Drug Interactions. There are few in vivo studies. In vitro, ketoconazole and quinidine decrease donepezil metabolism; enzyme inducers might increase its metabolism. Although extensively bound to plasma proteins, donepezil does not interact with warfarin or furosemide or with cimetidine or digoxin. Donepezil can increase the risk of GI side effects from NSAIDs because of the possible increase in stomach acid production.

Parameters to Monitor. Monitor mental status and improvements in activities of daily living initially and then periodically during therapy. Since cholinesterase increase production of gastric acid, patients should be monitored for symptoms of occult GI bleeding.

Notes. Because Alzheimer's disease is a neurodegenerative disorder, patients might improve or show no change in their cognitive functions.

DOPAMINE AGONISTS	
APOMORPHINE	Apokyn
BROMOCRIPTINE	Parlodel
PRAMIPEXOLE	Mirapex
ROPINIROLE	Requip

Pharmacology. Bromocriptine is an ergot-derived dopamine agonist that stimulates dopamine D_2 receptors partly antagonizes D_1 receptors. Pramipexole and ropinirole are non–ergot-derived dopamine subtype selective agonists that exert activity in the CNS at D_2 and D_3 receptors but have no activity at the D_1 receptor.[15–17] Apomorphine is a non-ergot dopamine agonist that is used to treat "off episodes." It has high affinity for the dopamine D_4 receptor and moderate affinity for D_2, D_3, and D_5.[18] D_2 receptors are thought to play an important role in improving the akinesia, bradykinesia, rigidity, and gait disturbances of Parkinson's disease. Pramipexole, unlike other dopamine agonists, binds with 7-fold greater affinity to D_3 receptors than to D_2 receptors and can improve mood. Although bromocriptine also can inhibit prolactin secretion, it is no longer indicated for the prevention of postpartum lactation. Other uses of bromocriptine are the treatment of acromegaly, prolactin-secreting pituitary adenomas, and amenorrhea/galactorrhea secondary to hyperprolactinemia without a primary tumor.[19] (*See* Dopamine Agonists Comparison Chart.)

Administration and Adult Dosage. (Bromocriptine) **PO for acromegaly**—1.25 mg/d or 2 times daily with food initially and then increasing in 1.25–2.5 mg/d increments every 3–7 days to a **usual maintenance dosage** of 2.5 mg 2–3 times daily, to a maximum of 100 mg/d. **PO for hyperprolactinemia**—1.25–2.5 mg/d initially, titrate in 2.5-mg increments every 2–7 days until optimal response. **PO for Parkinson's disease**—(*see* Dopamine Agonists Comparison Chart). **PO for moderate-to-severe restless leg syndrome**—(pramipexole) 0.125 mg nightly 2–3 h before bedtime. May be increased every 4–7 days to 0.5–0.75 mg nightly; (ropinirole, immediate-release tablets only) 0.25 mg nightly, 1–3 h before bedtime. After 2 days, may increase to 0.5 mg nightly and to 1 mg nightly at the end of the first week, if needed.

Special Populations. *Pediatric Dosage.* (Bromocriptine) Safety and efficacy not established. **PO for treatment of prolactin-secreting pituitary adenomas**—(≥11 years) 1.25–2.5 mg daily; increase in 2.5 mg/d increments every 2–7 days as tolerated until therapeutic response is achieved.

Geriatric Dosage. Same as adult dosage.

Other Conditions. *Renal Impairment*: (Pramipexole) Cl_{Cr} 35–59 mL/min, give 1.5 mg initially, to a maximum of 1.5 mg twice daily; Cl_{Cr} 15–34 mL/min, give 0.125 mg initially, to a maximum of 1.5 mg/d.

Dosage Forms. *See* Dopamine Agonists Comparison Chart.

Patient Instructions. This medication might improve the symptoms of Parkinson's disease but will not cure it. Take this drug with food to minimize stomach upset. This drug can cause dizziness, drowsiness, or fainting, especially after the first dose. Until the extent of these effects is known, use caution when driving, operating machinery, or performing tasks requiring mental alertness. Mental disturbances, including vivid dreams, confusion, and paranoid delusions, can occur even with low doses, especially when added to levodopa therapy. Avoid concurrent use of alcohol. Inform your physician and pharmacist of any other prescription or over-the-counter medications you might be taking because these can interact with your antiparkinson medications. Do not abruptly stop taking this medication or change your dosage without medical supervision. (Bromocriptine) women taking this drug to induce ovulation should use a barrier contraceptive. (Pramipexole and ropinirole) some patients have reported sudden excessive drowsiness, causing them to fall asleep during activities of daily living, including driving. Notify your doctor immediately if you notice significant daytime drowsiness. Avoid use of other sedating medications. Report any changes in behavior or compulsive urges (gambling, sexual) to your doctor. (Apomorphine) read the Apokyn "Instructions for Use." Do not administer unless you and your caregiver have been instructed on the proper procedure.[18]

Missed Doses. Take this drug at regular intervals. If you miss a dose, take it as soon as you remember. If it is about time for the next dose, take that dose only. Do not double the dose or take an extra dose.

Pharmacokinetics. ***Onset and Duration.*** (Bromocriptine) onset 0.5–1 h;[9,20,21] (pramipexole) 2 h on an empty stomach, 3 h with food;[15] (ropinirole) 1–2 h on an empty stomach, 3–4 h with food.[17] (Bromocriptine, ropinirole) duration 3–6 h; (pramipexole) 8–12 h. (Bromocriptine) in amenorrhea, normal menstrual function usually returns within 6–8 weeks.

Fate. (Bromocriptine) bioavailability is approximately 28%; it is 90% bound to plasma proteins. Peak serum concentrations occur in 1.2 ± 0.4 h, and detectable concentrations are found for up to 12 h after discontinuation of drug;[20] clearance is 4.4 ± 2.6 L/h/kg.[21] The majority (98%) is excreted in the feces via bile.[20] (Pramipexole) bioavailability is approximately 90%; it is 15% bound to plasma proteins. V_d is 7 L/kg; renal clearance is approximately 0.4 L/h/kg and markedly exceeds the GFR. Approximately 90% of a dose is excreted unchanged in urine. (Ropinirole) although completely absorbed, bioavailability is 55% because of first-pass metabolism. It is 36% bound to plasma proteins and undergoes extensive metabolism in the liver to inactive metabolites. The *N*-despropyl metabolite is the major metabolite; the drug also is hydroxylated and glucuronidated. **Half-life.** (*See* Dopamine Agonists Comparison Chart.)

Adverse Reactions. Nausea, headache, hallucinations, dyskinesias, somnolence, vomiting, symptomatic hypotension, dizziness, fatigue, constipation, and light-headedness occur frequently. Occasionally, abdominal cramps and diarrhea occur. (Apomorphine) angina and cardiac arrest (4% in clinical development). Use with caution in patients with known cardiac or cerebrovascular disease. (Bromocriptine) rarely, hypertension, stroke, seizures, rhinorrhea, or erythromelalgia are reported. Pleuropulmonary disease is rare and usually occurs in men, especially in smokers receiving 20–100 mg/d of bromocriptine for 6–36 months; it presents with dyspnea and improves with drug discontinuation.[19] Compulsive behaviors, including intense urges to gamble and hypersexuality, have occurred in patients taking ropinirole and pramipexole.[15–17]

Contraindications. (Apomorphine) because of episodes of profound hypotension and loss of consciousness when given with ondansetron, the concomitant use of apomorphine with 5-HT$_3$ antagonist antiemetics (such as ondansetron, granisetron, dolasetron, palonosetron, and alosetron) is contraindicated. Apomorphine injection is contraindicated in patients who have demonstrated hypersensitivity to the drug or its ingredients (notably sodium metabisulfite).[18] (Bromocriptine) pregnancy; lactation; uncontrolled hypertension; preeclampsia; concurrent use of other ergot alkaloids; hypersensitivity to ergot alkaloids.

Precautions. (Apomorphine) should not be administered intravenously. Serious adverse events (i.e., crystallization of apomorphine leading to thrombus formation and pulmonary embolism) have followed intravenous administration. Because of severe nausea and vomiting due to apomorphine, patients should be started on trimethobenzamide for 3 days before starting apomorphine and should continue trimethobenzamide for at least 6 seeks. Trimethobenzamide was the antiemetic used in premarketing studies. Antiemetics and other drugs with antidopamine activity (metoclopramide, phenothiazines, haloperidol) should be avoided. The risks of hypotension and falling are increased by concomitant administration of antihypertensives, vasodilators (especially nitrates), and alcohol. Use extra caution in patients with cardiovascular or cerebrovascular disease, as decreased blood pressure may increase the risk of ischemia. Since apomorphine solution contains sodium metabisulfite, serious allergic reactions may occur in sensitive patients and in those with asthma. Since apomorphine can prolong the QT interval, use with caution in patients who are receiving other QT prolonging drugs. Apomorphine injection is dosed in milliliters, not milligrams. Patients should be instructed in proper administration. (Bromocriptine) use with caution in patients with symptoms of peptic ulcer disease, history of pulmonary disease, MI, liver disease, severe angina, peripheral vascular disease or psychiatric disease. Hypotension and hypertension sometimes occur, especially in the first 2 weeks of therapy. Seizures and stroke (mostly in women taking the medication to inhibit lactation) have occurred in patients taking bromocriptine, often following a severe headache. Use a barrier contraceptive during treatment for amenorrhea, galactorrhea, or infertility. If pregnancy is detected, discontinue the drug. (Pramipexole, ropinirole) several patients have reported "sleep attacks," or falling asleep during activities of daily living. These sudden occasions of sleepiness have resulted in motor vehicle accidents. Advise patients of this possibility and assess them regularly for symptoms of drowsiness. Instruct patients to avoid other sedating medications and drugs that can increase blood levels of these agents (e.g., cimetidine with pramipexole, ciprofloxacin with ropinirole). Sudden episodes of falling asleep might necessitate discontinuation of the dopamine agonist. If pramipexole or ropinirole is continued after such an incident, instruct the patient not to drive or use dangerous machinery.

Drug Interactions. When used with carbidopa/levodopa, it might be necessary to reduce the dosage of levodopa by as much as 30% to reduce the potential for developing dyskinesias. Drugs that antagonize dopamine (e.g., phenothiazines, butyrophenones, metoclopramide) can reduce the effectiveness of these drugs. (Bromocriptine) erythromycin can increase bromocriptine serum levels. Other ergot alkaloids can exacerbate cardiotoxic effects. (Pramipexole) can result in an earlier and higher peak serum level of levodopa. Drugs that interfere with renal tubular secretion of cations (e.g., cimetidine, ranitidine, verapamil, quinidine) can decrease pramipexole renal elimination. (Ropinirole) metabolized by CYP1A2; therefore, it might interact with inhibitors or inducers of this isozyme; ciprofloxacin markedly increases AUC and peak serum concentrations. Ropinirole might require dosage reduction with coadministration of estrogen.

Parameters to Monitor. (Bromocriptine) monitor blood pressure frequently during the first few days of therapy and periodically thereafter. Periodically evaluate hepatic, hematopoietic, cardiovascular, and renal function during long-term therapy. Monitor symptoms of Parkinson's disease periodically. Discontinue and seek medical help if hypertension, severe headache, or CNS toxicity develops. Patients with Parkinson's disease are at increased risk for melanoma; dermatological screening is recommended for all patients taking dopamine agonists.

Notes. Bromocriptine, pramipexole, and ropinirole can be used as single agents for the treatment of early Parkinson's disease and as adjunctive agents in moderate- to late-stage disease.[9,22] As first-line agents, dopamine agonists may offer neuroprotection by delaying the introduction of levodopa. However, as single agents, they are less effective than **levodopa**.[22] A new formulation of bromocriptine is currently approved for the treatment of type 2 diabetes.

ENTACAPONE	Comtan

Pharmacology. Entacapone is a peripheral acting, selective, and reversible inhibitor of COMT, similar in mechanism to tolcapone. Entacapone is indicated as an adjunct to levodopa/carbidopa to treat patients with Parkinson's disease who experience end-of-dose "wearing-off."[23]

Administration and Adult Dosage. PO for Parkinson's disease—200 mg, taken with each levodopa/carbidopa dose, to a maximum of 8 times daily (1600 mg/d). The 200-mg dose is optimal and is more efficacious than higher doses, possibly because of interference with carbidopa absorption at doses ≥400 mg.[24]

Special Populations. *Geriatric Dosage.* Same as adult dosage.

Dosage Forms. Tab 200 mg.

Patient Instructions. Take one tablet of entacapone with each dose of levodopa/carbidopa. Be aware of the possibility of developing dizziness and hypotension when rising from a sitting or supine position. This effect is more likely to occur when the drug is first started. Nausea is another potential side effect in early therapy. Entacapone can cause a brownish orange discoloration of the urine that is harmless. Dyskinesias and hallucinations can occur with entacapone, which can necessitate the reduction of the carbidopa/levodopa dose. Do not drive a car or operate machinery until you know how entacapone will affect your mental alertness or motor abilities.

Missed Doses. Take this drug at regular intervals. If you miss a dose, take it as soon as you remember. If it is close to the time of the next dose, take that dose only. Do not double the dose or take an extra dose.

Pharmacokinetics. *Onset and Duration.* Onset is rapid and occurs with first dose. Peak effect is 0.7–1.3 h after oral administration. Entacapone can prolong the effects of a carbidopa/levodopa dose by approximately 30 min.[24]

Fate. Oral bioavailability is 35%. Food does not affect entacapone pharmacokinetics, but bioavailability is doubled with liver cirrhosis. Peak after a single 200-mg dose is ~1.2 μg/mL. Plasma binding is 98%, mainly to serum albumin. Entacapone does not distribute widely into tissues or CNS; V_{dss} is 0.4 ± 0.16 L/kg. Clearance is 0.6 ± 0.1 L/kg/h. Entacapone is metabolized almost completely before elimination, mainly by isomerization followed by glucuronidation. Metabolites are eliminated primarily by biliary excretion, with 90% of the metabolized dose found in the feces and 10% in urine. Only approximately 0.2% of the dose is eliminated unchanged in urine.[25] **Half-life.** β phase 0.4–0.7 h; γ phase 2.4 h, which accounts for approximately 10% of the total AUC.

Adverse Reactions. Orthostatic hypotension, diarrhea, dyskinesias, and hallucinations can occur with entacapone therapy, especially during the initial days of therapy. Dopaminergic side effects, including dyskinesias, nausea, dizziness, hallucinations, and insomnia, can occur. Dyskinesias are the most common side effect, usually early in therapy. Their frequency is reduced with lowering of the levodopa/carbidopa dose. Diarrhea is a frequent side effect that is mild to moderate in 4%–10% of patients but severe in 1.3%. Orthostatic hypotension, urine discoloration, abdominal pain, and constipation occur occasionally. Elevation of liver enzymes was the same as that with placebo (0.8%). Rarely, rhabdomyolysis, hyperpyrexia, and confusion, resembling neuroleptic malignant syndrome, occur.

Contraindications. Hypersensitivity to the drug or its ingredients; concurrent use with nonselective MAOIs, but it can be taken with a selective MAO-B inhibitor (e.g., selegiline).

Precautions. Because 90% of drug elimination is by biliary excretion, use with caution in patients with biliary obstruction, and in patients taking drugs that interfere with biliary excretion, glucuronidation, or intestinal β-glucuronidase (probenecid, cholestyramine) and antibiotics such as erythromycin, ampicillin, rifampicin, and chloramphenicol. Since entacapone increases levodopa bioavailability, anticipate an increase in levodopa side effects, such as orthostatic hypotension and hallucinations. COMT inhibitors should not be used with nonselective monoamine oxidase inhibitors, but may be used with selegiline, a selective (MAO-B) inhibitor. COMT inhibitors should be used with caution in patients receiving drugs metabolized by COMT (epinephrine, isoproterenol, norepinephrine, dopamine, dobutamine, methyldopa, apomorphine, isoetharine, and bitolterol), because of the risk of tachycardia, arrhythmias, and excessive blood pressure changes. Rhabdomyolysis is a risk possibly associated with a symptom complex resembling neuroleptic malignant syndrome; may occur with rapid withdrawal of antiparkinson medications; for this reason, withdraw entacapone slowly.[23]

Drug Interactions. Entacapone does not inhibit cytochrome P450 enzymes at doses used for Parkinson's disease. Despite its extensive protein binding, in vitro studies have not shown binding displacement between entacapone and other highly bound drugs such as warfarin, salicylic acid, and diazepam. Drugs that interfere with biliary excretion, glucuronidation, and intestinal β-glucuronidase, such as probenecid, cholestyramine, erythromycin, ampicillin, rifampin, and chloramphenicol, have the potential to interfere with entacapone elimination. Drugs that are metabolized by COMT, such as methyldopa, dobutamine, isoproterenol, and epinephrine, can have enhanced effects when given with entacapone.[23]

Parameters to Monitor. Monitor symptoms of Parkinson's disease and excessive dopaminergic activity. The dose of carbidopa/levodopa might need to be reduced if side effects such as dyskinesias and hallucinations are excessive or intolerable.

Notes. Stalevo incorporates carbidopa, levodopa, and entacapone with 200 mg of entacapone in each dose and carbidopa and levodopa in a 1:4 ratio. Doses with amounts of carbidopa, levodopa, and entacapone, respectively: Stalevo 50 (12.5, 50, 200 mg), Stalevo 75 (18.75, 75, 200 mg), Stalevo 100 (25, 100, 200 mg), Stalevo 125 (31.25, 125, 200 mg), Stalevo 150 (37.25, 150, 200 mg), and Stalevo 200 (50, 200, 200 mg).[12]

GALANTAMINE HYDROBROMIDE   Razadyne

Pharmacology. Galantamine is a competitive, reversible AChE inhibitor similar to donepezil and rivastigmine.[26]

Administration and Adult Dosage. PO for mild-to-moderate Alzheimer's disease—4 mg twice a day initially with a meal, increasing in 4-mg increments at 4-week intervals to a maximum of 12 mg twice daily. In moderate hepatic (Child-Pugh 7–9) or moderate renal dysfunction, the maximum dosage is 8 mg twice daily. Use not recommended in severe hepatic (Child-Pugh 10–15) or renal ($Cl_{Cr} < 9$ mL/min) impairment. If more than a few days of therapy are missed, resume therapy at 4 mg twice daily. **Extended-release**—8 mg daily. Increase to 16 mg daily after a minimum of 4 weeks. If 16 mg daily is tolerated, attempt to increase to 24 mg daily after at least 4 weeks at 16 mg daily.[26]

Dosage Forms. Cap 4, 8, 12 mg; **ER Cap** 8, 16, 24 mg; **Soln** 4 mg/mL.

Pharmacokinetics. Oral bioavailability is ≥90%; food decreases peak concentration and rate, but not extent of absorption. Peak cholinesterase inhibition occurs 1 h after a dose. It is 18% plasma protein bound and distributed extensively into RBCs. V_{dss} is 2.6 L/kg; clearance is 0.34 L/h/kg. Metabolism is primarily by CYP2D6 and 3A4. CYP2D6 poor metabolizers, approximately 7% of the population, have decreased clearance. Approximately 20%–25% is excreted unchanged in urine in 24 h. **Half-life.** 5–7 h.[27]

Adverse Reactions. GI side effects (e.g., nausea, vomiting, diarrhea, anorexia, weight loss), are most prominent during dosage escalation. Dizziness, headache, chest pain, tremor, depression, rhinitis, urinary incontinence, flatulence, and bradycardia also occur frequently. Various cardiac arrhythmias, increased alkaline phosphatase, thrombocytopenia, GI bleeding, hyperglycemia, and psychiatric symptoms occur occasionally. Esophageal perforation, dehydration, aggression, GI bleeding, elevated liver enzymes, hypokalemia, dysgeusia, hypersomnia, and blurred vision have been reported.

Contraindications. Known hypersensitivity to galantamine or any excipients used in the formulation.

Precautions. Effects of neuromuscular blocking drugs such as succinylcholine may be exaggerated due to cholinesterase inhibition. Bradycardia and heart block risks are increased with galantamine therapy. Use caution in dose escalation in patients with impaired liver or kidney function. Not recommended for patients with creatinine clearance < 9 mL/min. Other precautions as with donepezil and rivastigmine.[26]

Drug Interactions. Cholinesterase inhibitors may interfere with the activity of anticholinergic drugs. Expect a synergistic effect when administered with neuromuscular blockers or cholinergic agonists such as bethanechol. Cimetidine increases the bioavailability of galantamine by 16%. Ketoconazole, by inhibiting CYP 3A4, increases the AUC of galantamine by 30%. Erythromycin causes a 10% increase in galantamine AUC. Paroxetine, an inhibitor of CYP2D6, increases galantamine bioavailability by approximately 40%.[26]

Notes. In two placebo-controlled trials, patients with mild cognitive impairment who took galantamine had higher rates of death from all causes than patients taking placebo. This effect was not seen in Alzheimer's disease patients in premarket testing.[26]

| **MEMANTINE** | Namenda |

Pharmacology. Memantine is an uncompetitive antagonist with moderate activity at N-methyl-D-aspartate receptors. Glutamate activation of CNS NMDA receptors is believed to contribute Alzheimer's disease symptoms. Memantine is also moderately antagonistic at 5-HT$_3$ receptors and has low antagonistic potency at nicotinic acetylcholine receptors.[28]

Administration and Adult Dosage. **PO for moderate to severe Alzheimer's disease**—5 mg daily initially. Increase by 5-mg increments to 10 mg twice daily. The interval between dose increases should be at least 1 week.

Special Populations. *Pediatric Dosage.* Safety and efficacy not established.

Geriatric Dosage. Same as adult dosage.

Other Conditions. Reduce the target dosage in severe renal impairment (Cl$_{Cr}$ of 5–29 mL/min) to 5 mg twice daily.[28]

Dosage Forms. **Tab** 5, 10 mg. **Oral Soln** 2 mg/mL.

Patient Instructions. Take this medication with or without food. A low dose is given initially allowing you to adjust to the effects of the drug. Wait at least 1 week between dosage increases. Avoid usage with amantadine, ketamine, and dextromethorphan. Let your physician know of any dizziness, fainting, headache, or confusion. This medicine may cause constipation. Let your doctor and pharmacist know of any other medications you are using, including herbal products.

Missed Doses. Take this drug at regular intervals. If you miss a dose, take it as soon as you remember. If it is about time for the next dose, take that dose only. Do not double the dose or take extra.

Pharmacokinetics. *Onset and Duration.* Clinical improvement may begin within 2–4 weeks. Improvement is not dramatic, but measures of activities of daily living improve modestly. Patients on memantine declined less rapidly over 6 months than patients taking placebo.[28]

Fate. Memantine is completely absorbed from the GI tract, with a peak between 3 and 8 h; 45% is bound to plasma proteins. Approximately 50% of the dose is eliminated unchanged in the urine, in part by tubular secretion. The balance is metabolized by the liver to memantine glucuronide conjugate, 6-hydroxy memantine, and 1-nitroso-deaminated memantine, which also has minor activity as an NMDA receptor antagonist; V_{dss} is $14.4 \pm 0.9.7$ L/kg. Clearance is 0.16 ± 0.03 L/kg/h. After 22 days at doses of 10 mg once daily in young healthy men, mean trough serum levels of memantine are 25.9 ± 4.1 mg/L and peaks are 35.2 ± 4.5 mg/L. Pharmacokinetics are linear after investigated doses of 5–40 mg. Elimination is prolonged in patients with severe renal impairment.[28–31] **Half-Life.** 60–80 h.

Adverse Reactions. Headache, dizziness, fainting, confusion, hallucinations, insomnia, diarrhea, and constipation are the most frequent adverse effects reported in patients with moderately severe to severe dementia.

Contraindications. Memantine is contraindicated in patients with known hypersensitivity to memantine or any excipients in the formulation.

Precautions. Patients and caregivers should follow the recommended titration schedule. Seizures have rarely occurred in patients taking memantine, but at no greater frequency (0.2%) than in patients taking a placebo. Conditions or medications that raise urine pH may decrease renal elimination of memantine, resulting in increased plasma levels of the drug. This event may increase the risk of adverse reactions. Conversely, conditions that lower urine pH may cause lower plasma levels. Use with other NMDA antagonists (e.g., ketamine, amantadine, dextromethorphan) has not been studied and should be undertaken cautiously.

Drug Interactions. Urine alkalinizers (carbonic anhydrase inhibitors, sodium bicarbonate) may reduce the clearance of memantine and increase plasma levels and adverse reactions. At a urine pH of 8, the clearance of memantine was reduced approximately 80%.[28] Acidification of the urine with ammonium chloride caused increase in renal excretion of memantine.[28–30] Coadministration with other drugs that are eliminated by tubular secretion (hydrochlorothiazide, triamterene, metformin, cimetidine, ranitidine, quinidine, nicotine) may theoretically alter plasma concentrations of memantine or the other drug. Coadministration of memantine and hydrochlorothiazide decreased the bioavailability of hydrochlorothiazide by 20%, but coadministration of memantine has not altered levels of either triamterene or metformin. One case of myoclonus and delirium was reported when memantine was administered along with trimethoprim in a 78-year-old woman with Alzheimer's disease.[32] No interactions have been reported with cholinesterase inhibitors.

Parameters to Monitor. Monitors of cognitive function, activities of daily living, and caregiver impression may assist evaluation of memantine effectiveness.

MONOAMINE OXIDASE INHIBITORS

RASAGILINE	Azilect
SELEGILINE	Eldepryl, Emsam, Zelapar

Pharmacology. Rasagiline and selegiline (formerly L-deprenyl) are irreversible monoamine oxidase inhibitors. Selegiline is selective for MAO-B; rasagiline inhibits MAO-B, but its selectivity for MAO-B has not been determined.[33,34] Both are used as adjunctive therapy in the management of Parkinson's disease.

In addition, rasagiline is approved for monotherapy for Parkinson's disease. MAO-B is found in the brain and plays a role in the catabolism of dopamine. By preventing the breakdown of dopamine by MAO-B, selegiline and rasagiline increase the net amount of dopamine available in the brain.

Administration and Adult Dosage. **PO for adjunctive therapy to levodopa in Parkinson's disease**—(selegiline) 5 mg twice daily taken at breakfast and lunch. Alternatively, give an initial dosage of 2.5 mg/d and slowly increase to 10 mg/d over several weeks to minimize side effects.[35] There is no evidence that dosages >10 mg/d increase efficacy, and they can lead to nonspecific inhibition of MAO-A. (Rasagiline) 0.5 mg once daily. If response is not adequate, may be increased to 1 mg daily. **PO for monotherapy in Parkinson's disease**—(rasagiline) 1 mg once daily.

Special Populations. *Pediatric Dosage.* Safety and efficacy not established.

Geriatric Dosage. Same as adult dosage.

Other conditions. (Rasagiline) patients with mild liver impairment (Child-Pugh score 5 and 6) should take a maximum dose of 0.5 mg daily. Do not use in moderate or severe liver impairment. Patients taking ciprofloxacin or other CYP1A2 inhibitors should take a maximum of 0.5 mg daily.

Dosage Forms. (Selegiline) **Cap** 5 mg; **Tab** 5 mg; **Orally Disintegrating Tab** 1.25 mg; **Patch** 6 mg/24 h, 9 mg/24 h, 12 mg/24 h (Emsam). (Rasagiline) **Tab** 0.5, 1 mg.

Patient Instructions. Take this medication early in the day (morning to midday) to minimize nighttime insomnia. At a selegiline dosage of 10 mg/d or less, tyramine-containing foods and medications containing amines are safe to consume. Initiation of selegiline might require a reduction of carbidopa/levodopa dosage. Take selegiline with food to reduce nausea. Report immediately any severe headache or other unusual or unexpected symptoms. Patients taking rasagiline should avoid foods containing tyramine (aged, dried, fermented meats; aged cheeses; red wine; tap beer and no-pasteurized beer; fava bean pods; concentrated yeast extract; sauerkraut; most soybean products, including soy sauce and tofu) and OTC medications containing sympathomimetic drugs such as pseudoephedrine and phenylephrine.[34]

Missed Doses. Take this drug at regular intervals. If you miss a dose, take it as soon as you remember. If it is about time for the next dose, take that dose only. Do not double the dose or take an extra dose. Do not take late in the evening.

Pharmacokinetics. *Onset and Duration.* (Selegiline) recovery of platelet MAO-B activity after a single oral dose of selegiline is 2–4 days; after long-term treatment, >90% of platelet MAO-B remains inhibited after 5 days.[36] (Rasagiline) 90% inhibition of MAO-B was achieved after 3 days of dosing. Inhibition of MAO-B lasts at least 1 week after last dose.[34]

Fate. (Selegiline) readily absorbed from the GI tract, with a peak at 0.5–2 h; 85% is bound to plasma proteins.[33] It is metabolized by the liver to N-desmethylselegiline, L-amphetamine, and L-methamphetamine; these isomers, however, are only 10% as potent as the D-isomers. After long-term therapy with 10 mg/d in 2 divided doses, mean trough serum levels of selegiline and N-desmethylselegiline are undetectable; L-amphetamine is 5.9 ± 2.7 µg/L (22 ± 10 nmol/L) and L-methamphetamine is 14.9 ± 6.8 µg/L (100 ± 45 nmol/L). The concentrations of these metabolites are probably too low to contribute to the drug's clinical efficacy but can contribute to adverse effects. Approximately 86% is excreted in urine as inactive metabolites.[35,36] (Rasagiline) T_{max} approximately 1 h after dosing; bioavailability is ~36%. Plasma protein binding is 88%–94%. Rasagiline is metabolized in the liver, with CYP1A2 being the major isoenzyme involved. Elimination is via urinary excretion after glucuronide conjugation of rasagiline and its metabolites.[34] **Half-life.** (N-desmethylselegiline) 2 ± 1.2 h; (L-amphetamine) 17.7 ± 16.3 h; (L-methamphetamine) 20.5 ± 11.4 h.[35,36] (Rasagiline) 3 h.

Adverse Reactions. Nausea, abdominal pain, dry mouth, confusion, hallucinations, dizziness, insomnia, lightheadedness, and/or fainting occur frequently. Vivid dreams, dyskinesias, and headache occur occasionally. In decreasing order of frequency—nausea, hallucinations, confusion, depression, loss of balance, and insomnia—can lead to discontinuation. Mild, asymptomatic elevations in liver function tests can occur.

Contraindications. Rasagiline and selegiline are contraindicated for use with meperidine. Concomitant use of meperidine has precipitated coma, severe hypertension or hypotension, respiratory depression, seizures, malignant hyperpyrexia, peripheral vascular collapse, and death. At least 14 days should elapse between discontinuation of rasagiline or selegiline and treatment with meperidine. Likewise, rasagiline and selegiline should not be used with tramadol, methadone, and propoxyphene. Dextromethorphan should not be used in combination with MAO inhibitors because of reports of psychotic behavior. Use along with other MAO inhibitors is also contraindicated.[36] Rasagiline is also contraindicated with St. John's wort, mirtazapine, cyclobenzaprine, and sympathomimetic amines such as amphetamines, pseudoephedrine, and phenylephrine. Patients taking rasagiline should discontinue the drug at least 14 days prior to elective surgery. If surgery is necessary sooner, benzodiazepines, mivacurium, rapacuronium, fentanyl, morphine, and codeine may be used cautiously, but cocaine or local anesthetics containing epinephrine should not be used.[36] MAOIs should not be used in patients with pheochromocytoma.

Precautions. Pregnancy; lactation. Do not use at dosages exceeding 1 mg/d of rasagiline or 10 mg/d of selegiline. Patients with Parkinson's disease are at increased risk for melanoma; dermatological screening is recommended. Use with levodopa increases the risk of hypotension and may exacerbate preexisting dyskinesia. (Rasagiline) avoid tyramine-rich foods. Use with caution in mild hepatic impairment; do not use in moderate to severe hepatic impairment.

Drug Interactions. Concurrent administration of selegiline or rasagiline and serotonin reuptake inhibitors (e.g., SSRIs, nefazodone, venlafaxine) can cause serotonin syndrome; do not give them within 1–2 weeks of each other (5 weeks after stopping fluoxetine). Tricyclic antidepressants also pose a risk that increases with higher doses. (Rasagiline) metabolism is inhibited by CYP1A2 inhibitors such as ciprofloxacin.

Parameters to Monitor. Evaluate cardiovascular status and monitor liver function tests periodically. Monitor Parkinson's disease symptoms periodically. Monitor for development of melanoma, which occurs more often in patients with Parkinson's disease.[36]

Notes. **Emsam** is selegiline in a transdermal patch with an indication for major depressive disorder. It is dosed at 6 mg (initially), 9 mg, or 12 mg daily.[37]

RILUZOLE
Rilutek

Pharmacology. In the treatment of amyotrophic lateral sclerosis, riluzole is hypothesized to protect motor neurons from degeneration and death. Although the exact mechanism of action is unknown, there are 3 pharmacologic properties of the drug that are thought to be relevant: inhibition of glutamate release, inactivation of voltage-dependent sodium channels, and interference with intracellular events that follow activation of excitatory amino acid receptors.[38]

Administration and Adult Dosage. **PO for amyotrophic lateral sclerosis**—50 mg every 12 h, 1 h before or 2 h after a meal.

Special Populations. *Geriatric Dosage.* Same as adult dosage.

Dosage Forms. **Tab** 50 mg.

Patient Instructions. Take this medication at the same time each day on an empty stomach. It can cause dizziness, drowsiness, or vertigo. Until the extent of these effects is known, use caution when driving, operating machinery, or performing tasks requiring mental alertness. Do not drink alcohol while taking this medication. Contact your doctor if fever or flulike symptoms occur. Protect the drug from exposure to light.[38]

Missed Doses. Take this drug at regular intervals. If you miss a dose, take it as soon as you remember. If it is about time for the next dose, take that dose only. Do not double the dose or take an extra dose.

Pharmacokinetics. *Fate.* Riluzole is rapidly absorbed, with approximately 90% absorbed, but absolute bioavailability is $60 \pm 9\%$ because of a first-pass effect. Peak serum concentrations occur within 60–90 min.[39] A high-fat meal decreases the AUC by approximately 20%. Approximately 96% is bound to serum proteins, mainly albumin and lipoproteins; it is distributed extensively throughout the body, with a V_d of approximately 3.4 L/kg; clearance is 0.7 L/h/kg in white males. Riluzole is metabolized extensively in the liver to at least 6 major metabolites, mainly by CYP1A2 (hydroxylated derivatives) and P450-dependent glucuronidation.[40] Its metabolism is slower by 32% in women and by 50% in subjects native to Japan than in white males. Glucuronides account for approximately 85% of urine metabolites.[40–42] **Half-life.** 12 ± 1.8 h.

Adverse Reactions. Nausea, constipation, vomiting, abdominal pain, elevations in AST and ALT (50% experience levels above the upper limit of normal), asthenia, dizziness, diarrhea, vertigo, and circumoral paresthesia occur frequently. Decreased lung function, pneumonia, somnolence, and neutropenia occur occasionally (3 cases of neutropenia in 4000 during clinical trials).

Contraindications. Riluzole is contraindicated in patients with a history of hypersensitivity reactions to the drug or any tablet excipients.

Precautions. Use with caution in patients with renal or hepatic disease, especially the elderly. Also, females and Japanese patients may possess a lower metabolic capacity to eliminate riluzole. Because of the risk of neutropenia, patients should report febrile illness to their physicians immediately.

Drug Interactions. Riluzole might interact with other drugs that also are metabolized by CYP1A2, including theophylline, caffeine, fluoroquinolones, and amitriptyline. Enzyme inducers of CYP1A2 and cigarette smoking increase the metabolism of riluzole.[38]

Parameters to Monitor. Monitor liver function tests every month for the first 3 months of therapy, then every 3 months for the rest of the first year. Approximately 8% of patients on riluzole will have ALT elevations >3 times the upper limit of normal.[38]

RIVASTIGMINE Exelon

Pharmacology. Rivastigmine is an intermediate-acting (pseudoirreversible) AChE inhibitor that binds to AChE, resulting in a carbamated form of AChE that cannot hydrolyze acetylcholine. This action increases CNS acetylcholine activity. It is indicated for treatment of mild-to-moderate symptoms of dementia of the Alzheimer's type and for mild-to-moderate dementia associated with Parkinson's disease.[42,43]

Administration and Adult Dosage. **PO for mild-to-moderate dementia in Alzheimer's disease or Parkinson's disease**—1.5 mg twice daily initially. After at least 2 weeks, increase in 1.5-mg increments every 2 weeks as tolerated, to a maximum of 6 mg twice daily. If more than a few days of therapy are missed, resume therapy at the initial dose of 1.5 mg twice daily. **Patch for mild-to-moderate dementia in Alzheimer's disease or Parkinson's disease**—4.6 mg/24 h initially. After at least 4 weeks and if well tolerated, increase to 9.5 mg/24 h.

Special Populations. *Geriatric Dosage.* No specific dosage adjustment is needed because the dose is adjusted to patient tolerance.

Dosage Forms. **Cap** 1.5, 3, 4.5, 6 mg; **Soln** 2 mg/mL; **Patch** 4.6 mg/24 h (9 mg rivastigmine in 5 cm^2 patch) 9.5 mg/24 h (18 mg rivastigmine in 10 cm^2 patch).

Patient Instructions. **Oral**—take this drug with food in the morning and evening. **Patch**—apply patch to skin and rotate application site to minimize irritation of skin.[42] The same site should not be used again for 2 weeks. To discard, fold patch in half and return to original pouch before throwing away. Keep away from children and pets. The patch will still contain some drug after removal.[43]

Dosage will be increased approximately every 2 weeks until the maximum tolerable dose is reached. If you experience adverse effects, such as loss of appetite, nausea, vomiting, or abdominal pain, stop treatment for several doses and then resume at the same or next lower dose level. Inform your physician if these symptoms occur.

Missed Doses. Take this drug at regular intervals. If you miss a dose, take it as soon as you remember. If it is within a few hours of the next dose, take that dose only. Do not double the dose or take an extra dose. If you miss more than a few doses, do not resume the same dosage. Inform your physician.

Pharmacokinetics. *Onset and Duration.* After 6 mg, anticholinesterase activity is present in the CSF for approximately 10 h, with a maximum inhibition of approximately 60% 5 h after a dose.

Fate. Rivastigmine is rapidly and completely absorbed with bioavailability of approximately 36% after a 3-mg dose. Peak plasma concentrations occur within 1 h, with peak CSF concentrations achieved in 1.4–2.6 h. Food delays plasma peak time by 90 min, lowers the peak by 30%, and increases bioavailability by 30%.

Rivastigmine is 40% bound to plasma proteins; V_d is 1.8–2.7 L/kg.[44] Clearance is 108 ± 36 L/h after 6 mg twice daily. Pharmacokinetics are nonlinear at doses above 3 mg 2 times a day. Metabolism is mainly by cholinesterase-mediated hydrolysis. It is then eliminated renally, with 97% of the dose detected in the urine as metabolites, most commonly as the sulfate conjugate of the decarbamylated metabolite (40%). Clearance is reduced in the elderly (by 30%) and in patients with renal (by 64%) or hepatic (by 60%) disease. Only 0.4% is eliminated in the feces. **Half-life.** 1.5 h.[42]

Adverse Reactions. Nausea (47%) and vomiting (31%) are frequent occurrences in patients, especially women, treated with 6–12 mg/d and are more likely during the titration phase rather than the maintenance phase. Anorexia and weight loss also occur more frequently in women. Other side effects are dizziness, headache, tremor, abdominal pain, dyspepsia, hypotension, orthostatic hypotension, insomnia, tinnitus, palpitations, confusion, anemia, and rash.[42,43] Resumption of a high dose after a few days without taking the drug can result in severe vomiting and esophageal perforation.

Contraindications. Hypersensitivity to rivastigmine, other carbamate derivatives, or other components of the formulation.[42]

Precautions. (*See* Donepezil.) Induction of extrapyramidal symptoms and worsening of Parkinson's symptoms have been seen. Patients and/or caregivers should be instructed on the proper administration of the oral solution. Increased risk of adverse effects in patient with low body weight (<50 kg) on patch, particularly when titrating above 9.5 mg/24 h.

Drug Interactions. Excessive cholinergic effect can occur if rivastigmine is given with cholinergic drugs (e.g., succinylcholine, bethanechol). Rivastigmine can antagonize the effects of anticholinergic drugs and antiparkinson's drugs. On the basis of in vitro studies, rivastigmine does not interact with digoxin, warfarin, diazepam, or fluoxetine. Rivastigmine pharmacokinetics are not altered by antacids, antihypertensives, calcium channel blockers, antidiabetics, NSAIDs, salicylates, antianginals, antihistamines, estrogens, or β-blockers. Rivastigmine can increase the risk of GI side effects from NSAIDs because of the possible increase in stomach acid production.

Parameters to Monitor. Because of the high frequency of nausea, vomiting, and anorexia, monitor patients for these reactions and for possible weight loss.

Notes. In switching from capsules or oral solution to patch: An oral total daily dose of <6 mg rivastigmine can be switched to 4.6 mg/24 h patch. For oral total-daily dose of 6–12 mg rivastigmine, switch to 9.5 mg/24 h patch. Apply the first patch on the day following the last oral dose.[43]

TETRABENAZINE	Xenazine

Pharmacology. Tetrabenazine is a reversible inhibitor of human vesicular monoamine transporter type 2 (VMAT2) and is approved for the chorea symptoms of Huntington's disease. The mechanism is unknown but is considered to be related to its effect in reversibly depleting monoamines (e.g., dopamine, histamine, norepinephrine, and serotonin) from nerve terminals. Tetrabenazine also has weak binding at the dopamine D_2 receptor in vitro.[45]

Administration and Adult Dosage. **PO for Huntington's disease**—initially, 12.5 mg once daily in the morning. After 1 week increase to 12.5 mg twice daily, and titrate by 12.5 mg increases every week. The maximum single dose is 25 mg. Doses of 37.5 mg or higher should be given as a 3 times daily regimen. Stop titration and reduce the dose if adverse effects such as parkinsonism, depression, akathisia, or intolerable sedation occur. Patients who need doses over 50 mg daily should be genotyped for CYP2D6. Poor metabolizers (patients who do not express CYP2D6) should not be increased beyond 50 mg daily. For extensive and intermediate metabolizers, continue to a maximum dose of 100 mg and maximum single dose of 37.5 mg. Tetrabenazine may be discontinued without tapering. After more than 5 days of treatment interruptions, tetrabenazine should be retitrated if resumed.[45]

Dosage Forms. **Tab** 12.5, 25 mg.

Pharmacokinetics. Oral bioavailability is $\geq$ 75%; food has no effect on absorption. Tetrabenazine is rapidly transformed into active metabolites by the liver, which peak within 90 min after dosing. Protein binding of tetrabenazine and its metabolites is 60%–85%. Metabolism is primarily by CYP2D6. Urinary excretion of metabolites accounts for 75% of the dose. **Half-life.** Major metabolites are 2–8 h, but prolonged in patients who have liver disease or who lack CYP2D6.[45]

Adverse Reactions. Sedation, depression, anxiety, insomnia, fatigue, akathisia, nausea, hypotension, falls, and upper respiratory tract infections occur frequently (>10%). Suicidal thoughts and actions and changes in behavior have occurred in patients taking this drug. Tetrabenazine dramatically increases prolactin levels (4-fold or greater). Use caution in patients with prolactin-dependent breast cancer. Since tetrabenazine may cause extrapyramidal symptoms as neuroleptics do, tardive dyskinesia is believed to be a possibility with this drug, but as yet it has not been reported.[45]

Contraindications. Patients with liver impairment, patients with suicidal ideation or inadequately treated for depression, patients taking MAOIs or reserpine. Patients who have untreated or inadequately treated depression and impaired hepatic function. Use of tetrabenazine within 20 days of reserpine discontinuation.

Precautions. Avoid in combination with other drugs known to prolong the QT interval. Monitor for symptoms such as akathisia, parkinsonism, sedation, somnolence, and dysphagia, hypotension, and orthostatic hypotension.

Drug interactions. Increased risk of neuroleptic malignant syndrome with concomitant use of neuroleptic drugs. Worsening of sedation with alcohol and other sedatives. Reserpine should be discontinued for >20 days before initiating tetrabenazine. It should not be used concomitantly with MAOIs.

Notes. Tetrabenazine is only available from specialty pharmacies.

TOLCAPONE	Tasmar

Pharmacology. Tolcapone reversibly inhibits at least 80% of the activity of COMT. This action prevents the metabolism of levodopa to 3-O-methyldopa and thus prolongs its duration of action, especially with coadministration of carbidopa.[46,47] Tolcapone increases plasma levodopa bioavailability by approximately 2-fold and variably prolongs the terminal half-life of levodopa (given with carbidopa) in the elderly from 2 h to as long as 3.5 h, but has no effect on the peak serum levels of levodopa or the time at which they occur. (*See* Notes.)

Administration and Adult Dosage. **PO for Parkinson's disease**—100 mg 3 times a day initially, always as an adjunct to levodopa/carbidopa therapy, increasing to a maximum of 200 mg 3 times daily. If the patient shows no substantial clinical benefit after 3 weeks of therapy, discontinue tolcapone. (*See* Parameters to Monitor.)

Special Populations. *Geriatric Dosage.* Same as adult dosage.

Dosage Forms. **Tab** 100, 200 mg.

Patient Instructions. This drug can lower blood pressure and cause unsteadiness, nausea, or sweating initially. Do not rise rapidly after sitting or lying down. It also can cause drowsiness. Until the extent of these effects is known, use caution when driving, operating machinery, or performing tasks that require mental alertness. This drug also can worsen dyskinesias or dystonia when it is first started and might require adjustment of the amount of carbidopa/levodopa you are taking. Because of the risk of liver damage with this drug, you will require regular liver enzyme tests. Notify your physician immediately if signs of liver toxicity develop.

Missed Doses. Take this drug at regular intervals. If you miss a dose, take it as soon as you remember. If it is about time for the next dose, take that dose only. Do not double the dose or take an extra dose.

Pharmacokinetics. *Onset and Duration.* Onset 1–2 h; duration 12–24 h.

Fate. Approximately 65% is orally absorbed. A peak serum concentration of 6.3 ± 2.9 mg/L occurs 1.8 ± 1.3 h after a 200-mg dose. Food increases the peak time and decreases the peak and AUC of tolcapone. Approximately 99.9% is bound to plasma proteins, mainly albumin. The predominant metabolic pathway is glucuronidation. Major metabolites that are a product of oxidative processes include 3-*O*-methyltolcapone and carboxylic acid derivatives metabolized by CYP2A6 and CYP3A4. Those that are a product of reductive processes include amines and N-acetyl derivatives. Clearance is approximately 0.1 L/kg/h. Approximately 40% of an orally administered dose is excreted in the urine and feces in 24 h and >95% in 7–9 days. Less than 0.5% of tolcapone is excreted unchanged in urine.[47,48]

Half-life. (tolcapone) 2 ± 0.8 h (3-*O*-methyltolcapone) 32 ± 7 h.[47,48]

Adverse Reactions. Tolcapone has caused several cases of severe, fulminant liver failure that were sometimes fatal. Monitor liver function carefully. Adverse reactions consistent with increased levodopa exposure include worsening dyskinesia, nausea, sleep disorders, dystonia, somnolence, anorexia, hallucinations, and postural hypotension. They might be lessened by reducing levodopa dosage. Urine discoloration also occurs and is attributable to the yellow color of tolcapone and its metabolites. Other tolcapone-related side effects include headache, abdominal pain, and diarrhea. The most common reason for drug discontinuation from clinical studies was severe diarrhea in 3% of patients. The onset is often delayed and usually occurs within 0.5–3 months after initiation of therapy.

Contraindications. Liver disease or in patients who have discontinued tolcapone therapy because of liver toxicity; history of rhabdomyolysis caused by any medication; history of hyperpyrexia and confusion related to medication use or to medication discontinuation.

Precautions. Because of the risk of liver failure, tolcapone should be used only in Parkinson's disease patients on carbidopa/levodopa who are not appropriate candidates for other adjunctive therapies. Any patient who fails to have substantial benefit after 3 weeks of tolcapone therapy should have the drug withdrawn.[46] Orthostatic hypotension, hallucinations, diarrhea, or dyskinesias can occur at the initiation of therapy. Use with caution in patients with renal impairment. Follow recommended plan for monitoring liver enzymes. Discontinue tolcapone if ALT or AST exceeds the upper limit of normal or if the patient develops signs and symptoms of liver failure (jaundice, anorexia, dark urine, pruritus, nausea, and right upper quadrant tenderness). The patient should sign a consent form before therapy is initiated.

Drug Interactions. Tolcapone can inhibit the metabolism of other drugs also metabolized by COMT (e.g., dobutamine, isoproterenol) and exacerbate the dopaminergic side effects of other antiparkinsonian agents. It does not interact with ephedrine or desipramine (a substrate for CYP2D6) but has in vivo affinity for CYP2C9 (although the clinical relevance is undetermined).

Parameters to Monitor. Before starting treatment, conduct tests to exclude the presence of liver disease. Obtain ALT and AST levels at baseline and then every 2 weeks for the first year of therapy, every 4 weeks for the next 6 months, and every 8 weeks thereafter. Tolcapone should be discontinued if ALT or AST levels exceed 2 times the upper limit of normal or if signs or symptoms of liver dysfunction occur.[46] If the dose is increased, begin liver enzyme monitoring again as when the drug was initiated.

Notes. Tolcapone can be administered on a schedule (3 times daily) and does not need to be administered with each dose of levodopa. In clinical trials, the average decrease in daily levodopa dosage was approximately 30% in ~70% of patients. Tolcapone has no benefit when used alone. It should only be used in Parkinson's patients who have symptom fluctuations and have not responded to other adjunctive therapy.[2]

TRIHEXYPHENIDYL HYDROCHLORIDE   Various

Pharmacology. Trihexyphenidyl is a competitive antagonist of acetylcholine at central muscarinic receptors. In Parkinson's disease, it is an adjunctive treatment that balances cholinergic and dopaminergic activities in cerebral synapses.

Administration and Adult Dosage. **PO for Parkinson's disease**—1 mg/d initially, increasing in 2 mg/d increments every 3–5 days, to a maximum of 12–15 mg/d. **Usual maintenance dosage**—6–10 mg/d in 3 divided doses or 3–6 mg/d in 3 divided doses concurrent with levodopa. **PO for drug-induced extrapyramidal disorders**—1 mg initially, increasing in 1-mg increments every few hours until symptoms are controlled, usually 5–15 mg/d in 3–4 divided doses.[49,50]

Dosage Forms. **Elxr** 0.4 mg/mL; **Tab** 2, 5 mg.[49]

Pharmacokinetics. The onset of action is within 1 h, and the peak effect lasts 2–3 h; the duration of action is 6–12 h. The majority of the drug is excreted in the urine, probably unchanged. **Half-Life.** 10.2 ± 4.7 h.[7]

Adverse Reactions. Adverse reactions, precautions, contraindications, and drug interactions are the same as those for benztropine. When trihexyphenidyl is used concurrently with levodopa, the dosages of both drugs might require reduction.

Precautions. Use with great caution in patients >65 years because they are more sensitive to the effects of anticholinergic agents.

DOPAMINE AGONISTS COMPARISON CHART

DRUG	DOSAGE FORMS	ADULT DOSAGE	DOPAMINE RECEPTOR SELECTIVITY				EFFECT ON CYTOCHROME P450 ISOZYMES	HALF-LIFE (h)
			D_1	D_2	D_3	D_4		
Apomorphine[a] Apokyn	SQ Inj 10 mg/mL in 3 mL cartridge	SQ for "off" episodes 0.2 mL (2 mg) initially[a], up to maximum 0.6 mL (6 mg)	0/+	++	++	++++	No effect	0.5–1
Bromocriptine Parlodel	Cap 5 mg Tab 2.5 mg	PO 1.25 mg twice daily initially, increasing in 2.5 mg/d increments every 2 weeks to a usual dosage of 10–40 mg/d	0/+	++	+	0/+	*Inhibits CYP3A4*	4
Pramipexole Mirapex	Tab 0.125, 0.25, 1, 1.5 mg	PO 0.125 mg 3 times daily initially, increasing in increments of 0.75 mg/d at weekly intervals to a usual dosage of 1.5–4.5 mg/d in 3 divided doses	0	++	++++	++	No effect	12

(continued)

DOPAMINE AGONISTS COMPARISON CHART (*continued*)

DRUG	DOSAGE FORMS	ADULT DOSAGE	DOPAMINE RECEPTOR SELECTIVITY D_1	D_2	D_3	D_4	EFFECT ON CYTOCHROME P450 ISOZYMES	HALF-LIFE (h)
Ropinirole Requip Requip XL	Tab 0.25, 0.5, 1, 2, 3, 4, 5 mg Extended-release Tab 2, 4, 8, 12 mg	PO 0.25 mg 3 times daily initially, increasing in increments of 0.75 mg/d at weekly intervals for 4 weeks, then in increments of 1.5–3 mg/d at weekly intervals to a usual dosage of 3–12 mg/a in 3 divided doses	0	++	+++	++	*Inhibits CYP2D6*	4–6

0, none; 0/+, minimal; +, mild; ++, moderate; +++, potent; ++++, very potent.
[a]Pretreat with oral trimethobenzamide.
From Refs. 15–22.

■ REFERENCES

1. Product information. Symmetrel® amantadine hydrochloride. Chadds Ford, PA: Endo Pharmaceuticals, Inc.; 2007.
2. Pahwa R et al. Practice parameter: treatment of Parkinson disease with motor fluctuations and dyskinesia (an evidence-based review). *Neurology.* 2006;66:283-295.
3. Hordam VW et al. Pharmacokinetics of amantadine hydrochloride in subjects with normal and impaired renal function. *Ann Intern Med.* 1981;94(pt 1):454-458.
4. Aoki FY, Sitar DS. Amantadine kinetics in healthy elderly men: implications for influenza prevention. *Clin Pharmacol Ther.* 1985;37:137-144.
5. Product information. Cogentin® benztropine mesylate. Whitehouse Station, NJ: Merck & Co, Inc.; 2001.
6. Product information. Benztropine mesylate. Allendale, NJ: Rising Pharmaceuticals, Inc.; 2007.
7. Stanilla JK, Simpson GM. Drugs to treat extrapyramidal side effects. In: Schatzberg AF, Nemeroff CB, eds. *Textbook of Psychopharmacology.* 3rd ed. Arlington, VA: American Psychiatric Publishing, Inc.; 2004:chap 34.
8. Product information. Sinemet CR®, carbidopa-levodopa. Whitehouse Station, NJ: Merck & Co, Inc.; 2009.
9. Nyholm D. Pharmacokinetic optimisation in the treatment of Parkinson's disease, an update. *Clin Pharmacokinet.* 2006;45:109-136.
10. Koller WC, Hubble JP. Levodopa therapy in Parkinson's disease. *Neurology.* 1990;40(suppl 3):S40-S47.
11. Cedarbaum JM. Pharmacokinetic and pharmacodynamic considerations in management of motor response fluctuations in Parkinson's disease. *Neurol Clin.* 1990;8:31-49.
12. Product information: Stalevo®, carbidopa, levodopa, and entacapone. East Hanover, NJ: Novartis Pharmaceuticals Corporation; 2008.
13. Product information: Aricept® and Aricept® ODT, donepezil hydrochloride. New York: Pfizer, Inc.; 2006.
14. Sunderland T et al. Cognitive enhancers. In: Schatzberg AF, Nemeroff CB, eds. *Textbook of Psychopharmacology.* 3rd ed. Arlington, VA: American Psychiatric Publishing, Inc.; 2004:chap 41.
15. Product information: Mirapex®, pramipexole dihydrochloride. Ridgefield, CT: Boehringer Ingleheim Pharmaceuticals, Inc.; 2009.
16. Product information: Requip® XL, ropinirole hydrochloride. Research Triangle Park, NC: GlaxoSmithKline; 2008.
17. Product information: Requip®, ropinirole hydrochloride. Research Triangle Park, NC: GlaxoSmithKline; 2006.
18. Product information: Apokyn®, apomorphine hydrochloride. Morristown, NJ: Vernalis Pharmaceuticals, Inc.; 2006.
19. Product information: Parlodel®, bromocriptine mesylate. East Hanover, NJ: Novartis Pharmaceuticals Corporation; 2003.
20. Schran HF et al. The pharmacokinetics of bromocriptine in man. In: Goldstein M et al., eds. *Ergot Compounds and Brain Function.* New York: Raven Press; 1980:125-139.
21. Friis ML et al. Pharmacokinetics of bromocriptine during continuous oral treatment of Parkinson's disease. *Eur J Clin Pharmacol.* 1979;15:275-280.
22. Bonucelli U, Pavese N. Role of dopamine agonists in Parkinson's disease: an update. *Expert Rev Neurother.* 2007;7:1391-1399.
23. Product information: Comtan®, entacapone. East Hanover, NJ: Novartis Pharmaceuticals Corporation; 2000.
24. Bonifati V, Meco G. New, selective catechol-*O*-methyltransferase inhibitors as therapeutic agents in Parkinson's disease. *Pharmacol Ther.* 1999;81:1-36.
25. Keränen T et al. Inhibition of soluble catechol-*O*-methyltransferase and single-dose pharmacokinetics after oral and intravenous administration of entacapone. *Eur J Clin Pharmacol.* 1994;46:151-157.
26. Product information: Razadyne® and Razadyne® ER, galantamine hydrobromide. Titusville, NJ: Ortho-McNeil Neurologics; 2008.
27. Scott LJ, Goa KL. Galantamine. A review of its use in Alzheimer's disease. *Drugs.* 2000;60:1095-1022.
28. Product information: Namenda®, memantine hydrochloride. St. Louis, MO: Forest Pharmaceuticals, Inc.; 2006.
29. Chladek J et al. Steady-state bioequivalence studies of two memantine tablet and oral solution formulations in healthy volunteers. *J Appl Biomed.* 2007;6:39-45.
30. Kornhuber J et al. Memantine pharmacotherapy—a naturalistic study using a population pharmacokinetic approach. *Clin Pharmacokinet.* 2007;46:599-612.
31. Liu Ming-Yan et al. Pharmacokinetics of single-dose and multiple-dose memantine in healthy Chinese volunteers using an analytic method of liquid chromatography-tandem mass spectrometry. *Clin Ther.* 2008;30:641-653.
32. Moellentin D et al. Memantine-induced myoclonus and delirium exacerbated by trimethoprim. *Ann Pharmacother.* 2008;42:443-447.
33. Product information: Zelapar®, selegiline hydrochloride. Costa Mesa, CA: Valeant Pharmaceuticals International, 2006.

34. Product information: Azilect®, rasagiline. Kansas City, MO: Teva Neuroscience, Inc.; 2006.

35. Youdim MBH, Finberg JPM. Pharmacological actions of l-deprenyl (selegiline) and other selective monoamine oxidase B inhibitors. *Clin Pharmacol Ther.* 1994;56:725-733.

36. Mahmood I. Clinical pharmacokinetics and pharmacodynamics of selegiline. *Clin Pharmacokinet.* 1997;33:99-102.

37. Product information: Emsam®, selegiline transdermal system. Tampa, FL: Somerset Pharmaceuticals, Inc., 2008.

38. Product information: Rilutek®, riluzole. Bridgewater, NJ: Sanofi-Aventis U.S. LLC; 2006.

39. Bryson HM et al. Riluzole. A review of its pharmacodynamic and pharmacokinetic properties and therapeutic potential in amyotrophic lateral sclerosis. *Drugs.* 1996;52:549-563.

40. Sanderink GJ et al. Involvement of human CYP1A isoenzymes in the metabolism and drug interactions of riluzole in vitro. *J Pharmacol Exp Ther.* 1997;282:1465-1472.

41. Bruno E et al. Population pharmacokinetics of riluzole in patients with amyotrophic lateral sclerosis. *Clin Pharmacol Ther.* 1997;62:518-526.

42. Product information: Exelon®, rivastigmine. East Hanover, NJ: Novartis Pharmaceuticals Corporation; 2006.

43. Product information: Exelon Patch ®, rivastigmine transdermal system. East Hanover, NJ: Novartis Pharmaceuticals Corporation, 2009.

44. Jann MW. Rivastigmine, a new-generation cholinesterase inhibitor for the treatment of Alzheimer's disease. *Pharmacotherapy.* 2000;20:471-512.

45. Product information: Xenazine®, tetrabenazine. Deerfield, IL: Ovation Pharmaceuticals, Inc.; 2008.

46. Product information: Tasmar®, tolcapone. Aliso Viejo, CA: Valeant Pharmaceuticals North America; 2008.

47. Dingemanse J et al. Integrated pharmacokinetics and pharmacodynamics of the novel catechol-*O*-methyltransferase inhibitor tolcapone during first administration to humans. *Clin Pharmacol Ther.* 1995;57:508-517.

48. Jorga KM et al. Optimizing levodopa pharmacokinetics with multiple tolcapone doses in the elderly. *Clin Pharmacol Ther.* 1997;62:300-310.

49. Product information: Trihexyphenidyl hydrochloride. Corona, CA: Watson Laboratories, Inc.; 2006.

50. Product information: Trihexyphenidyl hydrochloride oral solution. Marietta, GA: VersaPharm, Inc.; 2005.

Chapter 42

Ophthalmic Drugs for Glaucoma

Mikael D. Jones

Class Instructions. *Ophthalmic Solutions.* Proper instillation of eye drops improves absorption of the drug into the eye and minimizes systemic absorption and adverse effects. If you wear contact lenses, remove them. Wash your hands before instilling eye drops. Tilt the head back and pull down the lower lid. Place one drop into the lower lid. Once medication has been placed in the eye(s), close the eye(s) and press lightly on the inside corner of each eye. Keep the eye(s) closed and continue pressure to the inside corner of the eye(s) for 2–5 min. Wash your hands to remove medication. If you miss a dose, apply it as soon as possible. If it is almost time for your next dose, skip the missed dose and go back to your regular schedule. Do not double doses.[1]

Ophthalmic Ointments. If you wear contact lenses, remove them. Wash your hands. Tilt the head back and pull down the lower lid. Unless told to use a different amount, squeeze a thin strip (approximately 0.5 cm) of ointment into the lower lid. Let go of the eyelid and close the eye(s) for 1–2 min. Wash your hands to remove any medication. To keep the medication as sterile as possible, do not touch the tip to any surface. Wipe the tip with a clean tissue before closing. If you miss a dose, take it as soon as possible. If it is almost time for your next dose, skip the missed dose and go back to your regular dosage schedule. Do not double doses.[1] If multiple eye preparations are used, they should be separated by 5–10 min. Solutions and suspensions should be applied 5–10 min before applying a gel.

Pharmacology. The only medical treatment for primary open-angle glaucoma is to decrease intraocular pressure (IOP), the only treatable risk factor. Glaucoma drugs lower IOP by reducing production of aqueous humor, decreasing the resistance to the outflow of aqueous humor through the trabecular meshwork, and improving flow through uveoscleral pathway.[2,3]

Administration and Dosage. The ocular cul-de-sac has a capacity of only approximately 7–9 μL. After instillation of an eye drop, this capacity temporarily increases to 30 μL.[4] The drop size of glaucoma medications range from 25.1 to 56.4 μL, which exceeds the capacity of the cul-de-sac.[4] Control dosage by changing the concentration of the solution rather than instilling multiple drops. Ophthalmic solutions are generally administered at a frequency that is determined by their duration of action. Gels provide a sustained-release of active drug from the vehicle, allowing some products to be administered less frequently than solutions of the same drug. Because they are effective and have relatively fewer adverse effects, begin treatment with a β-adrenergic blockers or prostaglandin analogues with a goal of decreasing IOP by 20%.[5] To slow progression of visual field loss, patients with normal tension glaucoma or patients with severe disease require greater reductions, possibly to as low as 30%–50% from baseline.[5,6] If monotherapy alone lowers IOP without reaching target pressure, then combination therapy or switching to alternative first-line agent, or a carbonic anhydrase inhibitor (CAI), or brimonidine is appropriate. Increasing the concentration or dose frequency can also be tried when possible. Frequency should not be increased with the prostaglandin analogues.[2,5,6]

Patient Instructions. Patient adherence to glaucoma regimens is poor with up to 80% of patients deviating from prescribed regimen.[7] Use adherence aids, the least complex regimen, and educate patients about their glaucoma and administration of their glaucoma medications. (*See* Class Instructions.)

Pharmacokinetics. The eye is mostly secluded from systemic access. A majority of glaucoma medications are administered topically to the cornea, and therefore the following overview of ocular pharmacokinetics is from the prespective of topically administered medications.[8] Absorption is the process by which a drug enters the aqueous humor, and bioavailability refers to the rate and extent of absorption into the aqueous humor. After transcorneal absorption, drug is distributed to intraocular structures (ciliary body and iris) via the aqueous humor.[9]

Fate. Ophthalmic preparations must have both hydrophilic and lipophilic properties to penetrate the cornea. The epithelium and endothelium of the cornea are lipophilic. The inner layer, the stroma, is hydrophilic. The lipophilic epithelium is penetrated by the undissociated drug. Then the stroma is penetrated by the dissociated, hydrophilic drug. Corneal penetration is enhanced when the epithelium is injured or otherwise compromised.[4,9,10] Drug that does not penetrate the cornea can be spilled onto the check or systemically absorbed through the conjunctival vessels or through nasolacrimal drainage. Any remaining drug in the cul-de-sac is drained in 3–6 min.[4,10] Drugs that are systemically absorbed after ophthalmic administration do not pass through the liver; therefore, a relatively small amount of absorbed drug can result in adverse systemic effects.[11] Nasolacrimal occlusion increases drug–corneal contact time, thereby enhancing ocular absorption and decreasing systemic absorption.[4] Drugs that pass through the cornea and reach their sites of action can be metabolized by esterases, peptidases, catechol-*O*-methyl-transferase and a variety of other enzymes but mostly are eliminated from the eye by aqueous humor turnover, which is 1.5–3.4 µL/min.[12]

Half-life. For ophthalmic solutions, half-life is determined primarily by tissue binding. Many medications are eliminated by aqueous humor outflow and therefore for drugs that are not strongly bound to pigments in the iris or other tissues; half-life is determined by the aqueous humor turnover rate of 52 min.[13]

Parameters to Monitor. *General.* An ophthalmologist or optometrist should perform slit-lamp biomicroscopy, monitor IOP, and visual acuity every 2–4 weeks during initial treatment and stabilization. The patient also needs periodic evaluation of the optic nerve head and visual fields. Follow-up can range from every 1–12 months and is determined by the severity and progression of glaucoma along with level and duration of control. Decreasing the progression of the disease rather than achievement of a goal IOP is the preferred goal of therapy. Pharmacist monitoring is limited to noncompliance and detection of adverse effects.

α₂-ADRENERGIC AGONISTS	
APRACLONIDINE HYDROCHLORIDE	Iopidine
BRIMONIDINE HYDROCHLORIDE	Alphagan, Alphagan P

Pharmacology. Apraclonidine and brimonidine act at α_2-adrenergic sites in the ciliary body to inhibit norepinephrine release, causing a decrease in aqueous humor production. Brimonidine also increases uveoscleral outflow and may have neuroprotective properties.[2,3] Apraclonidine is more hydrophilic than clonidine, resulting in less permeability of the blood–brain barrier.[2,3] Apraclonidine has a high rate of tachyphylaxis, limiting it to short-term use. Brimonidine is more α_2-selective and more lipophilic than apraclonidine, allowing the use of lower concentrations.[2]

Administration and Adult Dosage. (Apraclonidine) **Ophthalmic in laser surgery**—1 drop of 1% solution in the affected eye 1 h before surgery and then 1 drop immediately after surgery to prevent the IOP spikes that occur. **Ophthalmic in open-angle glaucoma as a short-term adjunct**—1–2 drops of 0.5% solution 3 times daily. (Brimonidine) **Ophthalmic for primary open-angle glaucoma**—1 drop of 0.2% solution 3 times daily, approximately 8 h apart. (*See* Notes.)

Special Populations. *Pediatric Dosage.* (Apraclonidine) Same as adult dosage; (Brimonidine) (>2 years) Same as adult dosage. Not recommended because of concerns with CNS and respiratory depression.[2,14]

Geriatric Dosage. Same as adult dosage.

Dosage Forms. (Apraclonidine) **Ophth Soln** 0.5 and 1%. (Brimonidine) **Ophth Soln** 0.15 and 0.2%. Brimonidine 0.15% preserved with an oxychloro complex (Alphagan P) is equivalent to the 0.2% solution preserved with benzalkonium chloride (Alphagan).

Patient Instructions. *See* Ophthalmic Solutions, Class Instructions.

Pharmacokinetics. *Onset and Duration.* (Apraclonidine) onset 1 h; peak 3 h. (Brimonidine) onset 1 h; peak 2 h.

Fate. (*See* Ophthalmic Solutions, Fate.) Brimonidine, which is systemically absorbed, is metabolized primarily in the liver; 74% is eliminated in the kidney within 120 h. **Half-life.** (apraclonidine) 8 h; (brimonidine) 2.1 h. (*See* Ophthalmic Solutions, Half-life.)

Adverse Reactions. (Apraclonidine) causes adverse ocular effects in 15%–48% of patients, especially allergic reactions and rarely upper eyelid retraction. Frequent systemic effects are dry mouth and dry nose. Cardiovascular effects have not been reported.[2] (Brimonidine) has similar but less frequent ocular adverse effects. Frequent ocular effects are allergic conjunctivitis, conjunctival hyperemia, burning sensation, blepharitis, blepharoconjunctivitis, conjunctival follicles, blurred vision, and headache. Similar to apraclonidine, it frequently causes dry mouth and dry nose. Brimonidine does not decrease heart rate. It can mildly decrease blood pressure in some patients, although it frequently causes lethargy.[2,14] Several severe adverse systemic effects have been reported in children between 28 days and 3 months of age, including bradycardia, hypotension, hypothermia, hypotonia, apnea, dyspnea, hypoventilation, cyanosis, and lethargy. This is believed to be caused by immaturity of the blood–brain barrier and higher systemic concentrations because of low body weight.[15]

Precautions. Severe cardiovascular disease, cerebrovascular disease, chronic renal failure, Raynaud's diease.

Parameters to Monitor. Monitor for conjunctivitis and lethargy. (*See* Ophthalmic Solutions, Parameters to Monitor.)

Notes. Generic brimonidine 0.15% is preserved with polyquaternium-1. Brimonidine twice daily is equivalent to **timolol** 0.5% in lowering peak IOP, but much less effective in lowering trough IOP.[2,16] Brimonidine twice daily is less effective in decreasing IOP over 24 h compared to prostaglandin analogues, timolol, and dorzolamide.[17] Brimonidine twice daily is more effective than **betaxolol** 0.25% suspension at peak but similar at trough.[2] As adjunct therapy in patients who fail to reach target IOP with other therapy, brimonidine twice daily decreases IOP by an additional 4.7 ± 5.3 mm Hg, or 20%.[15] (*See* Glaucoma Drugs Comparison Chart.)

β-ADRENERGIC BLOCKING DRUGS	
BETAXOLOL HYDROCHLORIDE	Betoptic, Betoptic-S
CARTEOLOL HYDROCHLORIDE	Ocupress, Various
LEVOBUNOLOL HYDROCHLORIDE	Betagan, Various
METIPRANOLOL	Optipranolol, Various
TIMOLOL MALEATE	Timoptic, Timoptic-XE, Various

Pharmacology. β-adrenergic blocking drugs downregulate adenylate cyclase by blocking β_2-adrenergic receptors in the ciliary body, resulting in a decrease in aqueous production and IOP. Although **betaxolol** is a β_1-selective adrenergic blocker, it is effective in treating glaucoma. Betaxolol might have more β_2 activity than previously thought since small concentrations of β_2-blockade might be sufficient to curb aqueous production. β_2-receptors in the eye might be different from those in other tissues; or betaxolol's IOP-lowering effect might be caused by a calcium channel antagonistic effect.[2,18] **Carteolol** has intrinsic sympathomimetic activity (ISA) that theoretically make it less likely to cause adverse pulmonary or cardiovascular effects and possibly provide increased blood flow to the retina.[2,18,19] However, ISA does not seem to make a clinical difference in cardiac and pulmonary effects in most studies.[18,19] Retinal and optic nerve head circulations are improved by β-adrenergic blocking agents without ISA.[2,18,19]

Administration and Adult Dosage. Ophthalmic—(betaxolol) 1 drop twice daily; (carteolol) 1 drop twice daily; (levobunolol) 1 drop/d, increase to twice daily; (metipranolol) 1 drop twice daily; (timolol solution) 1 drop twice daily of 0.25% solution initially; if target IOP is not reached in 4 weeks, increase to 0.5%; (timolol gel forming solution) 1 drop/d of 0.25% solution initially; if target IOP is not reached in 4 weeks, increase to 0.5%. (*See* Notes.)

Special Populations. *Pediatric Dosage.* Same as adult dosage.

Geriatric Dosage. Same as adult dosage.

Dosage Forms. (Betaxolol) **Ophth Soln** 0.5%; **Ophth Susp** 0.25%. (Carteolol) **Ophth Soln** 1%. (Levobunolol) **Ophth Soln** 0.25% and 0.5%. (Metipranolol) **Ophth Soln** 0.3%. (Timolol) **Ophth gel-forming Soln** 0.25% and 0.5%; **Ophth Soln** 0.25% and 0.5%.

Patient Instructions. *See* Class Instructions.

Pharmacokinetics. *Onset and Duration.* (Betaxolol) onset 30 min; peak 2 h; duration 12 h. (Carteolol) onset 1 h; peak 2 h; duration 12 h. (Levobunolol) onset 1 h; peak 2–6 h; duration 24 h. (Metipranolol) onset 30 min; peak 2 h; duration 24 h. (Timolol drops) onset 30 min; peak 1–2 h; duration 24 h.

Fate. (*See* Ophthalmic Solutions, Fate.) **Half-life.** (betaxolol) 12–20 h; (carteolol) 3–7 h; (levobunolol) 6 h; (metipranolol) 3–4 h; (timolol) 3–5 h.[18] (*See* Ophthalmic Solutions, Half-life.)

Adverse Reactions. Frequent, but mild, ocular adverse effects include burning and stinging at instillation. Betaxolol ophthalmic suspension and timolol gel-forming solution frequently cause temporary blurred vision. Occasional, but serious, granulomatous anterior uveitis is caused by metipranolol.[2] Occasional, but serious, systemic reactions include bronchospasm, bradycardia, heart failure, heart block, cerebral vascular ischemia, mask symptoms of hypoglycemia and depression.[2,18,20]

Contraindications. Sinus bradycardia; greater than first-degree AV block; cardiogenic shock; overt cardiac failure. Nonselective drugs are also contraindicated in patients with histories of bronchial asthma or severe COPD.

Precautions. Diabetes mellitus; cerebrovascular insufficiency; myasthenia gravis.

Drug Interactions. Oral β-adrenergic blocking agents, calcium channel blockers, and digoxin can cause additive effects on AV conduction. Quinidine can inhibit the metabolism of β-adrenergic blocking agents by CYP2D6, causing bradycardia.

Parameters to Monitor. (*See* Ophthalmic Solutions, Parameters to Monitor.) Monitor for complaints of ocular adverse effects such as burning or stinging. Monitor heart rate, shortness of breath, nervousness, and depression.[2,18,20]

Notes. Timolol reduces the mean 24-h IOP reduction by 19% and is similar to dorzolamide.[17] With the exception of betaxolol, β-blockers are not effective when combined with **epinephrine** or **dipivefrin**. (*See* Glaucoma Drugs Comparison Chart.)

CARBONIC ANHYDRASE INHIBITORS	
ACETAZOLAMIDE	Diamox
BRINZOLAMIDE	Azopt
DORZOLAMIDE HYDROCHLORIDE	Trusopt
METHAZOLAMIDE	Neptazane

Pharmacology. CAIs inhibit the carbonic anhydrase II isoenzyme in the ciliary epithelium, thereby blocking the formation of bicarbonate. This causes a decrease in sodium and water outflow from the ciliary body. More than 99% of carbonic anhydrase must be inhibited to be effective.[2,3,20] Orally administered CAIs also inhibit carbonic anhydrase in the kidney, red blood cells, and other tissues, causing diuresis and often acidosis and other serious adverse effects that limit their use.[2,13,20]

Administration and Adult Dosage. Ophthalmic for primary open-angle glaucoma—(brinzolamide) 1 drop 3 times daily; (dorzolamide) 1 drop 3 times daily. When used adjunctively, dorzolamide is administered twice daily.[2] **PO for primary open-angle glaucoma**—(acetazolamide) **SR capsule** 500 mg twice daily has been better tolerated than tablets; **Tablet** 125 mg every 4 h to 250 mg 4 times daily. Dosages >1 g/d are not more effective. (Methazolamide) 50–100 mg 2–3 times daily. **PO for prevention of altitude sickness**—(acetazolamide) 500–1000 mg/d. (*See* Notes.)

Special Populations. *Pediatric Dosage.* (Dorzolamide) Safety and efficacy has been established for dorzolamide in children aged 3 months to 6 years. Same as adult dosage.[14,21] Safety and efficacy has been established in children 4 weeks to 5 years in age using twice-daily administration. (Acetazolamide) (1 month–12 years) 10–20 mg/kg daily in 2–4 divided doses. Maximum dose is 750 mg daily. (12–18 years) 0.5–1 g daily in 2 divided doses.[14]

Geriatric Dosage. Same as adult dosage.

Dosage Forms. (Acetazolamide) **Tab** 125 and 250 mg; **SR Cap** 500 mg; **Inj** 500 mg. (Brinzolamide) **Ophth Susp** 1%. (Dorzolamide) **Ophth Soln** 2%. (Methazolamide) **Tab** 25 and 50 mg.

Patient Instructions. *See* Class Instructions.

Pharmacokinetics. *Onset and Duration.* (Acetazolamide tablet) onset 1 h; peak IOP reduction 2–4 h; duration 6–8 h. (Acetazolamide SR capsule) onset 2 hours; peak 4–6 h; duration 18–24 h. IV—onset 3 min; peak 15 min; duration 4-5 h.[22] (Brinzolamide) onset <2 h; peak 2 h; duration >12 h.[23] (Dorzolamide) peak 2 h; duration 8 h.[22] (Methazolamide) onset 2–4 h; peak 6–8 h; duration 10–18 h.

Fate. (Acetazolamide tablet) plasma concentrations peak 1–4 h; (acetazolamide SR capsule) plasma concentrations peak 3–6 h. Ninety-five percent bound to plasma proteins; elimination is by active renal tubular secretion.[22] (Methazolamide) well absorbed and distributed in plasma, CSF, aqueous humor, red blood cells, bile, and extracellular fluid. Peak serum concentrations after 50 and 100 mg twice-daily dosages are 5.1 and 10.7 mg/L, respectively. V_{dss} is 17–23 L. Renal clearance accounts for 20%–25% of the total clearance, with approximately 25% of the drug eliminated in the urine unchanged. **Brinzolamide** and **dorzolamide** are systemically absorbed and bind to carbonic anhydrase in erythrocytes with terminal half-lives of 111 days and 4 months, respectively. Systemic inhibition of carbonic anhdyrase is below the degree of necessary inhibition to have effect on renal function or respiration. **Half-life.** (acetazolamide) 4 h; (methazolamide) 15 h.[22] (*See* Ophthalmic Solutions, Half-life).

Adverse Reactions. Topical ophthalmic solutions frequently cause ocular burning, stinging, foreign-body sensation, ocular pain, or allergic ocular reactions.[2,20] Frequent systemic effects of topical ophthalmic solutions consist of bitter taste, occasional headache, nausea, fatigue, and, rarely, urolithiasis and iridocyclitis. Oral administration frequently causes paresthesias, gastrointestinal disturbances, anorexia, drowsiness, and confusion. Occasionally, metabolic acidosis, hypokalemia, or urolithiasis occurs. Rare, but possibly fatal, reactions include aplastic anemia, agranulocytosis, and thrombocytopenia.

Contraindications. (Oral) sulfonamide allergy, hypokalemia; hyponatremia; hyperchloremic acidosis; adrenocortical insufficiency; marked renal or hepatic impairment; severe COPD. Long-term use of oral CAIs is contraindicated in angle-closure glaucoma.

Precautions. Because all CAIs are sulfonamides, avoid their use in patients with histories of sulfonamide allergy. Corneal decompensation has been reported in patients with marked endothelial compromise.[2,20] Neither topical nor oral CAIs are recommended in patients with severe renal impairment; use caution in patients with hepatic impairment. Acidosis can cause sickling of RBC in patients with sickle cell anemia.

Drug Interactions. Do not use topical CAIs with oral CAIs, because the combination is no more effective and adverse effects are additive, particularly in causing corneal endothelial dysfunction. Oral CAIs can cause salicylate toxicity in patients taking high doses of aspirin.

Parameters to Monitor. (Oral) malaise or fatigue, serum creatinines, serum potassium, serum carbon dioxide. Baseline CBC and platelet count with monitoring at regular intervals.

Notes. Because of their severe adverse effects and poor tolerability, use oral CAIs in primary open-angle glaucoma only as a last resort.[20] (Brinzolamide) Relative IOP reductions from baseline after 1 month of therapy is 15%–19% 2 h after morning dose and 12 h after evening dose.[16] Brinzolamide twice daily added to travoprost reduces mean diurnal IOP by an additional 15%.[24] (Dorzolamide) Relative IOP reductions from baseline after 1 month of therapy is 20%–24% 2 h after morning dose and 15%–19% 12 h after evening dose.[16] Dorzolamide twice daily added to latanoprost decreases diurnal curve IOP 11%–14%.[24] Adding topical CAIs to a topical β-blocker reduces IOP by an additional 11%–23%.[24] (*See* Glaucoma Drugs Comparison Chart.) For PO prophylaxis of acute altitude sickness. 24–48 h before ascent and continue for 48 h while at high altitude or longer to control symptoms.

CHOLINERGICS AND CHOLINESTERASE INHIBITORS

CARBACHOL	Isopto Carbachol, Miostat
ECHOTHIOPHATE IODIDE	Phospholine Iodide
PILOCARPINE SALTS	Various

Pharmacology. Carbachol and pilocarpine are direct cholinergic agonists that act at acetylcholine receptors to stimulate the ciliary muscle. Carbachol is also a weak cholinesterase inhibitor. Echothiophate iodine, and other cholinesterase inhibitors, acts indirectly by inhibiting Acetylcholinesterase (AChE). Ciliary body contraction causes pupillary constriction and eases the restriction of outflow of aqueous humor through the trabecular meshwork. Echothiophate is an irreversible cholinesterase inhibitor with long durations of action.[2]

Administration and Adult Dosage. Ophthalmic for glaucoma—(carbachol) 1 drop 3 times daily of the 0.75% solution; (echothiophate) 1 drop once to twice daily; (pilocarpine ophthalmic solution) 1 drop of 1%–2% solution every 6–8 h. Most patients eventually require 4 times daily administration. Because pilocarpine is bound to pigments in the iris and the ciliary body, patients with dark eyes sometimes require 4% and occasionally 6% solutions; (pilocarpine gel) apply a thin (1/4 in. strip) at bedtime. **Ophthalmic for treatment of accommodative esotropia**—(echothiophate) 1 drop every 1–2 days.

Special Populations. *Pediatric Dosage.* Same as adult dosage.[14]

Geriatric Dosage. Same as adult dosage.

Dosage Forms. (Carbachol) **Ophth Soln** 0.75, 1.5, 2.25, 3%. (Echothiophate iodide) **Pwdr for reconstitution** 0.03, 0.06, 0.125, 0.25%. (Pilocarpine) **Ophth Gel** 4%. (Pilocarpine HCl) **Ophth Soln** 0.25, 0.5, 1, 2, 3, 4, 5, 6, 8, 10%. (Pilocarpine nitrate) **Ophth Soln** 1, 2, 4%.

Patient Instructions. *See* Glaucoma Drugs, Class Instructions.

Pharmacokinetics. *Onset and Duration.* (Carbachol ophthalmic solution) onset 13 ± 2.2 min; peak 4 h; duration 8 h. (Echothiophate solution) onset within minutes, peak 2–7 weeks; duration several weeks. (Pilocarpine ophthalmic solution) onset within minutes; peak 2 h; duration 8 h. (Pilocarpine ophthalmic gel) 4% maintains IOP reductions of 30% or more for 24 h.[75]

Fate. Absorption characteristics. (*See* Glaucoma Drugs, Fate.) Cholinergic and cholinesterase inhibitors are hydrolyzed by acetylcholine. **Half-life.** (*See* Ophthalmic Solutions, Half-life.)

Adverse Reactions. Reduced visual acuity in poor lighting occurs frequently because of papillary constriction and accommodative spasm. Occasional effects include ciliary spasm, headache, lacrimation, myopia, blurred vision, retinal detachment, and iris cysts. Cataracts have been reported with echothiophate.[2] Cholinergic syndrome consisting of weakness, nausea, diaphoresis, and dyspnea occurs rarely. Patients with myopia of >6 diopters or greater and those with histories of retinal detachment are at greater risk of developing retinal detachment.[26]

Contraindications. Acute iritis, uveal inflammation, and other conditions in which papillary constriction is undesirable.

Precautions. Pregnancy, lactation; night driving or other activities in poor light. Use cholinesterase inhibitors cautiously in patients with histories of retinal detachment, asthma, bradycardia, hypotension, epilepsy, parkinsonism, recent MI, or patients using systemic cholinesterase inhibitors for myasthenia gravis. Cholinesterase inhibitors can cause prolonged respiratory paralysis if succinylcholine is utilized during general ananesthesia.[1]

Drug Interactions. Antihistamine, antidepressants, antipsychotics, and other anticholinergics can decrease the effects of cholinergics and cholinesterase inhibitors.

Parameters to Monitor. Monitor compliance, pulse for bradycardia, and complaints of visual blurring, nausea, vomiting, diarrhea, and headache.

Notes. Use long-acting AChE inhibitors in patients who are not controlled with pilocarpine. Longer-acting agents are also used to diagnose and treat accommodative esotropia. Refrigerate echothiophate iodide before reconstitution. Once reconstituted, store at room temperature for no more than 4 weeks. (*See* Glaucoma Drugs Comparison Chart.)

PROSTAGLANDINS	
BIMATOPROST	Lumigan
LATANOPROST	Xalatan
TRAVOPROST	Travatan, Travatan Z

Pharmacology. Latanoprost and travoprost are analogues of prostaglandin $F_{2\alpha}$ and are agonists of the prostanoid FP receptor, which appears to lower IOP by increasing aqueous humor outflow through the uveoscleral pathway. Bimatoprost is a prostamide analogue and appears to lower IOP by activating prostamide receptors in the uveoscleral pathway and possibly through increasing outflow through the trabecular meshwork. Stimulation of prostanoid FP receptors and prostamide receptors in the ciliary body cause remodeling of the extracelluar matrix making it more permeable to aqueous humor, thus increasing aqueous humor outflow through the ciliary muscles.[2,3] These agents lower IOP by 25%–35%.

Administration and Adult Dosage. **Ophthalmic for glaucoma**—(bimatoprost) 1 drop daily in the evening; (latanoprost) 1 drop daily in the evening; (travoprost) 1 drop daily in the evening. For all ocular prostaglandin analogues, once daily administration is more effective than twice daily. Evening administration is more effective than morning administration.[2,17]

Special Populations. *Pediatric Dosage.* Safety and efficacy not established.

Geriatric Dosage. Same as adult dosage.

Dosage Forms. **Ophth Soln**—(bimatoprost) 0.03%; (latanoprost) 0.005%; (travoprost, travoprost Z) 0.004%.

Patient Instructions. (*See* Class Instructions.) (Latanoprost) protect from light, store unopened bottles in refrigerator. Once opened it may be stored at room temperature for 6 weeks.

Pharmacokinetics. *Onset and Duration.* (Bimatoprost) onset 4 h; peak 8–12 h; duration 24 h. (Latanoprost) onset 3–4 h; peak 8–12 h; duration 24 h. (Travoprost) onset 2 h; peak 12 h; duration 24 h.

Fate. (Bimatoprost) after ocular administration, plasma concentration peak within 10 min. Blood concentration was below lower limit of detection in most subjects within 1.5 h after dosing. (Latanaprost) once absorbed through the cornea, it is hydrolyzed to the active free acid. Peak concentrations in aqueous humor occur 2 h after administration and is measurable for approximately 4 h. Plasma concentrations are undetectable 1 h after administration. Primarily metabolized in the liver via β-oxidation. (Travoprost) once absorbed through the cornea, it is hydrolyzed to the active free acid. Peak plasma levels of 0.18 ng/L are reached in 30 min and rapidly eliminated. Many patients will have plasma levels less than 0.01 ng/mL.

Half-life. (*See* Ophthalmic Solutions, Half-life.) Plasma half-lives are (bimatoprost) 45 min; (latanoprost) 17 min; (travoprost) 45 min.

Adverse Reactions. Ocular reactions frequently include burning, stinging, conjunctival hyperemia, foreign-body sensation, blurred vision. The major limitation is increased pigmentation of the iris in patients with green-brown, yellow-brown, and blue/gray-brown eyes that occurs from months to years in approximately 5%–15% of patients.[27] The darkening is irreversible. Reversible darkening of the eyelids and increase in eyelashes and eyelash length after use can occur. Diplopia occasionally occurs; retinal artery embolus, retinal detachment, and vitreous hemorrhage occur rarely.

Precautions. Infections occur from contamination of multiple-dose containers. Instruct patients to avoid touching the tip of the container to the eye. Patients with diabetic retinopathy or complicated ocular surgery have a greater risk of developing cystoid macular edema, anterior uveitis, or vitreous hemorrhage.[26]

Drug Interactions. Precipitate occurs when used with thimerosal-containing eye drops. Separate doses of different ophthalmic solutions by at least 5 min.

Parameters to Monitor. Darkening of iris, eye pain, eye lid darkening. (*See* Ophthalmic Solutions, Parameters to Monitor.)

Notes. Prostaglandins have the greatest 24-h IOP reduction compared to timolol, dorzolamide, and brimonidine.[17] (Bimatoprost) relative IOP reductions from baseline after 1 month of therapy is 31%–35% 12 h after evening dose and 27%–29% before next dose.[16] (Latanoprost) relative IOP reductions from baseline after 1 month of therapy is 29%–33% 12 h after evening dose and 26%–30% before next dose.[16] An eye drop applicator (Xal-Ease) is available to patients through the manufacturer. (Travoprost) it is available in 2 formulations. Travatan uses benzalkonium chloride as a preservative, while Travatan Z uses a proprietary ionic buffer system (SofZia). Relative IOP reductions from baseline after 1 month of therapy is 29%–32% 12 h after evening dose and 25%–32% before next dose.[16] A dosing aid with a programmable reminder is available through the manufacturer. Dosing aid tracks medication use and can be downloaded by practitioner.

SYMPATHOMIMETICS	
DIPIVEFRIN HYDROCHLORIDE	AKPro, Propine
EPINEPHRINE AND SALTS	Various

Pharmacology. Epinephrine stimulates α- and β₂-adrenergic receptors in the ciliary body, increasing outflow. Dipivefrin is an epinephrine prodrug that is enzymatically converted into epinephrine in the eye. IOP is reduced by 15%–25%.[2]

Administration and Adult Dosage. **Ophthalmic for glaucoma**—(epinephrine) 1 drop (usually 2%) twice daily; (dipivefrin) 1 drop of 0.1% solution twice daily.

Special Populations. *Pediatric Dosage.* Same as adult dosage.

Geriatric Dosage. Same as adult dosage.

Dosage Forms. (Dipivefrin) **Ophth Soln** 0.1%; (epinephrine HCl) **Ophth Soln** 0.5, 1, 2%.

Patient Instructions. *See* Class Instructions.

Pharmacokinetics. (Dipivefrin) onset 30 min, peak 1 h; (epinephrine HCl) onset <1 h, peak 4–8 h, duration 24 h.

Fate. Dipivefrin is absorbed 17 times more than epinephrine. Upon entry into the cornea, the 2 pivalic acid groups are removed by esterases, yielding epinephrine. Because of the better absorption, it can be administered as a 0.1% solution, decreasing the amount of epinephrine exposure to the conjunctiva and available for systemic absorption, thereby decreasing adverse effects. Epinephrine, which is absorbed systemically, is metabolized by MAO and COMT.

Adverse Reactions. Intolerance to ocular adverse effects leads to discontinuation of epinephrine in most of patients. Dipivefrin is associated with less ocular side effects than epinephrine. Burning, tearing, reactive conjunctival hyperemia, allergic blepharoconjunctivitis, and mydriasis resulting in blurring of vision occur frequently. Adrenochrome deposits in palpebral conjunctiva and the superficial cornea occur occasionally. Rare systemic adverse effects include tachycardia, hypertension, anxiety, and arrhythmia.[2]

Precautions. Epinephrine may induce acute angle-closure glaucoma in patients with narrow angles.[28] Cystoid macular edema with epinephrine treatment has occurred in patients after cataract surgery.[2]

Parameters to Monitor. (*See* Ophthalmic Solutions, Parameters to Monitor.) Monitor for blurring of vision, mydriasis, conjunctival irritation, hypertension, and rapid pulse.

Notes. Do not use epinephrine solutions that are cloudy or have become pinkish or brownish. (*See* Glaucoma Drugs Comparison Chart.)

GLAUCOMA DRUGS COMPARISON CHART[a]

MEDICATIONS	DOSAGE FORMS	ADULT DOSAGE	ONSET	PEAK	DURATION
α2-ADRENERGIC AGONISTS					
Apraclonidine HCl	Ophth Soln 0.5, 1%	0.5% 3 times daily for short term; 1% 1 h	1 h	3 h	—
Iopidine		before and immediatel] after surgery			
Brimonidine Tartrate	Ophth Soln 0.15%	3 times daily	1 h	2 h	—
Alphagan	(Alphagan P); 0.2%				
Alphagan P	(Alphagan)				
β-ADRENERGIC BLOCKERS					
Betaxolol HCl	Ophth Soln 0.5%	Twice daily	30 min	2 h	12 h
Betoptic	Ophth Susp 0.25%	Twice daily	30 min	2 h	24 h
Betoptic-S					
Carteolol HCl	Ophth Soln 1%	Twice daily	1 h	2 h	12 h
Ocupress					
Levobunolol HCl	Ophth Soln 0.25, 0.5%	Once to twice daily	1 h	2–6 h	24 h
Betagan					
Various					
Metipranolol	Ophth Soln 0.3%	Twice daily	30 min	2 h	24 h
Optipranolol					
Timolol Maleate	Ophth Soln 0.25, 0.5%	Twice daily	30 min	1–2 h	24 h
Timoptic	Ophth gel-forming Soln	Once daily	30 min	1–2 h	24 h
Timoptic-XE	0.25, 0.5%				

(continued)

651

GLAUCOMA DRUGS COMPARISON CHART[a] (*continued*)

MEDICATIONS	DOSAGE FORMS	ADULT DOSAGE	ONSET	PEAK	DURATION
CAI TOPICAL					
Brinzolamide Azopt	Ophth Susp 1%	3 times daily	<2 h	2 h	>12 h
Dorzolamide Trusopt	Ophth Soln 2%	3 times daily	<2 h	2–4 h	6–8 h
CAI ORAL					
Acetazolamide Diamox	Tab 125, 250 mg	125–250 mg every 4 h to 250 mg 4 times daily	1–1.5 h	2–4 h	6–8 h
Diamox Sequels	SR Cap 500 mg	500 mg twice daily	2 h	4–6 h	18–24 h
Methazolamide Naptazane	Tab 25, 50 mg	50–100 mg 2–3 times daily	2–4 h	6–8 h	10–18 h
CHOLINERGICS					
Carbachol Isopto Carbachol	Ophth Soln 0.75, 1.5, 2.25, 3%	3 times daily	13 min	4 h	8 h
Pilocarpine HCl Pilocar	Ophth Soln (HCl) 0.25, 0.5, 1, 2, 3, 4, 5, 6, 8, 10%	4 times daily	10–30 min	2 h	8 h
Various	Ophth gel 4%	Once daily	10–30 min	2 h	24 h
Pilocarpine Nitrate Pilagan	Ophth Soln (nitrate) 1, 2, 4%	4 times daily	10–30 min	2 h	8 h

(continued)

GLAUCOMA DRUGS COMPARISON CHART[a] (*continued*)

MEDICATIONS	DOSAGE FORMS	ADULT DOSAGE	ONSET	PEAK	DURATION
CHOLINESTERASE INHIBITORS					
Echothiophate Iodide Phospholine Iodide	Pwdr 0.03, 0.06, 0.125, 0.25%	Once to twice daily	<1 h	2–7 wk	Several weeks
PROSTAGLANDIN ANALOGUES					
Bimatoprost Lumigan	Ophth Soln 0.03%	In the evening	4 h	8–12 h	24 h
Latanoprost Xalatan	Ophth Soln 0.005%	In the evening	3–4 h	8–12 h	24 h
Travoprost Travatan Travatan Z	Ophth Soln 0.004%	In the evening	2 h	12 h	24 h
SYMPATHOMIMETICS					
Epinephrine Various	Ophth Soln 0.5, 1, 2%	Twice daily	<45 min	4–6 h	24 h
Dipivefrin Propine	Ophth Soln 0.1%	Twice daily	<45 min	4–6 h	24 h

CAI, carbonic anhydrase inhibitor.
[a]Dosages in this chart are for primary open-angle glaucoma.

■ REFERENCES

1. United States Pharmacopeial (USP) Convention. *United States Pharmacopeia Dispensing Information. Advice for the Patient.* 27 ed. Greenwood Village, CO: Thomson Micromedex; 2007.
2. Marquis RE, Whitson JT. Management of glaucoma: focus on pharmacological therapy. *Drugs Aging.* 2005;22:1-21.
3. Woodward DF, Gil DW. The inflow and outflow of anti-glaucoma drugs. *Trends Pharmacol Sci.* 2004;25:238-241.
4. Ghate D, Edelhauser HF. Barriers to glaucoma drug delivery. *J Glaucoma.* 2008;17:147-156.
5. American Academy of Opthalmology. *Preferred Practice Pattern: Primary Open Angle.* San Francisco, CA: American Academy of Opthalmology; 2005.
6. Weinreb RN, Khaw PT. Primary open-angle glaucoma. *Lancet.* 2004;363:1711-1720.
7. Olthoff CM et al. Noncompliance with ocular hypotensive treatment in patients with glaucoma or ocular hypertension: an evidence-based review. *Ophthalmology.* 2005;112:953-961.
8. Schoenwald R. Ocular pharmacokinetics. In: Zimmerman TJ, ed. *Textbook of Ocular Pharmacology.* Philadelphia, PA: Lippincott–Raven; 1999:119-138.
9. Brunton LL, Parker KL, Blumenthal DK, Buxton IL, eds. *Goodman and Gilman's Manual of Pharmacology and Therapeutics.* 1st ed. New York: McGraw-Hill; 2008.
10. Kaur IP, Kanwar M. Ocular preparations: the formulation approach. *Drug Dev Ind Pharm.* 2002;28:473-493.
11. Vander Zanden JA, Valuck RJ, Bunch CL, et al. Systemic adverse effects of ophthalmic beta-blockers. *Ann Pharmacother.* 2001;35:1633-1637.
12. Ramos RF et al. Schlemm's canal endothelia, lymphatic, or blood vasculature? *J Glaucoma.* 2007;16:391-405.
13. Law S, Lee D. Ocular Pharmacology. In: Netland PA, ed. *Glaucoma Medical Therapy: Principles and Management.* 2nd ed. New York: Oxford University Press; 2008:3-11.
14. Moore W, Nischal KK. Pharmacologic management of glaucoma in childhood. *Paediatr Drugs.* 2007;9:71-79.
15. Thoe Schwartzenberg GWS, Buys YM. Efficacy of brimonidine 0.2% as adjunctive therapy for patients with glaucoma inadequately controlled with otherwise maximal medical therapy. *Ophthalmology.* 1999;106:1616-1620.
16. van der Valk R et al. Intraocular pressure-lowering effects of all commonly used glaucoma drugs: a meta-analysis of randomized clinical trials. *Ophthalmology.* 2005;112:1177-1785.
17. Stewart WC et al. Meta-analysis of 24-hour intraocular pressure studies evaluating the efficacy of glaucoma medicines. *Ophthalmology.* 2008;115:1117-1122, e1.
18. Han JA et al. Cardiovascular and respiratory considerations with pharmacotherapy of glaucoma and ocular hypertension. *Cardiol Rev.* 2008;16:95-108.
19. Henness S et al. Ocular carteolol: a review of its use in the management of glaucoma and ocular hypertension. *Drugs Aging.* 2007;24:509-528.
20. Singh A. Medical therapy of glaucoma. *Ophthalmol Clin North Am.* 2005;18(3):397-408, vi.
21. Ott EZ et al. A randomized trial assessing dorzolamide in patients with glaucoma who are younger than 6 years. *Arch Ophthalmol.* 2005;123:1177-1186.
22. Amin AR, Remis LL. Carbonic anhydrase inhibitors. In: Daniel M. Albert FAJ, eds. *Principles and Practice of Ophthalmology.* 2nd ed. Philadelphia, PA: WB Saunders; 2000:340-345.
23. Silver LH. Dose-response evaluation of the ocular hypotensive effect of brinzolamide ophthalmic suspension (Azopt). Brinzolamide Dose-Response Study Group. *Surv Ophthalmol.* 2000;44(suppl 2):S147-S153.
24. Webers CA et al. Pharmacological management of primary open-angle glaucoma: second-line options and beyond. *Drugs Aging.* 2008;25:729-759.
25. Gabelt B, Kaufman P. Cholinergic drugs. In: Netland PA, ed. *Glaucoma Medical Therapy: Principles and Management.* 2nd ed. New York: Oxford University Press; 2008:103-119.
26. Hoyng PF, van Beek LM. Pharmacological therapy for glaucoma: a review. *Drugs.* 2000;59:411-434.
27. Ishida N, Odani-Kawabata N, Shimazaki A, Hara H. Prostanoids in the therapy of glaucoma. *Cardiovasc Drug Rev.* 2006;24:1-10.
28. Lachkar Y, Bouassida W. Drug-induced acute angle closure glaucoma. *Curr Opin Ophthalmol.* 2007;18:129-133.

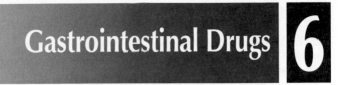

Gastrointestinal Drugs | 6

Daniel M. Riche

Chapter 43

Acid-Peptic Therapy

P. Shane Winstead and George A. Davis

ANTACIDS

Pharmacology. Antacids are weak basic inorganic salts whose primary action is to neutralize gastric acid; pH >4 inhibits the proteolytic activity of pepsin. However, there is also evidence to support that the healing of peptic ulcerations may be independent of gastric acid neutralization. Although the exact mechanism is unknown, these agents can enhance mucosal defense through a variety of cytoprotective effects.[1] This is especially true for the aluminum salts, which also bind phosphate and bile salts in the gastrointestinal (GI) tract, decreasing serum phosphate and serum bile salt levels. Antacids are salts of aluminum, calcium, magnesium, or sodium or a combination of these. (*See* Acid Neutralizing Capacity of Common Organic Salts Used in Antacid Products Table.)

Administration and Adult Dosage. **PO for symptomatic relief of indigestion, nonulcer dyspepsia, epigastric pain in peptic ulcer disease (PUD), or heartburn in gastroesophageal reflux disease (GERD)**—[HCl-neutralizing capacity, 25 mEq/5 mL] 15 mL as needed; or four times daily, 1 h after meals and at bedtime; or 2–4 tab four times daily, at bedtime, or as needed.[2]

Special Populations. *Pediatric Dosage.* **PO for treatment of PUD or GERD**— (≤12 years), 5–15 mL every 1–3 hours; (>12 years) Same as adult dosage.

Geriatric Dosage. Avoid using magnesium-containing antacids in renal impairment.

Other Conditions. Use with caution in renal insufficiency, particularly magnesium-containing products. Magnesium products may cause hypermagnesemia and calcium-containing products may cause hypercalcemia, alkalosis, and milk-alkali syndrome. Aluminum-containing products may cause aluminum neurotoxicity.[1]

Dosage Forms. Antacids may be marketed as liquid or tablet formulations. Products vary in which organic salt is used and many contain combinations of more

655

than one salt. Additionally, medications such as simethicone or alginate may be included in formulations.

Patient Instructions. If antacids do not relieve symptoms of indigestion, upset stomach, or heartburn within 2 weeks, contact your health care practitioner. Diarrhea can occur with magnesium-containing antacids; decrease the daily dosage, alternate doses with, or switch to, an aluminum- or calcium-containing antacid. Constipation can occur with aluminum-containing antacids; decrease the daily dosage, alternate doses with, or switch to, a magnesium-containing antacid. Refrigerating liquid antacids or flavored antacids can improve their palatability. Antacids can interfere with other medications; take other medications 1–2 h before or after antacids unless otherwise directed. If tablets are used, chew thoroughly before swallowing, and follow administration with a glass of water.

Missed Doses. If your health care practitioner has told you to take this medicine on a regular schedule and you miss a dose, take it as soon as possible. If it is almost time for your next dose, skip the missed dose and return to your usual dosage schedule. Do not double doses.

Pharmacokinetics. *Onset and Duration.* Onset of acid neutralizing is immediate; duration is 30 ± 10 min in the fasted state and 1–3 h if ingested with or within 1 h of a meal.

Fate. Antacid cations are absorbed to different degrees. Sodium is highly soluble and readily absorbed; calcium absorption is generally less than 30% but can decrease with advancing age, intake, achlorhydria, and estrogen loss at menopause; magnesium is generally absorbed approximately 30%, but the percentage of absorption changes inversely with intake; aluminum is slightly absorbed. Calcium, magnesium, and aluminum are excreted renally with normal renal function.[1] The unabsorbed portion is excreted in the feces.

Adverse Reactions. Long-term use of sodium- or calcium-containing antacids can cause systemic alkalosis. Hypercalcemia can occur with the ingestion of large amounts of calcium; soluble antacids plus a diet high in milk products can result in milk-alkali syndrome, which can lead to nephrolithiasis and, in severe cases, neurologic abnormalities.[1] Magnesium-containing antacids cause dose-related laxative effects. Aluminum-containing antacids cause dose-related constipation, especially in the elderly. Prolonged administration or large dosages of aluminum hydroxide or carbonate can result in hypophosphatemia, particularly in the elderly and alcoholics; encephalopathy has been reported in dialysis patients receiving aluminum-containing antacids alone or with sucralfate.

Precautions. Use caution with aluminum and calcium salts and avoid magnesium-containing products in patients with renal insufficiency. Use caution when using sodium bicarbonate in patients with chronic renal failure, edema, hypertension, or heart failure.

Drug Interactions. Antacids reduce the absorption of numerous drugs by three different mechanisms: altering GI pH, altering urinary pH, and binding to drugs in the GI tract. Factors that affect the likelihood of drug interactions are the drug's dose, valence of cations (e.g., tetracycline is polyvalent), and timing of the doses of antacid and drug. Some clinically important interactions include digoxin, oral iron, isoniazid, ketoconazole, oral quinolones, and oral tetracyclines. Antacids can reduce salicylate levels and increase quinidine levels because of urinary pH changes. Large dosages of calcium antacids can produce hypercalcemia in the presence of thiazides. Sodium polystyrene sulfonate resin can bind magnesium and calcium ions from the antacid in the gut, resulting in systemic alkalosis.

Parameters to Monitor. Monitor for relief of dyspepsia, epigastric pain or heartburn, and diarrhea or constipation. Monitor serum phosphate during long-term use of aluminum-containing products in patients with chronic renal impairment. Monitor for drug interactions.

Notes. Amongst the pharmacologic classes that inhibit the production of acid, antacids are used for symptomatic relief of dyspepsia and rarely utilized as primary treatment for acid-related illnesses.[1] Most antacid products have been reformulated to contain low amounts of sodium; some antacid products contain considerable amounts of sugar or artificial sweetener. Antacid tablets, if chewed and swallowed, can be as effective as equivalent doses of liquid formulations. Although gastrin is stimulated by calcium, gastric acid rebound with calcium-containing antacids is of questionable clinical importance.

BISMUTH PREPARATIONS Pepto-Bismol, Various

Pharmacology. Bismuth salts are used to treat nausea, indigestion, diarrhea, gastritis, and peptic ulcers. The precise method by which bismuth heals gastritis and ulcers is uncertain, but possible mechanisms are local gastroprotective effect, stimulation of endogenous prostaglandins, and antimicrobial activity against *Helicobacter pylori*.[1] Given alone, bismuth salts suppress *Heliobacter pylori*, but longterm eradication requires combination therapy with antibiotics.

Administration and Adult Dosage. PO for the control of nausea, abdominal cramps, and diarrhea—Bismuth subsalicylate (BSS) 525 mg/30 mL. Administer dosage every 30–60 min, if needed, to a maximum of 4.2 g/d; **PO with antibiotics to eradicate *Heliobacter pylori*—**(BSS) 2 tab or 524 mg twice daily, treatment is usually limited to 1–2 weeks. (*See* Eradication of *Helicobacter pylori* Infection.)

Special Populations. *Pediatric Dosage.* (<12 years) Not recommended. As of spring 2004, child dosing directions were removed from the label of all anti-diarrheal products containing bismuth subsalicylate.[4]

Geriatric Dosage. Same as adult dosage.

Dosage Forms. (BSS) **Susp** 17.5 mg/mL and 35 mg/mL; **Chew Tab** 262 mg; **Tab** 262 mg.

Pharmacokinetics. After oral administration, BSS (58% bismuth, 42% salicylate) is converted in the GI tract to bismuth oxide and salicylic acid. Bismuth is less than 0.2% absorbed, with more than 99% of an oral dose excreted in the feces. Over 90% of the salicylate dose is absorbed and excreted in the urine.

Adverse Reactions. BSS can temporarily darken the tongue and stool. Use BSS with caution in the elderly; in patients with renal impairment, salicylate sensitivity, or bleeding disorders; in those receiving high-dosage salicylate therapy; or in those taking potentially interacting medications. Salicylic acid is less likely than aspirin to cause gastric mucosal damage and blood loss. Prolonged use, dosages higher than those recommended, and the use of other salts (subgallate and subnitrate) have been associated with neurotoxicity. Bismuth concentrations can be elevated in the elderly and patients with renal impairment because of decreased renal elimination. There is an increased risk in children and teenagers who are experiencing or recovering from nausea and vomiting symptoms because these might be early sign of Reye's syndrome. Changes were required in package labeling to note this risk and remove dosing recommendations for children younger than 12 years.[4] Avoid BSS in patients who are hypersensitive to aspirin or nonaspirin salicylates.

Notes. BSS is the bismuth salt used most frequently in the United States.

HISTAMINE H2-RECEPTOR ANTAGONISTS	
CIMETIDINE	Tagamet, Various
RANITIDINE	Zantac, Various
FAMOTIDINE	Pepcid, Various

Pharmacology. Histamine H2-receptor antagonists (H2RA) competitively inhibit the actions of histamine at the H2-receptors of the parietal cell and reduce basal as well as food-stimulated gastric acid.[1] (*See* Histamine H2-Receptor Antagonists Structures Table.)

Administration and Adult Dosage. (*See* Histamine H2-Receptor Antagonists Adult Indications and Dosage Table.) Data support the superiority of proton pump inhibitors (PPI) in the treatment of most acid related illnesses.[5] Therefore, the use of H2RA is primarily as symptomatic relief of dyspepsia symptoms (e.g., using OTC products) and as PO or IV prevention of stress ulcers in the hospitalized patient.

Special Populations. *Pediatric Dosage.* There is lack of large controlled trials in this population; the majority of data is generated through case reports. The clinical experience with ranitidine in children is superior to any other H2RA.[12]

Geriatric Dosage. Reduce dosage based on renal function.

Other Conditions. Renal Impairment. The dose should be reduced by half if Cl_{Cr} is 15–30 mL/min with cimetidine and famotidine or < 50 mL/min with ranitidine. Dialysis does not remove a sufficient amount to require adjustment in these patients.[1]

Dosage Forms. *See* Histamine H2-Receptor Antagonists Dosage Forms Table.

Patient Instructions. The effectiveness of H2RA in PUD might be decreased by cigarette smoking. Discontinue or decrease smoking or avoid smoking after the last dose of the day. Antacids can be used as needed for relief of epigastric pain. Even though ulcer or GERD symptoms might improve, continue treatment for the duration of therapy unless instructed otherwise. If symptomatic relief is not obtained in 2 weeks with over-the-counter medication, contact your health care practitioner. Report any bleeding, vomiting, or severe esophageal or abdominal pain.

Missed Doses. If you miss a dose, take it as soon as possible. If it is almost time for your next dose, skip the missed dose and return to your usual dosage schedule. Do not double doses.

Pharmacokinetics. *See* Histamine H2-Receptor Antagonists Pharmacokinetics Table.

Adverse Reactions. Adverse reactions are generally mild. A published meta-analysis of randomized trials concluded that the adverse event profile for H2RA is similar to placebo.[13] Reversible CNS manifestations including headaches, restlessness, and somnolence can occur occasionally with any H2RA.[1] In addition, mild, reversible increases in hepatic aminotransferases have been reported. These are generally asymptotic and may resolve, even if the agent is continued.[1] Myelosuppression may occur with H2RA and include leukopenia, neutropenia, thrombocytopenia, and pancytopenia; agranulocytosis and aplastic anemia occur rarely.[1] Gynecomastia develops rarely in patients receiving cimetidine.

Precautions. H2RA are used safely during pregnancy, and ranitidine is the preferred drug.[14] Dosage reduction might be required in severe renal and/or hepatic failure. Symptomatic response to therapy does not preclude the possibility of gastric or esophageal malignancy.

Drug Interactions. Cimetidine inhibits hepatic CYP1A2, CYP2C8–10, CYP2D6, and CYP3A3–5; ranitidine inhibits CYP2D6 and CYP3A3–5 to a much lesser extent. Clinically important interactions with drugs metabolized by these isoenzymes can occur (the most important of which are carbamazepine, chlordiazepoxide, clozapine, diazepam, glipizide, lidocaine, phenytoin, propranolol, theophylline, tolbutamide, tricyclic antidepressants, quinidine, tacrine, and warfarin). Elevations in gastric pH can alter the rate or extent of absorption of ketoconazole, itraconazole, and other drugs including anti-retroviral agents whose dissolution and absorption are pH dependent.

Parameters to Monitor. Improvement in epigastric pain or heartburn. However, pain relief in PUD and GERD does not correlate directly with endoscopic evidence of healing. Monitor serum creatinine, CBC, AST, ALT, and CNS status periodically. In patients receiving IV doses of cimetidine (>2.4 g/d) or ranitidine (≥ 400 mg/d), it is advisable to monitor serum transaminases routinely throughout IV therapy. Monitor for potential drug interactions.

Notes. Although the cause is unclear, tolerance to the antisecretory effects of the H2RA may occur. This tolerance can appear quickly and frequently and may not be overcome with increased doses.[1] Usual dosages of H2RA are less effective than **misoprostol** or **PPI** in preventing NSAID-induced gastric ulcer. Published studies consistently show more rapid healing of gastric and duodenal ulcers with PPIs than H2RA. Although all H2RA provide symptomatic relief and esophageal healing, higher dosages are required in patients with moderate to severe esophagitis than those used in patients with mild GERD symptoms. The maintenance of intragastric pH above 4.0 does not conclusively prevent upper GI bleeding.[10,11] Although it is easier to maintain the intragastric pH above 4.0 by continuous infusion, the superiority of continuous infusion of the H2RA in preventing upper GI bleeding in a patient who is critically ill has not been established.[10] Combination of an H2RA with sucralfate provides two different mechanisms of drug action and might be beneficial. However, enhanced efficacy of two drugs compared with single-drug therapy has not been substantiated in controlled trials in patients with duodenal ulcer, gastric ulcer, or GERD or when used to prevent or treat upper GI bleeding. Coadministration of an H2RA with a PPI is without established benefit and might compromise the action of the PPI. Controlled trials have not demonstrated that H2RA are of benefit in patients with active upper GI bleeding.[15] The relation of H2RA therapy to the development of nosocomial pneumonia, in patients who are critically ill, is inconclusive.[10] Nitazdine (Axid) is no longer readily available in the U.S.

MISOPROSTOL
Cytotec, Various

Pharmacology. Misoprostol is a synthetic prostaglandin E_1 analogue that inhibits gastric acid secretion and enhances gastric mucosal defense.[1] Since the ulcerogenic effects of NSAIDs are thought to be related to the suppression of prostaglandin production, misoprostol is used to reduce the frequency of NSAID-induced complications, including GI perforation, obstruction, and bleeding.[1] Misoprostol also causes uterine contraction.

Administration and Adult Dosage. PO for GI protection during NSAID therapy— 200 μg four times daily with food; if this dosage is not tolerated, 100 μg four times daily can be used. Lower-dosage regimens of misoprostol 200 μg two to three times daily appear similar in efficacy and better tolerated for protection against NSAID-induced gastric and duodenal ulcers than the 200 μg four times daily dosage. Dosage reduction is not required in renal impairment, hepatic failure, or the elderly. (*See* Notes.)

Special Populations. *Pediatric Dosage.* Safety and efficacy not established.

Dosage Forms. Tab 100, 200 μg. Misoprostol is also available in combination with diclofenac (Arthrotec). (*See* Nonsteroidal Anti-Inflammatory Drugs.)

Pharmacokinetics. After oral administration, misoprostol is extensively absorbed and rapidly de-esterified to the active drug, misoprostol acid. Peak serum concentrations of misoprostol acid are reduced when the drug is taken with food. Plasma protein binding of misoprostol acid is <90%. Misoprostol acid undergoes further metabolism, but ~80% is excreted unchanged in urine.

Adverse Reactions. Diarrhea is reported to occur in up to 30% of patients and may limit its use in some patients.[1] Diarrhea is dose-related and is seen more frequently in patients receiving 800 μg/d than with 400–600 μg/d. Diarrhea usually resolves in approximately 1 week with continued treatment. Abdominal pain occurs in 13%–20% of patients on NSAIDs receiving misoprostol 800 μg/d, but there is no consistent difference from placebo. Nausea, flatulence, headache, dyspepsia, vomiting, and constipation occur occasionally. Women who receive misoprostol occasionally develop gynecologic disorders including cramps or vaginal bleeding.

Precautions. Advise patients (especially those receiving concurrent corticosteroids or anticoagulants) to report bleeding, vomiting, severe abdominal pain, and diarrhea. For GI protective uses, misoprostol is contraindicated in pregnancy because of the risk of abortion. Women of childbearing potential should have a negative serum pregnancy test within 2 weeks of beginning therapy, should begin treatment on the second or third day of the next menstrual period, should comply with effective contraceptive measures, and should receive oral and written warnings of the hazards of misoprostol therapy and the risk of contraceptive failure. Warn patients not to give misoprostol to others.

Drug Interactions. Misoprostol does not affect the hepatic cytochrome P450 microsomal enzyme system and does not interfere with the beneficial effects of NSAIDs in rheumatoid arthritis.

Notes. Although misoprostol demonstrates efficacy as a gastroduodenal protective strategy, it does not relieve GI pain or discomfort associated with NSAID use.[16] **Omeprazole** 20 mg/d is associated with a lower relapse rate and is better tolerated than misoprostol 200 μg twice daily for prophylactic treatment of NSAID-induced ulcers.[17] Misoprostol has been used as an abortifacient and is labor inducer.

PROTON PUMP INHIBITORS	
DEXLANSOPRAZOLE	Kapidex
ESOMEPRAZOLE	Nexium
LANSOPRAZOLE	Prevacid
OMEPRAZOLE	Prilosec, Zegerid, Various
PANTOPRAZOLE	Protonix, Various
RABEPRAZOLE	Aciphex

Pharmacology. PPIs are inactive substituted benzimidazoles that, when protonated in the secretory canaliculi of the parietal cells, covalently bind to H^+/K^+-ATPase (proton pump), which is the final pathway for acid secretion. PPIs produce a profound and prolonged antisecretory effect and inhibit all phases of gastric acid secretion.[18] Serum gastrin levels increase during treatment but return to pretreatment levels within 1–2 weeks of discontinuing therapy.

Administration and Adult Dosage. (*See* Proton Pump Inhibitor Adult Indications and Dosage Table.) Administer the PPI at least 30–60 min before meals, preferable in the morning, because these agents inhibit only those proton pumps that are actively secreting acid.[18] The design of the tablet and capsule formulations protect the acid-labile product allows it to pass through the stomach, since gastric acid will rapidly neutralize the medication. The immediate release omeprazole packets contain sodium bicarbonate to raise the pH and prevent acid degradation.[19] Omeprazole and lansoprazole can be mixed with sodium bicarbonate to make a simplified suspension for administration through feeding tubes. The IV formulations are approved for treatment of erosive esophagitis in patients unable to tolerate oral administration. The majority of the use, however, is for bleeding peptic ulcers or for stress ulcer prophylaxis (SUP). The oral and IV formulations are generally thought to be equivalent.[19]

Special Populations. *Pediatric Dosage.* (*See* Proton Pump Inhibitor Pediatric Indications and Dosage Table.) The use of PPIs has become widespread in children and infants for the management of pediatric acid-related disease.[20] Omeprazole appears to be safe in children if used for more than 2 years. Additional data on the safety of long-term omeprazole treatment in children are necessary.

Geriatric Dosage. Dosage reduction is not usually necessary; reduce only if the drug is not well tolerated.[16]

Other Conditions. Dosage adjustments of PPIs are unnecessary in renal impairment or mild to moderate liver disease.[19] PPIs are not readily dialyzable. There are identified variations in polymorphisms of CYP2C19 which will impact the rate of hepatic elimination of various products.[5] Since this genotype-dependant difference may impact the amount of acid suppression and anticipated clinical response, it could be beneficial to consider genotype-adjusted dosing as a method to optimize response in patients receiving PPI therapy.[5]

Dosage Forms. *See* Proton Pump Inhibitor Availability Table.

Patient Instructions. Swallow capsule (dexlansoprazole, lansoprazole, omeprazole, esomeprazole) or tablet (pantoprazole, rabeprazole) whole; do not crush or chew. Take medication 30–60 min before meals, preferably in the morning. Capsules can be opened and the granules sprinkled on applesauce, yogurt, or apple or orange juice if you have difficulty swallowing. Do not chew, and do swallow the preparation immediately after sprinkling the content onto food. (*See* Notes.) Cigarette smoking can decrease the effectiveness of PPIs in PUD. Even though symptoms can improve quickly, continue treatment for the duration of therapy unless instructed otherwise.

Missed Doses. If you miss a dose, take it as soon as possible. If it is almost time for the next dose, skip the missed dose and return to your usual dosage schedule. Do not double doses.

Pharmacokinetics. *See* Proton Pump Inhibitor Pharmacokinetics Table.

Onset and Duration. PO onset of antisecretory activity is rapid and duration is dose dependent. Gastric acid inhibition increases with repeated daily doses with achievement of maximum acid suppression around day 3 of therapy.[18] Upon discontinuing the PPI, gastric secretory activity gradually returns to pretreatment level within 2–7 days. There is no indication that rebound gastric acidity occurs.

Adverse Effects. All PPIs have similar side effect profiles. The most frequent short-term adverse effects are headache, diarrhea, nausea, skin rashes and abdominal pain.[5,19] In addition, there have been rare reports of topic hepatitis and visual disturbances.[5] Patients infected with *H. pylori* are at greater risk for atrophic gastritis.[19] Through gastric acid secretion, PPIs may cause hypergastrinemia, which is usually modest. Although gastrin levels return to normal after discontinuation of the medication, there is concern that prolonged use and protracted hypergastrinemia may lead to ECL cell hyperplasia and gastric carcinoid tumors. These events have been reported in animals, but human data does not support this increased risk.[1] There is significant concern over the long-term use of PPI and the association with increased infectious risk, such as community-acquired pneumonia, *Clostridium difficile* diarrhea and colitis.[21,22] The potential mechanism for this is increase in chronic hypochlorhydria, which can allow microbial translocation. Another long-term risk is the potential for a decrease in bone density, which has been connected with hip fractures in elderly patients.[23]

Precautions. Experience with PPI use during gestation is limited. Although they appear to be safe, their use is reserved for those whose symptoms fail to be relieved with histamine H2-receptor antagonists.[14] There are sporadic reports of congenital abnormalities in infants born to women who took omeprazole during pregnancy. Symptomatic response to PPI therapy does not preclude the possibility of gastric malignancy.

Drug Interactions. Elevations in gastric pH can affect the absorption of a number of medications. The use of these agents may decrease the rate or extent of absorption of digoxin, itraconazole, ketoconazole, and other drugs or dosage forms that are pH dependent.[1] PPIs are metabolized to different degrees via the cytochrome P450 system. Although lansoprazole, pantoprazole, and rabeprazole do not increase diazepam, warfarin, digoxin, carbamazepine or phenytoin concentrations, these medications are affected by omeprazole and esomeprazole because of its extensive metabolism via the hepatic CYP2C19 isoenzyme.[19] Absorption of PPIs is not affected by coadministration with antacids.[1] Isoenzyme breakdown of clopidogrel to active metabolites may be impaired by PPIs, possibly decreasing efficacy.

Parameters to Monitor. Improvement in epigastric pain or heartburn; however, pain relief in PUD and GERD does not correlate directly with endoscopic evidence of healing. Monitor for potential drug interactions and adverse effects. Monitor laboratory values, including liver function tests, CBC, and SMA-7. Assess the indication, dosage, and duration of PPI therapy, especially as it relates to the need for treatment beyond 16 weeks. Monitor serum vitamin B_{12} concentrations every few years in patients on long-term PPI therapy, especially the elderly.

Notes. Standard dosages provide more rapid relief of symptoms and ulcer or esophageal healing than standard dosages of **H2RA**. This makes them preferred over **H2RA** for PUD, GERD, and for most acid related illnesses.[5] PPIs are the drugs of choice for erosive esophagitis and Zollinger–Ellison syndrome. Patients with gastric or duodenal ulcers or esophagitis refractory to H2RA are likely to respond to PPIs, but the rate of recurrence after discontinuation is similar to that of H2RA. **NSAID**-induced gastric and duodenal ulcers can be prevented or treated by PPIs and are superior to and have a better side effect profile than **misoprostol** 200 µg twice or **ranitidine** 150 mg twice daily.[17,19,24] Dexlansoprazole (Kapidex) is *R*–enantiomer of lansoprazole (a racemic mixture of the *R*– and *S*–enantiomers).

Coadministration of a PPI with an histamine H_2-receptor antagonist or sucralfate is without established benefit. IV PPI therapy can be used for patients with active bleeding and high-risk endoscopic stigmata. The goal of medical management with aggressive acid suppression in this patient population is to prevent re-bleeding following endoscopic stabilization. The regimen is administered as bolus dose followed by continuous infusion. For all other uses, IV PPI formulations are no more effective than oral PPIs.[19]

SUCRALFATE
Carafate, Various

Pharmacology. Sucralfate is an aluminum hydroxide salt of a sulfated disaccharide. Its exact mechanism of action is not known. It forms an ulcer-adherent complex with proteinaceous exudates at the ulcer site, thereby protecting against further attack by acid, pepsin, and bile salts.[1] Adherence to the ulcer crater is enhanced at pH <3.5. The aluminum moiety stimulates endogenous prostaglandins and binds bile salts and phosphate in the GI tract.[1]

Administration and Adult Dosage. **PO for short-term treatment of duodenal ulcer**—1 g four times daily on an empty stomach, 1 h before meals and at bedtime, or 2 g twice daily for 4–8 weeks;[25,26] **PO for maintenance of healed duodenal ulcer**—1 g twice daily; **PO for short-term treatment of active benign gastric ulcer**—1 g four times daily; **PO for treatment of symptomatic GERD or erosive esophagitis**—1 g four times daily; **PO or NG for prevention of upper GI bleeding in patients who are critically ill**—1 g every 4–6 h.[10]

Special Populations. *Pediatric Dosage.* Safety and efficacy not well established. **PO**—40–80 mg/kg/d in 4 divided doses. Alternatively, (<10 kg) 0.5 g every 6h; (>10 kg) 1 g every 6h.[27]

Geriatric Dosage. Dosage reduction usually not necessary.

Dosage Forms. **Tab** 1 g, **Susp** 100 mg/mL.

Patient Instructions. Take this drug with water on an empty stomach 1 hour before each meal and at bedtime. Antacids can be used as needed for pain relief but do not take them within 30 min before or after taking sucralfate. Take potentially interacting drugs 2 h before taking sucralfate to avoid or minimize drug interactions. Even though symptoms can decrease, continue treatment for the duration of therapy unless instructed otherwise.

Missed Doses. If you miss a dose, take it as soon as possible. If it is almost time for your next dose, skip the missed dose and return to your usual dosage schedule. Do not double doses.

Pharmacokinetics. *Onset and Duration.* Onset (attachment of sucralfate to ulcer site) is within 1 h; duration is approximately 6 h.

Fate. Sucralfate is only minimally absorbed from the GI tract and is excreted primarily in the feces. Less than 5% (primarily aluminum) is absorbed and excreted in urine.[1] Aluminum excretion is decreased in uremia.

Adverse Reactions. Because of the minimal absorption, systemic adverse reactions are rare and usually minor in nature. Constipation occurs in ~2% of patients. Other effects, including diarrhea, nausea, gastric discomfort, indigestion, dry mouth, rash, pruritus, backache, dizziness, drowsiness, vertigo, and a metallic taste, occur occasionally. Aluminum accumulation and neurotoxicity, have been reported in patients with chronic renal failure.[1] Hypophosphatemia can develop in patients who are critically ill and those on prolonged sucralfate therapy. Bezoar formation in the esophagus and GI tract and intestinal obstruction and perforation have been reported.[25]

Precautions. Use with caution in patients receiving other aluminum-containing drugs or in chronic renal failure and dialysis. Avoid administration through feeding tubes because the drug can occlude the tube.

Drug Interactions. Sucralfacte can bind a number of medications and may reduce absorption. Sucralfate can inhibit the absorption of drugs including digoxin, ketoconazole, levothyroxine, phenytoin, quinidine, oral fluoroquinolones, tetracyclines, theophylline, and warfarin. In most cases, drug interactions can be avoided if the drug is given 2 h before sucralfate administration, especially in patients receiving tube feedings.

Parameters to Monitor. Improvement in epigastric pain or heartburn; however, pain relief in PUD and GERD does not correlate directly with endoscopic evidence of healing. Monitor for constipation and signs of aluminum toxicity in the elderly, in chronic renal failure, or in patients receiving other aluminum-containing drugs. Obtain serum phosphate levels periodically in patients receiving concurrent aluminum-containing drugs or with prolonged use. Monitor for potential drug interactions.

Notes. Sucralfate can overcome the negative effect of cigarette smoking on duodenal ulcer healing and recurrence.[25] Its efficacy in healing erosive esophagitis and maintaining esophageal healing is inferior to the **H2RA** or PPI. Its efficacy as a single agent in preventing NSAID-induced gastric and duodenal ulcers, chemotherapy-induced stomatitis, and stress-related bleeding in high-risk critically ill surgical patients is unsubstantiated. Whether sucralfate is associated with a lower frequency of nosocomial pneumonia than histamine H2-receptor antagonists or antacids in patients who are critically ill remains controversial.[10] Although therapy with sucralfate and an H2RA or PPI provides two different mechanisms of drug action, enhanced efficacy of two drugs has not been substantiated for any indication.

ERADICATION OF *HELICOBACTER PYLORI* INFECTION

After excluding the use of NSAIDs, the primary cause of PUD is associated with *H. pylori* infections. *H. pylori* is a fastidious, micro-aerophilic, gram-negative flagellate first described in 1984.[28] Risk factors for infection with *H. pylori* are birth outside the United States and lower socioeconomic status.[29] However, it is estimated that 20–50% of the population in developed countries is infected with *H. pylori*.[30,31] Patients infected or colonized with *H. pylori* are at increased risk for developing PUD, chronic gastritis, gastric carcinoma, atrophic gastric and gastric mucosa-associated lymphoid tissue (MALT) lymphoma.[31]

Diagnosis and treatment for *H. pylori* infection is indicated in patients with active peptic acid disease, confirmed history of documented peptic ulcer (not previously treated for *H. pylori*), post-endoscopic resection of early gastric cancer, or gastric MALT lymphoma. The value of *H. pylori* diagnosis and treatment in patients with dyspepsia or nonulcer dyspepsia, GERD, active NSAID use, unexplained iron deficiency anemia, and high risk for gastric cancer remains controversial.[32–34] The goal of therapy is to promote rapid ulcer healing and prevent relapse by eradicating the infection.

The American College of Gastroenterology Guidelines published in 2007 recommend that the initial choice in antimicrobial and acid suppression therapy utilize a PPI, clarithromycin, and either amoxicillin or metronidazole. This triple drug regimen can be substituted for a regimen containing a H2RA, bismuth, metronidazole, and tetracycline. This regimen would be an option for penicillin-allergic patients as one triple therapy regimen contains amoxicillin. Duration of therapy generally recommended is 10–14 days. Sequential therapy (5 days of PPI + amoxicillin; 5 days of PPI + clarithromycin + tinidazole) is favored in Europe, and implies that two separate regimens are used in combination to increase likelihood of successful eradication.[31,35] Further validation is required in the United States before it can be recommended as first-line therapy.[31,35]

Factors to consider when choosing a *H. pylori* regimen include eradication rates, patient compliance, and minimizing drug resistance and adverse effects associated with the drug therapy. Dual therapy (PPI and one antibiotic) is rarely used because eradication rates are often poor (<70%), but triple therapy is used because it obtains an eradication rate of at least 80%–90%. The eradication rate for quadruple therapy is >90%.[31] Even though quadruple therapy is effective in eliminating the infection, it is not ideal because of the complicated dosage regimen that can lead to decreased patient adherence. Adverse effects can decrease patient adherence, especially those treated with metronidazole.

Eradication of the organism occurs in ~80% of patients treated with the recommended therapy; however, a proportion of patients will fail initial therapy. If the initial regimen contained clarithromycin then the second-line regimen should not include this drug. It has been suggested that if the patient does not respond to initial triple therapy, then quadruple drug regimens should be considered.[31,35,36] It should be noted that in European studies, a shorter duration of therapy is utilized; however, the regimens are associated with higher rates of treatment failures.[31] Resistance is a significant issue in regard to *H. pylori*. When choosing antibiotics, resistance is always an issue. Metronidazole resistance to *H. pylori* infections is ~40% in the U.S. and higher in other countries. It is also more frequent in women. Macrolide resistance is less common (up to 10%) and is less frequent with tetracycline and amoxicillin.[33]

Antibiotics should not be used for longer than 2 weeks. If treatment fails, an alternative antibiotic regimen should be considered. Although any PPI can be used in the various regimens, there are some substitutions that should not be done (e.g., ampicillin for amoxicillin, doxycycline for tetracycline, azithromycin for clarithromycin, or an H2RA for a PPI).[37–40] There are studies that support the use of levofloxacin-containing regimens as third-line therapies. These studies have demonstrated that levofloxacin could be a viable alternative to standard regimens, as levofloxacin is well tolerated by most patients and offers ease of administration when compared to other regimens with greater pill burden.[41,42] At this time, regimenscontaining levofloxacin should NOT be utilized as a first-line treatment as they require further study in the United States.

ACID NEUTRALIZING CAPACITY OF COMMON ORGANIC SALTS USED IN ANTACID PRODUCTS

ORGANIC SALT[a]	ACID NEUTRALIZING CAPACITY mEq/15 mL
Aluminum Carbonate, Basic	36
Aluminum Hydroxide	29
Magnesium Carbonate	Low[b]
Aluminum Hydroxide with Magnesium Hydroxide	63
Sodium Bicarbonate	17
Calcium Carbonate	58
Magnesium Hydroxide	35
Magaldrate	36

[a]These compounds are often marketed as combination products.
[b]Due to low acid neutralizing capacity, should be combined with other compounds.
From Ref. 3.

HISTAMINE H2-RECEPTOR ANTAGONISTS ADULT INDICATIONS AND DOSAGE

INDICATION	CIMETIDINE	FAMOTIDINE	RANITIDINE
PO for prevention or symptomatic relief of heartburn or indigestion (OTC)	200 mg/d or 200 mg twice daily	10–20 mg/d or 10–20 mg twice daily	75–150 mg/d or 75–150 mg twice daily
PO for short-term treatment of active duodenal or gastric ulcer (4–8 wk)	300 mg four times daily, 400 mg twice daily, 800 mg at bedtime, or 1600 mg at bedtime[a]	20 mg twice daily or 40 mg at bedtime	150 mg twice daily or 300 mg at bedtime
PO for maintenance of healed duodenal or gastric ulcer	400–800 mg at bedtime	20 mg at bedtime	150–300 mg at bedtime
IV intermittent	300 every 6–8 h, up to 2.4 g/d[d]	20 mg every 12 h[c]	50 mg every 6–8 h, up to 400 mg/d[c]

(continued)

HISTAMINE H2-RECEPTOR ANTAGONISTS ADULT INDICATIONS AND DOSAGE (*continued*)

INDICATION	CIMETIDINE	FAMOTIDINE	RANITIDINE
IV intermittent bolus	Dilute to 20 mL; Inject over not less than 5 min[c]	Dilute to 5–10 mL; Inject over not less than 2 min[c]	Dilute to 20 mL; Inject over not less than 5 min[c]
IV intermittent infusion	Dilute to 50 mL; infuse over 15–20 min[c]	Dilute to 100 mL; infuse over 15–30 min[c]	Dilute to 100 mL; infuse over 15–20 min[c]

IV for prevention of upper GI bleeding in critically ill patients. (cimetidine) 50 mg/h by continuous infusion OR cimetidine, famotidine, or ranitidine use standard dosages given enterally or by intermittent or continuous infusion.[b]

[a]Heavy smokers with ulcers larger than 1 cm in diameter.
[b]Unapproved indication and dosage.
[c]Pathologic hypersecretory states, intractable ulcers, or patients unable to take oral medication.
[d]Unapproved route of administration.
From Refs. 6–11.

HISTAMINE H2-RECEPTOR ANTAGONISTS DOSAGE FORMS

CIMETIDINE	FAMOTIDINE	RANITIDINE
Tab 100, 200, 300, 400, 800 mg	Tab 10, 20, 40 mg	Tab 75, 150, 300 mg
	Chew Tab 10 mg	Effervescent Tab 150 mg[a]
Soln 60 mg/mL	Chew Tab	Effervescent Granules
Inj 6 mg/mL (premixed)	10 mg (Pepcid Complete)[b]	150 mg[a]
Inj 150 mg/mL	Rapid Dissolving Tab	Cap 150, 300 mg
	20, 40 mg	Syrup 15 mg/mL
	Susp 8 mg/mL [c]	Inj 0.5 (premixed), 25 mg/mL
	Inj 0.4 mg/mL (premixed)	
	Inj 10 mg/mL[d]	

[a]Dissolve dose in approximately 180–240 mL (6–8 fl oz) of water before drinking.
[b]Contains calcium carbonate 800 mg and magnesium hydroxide 165 mg.
[c]Discard reconstituted suspension after 30 days.
[d]Store at 2°C–8°C (36–46°F).

HISTAMINE H2-RECEPTOR ANTAGONISTS STRUCTURES

	CIMETIDINE	FAMOTIDE	RANITIDINE
Ring structure	Imidazole	Thiazole	Furan
Relative potency	1	20–50	4–8
Neonates	5–10 mg/kg/d	1–1.2 mg/kg/d	0.5–3 mg/kg/d
Children	20–40 mg/kg/d twice daily	1–1.2 mg/kg/d two to three time daily	2–4 mg/kg/d[a] 5–10 mg/kg/d twice daily[b]

[a]Duodenal ulcer and gastric ulcer.
[b]GERD and esophagitis.
From Ref. 12.

HISTAMINE H2-RECEPTOR ANTAGONISTS PHARMACOKINETICS

	CIMETIDINE	FAMOTIDINE	RANITIDINE
Onset			
All agents have an oral onset of 1 h and a IV onset of 15 min.			
Serum Levels			
EC_{50}[a]	625 ± 375 μg/L	11 ± 2 μg/L	112 ± 52 μg/L
Fate			
Oral bioavailability	$60 \pm 20\%$	$41 \pm 4\%$	$55 \pm 25\%$
V_d	1 ± 0.2 L/kg	1.2 ± 0.3 L/kg	1.6 ± 0.4 L/kg
Protein binding	$20 \pm 6\%$	16%	15%
Excreted unchanged in urine	75%	65–70%	68–79%
Half-life			
Normal	1.9 ± 0.4 h	3 ± 0.5 h	2 ± 0.4 h
Anuric	4.5 ± 0.5 h	20 ± 4 h	7 ± 3 h

[a]EC_{50} is the serum concentration necessary to inhibit pentagastrin-stimulated secretion of acid by 50.
From Refs. 6–12.

PROTON PUMP INHIBITOR ADULT INDICATIONS AND DOSAGE

INDICATION	ESOMEPRAZOLE	LANSOPRAZOLE	OMEPRAZOLE	PANTOPRAZOLE	RABEPRAZOLE
Treatment of active duodenal ulcer (4 wk)	–	15 mg/d[a]	20 mg/d[a]	40 mg/d[b]	20 mg/d[a]
Maintenance of duodenal ulcer healing (1 y)	–	15 mg/d[a]	20 mg/d[b]	20 mg/d[b]	20 mg/d[a]
Treatment of active gastric ulcer (4–8 wk)	–	30 mg/d[a]	40 mg/d[a]	40 mg/d[b]	20–40 mg/d[b]
Maintenance of gastric ulcer healing	–	15–30 mg/d[b]	20–40 mg/d[b]	40 mg/d[b]	20–40 mg/d[b]
Treatment of symptomatic GERD (4–8 wk)	20–40 mg/d[a]	15 mg/d[a]	20 mg/d[a]	20 mg/d[b]	20 mg/d[a]
Treatment of erosive esophagitis (4–8 wk)	20–40 mg/d[a]	30 mg/d[a]	20 mg/d[a]	40 mg/d[a]	20 mg/d[a]
Maintenance of erosive esophagitis	20 mg/d[a]	15 mg/d[a]	20 mg/d[a]	40 mg/d[a]	20 mg/d[a]

(continued)

PROTON PUMP INHIBITOR ADULT INDICATIONS AND DOSAGE (*continued*)

INDICATION	ESOMEPRAZOLE	LANSOPRAZOLE	OMEPRAZOLE	PANTOPRAZOLE	RABEPRAZOLE
PO for treatment of pathologic hypersecretory conditions	40 mg twice daily[a]	60 mg/d,[a] up to 90 mg twice daily[c]	60 mg/d,[a] up to 120 mg three times daily[c]	40 mg twice daily[a] up to 240 mg/d[c]	60 mg/d,[a] up to 120 mg three times daily[c]
Risk reduction of NSAID-induced gastric ulcers	20–40 mg/d	15 mg/d[a]	20 mg/d[b]	40 mg/d[b]	–

[a]Approved indication and dosage.
[b]Unapproved indication and dosage.
[c]Adjust dosage to patient's needs and continue as long as clinically indicated.
From Ref. 19.

PROTON PUMP INHIBITOR PEDIATRIC INDICATIONS AND DOSAGE

MEDICATION	INDICATION	STARTING DOSE	MAXIMUM DOSE
Omeprazole	GERD	1 mg/kg/d daily or twice daily	60–80 mg/d
	PUD[a]	1 mg/kg/d twice daily	
Lansoprazole	GERD[b]	(≤30kg) 15 mg once daily	30 mg/d
		(>30 kg) 30 mg once daily	60 mg/d
	PUD[a]	1 mg/kg/d twice daily	60 mg/d

[a]Used in combination with antimicrobial therapy for treatment of *H. pylori*.
[b]Short-term treatment up to 12 weeks.
From Ref. 20.

PROTON PUMP INHIBITOR AVAILABILITY

DEXLANSOPRAZOLE	ESOMEPRAZOLE	LANSOPRAZOLE	OMEPRAZOLE	PANTOPRAZOLE	RABEPRAZOLE
Delayed-release Cap 30 mg, 60 mg	Delayed-release Cap 20 mg, 40 mg	Enteric-coated granule Cap 15[a], 30[b] mg	Enteric-coated granules Cap 10, 20, 40 mg	Enteric-coated Tab 20 mg, 40 mg	Delayed-release Tab 20 mg
	Susp packets 10 mg, 20 mg, 40 mg Inj 20 mg/vial, 40 mg/vial	Solu Tab® 15 mg	Pwdr for PO Susp 20 mg, 40 mg[c]	Delayed release PO Susp packet 40 mg Inj 40 mg	

[a]Naprapac consists of lansoprazole delayed-release 15 mg capsules and naproxen 500 mg tablets kit.

[b]Prevpac for *H. pylori* therapy consists of two lansoprazole 30 mg capsules, four amoxicillin 500 mg capsules, and two clarithromycin 500 mg tablets in an individual daily administration pack.

[c]Contains sodium bicarbonate.

PROTON PUMP INHIBITOR PHARMACOKINETICS

	DEXLANSOPRAZOLE	ESOMEPRAZOLE	LANSOPRAZOLE	OMEPRAZOLE	PANTOPRAZOLE	RABEPRAZOLE
Oral Bioavailability (%)	N/A	64	80	30–40	77	52
Protein Binding (%)	96–98	97	97	95	98	96
T_{max} (h)	1–2 and 4–5	1.6	1.7	0.5–3.5	2.0–4.0	1.6–5.0
Half-life (h)	1–2	1.2–1.5	1.5	0.5–1	1.9	0.7–1.5

From Ref. 19.

DRUG TREATMENT REGIMENS USED TO ERADICATE *HELICOBACTER PYLORI*

DRUGS	DOSE	FREQUENCY	DURATION	EFFICACY[a]	ADVERSE EFFECTS[b]	COMPLIANCE[c]
Amoxicillin Omeprazole[d,e]	1 g 20 mg	two to three times daily two to three times daily	14 d 14 d	Poor–fair	Low–medium	Likely
Clarithromycin Omeprazole[d,e,f]	500 mg 40 mg	three times daily qd	14 d 14 d	Fair–good	Low–medium	Likely
Amoxicillin Lansoprazole[d,e,f,]	1 g 30 mg	three times daily three times daily	10–14 d 10–14 d	Poor–Fair	Low–medium	Likely
Clarithromycin RBC	500 mg 400 mg	three times daily twice daily	14 d 28 d	Fair–good	Low–Medium	Likely
Clarithromycin Metronidazole Omeprazole[d,e]	500 mg 500 mg 20 mg	twice daily twice daily twice daily	10–14 d 10–14 d 10–14 d	Good–excellent	Medium	Likely
Clarithromycin Amoxicillin Lansoprazole[d,e,f]	500 mg 1 g 30 mg	twice daily twice daily twice daily	10–14 d 10–14 d 10–14 d	Good–excellent	Low–medium	Likely
Amoxicillin Metronidazole Omeprazole[d,e]	1 g 500 mg 20 mg	twice daily twice daily twice daily	14 d 14 d 14 d	Fair–good	Medium	Likely

(continued)

DRUG TREATMENT REGIMENS USED TO ERADICATE *HELICOBACTER PYLORI* (*continued*)

DRUGS	DOSE	FREQUENCY	DURATION	EFFICACY[a]	ADVERSE EFFECTS[b]	COMPLIANCE[c]
Clarithromycin	500 mg	twice daily	14 d	Good	Medium	Unlikely
Metronidazole	500 mg	twice daily	14 d			
RBC	400 mg	twice daily	14–28 d			
BSS	525 mg	four times daily	14 d	Good–excellent	Medium–high	Unlikely
Metronidazole	150 mg	four times daily	14 d			
Tetracycline	500 mg	four times daily	14 d			
H2RA[f]	Conventional ulcer healing dosage regimen for ≥8 c					
BSS	525 mg	four times daily	14 d	Fair–good	Medium–high	Unlikely
Metronidazole	250 mg	four times daily	14 d			
Amoxicillin	500 mg	four times daily	14 d			
H2RA[f]	Conventional ulcer healing dosage regimen for ≥8 c					
BSS	525 mg	four times daily	7 d	Good–excellent	Medium–high	Unlikely
Metronidazole	500 mg	four times daily	7 d			
Tetracycline	500 mg	four times daily	7 d			
Omeprazole[d,e]	20 mg	twice daily	7 d			
BSS	525 mg	four times daily	7 d	Good–excellent	Medium–high	Unlikely
Metronidazole	500 mg	four times daily	7 d			
Clarithromycin	500 mg	twice daily	7 d			
Omeprazole[d,e]	20 mg	twice daily	7 d			

(*continued*)

DRUG TREATMENT REGIMENS USED TO ERADICATE *HELICOBACTER PYLORI* (continued)

DRUGS	DOSE	FREQUENCY	DURATION	EFFICACY[a]	ADVERSE EFFECTS[b]	COMPLIANCE[c]
BSS	525 mg	four times daily	7–14 d	Good–excellent	Medium	Unlikely
Clairthromycin	500 mg	three times daily	7–14 d			
Tetracycline	500 mg	four times daily	7–14 d			
Omeprazole[d,e]	20 mg	twice daily	7–14 d			

BSS = bismuth subsalicylate; H2RA = Histamine H2-receptor antagonist; PPI = proton pump inhibitor; RBC = ranitidine bismuth citrate.

[a]Efficacy (eradication rate): excellent >90%; good 80–90%; fair 70–80%; poor <70%.

[b]Adverse Effects = frequency of clinically important adverse effects.

[c]Compliance = estimate based on total number of tablets/capsules, frequency of administration, and clinically important adverse effects.

[d]Any PPI can be used (esomeprazole 40 mg, lansoprazole 30 mg, omeprazole 20 mg, pantoprazole 20–40 mg, rabeprazole 40 mg).

[e]PPI therapy can be extended to 28 days in patients with active ulcer.

[f]Approved regimen.

■ REFERENCES

1. Chan F, Lau J. Treatment of Peptic Ulcer Disease. In: Feldman M, Friedman LS, Brandt LJ, eds. *Sleisenger & Fordtran's Gastrointestinal and Liver Disease*, Philadelphia: WB Saunders; 1111-1115.

2. Orlando R. Diseases of the Esophagus. In: Goldman L, Ausiello DA, eds. *Cecil Medicine* 23rd ed. Philadelphia: Saunders Elsevier; 2008:998-1009.

3. Maton P, Burton M. Antacids revisited: a review of their clinical pharmacology and recommended therapeutic use. *Drugs*. 1999;57:855-870.

4. Labeling of drug preparations containing salicylates. Food and Drug Administration. http://www.fda.gov/cder/otcmonographs/Antidiarrheal/antidiarrheal_FM_20030417.pdf. Accessed April 29, 2009.

5. Shi S, Klotz U. Proton pump inhibitors: an update of their clinical use and pharmacokinetics. *Eur J Clin Pharmacol*. 2008;64:935-951.

6. Product Information: Tagamet, cimetidine. Miami, FL. IVAX Pharmaceuticals, Inc. 08/2008.

7. Product Information: Pepcid AC®, famotidine. Johnson & Johnson—Merck Consumer Pharmaceuticals Co. Available at: http://www.pepcid.com/page.jhtml?id=pepcid/relief/relief_2.inc Accessed April 29, 2009.

8. Product Information: Zantac, ranitidine. Boehringer Ingelheim Pharmaceuticals. http://www.zantacotc.com/product_info_CD.aspx Accessed April 29, 2009.

9. Hatlebakk JG, Berstad A. Pharmacokinetic optimisation in the treatment of gastro-oesophageal reflux disease. *Clin Pharmacokinet*. 1996;31:386-406.

10. ASHP Therapeutic Guidelines on stress ulcer prophylaxis. *Am J Health-Syst Pharm*. 1999;15(56):347-379.

11. Welage LS. Overview of pharmacologic agents for acid suppression in critically ill patients *Am J Health-Syst Pharm*. 2005;62(Suppl 10):S4-S10.

12. Guimarães EV et al. Treatment of gastroesophageal reflux disease. *Jornal de Pediatria*. 2006;82(Suppl 5): S133-S144.

13. Richter JM et al. Cimetidine and adverse reactions: a meta-analysis of randomized clinical trials of short-term therapy. *Am J Med*. 1989;87:278-284.

14. Eliot D. Pregnancy, hypertension and other common medical problems. In: Goldman L, Ausiello DA, eds. *Cecil Medicine*. 23rd ed. Philadelphia: Saunders Elsevier; 2008:1840-1850.

15. Gralnek IM et al. Management of acute bleeding from a peptic ulcer. *N Engl J Med*. 2008;359:928-937.

16. Pilotto A at al. Recent advances in the treatment of GERD in the elderly: focus on proton pump inhibitors. *Int J Clin Pract*. 2005;59:1204-1209.

17. Hawkey CJ et al. Omeprazole compared with misoprostol for ulcers associated with nonsteroidal anti-inflammatory drugs. *N Engl J Med*. 1998; 338:727-734.

18. Sachs G et al. Review article: the clinical pharmacology of proton pump inhibitors. *Aliment Pharmacol Ther* 2006;23(Suppl 2):2-8.

19. Boparai V et al. Guide to the use of proton pump inhibitors in adult patient. *Drugs*. 2008;68:925-947.

20. Litalien C. Pharmacokinetics of proton pump inhibitors in children. *Clin Pharmacokinet*. 2005;44:441-466.

21. Laheij RJ et al. Risk of community-acquired pneumonia and use of gastric acid suppressive drugs. *JAMA*. 2004;292:1955-1960.

22. Dial S et al. Risk of *Clostridium difficile* diarrhea among hospital patients prescribed proton pump inhibitors: cohort and case-control studies. *CMAJ* 2004;171:33-38.

23. Yang YX et al. Long-term proton pump inhibitor therapy and risk of hip fracture. *JAMA*. 2006;286:2947-2953.

24. Zullo A et al. Bleeding peptic ulcer in the elderly. *Drugs Aging*. 2007;24:815-828.

25. McCarthy DM. Sucralfate. *N Engl J Med*. 1991;325:1017-1025.

26. Jensen SL, Funch Jensen P. Role of sucralfate in peptic disease. *Dig Dis*. 1992;10:153-161.

27. Crill CM, Hak EB. Upper gastrointestinal tract bleeding in critically ill pediatric patients. *Pharmacotherapy*. 1999;19:162-180.

28. Marshall BJ, Warren JR. Unidentified curved bacilli in the stomach of patients with gastritis and peptic ulceration. *Lancet*. 1984;1:1311-1315.

29. Everhart JE et al. Seroprevalence and ethnic differences in *Helicobacter pylori* infection among adults in the United States. *J Infect Dis*. 2000;181:1359-1363.

30. Suerbaum S, Michetti P. *Helicobacter pylori* infection. *N Engl J Med*. 2002;347:1175-1186.

31. Chey WD, Wong BC. American College of Gastroenterology guideline on the management of *Helicobacter pylori* infection. *Am J Gastroenterol* 2007;102:1808-1825.

32. Talley NJ. How should *Helicobacter pylori* positive dyspeptic patients be managed? *Gut* 1999;45(Suppl 1): I28-I31.

33. Peitz U et al. A practical approach to patients with refractory *Helicobacter pylori* infection, or who are reinfected after standard therapy. *Drugs*. 1999;57:905-920.

34. Stanghellini V et al. How should *Helicobacter pylori* negative patients be managed? *Gut*. 1999;45(Suppl 1): I32-I35.

35. Egan BJ et al. Treatment of *Helicobacter pylori* infection. *Helicobacter.* 2008;13(Suppl 1):35-40.

36. Gisbert JP. "Rescue" regimens after *Helicobacter pylori* treatment failure. *World J Gastroenterol.* 2008;14: 5385-5402.

37. Welage LS, Berardi RR. Evaluation of omeprazole, lansoprazole, pantoprazole, and rabeprazole in the treatment of acid-related diseases. *J Am Pharm Assoc.* 2000;40:52-62.

38. Klotz U. Pharmacokinetic considerations in the eradication of *Helicobacter pylori. Clin Pharmacokinet* 2000;38:243-270.

39. Stack WA et al. Safety and efficacy of rabeprazole in combination with four antibiotic regimens for the eradication of *Helicobacter pylori* in patients with chronic gastritis with or without peptic ulceration. *Am J Gastroenterol.* 1998;93:1909-1913.

40. Dajani AI et al. One-week triple regime therapy consisting of pantoprazole, amoxicillin and clarithromycin for cure of *Helicobacter pylori*-associated upper gastrointestinal diseases. *Digestion* 1999;60:298-304.

41. Gisbert JP et al. Second-line rescue therapy with levofloxacin after *H. pylori* treatment failure: a Spanish multi-center study of 300 patients. *Am J Gastroenterol.* 2008;103:71-76.

42. Kuo CH et al. Efficacy of levofloxacin-based rescue therapy for *Helicobacter pylori* infection after standard triple therapy: a randomized controlled trial. *J Antimicrob Chemother* 2009;63:1017-1024.

Chapter 44

Antiemetics

Mark T. Holdsworth

APREPITANT Emend

Pharmacology. Aprepitant is an antagonist at the substance P/neurokinin 1 (NK_1) receptor. It has antiemetic activity in both the acute (e.g., during chemotherapy) and delayed (e.g., following chemotherapy) phases of chemotherapy-induced emesis. It is indicated for the prevention of acute and delayed nausea and vomiting due to either moderately or highly emetogenic chemotherapy. It is also indicated for the prevention of postoperative nausea/vomiting.[1]

Administration and Adult Dosage. **PO for chemotherapy-induced nausea and vomiting**—125 mg on day 1, followed by 80 mg on days 2 and 3. **IV for chemotherapy-induced nausea and vomiting**—115 mg on day 1 only. **PO for postoperative nausea and vomiting**—40 mg within 3 h prior to induction.

Pediatric Dosage. Safety and efficacy not established.

Dosage Forms. **Cap** 40 mg, 80 mg, 125 mg; **Inj** 115 mg.

Pharmacokinetics. *Fate.* Aprepitant undergoes extensive hepatic metabolism, mainly by CYP3A4 and to a lesser degree by CYP1A2 and CYP2C19. The IV formulation, fosaprepitant, is a prodrug that is rapidly converted to aprepitant following IV administration. V_{dss} is ~70 L and Cl is 60–90 mL/min. The pharmacokinetics of aprepitant within the approved dosage range are nonlinear, such that the AUC was 26% greater than what would be dose proportional between the 80 mg and 125 mg doses. Absolute oral bioavailability is approximately 60%–65% and is not influenced by food. Time to C_{max} is ~4 h. No dosage adjustment is necessary for patients with mild-moderate hepatic dysfunction or in patients with severe renal dysfunction, including those requiring hemodialysis.[1] **Half-life.** 9–13 h.

Adverse Reactions. The most commonly reported adverse effect is asthenia/fatigue and occurred to a greater extent on study arms employing aprepitant versus standard therapy (~17% vs 10%). Other commonly reported adverse reactions included anorexia, constipation, diarrhea, nausea, and hiccups; although there was not a substantial difference in these events between aprepitant arms and arms that did not contain aprepitant.

Drug Interactions. As a substrate and a moderate inhibitor and inducer of CYP3A4, and an inducer of CPY2C9, aprepitant does have the potential to either cause or be impacted by drug interactions. It has been demonstrated that aprepitant will increase systemic exposure to dexamethasone, methylprednisolone and midazolam. The interaction with dexamethasone is substantial, with an approximate 2-fold increase in dexamethasone AUC following oral administration.[1] The interaction with IV dexamethasone also appears to be of a similar magnitude.[2] This is of particular importance since dexamethasone is very likely to be employed in combination with aprepitant as a component of antiemetic therapy. As such, it is recommended that the dexamethasone dose be reduced by ~50% when it is combined with aprepitant. In a study where aprepitant was associated with a higher incidence of febrile neutropenia in patients, the dexamethasone dose was not reduced to account for the interaction and thus these patients were exposed to double the systemic exposure, which likely accounted for the greater risk of febrile neutropenia.[1] It is also important to acknowledge that some of the potential drug interactions between aprepitant and chemotherapy agents have not actually been demonstrated in carefully conducted trials. In particular, despite potential interactions between aprepitant and both vinorelbine and docetaxel, which are both primarily 3A4 substrates, no significant interactions were demonstrated.[3,4]

Notes. Studies to date have demonstrated a greater impact of aprepitant on reducing vomiting versus reducing nausea scores among patients receiving chemotherapy.

DOLASETRON MESYLATE   Anzemet

Pharmacology. Dolasetron and its active metabolite, hydrodolasetron, are selective serotonin$_3$ (5-HT$_3$) antagonists. Its use is similar to those of ondansetron and granisetron.[5] (*See* Antiemetic Drugs Comparison Chart.)

Administrxation and Adult Dosage. **PO or IV for chemotherapy-induced nausea and vomiting**—100 mg or 1.8 mg/kg; **IV for postoperative nausea and vomiting**—12.5 mg. **PO for postoperative nausea and vomiting**—100 mg.

Pediatric Dosage. **PO or IV for chemotherapy-induced nausea and vomiting**—(≤2 years) Safety and efficacy not established; (2–16 years) 1.8 mg/kg, to a maximum of 100 mg; **IV for postoperative nausea and vomiting**—(2–16 years) 0.35 mg/kg, to a maximum of 12.5 mg; **PO for postoperative nausea and vomiting**—(2–16 years) 1.2 mg/kg, to a maximum of 100 mg.

Dosage Forms. **Inj** 20 mg/mL; **Tab** 50 and 100 mg.

Pharmacokinetics. Approximately 75% of dolasetron mesylate is dolasetron base. The apparent absolute bioavailability of oral dolasetron is approximately 75%. Little dolasetron is detected in the plasma because of rapid conversion to hydrodolasetron by the ubiquitous enzyme, carbonyl reductase. Hydrodolasetron is partly metabolized in the liver and 61% is excreted unchanged in the urine. Hydrodolasetron has a V_d of 5.8 ± 1.5 L/kg and Cl of 0.56 ± 0.16 L/h/kg. **Half-life.** 7.3 ± 1.8 h.

Adverse Reactions. Acute, reversible ECG changes (PR and QT$_c$ prolongation, and QRS widening) have occurred in clinical trials and in healthy volunteers. Other adverse effects are similar to those of ondansetron and granisetron.

Notes. Dolasetron can be prepared extemporaneously as an oral solution by mixing the injectable form in apple or apple–grape juice. The diluted product can be kept up to 2 h at room temperature before use. IV doses can be administered over a minimum of 30 s or further diluted in 50 mL of NS or D5W and infused over a period of up to 15 min. In some dose-finding trials in adults, higher response rates were obtained with 200 mg PO and 2.4 mg IV than with lower doses by the respective routes.[5]

DRONABINOL
Marinol

Pharmacology. Dronabinol (Δ-9-tetrahydrocannabinol) is an active antiemetic component of *Cannabis*. Its mechanism of action as an antiemetic is complex and poorly understood, but it probably inhibits the chemoreceptor trigger zone in the medulla.

Administration and Adult Dosage. **PO for chemotherapy-induced nausea and vomiting**—5 mg/m^2 1–3 h before chemotherapy and then every 2–4 h after chemotherapy, for a total of 4–6 doses/d. Dosage can be increased in 2.5 mg/m^2 increments, to a maximum of 15 mg/m^2/dose.[6–8] **PO for appetite stimulation in AIDS patients**—2.5 mg before lunch and dinner or 2.5 mg at bedtime if unable to tolerate daytime administration, to a maximum of 20 mg/d.

Special Populations. *Pediatric Dosage.* **PO as an antiemetic during cancer chemotherapy**—Same as adult dosage in mg/m^2.

Geriatric Dosage. Same as adult dosage. (*See* Adverse Reactions.)

Dosage Forms. Cap 2.5, 5, 10 mg.

Patient Instructions. This drug can cause drowsiness or changes in mood. Until the extent of this effect is known, use caution when driving, operating machinery, or performing other tasks requiring mental alertness. Avoid excessive concurrent use of alcohol or other drugs that cause drowsiness. Store this medication in the refrigerator.

Missed Doses. Take this drug at regular intervals. If you miss a dose, take it as soon as you remember. If it is about time for the next dose, take that dose only. Do not double the dose or take an extra dose.

Pharmacokinetics. *Onset and Duration.* Oral onset 30–60 min; peak 2–4 h; duration is 4–6 h, but can be longer in those who have not previously used the drug.[9,10] *Cannabis* smoking onset 15 sec–2 min; peak 8–16 min; duration 3–12 h.[11]

Fate. Bioavailability is 4%–12% orally, 2%–50% by smoking. About 95% bound to plasma proteins. V_d is 8.9 $\pm$ 4.2 L/kg; CL is 0.21 $\pm$ 0.054 L/h/kg. Primarily metabolized by hydroxylation to active and inactive metabolites. Ultimately, 35% of metabolites are found in feces and 15% in urine, with <1% excreted unchanged in urine.[12–14] **Half-life.** Terminal phase 32 $\pm$ 12 h, although time course of effects more closely parallels initial distribution phase.[12]

Adverse Reactions. Euphoria, dizziness, paranoia, or drowsiness occur frequently and might be accompanied by ataxia, loss of balance, and disorientation to the point of being disabling. Other frequent side effects are dry mouth, orthostatic hypotension, and conjunctival infection.[15] The "high" experienced by some is not always well tolerated, especially by older patients.[16]

Contraindications. Allergy to dronabinol, marijuana, or sesame oil; mentally ill patients.

Precautions. Avoid during lactation. Use with caution in patients with hypertension or heart disease. Use with caution in patients with epilepsy.[6]

Drug Interactions. Not well studied, but some apparent interactions have been reported after *Cannabis* use: additive or supra-additive sedation with alcohol and other CNS depressants; additive hypertension and tachycardia with anticholinergics, antihistamines, sympathomimetics, or tricyclic antidepressants; and hypomania with disulfiram or fluoxetine.

Parameters to Monitor. Observe for frequency of emesis, drowsiness, or disorientation.

Notes. Dronabinol is at least as effective as **phenothiazines** for chemotherapy-induced nausea and vomiting,[8] but not as effective as **serotonin antagonists** or IV **metoclopramide.**[17,18] It is not particularly effective for cisplatin-induced nausea and vomiting. It might not be as effective as smoking *Cannabis*, which is easier to titrate.[18] (*See* Antiemetic Drugs Comparison Chart.)

DROPERIDOL
Inapsine, Various

Pharmacology. Droperidol is a butyrophenone derivative and a dopamine D2 receptor antagonist. It also has a lower affinity for α_{1A} adrenergic receptors and can produce a decrease in blood pressure. It has demonstrated antiemetic activity in patients undergoing general anesthesia. Studies have demonstrated a lower duration of activity on preventing nausea versus vomiting, perhaps due to its short half-life.[19]

Administration and Adult Dosage. **IV for prevention and treatment of postoperative nausea and vomiting**—0.625–1.25 mg (up to a maximum of 2.5 mg) at the end of anesthesia.

Special Populations. *Pediatric Dosage.* **IV for prevention and treatment of postoperative nausea and vomiting**—(>2 years and >10 kg) 0.02–0.075 mg/kg.

Geriatric Dosage. Same as adult dosage. (*See* Adverse Reactions.)

Other conditions. Renal and Hepatic Impairment. Lower doses are preferred.

Dosage Forms. Inj. 2.5 mg/mL.

Pharmacokinetics. *Fate.* Droperidol has rapid distribution to the brain. V_{DSS} 1.5 L/kg in adults and 0.6 L/kg for children. Cl is 0.66 L/h/kg. Droperidol is metabolized by the liver and excreted by the kidney. **Half-life.** 2 h.

Adverse Reactions. The most common adverse effect is sedation, which is dose-related. Headache and dizziness are also reported. Droperidol can produce a dose-related increase in the QT_c interval. A black box warning was issued regarding the association of droperidol with fatal cardiac arrhythmias. Many studies exist to challenge the association between droperidol and cardiac problems at doses employed for postoperative nausea and vomiting. Droperidol can also produce extrapyramidal symptoms at doses greater than those used for postoperative nausea and vomiting. In single dose studies, the incidence of adverse effects of droperidol were similar to placebo.[19]

Contraindications. Hypersensitivity; pheochromocytomia inducing hypertensive crisis.

Precautions. Pregnancy category C; potential for increased plasma concentrations in patients with renal or hepatic impairment; QT_c prolongation.

Drug Interactions. Concomitant CNS depressants will potentiate sedation; use concomitant administration with medications known to cause QT_c interval prolongation with caution.

Parameters to Monitor. Observe for frequency of emesis and assess severity of nausea.

Notes. Droperidol has also been used for chemotherapy-induced nausea and vomiting, agitation related to psychosis, and migraine headaches. Concomitant administration with halothane or isoflurane does not affect the pharmacokinetics of droperidol. For postoperative nausea and vomiting, droperidol has similar efficacy to that of ondansetron or dexamethasone.[19] Concomitant administration with ondansetron has not resulted in greater QT_c interval prolongation than that associated with either agent alone. Droperidol appears to have an antipruritic effect that may help to mitigate pruritus from opioids.[19]

GRANISETRON
Kytril, Sancuso

Pharmacology. Granisetron is a selective antagonist at the 5-HT_3 receptor used for the prevention of nausea and vomiting associated with cancer chemotherapy. Its use in cancer chemotherapy is similar to that of ondansetron, and its efficacy and side effects are comparable to those of ondansetron.[5,20] (*See* Antiemetic Drugs Comparison Chart.)

Adult Dosage. **IV for cancer chemotherapy-induced nausea and vomiting**— 10 μg/kg administered in 20–50 mL NS or D5W over 5 min, 30 min before the start of chemotherapy. **Transdermal for the prevention of chemotherapy-induced nausea and vomiting for up to 5 consecutive days**—Apply 34.3 mg patch to the upper outer arm at least 24 h prior to chemotherapy and remove a minimum of 24 h after completion of chemotherapy. May be worn for up to 7 days. **PO for cancer chemotherapy-induced and radiation-induced nausea and vomiting**—1 mg up to 1 h before chemotherapy and additional 1 mg doses at 12-h intervals thereafter while receiving chemotherapy. **IV for prophylaxis for postoperative nausea and vomiting**—1 mg before induction of anesthesia or immediately before reversal of anesthesia.

Special Populations. *Pediatric Dosage.* **IV** (>2 years) Same as adult dosage, but children may require up to 40 μg/kg.[20]

Dosage Forms. **Inj** 1 mg/mL; **Tab** 1 mg; **Transdermal** 34.3 mg (3.1 mg/24-h).

Pharmacokinetics. *Fate.* Oral absorption is approximately 60%. V_d is 30 ± 1.5 L/kg; Cl is 0.060 ± 0.54 L/h/kg. Elimination is mostly by hepatic metabolism, with 16 ± 14% appearing in the urine as unchanged drug. **Half-life.** 5.3 ± 3.5 h (can be longer in cancer patients than in non-cancer patients). The metabolism of granisetron might be changed by inducers or inhibitors of the cytochrome P450 system, but dosage adjustment is not recommended.

Adverse Reactions. Headache, somnolence, and abdominal pain occur frequently.

ONDANSETRON HYDROCHLORIDE
Zofran, Various

Pharmacology. Ondansetron is a selective antagonist at the 5-HT_3 receptor used for the prevention of nausea and vomiting associated with cancer chemotherapy, especially cisplatin, and for postoperative nausea and vomiting. It is also useful for radiotherapy-induced nausea and vomiting. Ondansetron is thought to block these receptors at both peripheral sites in the GI tract and within the area postrema in the CNS.[21] It is not a dopamine receptor antagonist, so it has no extrapyramidal side effects. (*See* Notes.)

Administration and Adult Dosage. **IV for chemotherapy-induced nausea or vomiting**—0.15 mg/kg for 3 doses (30 min before chemotherapy and then 4 and 8 h after) or 0.45 mg/kg, to a maximum of 32 mg as a single dose or 8 mg IV as a single dose for cisplatin doses <100 mg/m². [5] (*See* Notes.) Infuse slowly over 15 min in 50 mL D5W or NS. **IV bolus for postoperative nausea or vomiting**—4 mg over 2–5 min before induction or postoperatively. **PO for chemotherapy-induced nausea or vomiting**—8 mg 2–3 times daily or 24 mg once daily. **PO for radiation-induced nausea or vomiting**—8 mg 1–3 times daily. **PO for postoperative nausea or vomiting**—8–16 mg 1 h before surgery.[5]

Special Populations. *Pediatric Dosage.* **IV for chemotherapy-induced nausea or vomiting**—(<2 years) Safety and efficacy not established. (2–18 years). Same as adult dosage or 0.15 mg/kg for 2 doses or 0.3 mg/kg for 1 dose for moderately emetogenic chemotherapy.[22–24] **IV for postoperative nausea or vomiting**—0.05–0.1 mg/kg, to a maximum of 4 mg as a single dose more than 30 sec before the surgical incision.[5] **PO for chemotherapy-induced nausea and vomiting**—(4–11 years) 4 mg every 8h. **PO for postoperative nausea or vomiting**—0.15 mg/kg 30–45 min before IV catheter placement.[25]

Geriatric Dosage. Same as adult dosage.

Other Conditions. In hepatic function impairment, do not exceed a single oral dose of 8 mg or a total daily IV dosage of 8 mg.

Dosage Forms. **Inj** 0.64 and 2 mg/mL; **Tab** 4, 8, 24 mg; **Oral Disintegrating Tab** 4 and 8 mg; **Soln** 0.8 mg/mL.

Pharmacokinetics. *Fate.* Oral absorption is $62 \pm 15\%$. V_d is 1.9 ± 0.5 L/kg; Cl is 0.35 ± 0.16 L/h/kg in adults and can be higher in children. The drug is extensively metabolized to glucuronide and sulfate conjugates. About 5% appears in urine as unchanged ondansetron.[12] **Half-life.** 3.5 ± 1.9 h in normal adults, increased in the elderly.[12] However, the duration of activity is not related to the half-life.[5]

Adverse Reactions. Headache occurs frequently. Transient increased serum levels of hepatic enzymes also occur frequently, but these are probably caused by chemotherapy rather than by ondansetron.[5,26–28]

Contraindications. None known.

Precautions. Pregnancy; lactation; suspected ileus. Patients who are hypersensitive to other 5-HT₃ antagonists might cross-react with ondansetron.[29]

Drug Interactions. The metabolism of ondansetron can be changed by inducers or inhibitors of the cytochrome P450 system, but dosage adjustment is not recommended.

Parameters to Monitor. Frequency of vomiting.

Notes. Protect vials from light; inspect for discoloration and particulate matter before using. **Dexamethasone** enhances the antiemetic effect of the 5-HT₃ antagonists.[5,30] The combination of ondansetron and dexamethasone is more effective than **metoclopramide** and dexamethasone for the acute component but not for the delayed phase of severely emetogenic chemotherapy.[5] Several studies have documented the lack of additional efficacy beyond that achieved with a total daily ondansetron dosage of 0.45 mg/kg.[30,31] (*See* Antiemetic Drugs Comparison Chart.)

PALONOSETRON HYDROCHLORIDE — Aloxi

Pharmacology. Palonosetron is a highly selective antagonist at the 5-HT$_3$ receptor used for the prevention of nausea and vomiting associated with cancer chemotherapy, especially cisplatin. Palonosetron is thought to block these receptors at both peripheral sites in the GI tract and within the area postrema in the CNS. Palonosetron has a greater affinity for 5-HT$_3$ receptors than that of ondansetron in cell binding studies.[31]

Administration and Adult Dosage. IV for chemotherapy-induced nausea and vomiting—0.25 mg as a 30-s IV infusion 30 min prior to chemotherapy initiation. **PO for chemotherapy-induced nausea and vomiting**—0.5 mg 1 h prior to chemotherapy. **IV for postoperative nausea and vomiting** —0.075 mg over 10 sec immediately prior to anesthesia induction.

Special Populations. *Pediatric Dosage.* (<18 years) Safety and efficacy not established for any indication.

Geriatric Dosage. Same as adult dosage.

Other Conditions. No dosage adjustments are required for hepatic or renal impairment.

Dosage Forms. Inj 0.25 mg/5 mL and 0.075 mg/1.5 mL; **Cap** 0.5 mg.

Pharmacokinetics. *Fate.* Oral absorption is 97%. V$_d$ is 8.3 ± 2.5 L/kg; Cl is 0.16 ± 0.035 L/h/kg in adults. The drug is eliminated by multiple routes and approximately 50% is metabolized to two metabolites with very little 5-HT$_3$ receptor antagonist activity. Metabolic routes include CYP2D6 and to a lesser extent 3A4 and 1A2, although pharmacokinetics are not significantly different between extensive and poor metabolizers of CYP2D6. About 40± appears in urine as unchanged palonosetron by 144 h. **Half-life.** ~40 h.

Adverse Reactions. Headache and constipation occur most commonly, but are not similar in frequency to that of other serotonin antagonists.

Contraindications. For patients with known hypersensitivity.

Precautions. None known other than hypersensitivity, although there is no experience in pregnancy or breast feeding.

Drug Interactions. The potential for clinically significant drug interactions appears to be low.

Parameters to Monitor. Frequency of vomiting and nausea severity.

Notes. Protect vials from freezing and light. While palonosetron has demonstrated greater efficacy than both dolasetron and ondansetron for delayed nausea/vomiting from moderately emetogenic chemotherapy,[32] these studies did not incorporate standard antiemetic therapy with dexamethasone, thus it is unclear whether this represents a substantial advantage for palonosetron. One dose of palonosetron would offer antiemetic protection for multiple days (e.g., 1 course) of chemotherapy, as the antiemetic effect persists for >120 h.

PROCHLORPERAZINE SALTS   Compazine, Various

Pharmacology. Prochlorperazine is a phenothiazine tranquilizer with antidopaminergic and weak anticholinergic activities. It suppresses the chemoreceptor trigger zone in the CNS and is used mainly for its antiemetic properties. It is not effective for the treatment of motion sickness or vertigo.

Administration and Adult Dosage. PO as an antiemetic—5–10 mg 3–4 times daily; **PR as an antiemetic**—25 mg twice daily. **IM as an antiemetic**—(deep in upper outer quadrant of buttock) 5–10 mg every 4–6 h, to a maximum of 40 mg/d; **IM presurgically**—(deep in upper outer quadrant of buttock) 5–10 mg 1–2 h before induction, can repeat once before or after surgery. **IV presurgically**—5–10 mg 15–30 min before induction or as infusion (20 mg/L) started 15–30 min before induction. **SQ**—Not recommended.

Special Populations. *Pediatric Dosage.* Not to be used in surgery, in patients <9 kg, or <2 years. **PO or PR as an antiemetic**—(9–13 kg) 2.5 mg once to twice daily; (14–18 kg) 2.5 mg 2–3 times daily; (19–39 kg) 2.5 mg 3 times daily OR 5 mg twice daily. (*See* Notes.) **IM as an antiemetic**—(deep in upper outer quadrant of buttock) 0.13 mg/kg. **SQ**—Not recommended.

Geriatric Dosage. Use the lower end of the recommended dosage range in elderly patients.

Dosage Forms. Inj 5 mg/mL; **Supp** 2.5, 5, 25 mg; **Syrup** 1 mg/mL; **Tab** 5, 10, 25 mg. Higher-dose tablets are available for psychiatric use.

Patient Instructions. This drug can cause drowsiness. Until the extent of this effect is known, use caution when driving, operating machinery, or performing other tasks requiring mental alertness. Avoid excessive concurrent use of alcohol or other drugs that cause drowsiness.

Missed Doses. Take this drug as prescribed. If you miss a dose, take it as soon as you remember. If it is about time for the next dose, take that dose only. Do not double the dose or take an extra dose.

Pharmacokinetics. *Onset and Duration.* PO onset 30–40 min; PR onset 60 min; IM onset 10–20 min. Duration for all routes 3–4 h.

Fate. The drug is well absorbed, but extensive and variable presystemic metabolism in the gut wall and liver limits bioavailability. Eliminated primarily by hepatic metabolism and biliary excretion. **Half-Life.** 23 h.[33]

Adverse Reactions. Extrapyramidal reactions, especially dystonias and dyskinesias, occur occasionally in adults and frequently in children (other extrapyramidal reactions are less likely because of the short duration of therapy when used as an antiemetic). Anticholinergic effects such as dry mouth, mydriasis, cycloplegia, urinary retention, decreased GI motility, and tachycardia occur occasionally. SQ administration can cause local reactions at injection site.

Contraindications. Pediatric surgery; children <9 kg or <2 years; coma or greatly depressed state caused by CNS depressants.

Precautions. Antiemetic action can mask signs and symptoms of overdose with other drugs and can mask the diagnosis and treatment of other conditions such as intestinal obstruction, brain tumor, or Reye's syndrome. Use with caution in conditions in which the drug's anticholinergic effects might be detrimental, in children with acute illnesses or dehydration, or in patients with histories of allergy to phenothiazine derivatives (e.g., blood dyscrasias, jaundice). Avoid exposure to concentrate on hands or clothing because of the possibility of contact dermatitis.

Drug Interactions. Phenothiazines can decrease the efficacy of guanethidine or guanadrel or have additive hypotensive effects with hypotensive drugs. Phenothiazines can inhibit the antiparkinson activity of levodopa.

Parameters to Monitor. Monitor for extrapyramidal side effects and drug efficacy.

Notes. Protect the solution from light; a slight yellowish discoloration does not indicate altered potency, but markedly discolored solution should be discarded. Protect suppositories from heat. Sustained-release products have no demonstrated advantage over rapid-release products. Prochlorperazine does not predictably reduce chemotherapy-induced nausea and vomiting in children and might be associated with an increase in symptoms.[34] (*See* Antiemetic Drugs Comparison Chart.)

SCOPOLAMINE TransDerm Scop

Pharmacology. Scopolamine is a naturally occurring parasympatholytic and is a nonselective acetylcholine antagonist with peripheral anticholinergic activities and central activities encompassing sedation, amnesia and antiemesis. The antiemetic effect of scopolamine is believed to be due to its interference with vestibular transmission to the CNS and by interfering with transmission from the reticular formation to the vomiting center.

Administration and Adult Dosage. Transdermal for postoperative nausea and vomiting—Apply to the hairless area behind the ear in the evening prior to the scheduled surgery or 1 h prior to cesarean section and leave in place for 24 h. **Transdermal for motion sickness**—Apply the patch to the hairless area behind the ear at least 4 h prior to desired antiemetic effect. If treatment is needed for >72 h, the first patch can be discontinued and a second patch applied behind the opposite area at 72 h.

Special Populations. *Pediatric Dosage.* (<18 years) Not recommended.

Geriatric Dosage. Same as adult dosage but use with caution due to the increased likelihood of CNS effects.

Other Conditions. No dosage adjustments are required for hepatic or renal impairment.

Dosage Forms. Transdermal TTS Patch—Patch reservoir contains 1.5 mg and when applied delivers a 140 μg priming dose and then releases 1 mg over 3 days at a rate of 5 μg /h.

Pharmacokinetics. *Fate.* With transdermal administration scopolamine is well absorbed with plasma levels detected in 4 h and peak plasma concentrations are achieved in approximately 24 h. V_d (IV) is 141 ± 1.6 L; Cl (IV) is 81 ± 1.5 L/h in adults. Scopolamine metabolism in man is still not completely elucidated. The drug is metabolized in the liver and metabolites from glucuronide or sulfate conjugation are excreted in the urine.[35] **Half-life.** (transdermal following patch removal) 9.5 h.

Adverse Reactions. The transdermal patch was developed to minimize the adverse reactions that occur with oral and parenteral administration of scopolamine. Typically anticholinergic adverse reactions occur (dry mouth and skin, drowsiness, blurred vision and dizziness). Rarely, idiosyncratic reactions can occur at therapeutic doses including confusion, agitation, and acute psychotic reactions. Skin burns are reported with aluminized patches worn during magnetic resonance imaging (MRI), and the Transderm Scop patch contains aluminum and should therefore be removed prior to any MRI procedures.

Contraindications. Hypersensitivity; plaster allergy; narrow angle glaucoma.

Precautions. Pregnancy Category C; excreted in human breast milk and should be used with caution in women who are nursing; intestinal obstruction; impaired hepatic or renal function; urinary bladder neck obstruction; psychosis; history of seizures.

Drug Interactions. Other medications that cause drowsiness or that have anticholinergic effects.

Parameters to Monitor. Frequency of vomiting and nausea severity.

Notes. The effect on motion sickness is not achieved until 4–6 h following transdermal application. Disturbances in equilibrium can occur following discontinuation of the transdermal patch. The patch should not be cut and only one patch should be worn at a time. If a patch should become displaced, it should be discarded and an additional patch should be applied to the area behind the opposite ear.

ANTIEMETIC DRUGS COMPARISON CHART

| MEDICATION | DOSAGE FORMS | INITIAL DOSE[a,b] | | INDICATIONS | | |
		Adult	Pediatric	Nausea/Vomiting	Motion Sickness	Vertigo
ANTIHISTAMINES						
Bucladin-S (buclizine)	Chew Tab 50 mg	PO 50 mg	N/A		X	
Marezine (cyclizine)	Tab 50 mg	PO 50 mg	PO (6–12 y) 25 mg		X	
Dramamine (dimenhydrinate)	Tab 50 mg Chew Tab 50 mg Liquid 2.5, 3.1 mg/mL Inj 50 mg/mL	PO 50–100 mg PO 50 mg PO 50 mg IM, IV 50 mg	PO (2–6 y) 12.5–25 mg PO (6–12 y) 25–50 mg PO (6–12 y) 25–50 mg PO (2–6 y) 12.5–25 mg; PO (6–12 y) 25–50 mg IM, IV (>2 years) 1.25 mg/kg	X	X	X
Benadryl (diphenhydramine)	Cap 25, 50 mg Tab 25, 50 mg Chew Tab 12.5 mg Elixir 2.5 mg/mL Soln 1.25, 2.5 mg/mL Syrup 2.5 mg/mL Inj 50 mg/mL	PO 50 mg N/A PO 50 mg IM, IV 10–50 mg	PO (2–6 y) 6.25 mg PO 1.25 mg/kg PO (6–12 y) 12.5–25 mg PO (2–6 y) 6.25 mg PO (6–12 y) 12.5–25 mg PO (2–6 y) 6.25 mg PO (6–12 y) 12.5–25 mg IM, IV (>9 kg) 1.25 mg/kg			

(continued)

ANTIEMETIC DRUGS COMPARISON CHART (continued)

| MEDICATION | DOSAGE FORMS | INITIAL DOSE[a,b] | | INDICATIONS | | |
		Adult	Pediatric	Nausea/Vomiting	Motion Sickness	Vertigo
Antivert (meclizine)	Cap 25 mg Tab 12.5, 25, 50 mg	PO 25–50 mg PO 25–50 mg	N/A N/A	X	X	C
Bonine (meclizine)	Chew Tab 25 mg	PO 25 mg	N/A			
CANNABINOIDS						
Marinol (dronabinol)[d]	Cap 2.5, 5, 10 mg	PO 5 mg/m^2	PO 5 mg/m^2	X		
NEUROKININ ANTAGONISTS						
Emend (aprepitant)	Cap 40, 80, 125 mg Inj 115 mg	PO Day 1: 125 mg Day 2 and 3: 80 mg IV 115 mg	N/A	X		
PHENOTHIAZINES						
Thorazine (chlorpromazine)	Tab 10, 25, 50 mg Suppository 25, 100 mg Inj 25 mg/mL Liquid 30 and 100 mg/mL Syrup 2 mg/mL	PO 10–25 mg PR 50–100 mg IM 25 mg PO 10–25 mg PO 10–25 mg	PO (≥6 mo) 0.5–1 mg/kg PR (≥6 mo) 1 mg/kg IM (≥6 mo) 0.55 mg/kg PO (≥6 mo) 0.5–1 mg/kg? PO (≥6 mo) 0.5–1 mg/kg	X		

(continued)

ANTIEMETIC DRUGS COMPARISON CHART (*continued*)

MEDICATION	DOSAGE FORMS	INITIAL DOSE[a,b] Adult	INITIAL DOSE[a,b] Pediatric	INDICATIONS Nausea/Vomiting	INDICATIONS Motion Sickness	INDICATIONS Vertigo
Trilafon (perphenazine)	Tab 2, 4, 8, 16 mg Liquid 3.2 mg/mL Inj 5 mg/mL	PO 2–4 mg PO 2–4 mg IM 5 mg	N/A N/A N/A	X		
Compazine (prochlorperazine)	Tab 5, 10 mg Syrup 1 mg/mL Inj 5 mg/mL Suppository 2.5, 5, 25 mg	PO 5–10 mg PO 5–10 mg IV 2.5–10 mg IM 5–10 mg PR 25 mg	PO (>10 kg OR >2 y) 2.5 mg OR 0.4 mg/kg/24 h in 3–4 divided doses PO 2.5 mg OR 0.4 mg/kg/24 hr in 3–4 divided doses IM (>13 kg OR >2 y) 0.13 mg/kg PR (>10 kg OR >2 y) 2.5 mg OR 0.4 mg/kg/ 24 h in 3–4 divided doses	X		
Phenergan (promethazine)	Syrup 1.25, 5 mg/mL Tab 12.5, 25, 50 mg Suppository 12.5, 25, 50 mg Inj 25, 50 mg/mL	PO 25 mg PO 25 mg PR 25 mg IM, IV 12.5–25 mg	PO (>2 yr) 0.25–0.5 mg/kg PO (>2 y) 0.25–0.5 mg/kg PR (>2 y) 0.25–0.5 mg/kg IM (>2 y) 0.25–0.5 mg/kg	X	X	
Torecan (thiethylperazine)	Tab 10 mg Inj 5 mg/mL	PO 10 mg IM 10 mg	N/A N/A	X		

(continued)

ANTIEMETIC DRUGS COMPARISON CHART (*continued*)

| MEDICATION | DOSAGE FORMS | INITIAL DOSE[a,b] | | INDICATIONS | | |
		Adult	Pediatric	Nausea/Vomiting	Motion Sickness	Vertigo
Vesprin (triflupromazine)	Inj 10, 20 mg/mL	IM 5–15 mg IM (elderly) 2.5 mg IV 1 mg	IM (>2.5 y) 0.2–0.25 mg/kg	X		
SEROTONIN 5-HT₃ ANTAGONISTS						
Anzemet (dolasetron)	Tab 50, 100 mg Inj 20 mg/mL	PO 100 mg IV 1.8 mg/kg	PO 1.8 mg/kg IV 1.8 mg/kg	X		
Kytril (granisetron)	Tab 1 mg Soln 0.2 mg/ml Inj 1 mg/mL	PO 1–2 mg IV 10 μg/kg	N/A IV (>2 y) 10 μg/kg	X		
Zofran (ondansetron)	Tab 4, 8, 24 mg Inj 2 mg/mL Oral Disintegrating Tab 4, 8 mg Soln 0.8 mg/mL	PO 8 or 16 mg IV 0.15–0.45 mg/kg (MAX 32 mg) PO 8 or 16 mg PO 8 or 16 mg	PO (>4 y) 4 mg IV (>2 y) 0.15 mg/kg PO (>4 y) 4 mg PO (>4 y) 4 mg	X		
Aloxi (palonosetron)	Cap 0.5 mg Inj 0.25 mg and 0.075 mg/1.5 ml	PO 0.5 mg IV 0.25 mg	N/A	X		

(continued)

ANTIEMETIC DRUGS COMPARISON CHART (*continued*)

MEDICATION	DOSAGE FORMS	INITIAL DOSE[a,b] Adult	INITIAL DOSE[a,b] Pediatric	INDICATIONS Nausea/Vomiting	INDICATIONS Motion Sickness	INDICATIONS Vertigo
MISCELLANEOUS						
Decadron (dexamethasone)	Elixir 0.1 mg/mL Soln 0.1, 1 mg/mL Tab 0.25, 0.5, 0.75, 1, 1.5, 2, 4, 6 mg Inj 4, 10, 20, 24 mg/mL	PO 10–20 mg PO 10–20 mg PO 10–20 mg	PO 10 mg/m^2 PO 10 mg/m^2 PO 10 mg/m^2	F		
Inapsine (Droperidol)	Inj 2.5 mg/mL	IV 10–20 mg IM, IV 0.625–1.25 mg	IV 10 mg/m^2 IV 0.015–0.075 mg/kg	F		
Ativan (lorazepam)[d]	Tab 0.5, 1, 2 mg Soln 2 mg/mL Inj 2 and 4 mg/mL	PO 0.5–2 mg PO 0.5–2 mg IV 0.5–2 mg	PO 0.05 mg/kg PO 0.05 mg/kg IV 0.05 mg/kg			
Solu-Medrol (methylprednisolone)	Inj 40, 125, 500 mg	IV up to 100 mg	IV 2–4 mg/kg	E		
Reglan (metoclopramide)	Inj 5 mg/mL	IV 1–2 mg/kg	IV 1–2 mg/kg	X		
Scopace (scopolamine)	Tab 0.4 mg	PO 0.4 mg	N/A		X	
Transderm Scop (scopolamine)	Transdermal Patch 1.5 mg	1 disk behind ear over 3 d	N/A		X	

(continued)

ANTIEMETIC DRUGS COMPARISON CHART (*continued*)

| MEDICATION | DOSAGE FORMS | INITIAL DOSE[a,b] | | INDICATIONS | | |
		Adult	Pediatric	Nausea/Vomiting	Motion Sickness	Vertigo
Tigan (trimethobenzamide)	Cap 300 mg Suppository 100, 200 mg Inj 100 mg/mL	PO 300 mg PR 200 mg IM 200 mg	PO (14–40 kg) 00–200 mg PR (<14 kg) 100 mg PR (14–40 kg) 100–200 mg N/A	X		

[a]Initial dose only; check prescribing information for subsequent dosage.
[b]Doses of serotonin antagonists are for chemotherapy-induced nausea and vomiting. (See monograph for doses in postoperative nausea and vomiting.)
[c]Possibly effective.
[d]Controlled substance.
[e]Not labeled for this use: used as adjunctive for cancer chemotherapy-induced nausea and vomiting.
[f]Effective, but not labeled for this use.
References from product information.

■ REFERENCES

1. Dando TM, Perry CM. Aprepitant: a review of its use in the prevention of chemotherapy-induced nausea and vomiting. *Drugs.* 2004;64:777-794.
2. Nakade S et al. Population pharmacokinetics of aprepitant and dexamethasone in the prevention of chemotherapy-induced nausea and vomiting. *Cancer Chemother Pharmacol.* 2008;63:75-83.
3. Nygren P et al. Lack of effect of aprepitant on the pharmacokinetics of docetaxel in cancer patients. *Cancer Chemother Pharmacol.* 2005;55:609-616.
4. Loos WJ et al. Aprepitant when added to a standard antiemetic regimen consisting of ondansetron and dexamethasone does not affect vinorelbine pharmacokinetics in cancer patients. *Cancer Chemother Pharmacol.* 2007;59:407-412.
5. ASHP Commission on Therapeutics. ASHP therapeutic guidelines on the pharmacologic management of nausea and vomiting in adult and pediatric patients receiving chemotherapy or radiation therapy or undergoing surgery. *Am J Health Syst Pharm.* 1999;56:729-764.
6. Poster DS et al. Delta-9-tetrahydrocannabinol in clinical oncology. *JAMA.* 1981;245:2047-2051.
7. Cocchetto DM et al. A critical review of the safety and antiemetic efficacy of delta-9-tetrahydrocannabinol. *Drug Intell Clin Pharm.* 1981;15:867-875.
8. Voth EA, Schwartz RH. Medicinal applications of delta-9-tetrahydrocannabinol and marijuana. *Ann Intern Med.* 1997;126:791-798.
9. Lemberger L et al. Delta-9-tetrahydrocannabinol. Temporal correlation of the psychologic effects and blood levels after various routes of administration. *N Engl J Med.* 1972;286:685-688.
10. Hollister LE et al. Do plasma concentrations of delta-9-tetrahydrocannabinol reflect the degree of intoxication? *J Clin Pharmacol.* 1981;21(suppl 8-9):171S-177S.
11. Huestis MA et al. Characterization of the absorption phase of marijuana smoking. *Clin Pharmacol Ther.* 1992;52:31-41.
12. Benet LZ et al. Design and optimization of dosage regimens; pharmacokinetic data. In, Hardman JG et al., eds. *Goodman and Gilman's the pharmacological basis of therapeutics.* 9th ed. New York: McGraw-Hill; 1996:1707-1792.
13. Wall ME et al. Metabolism, disposition, and kinetics of delta-9-tetrahydrocannabinol in men and women. *Clin Pharmacol Ther.* 1983;34:352-363.
14. Agurell S et al. Pharmacokinetics and metabolism of delta 1-tetrahydrocannabinol and other cannabinoids with emphasis in man. *Pharmacol Rev.* 1986;38:21-43.
15. Devine ML et al. Adverse reactions to delta-9-tetrahydrocannabinol given as an antiemetic in a multicenter study. *Clin Pharm.* 1987;6:319-322.
16. Anon. Synthetic marijuana for nausea and vomiting due to cancer chemotherapy. *Med Lett Drugs Ther.* 1985; 27:97-98.
17. Gralla RJ et al. Antiemetic therapy: a review of recent studies and a report of a random assignment trial comparing metoclopramide with delta-9-tetrahydrocannabinol. *Cancer Treat Rep.* 1984;68:163-172.
18. Doblin RE, Kleiman MA. Marijuana as antiemetic medicine: a survey of oncologists' experiences and attitudes. *J Clin Oncol.* 1991;9:1314-1319.
19. McKeage K et al. Intravenous Droperidol. a review of its use in the management of postoperative nausea and vomiting. *Drugs.* 2006;66:2123-2147.
20. Adams VR, Valley AW. Granisetron: the second serotonin-receptor antagonist. *Ann Pharmacother.* 1995;29: 1240-51.
21. Freeman AJ et al. Selectivity of 5-HT3 receptor antagonists and anti-emetic mechanisms of action. *Anticancer Drugs.* 1992;3:79-85.
22. Holdsworth MT et al. Assessment of chemotherapy-induced emesis and evaluation of a reduced-dose intravenous ondansetron regimen in pediatric outpatients with leukemia. *Ann Pharmacother.* 1995;29:16-21.
23. Billett AL, Sallan SE. Antiemetics in children receiving cancer chemotherapy. *Support Care Cancer.* 1994;2:279-285.
24. Foot AB, Hayes C. Audit of guidelines for effective control of chemotherapy and radiotherapy induced emesis. *Arch Dis Child.* 1994;71:475-480.
25. Rose JB et al. Preoperative oral ondansetron for pediatric tonsillectomy. *Anesth Analg.* 1996;82:558-562.
26. Blackwell CP, Harding SM. The clinical pharmacology of ondansetron. *Eur J Cancer Clin Oncol.* 1989;25(suppl 1): S21-S24.
27. Hesketh PJ et al. GR 38032F (GR-C507/75): a novel compound effective in the prevention of acute cisplatin-induced emesis. *J Clin Oncol.* 1989;7:700-705.
28. Grunberg SM et al. Dose ranging phase I study of the serotonin antagonist GR38032F for prevention of cisplatin-induced nausea and vomiting. *J Clin Oncol.* 1989;7:1137-1141.
29. Kataja V, de Bruijn KM. Hypersensitivity reactions associated with 5-hydroxytryptamine3-receptor antagonists: a class effect? *Lancet.* 1996;347:584-585.

30. Chaffee BJ, Tankanow RM. Ondansetron—the first of a new class of antiemetic agents. *Clin Pharm.* 1991;10:430-446.

31. Grunberg SM et al. Randomized double-blind comparison of three dose levels of intravenous ondansetron in the prevention of cisplatin-induced emesis. *Cancer Chemother Pharmacol.* 1993;32:268-272.

32. Siddiqui MA, Scot LJ. Palonosetron. *Drugs.* 2004;64:1125-1132.

33. Vozeh S et al. Pharmacokinetic drug data. *Clin Pharmacokinet.* 1988;15:254-282.

34. Zeltzer L et al. Paradoxical effects of prophylactic phenothiazine antiemetics in children receiving chemotherapy. *J Clin Oncol.* 1984;2:930-936.

35. Renner UD et al. Pharmacokinetics and pharmacodynamics in clinical use of scopolamine. *Ther Drug Monit.* 2005;27:655-665.

Chapter 45

Gastrointestinal Motility and Miscellaneous Gastrointestinal Drugs

Scott S. Malinowski

LAXATIVES

PSYLLIUM HUSK   Metamucil, Konsyl, Various

Pharmacology. Psyllium is a bulk-forming cathartic that absorbs water and provides an emollient mass.

Administration and Adult Dosage. **PO for constipation**—2.5–12 g 1–3 times daily, stirred in a full glass of fluid, followed by an additional glass of liquid. **PO for mild diarrhea**—Usual doses titrated to effect can be used to improve consistency. **PO to lower cholesterol**—10–30 g/d in divided doses in combination with diet can decrease cholesterol in patients with mild-to-moderate hypercholesterolemia.[1–3]

Special Populations. *Pediatric Dosage.* **PO for constipation**—(≤6 years) safety and efficacy not established; (6–12 years) 2.5–3 g (psyllium) 1–3 times daily with fluid as above.

Geriatric Dosage. Same as adult dosage.

Dosage Forms. **Pwdr** Konsyl (sugar-free, containing 100% psyllium) 6-g packet, 200–660 g; Metamucil (sugar-free orange flavor, containing 65% psyllium); **Pwdr** Metamucil (orange flavor, 50% or 65% sucrose), Konsyl-Orange (28% psyllium, 72% sucrose) 7-, 11-, 12-g packet, 210, 420, 538, 630, 960 g; **Wafer** Metamucil (containing 5 g fat) 3.4 g of psyllium per wafer.

Patient Instructions. Mix powder with a full glass of fluid before taking and follow with another glass of liquid.

Pharmacokinetics. *Onset and Duration.* Onset 12–24 h, but 2–3 days might be required for full effect.[4]

Fate. Not absorbed from gastrointestinal (GI) tract; eliminated unchanged in feces.

Adverse Reactions. Flatulence occurs frequently. Serious side effects are rare, but esophageal, gastric, intestinal, and rectal obstructions have been reported. Allergic reactions and bronchospasm have occurred after inhalation of dry powder.[1,4,5]

Contraindications. Acute surgical abdomen; fecal impaction; intestinal obstruction; abdominal pain of unknown origin; nausea; vomiting.

Precautions. Rectal bleeding or failure to respond to therapy might indicate a serious condition and the need for medical attention. Use with caution in patients who require fluid restriction because constipation can occur unless fluid intake is adequate. Psyllium can be hazardous in patients with intestinal ulcerations, stenosis, or disabling adhesions. Use effervescent Metamucil formulations (packet) with caution in patients who require potassium restriction (7.4 and 7.9 mEq potassium/packet). Use the noneffervescent formulations of Metamucil cautiously in patients with diabetes because they contain 50% or 65% sucrose. Sugar-free preparations include Konsyl and Metamucil.

Drug Interactions. None known.

Notes. Psyllium is useful in lessening the strain of defecation and for inpatients that are on low-residue diets or constipating medications. It is safe to use during pregnancy.[1,4]

DOCUSATE SALTS	Colace, Surfak, Dialose, Various

Pharmacology. Docusate is an anionic surfactant that lowers the surface tension of the oil–water interface of the stool, allowing fecal material to be penetrated by water and fat, thereby softening the stool, and facilitating bowel movements. The emulsifying action also enhances the absorption of many fat-soluble drugs and mineral oil. These agents also can cause subtle effects on fluid absorption and secretion in the GI tract.[1,4]

Administration and Adult Dosage. **PO as a stool softener**—(sodium salt) 50–500 mg/d in single or divided doses (give solution/syrup in milk or fruit juice to mask taste); begin therapy with up to 500 mg/d and adjust after maximal effects occur (approximately 3 days); (calcium salt) 240 mg/d; (potassium salt) 100–300 mg/d. **PR as enema**—50–100 mg in water.

Special Populations. *Pediatric Dosage.* **PO**—(sodium salt) (<3 years) 10–40 mg/d; (3–6 years) 20–60 mg/d; (6–12 years) 40–120 mg/d; (>12 years) same as adult dosage; give solution/syrup in milk, fruit juice, or formula to mask taste; (calcium salt) (≥6 years) 50–150 mg/d; (potassium salt) (≥6 years) 100 mg/d.

Geriatric Dosage. Same as adult dosage. Use of these agents in elderly, bedridden patients might be ineffective in altering the prevalence of constipation.[1,6] (*See* Notes.)

Dosage Forms. (Sodium salt: Colace, various) **Cap** 50, 100, 240, 250 mg; **Soln** 10, 50 mg/mL; **Syrup** 3.3, 4 mg/mL; **Tab** 100 mg. (Calcium salt: Surfak, various) **Cap** 50, 240 mg. (Potassium salt: Dialose, various) **Cap** 240 mg; **Tab** 100 mg.

Patient Instructions. Take this with a full glass of fluid; take the liquid or solution forms in milk, fruit juice, or infant formula to mask the bitter taste.

Pharmacokinetics. *Onset and Duration.* Onset of effect on stools is 2–3 days after first dose with continuous use.

Fate. Drug action is local to the gut, but docusate can be partially absorbed in the duodenum and jejunum and secreted in the bile.[7]

Adverse Reactions. Bitter taste, throat irritation, and nausea (more common with syrup and liquid) occur frequently; abdominal cramps occasionally. Docusate can change intestinal morphology and cellular function and cause fluid and electrolyte accumulation in the colon.[7]

Contraindications. Undiagnosed abdominal pain; intestinal obstruction; concomitant use with mineral oil.

Precautions. Rectal bleeding or failure to respond to therapy might indicate a serious condition and the need for medical attention.

Drug Interactions. Concomitant use with mineral oil can enhance mineral oil systemic absorption, resulting in uptake into the lymph nodes, intestinal mucosa, liver, and spleen.[4]

Parameters to Monitor. Frequency and consistency of stools; ease of defecation.

Notes. Surfactant stool softeners are useful for softening hard, dry stools in painful anorectal conditions and in cardiac and other conditions to lessen the strain of defecation. They are more useful in preventing than in treating constipation but they might not be effective for long-term prevention of constipation in institutionalized, elderly patients. Docusate has not been proven to be effective in the treatment of chronic constipation.[1,4,8,9]

BISACODYL
Dulcolax, Various

Pharmacology. Bisacodyl is a stimulant laxative, structurally similar to phenolphthalein, that produces its effect by direct contact with colonic mucosa, resulting in stimulation of colonic peristalsis. It can inhibit water reabsorption in the small bowel and colon.[1,4]

Administration and Adult Dosage. PO for constipation and bowel preparation— 10–30 mg/d; rectally for constipation and bowel preparation—10 mg once daily. Adjust dosage based on response.

Special Populations. *Pediatric Dosage.* **PO for constipation**—(≤6 years) safety and efficacy not established; (>6 years) 5–10 mg or 0.3 mg/kg once daily. **PR**—(≤6 years) safety and efficacy not established; (6–12 years) 5 mg; (>12 years) 10 mg.

Geriatric Dosage. Same as adult dosage.

Dosage Forms. EC Tab 5 mg; Enema (adult) 10 mg; Supp 10 mg.

Patient Instructions. Remove foil or plastic wrapping before inserting suppository into rectum. Swallow tablets whole (not chewed or crushed) and do not take within 1 h after having antacids or dairy products. Daily use beyond 7 days is NOT recommended. Do NOT use oral products in children ≤6 years of age.

Pharmacokinetics. *Onset and Duration.* Onset PO—6–12 h; PR 15 min–1 h.[1,4]

Fate. Absorption is less than 5% by oral or rectal route, with subsequent conversion to the glucuronide salt and excretion in urine. Requires hydrolysis by endogenous esterases to its active metabolite.[10]

Adverse Reactions. Abdominal cramps occur frequently; diarrhea; with long-term use, metabolic acidosis or alkalosis, hypocalcemia, tetany, loss of enteric protein, and malabsorption occur occasionally; suppositories can cause proctitis and rectal inflammation and are not recommended for long-term use.

Drug Interactions. Antacids or milk can dissolve the enteric coating of oral bisacodyl tablets, causing drug release in the stomach, resulting in gastric irritation.

Contraindications. Acute surgical abdomen; nausea, vomiting, or other symptoms of appendicitis; fecal impaction; intestinal or biliary tract obstruction; abdominal pain of unknown origin.

Notes. Useful for preoperative or preradiographic bowel preparation. Bisacodyl has been used in combination with **polyethylene glycol (PEG) electrolyte lavage solution** to decrease the amount of solution required.[1,4,11] (*See* PEG 3350/Electrolytes Lavage Solution.)

PEG 3350/ELECTROLYTES LAVAGE SOLUTION   GoLYTELY, Various

Pharmacology. PEG with electrolytes lavage solution is an isosmotic solution containing approximately 5.69 g/L sodium sulfate, 1.68 g/L sodium bicarbonate, 1.46 g/L sodium chloride, 745 mg/L potassium chloride, and 60 g/L PEG 3350; it is used for total bowel cleansing before GI examination. A solution lacking sodium sulfate, with a slight variation in other salts and PEG (NuLYTELY), and flavored solutions are available with improved palatability. PEG acts as an osmotic cathartic, and the electrolyte concentrations are such that there is little net fluid or electrolyte movement into or out of the bowel.[1,11,12]

Administration and Adult Dosage. PO or NG for bowel preparation for colonscopy—200–300 mL orally every 10 min or by NG tube at a rate of 20–30 mL/min until approximately 4 L are consumed or the rectal effluent is clear. Use a 1-L trial before the full dosage in patients suspected of having bowel obstruction. Use the solution at least 4 h before the examination, allowing the patient 3 h for drinking and a 1-h period to complete bowel evacuation. Another method is to give the solution the evening before the examination. Chilling the solution might improve its palatability but do not add other ingredients. Withhold solid food for 2 h and medication for 1 h before the solution is administered.

Pediatric Dosage. PO or NG for bowel preparation for colonscopy—25–40 mL/kg/h for 4–10 h appears safe and useful for bowel evacuation.

Dosage Forms. Available as powder for reconstitution and oral solution.

Pharmacokinetics. The first bowel movement usually occurs after 1 h, with total bowel cleansing 3–4 h after starting.

Adverse Reactions. Frequent side effects are nausea, abdominal fullness, bloating (in up to 50% of patients), cramps, anal irritation, and vomiting. Urticaria, rhinorrhea, and dermatitis occur occasionally. Do not use PEG electrolyte lavage solution in patients with GI obstruction, gastric retention, toxic colitis, toxic megacolon, ileus, or bowel perforation; the solution seems to be safe for patients with liver, kidney, or heart disease.

Notes. This product is well suited for bowel cleansing before colonoscopy, but, because of some residual lavage fluid retained in the colon, other cleansing methods might be preferred before barium enema. Colonic cleaning with **bisacodyl** 15 mg orally followed by 2 L of PEG lavage solution 8 h later has been found to be equally effective and more acceptable to patients than 4 L of solution used alone. Similar results were obtained using 300 mL of magnesium citrate solution 2 h before PEG lavage solution that was continued until stool return was clear.[13] The drug might be useful as a GI evacuant in ingestions and overdoses with iron and some EC and SR drug products.[1,11–14]

POLYETHYLENE GLYCOL 3350   MiraLax

Pharmacology. PEG 3350 creates an osmotic gradient in the bowel, drawing fluid into the lumen, causing water to be retained in the stool, therefore promoting stool softening and laxation. PEG 3350 has demonstrated safety effectiveness for the treatment of both occasional and chronic constipation. PEG 3350 is similar to PEG electrolyte lavage solution except that it does not contain electrolytes and has no taste.

Administration and Adult Dosage. **PO for acute or chronic constipation**—17 g (approximately 1 heaping tablespoon) once daily. The product MiraLax provides a bottle cap that also serves as a measuring cup (marked with a measuring line). When filled to the measuring line (white section in cap), it provides approximately 17 g of PEG 3350. Powder must be mixed with 4–8 oz of water or other beverage.

Special Populations. *Pediatric Dosage.* **PO for constipation**—0.8 g/kg/d OR 10 g/m^2/d divided into 2 doses.[15-17]

Geriatric Dosage. Same as adult dosage. Efficacy and safety in elderly is established. Elderly patients may be more susceptible to the diarrhea adverse effect of PEG 3350.[18]

Dosage Forms. **Pwdr** 238-g bottle and 510-g bottle. Bottles of the product MiraLax come with a cap that serves as a measuring cup (marked with a measuring line). MiraLax is available over-the-counter (OTC).

Patient Instructions. Fill to the top of the white section of cap (measuring cup). Mix powder with 4–8 oz of water or other beverage. Stir well. Onset of action may occur in 1–3 days (with repeated use). Use may result in loose, watery, and/or more frequent bowel movements. Do not use beyond 7 days without consulting your health care professional. Report any nausea, vomiting, abdominal distention/pain, or blood in the stool. Lifestyle changes to promote normal, regular bowel movements should be discussed with health care provider.

Pharmacokinetics. *Onset and Duration.* PO onset of activity is usually within 1–3 days with repeated dosing.[19]

Fate. PEG 3350 plasma concentration peaks occurr 2–4 h after administration and declines to undetectable levels within 18 h after single and multiple doses. **Half-life.** 4–6 h. Steady state is reached within 5 days of dosing. Mean urinary excretion of the administered dose ranged from 0.19% to 0.25%. The pharmacokinetics of PEG 3350 were not affected by age, gender, or mild renal impairment.[19]

Adverse Reactions. Nausea, abdominal cramping, flatulence.

Contraindications. Do not use PEG 3350 solution in patients with GI obstruction, gastric retention, toxic colitis, toxic megacolon, ileus, or bowel perforation; the solution seems to be safe for patients with liver, kidney, or heart disease.

Drug Interactions. None demonstrated.

LACTULOSE	Cephulac, Chronulac, Enulose, Kristalose, Various

Pharmacology. Lactulose is a synthetic disaccharide analogue of lactose that contains galactose and fructose and is metabolized by colonic bacteria to lactic acid, and small amounts of acetic and formic acids. These acids result in acidification of colonic contents, conversion of ammonia to ammonium (not well absorbed), and an osmotic catharsis.[20]

Administration and Adult Dosage. **PO as a cathartic**—15–30 mL (10–20 g), to a maximum of 60 mL. **PO for hepatic encephalopathy and portal systemic**

encephalopathy—30–45 mL (20–30 g) every hour until laxation, then 30–45 mL 3–4 times daily, titrated to produce approximately 2 or 3 soft stools/d. **PR for hepatic encephalopathy as an enema**—300 mL with 700 mL water or NS retained for 30–60 min, can repeat every 4–6 h. Repeat immediately if evacuated too promptly.

Special Populations. *Pediatric Dosage.* **PO for hepatic encephalopathy**—(infants) 2.5–10 mL/d in divided doses; (older children and adolescents) 40–90 mL/d in divided doses, titrated to produce 2 or 3 soft stools daily. If initial dose causes diarrhea, reduce dose immediately; if diarrhea persists, discontinue.

Geriatric Dosage. Same as adult dosage. (*See* Notes.)

Dosage Forms. **Syrup** 667 mg/mL (10 g/15 mL); **Pwdr** 10 or 20 g per packet.

Patient Instructions. This syrup can be mixed with fruit juice, water, or milk to improve its palatability. Mix powder in 4 fl oz of water. In the treatment of hepatic encephalopathy, 2–3 loose stools/d are common, but report any worsening of diarrhea. Report belching, flatulence, or abdominal cramps if they are bothersome.

Pharmacokinetics. *Onset and Duration.* (Catharsis) Onset 24–48 h; duration 24–48 h. (Hepatic encephalopathy) Onset and duration variable; however, reversal of coma can occur within 2 h of the first enema.

Fate. After oral administration, less than 3% is absorbed and most reaches the colon unabsorbed and unchanged. Unabsorbed drug is metabolized in the colon by bacteria to low-molecular-weight acids and carbon dioxide. The small amount of absorbed drug is excreted in the urine unchanged.

Adverse Reactions. Flatulence, belching, and abdominal discomfort are frequent initially. Colonic dilation occurs occasionally. Excessive diarrhea and fecal water loss can result in hypernatremia.[21]

Contraindications. Patients who require a low-galactose diet.

Precautions. Use with caution in patients with diabetes because the drug contains small amounts of free lactose and galactose. Rectal bleeding or failure to respond to therapy might indicate a serious condition and the need for medical attention.

Drug Interactions. Do not use other laxatives concomitantly because their induction of loose stools might confound proper lactulose dosage titration for hepatic encephalopathy. Nonabsorbable antacids can interfere with the colonic acidification of lactulose. Theoretically, some antibacterials might interfere with the intestinal bacteria that metabolize lactulose; however, oral neomycin has been used concurrently in hepatic encephalopathy.

Parameters to Monitor. (Hepatic encephalopathy) Observe for changes in hepatic encephalopathy and number of stools per day. Periodically obtain serum sodium, chloride, potassium, and bicarbonate levels during prolonged use, especially in elderly or debilitated patients.

Notes. Lactulose is effective in hepatic encephalopathy, but as a general laxative it offers no advantage over less expensive drugs.[21] One study of constipation in the elderly found that up to 60 mL/d of 70% **sorbitol** was equivalent in laxative effects and caused less nausea than the same dosage of lactulose syrup.[22]

MAGNESIUM SALTS
Various

Pharmacology. Magnesium salts act as saline laxatives that inhibit fluid and electrolyte absorption by increasing osmotic forces in the gut lumen. Part of the action might be caused by cholecystokinin release, which stimulates small bowel motility and inhibits fluid and electrolyte absorption from the small intestine.[4,23]

Administration and Adult Dosage. PO as a laxative/cathartic—(citrate) 240 mL; (sulfate) 20–30 mL of 50% solution (10–15 g) in a full glass of water; (hydroxide; milk of magnesia) 30–60 mL with liquid; (concentrate) 10–30 mL. (*See* Notes.)

Special Populations. *Pediatric Dosage.* PO as a laxative/cathartic—(citrate) one-half the adult dosage; (sulfate) (2–5 years) 2.5–5 g, (≥6 years) 5–10 g in one-half glass or more of water; (hydroxide; milk of magnesia) 0.5 mL/kg.[4]

Geriatric Dosage. Same as adult dosage.

Other Conditions. Avoid use in patients with impaired renal function.[7,23]

Dosage Forms. Soln (citrate) 77 mEq/dL magnesium, 300 mL; (sulfate); **Susp** (hydroxide; milk of magnesia) 7%–8.5%, many sizes, (*see* Notes) (also available as concentrates with 10 mL equivalent to 20 or 30 mL of Susp); **Tab** (hydroxide; milk of magnesia) 311 mg; **Pwdr** (sulfate) 150, 240, 454 g.

Patient Instructions. Take milk of magnesia or magnesium sulfate with at least one full glass of liquid. You can take magnesium sulfate with fruit juice to partly mask its bitter taste. Refrigerating magnesium citrate improves its palatability.

Pharmacokinetics. *Onset and Duration.* Onset is dose dependent: (high end of dosage range) 1–3 h; (low end of dosage range) approximately 6 h.[10]

Fate. Slow absorption of approximately 10% of a dose from the GI tract. Absorbed magnesium is rapidly excreted in the urine in normal renal function.[4]

Adverse Reactions. Abdominal cramping, excessive diuresis, nausea, vomiting, and diarrhea occur frequently. Excessive use can lead to electrolyte abnormalities; dehydration can occur if taken with insufficient fluids. Use in patients with renal impairment can lead to hypermagnesemia, CNS depression, and hypotension.[4,7,23]

Contraindications. Acute surgical abdomen; fecal impaction; intestinal obstruction; abdominal pain of unknown origin; nausea; vomiting.

Precautions. Rectal bleeding or failure to respond to therapy might indicate a serious condition and the need for medical attention. Avoid use in patients with impaired renal function.[4,7,23]

Drug Interactions. Decreased absorption of tetracycline and quinolone antibiotics.

Parameters to Monitor. Periodically check serum magnesium levels in patients with impaired renal function who are receiving long-term daily administration.

Notes. Magnesium salts are useful for preparing the bowel for radiologic examination and surgical procedures. One regimen used magnesium citrate solution 300 mL 2 h before PEG electrolyte lavage solution that was continued until the stool return was clear.[13] The following amounts of various magnesium salts are approximately equivalent to 80 mEq of magnesium: 100 mL citrate, 2.4 g (30 mL) milk of magnesia, and 10 g sulfate. The sulfate salt is the most potent but the least palatable cathartic. (*See* Magnesium Salts in the Section "Renal and Electrolytes.")

ALVIMOPAN
Entereg

Pharmacology. Peripherally acting μ-opioid receptor antagonist that accelerates the time to upper and lower GI recovery following partial large or small bowel resection with primary anastomosis. Following oral administration, alvimopan antagonizes the peripheral effects of opioids on GI motility and secretion by competitively binding to GI tract μ-opioid receptors. Alvimopan achieves this selective GI opioid antagonism without reversing the central analgesic effects of μ-opioid agonists.

Administration and Adult Dosage. PO for postoperative ileus following partial large or small bowel resection surgery with primary anastamosis—12 mg (1 capsule) 30 min to 5 h before surgery, then 12 mg twice daily for up to 7 days, or a maximum of 15 doses.

Special Populations. *Pediatric Dosage.* Safety and efficacy not established.

Geriatric Dosage. Same as adult dosage.

Renal Impairment. Not recommended in end-stage renal disease.

Hepatic Impairment. Mild to moderate: dosage adjustments not necessary. Severe: use not recommended.

Dosage Forms. Cap 12 mg.

Patient Instructions. Patients should be informed that they must disclose long-term or intermittent opioid pain therapy, including any use of opioids in the week prior to receiving alvimopan. They should understand that recent use of opioids may make them more susceptible to adverse reactions to alvimopan, primarily those limited to the GI tract (e.g., abdominal pain, nausea and vomiting, diarrhea).

Pharmacokinetics. *Onset and Duration.* GI recovery from postoperative ileus began around 48 h after surgery, on average. Resolution occurred 92–116.4 h after surgery, and was 10.7–26.1 h quicker with alvimopan versus placebo.

Fate. Renal excretion and biliary secretion. **Half-life.** 10–17 h.

Adverse Reactions. Constipation, dyspepsia, flatulence, back pain, and urinary retention.

Contraindications. Alvimopan is contraindicated in patients who have taken therapeutic doses of opioids for more than 7 consecutive days immediately prior to taking alvimopan.

Precautions. A higher number of myocardial infarctions was reported in patients treated with alvimopan 0.5 mg twice daily compared with placebo in a 12-month study in patients treated with opioids for chronic pain, although a causal relationship has not been established; patients recently exposed to opioids are expected to be more sensitive to the effects of alvimopan and therefore may experience abdominal pain, nausea and vomiting, and diarrhea; not recommended in patients with severe hepatic impairment; not recommended in patients with end-stage renal disease.

Drug Interactions. None demonstrated.

Notes. Alvmiopan is intended for short-term, hospital use only. In order for hospital pharmacies to order, stock, and dispense alvimopan, hospitals must be enrolled in the Entereg Access Support and Education (EASE) program. This program requires the following:

1. The EASE program enrollment kit has been received by the hospital and provided to the health care practitioners who are responsible for the ordering, dispensing, and administering of alvimopan.
2. The hospital has systems, order sets, protocols, or other measures in place to limit the use of alvimopan to no more than 15 doses per patient for administration in the hospital only.
3. The hospital will not dispense alvimopan for outpatient use and will not transfer alvimopan to any hospital not registered with the EASE program.

METHYLNALTREXONE BROMIDE — Relistor

Pharmacology. Methylnaltrexone bromide demonstrates selective antagonism of the μ-opioid receptors in the peripheral nervous system. Since methylnaltrexone bromide is a quaternary amine, its ability to cross the blood–brain barrier is restricted. This allows methylnaltrexone bromide to function as a peripherally acting μ-opioid receptor antagonist in tissues such as the GI tract, thereby decreasing the constipating effects of opioids without impacting opioid mediated analgesic effects on the central nervous system. Methylnaltrexone bromide is indicated for the treatment of opioid-induced constipation in patients with advanced illness who are receiving palliative care, when response to laxative therapy has not been sufficient.

Adminstration and Adult Dosage. SQ treatment of opioid-induced constipation—8 mg every 24–48 h as needed for patients weighing 38–62 kg (84–136 lb); 12 mg every 24–48 h as needed for patients weighing 62–114 kg (136–251 lb). Patients whose weights fall outside of these ranges should be dosed at 0.15 mg/kg.

Special Populations. *Pediatric Dosage.* Not established.

Geriatric Dosage. Same as adult dosage.

Dosage Forms. **Inj** 12 mg/0.6-mL single-use vial.

Pharmacokinetics. *Onset and Duration.* In clinical trials, $\sim$30% of patients experienced laxation within 30 min of the first dose.

Fate. Approximately half of the dose is excreted in the urine and somewhat less in feces. **Half-life.** 8 h.

Adverse Reactions. Abdominal pain, flatulence, nauseas, dizziness, diarrhea.

Contraindications. Known or suspected mechanical GI obstruction.

Precautions. Discontinue therapy if severe or persistent diarrhea occurs.

Drug Interactions. None demonstrated.

LUBIPROSTONE — Amitiza

Pharmacology. Lubiprostone activates type-2 chloride channels (ClC-2) in the apical membrane of the intestine resulting in increased chloride concentration in the intestinal fluid. This in turn causes an increase in intestinal fluid secretion (without altering sodium and potassium serum concentrations). This increase in intestinal fluid increases intestinal motility, which facilitates the passage of stool.

Administration and Adult Dosage. **PO for chronic constipation**—24 μg twice daily with food and water; **PO for IBS-C** (irritable bowel syndrome—constipation)—8 μg twice daily with food and water.

Special Populations. *Pediatric Dosage.* Not established.

Geriatric Dosage. Same as adult dosage.

Dosage Forms. Cap 8, 24 μg.

Patient Instructions. Swallow capsule whole, do not break apart or chew. Patients who experience severe nausea, diarrhea, or dyspnea should inform their physician. Patients taking lubiprostone may experience dyspnea within an hour of the first dose. This symptom generally resolves within 3 h, but may recur with repeat dosing.

Pharmacokinetics. *Onset and Duration.* Systemic absorption following oral administration is undetectable. In clinical trials, 56.7%–62.9% of patients experienced a bowel movement within 24 h after the first dose of lubiprostone.

Fate. Animal studies have shown that metabolism of lubiprostone rapidly occurs within the stomach and jejunum; highly protein bound (94%) and rapid metabolism to M3 metabolite.

Adverse Reactions. Nausea, diarrhea, headache, abdominal pain, abdominal distention, and flatulence. Nausea may decrease when taken with food. Dyspnea may occur within 1 h of first dose and resolves within 3 h, but may recur with repeat dosing.

Contraindications. Patients with a known or suspected mechanical GI obstruction.

Precautions. Preganancy; severe diarrhea; mechanical GI obstruction.

Drug Interactions. None demonstrated.

ANTIDIARRHEALS

DIPHENOXYLATE HYDROCHLORIDE AND ATROPINE SULFATE   Lomotil, Various

Pharmacology. Diphenoxylate is a synthetic meperidine analogue without analgesic activity that inhibits peristalsis via stimulation of μ- and δ-opiate receptors in the bowel, resulting in increased water reabsorption in the colon. Since high doses of diphenoxylate (40–60 mg) cause central nervous system effects, including euphoria, atropine is added in subtherapeutic amounts to decrease abuse potential.

Administration and Adult Dosage. **PO for diarrhea**—2 tablets or 10 mL 4 times daily initially and then, if control is achieved (usually within 48 h), decrease to a **maintenance dosage** as low as 2 tablets or 10 mL daily as needed, to a maximum of 20 mg/d. If chronic diarrhea is not controlled in 10 days at the full dosage, then symptoms are unlikely to be controlled by further administration.

Special Populations. *Pediatric Dosage.* **Use liquid only**—(<2 years) not recommended. **PO for diarrhea**—0.3–0.4 mg/kg/d of diphenoxylate in 4 divided doses initially, not to exceed adult dosage. Reduce dosage once diarrhea is controlled.

Geriatric Dosage. Same as adult dosage.

Dosage Forms. **Syrup** 500 μg diphenoxylate and 5 μg atropine/mL; **Tab** 2.5 mg diphenoxylate and 25 μg atropine.

Patient Instructions. This drug can cause dry mouth, blurred vision, drowsiness, or dizziness; use caution while driving or performing other tasks requiring alertness, coordination, or physical dexterity. Avoid alcohol and other CNS depressants. Seek medical attention if diarrhea persists or if fever, palpitations, or abdominal distention occurs.

Pharmacokinetics. *Onset and Duration.* Onset 45–60 min; duration 3–4 h. Improvement in diarrhea usually occurs within 48 h.

Fate. Diphenoxylate is well absorbed from the GI tract and metabolized to an active metabolite, diphenoxylic acid. Drug and metabolite attain peak serum levels in 2 h. Diphenoxylate V_d is 3.8 ± 1.1 L/kg; clearance is 1.04 ± 0.14 L/h/kg.[24] Conjugates of the drug and metabolite are excreted primarily in the urine. **Half-life.** (diphenoxylate) 2.5 ± 0.6 h; (diphenoxylic acid) 7.2 ± 0.7 h.[25]

Adverse Reactions. Anticholinergic symptoms such as dry mouth, urinary retention, blurred vision, fever, or tachycardia occur frequently with high daily dosages and occasionally with usual dosages in children.[7] Drowsiness, dizziness, and headache occur occasionally. The potential for addiction and/or opiate withdrawal symptoms exists.

Contraindications. Children <2 years; obstructive jaundice; diarrhea associated with pseudomembranous enterocolitis or enterotoxin-producing bacteria. (*See* Notes.)

Precautions. Use with caution in children because of variable response and potential for toxicity (atropinism) with recommended dosages (particularly in children with Down's syndrome) and in patients with acute ulcerative colitis, hepatic dysfunction, or cirrhosis.

Drug Interactions. Because of its chemical similarity to meperidine, avoid diphenoxylate use with MAOIs. Use with caution in combination with CNS depressants.

Parameters to Monitor. Frequency and volume of bowel movements; body temperature; blood in stool. Watch for signs of atropine toxicity. Monitor for abdominal distention.

Notes. In chronic diarrhea, diphenoxylate 5 mg is about equipotent with **loperamide** 2 mg or **codeine** 30–45 mg. It might provide temporary symptomatic relief of infectious traveler's diarrhea (although loperamide is preferred) if used cautiously with an antibiotic, but discontinue if fever occurs, symptoms persist beyond 48 h, or blood or mucus appears in the stool.[26,27]

LOPERAMIDE   Imodium

Pharmacology. Loperamide is a synthetic antidiarrheal with μ-opioid receptor agonist properties that does not cross the blood–brain barrier. It causes a dose-related inhibition of colonic motility and affects water and electrolyte movement through the bowel. Tolerance has not been observed.

Administration and Adult Dosage. **PO for acute diarrhea or traveler's diarrhea (OTC)**—4 mg initially and then 2 mg after each unformed stool (often with an antibiotic for traveler's diarrhea), to a maximum of 16 mg/d (8 mg/d for no more than 2 days with OTC product).[26,27,28] **PO for chronic diarrhea**—Initiate therapy as above and then individualize dosage. **Usual maintenance dosage** is 4–8 mg/d in single or divided doses. If clinical improvement does not occur after treatment with 16 mg/d for at least 10 days, symptoms are unlikely to be controlled by further use.

Special Populations. *Pediatric Dosage.* (<2 years) safety and efficacy not established. **PO for acute diarrhea**—(2–5 years) up to 1 mg 3 times daily as liquid; (6–8 years) 2 mg twice daily; (8–12 years) 2 mg 3 times daily. After the first day of therapy, give 1 mg/10 kg after each loose stool, to a maximum daily dosage equal to the initial daily dosage. **PO for acute or traveler's diarrhea (OTC)**—(2–5 years) not recommended; (6–8 years) 1 mg initially and then 1 mg after each loose stool, to a maximum of 4 mg/d for 2 days; (9–11 years) 2 mg initially and then 1 mg after each loose stool, to a maximum of 6 mg/d for 2 days. **PO for chronic diarrhea**—Dosage not established.

Geriatric Dosage. Same as adult dosage.

Dosage Forms. **Cap** 2 mg; **Chew Tab** 2 mg; **Tab** 2 mg; **Soln** 0.2, 1 mg/mL; **Chew Tab** 2 mg plus simethicone (Imodium Advanced).

Patient Instructions. This drug can cause drowsiness or dizziness. Until the severity of these reactions is known, use caution when performing tasks that require mental alertness. It can cause dry mouth. Drink plenty of clear fluids to prevent the dehydration that can accompany diarrhea. If diarrhea does not stop after a few days, or if abdominal pain, distention, or fever occurs, seek medical attention.

Pharmacokinetics. *Onset and Duration.* Onset 45–60 min; duration 4–6 h.

Fate. GI absorption is approximately 40%; ≥25% is excreted in the stool unchanged; <2% of a dose is recovered in the urine.[29,30] **Half-life.** 10.8 ± 1.7 h.[29,30]

Adverse Reactions. Abdominal cramping, constipation, distention, headache, rash, tiredness, drowsiness, dizziness, and dry mouth occur frequently.[7]

Contraindications. Patients who must avoid constipation; children <2 years; bloody diarrhea; body temperature above 38°C (101°F); diarrhea associated with pseudomembranous colitis; or enterotoxin-producing bacteria. (*See* Notes.)

Precautions. Use with caution in patients with ulcerative colitis. Discontinue if improvement is not observed within 48 h. Use cautiously in patients with hepatic dysfunction.

Drug Interactions. Absorption of loperamide can be decreased by cholesterol-binding resins.

Parameters to Monitor. Frequency and volume of bowel movements; body temperature; blood in stool. Monitor for abdominal distention.

Notes. Adverse reactions might be less frequent and efficacy might be greater than with **diphenoxylate** with atropine. Loperamide can provide temporary symptomatic relief of infectious traveler's diarrhea if used cautiously with an antibiotic, but discontinue if fever occurs or other symptoms persist beyond 48 h, or blood or mucus in stool develops.[20,26,27]

PROKINETIC AGENTS

METOCLOPRAMIDE
Reglan, Various

Pharmacology. Metoclopramide stimulates the release of acetylcholine from the gastric myenteric plexus by antagonizing peripheral and central dopamine receptors, specifically the D_2 subtype receptors. Metoclopramide also acts as a partial agonist at the 5-HT_4 receptors, thereby facilitating the release of acetylcholine in the GI tract; however, it acts as an antagonist at the 5-HT_3 receptor site.[31] It increases peristalsis of the gastric antrum, duodenum, and jejunum; relaxes the pyloric sphincter and duodenal bulb; and has little effect on the colon or gallbladder. In patients with GERD, metoclopramide produces a dose-dependent increase and duration of action in lower esophageal sphincter pressure. Its antiemetic action results from a direct antidopaminergic effect on the chemoreceptor trigger zone and vomiting center and from 5-HT_3 receptor blocking effects. Metoclopramide increases prolactin secretion and serum prolactin. It also produces a transient increase in aldosterone secretion, thought to be related to direct stimulation of the adrenal gland via stimulation of the 5-HT_4 receptor.[32]

Administration and Adult Dosage. **PO for short-term treatment of symptomatic GERD in patients who fail to respond to conventional therapy**—up to 15 mg 4 times daily 30 min before each meal and at bedtime for 4–12 weeks or intermittent single doses of up to 20 mg. **PO for symptomatic diabetic gastroparesis**—10 mg 4 times daily 30 min before each meal and at bedtime for 2–8 weeks. **IM or IV for severe symptoms associated with gastroparesis**—10 mg 4 times daily for up to 10 days. **IV to facilitate small bowel intubation or to aid in radiologic examination**—10 mg over 1–2 min, 10–30 min before tube placement.[33,34] **PO to increase maternal milk supply**—10 mg 3 times daily for 10–14 days.[35] **PO, IM, or IV for the treatment of hiccups**—(PO) 10 mg every 6 h for 10 days, (IM, IV) 5–10 mg every 8 h for 24–48 h and then switch to PO.[36] **IV for prevention of chemotherapy-induced emesis**—2 mg/kg every 2–4 h for 2–5 doses. **IV for delayed nausea and vomiting**—0.5 mg/kg or 30 mg IV every 4–6 h for 3–5 days. **IM for prevention of postoperative nausea and vomiting**—10–20 mg near the end of surgery. **IV for treatment of postoperative nausea and vomiting**—10 mg every 4–6 h as needed postoperation. Administer undiluted IV metoclopramide slowly (at least 1–2 min for a 10-mg dose); infuse diluted IV doses over at least 15 min. (*See* Notes.)

Special Populations. *Pediatric Dosage.* **IV to facilitate small bowel intubation or aid radiologic examination**—(<6 years) 0.1 mg/kg; (6–14 years) 2.5–5 mg; (>14 years) Same as adult dosage. **IV for postoperative nausea and vomiting**—0.1–0.2 mg/kg.

Geriatric Dosage. Begin at one-half the initial dose (usually 5 mg) and increase or decrease based on efficacy and side effects.

Other Conditions. With Cl_{Cr} <40 mL/min, begin at one-half the initial dose (usually 5 mg) and increase or decrease based on efficacy and side effects.

Dosage Forms. **Tab** 5, 10 mg; **Soln** 1 mg/mL; **Syrup** 1 mg/mL; **Inj** 5 mg/mL.

Patient Instructions. Take each dose 30 min before meals and at bedtime. This drug can cause drowsiness. Until the degree of drowsiness is known, use caution when driving, operating machinery, or performing other tasks requiring mental alertness. Avoid excessive concurrent use of alcohol or other drugs that cause drowsiness. Report any involuntary movements (e.g., muscle spasms and jerky movements of the head and face) that occur, especially in children and the elderly.

Missed Doses. If you miss a dose, take it as soon as possible. If it is almost time for your next dose, skip the missed dose and return to your usual dosage schedule. Do not double doses.

Pharmacokinetics. *Onset and Duration.* (GI effects) PO onset 45 ± 15 min, IM 12.5 ± 2.5 min, IV 2 ± 1 min; duration 1–2 h.

Fate. Bioavailabilities are PO 80 ± 15.5% and IM 85 ± 11%. Peak-serum concentration after a PO dose occurs in 1–2 h but can be delayed with impaired gastric emptying. The drug is approximately 30% bound to plasma proteins. V_d is 3.4 ± 1.3 L/kg, increased in uremia and in cirrhosis; clearance is 0.37 ± 0.08 L/h/kg, decreased in uremia and in cirrhosis. Approximately 85% of orally administered drug is recovered in the urine after 72 h as unchanged drug; 20% of an IV dose is excreted unchanged in urine. **Half-life.** α phase 5 min; β phase 5.5 ± 0.5 h, increasing to approximately 14 h in severe renal failure. Half-life also can be prolonged in cirrhosis.

Adverse Reactions. Most side effects are related to dosage and duration of use. Drowsiness, restlessness, fatigue, and lassitude occur in 10% of patients with a dosage of 10 mg 4 times daily and in 70% with IV doses of 1–2 mg/kg. Acute dystonic reactions occur in 0.2% of patients receiving 30–40 mg/d, 2% in cancer chemotherapy–treated patients >35 years receiving doses of 1–2 mg/kg, and 25% in cancer chemotherapy-treated children without prior diphenhydramine treatment. Parkinsonian symptoms, tardive dyskinesia, and akathisia occur less frequently. Rapid IV push produces transient, intense anxiety, and restlessness followed by drowsiness. Transient flushing of the face and/or diarrhea occur frequently after large IV doses. Hyperprolactinemia can occur, resulting in gynecomastia and impotence in males and galactorrhea and amenorrhea in females. Fluid retention can result from transient elevation of aldosterone secretion that occurs after parenteral, but not oral, administration.[32] Diarrhea, hypertension, and mental depression have been reported. Neuroleptic malignant syndrome is a rare, but potentially fatal, adverse effect reported to occur with metoclopramide.[37]

Contraindications. GI hemorrhage; mechanical obstruction or perforation; pheochromocytoma; epilepsy; concurrent use of drugs that cause extrapyramidal effects.

Precautions. Pregnancy; lactation; elderly;[38] patients with hypertension, renal failure, or Parkinson's disease; history of depression or attempted suicide; and after gut anastomosis. In patients with diabetic gastroparesis, insulin dosage or timing might require adjustment.

Drug Interactions. Absorption of drugs from the stomach or small bowel can be altered by metoclopramide (e.g., digoxin and cimetidine absorption is decreased; cyclosporine absorption is increased). Anticholinergics and narcotics may antagonize GI effects of metoclopramide. Use with an MAOI can result in hypertension, and the combination should be avoided. Additive sedation can occur with alcohol or other CNS depressants.

Parameters to Monitor. Monitor periodically for CNS effects, extrapyramidal reactions, and changes in serum creatinine, blood glucose, or blood pressure. (GERD or diabetic gastroparesis) observe for symptomatic relief.

Notes. Tolerance to the drug's gastrokinetic effect can develop with long-term therapy. Metoclopramide has been used in the treatment of neurogenic bladder, orthostatic hypotension, Tourette's syndrome, adynamic or chemotherapy-induced ileus, anorexia, and complications of scleroderma. If extrapyramidal symptoms occur, administer **diphenhydramine** 50 mg IM or **benztropine** 1–2 mg IM.

Cisapride (Propulsid) was available for the symptomatic treatment of adults with nighttime heartburn due to GERD. Cisapride is no longer marketed in the United States, but will be available through an investigational limited-access program because of serious cardiovascular effects (e.g., prolonged QT interval, torsades de pointes) in patients taking interacting medications or with certain underlying health conditions. For patients to be considered for the Propulsid investigational limited-access program, they must have failed all standard therapies and have baseline laboratory tests and ECG, and undergone an appropriate diagnostic evaluation including radiologic examinations or endoscopy. Contact Janssen Pharmaceutica at 1–800-JANSSEN to determine whether a patient qualifies for the program.

Domperidone (Motilium) is a prokinetic agent available outside the United States for the treatment of diabetic gastroparesis. It selectively blocks peripheral dopamine D_2 receptors in the GI tract; it has antiemetic effects related to its action at the chemoreceptor trigger zone; and it stimulates pituitary prolactin release in humans but has no cholinergic activity. The drug does not cross the blood–brain barrier and thus does not produce CNS and extrapyramidal effects. Domperidone improves delayed gastric emptying and enhances antral and duodenal peristalsis but does not affect esophageal or colonic motility. Proton pump inhibitors (PPIs), histamine H2-receptor antagonists, and antacids should not be coadministered with domperidone because the drug requires an acidic environment for activity. Dosages of 10–20 mg 3 times daily have been studied for dyspepsia and 20 mg 4 times daily is being studied for the treatment of diabetic gastroparesis. The most frequent side effects of domperidone are headache, dry mouth, anxiety, and elevation in serum prolactin concentrations.[39]

Erythromycin is a macrolide antibiotic that has prokinetic activity by acting as a motilin receptor agonist in the GI tract to stimulate GI contractility.[40] In gastroparesis, doses of 200–250 mg IV given over 15–30 min of the lactobionate salt, 250 mg PO 3 times daily of the ethylsuccinate salt, or 500 mg PO of the stearate salt 15–120 min before meals and at bedtime appear to be effective.[40,41] Erythromycin ethylsuccinate suspension formulation has a faster prokinetic action than erythromycin stearate tablets.[41]

MISCELLANEOUS GASTROINTESTINAL DRUGS

ACTIVATED CHARCOAL   Various

Pharmacology. Activated charcoal is a nonspecific GI adsorbent with a surface area of 900–2000 m^2/g that is used primarily in the management of acute poisonings.[42]

Administration and Adult Dosage. **PO or via gastric tube for poisoning—** 50–120 g dispersed in liquid as soon as possible after ingestion of poison (the

U.S. Food and Drug Administration suggests 240 mL diluent/30 g activated charcoal). Repeat administration of activated charcoal after gastric lavage. (*See* Notes.)

Special Populations. *Pediatric Dosage.* **PO or via gastric tube for poisoning**— (≤12 years) 25–50 g or 1–2 g/kg dispersed in liquid; (>12 years) same as adult dosage.[43]

Geriatric Dosage. Same as adult dosage.

Dosage Forms. **Pwdr** plain or dispersed in water or sorbitol–water.

Patient Instructions. This drug causes stools to turn black.

Pharmacokinetics. *Onset and Duration.* Onset is immediate; duration is continual while it remains in the GI tract.

Fate. Not orally absorbed; eliminated unchanged in the feces.

Adverse Reactions. Black stools; gritty consistency can cause emesis in some patients.

Precautions. Insufficient hydration or use in patients with decreased bowel motility can result in intestinal bezoars.

Drug Interactions. Activated charcoal can decrease the oral absorption and efficacy of many drugs. (*See* Notes.)

Parameters to Monitor. Passage of activated charcoal in the stools. If sorbitol or other cathartics are administered, limit their dosages to prevent excessive fluid and electrolyte losses.

Notes. A suspension of activated charcoal in 25%–35% **sorbitol** can increase palatability of the drug; total dosage of sorbitol should not exceed 1 g/kg. Substances *not* adsorbed by activated charcoal are mineral acids, alkalis, iron, cyanide, lithium and other small ions, and alcohols. Repeated oral doses of activated charcoal (e.g., 15–30 g every 4–6 h) have been used to enhance the elimination of some drugs, most notably **carbamazepine, phenobarbital, salicylates,** and **theophylline.**

OCTREOTIDE ACETATE   Sandostatin, Sandostatin LAR Depot, Various

Pharmacology. Octreotide is a synthetic octapeptide with pharmacologic actions similar to those of somatostatin. The actions of somatostatin are regulated by somatostatin receptors (5 known subtypes) located in regions of the brain, leptomeninges, anterior pituitary, endocrine and exocrine pancreas, GI mucosa, and cells of the immune system. Octreotide binds primarily to somatostatin-receptor subtype 2, to a lesser extent to subtype 5, and to an even lesser extent to subtype 3; it does not bind to subtypes 1 and 4. It suppresses the secretion of numerous substances including serotonin, gastrin, vasoactive intestinal peptide (VIP), cholecystokinin, insulin, glucagon, secretin, motilin, pancreatic polypeptide, and growth hormone (GH). It suppresses the luteinizing hormone response to gonadotropin-releasing hormone and the secretion of thyroid stimulating hormone. It also decreases splanchnic and venous blood flow.[44,45]

Administration and Adult Dosage. (*See* Notes.) **SQ or IV for treatment of diarrhea associated with VIP-secreting tumor**—200–300 μg/d in 2–4 divided doses for 2 weeks. **SQ or IV for treatment of metastatic carcinoid syndrome**—initially 100–600 μg/d in 2–4 divided doses for 2 weeks. **Usual maintenance** is 450 μg/d.

SQ or IV for treatment of drug and surgery-resistant acromegaly—initially 50 μg 3 times daily. **Usual maintenance**—100–500 μg 3 times daily. **IV (immediate injection only)**—same dosage as SQ, dilute in 50–200 mL of NS or D5W and infuse over 15–30 min or give by IV push over 3 min. In emergency situations (e.g., carcinoid crisis), give by rapid IV bolus.

Special Populations. *Pediatric Dosage.* **SQ (immediate)**—(≥1 month) 1–10 μg/kg are well tolerated, and studies of various GI disorders have used widely different dosages in children aged 3 days–16 years.[46] Octreotide is not approved, but has been studied in the treatment of hyperinsulinemic hypoglycemia in neonates in different dosages.[46,47] **SQ for anti-VIP effects**—3.5 μg/kg/d divided every 8 h.[48] **SQ for chronic GI bleeding**—4–8 μg/kg/d.[49]

Geriatric Dosage. Dosage reduction is recommended because of decreased renal clearance, but specific guidelines are not established.

Other Conditions. The effect of hepatic disease on the disposition of octreotide is unknown. Reduction of maintenance dosages might be required in patients with renal impairment and those undergoing dialysis.[45]

Dosage Forms. **Inj (immediate)** 50, 100, 200, 500, 1000 μg/mL; **Inj (depot)** 2, 4, 6 mg/mL.

Patient Instructions. (Immediate-release) instruct patient in sterile SQ injection technique. Avoid multiple SQ injections at the same site within a short period. Systematically rotate injection sites. Do not use solution if particulates and/or discoloration are present. Store medication in refrigerator but do not allow it to freeze; individual ampules can remain at room temperature for up to 24 h. Octreotide is stable at room temperature for 14 days if protected from light. Pain at injection site can be minimized by using the smallest volume necessary to obtain the desired dose and by bringing the solution to room temperature before injection, but do not warm artificially. Stop medication and report if symptoms worsen or you have abnormal blood sugar levels or abnormal blood pressure. Inspect the vial for particulate matter or discoloration of the solution; do not use if either is present.

Missed Doses. (Immediate-release) If you miss a dose, take it as soon as possible. If it is almost time for your next dose, skip the missed dose and return to your usual dosage schedule. Do not double doses. Although you will not be harmed by forgetting a dose, the symptoms that you are trying to control might reappear. To control your symptoms, your doses should be evenly spaced over 24 h.

Pharmacokinetics. *Onset and Duration.* (Immediate-release) SQ peak concentrations occur in 0.4 h (0.7 h in acromegaly). Duration is up to 12 h, depending on tumor type. (Depot) IM initial peak occurs at 1 h and then slowly decreases over 3–5 days; a second peak appears 2–3 weeks postinjection. Duration is up to 2–3 weeks. Steady-state levels are usually attained after approximately 12 weeks.

Fate. Oral absorption is poor; SQ and IV routes are bioequivalent. The drug is 65% protein bound (41% in acromegaly), primarily to lipoprotein and, to a lesser extent, albumin. V_d is 0.35 ± 0.22 L/kg; clearance is 0.16 ± 0.08 L/h/kg. V_d and clearance are both increased in acromegaly; clearance is decreased in the elderly by 26% and in those with renal impairment. Octreotide exhibits nonlinear pharmacokinetics at dosages of 600 μg/d. Approximately 32% is excreted unchanged in urine. **Half-life.** 1.5 ± 0.4 h; increased by 46% in the elderly.

Adverse Reactions. Single doses of octreotide acetate can inhibit gallbladder contractility and decrease bile secretion. Approximately half of patients treated for at least 12 months experience cholesterol gallstones or sludge unrelated to age, sex, or dosage. Approximately 22% of patients with acromegaly treated with the depot formulation developed new cholelithiasis, 7% of which were microstones. Approximately 24% of patients with malignant carcinoid who received 18 months of depot therapy developed gallstones; 1% might require cholecystectomy. Five to ten percent of nonacromegalic patients and 34%–61% of acromegalic patients experience diarrhea, loose stools, nausea, and abdominal discomfort. The severity, but not frequency, is dose dependent and usually occurs with the initial dose, with the symptoms spontaneously resolving within 10–14 days.[44] Hypoglycemia (in 3%) and hyperglycemia (in 16%) are more common in acromegalic patients than in nonacromegalic patients. The frequencies of hypoglycemia (4%) and hyperglycemia (27%) are higher in carcinoid patients treated with the depot formulation. Octreotide suppresses secretion of TSH; alters the balance between insulin, glucagon, and GH; and might be responsible for cardiac conduction abnormalities, which are particularly frequent in acromegaly—bradycardia (25%), conduction abnormalities (10%), and arrhythmias (9%). Pain on injection occurs frequently with the immediate-release formulation and can be minimized by warming the solution before injection and using the smallest possible volume of solution to obtain the appropriate dose. Pain on injection is more frequent with the depot injection, from 2% to 11% in acromegalic patients to 20%–50% in carcinoid patients. Flulike symptoms, vomiting, flatulence, constipation, and headaches occur in 1%–10%. Several cases of pancreatitis have been reported. Steatorrhea also can occur while on long-term therapy.[45] Abnormal Schilling's tests and decreased vitamin B_{12} levels have been reported.

Precautions. Pregnancy; lactation. Never give depot formulation by the IV or SQ route. Use with caution in patients with diabetic gastroparesis because octreotide slows GI transit time;[50] insulin-dependent patients with diabetes might require a reduction in insulin dosage.

Drug Interactions. In acromegaly, reducing the dosage of medications that cause bradycardia (e.g., β-blockers) might be required. In all patients, the dosage of calcium channel blocking drugs, diuretics, insulin, or oral hypoglycemics might require an adjustment with concurrent octreotide. Octreotide can decrease the absorption of some orally administered nutrients and drugs (e.g., fat, cyclosporine).

Parameters to Monitor. Perform ultrasound of the gallbladder periodically during extended therapy. Obtain baseline and periodic total and/or free T_4 levels during long-term therapy. Monitor closely for hyper- or hypoglycemia, especially in patients with diabetes. Periodically monitor vitamin B_{12} during long-term therapy. Evaluate cardiac function at baseline and periodically during therapy, especially in acromegalic patients. Monitor serum concentrations of drugs whose absorption might be affected by octreotide (e.g., cyclosporine). To evaluate response, monitor GH or insulin-like growth factor-1 (IGF-I) concentrations in acromegalic patients; urinary 5-hydroxyindole acetic acid, plasma serotonin, plasma substance P in carcinoid patients; and plasma VIP in patients with VIPoma.

Notes. The absorption of dietary fats can decrease while on octreotide therapy. Zinc levels should be monitored periodically in patients receiving parenteral nutrition and octreotide. Store depot formulation at 2°C–8°C. Before administration, leave the drug at room temperature for 30–60 min. Octreotide must be administered immediately after mixing and should only be given IM intragluteally and not in the deltoid region to avoid injection site discomfort. Store the immediate-release formulation at 2°C–8°C and protected from light. If stored at room temperature (20°C–30°C) and protected from light, the product is stable for 14 days. Before SQ administration, the solution can be kept at room temperature to decrease injection site discomfort, but do not warm artificially. Octreotide 200 μg/mL is stable for up to 60 days in polypropylene syringes under refrigeration and protected from light.[51] Octreotide is not compatible with parenteral nutrition because of the formation of glycosyl octreotide conjugate.

URSODIOL
Actigall, Urso, Various

Pharmacology. Ursodiol (ursodeoxycholic acid) is a hydrophilic bile acid used to dissolve small (<20 mm), noncalcified, radiolucent cholesterol gallstones in mildly symptomatic patients with functioning gallbladders who cannot undergo a cholecystectomy. It is also used to treat primary biliary cirrhosis. The exact mechanism of action of ursodiol is unclear, but it is thought to have a hepatocytoprotective effect by displacing accumulated toxic bile acids with hydrophilic bile acids, to promote secretion of toxic bile acid salts from the bile ducts and suppress the synthesis of chenodeoxycholic acid, and to act as an immunosuppressive agent by downregulating the antigen expression in hepatocytes in patients with primary biliary cirrhosis or primary sclerosing cirrhosis. Ursodiol improves liver function tests, liver histology, and certain immune markers; relieves pruritus in some patients; and can extend the period before death or to liver transplantation.[52,53] Ursodiol also appears to be effective in decreasing episodes of rejection and improving 1-year survival rates after liver transplantation.[52] Patients undergoing bone marrow transplantation might benefit from ursodiol therapy through prevention of hepatic venoocclusive disease.[54]

Administration and Adult Dosage. All doses should be administered with food. **PO for gallstone dissolution**—8–10 mg/kg/d in 2–3 divided doses. Complete gallstone dissolution usually requires 6–24 months of treatment, and treatment should be continued for at least 3 months after stones or sludge are not apparent on ultrasound. **PO for prevention of gallstones in patients with rapid weight loss**—300 mg twice daily. **PO for primary biliary cirrhosis**—13–15 mg/kg/d in 4 divided doses.

Special Populations. *Pediatric Dosage.* Safety and efficacy not established; pediatric use has been reported. (*See* Notes.)

Geriatric Dosage. No dosage reduction is necessary.

Dosage Forms. **Cap** 300 mg; **Tab** 250 mg. Ursodiol can be formulated into a suspension.[55,56]

Adverse Reactions. Ursodiol is relatively safe, with minimal side effects. The most common adverse effects are diarrhea, nausea, vomiting, dyspepsia, abdominal pain, and arthritis.

Drug Interactions. Bile acid sequestering agents (e.g., cholestyramine, colestipol) and aluminum-containing antacids reduce ursodiol absorption; thus, the two drugs should be taken at least 2 h apart. Oral contraceptives, estrogens, and lipid-lowering agents (e.g., clofibrate) increase cholesterol secretion, thereby increasing the risk of developing cholesterol gallstones; using any of these agents can counteract the effectiveness of ursodiol.

Notes. Though unapproved in adults, ursodiol is also used PO for prevention of hepatic venoocclusive disease in bone marrow transplant (<90 kg) 300 mg twice daily; (>90 kg) 300 mg 3 times daily (or 300 mg every morning and 600 mg every evening),[54] and PO as an adjunct to immunosuppressants after liver transplantation 10–15 mg/kg/d in divided doses.[52,53] In pediatrics, ursodiol is used off-label PO for cystic fibrosis in patients with liver disease (5–20 mg/kg/d in divided doses or higher),[57] and PO for obese children with liver abnormalities (10–12.5 mg/kg/d in 2 divided doses).[58]

■ REFERENCES

1. AGA Governing Board. AGA technical review on constipation. *Gatroenterology.* 2000;119:1766-1778.
2. Chan EK, Schroeder DJ. Psyllium in hypercholesterolemia. *Ann Pharmacother.* 1995;29:625-626.
3. Anderson JW et al. Long-term cholesterol-lowering effects of psyllium as an adjunct to diet therapy in the treatment of hypercholesterolemia. *Am J Clin Nutr.* 2000;71:1433-1438.
4. Berardi RR et al., eds. *Handbook of Nonprescription Drugs.* 15th ed. Washington, DC: American Pharmacists Association; 2006.
5. Freeman GL. Psyllium hypersensitivity. *Ann Allergy.* 1994;73:490-492.
6. Hsieh C. Treatment of constipation in older adults. *Am Fam Physician.* 2005;72:2277-2284.
7. Gattuso JM, Kamm MA. Adverse effects of drugs used in the management of constipation and diarrhea. *Drug Saf.* 1994;10:47-65.
8. Tramonte SM et al. The treatment of chronic constipation in adults: a systematic review. *J Gen Intern Med.* 1997;12:15-24.
9. McRorie JW et al. Psyllium is superior to docusate sodium for treatment of chronic constipation. *Aliment Pharmacol Ther.* 1998;12:491-497.
10. Pasricha PJ. Treatment of disorders of bowel motility and water flux: antiemetics; agents used in biliary and pancreatic disease. In: Brunton LL, Lazo JS, Parker KL, eds. *Goodman & Gilman's the Pharmacological Basis of Therapeutics.* 11th ed. New York: McGraw-Hill; 2006:983-1008.
11. Adams WJ et al. Bisacodyl reduces the volume of polyethylene glycol solution required for bowel preparation. *Dis Colon Rectum.* 1994;37:229-233.
12. Goodale EP, Noble TA. Pediatric bowel evacuation with a polyethylene glycol and iso-osmolar electrolyte solution. *DICP.* 1990;23:1008-1009.
13. Sharma VK et al. Randomized, controlled study of pretreatment with magnesium citrate on the quality of colonoscopy preparation with polyethylene glycol electrolyte lavage solution. *Gastrointest Endosc.* 1997;46: 541-543.
14. Shannon M. Ingestion of toxic substances by children. *N Engl J Med.* 2000;342:186-191.
15. Gremse DA et al. Comparison of polyethylene glycol 3350 and lactulose for treatment of chronic constipation in children. *Clin Pediatr (Phila).* 2002;41:225-229.
16. Pashankar DS, Bishop WP. Efficacy and optimal dose of daily polyethylene glycol 3350 for treatment of constipation and encopresis in children. *J Pediatr.* 2001;139:428-432.
17. Bishop WP. Miracle laxative? *J Pediatr Gastroenterol Nutr.* 2001;32:514-515.

18. DiPalma JA et al. A randomized, multicenter, placebo-controlled trial of polyethylene glycol laxative for chronic treatment of chronic constipation. *Am J Gastroenterol.* 2007;102:1436-1441.

19. Pelham RW, Nix LC, Chavira RE, Cleveland MV, Stetson P. Clinical trial: single- and multiple-dose pharmacokinetics of polyethylene glycol (PEG-3350) in healthy young and elderly subjects. *Aliment Pharmacol Ther.* 2008;28:256-265.

20. Clausen MR, Mortensen PB. Lactulose, disaccharides and colonic flora: clinical consequences. *Drugs.* 1997;53: 930-942.

21. Kot TV, Pettit-Young NA. Lactulose in the management of constipation: a current review. *Ann Pharmacother.* 1992;26:1277-1282.

22. Lederle FA et al. Cost-effective treatment of constipation in the elderly: a randomized double-blind comparison of sorbitol and lactulose. *Am J Med.* 1990;89:597-601.

23. Swain R, Kaplan-Machlis B. Magnesium for the next millennium. *South Med J.* 1999;92:1040-1047.

24. Karim A et al. Pharmacokinetics and metabolism of diphenoxylate in man. *Clin Pharmacol Ther.* 1972;13: 407-419.

25. Jackson LS, Stafford JE. The evaluation and application of a radioimmunoassay for the measurement of diphenoxylic acid, the major metabolite of diphenoxylate hydrochloride (Lomotil), in human plasma. *J Pharmacol Methods.* 1987;18:189-197.

26. Ansdell VE, Ericsson CD. Prevention and empiric treatment of traveler's diarrhea. *Med Clin North Am.* 1999;83:945-973.

27. Ryan ET, Kain KC. Health advice and immunizations for travelers. *N Engl J Med.* 2000;342:1716-1725.

28. Anonymous. Advice for travelers. *Med Lett Drugs Ther.* 1999;41:39-41.

29. Killinger JM et al. Human pharmacokinetics and comparative bioavailability of loperamide hydrochloride. *J Clin Pharmacol.* 1979;19:211-218.

30. Lauritsen K et al. Clinical pharmacokinetics of drugs used in gastrointestinal disease (part II). *Clin Pharmacokinet.* 1990;19:94-125.

31. Hasler WL. Disorders of gastric emptying. In: Yamada T et al., eds. *Textbook of Gastroenterology.* 3rd ed. Philadelphia, PA: Lippincott Williams & Wilkins; 1999:1341-1369.

32. Rizzi CA et al. Regulation of plasma aldosterone levels by metoclopramide: a reappraisal of its mechanism from dopaminergic antagonism to serotonergic agonism. *Neuropharmacology.* 1997;36:763-768.

33. Heiselman DE et al. Enteral feeding tube placement success with intravenous metoclopramide administration in ICU patients. *Chest.* 1995;107:1686-1688.

34. Paz HL et al. Motility agents for the placement of weighted and unweighted feeding tubes in critically ill patients. *Intensive Care Med.* 1996;22:301-304.

35. Anderson PO, Valdés V. Increasing breast milk supply. *Clin Pharm.* 1993;12:479-480.

36. Friedman NL. Hiccups: a treatment review. *Pharmacotherapy.* 1996;16:986-995.

37. Nonino F, Campomori A. Neuroleptic malignant syndrome associated with metoclopramide. *Ann Pharmacother.* 1999;33:644-645.

38. Stewart RB et al. Metoclopramide: an analysis of inappropriate long-term use in the elderly. *Ann Pharmacother.* 1992;26:977-979.

39. Barone JA. Domperidone: a peripherally acting dopamine2-receptor antagonist. *Ann Pharmacother.* 1999;33: 429-440.

40. Weber FH et al. Erythromycin: a motilin agonist and gastrointestinal prokinetic agent. *Am J Gastroenterol.* 1993;88:485-490.

41. Ehrenpreis ED et al. Which form of erythromycin should be used to treat gastroparesis? A pharmacokinetic analysis. *Aliment Pharmacol Ther.* 1998;12:373-376.

42. Cooney DO. *Activated Charcoal in Medical Applications.* New York: Marcel Dekker; 1995.

43. Palatnick W, Tennenbein M. Activated charcoal in the treatment of drug overdose. *Drug Saf.* 1992;7:3-7.

44. Lamberts SWJ et al. Octreotide. *N Engl J Med.* 1996;334:246-254.

45. Beglinger C, Drewe J. Somatostatin and octreotide: physiological background and pharmacological application. *Digestion.* 1999;60(suppl 2):2-8.

46. Tauber MT et al. Clinical use of the long acting somatostatin analogue octreotide in pediatrics. *Eur J Pediatr.* 1994;153:304-310.

47. Barrons RW. Octreotide in hyperinsulinism. *Ann Pharmacother.* 1997;31:239-241.

48. Colon AR. Drug therapy in pediatric gastrointestinal disease. In: Lewis JH, ed. *A Pharmacologic Approach to Gastrointestinal Disorders.* Baltimore, MD: Williams & Wilkins; 1994:519-534.

49. Zellos A, Schwarz KB. Efficacy of octreotide in children with chronic gastrointestinal bleeding. *J Pediatr Gastroenterol Nutr.* 2000;30:442-446.

50. Chen JD et al. Effects of octreotide and erythromycin on gastric myoelectrical and motor activities in patients with gastroparesis. *Dig Dis Sci.* 1998;43:80-89.

51. Ripley RG et al. Stability of octreotide acetate in polypropylene syringes at 5 and 20°C. *Am J Health Syst Pharm.* 1995;52:1910-1911.

52. Kowdley KV. Ursodeoxycholic acid therapy in hepatobiliary disease. *Am J Med.* 2000;108:481-486.

53. Trauner M, Graziadei IW. Review article: mechanisms of action and therapeutic applications of ursodeoxycholic acid in chronic liver diseases. *Aliment Pharmacol Ther.* 1999;13:979-996.

54. Essell JH et al. Ursodiol prophylaxis against hepatic complications of allogeneic bone marrow transplantation. *Ann Intern Med.* 1998;128(12, pt 1):975-981.

55. Johnson CE, Nesbitt J. Stability of ursodiol in an extemporaneously compounded oral liquid. *Am J Health Syst Pharm.* 1995;52:1798-1800.

56. Mallett MS et al. Stability of ursodiol 25 mg/mL in an extemporaneously prepared oral liquid. *Am J Health Syst Pharm.* 1997;54:1401-1404.

57. Colombo C et al. Ursodeoxycholic acid therapy in cystic fibrosis-associated liver disease: a dose-response study. *Hepatology.* 1992;16:924-930.

58. Vajro P et al. Lack of efficacy of ursodeoxycholic acid for the treatment of liver abnormalities in obese children. *J Pediatr.* 2000;136:739-743.

Chapter 46

Inflammatory Bowel Disease

Juliana Chan and John Garofalo

ADALIMUMAB Humira

See Antirheumatic Drugs.

CERTOLIZUMAB PEGOL Cimzia

Pharmacology. Certolizumab pegol is a recombinant humanized FAB' fragment of anti-TNF-α monoclonal antibody. Anti-TNF-α agents are monoclonal antibodies that neutralize the inflammatory processes of the gastrointestinal mucosa by inhibiting TNF-α. Certolizumab's mechanism of action is similar to that of infliximab and adalimumab; but, because it lacks the Fc portion of the antibody, it does not cause complement activation, lacks apoptosis properties, and does not induce antibody-dependent cell breakdown.[1] Certolizumab is attached to a polyethylene glycol molecule, which results in a longer therapeutic half-life.[2]

Administration and Adult Dosage. **SQ for the treatment of reducing signs and symptoms of Crohn's disease and maintaining clinical response in adult patients with moderate to severe active disease who have had an inadequate response to conventional therapy**—400 mg initially, and at week 2 and 4. If a clinical response is achieved, then administer a maintenance dose of 400 mg every 4 weeks.

Special Populations. *Pediatric dosage.* Safety and efficacy not well established.

Geriatric dosage. Same as adult dosage.

Other Conditions. Pregnancy category B. Certolizumab pegol appears to be safe in animal studies and does not appear to affect fertility or harm the fetus in rats. No well-controlled trials have been conducted in pregnant women.

Dosage Forms. Pwdr for Inj 200 mg.

Patient Instructions. Certolizumab pegol is a medication that needs to be injected under the skin in either the stomach or the upper leg area. The health care provider will teach you how to inject the medication. Tell the doctor prior to starting certolizumab pegol if you have any history of infections, are currently experiencing flu or cold symptoms, or are currently receiving medications for an infection, including tuberculosis (TB) or human immunodeficiency virus (HIV). Also, tell the doctor if you have heart failure, seizures, multiple sclerosis, or cancer. Contact your health care provider immediately if during treatment you develop symptoms of the flu or other infections.

Pharmacokinetics. *Fate.* Subcutaneous administration of certolizumab pegol has a high bioavailability of about 80% (range 76%–88%). The time to peak plasma concentrations is quite variable ranging between 54 and 171 h after the subcutaneous administration. The apparent V_d is 45 mL/kg in healthy subjects.[2] Certolizumab pegol is a TNF-α blocker that has been pegylated with a polyethylene glycol molecule, which results in a decrease in drug clearance. **Half-life.** 14 days with a clearance rate of 0.17 mL/kg.[2] Primary route of elimination has not yet been determined.

Adverse Reactions. Adverse effects occurring in more than 5% of patients include headache, nasopharyngitis, abdominal pain, nausea, urinary tract infection, arthralgia, fevers, vomiting, cough, back pain, and injection site reactions.[3,4] Infections, primarily upper respiratory, developed in ~38% of patients while on treatment. Patients need to be tested negative for tuberculosis prior to treatment.

Precautions. Reactivation of tuberculosis has been observed in patients while being treated with certolizumab pegol. Infections including sepsis, opportunistic infections—fungal, viral, bacterial, and hepatitis B reactivation may occur and in some cases are fatal. Patients with an active infection should not be started on therapy until the infection resolves. Hematological events such as aplastic anemia, leukopenia, neutropenia, thrombocytopenia, and pancytopenia have been reported. Patients must be educated to recognize the signs and symptoms of infections and contact the health care provider immediately if these symptoms arise. Worsening heart failure has been reported while being treated with anti-TNF-α agents. Hypersensitivity reactions and new onset or exacerbation of demyelinating disease along with optic neuritis, peripheral neuropathy, and seizures have been reported. Hepatotoxicity and malignancies are rare yet have been associated with anti-TNF-α agents.

Drug Interactions. Anakinra administered with certolizumab pegol increases the risk of serious infections and neutropenia. Live vaccines may increase the risk of secondary transmission of infections.

Parameters to Monitor. Improvement in abdominal cramping, diarrhea, and rectal bleeding. Monitor for adverse effects, including infections, injection site reactions, and hypersensitivity reaction. Monitor for tuberculosis, CBC, Cl_{Cr}, liver function tests, and reactivation of hepatitis B, if the patient has a history of hepatitis B.

Notes. Treatment recommendations for the management of Crohn's disease are available and include biological agents such as Certolizumab pegol.[5–9] There is an ongoing debate as to whether a "step-down" or "step-up" approach should be used in the management of patients with Crohn's disease.[10] Step-down therapy uses biologic agents with or without immunosuppressives as first-line therapy. The traditional step-up approach calls for aminosalicylates as the initial treatment, followed by immunosuppressive agents and then biologic agents. There are 4 monoclonal antibody agents indicated for the treatment of Crohn's disease. Certolizumab pegol's role in the treatment of inflammatory bowel disease remains to be determined.

INFLIXIMAB	Remicade

See Antirheumatic Drugs.

MESALAMINE	Asacol, Apriso, Colazal, Canasa, Dipentum, Pentasa, Lialda, Rowasa, Various

Pharmacology. Mesalamine (5-aminosalicylic acid [5-ASA]) is thought to be the active moiety of sulfasalazine. The mechanism of action of 5-ASA in inflammatory bowel disease (IBD) is unknown, but it is thought to exhibit a localized effect on the gastrointestinal mucosa by inhibiting cyclooxygenase and 5-lipoxygenase, thereby down-regulating the production of inflammatory prostaglandins. An immunomodulatory response may also occur by inhibition and prevention of antibody and lymphocyte secretions during active disease. Mesalamine inhibits macrophage and neutrophil chemotaxis, reduces intestinal mononuclear cell production of immunoglobulin A and G antibodies, and is a scavenger of oxygen-derived free radicals, which are increased during active IBD.[11–14] **Balsalazide** disodium is a prodrug that is cleaved by bacterial azoreductase in the colon to release mesalamine and the inactive carrier, 4-aminobenzoyl-β-alanine.[12] Balsalazide 750 mg is equivalent to 267 mg of mesalamine. Each molecule of **olsalazine** that reaches the colon converts to 2 molecules of mesalamine.[12]

Administration and Adult Dosage. *See* Mesalamine Dosage.

Special Populations. *Pediatric Dosage.* Safety and efficacy not established for most of the 5-ASA agents, however pediatric use has been reported.[14,15] **Balsalazide**— (Colazal) 750–2250 mg tid is approved for children 5–17 years of age. **PO mesalamine**—(Asacol, Pentasa) 50 mg/kg/d in 2–3 divided doses (maximum dosages: Asacol 4.8 g/d, Pentasa 4 g/d) **PO olsalazine**— (Dipentum) 25–35 mg/kg/d in 2–3 divided doses.[14]

Geriatric Dosage. No dosage adjustments are necessary. Older patients are more likely to have renal impairment. (*See* Precautions.)

Other Conditions. Dosage reduction might be considered in severe renal and/or hepatic impairment (*See* Precautions.)

Dosage Forms. *See* Dosage Form and Site of Action.

Patient Instructions. (Oral) Take mesalamine with food and a full glass of water. Swallow tablets or capsules whole without crushing, breaking, or chewing. The tablet core (Asacol, Lialda) or small beads (Pentasa) might appear in the stool after mesalamine is released, but this does not mean there was a lack of effect. However, report intact or partly intact tablets or beads in the stool because this might indicate that the expected amount of mesalamine was not released. Report nausea, vomiting, abrupt change in character or volume of stools, or skin rashes to your doctor. (Rectal) empty bowel immediately before insertion of enema or suppository. Use enema at bedtime and retain for 8 h, if possible. Take foil off rectal suppository and insert pointed end first and retain for at least 3 h. Report signs of anal or rectal irritation. The rectal suspension can stain fabric, flooring, marble, granite, vinyl, and any painted surfaces that come into direct contact with them. The rectal suppository should be protected from light and heat.

Missed Doses. (Oral) If you miss a dose, take it as soon as possible. If it is almost time for your next dose, skip the missed dose and return to your usual dosage schedule. Do not double doses. (Rectal) if you miss a dose, use it as soon as possible if you remember it that same night. If you do not remember it until the next morning, skip the missed dose and return to your usual dosage schedule.

Pharmacokinetics. *Onset and Duration.* The onset of action of the various mesalamine agents (e.g., Asacol, Dipentum, Lialda, Apriso, and Pentasa) is delayed because of the release characteristics of their dosage forms; duration of action depends on intestinal transit time.[12] The onset of symptom relief is sooner with balsalazide than with delayed-release mesalamine.

Fate. About 70 ± 10% of oral mesalamine is absorbed in the proximal part of the gastrointestinal tract when administered as an uncoated product or unbound to a carrier molecule and is poorly absorbed from the colon. Various oral dosage forms have been formulated to deliver mesalamine topically to the more distal sites of inflammation. (*See* Dosage Form and Site of Action and Notes.) After oral administration, the control-released mesalamine microgranules (Pentasa) or delayed- and extended-release mesalamine (Apriso) is dispersed equally in the small as well as large bowel. About 20%–30% of released mesalamine is absorbed after oral administration of Asacol or Pentasa. About 98% of an oral olsalazine dose reaches the large bowel; less than 2% is absorbed.[12] The mean fecal excretion of Colazal, Dipentum, Asacol and Pentasa is estimated to be 46%, 14%–50%, 40%–64%, and 12%–51%, respectively.[12] Mesalamine absorption from the enema formulation is pH dependent; neutral solutions are better absorbed than acidic solutions. Rowasa (at pH 4.5) is less than 15% rectally absorbed. Plasma protein binding also is product specific: mesalamine (40%); *N*-acetylmesalamine (80%); balsalazide, olsalazine, and olsalazine-*O*-sulfate (>99%). Absorbed mesalamine is rapidly acetylated to *N*-acetyl-5-aminosalicylate (*N*-acetylmesalamine) in the intestinal mucosal wall and the liver. A small amount of olsalazine is metabolized to olsalazine-*O*-sulfate. *N*-acetylmesalamine is excreted in urine. Less than 1% of a dose of olsalazine is recovered unchanged in urine. The mean urinary excretion of mesalamine from balsalazide is approximately 12%–35%. **Half-life.** (PO mesalamine) 1 ± 0.5 h; (*N*-acetylmesalamine) 7.5 ± 1.5 h; (mesalamine suppository) 5 h; (olsalazine-*O*-sulfate) 7 days; (balsalazide) indeterminate.

Adverse Reactions. Adverse effects are usually less frequent than with oral sulfasalazine.[16,17] Headache, flatulence, abdominal pain, diarrhea, dizziness, anorexia, and dyspepsia are the most frequent side effects reported with oral formulations and, to a lesser extent, rectal formulations.[12,17,18] An acute intolerance syndrome (acute abdominal pain, bloody diarrhea, with or without fever, headache, and rash) associated with mesalamine occurs in approximately 3% of patients. About 15% of patients taking olsalazine experience secretory diarrhea.[14] Dermatologic reactions include rash (1%), acne, pruritus, urticaria, alopecia, and photosensitivity. Rare adverse effects include oral, esophageal, and duodenal ulcerations; hepatotoxicity; jaundice; cholestasis; cirrhosis; liver failure; pancytopenia; leukopenia; agranulocytosis; and anemia.[11,19] Pericarditis, fatal myocarditis, hypersensitivity pneumonitis, pancreatitis, nephrotic syndrome, and interstitial nephritis occur rarely.[11,14] Allergic cross-reactions can occur in sulfasalazine-allergic patients.

Contraindications. Pyloric stenosis; intestinal obstruction; salicylate hypersensitivity.

Precautions. Mesalamine is considered safe in pregnancy;[20] however, renal insufficiency has been reported in children. Monitor serum creatinine especially in those with preexisting renal impairments.[16,19] Use caution in patients with impaired hepatic function. Patients who experience rash or fever with sulfasalazine might have the same reaction to mesalamine or olsalazine; oral desensitization is an option for those who are allergic to mesalamine. Avoid Rowasa rectal suspension enemas in those with sulfite allergy.

Drug Interactions. In patients on warfarin, olsalazine can increase and mesalamine can decrease INR.[21] Mesalamine may increase 6-thioguanine nucleotide concentrations from the metabolism of azathioprine (AZA) and 6-mercaptopurine (6-MP). Leucopenia has been observed more frequently in patients on AZA and 6-MP while on mesalamine.[16]

Parameters to Monitor. Improvement in abdominal cramping, diarrhea, and rectal bleeding. Monitor for adverse effects, including diarrhea (olsalazine), acute intolerance syndrome, and hypersensitivity reaction. Monitor BUN, serum creatinine, and urinalysis before and periodically during therapy. Monitor INR in patients taking concurrent warfarin and WBC counts in patients also taking AZA or 6-MP.

Notes. The release characteristics of Pentasa are primarily time dependent, whereas those of Asacol are pH dependent; consequently, Asacol may not provide reliable site-specific release of 5-ASA, if the intestinal pH is inadequate. Balsalazide appears to more consistently distribute and liberate mesalamine in the colonic area, thus having greater effectiveness and less frequent side effects than sulfasalazine or olsalazine.[22] MMX mesalamine (Lialda), delayed-and extended-release mesalamine (Apriso) may be just as effective as other oral formulations of mesalamine without the excessive pill burden and therefore may increase medication compliance.[23] In 2%–3% of patients taking Asacol, intact or partly intact tablets were found in the stools.

There appears to be no clinically important advantage of one oral mesalamine product over another, or over **sulfasalazine**, in treating or maintaining remission of mild to moderate ulcerative colitis.[11–14,17] A mesalamine preparation might be beneficial in the sulfasalazine-sensitive patient and in men who wish to have children, because mesalamine does not alter sperm count, morphology, or motility.[17] The enema formulation of mesalamine is as effective as oral sulfasalazine or **hydrocortisone** enema in patients with active mild to moderate left sided ulcerative colitis and proctitis but is associated with a more rapid response and fewer and milder adverse effects.[12]

In patients with disease involving the ileum or proximal large bowel, oral formulations delivering mesalamine to the small bowel and colon are preferable to sulfasalazine, balsalazide, or olsalazine. Oral mesalamine preparations seem to be effective in treating active mild to moderate Crohn's disease (including ileal or ileal colonic) and maintaining remission.[17]

NATALIZUMAB   Tysabri

Pharmacology. Natalizumab is a recombinant humanized murine IgG4α monoclonal antibody that inhibits adhesion of leukocytes in the gut by binding α_4 integrins. In Crohn's disease, chronic inflammation has been associated with the interaction of integrins with the endothelial receptor mucosal addressin cell adhesion molecule-1 (MAdCAM-1), which is mainly expressed on gut endothelial cells.[24,25] The exact mechanism of action is still to be determined, however, it is theorized that the clinical effect of natalizumab in Crohn's disease may be attributed to the blockade of the molecular interaction of the integrin receptor with MAdCAM-1.

Administration and Adult Dosage. Intravenous infusion for the induction and maintenance of moderate-to-severe Crohn's disease who failed conventional

therapies and TNF-α inhibitors and are not on corticosteroids—300 mg over 1 h every 4 weeks for 12 weeks, then reevaluate for clinical response. (*See* Notes.) If on corticosteroids, 300 mg over 1 h every 4 weeks and taper off all corticosteroids. If corticosteroids cannot be completely discontinued by 6 months, natalizumab should be discontinued.

Special Populations. *Pediatric Dosage.* ($<$12 years) Safety and efficacy not established. Natalizumab 3 mg/kg by intravenous infusion at times 0, 4, and 8 weeks has been evaluated in adolescent individuals aged 12–17 years for active Crohn's disease.[26]

Geriatric Dosage. Same as adult dosage.

Other Conditions. Pregnancy category C. Risk versus benefit must be weighed when choosing to treat pregnant individuals with natalizumab. Animal studies using guinea pigs resulted in a reduced pup survival and hematological abnormalities were noted in monkey fetuses. There are no well-controlled studies in pregnant women using natalizumab.

Dosage Forms. **IV infusion** 300 mg/15 mL.

Patient Instructions. Natalizumab is a medication that needs to be administered in the doctor's office. Tell the doctor prior to starting natalizumab if you have any history of infections, are currently experiencing flu or cold symptoms, or currently receiving medications for an infection. The drug may cause progressive multifocal leukoencephalopathy (PML), a brain infection that may develop in individuals with a weak immune system. In most cases, PML is untreatable thereby causing severe disability that may lead to death.

Pharmacokinetics. *Fate.* Steady-state levels are attained in approximately 16–24 weeks after dosing every 4 weeks. V_d of natalizumab is 5.2 ± 2.8 L; Clearance is 22 ± 22 mL/hr. **Half-life.** 10 ± 7 days following repeated intravenous doses of 300 mg. The pharmacokinetic profiles of natalizumab in patients with renal or hepatic insufficiency have not been evaluated.

Adverse Reactions. Common adverse effects include flulike symptoms, infusion reactions, headache, fatigue, nausea, upper respiratory tract infections, and worsening of Crohn's disease.[27] Natalizumab carries a black box warning to emphasize the increased risk of PML, a fatal and untreatable brain infection associated with inflammation of the white matter, which occurs exclusively in immunocompromised patients.[28] Three cases of PML have occurred in patients on natalizumab, including one with Crohn's disease. Other serious adverse reactions include hypersensitivity, immunosuppression, and hepatotoxicity. Hepatotoxicity, marked by elevated serum hepatic enzymes and total bilirubin, occurs as early as 6 days after the initiation of natalizumab.[29] Formation of anti-natalizumab antibodies may occur and predispose patients to hypersensitivity reactions and decreased therapeutic effect.[25]

Contraindications. History of or existing PML or hypersensitivity to natalizumab.

Drug Interactions. Agents known to suppress the immune system should be avoided, as there is a potential increased risk of PML and other infections. Immunosuppressants (e.g., 6-MP, AZA, CSA (cyclosporine), MTX), TNFα inhibitors, chemotherapy, and corticosteroids should not be administered with natalizumab. (*See* Notes.)

Parameters to Monitor. Prior to initiating natalizumab, rule out all infections and PML. Monitor for signs and symptoms of infusion-related and hypersensitivity reactions. Obtain CBC and liver function tests to monitor for infections and hepatotoxicity, respectively. (*See* Notes.) In a Crohn's disease patient diagnosed with PML, JC virus DNA appeared in the serum 3 months after the start of natalizumab and 2 months before the presence of PML symptoms. (*See* Adverse Reactions.)[29]

Notes. Do not administer natalizumab as an intravenous push or bolus injection. After the infusion is complete, flush with 0.9% Sodium Chloride Injection, USP. Patients, prescribers, infusion centers, and pharmacies must be registered under the Tysabri Outreach: Unified Commitment to Health (TOUCH) Prescribing Program in order to administer natalizumab. (*See* Parameters to Monitor.) Natalizumab should be discontinued if no significant clinical response is seen after 12 weeks. It has been suggested that a washout period of at least 3 months is necessary prior to initiating natalizumab in patients previously treated with immunosuppressants, such as azathioprine and methotrexate, due to an increased risk of infectious diseases.[30] A study evaluating natalizumab with infliximab compared to infliximab alone found no difference in the rate of adverse events, including infections.[31] In addition, the only Crohn's disease patient diagnosed with PML had been off azathioprine for 8 months and off infliximab for 20 months prior to initiating natalizumab. Hence, implementation of a washout phase prior to initiation of natalizumab is still controversial.

Natalizumab was approved in November 2004 for the treatment of patients with relapsing forms of multiple sclerosis (MS). In February 2005, natalizumab was withdrawn from the market after three patients developed PML. It was not until March 2006 that natalizumab was reintroduced into the market under a strict monitoring protocol, TOUCH Prescribing Program, to help ensure the safe use of the drug. In January 2008, natalizumab was FDA approved for Crohn's disease. Similar to MS patients, Crohn's disease patients and caregivers must be part of the TOUCH program before natalizumab may be considered for the treatment. Considering there are several other treatment options for Crohn's disease that are associated with less risks, natalizumab should be reserved for patients who failed conventional immunomodulators and monoclonal antibody agents.

SULFASALAZINE   Azulfidine, Various

Pharmacology. Sulfasalazine is a conjugate of sulfapyridine linked to mesalamine by an azo bond. This bond is cleaved by colonic bacteria to sulfapyridine and mesalamine, the active moiety. (*See* Mesalamine.)

Administration and Adult Dosage. **PO for short-term treatment of active mild to moderate ulcerative colitis or Crohn's disease**—2–6 g/d and 3–6 g/d, respectively in equally divided doses; do not exceed an interval of 8 h between night and morning doses; administer with or after meals when feasible.[13] **PO for maintenance of remission of ulcerative colitis**—2–4 g/d in divided doses.[13] Dosages >4 g/d are associated with an increased frequency of adverse effects. Efficacy of sulfasalazine for Crohn's disease depends on the site of disease activity.[12] (*See* Notes.) **PO for desensitization of allergic patients**—Reinstitute sulfasalazine at a total daily dosage of 50–250 mg; thereafter, double the daily dosage every 4–7 days until the desired therapeutic effect is achieved. If symptoms of sensitivity recur, discontinue sulfasalazine. Do not attempt desensitization in patients who have histories of agranulocytosis or anaphylactic reactions during previous sulfasalazine therapy. Consider **mesalamine** instead of desensitization in sulfasalazine-sensitive patients.

Special Populations. *Pediatric Dosage.* (>6 years) **PO for short-term treatment of active mild to moderate ulcerative colitis**—40–60 mg/kg/d in 3–6 equally divided doses. Consider starting lower dose at 25 mg/kg/d in divided doses to minimize adverse effects.[14] Dosages up to 70 mg/kg/d in divided doses have been used.[14] **PO for maintenance of remission of ulcerative colitis**—30 mg/kg/d in 4 equally divided doses.

Geriatric Dosage. No dosage reduction is necessary. However, older patients may have renal impairment necessitating dosage adjustment.

Other Conditions. Pregnancy category B. Consider dosage reduction in severe renal or hepatic impairment. Reductions in dose may need to be considered in patients who are slow acetylators/metabolizers to minimize adverse effects. Sulfasalazine appears to be safe in animal studies and does not appear to affect female fertility or harm the fetus in rats and rabbits. No well-controlled trials have been conducted in pregnant women.

Dosage Forms. **Tab** 500 mg; **EC Tab** 500 mg.

Patient Instructions. Take each dose after meals or with food and drink at least 1 full glass of water with each dose; drink several additional glasses of water daily. This medication must be taken continually to be effective. It is often necessary to continue medication even when symptoms such as diarrhea and abdominal cramping have been controlled. Report any nausea, vomiting, abrupt change in character or volume of stools, or skin rashes to your doctor. Sulfasalazine can cause orange-yellow discoloration of the urine or skin. Reversible infertility can occur in males. Contact your health care provider if whole tablets appear in the stool.

Missed Doses. If you miss a dose, take it as soon as possible. If it is almost time for your next dose, skip the missed dose and return to your usual dosage schedule. Do not double doses.

Pharmacokinetics. *Onset of action:* Maximum effect is in 2–4 weeks.

Fate. Sulfasalazine is about 10%–15% absorbed from the small intestine. It is then metabolized in the large bowel by intestinal bacteria to sulfapyridine and mesalamine. Sulfapyridine is highly absorbed in the large intestines and metabolized by glucuronidation, hydroxylation, and polymorphic acetylation. An individual's acetylator status determines how fast sulfapyridine is eliminated; fast acetylators 6 h (150 mL/min), slow acetylators 15 h (40 mL/min).[12] Peak plasma level occurs approximately 10 h after initiating sulfasalazine. Acetylsulfapyridine is the principal metabolite of sulfapyridine. Acetylsulfapyridine is approximately 90% bound to plasma proteins, and sulfapyridine is ~70% bound to albumin. Both sulfapyridine and mesalamine are primarily eliminated in the urine. Renal clearance accounts for ~37% of the total clearance. Total mesalamine mean urinary excretion ranges between 10% and 35%.[12]

Adverse Reactions. Anorexia, nausea, vomiting, dyspepsia, and headache occur in about one-third of patients and are related to serum sulfapyridine concentrations.[11,12,14] These side effects usually resolve with dosage reduction or by initiating therapy at lower doses and titrating upward. Mild allergic reactions such as rash, pruritus, and fever are common. Decreased folate absorption leading to anemia can occur, so folic acid supplementation is recommended.[12] Rare toxic hypersensitivity reactions caused by sulfapyridine may occur and present as neutropenia, agranulocytosis, hepatitis, pancreatitis, pericarditis, pneumonitis, peripheral neuropathy, and severe hemolytic anemia.[11] Sulfasalazine can cause orange-yellow discoloration of the urine or skin and precipitate acute attacks of porphyria. In men, sulfasalazine frequently leads to a reversible decrease in sperm count and abnormal sperm morphology and motility; women's fertility is unaffected.[11,12]

Contraindications. Intestinal or urinary obstruction; porphyria; infants <2 years of age; hypersensitivity to sulfasalazine, its metabolites, sulfonamides, or salicylates.

Precautions. Pregnancy (despite reports of safety); lactation. Use with caution in patients with renal or hepatic impairment, blood dyscrasias, slow acetylators, bronchial asthma, G-6-PD deficiency, or severe allergies. Men who wish to father a child may have difficulty because sulfasalazine has been associated with infertility and oligospermia; this is reversible upon discontinuing treatment.

Drug Interactions. Decreased digoxin bioavailability has been reported when sulfasalazine is concurrently administered. Folic acid absorption is decreased with sulfasalazine administration. CSA levels may increase when initiating sulfasalazine; monitor CSA levels when initiating and discontinuing either medication.[32]

Parameters to Monitor. Monitor therapeutic response (e.g., decrease in degree and frequency of diarrhea, rectal bleeding, abdominal cramping) and adverse effects (e.g., headache, anorexia, dyspepsia, nausea, hypersensitivity reactions). Obtain baseline CBC with differential and liver function tests every second week for the first 3 months of therapy then monthly for 3 months and then every 3 months after that. Monitor renal function and serum folate levels periodically.[12,14] Monitor serum digoxin levels during initiation and after discontinuation of sulfasalazine.

Notes. Sulfasalazine has no therapeutic advantage over oral **mesalamine** when used to treat or maintain remission of ulcerative colitis; however, the higher sulfasalazine dosages used to treat active disease are associated with an increased frequency of adverse effects.[12,14] A lower initial dosage can decrease adverse gastrointestinal adverse effects. Crohn's disease patients with involvement of the ileum do not respond as well to sulfasalazine as those with only large bowel disease.[14] Combining sulfasalazine with an oral or rectal **corticosteroid** or with rectal mesalamine might be beneficial in patients with ulcerative colitis who do not respond to single-drug therapy. Sulfasalazine is also indicated for rheumatoid arthritis and polyarticular-course juvenile rheumatoid arthritis. EC tablet can appear whole in the stool; if this occurs, consider switching the patient to the uncoated form of sulfasalazine or to another mesalamine formulation. (*See* Mesalamine.)

MESALAMINE DOSAGE

BRAND NAME	ASACOL	APRISO	COLAZAL	DIPENTUM	LIALDA	PENTASA	CANASA, ROWASA
Generic Name	*Mesalamine*	*Mesalamine*	*Balsalazide*	*Olsalazine*	*Mesalamine*	*Mesalamine*	*Mesalamine*
INDICATION							
Short-term treatment of active mild to moderate ulcerative colitis	PO 800 mg tid OR 1.6 g tid[a] for 6 wk	a	PO 2.25 g tid for 8–12 wk	PO 500 mg tid,[a] 1 g bid,[a] OR 1 g tid[a] for 3–6 wk	2.4–4.8 g daily for 8 wk	PO 1 g qid for 8 wk	PR 2 g hs[a,b] OR 4 g hs[b] for 3–6 wk (enema)
Maintenance of ulcerative colitis remission	PO 800 mg bid	PO 1.5 g daily	PO 4 g daily	PO 500–1000 mg bid[c]	a	PO 1 g bid[a] OR 1 g qid[a]	PR 1–2 g hs[a,b] (enema)
Treatment or maintenance of Crohn's disease	PO 800 mg OR 1.6 g tid[a]	a	PO 2.25 g tid[a]	a	a	PO 1 g qid[a] for 8–16 wk	a
Maintenance of Crohn's disease remission	PO 800 mg–1.6 g tid[a]	a	a	a	a	PO 1 g bid[a] OR 1 g qid[a]	a
Treatment of active mild to moderate distal ulcerative colitis, proctosigmoiditis or proctitis	PO 800 mg tid[a]	a	a	a	a	PO 1 g qid[a]	PR 12 g hs[a,b] OR 4 g hs[b] (enema); 500 mg bid to tid[d]
Treatment of active proctitis	a	a	a	a	a	a	PR 1000 mg (suppository)

[a]Nonlabeled indication and dosage; optimal dosage regimen has not been determined.
[b]Retain enema for approximately 8 h.
[c]Patients intolerant to sulfasalazine.
[d]Retain suppository for 1–3 h or longer.
From Refs. 13, 14 and 18, and product information.

DOSAGE FORM AND SITE OF ACTION

DRUG	ASACOL	APRISO	COLAZAL	DIPENTUM	LIALDA	PENTASA	CANASA, ROWASA
	Mesalamine	*Mesalamine*	*Balsalazide*	*Olsalazine*	*Mesalamine*	*Mesalamine*	*Mesalamine*
Formulation	Tablet enteric coated pH dependent (pH 7), delayed release	Dual release capsule releasing mesalamine; delayed release and polymer matrix core	Capsule containing mesalamine prodrug cleaved by colonic bacterial azoreductases	Capsule containing 5-ASA[a] dimer; diazo bond is degraded by bacteria in colon[b]	Tablet containing mesalamine, gastroresistant polymer; outer layer dissolves at a pH of 7	Capsule containing ethylcellulose coated microgranules; controlled release	Rectal suspension, suppository
Site of action	Distal ileum to colon	Small bowel to colon	Colon	Colon	Terminal ileum and colon	Duodenum to colon	Rectum or splenic flexure (enema); rectum (suppository)
Dosage forms	Tab 400 mg	Cap 375 mg	Cap 750 mg	Cap 250 mg	Tab 1.2 g	Cap 250 mg Cap 500 mg	Enema 4 g/60 mL (Rowasa) Suppository 1000 mg (Canasa)

[a]5-ASA, 5-aminosalicylic acid.
[b]Each molecule of olsalazine that reaches the colon is converted to 2 molecules of mesalamine.

■ REFERENCES

1. Nesbitt A et al. Mechanism of action of certolizumab pegol (CDP870): in vitro comparison with other anti-tumor necrosis factor alpha agents. *Inflamm Bowel Dis.* 2007;13:1323-1332.
2. Blick SK, Curran MP. Certolizumab Pegol in Crohn's disease. *BioDrugs.* 2007;21:195-201.
3. Schreiber S et al. Maintenance therapy with certolizumab pegol for Crohn's disease. *N Engl J Med.* 2007;357: 239-250.
4. Sandborn WJ et al. Certolizumab pegol for the treatment of Crohn's disease. *N Engl J Med.* 2007;357:228-238.
5. Melmed GY et al. Certolizumab pegol. *Nat Rev Drug Discov.* 2008;7:641-642.
6. Lichtenstein GR et al. American Gastroenterological Association Institute technical review on corticosteroids, immunomodulators, and infliximab in inflammatory bowel disease. *Gastroenterology.* 2006;130:940-987.
7. Travis SP et al. European evidence based consensus on the diagnosis and management of Crohn's disease: Current management. *Gut.* 2006;55(suppl 1):i16-i35.
8. Kuhbacher T, Folsch UR. Practical guidelines for the treatment of inflammatory bowel disease. *World J Gastroenterol.* 2007;13:1149-1155.
9. Ouyang Q et al. Management consensus of inflammatory bowel disease for the Asia-Pacific region. *J Gastroenterol Hepatol.* 2006;21:1772-1782.
10. Löwenberg M, Peppelenbosch M, Hommes D. Biological therapy in the management of recent-onset Crohn's disease: why, when and how? *Drugs.* 2006;66:1431-1439.
11. Nielsen OH, Munck LK. Drug insight: aminosalicylates for the treatment of IBD. *Nat Clin Pract Gastroenterol Hepatol.* 2007;4:160-170.
12. Qureshi AI, Cohen RD. Mesalamine delivery systems: do they really make much difference? *Adv Drug Deliv Rev.* 2005;57:281-302.
13. Baumgart DC, Sandborn WJ. Inflammatory bowel disease: clinical aspects and established and evolving therapies. *Lancet.* 2007;369:1641-1657.
14. Rufo PA, Bousvaros A. Current therapy of inflammatory bowel disease in children. *Paediatr Drugs.* 2006;8:279-302.
15. Carvalho R, Hyams JS. Diagnosis and management of inflammatory bowel disease in children. *Semin Pediatr Surg.* 2007;16:164-171.
16. Cunliffe RN, Scott BB. Review article: monitoring for drug side effects in inflammatory bowel disease. *Aliment Pharmacol Ther.* 2002;16:647-662.
17. Tamboli CP. Current medical therapy for chronic inflammatory bowel diseases. *Surg Clin North Am.* 2007;87: 697-725.
18. Chan J. The pharmacologic management of Crohn's disease. *Formulary.* 2008;43:93-104.
19. Juillerat P et al. Drug safety in Crohn's disease therapy. *Digestion.* 2007;76:161-168.
20. Mottet C et al. Pregnancy and breastfeeding in patients with Crohn's disease. *Digestion.* 2007;76:149-160.
21. Marinella MA. Mesalamine and warfarin therapy resulting in decreased warfarin effect. *Ann Pharmacother.* 1998;32:841-842.
22. Prakash A, Spencer CM. Balsalazide. *Drugs.* 1998;56:83-89.
23. Lakatos PL, Lakatos L. Once daily 5-aminosalicylic acid for the treatment of ulcerative colitis; are we there yet? *Pharmacol Res.* 2008;58:190-195.
24. Lanzarotto F et al. Novel treatment options for inflammatory bowel disease. Targeting α4 Integrin. *Drugs.* 2006;66:1179-1189.
25. Sweet BV. Natalizumab update. *Am J Health Syst Pharm.* 2007;64:705-716.
26. Hyams J et al. Natalizumab Therapy for Moderate to Severe Crohn Disease in Adolescents. *J Pediatr Gastroenterol Nutr.* 2007;44:185-191.
27. Sandborn WJ et al. Natalizumab Induction and Maintenance Therapy for Crohn's Disease. *N Engl J Med.* 2005;353:1912-1925.
28. Van Assche G et al. Progressive Multifocal Leukoencephalopathy after Natalizumab Therapy for Crohn's Disease. *N Engl J Med.* 2005;353:362-368.
29. Tysabri (natalizumab) - Reports of Clinically Significant Liver Injury. FDA Medwatch. http://www.fda.gov/medwatch/safety/2008/safety08.htm#Tysabri. Accessed March 7, 2009.
30. Ilanjian H, Shane R. Washout period for immune-modifying drugs before natalizumab therapy. *Am J Health Syst Pharm.* 2008;65:18-19.
31. Sands BE et al. Safety and tolerability of concurrent natalizumab treatment for patients with Crohn's disease not in remission while receiving infliximab. *Inflamm Bowel Dis.* 2007;13:2-11.
32. Du Cheyron D et al. Effect of sulfasalazine on cyclosporin blood concentration. *Eur J Clin Pharmacol.* 1999;55:227-228.

Hematologic Drugs 7

Nickole N. Henyan

Chapter 47

Coagulants and Anticoagulants

Krista D. Riche and Paula Horn

ABCIXIMAB ReoPro

Pharmacology. Abciximab is a chimeric human-murine monoclonal antibody Fab fragment that binds to and irreversibly inhibits the platelet glycoprotein IIb/IIIa receptor. Blockade of the glycoprotein IIb/IIIa receptor prevents fibrinogen from binding, thereby inhibiting platelet aggregation. Abciximab also binds to the vitronectin receptor found on platelets, endothelial cells, monocytes, and smooth muscle cells; the clinical relevance of this is unknown. Abciximab inhibits platelet aggregation and prolongs bleeding time in a dose-dependent manner.[1,2]

Administration and Adult Dosage. IV for percutaneous coronary intervention (PCI)—0.25 mg/kg as a bolus 10–60 min before starting PCI and then 0.125 μg/kg/min (up to 10 μg/min) by continuous infusion for 12 h; **IV for unstable angina and planned PCI within 24 h**—0.25 mg/kg as a bolus and then 0.125 μg/kg/min (up to 10 μg/min) by continuous infusion for 18–24 h, concluding 1 h after the PCI. (*See* Parameters to Monitor and Notes.)

Special Populations. *Pediatric Dosage.* Safety and efficacy not established.

Geriatric Dosage. Same as adult dosage.

Dosage Forms. Inj 10 mg/5 mL.

Pharmacokinetics. *Onset and Duration.* Rapid inhibition of platelet function after IV administration. Platelet function gradually recovers after discontinuation of the IV infusion; bleeding time approaches baseline values within 24 h and ex vivo platelet aggregation approaches baseline levels within 48 h. Low levels of glycoprotein IIb/IIIa inhibition are detectable for up to 15 days after administration.[1]

Fate. Abciximab is rapidly cleared from the plasma after administration by rapid binding to the glycoprotein IIb/IIIa receptor.

Half-life. α phase <10 min; β phase 30 min.[1]

Adverse Reactions. Bleeding, particularly from vascular access sites, occurs frequently. To minimize bleeding complications, care of the femoral artery access site is important and lower doses of unfractionated heparin are necessary during PCI. (*See* Notes.) If serious bleeding complications occur, discontinue abciximab and transfuse platelets, if needed, to restore platelet function. Thrombocytopenia ($<100,000/\mu L$) has been reported in 2.6%–5.6% of patients; severe thrombocytopenia ($<50,000/\mu L$) has occurred in 0.9%–1.7% of patients. Thrombocytopenia can occur rapidly after administration and might require platelet transfusions if reversal is necessary.[1]

Contraindications. Hypersensitivity to any component of abciximab or murine proteins; active internal bleeding; recent (within 6 weeks) clinically significant gastrointestinal (GI) or genitourinary (GU) bleeding; history of cerebrovascular accident (CVA) within 2 years or CVA with significant residual neurologic deficit; bleeding diathesis; administration of oral anticoagulants within 7 days unless PT ≤ 1.2 times control; thrombocytopenia ($<100,000/\mu L$); recent (within 6 weeks) major surgery or trauma; intracranial neoplasm, AV malformation, or aneurysm; severe uncontrolled hypertension; presumed or documented history of vasculitis; use or planned use of IV dextran before or during PCI.

Precautions. Use with caution in patients being treated concomitantly with other antithrombotic drugs including thrombolytics, unfractionated heparin, low-molecular-weight heparin, oral anticoagulants; NSAIDs; and other drugs that increase bleeding risk.

Parameters to Monitor. Monitor CBC including platelet count; prothrombin time; aPTT; and activated clotting time at baseline. Maintaining the activated clotting time at 200–300 s during PCI minimizes the risk of bleeding complications.[1,3] Monitor platelet count 2–4 h after the IV bolus and again at 24 h OR before hospital discharge, whichever occurs first. If prolonged infusion of unfractionated heparin is necessary after PCI, maintain aPTT at 60–85 s.

Notes. Abciximab must be filtered using a sterile, nonpyrogenic, low protein-binding 0.2 or 0.22 μ filter either at admixture or during administration with an in-line filter. Abciximab should not be administered to patients in whom PCI is not planned. If a significant delay in PCI is likely, consider utilizing eptifibatide or tirofiban as the IIb/IIIa inhibitor. To minimize the risk of bleeding complications, the following care for the arterial access site is recommended: maintain patient on complete bed rest with the affected limb restrained in a straight position while vascular sheaths are in place; discontinue unfractionated heparin immediately after PCI; remove vascular sheaths within 6 h of completing the procedure if aPTT ≤ 50 s or activated clotting time ≤ 175 s; after sheath removal, apply pressure to the femoral artery for at least 30 min with manual compression or a mechanical device; and maintain bed rest for 6–8 h after sheath removal. To minimize bleeding complications, the following periprocedural heparin dosage is recommended: if baseline activated clotting time ≤ 150 s, administer 70 units/kg heparin IV bolus; if 150–199 s, administer 50 units/kg heparin IV bolus; if ≥ 200 s, do not administer heparin. During PCI, administer 20 units/kg heparin IV boluses as necessary to maintain activated clotting time at 200–300 s.[1,3]

ALTEPLASE
Activase, Cathflo

Pharmacology. Alteplase (recombinant tissue-type plasminogen activator [rt-PA]) is a 1-chain tissue plasminogen activator (fibrinolytic) produced by recombinant DNA technology. It has a high affinity for fibrin-bound plasminogen, allowing activation on the fibrin surface. Most of the plasmin formed remains bound to the fibrin clot, minimizing systemic effects.[4-6]

Administration and Adult Dosage. **Accelerated IV infusion for clot lysis after ST segment elevation myocardial infarction (STEMI) within 12 h of symptom onset**—(preferred) 15 mg as a bolus, followed by 0.75 mg/kg (up to 50 mg) over 30 min, and then 0.5 mg/kg (up to 35 mg) over the next 60 min. Start heparin infusion (titrated to an aPTT of 1.5–2.0 times control) with or at completion of the alteplase infusion and continue for at least 48 h; (*See* Notes.) **Alternatively, IV infusion for clot lysis after myocardial infarction (MI)**—60 mg over 1 h (6–10 mg in the first 1 2 min) and then 20 mg/h for 2 h to a total of 100 mg (for patients <65 kg, administer a dose of 1.25 mg/kg over 3 h). Begin as soon as possible after acute MI symptoms. Adjunctive heparin is also recommended.[5,7-9] **IV infusion for pulmonary embolism (PE)**—100 mg over 2 h. Initiate heparin infusion immediately after alteplase infusion when the aPTT or thrombin time returns to 2 times normal. Alternatively, 0.6 mg/kg as a single dose over 2 min in addition to heparin infusion has been used successfully;[10] **IV infusion for acute ischemic stroke within 90 min of symptom onset**—0.9 mg/kg, to a maximum of 90 mg; give 10% initially as a bolus, with the remainder given over the next 60 min. Avoid anticoagulants or antiplatelet drugs for 24 h after treatment.[11,12] **IV for catheter clearance**—Slowly inject 0.5 mg (1 mL) into the occluded catheter port. If catheter volume exceeds 1 mL, slowly inject a sufficient volume of NS to fill the catheter. Allow the solution to dwell for 60 min and then aspirate and flush the catheter with NS. If unsuccessful, repeat with escalating doses of alteplase (e.g., 1 mg, 2 mg) to a maximum of 2 mg.[13]

Special Populations. *Pediatric Dosage.* Safety and efficacy not established.

Geriatric Dosage. Same as adult dosage.

Dosage Forms. Inj 50, 100 mg.

Pharmacokinetics. *Onset and Duration.* Duration is several hours because of binding with fibrin. However, rethrombosis after reperfusion appears to be inversely proportional to serum half-life.[5]

Fate. There is rapid uptake by hepatocytes and fibrin binding. V_c is 3.8–6.6 L and $V_{d\beta}$ is 0.1 ± 0.01 L/kg; Clearance is 0.6 ± 0.24 L/h/kg.[5,14] **Half-life.** α phase 4.8 ± 2.4 min; β phase 26 ± 10 min.[14]

Adverse Reactions. Bleeding from GI and GU tracts and ecchymoses occur frequently. Retroperitoneal or gingival bleeding or epistaxis occurs occasionally. Superficial bleeding from trauma sites also can occur. The overall risk of intracranial hemorrhage is 0.1%–0.75%.[11] In ISIS-3, the rates for definite or possible cerebral bleed were: rt-PA (**duteplase**, a 2-chain form of alteplase), 0.5%; **streptokinase**, 0.2%; **anistreplase**, 0.7%.[15] Independent risk factors for thrombolytic-induced intracranial hemorrhage with alteplase are age >65 years, body weight <70 kg, and hypertension on hospitalization.[7] Cholesterol embolization, orolingual angioedema and reperfusion arrhythmias have also been reported. Extravasation may cause ecchymosis and/or inflammation.

Contraindications. (All patients) Active internal bleeding; history of CVA; recent (within 3 months) intracranial or intraspinal surgery or trauma; intracranial neoplasm, AV malformation, or aneurysm; bleeding diathesis (e.g., PO anticoagulation with INR >1.7 or PT >15 s, heparin within last 48 h with elevated aPTT, platelet count <100,000 mm^3); severe uncontrolled hypertension. (Stroke patients) recent head trauma (within 3 months); history of intracranial hemorrhage; seizure at onset of stroke; evidence or suspicion of intracranial hemorrhage in pretreatment evaluation; uncontrolled hypertension (systolic blood pressure [SBP] ≥180 mmHg, diastolic blood pressure [DBP] ≥110 mmHg).

Precautions. Use with caution in the following: pregnancy (category C); recent (within 10 days) major surgery, trauma, GI or GU bleeding; cerebrovascular disease; SBP ≥180 mmHg, DBP ≥110 mmHg; high likelihood of left heart thrombus; acute pericarditis; subacute bacterial endocarditis; hemostatic defects; significant liver dysfunction; septic thrombophlebitis; age >75 years; concurrent oral anticoagulants. Avoid IM injections and noncompressible arterial punctures; minimize arterial and venous punctures and excessive patient handling. Stop immediately if severe bleeding or anaphylactoid reaction occurs. Use cautiously in stroke patients with severe neurological deficits (NIHSS >22) or major early infarct signs on computerized cranial tomography because of increased bleeding incidence.

Drug Interactions. Preliminary data from a nonrandomized study suggest that concurrent IV nitroglycerin therapy impairs the thrombolytic effect of alteplase in acute MI.[16] Anticoagulants or antiplatelet drugs can increase the risk of bleeding.

Parameters to Monitor. For short-term thrombolytic therapy of MI, laboratory monitoring is of little value. No correlation has been made between clotting test results and likelihood of hemorrhage or efficacy.[5] Monitor for signs and symptoms of bleeding. Monitor the electrocardiogram (ECG) for reperfusion arrhythmias.

Notes. Other than cerebral hemorrhage, no clear differences in bleeding risk have been observed with the various thrombolytics.[5,7] Data from the ISIS-3 trial show the 5-week mortalities for **duteplase, streptokinase**, and **anistreplase** to be virtually identical.[15] Based on the GUSTO trial, some investigators have suggested that the accelerated alteplase regimen be used for patients <75 years with anterior or large infarctions presenting within 4 h of symptoms. The absolute survival advantage over streptokinase was 0.9%, representing a 14% risk reduction.[8,17] Double-bolus alteplase (50 mg IV over 1–3 min followed by 40–50 mg IV 30 min later) was compared with accelerated infusion alteplase to shorten and simplify administration. The double-bolus method was associated with a slightly higher rate of intracranial hemorrhage and is not recommended.[18] In a study on catheter clearance, 96.5% of catheters were cleared successfully, 86.2% with a dose of 0.5 mg, 8.6% with 1 mg, and 1.7% with 2 mg.[13] In STEMI patients, either PCI or thrombolysis is the primary therapy. In the case of thrombolytic failure, rescue PCI may be performed as clinically indicated. However, optimal anticoagulant and antiplatelet therapy has not been established under these circumstances.[5,9] Fibrinolytic therapy is NOT recommended for the treatment of non-ST segment elevation myocardial infarction (NSTEMI) because of the lack of demonstrated benefits in controlled clinical trials.[6–9]

ARGATROBAN

Pharmacology. Argatroban is a modified amino acid that is a reversible, competitive, direct thrombin inhibitor used as an anticoagulant in patients with heparin-induced thrombocytopenia.[19]

Administration and Adult Dosage. IV as a continuous infusion. Initial infusion rate is 2 μg/kg/min, titrating aPTT to 1.5–3 times control (maximum rate of 10 μg/kg/min). Initial infusion may need to be reduced to 0.5 μg/kg/min in renal or hepatic impairment or in the critically ill.[20]

Dosage Forms. **Inj** 100 mg/mL.

Pharmacokinetics. *Onset and Duration.* Onset <10 min after a bolus or 1–3 h after start of infusion without a bolus. **Half-life.** 18–41 min.[21] The half-life may be prolonged in hepatic impairment or the critically ill.

Fate. The drug is metabolized in the liver to three metabolites that are excreted renally.

Adverse Reactions. Bleeding is the most frequent complication but is usually minor. No specific reversal agent exists. Dose-related prolongation of PT occurs.[19] Other common side effects include dyspnea, hypotension, and fever. Repeat exposure does not appear to predispose to immunologic reactions or excessive anticoagulation.

Parameters to Monitor. Monitor aPTT 2 h after initiation of therapy or dosage adjustment and then once daily after stable anticoagulation has been achieved. Monitor the aPTT 3–4 h after initiation of therapy or dose adjustment in hepatic impairment or the critically ill due to prolonged half-life.[20]

Conversion to Oral Anticoagulation. Argatroban interferes with the prothrombin time test to artificially elevate the INR. Infusions at a rate up to 2 μg/kg/min may double the INR compared to that without argatroban influence. Warfarin should be started at typical starting doses. Once the INR is above 4 on combined therapy, argatroban infusion can be held, with repeat INR testing in 4 to 6 h. If the INR is not within the desired range, restart the argatroban infusion and repeat the process until the INR is within the desired range. The influence of argatroban on the INR at infusion rates above 2 μg/kg/min is less predictable. In this instance, temporarily decrease the infusion rate to 2 μg/kg/min and repeat the INR in 2 h. If the INR is above 4 on combined therapy, the process above can be continued. Alternatively, the effect of warfarin may be monitored using the chromogenic factor Xa test instead of the INR during argatroban therapy.

Notes. Argatroban has been used as an anticoagulant during extracorporeal circulation and percutaneous coronary intervention.[22]

BIVALIRUDIN   Angiomax

Pharmacology. Bivalirudin is a synthetic amino acid peptide that is a reversible direct thrombin inhibitor.

Administration and Adult Dosage. IV infusion for patients with unstable angina undergoing PCTA; for patients undergoing PCI with provisional use of a glycoprotein IIb/IIIa (GP IIb/IIIa) inhibitor; for patients with or at risk of HIT/HITTS undergoing PCI—Initial bolus dose of 0.75 mg/kg followed by an infusion of 1.75 mg/kg/h for the duration of PCI procedure. ACT should be monitored and an additional 0.3 mg/kg may be administered if needed. At the discretion of the treating physician, bivalirudin may be continued for up to 4 h after PCI and then decreased to a rate of 0.2 mg/kg/h for up to an additional 20 h. Avoid IM administration due to an increased risk of bleeding. Bivalirudin should be administered with aspirin (300–325 mg daily).

Special Populations. *Renal Impairment.* Cl_{Cr} *30–59 mL/min:* same as adult dosage. Monitor ACT and adjust if needed; Cl_{Cr} *<30 mL/min:* reduce infusion rate to 1 mg/kg/h; *Hemodialysis:* reduce infusion rate to 0.25 mg/kg/h. No reduction in bolus dose is needed in renal impairment

Pediatric Dosage. Safety and efficacy not established.

Geriatric Dosage. Same as adult dosage.

Dosage Forms. **Inj** 250 mg/vial for reconstitution.

Pharmacokinetics. *Onset and Duration.* Bivalirudin onset is immediate and effects persist for approximately 1 h after discontinuation of infusion.

Fate. Bivalirudin undergoes proteolytic cleavage in the plasma and is excreted renally.

$t_{1/2}$. 25 min.

Adverse Reactions. Adverse effects occur at different frequencies depending on whether bivalirudin is used alone or in combination with a GP IIb/IIIa inhibitor.[23] The most common adverse effect associated with bivalirudin use is back pain (>40% incidence in monotherapy and ~10% with GP IIb/IIIa inhibitor).[1] Other common adverse effects to be aware of include hypotension, nausea, headache, and pain. Major bleeding and other types of hemorrhage occur with bivalirudin use and may require transfusion. Other rare adverse effects include renal failure, nerve paralysis, and ventricular fibrillation.

Contraindications. Active major bleeding.

Precautions. Pregnancy category B; renal impairment; elderly; concurrent oral anticoagulants; or preexisting bleeding condition.

Drug Interactions. Use with caution in patients receiving thrombolytics, oral anticoagulants, or drugs that inhibit platelet function, including GP IIb/IIIa inhibitors.

Parameters to Monitor. ACT, blood pressure, hemoglobin/hematocrit, platelet count, signs and symptoms of bleeding.

Notes. Provisional GP IIb/IIIa inhibitor use should be considered if patients meet any of the criteria specified in the REPLACE-2 trial including: decreased TIMI flow (0–2) or slow reflow, dissection with decreased flow, new or suspected thrombus, persistent residual stenosis, distal embolization, enplaned stent, suboptimal stenting, side branch closure, abrupt closure, clinical instability, or prolonged ischemia.[23] Bivalirudin has also been studied in patients with ACS who are not undergoing PCI in the ACUITY trial.[24] Bivalirudin demonstrated noninferiority to bivalirudin plus GP IIb/IIIa inhibitors as well as to heparin plus GP IIb/IIIa inhibitors.[24] The FDA denied an application for an additional dosing regimen based on these findings in May 2008.[25]

CLOPIDOGREL BISULFATE   Plavix

Pharmacology. Clopidogrel is an antiplatelet agent that prevents platelet aggregation by direct inhibition of ADP binding to receptor sites, inhibiting subsequent activation of the glycoprotein IIb/IIIa complex. This action is irreversible; therefore, platelets exposed to clopidogrel are inhibited for their life spans.

Administration and Adult Dosage. **PO for recent stroke, recent MI, or established peripheral artery disease**—75 mg once daily; **PO for acute coronary syndrome (ACS)**—(NSTEMI) 300-mg loading dose followed by 75 mg daily; (STEMI) 75 mg daily with OR without a 300-mg loading dose.

Special Populations. *Pediatric Dosage.* Safety and efficacy not established.

Geriatric Dosage. Same as adult dosage.

Dosage Forms. **Tab** 75, 300 mg.

Pharmacokinetics. *Onset and Duration.* Clopidogrel is rapidly absorbed; bioavailability is ~50%; 98% is bound to plasma proteins. The parent compound has no platelet-inhibiting activity and undergoes extensive hepatic metabolism to a carboxylic acid derivative (main metabolite) and an unidentified active metabolite. Dose-dependent platelet inhibition is observable 2 h after PO administration. Platelet inhibition reaches steady state between day 3 and day 7. Platelet function normalizes 5 days after discontinuation of clopidogrel.

Fate. 50% Excretion of the drug is 50% renal, 46% in the feces. **Half-life.** (Carboxylic acid metabolite) ~8 h.

Adverse Reactions. The most frequent side effects are diarrhea in 4.5%, rash in 4.2%, GI hemorrhage in 2%, and GI ulcers in 0.7% of patients. Serious, but less frequent, side effects are intracranial hemorrhage in 0.4% and severe neutropenia in 0.04%. Clopidogrel has been associated with the development of thrombotic thrombocytopenic purpura.[26]

Contraindications. Hypersensitivity to drug or any component; active, pathological bleeding (e.g., peptic ulcer or intracranial hemorrhage).

Precautions. Use with caution in patients at increased risk of bleeding from trauma, surgery, or other conditions. Clopidogrel should be discontinued 5 days prior to surgery if an antiplatelet effect is not desired; Pregnancy category B.

Drug Interactions. Use with caution in patients receiving anticoagulants or drugs that inhibit platelet function including NSAIDs. Recent data suggest that clopidogrel's effects may be reduced by as much as 50% when administered with proton pump inhibitors (PPIs).[27] Platelet function was inhibited by omeprazole, but not the other PPIs in a single study. The Medco study combined prescription and medical claims data and found that pantoprazole and esomeprazole may have the largest impact in increased major adverse cardiovascular events (MACE).[28]

Parameters to Monitor. No specific monitoring is routinely recommended to assess antiplatelet effects. Monitor for signs and symptoms of bleeding.

Notes. The overall risk reduction for clopidogrel was 8.7% greater than that for **aspirin** in the CAPRIE study in patients at risk for ischemic events.[29] No additional benefit has been demonstrated when clopidogrel is added to aspirin therapy for patients with recurrent TIA or stroke. Combination antiplatelet therapy did result in a higher incidence of bleeding.[30]

DALTEPARIN

Pharmacology. Dalteparin is a low-molecular-weight heparin (average mass 3000–8000 daltons) prepared by depolymerization and chromatographic purification of unfractionated porcine intestinal mucosa heparin. Other pharmacologic properties are similar to those of enoxaparin.[31]

Administration and Adult Dosage. SQ for prevention of ischemic complications in unstable angina and non–Q-wave MI—120 International Units (IU)/kg (to a maximum of 10,000 IU) every 12 h with concurrent oral aspirin 81–160 mg once daily. Continue treatment until patient is clinically stable, usually 5–8 days; **SQ for prevention of deep vein thrombosis (DVT) and PE after abdominal surgery**—2500 IU 1–2 h before surgery and once daily for 5–10 days; **SQ for prevention of DVT and PE after abdominal surgery in high-risk patients (e.g., with malignancy)**—5000 IU the evening before surgery and then once daily postoperatively OR 2500 IU 1–2 h before surgery, 2500 IU 4–8 h postoperatively, and then 5000 IU once daily for 5–10 days; **SQ for prevention of DVT and PE after hip replacement surgery**—2500 IU 2 h before and 12 h after surgery, and then 5000 IU once daily for 6–13 days; or 5000 IU 10–14 h before surgery, 5000 IU 4–8 h postoperatively, and then 5000 IU once daily thereafter. For postoperative initiation, give 2500 IU 4–8 h postoperatively and then 5000 IU once daily. **Extended treatment of symptomatic DVT and PE in patients with cancer**—First month: 200 IU/kg SQ daily, not to exceed a daily dose of 18,000 IU[32] Month 2–6: approximately 150 IU/kg SQ daily, not to exceed a daily dose of 18,000 IU.

Special Populations. *Renal Insufficiency:* No specific dose reductions are recommended. Peak antifactor Xa levels may be used to monitor therapeutic dosing. *Obesity:* Doses above 18,000 IU are not recommended; however, data with other low-molecular-weight heparins suggest that dose capping causes increased risk of thromboembolism while weight-based dosing does not increase risk of bleeding.[33] *Pediatrics and Pregnancy:* Do not use the multiple dose vial to create dosing, and the preservative, benzyl alcohol, may cross the placenta and cause gasping syndrome in premature infants.

Dosage Forms. **Inj. Prefilled syringes:** 2,500 IU/0.2 mL, 5,000 IU/0.2 mL, 7,500 IU/0.3 mL, 10,000 IU/0.4 mL, 10,000 IU/1 mL, 12,500 IU/0.5 mL, 15,000 IU/0.6 mL, 18,000 IU/0.72 mL; **Multiple dose vial**: 95,000 IU/3.8 mL, 95,000 IU/9.5 mL

Pharmacokinetics. Bioavailability after SQ injection is about $87 \pm 6\%$. After SQ dose, V_d is 0.04–0.06 L/kg; after a single IV dose Clearance is 0.025 ± 0.0054 L/h/kg. **Half-life.** 2.1 ± 0.3 h; after SQ administration the apparent half-life is 3–5 h. Dalteparin is eliminated primarily by the kidney.

Adverse Reactions. Overall, rates of major and minor bleeding complications are similar to those with unfractionated **heparin**. Hematoma or pain at the injection site occurs frequently. Thrombocytopenia occurs in less than 1% of patients; however, dalteparin should be used with extreme caution in patients with a history of heparin-induced thrombocytopenia (in vitro platelet testing is recommended before use). Rash, fever, skin necrosis, and anaphylactoid reactions occur rarely.

Contraindications. (*See* Enoxaparin Sodium.) Patients undergoing regional anesthesia should not receive dalteparin for unstable angina or non–Q-wave MI. Patients with a current positive antiplatelet antibody in the presence of heparin or low-molecular-weight heparin should not receive dalteparin. Patients with sensitivity to pork products should not receive dalteparin.

Precautions. If epidural or spinal anesthesia or spinal puncture is used, patients receiving low-molecular-weight heparins for prevention of thromboembolic complications are at risk of developing epidural or spinal hematoma, which can result in permanent paralysis. The risk of these events can increase when postoperative indwelling epidural catheters are used. Use with caution in patients with renal impairment.

Drug Interactions. Use with caution in patients receiving thrombolytics, oral anticoagulants, or drugs that inhibit platelet function, including NSAIDs.

Parameters to Monitor. Monitor CBC, including platelet count, and stool for occult blood periodically; aPTT monitoring is not required. Antifactor Xa levels may be used to monitor the effects of dalteparin in renal insufficiency or extremes of weight. The Antifactor Xa level should be drawn 4–6 h after administration of the 4th and 5th dose. Peak therapeutic Antifactor Xa levels should be between 0.5 and 1.5 IU/mL[34].

Notes. Partial reversal of anticoagulant effects of dalteparin using protamine sulfate can occur. Initial dosing of protamine is 1 mg per 100 units of dalteparin. A maximum of 60%–75% reversal may be achieved.

ENOXAPARIN SODIUM
Lovenox

Pharmacology. Enoxaparin is a low-molecular-weight heparin (average mass 3500–5500 daltons) prepared by depolymerization of unfractionated porcine intestinal mucosa heparin. Like unfractionated heparin, enoxaparin binds with antithrombin III, accelerating the rate at which antithrombin III neutralizes several activated clotting factors. However, enoxaparin has many biologic properties that differ from those of unfractionated heparin. Enoxaparin has a higher ratio of antifactor Xa to antifactor IIa activity, reduced interactions with platelets, and less lipoprotein–lipase-releasing activity. It also has a lower affinity for platelet factor 4, von Willebrand factor (VIIIR), and vascular endothelium. At recommended dosages, single injections do not markedly affect platelet aggregation, prothrombin time, or aPTT.[35–38]

Administration and Adult Dosage. **SQ for prevention of DVT and PE after hip replacement surgery**—30 mg bid for 7–10 days started 12–24 h postoperatively or 40 mg once daily starting 12 h preoperatively; **SQ for prevention of DVT and PE after knee replacement surgery**—30 mg bid for 7–10 days started 12–24 h postoperatively; **SQ for prevention of DVT and PE after abdominal surgery**—40 mg once daily for 7–10 days started 2 h before surgery; **SQ for active DVT treatment with and without PE**—1 mg/kg every 12 h or 1.5 mg/kg daily initiated with warfarin therapy; continue for at least 5 days and until a warfarin target INR of 2.0 is achieved on 2 consecutive days; **SQ for unstable angina or non–Q-wave MI**—1 mg/kg every 12 h with concurrent aspirin 100–325 mg once daily. Continue treatment for at least 2 days or until patient is clinically stable, usually 2–8 days.

Special Populations. *Pediatric Dosage.* **SQ for treatment** (neonates) 1.6 mg/kg bid; (older infants and children) 1 mg/kg bid dosages have been used. These doses must be made from the preservative-free prefilled syringes. *Renal Impairment* (Cl_{Cr} <30 mL/min) **SQ for treatment**—1 mg/kg once daily. **SQ for prophylaxis**—30 mg once daily. *Morbid Obesity*—Dose capping is not recommended and twice-daily dosing is preferred [33] In patients undergoing bariatric surgery, increasing prophylactic dose 40 mg SQ every 12 h should be considered. *Geriatric Dosage.* Elderly patients might have reduced elimination; use with caution in these patients.

Dosage Forms. Inj. *Prefilled Syringes*—30 mg/0.3 mL; 40 mg/0.4 mL; 60 mg/0.6 mL; 80 mg/0.8 mL; 100 mg/mL; 120 mg/0.8 mL; 150 mg/mL. *Multiple Dose Vial*—300 mg/3 mL.

Pharmacokinetics. *Onset and Duration.* Peak antifactor Xa occurs 3–5 h after SQ injection and persists for about 12 h after a 40 mg SQ injection.

Fate. Mean absolute bioavailability after SQ injection is ~92%. V_d is about 6 L and Clearance is about 1.5 L/h after IV administration. Some hepatic desulfation and depolymerization occur, but most of the drug is eliminated renally. **Half-life.** 4.5 h.

Adverse Reactions. Overall, rates of major and minor bleeding complications in comparative studies with unfractionated heparin are similar. In clinical trials of enoxaparin in hip replacement surgery, major bleeding occurred in 4% of patients compared with 6% of patients treated with unfractionated heparin. Thrombocytopenia, fever, pain on injection, asymptomatic increases in transaminase levels, hypochromic anemia, and edema occur frequently. Skin necrosis occurs occasionally.

Contraindications. Hypersensitivity to heparin or pork-derived products; active major bleeding; thrombocytopenia associated with positive in vitro testing for antiplatelet antibody in the presence of heparin or a low-molecular-weight heparin.

Precautions. If epidural or spinal anesthesia or spinal puncture is used, patients receiving low-molecular-weight heparins for prevention of thromboembolic complications are at risk for developing epidural or spinal hematoma, which can result in permanent paralysis. The risk of these events can increase when postoperative indwelling epidural catheters are used. Use with caution in patients with renal impairment.

Drug Interactions. Use with caution in patients receiving thrombolytics, oral anticoagulants, or drugs that inhibit platelet function, including NSAIDs.

Parameters to Monitor. Monitor CBC, including platelet count, and stool for occult blood periodically; aPTT monitoring is not required. Antifactor Xa levels may be used to monitor the effects of enoxaparin in renal insufficiency or extremes of weight. Peak antifactor Xa levels should be drawn 4 h after the 3rd dose to target 0.6–1.0 IU/mL.

Notes. Partial reversal of anticoagulant effects of enoxaparin using protamine sulfate can occur[34]. If protamine is administered within 8 h of enoxaparin, the dose to neutralize 1 mg of enoxaparin is 1 mg of protamine. If enoxaparin administration occurred beyond 8 h, the dose of protamine should be decreased to 0.5 mg/1 mg of enoxaparin. A maximum of 60% reversal may be achieved.

EPTIFIBATIDE Integrilin

Pharmacology. Eptifibatide is a synthetic, cyclic heptapeptide that reversibly binds to and inhibits the platelet glycoprotein IIb/IIIa receptor, von Willebrand factor, and other adhesive ligands. Inhibition of the glycoprotein IIb/IIIa receptor prevents fibrinogen from binding, thereby preventing platelet aggregation. Eptifibatide reversibly inhibits platelet aggregation and prolongs bleeding time in a dose-dependent manner.[1]

Administration and Adult Dosage. **IV for unstable angina or NSTEMI (acute coronary syndrome, medical management, or in conjunction with PCI)**— 180 μg/kg as a bolus and then 2 μg/kg/min by continuous infusion. Continue infusion for up to 72 h, until hospital discharge or coronary artery bypass graft surgery, whichever occurs first. Should PCI be performed, continue infusion for 18–24 h after completing procedure (up to 96 h total in duration). Concomitant heparin therapy is recommended; (*See* Notes). **IV for PCI**—180 μg/kg as a bolus and then 2 μg/kg/min continuous infusion for 18–24 h. Give a second bolus of 180 μg/kg 10 min after the first.

Special Populations. *Pediatric Dosage.* Safety and efficacy not established.

Geriatric Dosage. Same as adult dosage.

Other Conditions. *Renal Impairment.* (Cl_{Cr} <50 mL/min) Give 180 μg/kg as a bolus and then 1 μg/kg/min continuous infusion. For PCI, give a second bolus of 180 μg/kg 10 min after the first.

Dosage Forms. Inj 75 mg/100 mL, 200 mg/100 mL.

Pharmacokinetics. *Onset and Duration.* Rapid inhibition of platelet function occurs after IV administration. Platelet function recovers soon after discontinuation of the IV infusion; bleeding time returns to baseline within 30 min and ex vivo platelet aggregation approaches baseline levels of >90% within 2–4 h.[1] Within 4 h of discontinuation of integrilin, inhibition of platelet aggregation drops to <50%.

Fate. Renal elimination accounts for about 50% of the total body clearance of eptifibatide. Clearance is 0.055–0.058 L/kg/h. **Half-life** is 2.5 h.[1]

Adverse Reactions. Bleeding, particularly from vascular access sites, occurs frequently. Oropharyngeal, GI, and GU bleeding also can occur. The frequency of thrombocytopenia is equal to that of placebo.[1,39,40] Hypotension is also reported.

Contraindications. Hypersensitivity; active internal bleeding within last 30 days; history of CVA within 30 days or any history of hemorrhagic CVA; bleeding diathesis; recent (within 6 weeks) major surgery or trauma; severe uncontrolled hypertension; current or planned use of another parenteral glycoprotein IIb/IIIa inhibitor; dependency on hemodialysis; severe hypertension (SBP >200 mm Hg or DBP >188 mm Hg).

Precautions. Pregnancy category B; use caution in elderly patients because eptifibatide clearance might be reduced, increasing risk of bleeding; thrombocytopenia (<100,000/μL), if it occurs discontinue eptifibatide and heparin; concomitant antithrombotic medications (e.g., thrombolytics, unfractionated heparin, low-molecular-weight heparin, and PO anticoagulants); NSAIDs; and other drugs that increase bleeding risk.

Drug Interactions. Anticoagulants or antiplatelet drugs can increase the risk of bleeding.

Parameters to Monitor. Monitor hemoglobin, hematocrit, platelet count, serum creatinine, PT, aPTT, and activated clotting time (if PCI performed). In clinical trials, the target activated clotting time (ACT) for patients treated with eptifibatide and undergoing percutaneous coronary intervention was 300–350 s.[39] If concomitant administration of unfractionated heparin is necessary, maintain aPTT at 50–70 s.[40]

Notes. (*See* Abciximab Notes for vascular access site care after percutaneous coronary intervention.) To minimize bleeding complications, discontinue anticoagulant therapy (e.g., heparin, LMWH, or bivalirudin) after PCI in uncomplicated cases.

FONDAPARINUX
Arixtra

Pharmacology. Fondaparinux is the modified synthetic analogue of the heparin pentasaccharide unit which binds to antithrombin III (AT)[34] When fondaparinux binds to AT, a conformational change occurs at the active site of AT, increasing its affinity for activated factor X inhibition. The small size of fondaparinux does not provide the bridge necessary to accelerate AT's inhibition of thrombin, giving fondaparinux the title as a factor Xa inhibitor.

Administration and Adult Dosage. **SQ for DVT/PE prophylaxis post-total hip or knee replacement**—2.5 mg daily starting 6–24 h after surgery. **SQ for DVT/PE prophylaxis post-hip fracture surgery**—2.5 mg daily starting 6–24 h after surgery for up to 32 days of extended prophylaxis. **SQ for DVT/PE prophylaxis post-abdominal surgery**—2.5 mg daily starting 6–8 h after surgery. **SQ for DVT or PE treatment**—Actual body weight <50 kg, 5mg daily; actual body weight 50–100 kg, 7.5 mg daily; actual body weight >100 kg, 10 mg daily.

Special Populations. *Pediatric dosage.* Safety and efficacy of fondaparinux in the pediatric population has not been established.

Dosage Forms. *Prefilled syringes*; 2.5 mg/0.5 mL; 5 mg/0.4 mL; 7.5 mg/0.6 mL; 10 mg/0.8 mg

Pharmacokinetics. *Onset and Duration.* Peak antifactor Xa occurs approximately 2–3 h after a 2.5 mg SQ injection.

Fate. Absolute bioavailability after SQ injection is 100%. V_d is about 7–11 L. Fondaparinux is eliminated renally as unchanged drug in the urine. **Half-life.** 17–21 h.

Adverse Reactions. Rates of major and minor bleeding complications in comparative studies with enoxaparin in hip fracture surgery and hip replacement surgery, versus dalteparin in abdominal surgery, and versus enoxaparin or IV heparin in the treatment of DVT and PE. Rates of major bleeding following knee replacement surgery were significantly higher in the fondaparinux group (2.1%) compared with enoxaparin (0.2%); however, a meta-analysis review indicated that the bleeding risk was associated with administration of fondaparinux in the 4–6 h time frame after surgery[41] Thrombocytopenia, fever, mild injection site irritation, asymptomatic increases in transaminase levels, and anemia occur frequently.

Contraindications. Patients with severe renal impairment (creatinine clearance <30 mL/min) should not receive fondaparinux. Patients with an actual body weight <50 kg should not receive prophylactic dose fondaparinux.

Precautions. If epidural or spinal anesthesia or spinal puncture is used, patients receiving fondaparinux for prevention of thromboembolic complications are at risk for developing epidural or spinal hematoma, which can result in permanent paralysis. The risk of these events can increase when postoperative indwelling epidural catheters are used. Use with caution in patients with renal impairment or low body weight.

Drug Interactions. Use with caution in patients receiving thrombolytics, oral anticoagulants, or drugs that inhibit platelet function, including NSAIDs.

Parameters to Monitor. Monitor CBC, including platelet count, and stool for occult blood periodically; aPTT monitoring is not required. Antifactor Xa levels specific to fondaparinux assays may be used to monitor fondaparinux, although the therapeutic range has not been established.[42]

Notes. Protamine sulfate does not bind to or reverse the effects of fondaparinux.[34] If serious bleeding occurs with fondaparinux, use of recombinant factor VIIa may be considered.

HEPARIN SODIUM	Various

Pharmacology. A heterogeneous, unfractionated group of mucopolysaccharides derived from the mast cells of animal tissues. It binds with antithrombin III, accelerating the rate at which antithrombin III neutralizes *activated forms* of factors XII, XI, IX, X, VII, and II. It is active in vitro and in vivo.

Administration and Adult Dosage. Express dosage in units only; dosage must be individually titrated to the institution-specific desired effect (usually 1.5–2.5 times aPTT).[4,8,43] Weight-based nomograms and computer-assisted dosages of heparin are effective, safe, and superior to "standard care" or empiric approaches.[44–46] **IV for thrombophlebitis or PE** 80 units/kg bolus followed by 18 units/kg/h continuous infusion; alternatively, 5000 units initially and then 1000 units/h.[4,8,43,44,47] Duration of therapy for thrombophlebitis or PE is 7–10 days, followed by oral anticoagulation (preferably initiated during the first 24 h of heparin therapy).[43,48] **SQ for thrombophlebitis or PE**—10,000–20,000 units initially (preceded by a 5000-unit IV loading dose) and then 8000–10,000 units q8h or 15,000–20,000 units q12h. **SQ for prophylaxis of DVT (low dose)**—5000 units 2 h before surgery, repeated q8–12h for 5–7 days or until patient is ambulatory.[49] **Cardiac indications**—60 units/kg bolus followed by a 12 units/kg/h continuous infusion. **IV for heparin lock flush**—inject sufficient solution (of 10 or 100 units/mL) into injection hub to fill the entire set after each heparin lock use. Some institutions reserve the 100 units/mL solution for flushing triple-lumen central catheters and use NS for all other catheters.

Special Populations. *Pediatric Dosage.* Same as adult dosage in units/kg.

Geriatric Dosage. Same as adult dosage.

Other Conditions. Patients with PE might require larger heparin doses than patients with thrombophlebitis.[47] (*See* Administration and Adult Dosage.) Patients with severe renal dysfunction might require lower dosages.[5] There is no good evidence that liver disease appreciably affects dosage requirements.

Dosage Forms. **Inj** 1000, 2000, 2500, 5000, 7500, 10,000 units/mL vials; 2, 50, 100 units/mL (prediluted); **Heparin Lock Flush** 10, 100 units/mL.

Patient Instructions. This drug is potentially harmful when taken with nonprescription or prescription drugs. Consult your physician or pharmacist when considering the use of other medications, in particular aspirin or NSAID-containing products.

Pharmacokinetics. *Onset and Duration.* Onset immediate after IV administration.

Serum Levels. The relation between heparin serum concentrations and aPTT response can change between reagents and reagent lots. Each laboratory should establish a therapeutic aPTT range corresponding to heparin serum concentrations of 0.3–0.7 units/mL using an Anti-Xa titration or 0.2–0.4 units/mL using protamine titration.[5,34] Circadian variation in heparin activity can occur, and aPTT response can change during the day at a given infusion rate.[50]

Fate. SQ bioavailability is 20%–40% and is dose dependent.[5] There is no biotransformation in plasma or liver; transfer and storage in reticuloendothelial cells have been suggested.[43,51] V_d is 0.058 ± 0.011 L/kg (approximates plasma volume).[14] Cl is dose dependent; Cl can be increased in PE, but this has not been a consistent finding.[43]

$t_{1/2}$. (Pharmacologic) 90 ± 60 min, dose related; higher doses lead to increased half-life; half-life can decrease in PE, but this has not been a consistent finding.[43,47,51,52] Shorter half-life has been reported in smokers versus nonsmokers.[5]

Adverse Reactions. Bleeding occurs in 3%–20% of patients receiving short-term, high-dose therapy.[43,53] Bleeding risk is increased by 3-fold when the aPTT is 2.0–2.9 and by 8-fold when the aPTT >3.0 times the control.[43] Heparin administration by continuous IV infusion can cause a lower frequency of bleeding complications than intermittent IV administration.[43] Renal dysfunction, liver disease, and other factors (serious cardiac illness, malignancy, age >60 years, and maximum aPTT >2.2 times control) can increase bleeding risk.[5,51,53] (*See* Precautions.) Thrombocytopenia occurs frequently (usually 1%–5%) and might be more common with heparin derived from bovine lung. (*See* Notes.) However, studies have suggested little difference and an overall decline in prevalence.[43,54,55] The decline might be related to improved manufacturing techniques and reduced therapy duration.[54] Osteoporosis and bone fractures occur rarely with doses of 15,000 units/d or more for longer than 5 months.[43] Patients receiving prolonged therapy or with diabetes or renal dysfunction rarely develop marked hyperkalemia.[56]

Heparin-Induced Thrombocytopenia (HIT). HIT is an antibody-mediated reaction to heparin and platelet factor-4 that causes platelet activation, thrombocytopenia, and potentially, arterial and venous thrombosis. HIT most commonly occurs within the first 2 weeks of heparin therapy and is detected by in vitro EIA antibody test, and platelet activation assay following a reduction in platelets by 50% from baseline. If HIT is suspected or diagnosed, all forms of heparin should be discontinued and treatment with a direct thrombin inhibitor (e.g., Argatroban, Lepirudin) should begin.

Contraindications. Active bleeding; thrombocytopenia; threatened abortion; subacute bacterial endocarditis; suspected intracranial hemorrhage; regional or lumbar block anesthesia; severe hypotension; shock; and after eye, brain, or spinal cord surgery.

Precautions. Risk factors for hemorrhage are IM injections, trauma, recent surgery, age >60 years, malignancy, peptic ulcer disease, potential bleeding sites, and acquired or congenital hemostatic defects.[43]

Drug Interactions. Thrombolytics, anticoagulants, or antiplatelet drugs including aspirin and other NSAIDs can increase risk of bleeding.

Parameters to Monitor. Baseline aPTT, PT/INR, hematocrit, and platelet count. Obtain aPTT (therapeutic range 1.5–2.5 times control) 3 or 4 times (or until therapeutic range is achieved) on day 1 and at least daily thereafter. Monitor platelets (for HIT) and hematocrit every other day and signs of bleeding (melena, hematuria, ecchymoses, hematemesis, epistaxis) daily.[4,8,43,57]

Notes. Heparin-induced thrombocytopenia is a potentially serious, and sometimes fatal, complication of heparin therapy. **Lepirudin and Argatroban** are approved for management of heparin-induced thrombocytopenia.

Protamine sulfate may be used to reverse the anticoagulant effects of heparin. For intravenous infusions of heparin, 1 mg of protamine will neutralize 100 units of heparin infused over the past 2.5 h[34] To reverse heparin administered SQ, an initial loading dose of 25–50 mg IV is given, then the remainder of the calculated dose is administered over 8–16 h.

LEPIRUDIN Refludan

Pharmacology. Lepirudin is a recombinant hirudin analogue that binds to thrombin in a 1:1 stoichiometric complex, thereby inhibiting the thrombogenic activity of thrombin, including clot-bound thrombin. Inhibition of thrombin occurs independently of antithrombin III.[58]

Administration and Adult Dosage. IV for heparin-induced thrombocytopenia and associated thromboembolic disease—0.4 mg/kg (up to 44 mg) as a bolus and then 0.15 mg/kg/h (up to 16.5 mg/h) by continuous infusion. In some cases where bleeding risk is elevated, lepirudin can be started without a bolus dose[34] **IV in patients being treated concomitantly with thrombolytics**—0.2 mg/kg as a bolus and then 0.1 mg/kg/h by continuous infusion. **Adjust dosage based on aPTT as follows:** for supratherapeutic aPTT, hold infusion for 2 h and then reduce infusion rate by 50%; for subtherapeutic aPTT, increase infusion in 20% increments, not to exceed 0.21 mg/kg/h.

Special Populations. *Other Conditions.* In renal insufficiency (Cr_s >1.5 mg/dL or Cl_{Cr} <60 mL/min), reduce the IV bolus to 0.2 mg/kg and base the initial IV infusion on renal function; Cl_{Cr} 45–60 mL/min or Cr_s 1.6–2 mg/dL, give 0.075 mg/kg/h; Cl_{Cr} 30–44 mL/min or Cr_s 2.1–3 mg/dL, give 0.045 mg/kg/h; Cl_{Cr} 15–29 mL/min or Cr_s 3.1–6 mg/dL, give 0.0225 mg/kg/h; Cl_{Cr} <15 mL/min or Cr_s >6 mg/dL, not recommended.

Dosage Forms. **Inj** 50 mg.

Pharmacokinetics. *Fate.* About 45% of the administered dose is eliminated in the urine, largely as unchanged drug (35%). Clearance is approximately 25% lower in women than in men and is also reduced about 20% in the elderly.

$t_{1/2}$. 60 min after IV injection.

Adverse Reactions. Bleeding complications are the most frequent adverse reactions. Hypersensitivity reactions, primarily allergic skin reactions, occur frequently.

Antihirudin antibodies form in almost 40% of patients with HIT treated with lepirudin. Antibodies may increase the anticoagulant effects of lepirudin, and rarely, may be related to severe anaphylactic reactions and death upon re-exposure[34]

Contraindications. Hypersensitivity to hirudins.

Precautions. Use with caution in patients with active internal bleeding, history of recent major bleeding, or known bleeding diathesis; history of CVA or any history of intracranial hemorrhage; history of intracranial neoplasm, AV malformation, or aneurysm; recent puncture of large blood vessel or organ biopsy; recent (within 1 month) major surgery or trauma; severe uncontrolled hypertension; bacterial endocarditis; poor renal function; receiving concomitant antithrombotic therapy including thrombolytics. Up to 40% of patients with heparin-induced thrombocytopenia treated with lepirudin develop antihirudin antibodies, which can increase the anticoagulant effects of lepirudin, necessitating strict monitoring of aPTT values.

Parameters to Monitor. Monitor aPTT 4 h after initiating lepirudin therapy, 4 h after each change in infusion rate, and daily-once target aPTT has been achieved. Maintain aPTT approximately 1.5–2.5 times the control aPTT.

PHYTONADIONE AquaMephyton, Mephyton

Pharmacology. Vitamin K is a required cofactor for the hepatic microsomal enzyme system that carboxylates glutamyl residues in precursor proteins to γ-carboxyglutamic residues. These proteins are present in vitamin K-dependent clotting factors (II, VII, IX, and X), anticoagulation proteins (proteins C and S), bone (osteocalcin), some plasma proteins (protein Z), and the proteins of several organs (kidney, lung, and testicular tissue).[59–61]

Administration and Adult Dosage. The normal daily nutritional requirement is about 0.03–1.5 μg/kg.[60,62,63] The adult RDAs are 70 μg/d for men 19–24 years and 80 μg/d for men >25 years; 60 μg/d for women 19–24 years and 65 μg/d for women >25 years.[64] **PO to reverse INR elevation—***INR > 5 but < 9.0 with no significant bleeding,* use 1–2.5 mg; if the INR is still elevated at 24–48 h, additional 1–2 mg can be given.[65] *INR > 9 with no significant bleeding,* use 2.5–5 mg with the expectation that the INR will be reduced substantially in 24–48 h. The IV solution can be administered orally to make doses <2.5 mg. **IV to reverse bleeding**—Use 10 mg by slow IV infusion (infuse no faster than 1 mg/min[66]). The initial dose can be repeated, based on PT and clinical response of 6–8 h if given parenterally. Use the smallest dosage possible to reverse anticoagulants and obviate possible refractoriness to additional anticoagulant therapy.[60,67] **IV**—do not give AquaMephyton intravenously unless it is *absolutely essential* (e.g., serious warfarin overdose or life-threatening bleeding) due to risk of anaphylaxis. The drug can be diluted in preservative-free dextrose or saline solution just before IV use. **PO for antenatal use in pregnant women receiving anticonvulsants**—20 mg/d throughout the last 4 weeks of pregnancy.[61]

Special Populations. *Pediatric Dosage.* RDAs are (<6 months) 5 μg/d; (6 months to –1 year) 10 μg/d; (1–3 years) 15 μg/d; (4–6 years) 20 μg/d; (7–10 years) 30 μg/d; (11–14 years) 45 μg/d; (15–18 years) 55 μg/d for females, 65 μg/d for males.[64] **IM for prophylaxis of hemorrhagic disease of the newborn**—0.5–1 mg within 1 h of birth. **SQ or IM for treatment of hemorrhagic disease of the newborn**—1 mg; more if mother has been receiving an oral anticoagulant.

Geriatric Dosage. (>55 years) RDAs are 65 µg/d for women and 80 µg/d for men.[64]

Dosage Forms. **Tab** (Mephyton) 5 mg; **Inj** (AquaMephyton) 1 mg/0.5 mL, 10 mg/mL ampules.

Pharmacokinetics. *Onset and Duration.* Reversal of anticoagulant effect is variable among individuals; parenteral onset is often within 6 h; peak and duration differ across individuals and doses. A 5-mg IV dose usually returns PT to normal in 24–48 h.[68] Large doses can cause prolonged refractoriness to oral anticoagulants.[60,67]

Fate. Absorbed from the GI tract via intestinal lymphatics only in the presence of bile; well absorbed after parenteral administration. Metabolized in the liver to hydroquinone and epoxide forms, which are interconvertible with the quinone.[59] Little storage occurs in the body. Without bile, hypoprothrombinemia develops over several weeks.[60,67,69]

Adverse Reactions. The drug itself appears to be nontoxic, but severe reactions (e.g., flushing, dyspnea, chest pain) and, occasionally, deaths have occurred after IV administration of AquaMephyton, possibly caused by the emulsifying agents.[60,63] This product should rarely be used IV, and used only when other routes of administration are not feasible. A transient flushing sensation, peculiar taste, and pain and swelling at the injection site can occur. Large parenteral doses in neonates have caused hyperbilirubinemia.

Precautions. Temporary refractoriness to oral anticoagulants can occur, especially with large doses of vitamin K. Reversal of anticoagulant activity can restore previous thromboembolic conditions. No effect or worsening of hypoprothrombinemia can occur in severe liver disease, and repeated doses are not warranted if response to the initial dose is unsatisfactory.[60,70]

Drug Interactions. Mineral oil and cholesterol-binding resins can impair phytonadione absorption.

Parameters to Monitor. Monitor PT before and at intervals after administration of the drug; the interval depends on the route of administration, the condition being treated, and the patient's status. (*See* Administration and Adult Dosage.)

Notes. Always protect the drug from light. Phytonadione reverses the effects of oral anticoagulant therapy but has no antagonist activity against heparin.

RETEPLASE
Retavase

Pharmacology. Reteplase (recombinant plasminogen activator) is a nonglycosylated mutant of wild-type tissue plasminogen activator, which converts plasminogen to plasmin. Plasmin then degrades the fibrin matrix of the thrombus. In animals, this modification results in less high-affinity fibrin binding, longer half-life, and greater thrombolytic potency than **alteplase** (rt-PA).

Administration and Adult Dosage. **IV for clot lysis in STEMI within 12 h of symptom onset**—Two 10 IU boluses 30 min apart, with adjunctive IV heparin given as a 5000-unit bolus followed by 1000 units/h (aPTT target 1.5–2.0 times control) for at least 24 h.

Special Populations. *Pediatric Dosage.* Safety and efficacy not established.

Geriatric Dosage. Same as adult dosage.

Dosage Forms. Inj 10.4 IU.

Pharmacokinetics. *Onset and Duration.* Onset of fibrinolytic activity is immediate after IV administration; duration is about 48 h as assessed by fibrinogen levels.

Fate. Elimination is primarily by the liver and kidneys. **Half-life** is 13–16 min

Adverse Reactions. Bleeding, cholesterol embolization, reperfusion arrhythmias, anaphylaxis reactions.

Contraindications. Active internal bleeding; history of cerebrovascular accident; recent intracranial or intraspinal surgery or trauma; intracranial or intraspinal surgery or trauma; known bleeding diathesis; severe uncontrolled hypertension.

Precautions. Pregnancy category B; recent major surgery; cerebrovascular disease; recent gastrointestinal or genitourinary bleeding; recent trauma; hypertension (SBP >180 mm Hg and/or DBP >110 mm Hg); high likelihood of left heart thrombus; acute pericarditis; subacute bacterial endocarditis; hemostatic defects; severe hepatic dysfunction; hemorrhagic ophthalmic conditions; septic thrombophlebitis or occluded AV cannula at a seriously infected site; elderly patients (increased bleeding risk); patients currently receiving oral anticoagulants.

Drug Interactions. Anticoagulants or antiplatelet drugs can increase the risk of bleeding. Heparin and reteplase are not compatible when combined in solution; infuse through separate lines.

Parameters to Monitor. For short-term thrombolytic therapy of MI, laboratory monitoring is of little value. No correlation has been made between clotting test results and likelihood of hemorrhage or efficacy.[5] Monitor for signs and symptoms of bleeding. Monitor the ECG for reperfusion arrhythmias. Monitor aPTT while on concomitant heparin therapy. Anticoagulation laboratory tests may be unreliable while on tenecteplase due to degradation of samples after removal for analysis.

Notes. In the Reteplase Angiographic Phase II International Dose-finding study (RAPID) open-label MI trial, reteplase achieved more rapid, complete, and sustained thrombolysis than did standard-dose rt-PA, with comparable bleeding risk.[71] The RAPID trial did not have sufficient power to detect differences in mortality between the groups. The GUSTO-III trial found reteplase equivalent to accelerated-infusion **alteplase** in MI for the combined endpoints of death or nonfatal, disabling stroke.[72] The International Joint Efficacy Comparison of Thrombolytics (INJECT) trial suggested that reteplase mortality rates were similar to those observed with streptokinase.[73] In STEMI patients, either PCI or thrombolysis is the primary therapy. In the case of thrombolytic failure, rescue PCI may be performed as clinically indicated; however, optimal anticoagulant and antiplatelet therapy has not been established under these circumstances.[5,9] Fibrinolytic therapy is NOT recommended for the treatment of NSTEMI because of lack of demonstrated benefits in controlled clinical trials.[6–9]

RIVAROXABAN   Xarelto

Pharmacology. Rivaroxaban is an oxazolidinone derivative that selectively and directly binds to activated factor X.[74]

Administration and Adult Dosage. **PO for prevention of DVT and PE post-hip and knee replacement**—10mg daily.

Dosage Forms. 10mg tab.

Pharmacokinetics. *Onset and Duration.* Peak antifactor Xa activity occurs 2–4 h after administration.

Fate. Highly bioavailable but absorption is influenced by administration with food. V_d is 50 L. Two-thirds is metabolized by CYP3A4, 2J2, and oxidation, with an overall 66% renal elimination as 33% unchanged drug and 33% inactive metabolite. The last third is eliminated as inactive metabolite via fecal route. *Half-life* is 5–9 h.

Adverse Reactions. Increased in transaminases (ALT, AST), anemia, nausea, postprocedural hemorrhage.

Contraindications. Hypersensitivity to the active substance or to any of the excipients; clinically significant active bleeding; hepatic disease associated with coagulopathy and clinically relevant bleeding risk, pregnancy, and lactation.

Precautions. Special consideration should be given when neuraxial anaesthesia or spinal/epidural puncture is employed. Patients with severe renal impairment (creatinine clearance <30 mL/min) may be at an increased risk of bleeding.

Drug Interactions. Rivaroxaban is metabolized by the CYP3A4 enzyme system and is transported by the P-glycoprotein efflux pump. Medications that are strong CYP3A4 and P-glycoprotein inhibitors will increase concentrations of rivaroxaban: azole antimycotics (ketoconazole, itraconazole, and voriconazole) or HIV protease inhibitors (ritonavir). Strong CYP3A4 inducers (rifampicin, phenytoin, carbamazepine, phenobarbital or St. John's Wort) should be used with caution since they may lead to reduced rivaroxaban plasma concentrations and thus may reduce efficacy. Rivaroxaban is a substrate of the P-glycoprotein system and is potentially susceptible to medications that alter P-glycoprotein efficiency. Other medications that affect hemostasis should be used with caution (NSAIDs, aspirin).

Parameters to Monitor. Monitor CBC and other signs of bleeding. Liver function test monitoring may be considered. Rivaroxaban may influence the prothrombin time and the anti-Xa test, but therapeutic targets are currently unknown.

Notes. Rivaroxaban received initial approval from the FDA in May 2009 for DVT and PE prophylaxis following hip and knee replacement. Other ongoing trials: Medically ill (Magellan), treatment of DVT and PE (Einstein trials), atrial fibrillation (Rocket), acute coronary syndrome (Atlas).

TENECTEPLASE   TNKase

Pharmacology. Tenecteplase is a recombinant tissue plasminogen activator, which converts plasminogen to plasmin. Plasmin then degrades the fibrin matrix of the thrombus. Tenecteplase is modified from human tissue plasminogen activator (t-PA). Genetic mutations of human t-PA resulted in greater thrombolytic potency, enhanced fibrin-specificity, decreased systemic activation of plasminogen, resistance to plasminogen activator inhibitor 1, and a longer half-life compared with t-PA.[75]

Administration and Adult Dosage. IV bolus for STEMI—(<60 kg) 30 mg; (60–69 kg) 35 mg; (70–79 kg) 40 mg; (80–89 kg) 45 mg; (≥90 kg) 50 mg. Give tenecteplase in combination with continuous IV heparin infusion. (*See* Notes.)

Special Populations. *Pediatric Dosage.* Safety and efficacy not established.

Geriatric Dosage. Same as adult dosage.

Dosage Forms. **Inj** 50 mg.

Pharmacokinetics. *Onset and Duration.* Rapid onset of thrombolysis occurs after IV administration.

Fate. Hepatic metabolism is the primary mode of clearance. Clearance is 5.94–7.14 L/h. **Half-life**—(α phase) 18–24 min; (β phase) 90–130 min.[75]

Adverse Reactions. Bleeding, cholesterol embolization, reperfusion arrhythmias, anaphylaxis reactions.

Contraindications. Active internal bleeding, history of cerebrovascular accident, intracranial or intraspinal surgery or trauma within 2 months, intracranial neoplasm, arteriovenous malformation or aneurysm, known bleeding diathesis, severe uncontrolled hypertension.

Precautions. Pregnancy category C; recent major surgery; cerebrovascular disease; recent gastrointestinal or genitourinary bleeding; recent trauma; hypertension (SBP >180 mm Hg and/or DBP >110 mm Hg); high likelihood of left heart thrombus; acute pericarditis; subacute bacterial endocarditis; hemostatic defects; severe hepatic dysfunction; hemorrhagic ophthalmic conditions; septic thrombophlebitis or occluded AV cannula at a seriously infected site; elderly patients (increased bleeding risk); patients currently receiving PO anticoagulants; recent administration of GP IIb/IIIa inhibitors.

Drug Interactions. Anticoagulants or antiplatelet drugs can increase the risk of bleeding.

Parameters to Monitor. For short-term thrombolytic therapy of MI, laboratory monitoring is of little value. No correlation has been made between clotting test results and likelihood of hemorrhage or efficacy.[5] Monitor for signs and symptoms of bleeding. Monitor the ECG for reperfusion arrhythmias. Monitor aPTT while on concomitant heparin therapy. Anticoagulation laboratory tests may be unreliable while on tenecteplase because of degradation of samples after removal for analysis.

Notes. In ASSENT-2, patients also were given concomitant IV heparin therapy as follows: (>67 kg) 4000 units as a bolus and then 800 units/h by continuous infusion; (>67 kg) 5000 units as a bolus and then 1000 units/h by continuous infusion. Heparin therapy was continued for 48–72 h. This study demonstrated comparable patency rates, mortality, intracranial hemorrhage, and stroke compared with front-loaded **alteplase**.[76] In STEMI patients, physicians should elect to utilize either PCI or thrombolysis as primary therapy. In the case of thrombolytic failure, rescue PCI may be performed as clinically indicated. However, optimal anticoagulant and antiplatelet therapy has not been established under theses circumstances.[5,9]

Fibrinolytic therapy is not recommended for the treatment of NSTEMI due to lack of demonstrated benefits in controlled clinical trials.[6–9]

TICLOPIDINE
Ticlid

Pharmacology. Ticlopidine is an antiplatelet agent that inhibits most known stimuli (e.g., ADP, collagen, epinephrine) for platelet aggregation. It prolongs bleeding time, normalizes shortened platelet survival, suppresses platelet growth factor release, and might block von Willebrand factor and fibrinogen interactions with platelets.[77–79]

Administration and Adult Dosage. **PO for thrombotic stroke reduction in patients with stroke or stroke precursors who are allergic to or have failed aspirin therapy, or those undergoing successful coronary stent implantation** 250 mg twice daily.

Special Populations. *Pediatric Dosage.* Safety and efficacy not established.

Geriatric Dosage. Same as adult dosage.

Dosage Forms. **Tab** 250 mg.

Pharmacokinetics. *Onset and Duration.* The onset of clinical effect is delayed, with maximum efficacy being achieved in 3–8 days. Approximately 80% of the drug is absorbed orally, with peak serum concentrations occurring in about 2 h. Steady state is reached at 14–21 days. Bleeding time and platelet function tests normalize approximately 2 weeks after discontinuation of therapy.

Fate. Ticlopidine undergoes extensive liver metabolism to possibly active metabolites, with only 2% excreted unchanged in urine. **Half-life** is 12.6 h with a single dose; 4–5 days with repeated dosages.

Adverse Reactions. Diarrhea and rash occur frequently. Minor bleeding such as bruising, petechiae, epistaxis, and hematuria occur occasionally. Severe neutropenia occurs in about 0.8% of patients and mild to moderate neutropenia in about 1.6% of patients during the first 3 months of therapy; neutropenia usually resolves within 3 weeks of discontinuation, although sepsis and death have been reported. Thrombocytopenia, thrombotic thrombocytopenic purpura (TTP), and cholestasis occur rarely.[79,80]

Contraindications. Hypersensitivity; presence of hematopoietic disorders, such as neutropenia, thrombocytopenia, or a history of TTP or aplastic anemia; history of a hemostatic disorder or active pathological bleeding; severe liver impairment.

Precautions. Black Box Warnings for neutropenia/agranulocytosis, TTP, and aplastic anemia. Use with caution in patients at increased risk of bleeding from trauma, surgery, or other conditions. Ticlopidine should be discontinued 10–14 days prior to surgery if an antiplatelet effect is not desired; pregnancy category B.

Drug Interactions. Use with caution in patients receiving anticoagulants or drugs that inhibit platelet function including NSAIDs. Antacids decrease ticlopidine bioavailability by 18%. Cimetidine decreases clearance of ticlopidine by 50%. Ticlopidine decreases digoxin levels by 15%. Ticlopidine increases theophylline half-life from 8.6 to 12.2 hours. Ticlopidine may increase phenytoin levels but has not been documented to effect phenobarbital or propranolol levels.

Parameters to Monitor. Obtain CBC and differential counts every 2 weeks during the first 3 months of therapy; more frequent monitoring is recommended if the ANC is consistently declining or is <30% of the baseline value or if patients demonstrate signs and symptoms of TTP (weakness, pallor, petechiae, or purpura), dark urine, jaundice, or neurologic changes. Cholesterol panel should be obtained 30 days after initiation of ticlopidine. No specific monitoring is routinely recommended to assess antiplatelet effects. Monitor for signs and symptoms of bleeding.

Notes. The Ticlopidine Aspirin Stroke Study trial found a 12% risk reduction in nonfatal stroke or cardiovascular death with ticlopidine compared with aspirin in high-risk (previous TIA or minor stroke) men and women. For secondary stroke prevention, the Canadian American Ticlopidine Study trial found that the risk of stroke, MI, or cardiovascular death was reduced by 23% with ticlopidine over placebo. Ticlopidine also was shown to markedly reduce MI, cardiovascular death, and ECG evidence of ischemia in patients with unstable angina.[81,82] Reserve ticlopidine for patients intolerant to aspirin and clopidogrel due to risk of TTP, neutropenia/agranulocytosis and aplastic anemia.

TINZAPARIN SODIUM	Innohep

Pharmacology. Tinzaparin is a low-molecular-weight heparin (average mass 2000–8000 daltons) prepared by depolymerization of unfractionated porcine intestinal mucosa heparin. Other pharmacologic properties are similar to those of enoxaparin.[31]

Administration and Adult Dosage. **SQ for treatment of DVT with or without PE.** 175 IU/kg once daily coadministered with warfarin until INR is therapeutic. **SQ for the prevention of DVT and PE.** 75 IU/kg once daily.

Special Populations. *Renal Impairment.* Severe renal impairment (Cl_{Cr} <30 mL/min) decreases elimination by almost 25%. No specific dose adjustments are recommended in this population. *Morbid Obesity.* Dose capping is not recommended; use weight-based dosing. *Geriatric Dosage.* Elderly patients might have reduced elimination; in a study of elderly patients with renal impairment (Cl_{Cr} < 30 mL/min), more patients died after treatment with tinzaparin than with unfractionated heparin.

Dosage Forms. **Inj.** *Multiple dose vial:* 40,000 IU/2 mL

Pharmacokinetics. *Onset and Duration.* Peak antifactor Xa occurs 4–5 h after SQ injection and may persist for almost 20 h.

Fate. Mean absolute bioavailability after SQ injection is ~87%. V_d is about 3–5 L and Clearance is about 1.7 L/h after IV administration. Some hepatic desulfation and depolymerization occur, but most of the drug is eliminated renally. **Half-life** is 3–4 h.

Adverse Reactions. Overall, rates of major and minor bleeding complications in comparative studies with unfractionated heparin are similar. Mild local irritation, hematoma, ecchymosis, and pain on injection; asymptomatic increases in transaminase levels may occur frequently. Thrombocytopenia occurs occasionally.

Contraindications. Hypersensitivity to heparin, pork-derived products, sulfite or benzyl alcohol; active major bleeding; thrombocytopenia associated with positive in vitro testing for antiplatelet antibody in the presence of heparin or a low-molecular-weight heparin.

Precautions. If epidural or spinal anesthesia or spinal puncture is used, patients receiving low-molecular-weight heparins for prevention of thromboembolic complications are at risk for developing epidural or spinal hematoma, which can result in permanent paralysis. The risk of these events can increase when postoperative indwelling epidural catheters are used. Use with caution in patients with renal impairment.

Drug Interactions. Use with caution in patients receiving thrombolytics, oral anticoagulants or drugs that inhibit platelet function, including NSAIDs.

Parameters to Monitor. Monitor CBC, including platelet count, and stool for occult blood periodically; aPTT monitoring is not required. Antifactor Xa levels may be used to monitor the effects of enoxaparin in renal insufficiency or extremes of weight. Peak Antifactor Xa levels should be drawn 4–5 h after administration to target levels of about 0.85 IU/mL.

Notes. Partial reversal of anticoagulant effects of tinzaparin using protamine sulfate can occur.[34] The dose to neutralize 100 units of tinzaparin is 1mg of protamine. A maximum 60% reversal may be achieved.

TIROFIBAN   Aggrastat

Pharmacology. Tirofiban is a nonpeptide, tyrosine derivative that reversibly binds to and inhibits the platelet glycoprotein IIb/IIIa receptor. Inhibition of the glycoprotein IIb/IIIa receptor prevents fibrinogen from binding, thereby preventing platelet aggregation. Tirofiban inhibits platelet aggregation and prolongs bleeding time in a dose-dependent manner.[1]

Administration and Adult Dosage. IV for unstable angina or NSTEMI (ACS medical management OR in conjunction with PCI). 0.4 μg/kg/min infusion for 30 min and then 0.1 μg/kg/min by continuous infusion. Continue infusion until patient has clinically stabilized; infusion can be continued for up to 108 h. Tirofiban can be administered to patients who undergo PCI. Should PCI be performed during tirofiban therapy, continue infusion for 12–24 h after completing the procedure. Give tirofiban in combination with continuous IV heparin infusion. (*See* Notes.)

Special Populations. *Pediatric Dosage.* Safety and efficacy not established.

Geriatric Dosage. Same as adult dosage.

Other Conditions. Renal Impairment. (Cl_{Cr} <30 mL/min) reduce maintenance infusion rate by 50%.

Dosage Forms. **Inj** 5 mg/100 mL, 12.5 mg/250 mL

Pharmacokinetics. *Onset and Duration.* Approximately 90% inhibition of platelet function occurs rapidly after IV administration. Platelet function recovers soon after discontinuation of the IV infusion; bleeding time and ex vivo platelet aggregation return to near baseline levels within 3–8 h.[1]

Fate. Renal elimination accounts for 39%–69% of the total body clearance. About 65% of a dose is excreted in the urine, largely as unchanged drug; about 25% of an administered dose is excreted in the feces. Clearance is 9.12–18.84 L/h. **Half-life** is 1.5–2 h.[1]

Adverse Reactions. Bleeding complications are the most frequent adverse reactions. Use care to minimize the risk of bleeding by minimizing vascular and other trauma and providing proper care of vascular access sites in patients having percutaneous coronary interventions performed. Thrombocytopenia occurs in <2% of patients and is reversible at discontinuation of the drug (discontinue tirofiban and heparin if platelet count is <90,000/mm³).[83] Edema, pelvic pain, leg pain, vasovagal reaction, coronary artery dissection, dizziness, sweating, nausea, headache, and fever are also reported.

Contraindications. Hypersensitivity; active internal bleeding or bleeding diathesis within the previous 30 days; history of CVA within 30 days or any history of intracranial hemorrhage; history of intracranial neoplasm, AV malformation, or aneurysm; history of hemorrhagic stroke; thrombocytopenia following previous exposure to tirofiban; recent (within 1 month) major surgery or trauma; history, symptoms, or findings suggestive of aortic dissection; severe uncontrolled hypertension (SBP >180 mm Hg or DBP >110 mm Hg); current or planned use of another parenteral glycoprotein IIb/IIIa inhibitor; acute pericarditis.

Precautions. Pregnancy category B; elderly patients, as eptifibatide clearance might be reduced thereby increasing the risk of bleeding; thrombocytopenia (platelet count <150,000/mm³); hemorrhagic retinopathy; hemodialysis patients; use with caution in patients being treated concomitantly with other antithrombotic drugs including thrombolytics, unfractionated heparin, low-molecular-weight heparin, oral anticoagulants; NSAIDs; and other drugs that increase bleeding risk.

Parameters to Monitor. Monitor hemoglobin, hematocrit, and platelets at baseline, 6 h after loading dose and then daily; prothrombin time; aPTT (maintain aPTT ~2 times control aPTT).[83]

Notes. (*See* Abciximab for vascular access site care after PCI.) **IV heparin during therapy**—5000 units as a bolus and then 1000 units/h continuous infusion adjusted to maintain aPTT 2 times control. **IV heparin if PCI was performed**—Discontinue IV infusion and give 5000–7500 units of heparin as a bolus and then 1000 units/h by continuous infusion.[83]

UROKINASE
Abbokinase

Pharmacology. Urokinase is a proteolytic enzyme produced by renal parenchymal cells that act to directly convert plasminogen to plasmin, with effects similar to those of streptokinase.[5]

Administration and Adult Dosage. **IV for PE**—4400 IU/kg loading dose over 10 min, followed by 4400 IU/kg/h for 12 h. Heparin therapy is initiated without a loading dose after discontinuation of the thrombolytic when the thrombin time or other coagulation test no longer exceeds 2 times normal control.

Special Populations. *Pediatric Dosage.* Safety and efficacy not established.

Geriatric Dosage. Same as adult dosage.

Dosage Forms. **Inj** 5000, 9000, 250,000 IU.

Pharmacokinetics. **Half-life** is 10–20 min.

Adverse Reactions. Bleeding, cholesterol embolization, reperfusion arrhythmias, anaphylaxis reactions and other infusion reactions, myocardial infarction, substernal chest pain, diaphoresis, stroke, hemiplegia, decreased hematocrit, thrombocytopenia, vascular emboli, pulmonary edema.

Contraindications. Active internal bleeding, cerebrovascular accident within 2 months; intracranial or intraspinal surgery within 2 months; recent trauma or cardiopulmonary resuscitation; intracranial neoplasm, arteriovenous malfunction, or aneurysm; known bleeding diathesis; severe uncontrolled hypertension.

Precautions. Pregnancy category B; elderly patients, due to limited data; recent (within 10 days) major surgery, obstetrical delivery, organ biopsy or puncture of noncompressible vessels; recent (within 10 days) serious gastrointestinal bleed; high likelihood of left heart thrombus; subacute bacterial endocarditis; homeostatic defects; cerebrovascular disease; diabetic hemorrhagic retinopathy.

Drug Interactions. Anticoagulants or antiplatelet drugs can increase the risk of bleeding.

Parameters to Monitor. Obtain a baseline hematocrit, platelet count, and aPTT. Monitor for signs and symptoms of bleeding. Monitor the ECG for reperfusion arrhythmias.

Notes. If patient is on heparin prior to initiation of urokinase therapy, discontinue heparin and wait for aPTT to decrease to less than 2 times the control before administering urokinase.

WARFARIN SODIUM   Coumadin, Various

Pharmacology. Warfarin prevents the conversion of vitamin K back to its active form from vitamin K epoxide. This impairs formation of the vitamin K-dependent clotting factors II, VII, IX, and X (prothrombin) and proteins C and S (physiologic anticoagulants). The (S)-warfarin enantiomer is approximately 4-fold more potent an anticoagulant than (R)-warfarin.[5,84]

Administration and Adult Dosage. PO or IV—average 5–7.5 mg/d (range 2–10 mg/d), titrating dosage to an INR of 2.0–3.0 for treatment or prophylaxis of venous thrombosis, PE, systemic embolism, tissue heart valves, valvular heart disease, aortic bileaflet mechanical prosthetic valve, atrial fibrillation, and recurrent systemic embolism. Adjust dosage to an INR of 2.5–3.5 for management of some mechanical prosthetic valves (caged-ball, tilting-disk, and mitral position valves);[85] adding **aspirin** 100 mg/d offers additional protection but increases the risk of mild bleeding.[7,43] For post-MI patients who are at increased risk of systemic or pulmonary embolism, maintain a warfarin dosage that achieves an INR of 2.5–3.5 for up to 3 months. *Genetic Factors.* Genetic mutations in hepatic metabolism of warfarin (CYP2C9) and in the ability for warfarin to inhibit vitamin K oxide reductase (VKORC1) have been able to explain some of the variability with initial warfarin dosing and response to dose changes.[65] Use of algorithms to predict initial warfarin dosing exist, but have not yet been linked to improved thromboembolic or hemorrhagic outcomes.

Special Populations. *Pediatric Dosage.* (<18 years) safety and efficacy not established. However, when used, dosage is titrated based on INR as in adult dosage. *Geriatric Dosage.* Same as adult dosage. (*See also* Precautions.)

Other Conditions. Large variability in response requires that dosage be carefully individualized to each patient. Patients with liver disease, CHF, hyperthyroidism, or fever might be particularly sensitive to warfarin. Renal failure does not enhance the hypoprothrombinemic response to warfarin, but these patients might have compromised hemostatic mechanisms that predispose to bleeding.[86]

Dosage Forms. **Tab:** 1, 2, 2.5, 3, 4, 5, 6, 7.5, 10 mg; **Inj:** 5 mg/2.5 mL vial.

Patient Instructions. Potentially harmful interactions may occur when taking warfarin with nonprescription or prescription drugs. Consult your physician or pharmacist when considering the use of other medications, in particular aspirin or NSAID-containing products. Alterations in vitamin K intake.

Missed Doses. Take this drug at the same time each day. It is important that you not miss any doses. If you do miss a dose, take it as soon as you remember. If it is closer to the time for the next dose, take that dose only. Do not double the dose or take extra.

Pharmacokinetics. *Onset and Duration.* Peak PT effect is in 36–72 h;[87] at least 4–6 days of warfarin therapy are required before full therapeutic effect is achieved.[4,43] Duration after discontinuation depends on resynthesis of vitamin K-dependent clotting factors II, VII, IX, and X (which require about 4–5 days).

Fate. Completely absorbed orally; well absorbed after small-bowel resection;[88] 99 $\pm$ 1% is bound to plasma proteins.[14] V_d (racemic) is 0.14 $\pm$ 0.06 L/kg; Cl (racemic) is 0.0027 $\pm$ 0.0014 L/h/kg.[14] It undergoes oxidative P450 enzyme biotransformation in the liver: (R)-warfarin, CYP1A2, and CYP34; (S)-warfarin, CYP2C9,[89] producing warfarin alcohols, which have minor anticoagulant activity.[90,91] Less than 2% is excreted unchanged in urine.[14]

$t_{1/2}$. 37 $\pm$ 15 h,[14,92] unchanged in acute hepatic disease.[93] Enantiomer half-lives: (R)-warfarin 43 $\pm$ 14 h; (S)-warfarin 32 $\pm$ 12 h.[14]

Adverse Reactions. Bleeding (major and minor) occurs frequently (6%–29%); fatal or life-threatening hemorrhage has been reported in 1%–8% of patients. Risk factors for increased bleeding are age >65 years, history of gastrointestinal bleeding, history of stroke, diabetes mellitus, renal insufficiency, recent myocardial infarction, and active cancer.[94,95] Skin necrosis (occurring early in therapy and involving the breast, buttocks, thigh, or penis), purple-toe syndrome (occurring after 3–8 weeks of therapy), and alopecia rarely occur.[4,43,53,96,97]

Contraindications. Pregnancy; threatened abortion; blood dyscrasias; bleeding tendencies; unsupervised patients with senility, alcoholism, psychosis, or lack of cooperation; anticipated spinal puncture procedure; regional or lumbar anesthesia.

Precautions. Several other factors can influence response: diet, travel, and environment. Monitor patients with liver disease, CHF, atrial fibrillation, hyperthyroidism, or fever especially carefully. The elderly have a greater risk of major trauma or falls (e.g., hip fractures) and physiologic changes in subcutaneous tissues and joint spaces, which can allow bleeding to expand unchecked.[97] IM injections should be limited because of risk of hematoma formation; they should occur when the INR is within or below range as needed.

Drug Interactions. There are many important interactions that have a potential clinical importance. Careful monitoring and appropriate dosage adjustment are recommended when any potential interacting drug is added or discontinued. Some agents commonly associated with increased warfarin effect are amiodarone, cimetidine, ciprofloxacin, clarithromycin, erythromycin, fluconazole, fluvoxamine, lovastatin, metronidazole, quinidine, and trimethoprim-sulfamethoxazole. Some agents commonly associated with decreased warfarin effect are barbiturates, carbamazepine, cholestyramine, griseofulvin, and rifampin. (*See* Refs. 98 and 99 for more comprehensive information regarding warfarin drug interactions.)

Parameters to Monitor. Monitor PT/INR daily while hospitalized and then 2–3 times weekly to monthly for therapeutic effect; hematocrit; stool guaiac; urinalysis (for hematuria) for toxicity. Also monitor for ecchymoses, hemoptysis, and epistaxis.

Notes. Loading dose has no therapeutic advantage and might be unsafe because of excessive depression of factor VII.[43] **Phytonadione** begins to restore the PT toward normal within 4–8 h, although large doses can induce subsequent resistance to anticoagulant effect lasting (≥ 1 week.[100] A small oral dose (e.g., 2.5 mg) or small slow IV injection (0.5–1 mg) of phytonadione can be used to bring an elevated PT/INR back into target range without resulting resistance.[7]

■ REFERENCES

1. Dobesh PP, Latham KA. Advancing the battle against acute ischemic syndromes: a focus on the GP IIb–IIIa inhibitors. *Pharmacotherapy.* 1998;18:663 685.

2. LeBreton H et al. Role of platelets in restenosis after percutaneous coronary revascularization. *J Am Coll Cardiol.* 1996;28:1643-1651.

3. The EPILOG Investigators. Platelet glycoprotein IIb/IIIa receptor blockade and low-dose heparin during percutaneous coronary revascularization. *N Engl J Med.* 1997;336:1689-1696.

4. Hyers TM et al. Antithrombotic therapy for venous thromboembolic disease. *Chest.* 1995;108:335S-351S.

5. Lutomski DM et al. Pharmacokinetic optimisation of the treatment of embolic disorders. *Clin Pharmacokinet.* 1995;28:67-92.

6. International Society and Federation of Cardiology and World Health Organization Task Force on Myocardial Reperfusion. Reperfusion in acute myocardial infarction. *Circulation.* 1994;90:2091 2102.

7. Becker RC, Ansell J. Antithrombotic therapy: an abbreviated reference for clinicians. *Arch Intern Med.* 1995; 155:149-161.

8. The GUSTO Investigators. An international randomized trial comparing four thrombolytic strategies for acute myocardial infarction. *N Engl J Med.* 1993;329:673-682.

9. Antman EM, Hand M, Armstrong PW, et al. 2007 Focused Update of the ACC/AHA 2004 Guidelines for the management of patients with ST-Elevation Myocardial Infarction. *J Am Coll Cardiol.* 2008;51:210-247.

10. Levine M et al. A randomized trial of a single bolus dosage regimen of recombinant tissue plasminogen activator in patients with acute pulmonary embolism. *Chest.* 1990;98:1473-1479.

11. Cairns JA et al. Coronary thrombolysis. *Chest.* 1995;108:401S-423S.

12. The National Institute of Neurological Disorders rt-PA Stroke Study Group. Tissue plasminogen activator for acute ischemic stroke. *N Engl J Med.* 1995;333:1581-1587.

13. Davis SN et al. Activity and dosage of alteplase dilution for clearing occlusions of venous access devices. *Am J Health Syst Pharm.* 2000;57:1039-1045.

14. Benet LZ et al. Design and optimization of dosage regimens; pharmacokinetic data. In: Hardman JG et al., eds. *Goodman and Gilman's the pharmacological basis of therapeutics.* 9th ed. New York, NY: McGraw-Hill; 1996:1707-1792.

15. Third International Study of Infarct Survival Collaborative Study. ISIS-3: a randomized comparison of streptokinase vs tissue plasminogen activator vs anistreplase and of aspirin plus heparin vs aspirin alone among 41,299 cases of suspected acute myocardial infarct. *Lancet.* 1992;339:753-770.

16. Nicolini FA et al. Concurrent nitroglycerin therapy impairs tissue-type plasminogen activator-induced thrombolysis in patients with acute myocardial infarction. *Am J Cardiol.* 1994;74:662-666.

17. Fuster V. Coronary thrombolysis—a perspective for the practicing physician. *N Engl J Med.* 1993;329:723-724.

18. The Continuous Infusion Versus Double-Bolus Administration of Alteplase (COBALT) Investigators. A comparison of continuous infusion of alteplase with double-bolus administration for acute myocardial infarction. *N Engl J Med.* 1997;337:1124-1130.

19. Januzzi JL Jr, Jang IK. Heparin induced thrombocytopenia: diagnosis and contemporary antithrombin management. *J Thromb Thrombolysis*. 1999;7:259-264.

20. Keegan SP, Gallagher EM, Ernst NE, et al. Effects of critical illness and organ failure on therapeutic argatroban dosage requirements in patients with suspected or confirmed heparin-induced thrombocytopenia. *Ann Pharmacother*. 2009;43(1):19-27.

21. Swan SK et al. Comparison of anticoagulant effects and safety of argatroban and heparin in healthy subjects. *Pharmacotherapy*. 2000;20:756-770.

22. Kawada T et al. Clinical application of argatroban as an alternative anticoagulant for extracorporeal circulation. *Hematol Oncol Clin North Am*. 2000;14:445-447.

23. Lincoff AM, Kleiman NS, Kereikes DJ, et al. Long-term efficacy of bivalirudin and provisional glycoprotein IIb/IIIa blockade vs heparin and planned glycoprotein IIB/IIIa blockade during percutaneous coronary revascularization: REPLACE-2. *JAMA*. 2004;292:696-703.

24. Stone GW, Ware JH, Bertrand ME. Antithrombotic strategies in patients with acute coronary syndromes undergoing early invasive management. One-year results from the ACUITY trial. *JAMA*. 2007;298:2497-2506.

25. The Medicines Company. The Medicines Company receives FDA review letter for Angiomax supplemental filing [press release]. May 28, 2008. http://ir.themedicinescompany.com/phoenix.zhtml?c=122204&p=irol-newsArticle&ID=1151111&highlight=.

26. Bennet CL et al. Thrombotic thrombocytopenic purpura associated with clopidogrel. *N Engl J Med*. 2000;342:1773-1777.

27. Sibbing D, Morath T, Stegherr J, et al. Impact of proton pump inhibitors on the antiplatelet effects of clopidogrel. *Thromb Haemost*. 2009;101:714-719.

28. Stanek EJ. Society for Cardiovascular Angiography and Interventions 2008 Scientific Sessions; May 6, 2009; Las Vegas, NV.

29. CAPRIE Steering Committee. A randomised, blinded, trial of clopidogrel versus aspirin in patients at risk for ischaemic events (CAPRIE). *Lancet*. 1996;348:1329-1339.

30. Bhatt DL, Fox KA, Hacke W, et al. Clopidogrel and aspirin verses aspirin alone for the prevention of atherothrombotic events. *N Engl J Med*. 2006;354:1706-1717.

31. Howard PA. Dalteparin: a low-molecular-weight heparin. *Ann Pharmacother*. 1997;31:192-203.

32. Lee AY, Levine MN, Baker RI, et al. Low-molecular-weight heparin versus coumarin for the prevention of recurrent venous thromboembolism in patients with cancer. *N Engl J Med*. 2003;349(2):146-153.

33. Nutescu EA, Spinler SA, Wittkowsky A, et al. Low-molecular-weight heparins in renal impairment and obesity: available evidence and clinical practice recommendations across medical and surgical settings. *Ann Pharmacother*. 2009;43(6):1064-1083.

34. Hirsch J, Bauer KA, Donati MB, et al. Parenteral anticoagulants. *Chest*. 2008;133(6):141S-159S.

35. Green D et al. Low molecular weight heparin: a critical analysis of clinical trials. *Pharmacol Rev*. 1994;46:89-109.

36. Noble S et al. Enoxaparin. A reappraisal of its pharmacology and clinical applications in the prevention and treatment of thromboembolic disease. *Drugs*. 1995;49:388-410.

37. Levine M et al. A comparison of low-molecular-weight heparin administered primarily at home with unfractionated heparin administered in the hospital for proximal deep-vein thrombosis. *N Engl J Med*. 1996;334:677-681.

38. Lensing AWA et al. Treatment of deep venous thrombosis with low-molecular-weight heparins. A meta-analysis. *Arch Intern Med*. 1995;155:601-607.

39. The IMPACT-II Investigators. Randomised placebo-controlled trial of effect of eptifibatide on complications of percutaneous coronary intervention: IMPACT-II. *Lancet*. 1997;349:1422-1428.

40. The PURSUIT Trial Investigators. Inhibition of platelet glycoprotein IIb/IIIa with eptifibatide in patients with acute coronary syndromes. *N Engl J Med*. 1998;339:436-443.

41. Turpie AG, Bauer KA, Eriksson BI, et al. Fondaparinux vs enoxaparin for the prevention of venous thromboembolism in major orthopedic surgery: a meta-analysis of 4 randomized double-blind studies. *Arch Intern Med*. 2002;162:1833-1840.

42. Weitz JI, Hirsh J, Samama MM. New antithrombotic drugs. *Chest*. 2008;133:234S-256S.

43. Carter BL. Therapy of acute thromboembolism with heparin and warfarin. *Clin Pharm*. 1991;10:503-518.

44. Raschke RA et al. The weight-based heparin dosing nomogram compared with a "standard care" nomogram. A randomized controlled trial. *Ann Intern Med*. 1993;119:874-881.

45. Kershaw B et al. Computer-assisted dosing of heparin. Management with pharmacy-based anticoagulation service. *Arch Intern Med*. 1994;154:1005-1011.

46. Gunnarsson PS et al. Appropriate use of heparin. Empiric vs nomogram-based dosing. *Arch Intern Med*. 1995;155:526-532.

47. Simon TL et al. Heparin pharmacokinetics: increased requirements in pulmonary embolism. *Br J Haematol*. 1978;39:111-120.

48. Kruchoski ME, Emory CE. Initiating heparin and warfarin therapy concurrently. *Hosp Pharm*. 1986;21:174.

49. Melamed AJ, Suarez J. Detection and prevention of deep venous thrombosis. *Drug Intell Clin Pharm.* 1988;22:107-114.

50. Cooke HM, Lynch A. Biorhythms and chronotherapy in cardiovascular disease. *Am J Hosp Pharm.* 1994;51: 2569-2580.

51. Estes JW. Clinical pharmacokinetics of heparin. *Clin Pharmacokinet.* 1980;5:204-220.

52. Hirsh J et al. Heparin kinetics in venous thrombosis and pulmonary embolism. *Circulation.* 1976;53:691-695.

53. Landefeld CS et al. A bleeding risk index for estimating the probability of major bleeding in hospitalized patients starting anticoagulant therapy. *Am J Med.* 1990;89:569-578.

54. Bailey RT et al. Heparin-associated thrombocytopenia: a prospective comparison of bovine lung heparin, manufactured by a new process, and porcine intestinal heparin. *Drug Intell Clin Pharm.* 1986;20:374-378.

55. Becker PS, Miller VT. Heparin-induced thrombocytopenia. *Stroke.* 1989;20:1449-1459.

56. Oster JR et al. Heparin-induced aldosterone suppression and hyperkalemia. *Am J Med.* 1995;98:575-586.

57. Warkentin TE, Greinacher A, Koster A, et al. Treatment and prevention of heparin-induced thrombocytopenia. *Chest.* 2008;133(6);340S-380S.

58. Verstraete M. Direct thrombin inhibitors: appraisal of the antithrombotic/hemorrhagic balance. *Thromb Haemost.* 1997;78:357-363.

59. Uotila L. The metabolic functions and mechanism of action of vitamin K. *Scand J Clin Lab Invest.* 1990;201 (suppl):109-117.

60. Hardman JG et al., eds. *Goodman and Gilman's the pharmacological basis of therapeutics.* 9th ed. New York, NY: McGraw-Hill; 1996:1583-1585.

61. Thorp JA et al. Current concepts and controversies in the use of vitamin K. *Drugs.* 1995;49:376-387.

62. Frick PG et al. Dose response and minimal daily requirement for vitamin K in man. *J Appl Physiol.* 1967;23: 387-389.

63. Mattea EJ, Quinn K. Adverse reactions after intravenous phytonadione administration. *Hosp Pharm.* 1981;16: 224-235.

64. Food and Nutrition Board, NRC. *Recommended dietary allowances.* 10th ed. Washington, DC: National Academy Press; 1989.

65. Ansell J, Hirsh J, Hylek E, et al. Pharmacology and management of the vitamin K antagonist. *Chest.* 133(6); 160S-198S.

66. Hirsch J et al. Oral anticoagulants. Mechanism of action, clinical effectiveness, and optimal therapeutic range. *Chest.* 1998;114(suppl):445S.

67. Koch-Weser J, Sellers EM. Drug interactions with coumarin anticoagulants (2 parts). *N Engl J Med.* 1971;285: 487-489, 547-558.

68. Zieve PD, Solomon HM. Variation in the response of human beings to vitamin K. *J Lab Clin Med.* 1969;73: 103-110.

69. Woolf IL, Babior BM. Vitamin K and warfarin. *Am J Med.* 1972;53:261-267.

70. O'Reilly RA et al. Intravenous vitamin K1 injections: dangerous prophylaxis. *Arch Intern Med.* 1995;155:2127.

71. Lopez LM. Clinical trials in thrombolytic therapy, Part 2: the open-artery hypothesis and RAPID-1 and RAPID-2. *Am J Health Syst Pharm.* 1997;54(suppl 1):S27-S30.

72. The Global Use of Strategies To Open Occluded Coronary Arteries (GUSTO III) Investigators. A comparison of reteplase with alteplase for acute myocardial infarction. *New Engl J Med.* 1997;337:1118-1123.

73. International Joint Efficacy Comparison of Thrombolytics (INJECT). Randomised, double-blind comparison of reteplase double-bolus administration with streptokinase in acute myocardial infarction: trial to investigate equivalence. *Lancet.* 1995;346:329-336.

74. Erikkson BI, Quinlan DJ, Weitz JI. Comparative pharmacodynamics and pharmacokinetics of oral direct thrombin inhibitors and factor Xa inhibitors in development. *Clin Pharmacokinet.* 2009;48(1):1-22.

75. Smalling RW. A fresh look at the molecular pharmacology of plasminogen activators: from theory to test tube to clinical outcomes. *Am J Health Syst Pharm.* 1997;54:S17-S22.

76. ASSENT-2 Investigators. Single-bolus tenecteplase compared with front-loaded alteplase in acute myocardial infarction: the ASSENT-2 double-blind randomised trial. *Lancet.* 1999;354:716-722.

77. Haynes RB et al. A critical appraisal of ticlopidine, a new antiplatelet agent. Effectiveness and clinical indications for prophylaxis of atherosclerotic events. *Arch Intern Med.* 1992;152:1376-1380.

78. Matchar DB et al. Medical treatment for stroke prevention. *Ann Intern Med.* 1994;121:41-53.

79. Carlson JA, Maesner JE. Fatal neutropenia and thrombocytopenia associated with ticlopidine. *Ann Pharmacother.* 1994;28:1236-1238.

80. Cassidy LJ et al. Probable ticlopidine-induced cholestatic hepatitis. *Ann Pharmacother.* 1995;29:30-32.

81. Hass WK et al. A randomized trial comparing ticlopidine hydrochloride with aspirin for the prevention of stroke in high-risk patients. *N Engl J Med.* 1989;321:501-507.

82. Gent M et al. The Canadian American Ticlopidine Study (CATS) in thromboembolic stroke. *Lancet.* 1989;1: 1215-1220.

83. The PRISM-PLUS Study Investigators. Inhibition of the platelet glycoprotein IIb/IIIa receptor with tirofiban in unstable angina and non–Q-wave myocardial infarction. *N Engl J Med.* 1998;338:1488-1497.

84. Breckenridge A et al. Pharmacokinetics and pharmacodynamics of the enantiomers of warfarin in man. *Clin Pharmacol Ther.* 1974;15:424-430.

85. Fihn SD. Aiming for safe anticoagulation. *N Engl J Med.* 1995;333:54-55. Editorial.

86. O'Reilly RA, Aggeler PM. Determinants of the response to oral anticoagulant drugs in man. *Pharmacol Rev.* 1970;22:35-96.

87. Nagashima R et al. Kinetics of pharmacologic effects in man: the anticoagulant action of warfarin. *Clin Pharmacol Ther.* 1969;10:22-35.

88. Lutomski DM et al. Warfarin absorption after massive small bowel resection. *Am J Gastroenterol.* 1985;80: 99-102.

89. Slaughter RL, Edwards DJ. Recent advances: the cytochrome P450 enzymes. *Ann Pharmacother.* 1995;29:619-624.

90. Yacobi A et al. Serum protein binding as a determinant of warfarin body clearance and anticoagulant effect. *Clin Pharmacol Ther.* 1976;19:552-558.

91. Lewis RJ et al. Warfarin metabolites: the anticoagulant activity and pharmacology of warfarin alcohols. *J Lab Clin Med.* 1973;81:925-931.

92. O'Reilly RA et al. Studies on the coumarin anticoagulant drugs: the pharmacodynamics of warfarin in man. *J Clin Invest.* 1963;42:1542-1551.

93. Williams RL et al. Influence of acute viral hepatitis on disposition and pharmacologic effect of warfarin. *Clin Pharmacol Ther.* 1976;20:90-97.

94. Byeth RJ, Quinn LM, Landefeld CS. Prospective evaluation of an index for predicting the risk of major bleeding in outpatients treated with warfarin. *Am J Med.* 1998;105:91-99.

95. Kuijer PMM, Hutten BA, Prins MH, et al. Prediction of the risk of bleeding during anticoagulation treatment for venous thromboembolism. *Arch Intern Med.* 1999;159:457-460.

96. Hirsh J. Drug therapy: oral anticoagulant drugs. *N Engl J Med.* 1991;324:1865-1875.

97. Landefeld CS, Goldman L. Major bleeding in outpatients treated with warfarin: incidence and prediction by factors known at the start of outpatient therapy. *Am J Med* .1989;87:144-152.

98. Hansten PD, Horn JR. *Drug interactions and updates quarterly* (updated quarterly). Vancouver, WA: Applied Therapeutics; 2001.

99. Tatro DS, ed. *Drug interaction facts* (updated quarterly). Philadelphia, PA: JB Lippincott; 2001.

100. Deykin D. Warfarin therapy (second of two parts). *N Engl J Med.* 1970;283:801-803.

Chapter 48

Hematopoietics

Catherine E. Ferara

EPOETIN ALFA Epogen, Procrit

Pharmacology. Epoetin alfa (erythropoietin) is a recombinant human glycoprotein produced from mammalian cells and stimulates production of RBC. The product contains the identical amino acid sequence and produces the same biologic effects as natural erythropoietin.[1-4]

Administration and Adult Dosage. IV or SQ for dialysis or nondialysis chronic renal failure patients—50–100 units/kg, 3 times/wk initially, increasing or decreasing by 25 units/kg to maintain a target hematocrit of 30%–36%. When the target hematocrit is reached (or when the increase >4% in any 2-week period), reduce the dosage to 25 units/kg, 3 times/wk. If at any time the hematocrit exceeds 36%, discontinue epoetin until the target hematocrit is achieved and then resume at a lower dosage. Individualize the maintenance dosage to maintain the target hematocrit. **IV or SQ for zidovudine-treated or HIV-infected patients**—100 units/kg, 3 times/wk for 8 weeks initially, increasing or decreasing by 50–100 units/kg based on response; maximum effective dosage is 300 units/kg, 3 times/wk. If hematocrit exceeds 40%, discontinue epoetin until the hematocrit returns to 36% and then reduce dosage by 25% adjust dosage to maintain desired hematocrit target. Patients with initial erythropoietin levels >500 units/L are unlikely to respond to epoetin. **SQ for anemia in chemotherapy-treated cancer patients**—150 units/kg, 3 times/wk for 8 weeks initially, increasing to 300 units/kg, 3 times/wk if there is an unsatisfactory reduction in transfusion requirement or an unsatisfactory increase in hematocrit. If hematocrit exceeds 40%, discontinue epoetin until the hematocrit returns to 36% and then reduce dosage by 25%; adjust dosage to maintain desired hematocrit target. **SQ for reduction of allogenic blood transfusion in surgery patients**—300 units/kg/d for 10 days before surgery, on day of surgery, and 4 days after surgery; alternatively, 600 units/kg/wk 21, 14, and 7 days before surgery and on day of surgery. For use in anemic patients (hemoglobin >10 g/dL and ≤13 g/dL) undergoing noncardiac, nonvascular surgery with an anticipated large blood loss.

Special Populations. *Pediatric Dosage.* Safety and efficacy not established. **SQ for anemia of prematurity**—(preterm neonates) 200 units (140 units/kg) every other day for 10 doses;[5] alternatively, 250 units/kg, 3 times/wk.[4] **SQ or IV for anemia of end-stage renal disease**—(newborns to 18-year olds) 50 units/kg, 3 times/wk has been used.[6,7,8]

Geriatric Dosage. Same as adult dosage.

Dosage Forms. Inj 2000, 3000, 4000, 10000, 20000, 40000 units/mL.

Pharmacokinetics. *Onset and Duration.* In response to administration 3 times/week, reticulocyte count increases within 10 days followed by increases in RBC count, hematocrit, and hemoglobin in about 2–6 weeks.

Fate. Not orally bioavailable. Peak serum levels occur 5–24 h after SQ administration. V_d is 0.033–0.055 L/kg; CL is about 0.00282 L/h/kg.[1]

Half-life is 9.3 ± 3.3 h initially; 6.2 ± 1.8 h during long-term therapy.[1]

Adverse Reactions. Hypertension, headache, tachycardia, nausea, vomiting, clotted vascular access, shortness of breath, hyperkalemia, and diarrhea occur frequently. Seizures occur occasionally; CVA, TIA, and MI occur rarely.[1-4]

Contraindications. Uncontrolled hypertension. Hypersensitivity to mammalian cell-derived products or albumin.

Precautions. Pregnancy. Use cautiously with a known history of seizure or underlying hematologic diseases such as sickle cell anemia, myelodysplastic syndromes, and hypercoagulable states.

Drug Interactions. None known.

Parameters to Monitor. Evaluate iron stores before and during therapy. Supplemental iron might be required to maintain a transferrin saturation of at least 20% and ferritin levels of at least 100 µg/L. Determine hematocrit twice a week for 2–6 weeks or until stabilized in the target range; monitor at regular intervals thereafter. Monitor CBC with differential platelet count, BUN, Cr_s, serum uric acid, serum phosphorus, and serum potassium at regular intervals.

Notes. Darbepoetin (Aranesp–Amgen) is a highly glycosylated form of erythropoetin that is absorbed slowly and can be given once weekly or every 2 weeks. The weekly dose in µg/kg equals the total weekly dosage of epoetin alfa in IV/week divided by 200.

FERROUS SALTS Various

Pharmacology. Ferrous salts are soluble forms of iron, an essential nutrient that functions primarily as the oxygen-binding core of heme in red blood cells (as hemoglobin) and muscles (as myoglobin) and in the respiratory enzyme cytochrome C.

Administration and Adult Dosage. PO as a dietary supplement—RDAs are 10 mg/d for men (19–51 years) and 15 mg/d for women (19–51 years).[5] **PO for treatment of iron deficiency**—2–3 mg/kg/d of elemental iron in divided doses. (*See* Ferrous Salts Comparison Chart for usual dosage ranges for individual salts.) Dose-related adverse effects can be decreased by using suboptimal dosages, increasing the daily dosage gradually, or administering with a small amount of food (although this latter method reduces absorption). After hemoglobin is normalized, continue oral therapy for 3–6 months to replenish iron stores.

Special Populations. *Pediatric Dosage.* **PO for prophylaxis**—RDA (infants) 6 mg/d; (1–10 years) 10 mg/d; (11–18 years, males) 12 mg/d; (11–18 years, females) 15 mg/d.[5] **PO for treatment**—(infants), 10–25 mg of elemental iron in 3–4 divided doses; (6 months to 2 years) up to 6 mg/kg/d of elemental iron in 3–4 divided doses; (2–12 years) 3 mg/kg/d of elemental iron in 3–4 divided doses.

Geriatric Dosage. Same as adult dosage, except dosage in women older than 51 years is 10 mg/d of elemental iron.

FERROUS SALTS COMPARISON CHART

DRUG	SOLID DOSAGE FORMS[a]	ADULT DOSAGE (CAP OR TAB/DAY)	ELEMENTAL IRON/CAP OR TAB (%)	ELEMENTAL IRON/CAP OR TAB (mg Fe)	OTHER DOSAGE FORMS[a]
Carbonyl Iron	Cap 50 mg iron	3	100	50	Susp 12 mg/mL iron
Ferrous Fumarate	Chew Tab 100 mg	1–4	33	33	Drp 75 mg/mL
	Tab 63, 200, 324, 325, 350 mg	1–4	33	20, 66, 106, 106, 115	Susp 20 mg/mL
Ferrous Gluconate	Tab 240, 325 mg	5–6	11	27, 36	Elxr 60 mg/mL
Ferrous Sulfate	SR Tab 160 mg	1–2	30	50	
Exsiccated	Tab 187, 200 mg	5–4	30	60, 65	
Ferrous Sulfate	SR Cap/Tab various	—	20	—	Drp 125 mg/mL
Hydrous	Cap 250 mg	3	20	50	Elxr 44 mg/mL
	Tab 195, 300, 324 mg	3–6	20	39, 60, 65	Syrup 18 mg/mL
Polysaccharide-	Cap 150 mg iron	1–2	—	150	Elxr 20 mg/mL iron
Iron Complex	Tab 50 mg iron	2–4	—	50	

[a]Doses listed represent total iron salt, not elemental iron, except for carbonyl iron and polysaccharide-iron complex.

Other Conditions. Iron requirement during pregnancy is approximately twice that of the normal, nonpregnant woman because of an expanding blood volume and the demands of the fetus and placenta. The RDA in pregnancy is 30 mg/d, and a prophylactic dose of 15–30 mg/d of elemental iron during the second and third trimesters has been recommended to prevent depletion of maternal iron stores. Iron-deficient patients might need higher doses.

Dosage Forms. *See* Ferrous Salts Comparison Chart.

Patient Instructions. Take this drug with a full glass of water on an empty stomach (1 h before or 2 h after meals) for best absorption. Take liquid preparations in water or juice and drink with a straw to minimize tooth staining. If gastric distress or nausea occurs, a small quantity of food can be taken with the drug but do not take with antacids because absorption is decreased. Iron preparations can cause constipation and black stools. Keep all iron products out of the reach of children.

Missed Doses. Take this drug at regular intervals. If you miss a dose, take it as soon as you remember. If it is about time for the next dose, take that dose only. Do not double the dose or take extra.

Pharmacokinetics. *Onset and Duration.* Responses to equivalent amounts of oral or parenteral therapy are essentially the same. Reticulocytes increase within 4–7 days and reach a peak on about the 10th day. An increase in hemoglobin of at least 2 g/dL and a 6% increase in hematocrit should occur in about 3–4 weeks. Three to six months of therapy is generally required for restoration of iron stores.[9,10]

Serum Levels. Normal levels are 65–170 μg/dL (12–30 μmol/L) in men, 50–170 μg/dL (9–30 μmol/L) in women, and 50–120 μg/dL (9–21 μmol/L) in children. A decrease in the transferrin saturation (serum iron ÷ total iron-binding capacity × 100) indicates preanemic iron deficiency. A transferrin saturation <16% or plasma ferritin concentration <12 μg/L indicates probable iron deficiency.[9,10] In overdosage, toxicity can occur at iron levels >350 μg/dL (63 μmol/L). Chelation therapy is indicated at these levels, especially if the patient is symptomatic.[9]

Fate. Iron is absorbed primarily from the duodenum at a rate that depends on the amount of iron in storage sites. About 10% of dietary iron is absorbed in normal subjects, 20% in iron-deficient patients, and as much as 70% of medicinal iron is absorbed during marked iron deficiency or increased erythropoiesis. In the plasma, iron is oxidized to the ferric state, combined with transferrin, and used or stored as ferritin (mostly in the reticuloendothelial system and hepatocytes). The average loss in the healthy adult male is about 1 mg/d. GI loss of extravasated red cells, iron in bile, and exfoliated mucosal cells accounts for two-thirds of this iron. The other one-third is lost in the skin and urine. Menstruating women have an additional loss of about 0.5 mg/d.

Adverse Reactions. Side effects are related primarily to the dose of elemental iron. Frequent GI irritation, constipation, and stained teeth (liquid preparations only—dilute and use a drinking straw). An increased risk of cancer associated with excessive iron stores has been reported.[11]

Contraindications. Hemochromatosis; hemosiderosis; hemolytic anemias in which no true iron deficiency exists.

Precautions. Use with caution in patients with peptic ulcer, regional enteritis, or ulcerative colitis. Serious acute poisoning (which can be fatal) occurs frequently in children: doses as low as 20 mg/kg of elemental iron can cause toxicity; 40 mg/kg is considered serious; and >60 mg/kg is potentially lethal.[12]

Drug Interactions. Food, calcium carbonate, sodium bicarbonate, and possibly magnesium trisilicate can reduce iron absorption. Vitamin E can reduce utilization of iron in iron-deficiency anemia. Iron salts can reduce oral absorption of carbidopa/levodopa, methyldopa, penicillamine, quinolones, tetracyclines, and thyroid hormones.

Parameters to Monitor. Periodic reticulocyte count, hemoglobin, and hematocrit. (*See* Onset and Duration.)

Notes. Ferrous salts are used to prevent and treat iron-deficiency anemias. Such anemias occur most frequently with exceptional blood losses (e.g., pathologic bleeding, menstruation) and during periods of rapid growth (e.g., infancy, adolescence, pregnancy). Iron is ineffective in hemoglobin disturbances not caused by iron deficiency. Concurrent administration of high doses of **vitamin C** can enhance absorption (particularly when given with SR formulations), but cost/benefit might not warrant its use. Wide variations in dissolution and absorption exist between SR and EC products, and the frequency of adverse effects, although negligible, probably reflects the small amount of ionic iron available for absorption because of transport of the iron past the duodenum and proximal jejunum.[13]

FILGRASTIM
Neupogen

Pharmacology. Filgrastim is an *Escherichia coli*–derived (nonglycosylated) recombinant human granulocyte colony-stimulating factor (G-CSF). G-CSF is one of many glycoprotein hormones that regulate the proliferation and differentiation of hematopoietic progenitor cells and the function of mature blood cells. Specifically, G-CSF promotes proliferation and maturation and enhances the function and migration of neutrophil granulocytes. G-CSF also promotes pre B cell activation and growth and acts in synergy with interleukin-3 to support megakaryocyte and platelet production.[2,14]

Administration and Adult Dosage. **SQ or IV for myelosuppressive cancer chemotherapy**—5 μg/kg/d as a single injection. The drug is usually discontinued once the postnadir ANC reaches 1500–2000/μL. Based on severity of ANC nadir, dosage can be increased in 5 μg/kg/d increments for each chemotherapy cycle. **SQ continuous infusion for chemotherapy-induced febrile neutropenia**—12 μg/kg/d beginning within 12 h of empiric antibiotic therapy and continued until ANC is >5000/μL and the patient is afebrile for 4 days.[15] **IV or SQ for bone marrow transplant patients**—10 μg/kg/d infused IV over 4 or 24 h or as a continuous SQ infusion and then decreasing to 5 μg/kg/d when ANC is >1000/μL for 3 consecutive days. Discontinue therapy if the ANC remains >1000/μL for 3 more consecutive days; resume at a dosage of 5 μg/kg/d when ANC becomes <1000/μL. **SQ for severe chronic neutropenia**—(congenital) 6 μg/kg bid; (idiopathic or cyclic) 5 μg/kg/d. Target ANC range is 1500–10,000/μL; decrease dosage if ANC is persistently >10,000/μL. **SQ with erythropoietin to decrease hematologic toxicity from zidovudine**—3.6 μg/kg/d initially, increasing or decreasing weekly by 1 μg/kg/d to maintain a target ANC of 1500–5000/μL.[16]

Special Populations. *Pediatric Dosage.* Safety and efficacy not established. **IV or SQ**—adult dosages in μg/kg are well tolerated.

Geriatric Dosage. Same as adult dosage.

Dosage Forms. Inj 300, 600 μg/mL.

Patient Instructions. Your pharmacist or physician should instruct you on proper dosage, administration, and disposal. Store vials in the refrigerator but do not freeze. Vials are designed for single use only; discard any unused portion. Bring vial to room temperature before administration; do not shake.

Pharmacokinetics. *Onset and Duration.* Increase in neutrophilic band forms occurs within about 60 min after administration. After therapy is discontinued, neutrophil counts return to baseline values in about 4 days.[14]

Fate. Not orally bioavailable. V_d is about 0.15 L/kg; CL is 0.03–0.042 L/h/kg. **Half-life** is 3.5–3.85 h.

Adverse Reactions. Mild to moderate bone pain responsive to nonnarcotic analgesics is reported frequently. Transient decreases in blood pressure occur occasionally. During long-term therapy, splenomegaly occurs frequently; occasional exacerbation of skin disorders, alopecia, hematuria, proteinuria, thrombocytopenia, and osteoporosis also are reported. Other adverse effects occur during administration of filgrastim that are likely the consequence of the underlying malignancy or cytotoxic chemotherapy. Acute reactions to sargramostim (e.g., febrile episodes, flushing, hypotension, tachycardia, and hypoxia) appear to be more common than with filgrastim.[2,14,16,17]

Contraindications. History of hypersensitivity to *E. coli*–derived proteins. Do not use 24 h before and 24 h after administration of cytotoxic chemotherapy.

Precautions. Use with caution in any malignancy with myeloid characteristics because of the possibility of tumor growth. The efficacy of filgrastim has not been established in patients receiving nitrosoureas, mitomycin, fluorouracil, or cytarabine.

Drug Interactions. None known.

Parameters to Monitor. Perform CBC and platelet counts before chemotherapy and twice a week during filgrastim therapy. Regular monitoring of WBC count at the time of recovery from the postchemotherapy nadir is recommended to avoid excessive leukocytosis.

Notes. Other potential uses for filgrastim include AIDS-related neutropenia, myelodysplastic syndromes, and drug-induced neutropenia or aplastic anemia. Further clinical trials are needed to prove that use of filgrastim for these and other indications is beneficial, safe, and cost effective.

IRON DEXTRAN	DexFerrum, InFeD, Various

Pharmacology. (*See* Ferrous Salts.) The overall response to parenteral iron is no more rapid or complete than the response to orally administered iron, so iron dextran is indicated only when oral iron therapy is determined to be ineffective or impossible.

Administration and Adult Dosage. The total cumulative amount required for restoration of hemoglobin (Hb) in g/dL and body stores of iron can be approximated using lean body weight (LBW) in kg (or actual body weight if less than LBW) from the formula:

$$\text{Total mg iron} = (0.0442 \times [\text{desired Hb} - \text{observed Hb}] \times \text{LBW} + [0.26 \times \text{LBW}]) \times 50$$

To calculate dose in mL, divide the result by 50. Usual Hb target for adults is 14.8 g/dL. The dose of iron required secondary to blood loss can be estimated from the formula:

$$\text{Total mg iron} = \text{blood loss (mL)} \times \text{hematocrit (observed, as decimal fraction)}$$

Deep IM—(in upper outer quadrant of buttock only with the Z-track technique) 25 mg (0.5 mL) test dose the first day and then, if no adverse reaction occurs, administer a maximum daily dose of 100 mg (2 mL) until the total calculated amount is reached. **Slow IV**—test dose of 25 mg (0.5 mL) over at least 30 s the first day; if no adverse reaction occurs after at least 1 h, proceed (until the total calculated amount is reached) by daily increments over 2–3 days, to a maximum dose of 100 mg/d at a rate not to exceed 50 mg/min.[16] **IV in erythropoietin-treated dialysis patients**—100–200 mg/wk after dialysis. **Total dose IV infusion**—is an off-label use and is discouraged by the FDA but is widely used. The total calculated dose of iron dextran is diluted in 500 mL of NS (dextrose solutions increase local phlebitis) and infused at a rate of 6 mg/min after a 30 mL test dose is delivered over 2 min.[18]

Special Populations. *Pediatric Dosage.* (<4 months) safety and efficacy not established; (5–15 kg) total cumulative amount required for restoration of Hb (in g/dL) and body stores of iron can be estimated using body weight (W) in kg from the formula:

$$\text{Total mg iron} = (0.0442 \times [\text{desired Hb} - \text{observed Hb}] \times W + [0.26 \times W]) \times 50$$

To calculate dose in mL, divide the result by 50. Usual Hb target for children ≤15 kg is 12 g/dL. Maximum daily dose is (infants <5 kg) 25 mg (0.5 mL), (children <10 kg) 50 mg (1 mL), (children >15 kg) same as adult dosage.

Geriatric Dosage. Same as adult dosage.

Dosage Forms. **Inj** 50 mg elemental iron/mL.

Pharmacokinetics. *Onset and Duration.* Hematologic response is the same as with oral therapy, although total body stores of iron are replaced when the above dosage regimens are used.

Serum Levels. See Ferrous Salts.

Fate. After IV administration, the inert complex is gradually cleared from the plasma by the reticuloendothelial cells of the liver, spleen, and bone marrow. With doses >500 mg, the rate of uptake is 10–20 mg/h. Iron dextran is then dissociated and released as free ferric iron (at a rate controlled by the serum iron level), which combines with transferrin and is incorporated into hemoglobin within the bone marrow.[18-20] Although all iron is eventually released in this manner, many months, often, are required for this process to be completed.[9]

Adverse Reactions. Hypotension and peripheral vascular flushing occur with too rapid IV administration. Mild, transient reactions including flushing, fever, myalgia, arthralgia, and lymphadenopathy usually occur only occasionally but have occurred in 80%–90% of patients with active rheumatoid arthritis or active SLE. Immediate anaphylactoid reactions, which can be life-threatening, occur in 0.1%–0.6% of patients.[21] A predictive test for predisposition to anaphylaxis is not available. IM administration has been associated with variable degrees of soreness, sterile abscess formation, tissue staining, and sarcoma formation.[19] Total dose infusion appears to be tolerated as well as divided doses.[18]

Contraindications. Anemias other than iron-deficiency anemia; hemochromatosis; hemosiderosis; SQ administration.

Precautions. Pregnancy. Use with extreme caution with serious liver impairment. Patients with rheumatoid arthritis might have an acute exacerbation or reactivation of joint pain and swelling after administration. History of allergies or asthma. Because of the potential for anaphylactoid reactions, have epinephrine, diphenhydramine, and methylprednisolone immediately available during iron dextran administration. Use parenteral iron only in patients in whom an iron-deficient state has been clearly established and who are not amenable to oral therapy.

Drug Interactions. None known.

Parameters to Monitor. *See* Ferrous Salts.

Notes. *Sodium ferric gluconate complex* (Ferrlecit) is an injectable iron product containing 12.5 mg/mL of elemental iron. It is indicated for iron-deficiency anemia in chronic hemodialysis patients receiving epoetin alfa. A test dose is not required, but a test dose of 2 mL in 50 mL of NS given IV over 1 h has been used. The standard dose is 10 mL/100 mL NS infused over 1 h. Most patients require a total dosage of 1 g of elemental iron in 8 doses on sequential dialysis sessions to replete iron stores. It might be better tolerated than iron dextran, but it is much more expensive. It is a good alternative in patients intolerant to iron dextran.

Iron sucrose (Venofer) is an injectable iron product containing 20 mg/mL of elemental iron. It is indicated for iron-deficiency anemia in chronic hemodialysis patients receiving epoetin alfa. A test dose is not required, but a test dose of 2.5 mL in 50 mL of NS over 3–10 min has been used. The drug can be given by direct IV injection at a rate of 1 mL (20 mg of iron) per minute or by slow infusion by diluting one vial (100 mg iron) in no more than 100 mL of NS and infusing it over at least 15 min. The recommended dosage is 100 mg of iron (1 vial) no more than 3 times per week to a total of 1 g in 10 doses. This regimen can be repeated if necessary.

SARGRAMOSTIM Leukine

Pharmacology. Sargramostim is a yeast-derived (glycosylated) recombinant human granulocyte–macrophage colony-stimulating factor (GM-CSF). GM-CSF is one of many glycoprotein hormones that regulate the proliferation and differentiation of hematopoietic progenitor cells and the function of mature blood cells. Specifically, GM-CSF promotes proliferation; maturation; and functions of neutrophils, eosinophils, monocytes, and macrophages. GM-CSF also stimulates production of cytokines such as interleukin-1 and tumor necrosis factor.[14,17,22]

Administration and Adult Dosage. **IV after autologous bone marrow infusion**— 250 μg/m²/d given as a 2-h infusion beginning 2–4 h after the autologous bone marrow infusion. Give the first dose no sooner than 24 h after the last chemotherapy dose or 12 h after the last dose of radiotherapy. Continue sargramostim until the ANC is >1500/μL for 3 consecutive days. **IV for bone marrow transplantation failure or delay in engraftment**—250 μg/m²/d for 14 days as a 2-h infusion; repeat in 7 days if engraftment has not occurred. If there is no improvement, a third course with 500 μg/m²/d given for 14 days can be tried. **IV for induction chemotherapy in acute myelogenous leukemia**—250 μg/m²/d over 4 h starting 4 days after completion of chemotherapy if bone marrow is hypoplastic (<5% blasts). Continue until ANC is >1500/μL for 3 consecutive days or at most 42 days. Discontinue or reduce dosage by 50% if ANC is >20,000/μL. Discontinue if leukemic regrowth occurs. **SQ for AIDS patients receiving ganciclovir**—1–15 μg/kg/d has been used investigationally.

Dosage Forms. Inj 250, 500 μg.

Adverse Reactions. Acute reactions (e.g., febrile episodes, flushing, hypotension, tachycardia, and hypoxia) appear to be more common than with filgrastim. Other adverse reactions that occur frequently with sargramostim are bone pain, lethargy, rash, and fluid retention.

Parameters to Monitor. Obtain CBC with differential twice weekly. In patients with renal or hepatic insufficiency, monitor renal and hepatic functions q2wk.

Notes. Sargramostim is indicated for myeloid reconstitution after autologous bone marrow transplantation. It has also been used with some success to maintain normal neutrophil counts in AIDS patients receiving **ganciclovir**. Other potential uses for sargramostim are AIDS-related neutropenia, myelodysplastic syndromes, and congenital, chronic, or drug-induced neutropenia, and aplastic anemia. Controlled clinical trials are needed to prove that use for these and other indications are beneficial, safe, and cost-effective. Clinical and laboratory evidence suggests that sargramostim enhances the effect of **zidovudine** against HIV.[2,14,17,22–24]

■ REFERENCES

1. Schwenk MH, Halstenson CE. Recombinant human erythropoietin. *DICP.* 1989;23:528-536.
2. Petersdorf SH, Dale DC. The biology and clinical applications of erythropoietin and the colony-stimulating factors. *Adv Intern Med.* 1995;40:395-428.
3. Erslev AJ. Erythropoietin. *N Engl J Med.* 1991;324:1339-1344.
4. Zachée P. Controversies in selection of epoetin dosages. Issues and answers. *Drugs.* 1995;49:536-547.
5. Food and Nutrition Board, NRC. *Recommended dietary allowances.* 10th ed. Washington, DC: National Academy Press; 1989.
6. Ohis RK, Christensen RD. Recombinant erythropoietin compared with erythrocyte transfusion in the treatment of anemia of prematurity. *J Pediatr.* 1991;119:781-788.
7. Ongkingco JR et al. Use of low-dose subcutaneous recombinant human erythropoietin in end-stage renal disease: experience with children receiving continuous cycling peritoneal dialysis. *Am J Kidney Dis.* 1991;18:446-450.
8. Rigden SP et al. Recombinant human erythropoietin therapy in children maintained by haemodialysis. *Pediatr Nephrol.* 1990;4:618-622.
9. Hardman JG et al., eds. *Goodman and Gilman's the pharmacological basis of therapeutics.* 9th ed. New York: McGraw-Hill; 1996.

10. Koeller JM, Van Den Berg C. Anemias. In: Koda-Kimble MA, Young LY, eds. *Applied therapeutics: the clinical use of drugs*. 6th ed. Vancouver, WA: Applied Therapeutics; 1995:88.3-88.17.

11. Stevens RG. Iron and the risk of cancer. *Med Oncol Tumor Pharmacother*. 1990;7:177-181.

12. Olson KR, ed. *Poisoning and drug overdose*. Norwalk, CT: Appleton & Lange; 1990.

13. Middleton EJ et al. Studies on the absorption of orally administered iron from sustained-release preparations. *N Engl J Med*. 1966;274:136-139.

14. Anon. G-CSF and GM-CSF: white blood cell growth factors. *Hosp Pharm* 1990;25:881-882.

15. Maher DW et al. Filgrastim in patients with chemotherapy-induced febrile neutropenia. *Ann Intern Med*. 1994;121:492-501.

16. Miles SA et al. Combined therapy with recombinant granulocyte colony-stimulating factor and erythropoietin decreases hematologic toxicity zidovudine. *Blood*. 1991;77:2109-2117.

17. Demuynck H et al. Comparative study of peripheral blood progenitor cell collection in patients with multiple myeloma after single-dose cyclophosphamide combined with rhGM-CSF or rhG-CSF. *Br J Haematol*. 1995; 90:384-392.

18. Auerbach M et al. A randomized trial of three iron dextran infusion methods for anemia in EPO-treated dialysis patients. *Am J Kidney Dis*. 1998;31:81-86.

19. Kumpf VJ, Holland EG. Parenteral iron dextran therapy. *DICP*. 1990;24:162-166.

20. Wood JK et al. The metabolism of iron-dextran given as a total-dose infusion to iron deficient Jamaican subjects. *Br J Haematol*. 1968;14:119-129.

21. Novey HS et al. Immunologic studies of anaphylaxis to iron dextran in patients on renal dialysis. *Ann Allergy*. 1994;72:224-228.

22. Hogan KR, Peters MD. Granulocyte-macrophage colony-stimulating factor in neutropenia. *DICP*. 1991;25:32-35.

23. Grossberg HS, Bonnem EM. GM-CSF with ganciclovir for the treatment of CMV retinitis in AIDS. *N Engl J Med*. 1989;320(letter):1560.

24. Groopman JE. Granulocyte-macrophage colony-stimulating factor in human immunodeficiency virus disease. *Semin Hematol*. 1990;27(suppl 3):8-14.

Hormonal Drugs | 8

Nickole N. Henyan

Chapter 49

Adrenal Hormones

Andrea N. Traina and Michael P. Kane

SYSTEMIC CORTICOSTEROIDS

Class Instructions. Endogenous corticosteroids exhibit a circadian rhythm, with the peak release occurring between 2 and 8 AM; therefore, single daily doses or alternate-day doses are given in the morning before 9 AM to mimic the circadian rhythm and minimize suppression of the hypothalamic pituitary–adrenal (HPA) axis. Take multiple daily doses at evenly spaced intervals during the day. To minimize GI upset, these drugs may be taken with food, milk, or antacids. Contact your physician if you experience any unusual weight gain, lower extremity swelling, muscle weakness, black tarry stools, vomiting of blood, facial swelling, menstrual irregularities, prolonged sore throat, fever, cold, infection, serious injury, fatigue, anorexia, nausea, vomiting, diarrhea, weight loss, dizziness, or low blood sugar. Consult your physician during periods of increased stress. If you have diabetes, you may have increased requirements for insulin or oral hypoglycemic agents. Carry appropriate identification (i.e., medical bracelet) if you are taking long-term corticosteroid therapy. Seek emergency department admission if you experience prolonged vomiting that prevents administration of corticosteroid doses. Do not discontinue this medication without medical approval; tell any new health care provider that you are taking a corticosteroid. Avoid immunizations with live vaccines.

Missed Doses. If a dose is missed and the proper schedule is *every other day*, take it as soon as possible and resume the schedule unless it is past noon. In that case, wait until the next morning and resume every-other-day administration. If the proper schedule is *once a day*, take the dose as soon as possible. If you do not remember until the next day, do not double that day's dose; skip the missed dose. If the proper schedule is *several times a day*, take the dose as soon as possible and resume the normal schedule. If you do not remember until the next dose is due, then take the regular and missed doses and resume the normal dosage schedule.

Stress Dosing. During times of medical or surgical stress, patients with adrenal insufficiency require supplemental steroid doses in addition to their maintenance steroid dose. The necessary amount of supplementation varies from the usual daily steroid dose to multiple times the usual daily dose based on the type of illness or surgery and the degree of associated stress.[1]

COSYNTROPIN
Cortrosyn

Pharmacology. Cosyntropin is a synthetic polypeptide containing the first 24 of the 39 amino acids of natural **corticotropin (adrenocorticotropic hormone; ACTH)** which retains the full activity of corticotropin with decreased antigenicity. Cosyntropin 250 μg is pharmacologically equivalent to corticotropin 25 units. Cosyntropin stimulates the adrenal cortex to produce and secrete gluco- and mineralocorticoids and androgens similar to corticotropin. Cosyntropin is used as a diagnostic agent to detect adrenocortical insufficiency; it is no longer used therapeutically as a replacement for corticotrophin or glucocorticoids.

Administration and Adult Dosage. **IM or IV** hold all exogenous corticosteroids (except dexamethasone) on the test day because of assay cross-reactivity and, if the patient is not taking spironolactone or an estrogen, a baseline cortisol level (which should exceed 5 g/dL) is drawn in the morning just before the dose. Then, cosyntropin 250 μg in 1 mL of NS is given IM, or 250 μg in 2–5 mL NS is given IV push over 2 min. Normal cortisol levels are >18 μg/dL (500 nmol/L) 30 min after the injection and 7 μg/dL (190 nmol/L) above baseline. The cortisol level is drawn 60 min post administration; doubling of the baseline cortisol value indicates a normal response. Alternatively, give an infusion of 250 μg in D5W or NS over 6 h in the morning, with serum cortisol levels drawn before and after. The second cortisol level should be >18 μ/dL (500 nmol/L) and ≥7 μg/dL (190 nmol/L) above baseline.[2,3]

Pediatric Dosage. **IM or IV as a diagnostic agent**—≤2 years of age 125 μg given as above; >2 years of age refer to adult dosing.

Geriatric Dosage. Refer to adult dosing.

Dosage Forms. **Inj** 250 μg.

Adverse Reactions. Rare reports of hypersensitivity.

DEXAMETHASONE
Decadron, Dexamethasone Intensol, Various

Pharmacology. Dexamethasone is a potent, long-acting glucocorticoid lacking sodium-retaining activity at low to moderate doses. (*See* Prednisone Pharmacology and the Systemic Corticosteroids Comparison Chart.)

Administration and Adult Dosage. Total daily dosage is variable depending on the clinical disorder and patient response. Not recommended for alternate-day administration because of prolonged duration of activity. **PO, IM, or IV for acute, self-limited allergic disorders or exacerbation of chronic allergic disorders**— 4–8 mg on the first day in 1 dose, 3 mg in 2 divided doses days 2 and 3, 1.5 mg in 2 divided doses day 4, 0.75 mg daily days 5 and 6, then discontinue. **IV for cerebral edema**—10 mg (as sodium phosphate) initially, followed by 4 mg IM or IV q6h for several days until maximal response occurs; then decrease the dosage over 5–7 days and discontinue. **PO, IM, or IV for palliative management of recurrent or inoperable brain tumors**—2 mg bid–tid. **PO or IV as an antiemetic with**

cancer chemotherapy (can be in combination with other antiemetics)—8–20 mg immediately before therapy; 8–16 mg daily for 2–4 days after chemotherapy depending on the chemotherapy emetogenic profile.[4] **PO as the dexamethasone suppression test to screen for Cushing's disease**—1 mg at 11 PM; a measured serum cortisol at 8 AM the next morning <5 μg/dL (140 nmol/L) indicates a normal response. Alternatively, PO 0.5 mg q6h for 48 h (8 doses); a positive response is indicated by a serum cortisol concentration of <2 μg/dL (50 nmol/L) following 48 h of dexamethasone administration.[5] **PO as a Cushing's syndrome test to distinguish pituitary origin from other causes**—2 mg q6h for 48 h (8 doses). At hours 0 and 48, serum cortisol levels are measured; >50% decrease from baseline indicates a positive response.[5] **IM (depot) for prolonged systemic effect**—8–16 mg every 1–3 weeks. **PO, IM, or IV (as sodium phosphate) for physiologic replacement**—0.03–0.15 mg/kg/d in divided doses every 6–12 h. **IM in women at high risk of preterm delivery between 24 and 34 weeks of gestation, and in over 34 weeks gestation when there is evidence of fetal pulmonary immaturity**—6 mg q12 h for 4 doses. (*IM Betamethasone 12 mg q24h for 2 doses is the treatment of choice in this setting.*) For complete recommendations, see guidelines for antenatal corticosteroid use.[6]

Special Populations. *Pediatric Dosage.* **PO, IM, or IV for airway edema or extubation**—0.5–2 mg/kg/dose q6h beginning 24 h before planned extubation, then for 4–6 doses[7]; **PO, IM, or IV as an anti-inflammatory or immunosuppressive**—0.08–0.3 mg/kg/d divided every 6–12 h[8]; **IV for *Haemophilus influenzae* type b bacterial meningitis**—(>6 weeks of age) 0.15 mg/kg/dose divided q6h, beginning 1–2 h before or with the first dose of antibiotics and continuing for 2 days.[9]

Geriatric Dosage. Refer to adult dosing; however, use cautiously with the smallest possible dose.

Patient Instructions. *See* Class Instructions: Systemic Corticosteroids.

Dosage Forms. **Elxr** 0.1 mg/mL; **Soln** 0.1, 1 mg/mL; **Tab** 0.25, 0.5, 0.75, 1, 1.5, 2, 4, 6 mg; **Inj** 4, 10, 20, 24 mg/mL (as sodium phosphate); **Depot Inj** 8, 16 mg/mL (as acetate).

Pharmacokinetics. *See* Systemic Corticosteroids Comparison Chart.

Adverse Reactions. (*See* Prednisone Adverse Reactions.) Perineal itching or burning can occur after IV administration.[10]

Contraindications. Systemic fungal infections (except as maintenance therapy in adrenal insufficiency); administration of live virus vaccines to patients receiving immunosuppressive doses of dexamethasone; IM use in idiopathic thrombocytopenic purpura.

Precautions. *See* Prednisone Precautions.

Drug Interactions. **Dexamethasone is a CYP 3A4 substrate:** *Azole antifungals* are CYP 3A4 inhibitors and can increase the serum concentration of dexamethasone. *Carbamazepine, phenytoin, and rifampin* are CYP 3A4 inducers and can decrease the serum concentration of dexamethasone. **Dexamethasone is a CYP 3A4 inducer:** Dexamethasone can decrease the serum concentration of *quetiapine*.

Parameters to Monitor. *See* Prednisone Parameters to Monitor.

HYDROCORTISONE
Cortef, Anusol-HC, Solu-Cortef, Various

Pharmacology. Hydrocortisone is a naturally occurring glucocorticoid with anti-inflammatory and sodium-retaining properties. It is typically used as replacement therapy in adrenocortical deficiency states. (*See* Prednisone Pharmacology and the Systemic Corticosteroids Comparison Chart.)

Administration and Adult Dosage. **IV (as sodium succinate) for acute adrenal insufficiency**—100 mg IV bolus, then continuous IV infusion of 50–100 mg every 8 h. When the patient is stable, decrease to IV or PO 25 mg every 6–8 h, and then titrate and manage as chronic adrenal insufficiency[3]; **PO for chronic/physiologic replacement for adrenal insufficiency**—15–30 mg/d (e.g., 10–20 mg q AM, and 5–10 mg q PM)[1]; **PO, IM, or IV as an anti-inflammatory or immuno-suppressive**—15–240 mg q12 h; **rectally for ulcerative colitis** 10–100 mg 1–2 times/d for 2–3 weeks.[11]

Special Populations. *Pediatric Dosage.*[12] Dosage depends on disease state and patient response rather than strict adherence to age or body weight. **IM or IV for acute adrenal insufficiency**—*infants* up to 10 mg every 6 h for the first 24 h, then titrate based on response; *young children* up to 25 mg every 6 h for the first 24 h, then titrate based on response; *older children* up to 50 mg every 6 h for the first 24 h, then titrate based on response; **PO as physiologic replacement**—10–15 mg/m^2/d in 3 divided doses.

Geriatric Dosage. Refer to adult dosing. Use the smallest effective dose for the shortest possible duration.

Patient Instructions. *See* Class Instructions: Systemic Corticosteroids.

Dosage Forms. **Inj** 100, 250, 500 mg, 1 g; **Rectal Supp** 25, 30 mg; **Tab** 5,10, 20 mg.

Pharmacokinetics. *See* Systemic Corticosteroids Comparison Chart.

Adverse Reactions. *See* Prednisone Adverse Reactions.

Contraindications. Systemic fungal infections (except as maintenance therapy in adrenal insufficiency); administration of live virus vaccines in patients receiving immunosuppressive doses of hydrocortisone. IM use in idiopathic thrombocytopenia purpura.

Precautions. *See* Prednisone Precautions.

Drug Interactions. Hydrocortisone is a CYP 3A4 substrate: *Azole antifungals* are CYP 3A4 inhibitors and can increase the serum concentration of hydrocortisone. *Azole antifungals* have also been shown to inhibit adrenal corticosteroid synthesis, leading to adrenal insufficiency with corticosteroid withdrawal. *Phenobarbital, phenytoin,* and *rifampin* are CYP 3A4 inducers and can decrease the serum concentration of hydrocortisone.

Parameters to Monitor. *See* Prednisone Parameters to Monitor.

METHYLPREDNISOLONE SODIUM SUCCINATE
Solu-Medrol, Various

Pharmacology. Methylprednisolone sodium succinate is an injectable glucocorticoid that has an anti-inflammatory potency 1.25 times greater than that of prednisone, with a similar duration of biologic activity. (*See* Prednisone Pharmacology and the Systemic Corticosteroids Comparison Chart.) It is commonly used when oral therapy is not possible and in situations in which large parenteral doses are necessary. Only the sodium succinate formulation of methylprednisolone can be given IV.

Administration and Adult Dosage. **IV as an anti-inflammatory or immunosuppressive**—10–40 mg given over several minutes, repeat as needed; when high-dose therapy is indicated, dosages up to 30 mg/kg given over ≥30 min every 4–6 h for up to 48 h; infuse large doses (≥500 mg) slowly over 30–60 min because arrhythmias and sudden death have occurred with rapid infusions[13]; **IV for aplastic anemia**—1 mg/kg/d for 2–4 weeks, or 2 mg/kg/d for 2 weeks, followed by dosage taper for 2 weeks.[14,15] **IV for acute spinal cord injury**—steroid use in this setting remains controversial.[16,17]

Special Populations. *Pediatric Dosage.* Dosages may need to be reduced for infants and children. Doses should be determined by severity of the condition and response to treatment, not the size or age of the patient. Doses should not be less than 0.5 mg/kg every 24 h. **IV as an anti-inflammatory or immunosuppressive**—0.5–1.7 mg/kg/d divided every 6–12 h.[8]

Geriatric Dosage. In the elderly, use the lowest effective adult dose.

Dosage Forms. **Inj** 40, 125, 500 mg, 1, 2 g; **Depot Inj** (as acetate) 20, 40, 80 mg/mL.

Pharmacokinetics. *See* Systemic Corticosteroids Comparison Chart.

Adverse Reactions. *See* Prednisone Adverse Reactions.

Contraindications. Administration of live virus vaccines while receiving methylprednisolone therapy. Methylprednisolone formulations containing the preservative benzyl alcohol are contraindicated in infants.

Precautions. *See* Prednisone Precautions.

Drug Interactions. **Methylprednisolone is a CYP 3A4 substrate:** *Azole antifungals* and some *macrolide antibiotics* are CYP 3A4 inhibitors and can increase the serum concentration of methylprednisolone. *Carbamazepine, phenytoin, and rifampin* are CYP 3A4 inducers and can decrease the serum concentration of methylprednisolone.

Parameters to Monitor. *See* Prednisone Parameters to Monitor.

PREDNISONE   Deltasone, Orasone, Various

Pharmacology. Prednisone is a synthetic glucocorticoid with less sodium-retaining activity than hydrocortisone. (*See* Systemic Corticosteroids Comparison Chart.) Prednisone is inactive until converted into prednisolone. At the cellular level, glucocorticoids act by controlling the rate of protein synthesis mediated through gene transcription. This action changes the types of proteins synthesized by specific target tissues. Because of the time required to change gene expression and protein synthesis, the effects of glucocorticoids are not apparent for several hours following administration. These drugs are used primarily for their anti-inflammatory and immunosuppressant effects.[3,18]

Administration and Adult Dosage. Total daily dosage is variable and must be individualized depending on the clinical disorder and patient response.[3,5] Dosages for prednisolone are the same as those for prednisone. Daily divided high-dose therapy for initial control of more severe disease states may be necessary until satisfactory control is obtained. Administration of a short-acting or intermediate-acting preparation given as a single dose in the morning (before 9 AM) is likely to produce fewer side effects and less HPA axis suppression than a divided dosage regimen with the same agent or an equivalent dosage of a long-acting agent. Alternate-day therapy (i.e., total 48-h dosage administered every other morning) with intermediate-acting agents (e.g., prednisone) further reduces the prevalence and degree of side effects. However, it might not be uniformly effective in treating all disease states. Adrenal suppression may not occur with single daily doses given in the morning if the prednisone dose is ≤7.5 mg, but Cushing's syndrome can still occur and patients should receive supplemental corticosteroids during periods of unusual stress.[1,5,18] **In times of stress** (e.g., surgery, severe trauma, serious illness), patients on long-term corticosteroid therapy (>5 mg/d prednisone or equivalent) should receive supplemental steroid doses. Depending on the type and degree of stress, these supplemental steroid doses range from normal PO replacement to several times the normal steroid dose given IV.[1] Guidelines for withdrawal from glucocorticoid therapy have been published.[2,5,18] Patients who have received daily glucocorticoid therapy for less than 2 weeks do not require dosage tapering to prevent acute adrenal insufficiency; however, dosage tapering may be required to maintain an adequate clinical response.[2,3,5]

   PO for acute asthma exacerbations in adults and adolescents[19]: *(Dosing applies to prednisone, methylprednisolone, and prednisolone)* 40–80 mg/d in 1 or 2 doses for 3–10 days or until peak expiratory flow is 70% of predicted or personal best; for outpatient "burst" therapy, 40–60 mg in a single or 2 divided doses for 5–10 days. For severe asthma exacerbations, there is no known advantage to higher doses or IV corticosteroid use over PO therapy (as long as GI transit time or absorption is not impaired). If corticosteroid treatment lasts less than 1 week, there is no need to taper the dose for reasons of adrenal insufficiency; for longer courses (up to 10 days), there is probably no need to taper the dose especially in patients currently using inhaled corticosteroids; **PO as an adjunct therapy for *Pneumocystis carinii* pneumonia in patients with substantial hypoxia** (arterial PO_2 ≤70 mmHg or an arterial–alveolar gradient ≥ 35 mmHg) begin within 72 h of PCP antimicrobial therapy 40 mg bid for 5 days, then 40 mg once daily for 5 days, and then 20 mg/d for 11 days or the duration of antimicrobial therapy;[20] **PO for rheumatoid arthritis**—5–10 mg/d[3]; **PO for SLE**—*mild* ≤10–20 mg/d, *refractory or severe organ-threatening* 1–2 mg/kg/d;[21] **PO for mild-moderate distal ulcerative colitis unresponsive to aminosalicylates**—40–60 mg/d or 1 mg/kg/d[11]; **PO for idiopathic thrombocytopenia purpura**—1–1.5 mg/kg/d.[3]

Special Populations. *Pediatric Dosage.* Dosage depends on disease state and patient response rather than strict adherence to age or body weight. **PO for acute asthma**[19]: *(Dosing applies to prednisone, methylprednisolone, and prednisolone)* 1–2 mg/kg in 2 divided doses to a maximum of 60 mg/d for 3–10 days or until peak expiratory flow is 70% of predicted or personal best; for outpatient "burst" therapy, 1–2 mg/kg/d to a maximum of 60 mg/d in 2 divided doses for 3–10 days. For severe asthma exacerbations, there is no known advantage to higher doses of corticosteroids or IV corticosteroid use over PO therapy (as long as GI transit time or absorption is not impaired). If corticosteroid treatment lasts less than 1 week, there is no need to taper the dose for reasons of adrenal insufficiency; for longer courses (up to 10 days), there is probably no need to taper the dose, especially in patients currently using inhaled corticosteroids. **PO as an anti-inflammatory or immunosuppressant**—0.05–2 mg/kg/d in 1–4 divided doses.[8]

Geriatric Dosage. Refer to adult dosing; use the lowest effective dose.

Dosage Forms. **Soln** 1, 5 mg/mL; **Tab** 1, 2.5, 5, 10, 20, 50 mg.

Patient Instructions. *See* Class Instructions: Systemic Corticosteroids.

Pharmacokinetics. *See* Systemic Corticosteroids Comparison Chart.

Adverse Reactions. Fluid and electrolyte disturbances (with possible edema and hypertension), hyperglycemia and glycosuria, accelerated atherosclerosis, peptic ulcer disease, insomnia, increased appetite, weight gain, osteoporosis, bone fractures, myopathy, menstrual irregularities, behavioral disturbances (most common with short-term therapy: euphoria and hypomania; long-term therapy: depressive symptoms [increased risk with dosages >40 mg/d]), poor wound healing, avascular necrosis, immunosuppression, cataracts, glaucoma, arrest of growth (in children), hirsutism, pseudotumor cerebri, pancreatitis, and cushingoid habitus (moon face, buffalo hump, central obesity, easy bruising, acne, hirsutism, and striae). Prolonged therapy (≥2 weeks) can lead to suppression of HPA axis. Rapid withdrawal of long-term therapy can cause acute adrenal insufficiency (e.g., fever, myalgia, arthralgia, and malaise); adrenally suppressed patients cannot adequately respond to stress by increasing endogenous glucocorticoid secretion. As corticosteroids supplementation is tapered, patients may remain adrenally suppressed for up to a year following discontinuation of glucocorticoid therapy.[1,3,18,22,23]

Contraindications. Systemic fungal infections (except as maintenance therapy in adrenal insufficiency); administration of live virus vaccines in patients receiving immunosuppressive doses of prednisone.

Precautions. Pregnancy and pediatrics (may affect growth velocity, monitor regularly). Use with caution in diabetes mellitus, osteoporosis, peptic ulcer, esophagitis, tuberculosis, and other acute and chronic bacterial, viral, and fungal infections, hypertension or other cardiovascular diseases, hypothyroidism, immunizations, hypoalbuminemia, psychosis, and liver disease. Suppression of PPD and other skin test reactions can occur.

Drug Interactions. **Prednisone is a CYP 3A4 substrate:** *Azole antifungals* and some *macrolide antibiotics* are CYP 3A4 inhibitors and can increase the serum concentration of prednisone. *Phenobarbital, phenytoin, and rifampin* are CYP 3A4 inducers and can decrease the serum concentration of prednisone.

Parameters to Monitor. Observe for behavioral disturbances and signs or symptoms of Cushing's syndrome. With short-term, high-dose therapy, frequently monitor serum electrolytes, blood glucose, blood pressure, and for signs and symptoms of infection. With long-term therapy, monitor these parameters and perform periodic eye examinations, bone mineral density, and possibly stool guaiac. Monitor growth in infants and children on prolonged therapy.

SYSTEMIC CORTICOSTEROIDS COMPARISON CHART

GLUCOCORTICOID	APPROXIMATE EQUIVALENT DOSE (mg)	ROUTES OF ADMINISTRATION	RELATIVE ANTI-INFLAMMATORY POTENCY	RELATIVE MINERALO-CORTICOID POTENCY	PROTEIN BINDING (%)	HALF-LIFE PLASMA (min)	HALF-LIFE BIOLOGIC (h)	METABOLISM	BIOAVAILABILITY (%)	EXCRETION	NOTES
Short-acting											
Cortisone	25	PO	0.8	2	90	30	8–12	Hepatic (to hydrocortisone)		Renal (>99% inactive)	
Hydrocortisone	20	PO, IM, IV, Rectal Supp	1	2	90	80–118	8–12	Hepatic	PO: 96 (dose dependent, BA ↓ with ↑ dose)	Renal (>99% inactive)	Active form of cortisone
Intermediate-acting											
Methylprednisolone	4	PO, IM, IV	5	0		78–188	18–36	Hepatic		Renal (mostly inactive)	
Prednisolone	5	PO	4	1	90–95	115–212	18–36	Hepatic	PO: ≥78	Renal (mostly active)	Active form of prednisone
Prednisone	5	PO	4	1	70	60	18–36	Hepatic (to prednisolone)	PO: 92	Renal (≈80% inactive)	
Triamcinolone	4	IM, IA, ID, IL, IS, ST Inj	5	0		≥200	18–36	Hepatic		Renal (15% unchanged)	
Long-acting											
Betamethasone	0.6–0.75	PO, IM, IA, IL, IS, ST Inj	25	0	64	≥300	36–54	Hepatic		Renal (<5% unchanged	

(continued)

SYSTEMIC CORTICOSTEROIDS COMPARISON CHART (*continued*)

GLUCOCORTICOID	APPROXIMATE EQUIVALENT DOSE (mg)	ROUTES OF ADMINISTRATION	RELATIVE ANTI-INFLAMMATORY POTENCY	RELATIVE MINERALO-CORTICOID POTENCY	PROTEIN BINDING (%)	HALF-LIFE PLASMA (min)	BIOLOGIC (h)	METABOLISM	BIOAVAILABILITY (%)	EXCRETION	NOTES
Dexamethasone	0.75	PO, IM, IV, IA, IL, ST Inj	25–3C	0		110–210	36–54	Hepatic	60–86	Hepatic (≈3% unchanged in urine)	
MINERALOCORTICOID											
Fludrocortisone	0.1	PO	10	125	42	≥210	18–36	Hepatic	100	Renal (mostly inactive)	No sig GC effect at usual daily doses

BA, bioavailability; GC, glucocorticoid; IA, intra-articular; ID, intradermal; IL, intralesional; IS, intrasyrovial; sig, significant; STInj, soft-tissue injection.
From Refs. 3, 5, 18, and 28.

777

TOPICAL CORTICOSTEROIDS

Pharmacology. Topical corticosteroids have nonspecific, local anti-inflammatory effects in the dermal and epidermal skin layers that occur by inhibiting mediators in the arachidonic acid pathway in cells, suppressing DNA synthesis at the cellular level, decreasing the production of cytokines along with numerous other effects on inflammatory cells, and by decreasing the influx of WBCs into the local area. Potency is dependent on the characteristics and concentration of the drug and the vehicle used and is usually measured by the assessment of the relative degree of skin blanching (vasoconstrictor assay).[24,25]

Administration and Adult Dosage. Uses for nonprescription hydrocortisone preparations (the only available over-the-counter topical corticosteroid; 0.5% and 1% strengths) include relief of itching, inflammation, and rashes caused by eczema, insect bites, poison oak, ivy, or sumac, soaps, detergents, or cosmetics, jewelry, seborrheic dermatitis, psoriasis, and external genital or anal itching. Prescription indications include relief of inflammatory and pruritic manifestations of corticosteroid-responsive dermatoses including contact or atopic dermatitis, nummular, stasis, or asteatotic eczema, lichen planus, lichen simplex chronicus, insect and arthropod bite reactions, and first-degree and second-degree localized burns and sunburns. These products are usually applied sparingly in a light film, 2–4 times/d; however, with continuous use, a repository effect may make 1–2 applications/d or intermittent courses as effective. High-potency agents should be reserved for short-term or intermittent use (e.g., every-other-day or weekend-only application) but may be more effective and cause fewer adverse effects than continuous therapy with lower potency products. Treatment with very high-potency agents should not exceed two consecutive weeks and the total dosage should not exceed 50 g or 50 mL/wk (60 g for fluocinonide), and treatment with medium-potency agents should not exceed 90–100 g/wk, because of the potential for HPA axis suppression.[24–27]

Dosage Forms. *See* Topical Corticosteroids Comparison Chart.

Patient Instructions. For external use only. Do not use in or around eyes, mucous membranes, open wounds, genital, or rectal areas, on the face, armpits, in skin creases, or with occlusive dressings unless directed by prescriber. Do not expose treated area to direct sunlight.

Missed Doses. Apply a missed dose as soon as you remember unless it is almost time for the regular application. If it is almost time for the regular application, then continue on the regular schedule. Do not apply a double dose.

Pharmacokinetics. The absorption of these drugs depends on the physical properties of the drug itself, the surface area of use, the thickness of the skin (greater absorption from the face, in skin folds, in the perineum, and on denuded skin; lesser absorption from the palms and soles), skin temperature or hydration status (greater with increased skin temperature or increased hydration), the age of the patient (children have a greater surface area: mass ratio increased systemic effects), the use of occlusive dressings, the vehicle, application frequency, and length of treatment.[24–26] (*See* Topical Corticosteroids Comparison Chart.)

Adverse Reactions. Adverse reactions occur more frequently with increasing product potency and include local burning, itching, irritation, erythema, dryness, folliculitis, hypertrichosis, acneiform eruptions, hypopigmentation, rosacea, skin atrophy, striae, telangiectasias, purpura, perioral dermatitis, overgrowth of skin bacteria and fungi, allergic contact dermatitis, and cataracts or glaucoma with prolonged application around the eye. Systemically, there can be enough absorption of potent steroids to cause suppression of the HPA axis, causing symptoms of Cushing's syndrome, and growth retardation, particularly in young children.[24–26]

TOPICAL CORTICOSTEROIDS COMPARISON CHART

CORTICOSTEROID	BRAND (GENERIC) NAMES	DOSAGE FORMS	STRENGTHS	NOTES
Low-potency				
Alclometasone dipropionate	Aclovate (Various)	Crm, Oint	0.05%	• Modest anti-inflammatory effects
Desonide	DesOwen, Tridesilon, Verdeso (Various)	Crm, Foam, Lot, Oint	0.05%	• Safest for chronic application, use on the face, or other areas most susceptible to corticosteroid damage
Fluocinolone acetonide	Capex, Synalar (Various)	Crm, Shampoo, Soln	0.01%	○ i.e., skin folds, groin, axilla
Hydrocortisone	Anusol-HC, Cortaid, Hytone, Various (Various)	Crm, Lot, Oint, Soln	0.5, 1, 2.5%	○ Safest for use on infants, children, and elderly • Hydrocortisone is available by prescription and OTC ○ 2.5% is prescription strength
Hydrocortisone acetate	Corticaine, Lanacort 10, Various (Various)	Crm, Oint	0.5, 1%	○ 1% some are prescription, and some are OTC ○ 0.5% is OTC strength
Medium-potency				
Betamethasone dipropionate	(Various)	Lot	0.05%	• Effective for moderate inflammatory dermatoses
Betamethasone valerate	Beta-Val (Various)	Crm, Lot	0.1%	○ i.e., chronic eczematous dermatoses
Clocortolone pivalate	Cloderm	Crm	0.1%	• May be used for ≤2 weeks on face or other sensitive areas
Desoximetasone	Topicort LP (Various)	Crm	0.05%	○ i.e., skin folds, groin, axilla
Fluocinolone acetonide	Synalar (Various)	Crm, Oint	0.025%	• May be used on scalp or extremities
Flurandrenolide	Cordran, Cordran SP	Crm, Lot, Tape	0.05%, 4 µg/cm^2 (tape)	• Flurandrenolide tape dressings have been associated with stripping of the epidermis and purpura
Fluticasone propionate	Cultivate (Various)	Crm, Oint	0.05, 0.005%	• Do NOT use occlusive dressings with Mometasone treatment
Hydrocortisone butyrate	Locoid, Locoid Lipocream (Various)	Crm, Oint, Soln	0.1%	• Treatment should not exceed 90–100 g/wk
Hydrocortisone valerate	Westcort (Various)	Crm, Oint	0.2%	
Mometasone furoate	Elocon (Various)	Crm, Lot, Oint	0.1%	
Triamcinolone acetonide	Aristocort, Kenalog (Various)	Crm, Lot, Oint	0.025, 0.1%	

(continued)

TOPICAL CORTICOSTEROIDS COMPARISON CHART (*continued*)

CORTICOSTEROID	BRAND (GENERIC) NAMES	DOSAGE FORMS	STRENGTHS	NOTES
High-potency				
Amcinonide	Cyclocort (Various)	Crm, Lot, Oint	0.1%	• Effective for more severe eczematous dermatoses
Betamethasone dipropionate (augmented)	Diprolene AF (Various)	Crm	0.05%	○ lichen simplex chronicus or psoriasis • May be used on scalp, trunk, hands, and feet
Betamethasone dipropionate	Diprosone (Various)	Crm, Oint	0.05%	• Avoid use on face or other sensitive areas (i.e., skin folds,
Betamethasone valerate	(Various)	Oint	0.1%	groin, axilla) due to risk of striae
Desoximetasone	Topicort (Various)	Crm, Gel, Oint	0.05, 0.25%	• Use for ≤2 consecutive weeks, and MAX 50 g or
Diflorasone diacetate	ApexiCon E, Florone, Psorcon E (Various)	Crm	0.05%	50 mL/wk (60 g/wk for fluocinonide)
Fluocinonide	Lidex, Lidex E (Various)	Crm, Gel, Oint, Soln	0.05%	Do NOT use occlusive dressings with augmented
Halcinonide	Halog	Crm, Oint, Soln	0.1%	betamethasone dipropionate or betamethasone dipropionate
Triamcinolone acetonide	Aristocort, Kenalog (Various)	Crm, Oint	0.5%	treatment
Very-high-potency				
Betamethasone dipropionate (augmented)	Diprolene (Various)	Gel, Lot, Oint	0.05%	• Used as an alternative to systemic corticosteroids when local areas are involved (Use ≤ 2 weeks, MAX 50 g
Clobetasol propionate	Clobex, Cormax, Olux, Olux E, Temovate, Temovate E (Various)	Crm, Foam, Gel, Lot, Oint, Shampoo, Spray	0.05%	or 50 mL/wk) • Effective for hyperkeratotic, chronic lesions of psoriasis, lichen simplex chronicus, or discoid lupus erythematosus
Diflorasone diacetate	ApexiCon, Psorcon (Various)	Oint	0.05%	• It is NOT recommended to discontinue use of these
Fluocinonide	Vanos	Crm	0.1%	agents abruptly, switch to a lower potency agent first
Halobetasol propionate	Ultravate (Various)	Crm, Oint	0.05%	• AVOID use on face, skin folds, groin, or axilla, and the use of occlusive dressings due to the risk of striae and atrophy • Clobetasol may cause HPA axis suppression with doses as low as 2 g daily (60 g/wk for fluocinonide)

From Refs. 24–26.

■ REFERENCES

1. Jung C, Inder WJ. Management of adrenal insufficiency during the stress of medical illness and surgery. *Med J Aust.* 2008;188(7):409-413.

2. Walsh JP, Dayan CM. Role of biochemical assessment in management of corticosteroid withdrawal. *Ann Clin Biochem.* 2000;37:279-288.

3. Schimmer BP, Parker KL. Adrenocorticotropic hormone: adrenocortical steroids and their synthetic analogs; inhibitors of the synthesis and action of adrenal hormones. In: Brunton LL, et al., eds. *Goodman and Gilman's the Pharmacological Basis of Therapeutics.* 11th ed. New York, NY: McGraw-Hill; 2006:1587-1612.

4. Hesketh PJ. Chemotherapy-induced nausea and vomiting. *N Engl J Med.* 2008;358(23):2482-2494.

5. Stewart PM. The adrenal cortex. In: Kronenberg HM, et al., eds. *Williams Textbook of Endocrinology.* 11th ed. Philadelphia, PA: Saunders Elsevier; 2008:445-503.

6. Miracle X et al. Guideline for the use of antenatal corticosteroids for fetal maturation. *J Perinat Med.* 2008;36(3):191-196.

7. Markovitz B, Randolph A, Khemani RG. Corticosteroids for the prevention and treatment of postextubation stridor in neonates, children and adults (review). *Cochrane Database Syst Rev.* 2008;2:CD001000.

8. Alt P et al. Pediatric endocrine medications. In: Alt P, et al., eds. *Clinical Handbook of Pediatric Endocrinology.* St. Louis, MO: Quality Medical Publishing, Inc.; 2003:294-345.

9. Prober CG. Central nervous system infections. In: Kliegman, et al., eds. *Nelson Textbook of Pediatrics.* 18th ed. Philadelphia, PA: Saunders Elsevier; 2007:2512-2524.

10. Perron G et al. Perineal pruritus after IV dexamethasone administration. *Can J Anaesth.* 2003;50(7):749-750.

11. Hemstreet BA, Dipiro JT. Inflammatory bowel disease. In: Dipiro JT, et al., eds. *Pharmacotherapy: a Pathophysiologic Approach.* 7th ed. New York, NY: McGraw-Hill; 2008:589-605.

12. White PC. Adrenocortical insufficiency. In: Kliegman, et al., eds. *Nelson Textbook of Pediatrics.* 18th ed. Philadelphia, PA: Saunders Elsevier; 2007:2355-2360.

13. Kamm GL, Hagmeyer KO. Allergic-type reactions to corticosteroids. *Ann Pharmacother.* 1999;33:451-460.

14. Whitby DH, Johns TE. Drug-induced hematologic disorders. In: Dipiro JT, et al., eds. *Pharmacotherapy: a Pathophysiologic Approach.* 7th ed. New York, NY: McGraw-Hill; 2008:1701-1714.

15. Rosenfeld S et al. Antithymocyte globulin and cyclosporine for severe aplastic anemia association between hematologic response and long-term outcome. *JAMA.* 2003;289:1130-1135.

16. Hurlbert RJ. Strategies of medical intervention in the management of acute spinal cord injury. *Spine.* 2006;31(suppl 11):S16-S21.

17. Sayer FT et al. Methylprednisolone treatment in acute spinal cord injury: the myth challenged through a structured analysis of published literature. *Spine J.* 2006;6(3):335-343.

18. Gums JG, Anderson S. Adrenal gland disorders. In: Dipiro JT, et al., eds. *Pharmacotherapy: A Pathophysiologic Approach.* 7th ed. New York, NY: McGraw-Hill; 2008:1265-1280.

19. National Institutes of Health. National asthma education and prevention program, expert panel report 3: guidelines for the diagnosis and management of asthma. 2007. NIH publication 08-4051. http://www.nhlbi.nih.gov/guidelines/asthma/asthgdln.htm. Accessed September 19, 2008.

20. Briel M et al. Adjunctive corticosteroids for *Pneumocystis jiroveci* pneumonia in patients with HIV-infection (review). *Cochrane Database Syst Rev.* 2006;3:CD006150.

21. Delafuente JC, Cappuzzp KA. Systemic lupus erythematosus and other collagen-vascular diseases. In: Dipiro JT, et al., eds. *Pharmacotherapy: A Pathophysiologic Approach.* 7th ed. New York, NY: McGraw-Hill; 2008:1431-1445.

22. Richards RN. Side effects of short-term oral corticosteroids. *J Cutan Med Surg.* 2008;12(2):77-81.

23. Warrington TP, Bostwick JM. Psychiatric adverse effects of corticosteroids. *Mayo Clin Proc.* 2006;81(10):1361-1367.

24. Fox LP et al. Dermatological pharmacology. In: Brunton LL, et al., eds. *Goodman and Gilman's the Pharmacological Basis of Therapeutics.* 11th ed. New York, NY: McGraw Hill; 2006:1679-1706.

25. Valencia IC, Kerdel FA. Topical corticosteroids. In: Wolff K, et al., eds. *Fitzpatrick's Dermatology in General Medicine.* 7th ed. New York, NY: McGraw-Hill; 2008:2102-2106.

26. Cupp M, Shields KM. Comparison of topical corticosteroids. Pharmacist's Letter/Prescriber's Letter 2006;22(3):220333.

27. Scott SA, Martin RW. Atopic Dermatitis and Dry Skin. In: Berardi RR, et al., eds. *Handbook of Nonprescription Drugs: an Interactive Approach to Self-Care.* 15th ed. Washington, DC: American Pharmacists Association; 2006:711-728.

28. Tsuei SE et al. Disposition of synthetic glucocorticoids. I. Pharmacokinetics of dexamethasone in healthy adults. *J Pharmacokinet Biopharm.* 1979;7:249-264.

Chapter 50

Antidiabetic Drugs

Stephen M. Setter, John R. White Jr., and R. Keith Campbell

ACARBOSE Precose

Pharmacology. Acarbose is an oral α-glucosidase inhibitor indicated for the management of hyperglycemia caused by type 2 diabetes mellitus. Inhibition of this gut enzyme system effectively reduces the rate of complex carbohydrate digestion and the subsequent absorption of glucose, thereby lowering postprandial glucose excursions in type 2 diabetes.[1] In obese and nonobese patients with type 2 diabetes, acarbose monotherapy is associated with a 0.5%–1% decrease in hemoglobin A_{1c}.[2]

Administration and Adult Dosage. PO for type 2 diabetes—(as monotherapy or with a sulfonylurea) 25 mg, tid initially, just before meals. Increase to 50 mg tid after 4–8 weeks and, if necessary, to 100 mg tid after 4–8 additional weeks. Dosages >100 mg tid are not recommended because of increased risk of hepatotoxicity, and patients weighing $\leq$ 60 kg should not receive >50 mg tid.

Special Populations. *Pediatric Dosage.* Safety and efficacy not established.

Geriatric Dosage. Same as adult dosage.

Dosage Forms. Tab 25, 50, 100 mg.

Patient Instructions. Take acarbose at the beginning of each meal. When a meal is skipped, also skip taking this medication. If a dose is missed, do not take it unless it is just before the next meal. If hypoglycemia occurs, dextrose (glucose) needs to be ingested; sucrose (table sugar) is not effective.

Pharmacokinetics. *Fate.* The drug is poorly absorbed from the GI tract (<2%). It undergoes extensive metabolism in the GI tract via intestinal flora and digestive enzymes. The clinical effect is not dependent on the serum level achieved. All absorbed acarbose and metabolites are renally excreted. In patients with renal impairment, plasma acarbose concentrations are elevated in relation to the degree of renal dysfunction.

$t_{1/2}$. approximately 2 h with normal renal function.

Adverse Reactions. The major side effects of acarbose are GI in nature and include flatulence, diarrhea, and abdominal pain. Acarbose monotherapy is not associated with hypoglycemia; however, patients managed with combination therapy (with a secretagogue or insulin) can experience hypoglycemia secondary to the action of the other drug. In this setting, manage hypoglycemia with oral glucose (if the patient is conscious) or IV glucose or glucagon (if the patient is unconscious) rather than with a complex carbohydrate (e.g., sucrose). Attempting to manage hypoglycemia with oral sugar sources other than glucose is not effective in acarbose-treated patients and might have grave consequences.

Contraindications. Inflammatory bowel disease; colonic ulceration; obstructive bowel disorders; cirrhosis; type 1 diabetes; history of diabetic ketoacidosis. Not recommended in patients with cirrhosis or patients with a $Cl_{Cr} \leq 24$ mL/min or in patients with $Cr_s > 2$ mg/dL.

Precautions. Use with caution in patients with disorders of digestion or absorption or with medical conditions that might deteriorate with increased intestinal gas formation.

Drug Interactions. Charcoal and other intestinal adsorbents as well as digestive preparations containing amylase, pancreatin, and related enzymes should not be taken concurrently with acarbose.

Parameters to Monitor. Monitor clinical symptoms of hyperglycemia (mainly polyphagia, polyuria, polydipsia, or numbing or tingling of feet) or hypoglycemia (hunger, nervousness, sweating, palpitations, headaches, confusion, drowsiness, anxiety, or blurred vision) when taken concurrently with insulin or insulin secretagogues (e.g., sulfonylureas). Self-monitoring of fasting and selected postprandial blood glucose levels by the patient is also helpful. (*See* Blood Glucose Monitors Comparison Chart.) Long-term diabetic control may best be monitored using hemoglobin A_{Ic}.[3]

Notes. Miglitol (Glyset, Bayer) is an α-glucosidase inhibitor that has similar indications, uses, and side effects as acarbose. The dosage of the two drugs is the same. The clinical benefits, if any, of miglitol over acarbose have not been determined.

ALDOSE REDUCTASE INHIBITORS

Prolonged hyperglycemia causes excess flux of glucose into tissues, and glucose is shunted to the polyol pathway, resulting in excess sorbitol production. Excess intracellular sorbitol causes a reduction in the uptake of myoinositol and ultimately a downregulation in the Na^+/K^+-ATPase system. This process is thought to be one of the biochemical mechanisms leading to the development of neuropathy, collagen disorders, cataracts, and possibly retinopathy in patients with diabetes. Because aldose reductase is the rate-limiting enzyme in this pathway, aldose reductase inhibitors are being studied as a possible means of decreasing the sorbitol-linked sequelae of diabetes.[4] Although this is a promising class of drugs, the side effects, dosage regimens, and long-term benefits are to be determined. Aldose reductase inhibitors currently under investigation are **ranirestat** and **fidarestat**.[5]

GLUCAGON   Glucagon Emergency Kit, Glucagon Diagnostic Kit

Pharmacology. Glucagon is a counterregulatory hormone that increases blood glucose levels by induction of glycogenolysis. It is indicated for the treatment of the unconscious hypoglycemic patient but is effective only in patients with adequate hepatic glycogen stores. Glucagon also has been used as a bowel relaxant during diagnostic procedures and in overdosage with β-**blockers** or **calcium channel blockers**.[6]

Adult Dosage. **IM, SQ, or IV for hypoglycemia**—0.5–1 mg. Response is usually observed in 10–20 min. Specifics for GlucaGen and Glucagon—parenteral dosage (GlucaGen) for adults and children weighing > 55 lb (25 kg) is 1 mg (1 IU) administered

IM, IV, or SQ and the recommended dose for children weighing < 55 lb (25 kg) or younger than 6–8 years old is 0.5 mg (0.5 IU) IM/IV/SQ. Dose should not exceed 1 mg. Parenteral dosage (Glucagon, recombinant by Lilly)—adults and children weighing ≥ 44 lb (20 kg) is 1 mg (1 IU) administered IM, IV, or SQ; for children weighing ≤ 44 lb (20 kg), the recommended dose is 0.5 mg (0.5 IU) or, alternatively, 0.02–0.03 mg/kg (IU/kg) IM, IV, or SQ. Dose should not exceed 1 mg.

Dosage Forms. Inj 1 mg.

Adverse Reactions. Glucagon occasionally causes nausea and vomiting, so position patients to prevent aspiration. Administration of glucagon rarely results in generalized allergic reactions such as urticaria, respiratory distress, and hypotension. Glucagon can precipitate hypertensive crisis in the patient with underlying pheochromocytoma (secondary to release of catecholamines).

INSULINS

Pharmacology. Insulin promotes cellular uptake of glucose, fatty acids, and amino acids and their conversion to glycogen, triglycerides, and proteins. Human insulin is produced by recombinant DNA technology.

Administration and Adult Dosage. SQ for type 1 diabetes usual initial dosage ranges of 0.6–0.75 unit/kg/d in divided doses.[7] During the first week of therapy, the dosage requirement might escalate to 1 unit/kg/d in divided doses because of insulin resistance and the usual age group (adolescents) being treated. The dosage requirement can temporarily decrease to 0.1–0.5 unit/kg/d if the patient experiences a "honeymoon phase." Dosage adjustments are made on the basis of clinical symptoms, blood glucose levels, and hemoglobin A_{1c} values. Insulin can be administered by various methods depending on a number of factors. Single daily SQ injections of intermediate-acting insulin are often used but should not usually be relied on to adequately control blood glucose levels in the type 1 patient, because they are not sufficient to prevent long-term complications even though they can offer protection from diabetic ketoacidosis. Intensive forms of insulin therapy, which may provide better glycemic control, include the split-and-mixed regimen (2 SQ injections daily of mixed short- and long-acting insulin), multiple daily SQ doses of short-acting insulin in combination with a single injection of long-acting insulin, and insulin pump therapy. **IV, SQ, or IM for diabetic ketoacidosis (IV preferred for patients in shock)**—0.1 unit/kg, followed by a continuous infusion of 0.1–0.2 unit/kg/h. If the serum glucose does not change in the first hour, double the insulin rate with further adjustments in insulin dosage based on glucose levels.[8] Fluid and electrolyte repletion must accompany insulin therapy. **SQ for type 2 diabetes**—(patients unresponsive to oral agent therapy or with extreme hyperglycemia—fasting serum glucose >200–225 mg/dL) may need as little as 5–10 units/d or >100 units/d.[8] Patients who require < 30 units/d may be well controlled with 1 injection/d of intermediate-acting insulin; patients who require >30 units/d should be treated with 2 injections/d. Insulin resistance in the type 2 population is usually associated with obesity. Weight reduction and improved glycemic control usually improve insulin response.

Special Populations. *Pediatric Dosage.* (*See* Administration and Adult Dosage.) **Common maintenance dosages** are 0.6–0.9 unit/kg/d in divided doses in prepubertal children, up to 1.5 units/kg/d during puberty, and <1 unit/kg/d after puberty. Requirements occasionally can be as high as 200 units/d during growth spurts.

Geriatric Dosage. Same as adult dosage.

Other Conditions. Insulin requirements may be decreased in patients with renal or hepatic impairment or hypothyroidism. Requirements may be increased during pregnancy (especially in the second and third trimesters); in patients with high fever, hyperthyroidism, or severe infections; and after trauma or surgery.

Dosage Forms. *See* Insulins Comparison Chart.

Patient Instructions. Instruct patients in the following areas: use of insulin syringes, needles, and insulin pens; storage, mixing, and handling of insulin; urine or blood ketone testing; blood glucose testing; adherence to proper diet and regular meals; personal hygiene (especially the feet); and recognition and treatment of hypoglycemia and hyperglycemia. (*See* Sulfonylurea Agents.)

Pharmacokinetics. *Onset and Duration.* *See* Insulins Comparison Chart.

Serum Levels. Patients with diabetes vary widely in their responses to insulin, and serum levels are not normally monitored clinically.

Fate. The rate of absorption depends on the insulin type. (*See* Insulins Comparison Chart.) Serum levels are affected by obesity, diet, degree of activity, pancreatic β-cell activity, growth hormone, and circulating antibodies. Insulin is metabolized primarily in the liver, although the kidneys are responsible for the metabolism of up to 40% of the daily insulin output.[9]

$t_{1/2}$. (regular insulin) 4–5 min after IV administration.

Adverse Reactions. Hypoglycemia is dose related. Patients being treated with intensive insulin regimens of ≥3 injections/d are more prone to hypoglycemic episodes than are patients treated with the conventional 1–2 injections/d.[10] Local allergic reactions, with an onset of 15 min–4 h, are usually caused by insulin impurities; 70% of these patients have histories of interrupted treatment. Immune or nonimmune insulin resistance occurs occasionally. Lipohypertrophy at the injection site can occur, especially with repeated use of the same site. Lipoatrophy also can occur at the injection site and be less frequent with human insulins.[11]

Contraindications. Hypoglycemic episodes.

Precautions. Use with caution in patients with renal or hepatic disease or hypothyroidism. Insulin requirements can change with exercise or infection, or when switching animal sources or to more purified products.

Drug Interactions. Alcohol can produce hypoglycemia, especially in fasting patients; moderate increases in blood glucose can occur in nonfasting patients. Oral contraceptives, corticosteroids, furosemide, niacin (large doses), diazoxide, thiazide diuretics, and thyroid hormones (large doses) can increase insulin requirements. Anabolic steroids can decrease the insulin requirement. Avoid MAOIs in patients with diabetes because they can interfere with the normal adrenergic response to hypoglycemia by prolonging the action of antidiabetic agents. β-blockers prolong hypoglycemic episodes and inhibit tachycardia and tremors, which are signs of hypoglycemia (sweating is not inhibited); hypertension can occur during hypoglycemia; cardioselective β-blockers (e.g., atenolol, metoprolol) are less likely than nonselective types (e.g., nadolol, propranolol) to cause problems. ACEIs may contribute to the hypoglycemic effects of insulin as can ARBs. Alterations in blood glucose can occur with quinolone antibiotics or retroviral protease inhibitors.

Parameters to Monitor. Monitor blood glucose routinely. (*See* Blood Glucose Monitors Comparison Chart.) Long-term diabetic control is best monitored using hemoglobin A_{1c}.[3] The patient should continually watch for subjective symptoms of hypoglycemia and hyperglycemia. Observe for signs of lipoatrophy, lipohypertrophy, and allergic reactions.

Notes. Insulin is the preferred treatment of choice for patients with severe insulin resistance, pregnancy, or allergy; new insulin-dependent patients; or any patient taking insulin intermittently. Insulin is stable for 1 month at constant room temperature and up to 24 months under refrigeration. Insulin is adsorbed by glass and plastic IV infusion equipment, with little difference between glass and plastic; maximal adsorption occurs within 15 s. Adsorption can be minimized by the addition of small amounts (1%–2%) of **albumin** to the infusion container; however, this may be costly and unnecessary because patient response is generally adequate without addition of albumin. Variation can be minimized by flushing all new IV administration equipment with 50 mL of the insulin-containing solution (thereby saturating "binding sites") before it is used.[12]

Pump devices are available to deliver insulin depending on or independent of a measured serum glucose level. "Open loop" devices can deliver insulin at a constant rate and be manually controlled. "Closed-loop" devices (the "artificial pancreas") can deliver insulin at variable rates in response to serum glucose but are used only in experimental settings.

INSULIN ANALOGUES

Insulin injected SQ does not result in serum insulin concentrations that mimic normal physiologic insulin response. More than 30 human insulin analogues with different pharmacokinetic profiles have been produced using recombinant DNA technology. The goal of insulin analogue research is to produce a human insulin analogue with a rapid action (to provide bolus postprandial insulin) and a slow, extended-release pattern (to provide basal insulin). **Insulin lispro** (Humalog) is a rapid-acting analogue with a pharmacokinetic profile between that of IV and SQ regular human insulin. It has an onset in ≤15 min, a peak at 1–2 h, and a duration of 2–4 h. Insulin lispro offers a pharmacokinetic profile that is superior to regular human insulin when used to cover postprandial glycemic excursions. Another short-acting analogue, **insulin aspart** (Novolog), has a pharmacokinetic profile similar to that of insulin lispro[13] as does **insulin glulisine**.[14] The long-acting analogue, **insulin glargine** (Lantus), has an onset of action of approximately 1 h, with a sustained peak activity beginning at 4–5 h and persisting for 24 h. Insulin glargine is a basal insulin that is administered once daily; it must be used in combination with a rapid-acting premeal insulin such as insulin lispro to achieve optimum results.[13,15] Insulin detemir (Levemir) is a once or twice daily insulin with an onset of action of 1–2 h with a duration that is dose dependent and up to 24 h. Duration of action varies as follows: 5.7 h when dosed 0.1 units/kg; 12.1 h when dosed 0.2 units/kg; 19.9 h when dosed 0.4 units/kg; 22.7 h when dosed 0.8 units/kg; and, 23.2 h when dosed 1.6 units/kg.[16]

INSULINS COMPARISON CHART[a]

PRODUCT	MANUFACTURER	STRENGTH
RAPID ACTING (ONSET, <0.25 h; PEAK, 1–2 h; DURATION 2–4 h)		
Biosynthetic		
Apidra (glulisine)	Aventis	U-100
NovoLog (aspart)	Novo Nordisk	U-100
Humalog (lispro)	Lilly	U-100
Humalog Cartridges (lispro)	Lilly	U-100
SHORT ACTING (ONSET, 0.5–2 h; PEAK, 3–4 h; DURATION, 4–8 h)		
Human		
Humulin R	Lilly	U-100, U-500
Humulin R Cartridges	Lilly	U-100
Novolin R	Novo Nordisk	U-100
Novolin R PenFill	Novo Nordisk	U-100
Velosulin	Novo Nordisk	U-100
INTERMEDIATE ACTING (ONSET, 2–4 h; PEAK, 8–14 h; DURATION, 14–24 h)		
Human		
Humulin N (NPH)	Lilly	U-100
Humulin N Cartridges	Lilly	U-100
Novolin N (NPH)	Novo Nordisk	U-100
Novolin N Penfill (NPH)	Novo Nordisk	U-100
Novolin N Prefilled (NPH)	Novo Nordisk	U-100
LONG ACTING (ONSET, 6–14 h; PEAK, NONE; DURATION, 20–30 h)		
Human		
Detemir (Levemir)[b]	Novo Nordisk	U-100
Lantus (glargine)[c]	Aventis	U-100
FIXED COMBINATIONS (ONSET, 0.5–1 h; PEAK, 3–10 h; DURATION, 14–18 h)		
Human		
Humalog Mix 75/25[c,d]	Lilly	U-100
Humalog 50/50[c,d]	Lilly	U-100
Humulin 70/30[c]	Lilly	U-100
Humulin 70/30 Cartridges[c]	Lilly	U-100
Novolin 70/30[c]	Novo Nordisk	U-100
Novolin 70/30 PenFill[c]	Novo Nordisk	U-100
Novolin 70/30 Prefilled[c]	Novo Nordisk	U-100
Novolog 70/30[e]	Novo Nordisk	U-100
Humulin 50/50[c]	Lilly	U-100

[a]There can be variations within the ranges of onset, peak, and duration among manufacturers. Onset and duration may be prolonged in long-standing diabetes, and large doses may have prolonged durations of action. Site of injection, depth of injection, and whether site is exercised, massaged, or has heat applied to it also affect rate of insulin absorption. Human insulins have a slightly more rapid onset and a shorter duration of action than animal-derived insulins.
[b]Onset of action is 1–3 h with a variable peak with the therapeutic duration of 5–24 h dependent upon the dose. [Ref. 17]
[c]These products contain isophane and regular insulin in the specified proportions; the first number designates the percentage of isophane insulin and the second designates the percentage of regular insulin.
[d]Suspension of insulin lispro protamine and soluble insulin lispro. Onset is within 0.25 h.
[e]Suspension of protamine aspart and aspart.
From Refs. 10, 11, and product information.

METFORMIN   Glucophage

Pharmacology. Metformin is a biguanide antihyperglycemic agent used in the management of type 2 diabetes mellitus. It does not affect insulin secretion; rather, it reduces hepatic glucose production and enhances glucose utilization by muscle. Reported increases in glucose utilization in muscle are 7%–35%. In addition to blood glucose reductions (mean 53 mg/dL), metformin may have beneficial effects on serum lipids.[18] (*See* Notes.)

Administration and Adult Dosage. **PO for type 2 diabetes**—(immediate-release) initiate 500-mg tablets with a dosage of 1 tablet bid with morning and evening meals. Increase dosage in 500 mg/d increments at weekly intervals, to a maximum of 2.5 g/d. Initiate 850-mg tablets with 1 tablet/d before the morning meal. Increase dosage in 850 mg/d increments q2wk, to a maximum of 850 mg tid. Individualize maintenance dosage based on glycemic response. Give all dosages up to 2 g/d in 2 divided doses; larger dosages require a tid regimen to reduce GI discomfort. **PO**—(SR Tab) 500 mg/d with the evening meal initially, increasing in 500 mg/d increments at weekly intervals to a maximum of 2 g/d with the evening meal. To switch from the immediate-release to the SR formulation, give the same daily dosage of SR as a single dose with the evening meal. Metformin is also available as a 500 mg/5 mL oral solution and as a combination product with one of the following: rosiglitazone, pioglitazone, glyburide, glipizide, or sitagliptin.

Special Populations. *Pediatric Dosage.* Safety and efficacy not established.

Geriatric Dosage. Initial and maintenance dosages should be lower in the elderly. Avoid usual maximum adult dosage. Do not start metformin in patients ≥80 years unless renal function is normal.

Dosage Forms. **Tab** 500, 850, 1000 mg; **SR Tab** 500, 750, 1000 mg; **Tab** 250 mg with glyburide 1.25 mg, 500 mg with glyburide 2.5 or 5 mg (Glucovance); 250 or 500 mg of metformin with glipizide 2.5 or 5 mg or 500 mg of metformin with 5 mg of glipizide (Metaglip); 500 or 850 of metformin with 15 mg pioglitazone (ActoPLUSMet); 500 or 1000 mg of metformin with 2 or 4 mg of rosiglitazone (Avandamet); 500 or 1000 mg with sitagliptin 50 mg (Janumet).

Patient Instructions. Take metformin just before meals to reduce gastrointestinal side effects (diarrhea, nausea, and heartburn). Contact your physician if gastrointestinal side effects persist. Do not take metformin if you develop a serious medical condition such as myocardial infarction, stroke, or serious infection; require surgery; consume excessive amounts of alcohol; or require X-ray procedures with contrast dyes. Discontinue metformin and contact your health care provider immediately if hyperventilation, muscle pain, malaise, unexplained drowsiness, or other unusual symptoms occur that might indicate the development of lactic acidosis.

Missed Doses. Take as soon as possible, unless the time for the next dose is near. Do not double doses.

Pharmacokinetics. *Fate.* Absorption half-life is 0.9–2.6 h for immediate-release tablets; peak levels occur at 4–8 h (median 7 h) with the SR formulation. Absolute bioavailability is 50%–60% for both products. With immediate-release tablets, peak serum levels are 1–2 mg/L in patients with type 2 diabetes; with the SR formulation, peak levels are 20% lower. Plasma protein binding is negligible; V_d is 654 ± 358 L after a single 850-mg oral dose; Cl is proportional to renal function. Metformin is excreted in the urine unchanged.[18]

$t_{1/2}$. (immediate-release) 1.7–4.5 h with normal renal function.[18]

Adverse Reactions. Acute side effects occur in as many as 30% of patients treated with metformin. Side effects include primarily GI complaints, such as diarrhea, abdominal discomfort, nausea, anorexia, and metallic taste. GI side effects are usually transient and dose related and can be mitigated by giving the drug just before meals, initiating therapy with small doses and slowly increasing the dosage. Metformin reduces serum **vitamin B$_{12}$** levels in approximately 7% of patients but is rarely associated with anemia. Vitamin B$_{12}$ deficiency anemia can be treated with vitamin B$_{12}$ supplementation or by discontinuing metformin. Diminished vitamin B$_{12}$ absorption and transport can be improved with oral **calcium** supplementation.[19] Lactic acidosis has been reported; however, almost all cases occur in patients in whom metformin was contraindicated or in patients who attempted suicide by overdose. Lactic acidosis occurs in 0.03 case/1000 patients per year, with fatalities in approximately 50% of cases.[18]

Contraindications. Acute or chronic metabolic acidosis; patients undergoing radiographic studies requiring contrast media (withhold metformin just before the radiographic study and do not reinstate for 48 h after contrast media administration and upon documentation of normal renal function); abnormal Cl_{Cr} or Cr_s >1.5 mg/dL in males or >1.4 mg/dL in females; any disease that can cause hypoxia and result in accumulation of lactate (e.g., CHF requiring pharmacologic treatment, MI, severe infections, stroke); hepatic dysfunction.

Precautions. Avoid during pregnancy and lactation.

Drug Interactions. Furosemide and nifedipine increase serum levels of metformin, the clinical relevance of which is unknown. Cimetidine reduces the tubular secretion of metformin and can increase peak serum concentrations by as much as 60%.[20] (*See also* Insulins, Drug Interactions.)

Parameters to Monitor. Monitor renal function, hepatic function, and CBC before initiation of therapy and at least annually thereafter. Monitor renal function more closely in the elderly because of the age-related changes in renal function and greater risk for acute renal failure. (*See* Contraindications.) The goal of therapy is to reduce fasting blood glucose and glycosylated hemoglobin levels to normal or near normal by using the lowest effective dosage of the drug.

Notes. Because of its effect on weight and lipids, metformin is an appropriate choice for initial monotherapy in obese, new-onset type 2 diabetic patients, whereas **sulfonylureas** are usually a better choice for nonobese patients. In patients who do not respond to metformin monotherapy, combination therapy with a sulfonylurea, thiazolidinedione, or sitagliptin might be effective. Weight loss has been associated with metformin therapy (mean 0.8 kg); weight gain (mean 2.8 kg) has been found in patients treated with sulfonylureas.[21] Reductions in total cholesterol, LDL cholesterol, and triglycerides of 5%, 8%, and 16%, respectively, and an increase of 2% in HDL cholesterol have been reported.

NATEGLINIDE Starlix

Pharmacology. Nateglinide is a meglitinide similar to repaglinide that is a rapid-acting oral insulin secretagogue that stimulates insulin secretion in relation to serum blood glucose levels.

Adult Dosage. PO for type 2 diabetes—(alone or in combination with metformin) 120 mg tid before each meal. For patients near their A_{1c} goals, a dose of 60 mg can be used. Dosage adjustment is not necessary in the elderly or those with mild-to-severe renal impairment or mild to moderate hepatic impairment.

Dosage Forms. Tab 60, 120 mg.

Pharmacokinetics. Oral bioavailability is 72%. Peak plasma concentrations occur within 0.5–1.9 h. Plasma protein binding is 97%; Cl is 8.4 L/h. The drug is metabolized in the liver primarily by CYP3A4 and somewhat by CYP2C9, with 80% of the parent drug and glucuronide metabolites eliminated in the urine. Mild-to-moderate hepatic cirrhosis does not markedly alter single-dose pharmacokinetics of nateglinide. Half-life is 1.4 h.[22] Administration with metformin does not alter the pharmacokinetics of either drug.[23]

Adverse Reactions. The most frequent side effect is mild hypoglycemia manifested by increased sweating, tremor, dizziness, and increased appetite. Headache has occurred. Because of nateglinide's hepatic metabolism and extensive protein binding, interactions with other drugs affecting CYP3A4 and CYP2C9 or drugs extensively protein bound might result in pharmacokinetic interactions.

Contraindications, Precautions, and Parameters to Monitor. *See* Repaglinide.

REPAGLINIDE Prandin

Pharmacology. Repaglinide is a meglitinide agent that stimulates insulin release from the pancreas, although it is structurally unrelated to sulfonylureas. Compared with the sulfonylureas, repaglinide has a quicker onset and shorter duration of action, resulting in a lower risk of prolonged hypoglycemia.[24]

Administration and Adult Dosage. PO for type 2 diabetes—newly treated patients with A_{1c} 8% should start with 0.5 mg within 30 min before each meal. Patients previously treated with antidiabetic agents should start with 1 or 2 mg within 30 min before each meal. Increase dosage based on glycemic response, to a maximum of 4 mg/dose or 16 mg/d. Starting doses of repaglinide are unchanged when taken concurrently with metformin.

Special Populations. *Pediatric Dosage.* Safety and efficacy not established.

Geriatric Dosage. Dosage adjustment is not needed unless renal function is compromised. However, the elderly are more sensitive to hypoglycemia and should be monitored closely with initiation of therapy.

Other Conditions. No adjustment of the initial dosage is required in renal impairment but use caution with subsequent dosage increases. In patients with hepatic abnormalities, wait longer before increasing the dosage.

Dosage Forms. Tab 0.5, 1, 2 mg.

Patient Instructions. Take each dose 0–30 min before each meal, usually 15 min. Recognize signs and symptoms of hypoglycemia and treat accordingly. Skip your dose if you will miss a meal. Add a dose when you eat an extra meal.

Missed Doses. If you miss a dose, take your regular dose at your next scheduled meal. Do not double the dose.

Pharmacokinetics. *Fate.* Oral bioavailability is 56%. Peak plasma concentrations occur within 1 h; food reduces mean peak concentration by 20%, although time to peak concentration is not altered. Serum concentrations are higher and prolonged in those with liver impairment. Plasma protein binding is > 98%. V_d is 31 L; Cl is 38 L/h. The drug is metabolized primarily in the liver by CYP3A4 to inactive metabolites excreted in the feces.

$t_{1/2}$. approximately 1 h.

Adverse Reactions. The most frequent side effect is hypoglycemia. Upper respiratory infections, sinusitis, nausea, diarrhea, constipation, arthralgia, and headache have been reported, but their frequencies are equal to or only slightly higher than that of placebo.

Contraindications. Diabetic ketoacidosis; type 1 diabetes.

Precautions. Pregnancy; lactation. Use cautiously in patients with renal impairment and those at increased risk of hypoglycemia, including those with hepatic or adrenal insufficiency and in debilitated, elderly, or malnourished patients. Hypoglycemia is more frequent in treatment of previously untreated patients and those with HbA_{1c} <8%.[25]

Drug Interactions. Inhibitors of CYP3A4 (e.g., ketoconazole, miconazole, erythromycin) inhibit the metabolism of repaglinide. CYP3A4 inducers (e.g., rifampin, barbiturates, carbamazepine) might reduce serum levels of repaglinide.

Parameters to Monitor. Monitor fasting and selected postprandial blood glucose levels regularly and HbA_{1c} periodically.

SULFONYLUREA AGENTS

Pharmacology. Sulfonylureas enhance insulin secretion from pancreatic β cells and potentiate insulin action on several extrahepatic tissues. Long-term, sulfonylureas increase peripheral utilization of glucose, suppress hepatic gluconeogenesis, and possibly increase the sensitivity and/or number of peripheral insulin receptors. Second-generation sulfonylureas (e.g., **glyburide, glipizide, glimepiride**) are more potent than first-generation agents and are used in much smaller dosages, with lower resultant blood levels. These lower serum concentrations decrease the likelihood of protein-binding displacement and hepatic metabolic interference.

Administration and Adult Dosage. *See* Sulfonylurea Agents Comparison Chart.

Special Populations. *Pediatric Dosage.* Safety and efficacy not established.

Geriatric Dosage. Start at the lower end of the dosage range and slowly titrate upward if needed. Observe precautions with renal or hepatic impairment.

Other Conditions. Dosage alterations may be necessary with all sulfonylureas in patients with severe hepatic dysfunction. With renal disease, especially in geriatric patients, there is an increased duration of action with **chlorpropamide, acetohexamide,** and possibly **glyburide.**[26]

Dosage Forms. *See* Sulfonylurea Agents Comparison Chart.

Patient Instructions. Eat a recommended diet consistently on a day-to-day basis. Take this medication at the same time each day (in the morning for once-daily medications). Report factors that might alter blood glucose levels (e.g., infection, fasting states) and any side effects.

Missed Doses. Take a missed dose as soon as you remember unless it is near time of the next dose. Do not double doses.

Pharmacokinetics. *See* Sulfonylurea Agents Comparison Chart.

Adverse Reactions. Hypoglycemic reactions (especially with **chlorpropamide**), anorexia, nausea, vomiting, diarrhea, allergic skin reactions, and cholestatic jaundice occur occasionally. Hematologic disorders, mild disulfiram-like reaction to alcohol, hyponatremia (most common with **chlorpropamide** but can occur with **tolbutamide**), and bone marrow suppression occur rarely.[27]

Contraindications. Pregnancy; type 1 diabetes; juvenile, unstable, or brittle diabetes; diabetes complicated by acidosis, ketosis, diabetic coma, major surgery, severe infection, or severe trauma.

Precautions. Patients sensitive to one sulfonylurea might experience cross-sensitivity to other sulfonylureas. **Chlorpropamide** can cause hyponatremia, particularly in elderly women taking diuretics.[28]

Drug Interactions. Drugs that have been reported to enhance sulfonylurea effects include chloramphenicol (chlorpropamide and tolbutamide), dicumarol, fluconazole (glipizide, glyburide, tolbutamide, and possibly others), sulfonamides, and high-dose salicylates. Rifampin stimulates the metabolism of tolbutamide and possibly other sulfonylureas. Drugs that impair glucose tolerance include oral contraceptives, corticosteroids, thiazide diuretics, furosemide, thyroid hormones (large doses), and niacin.[29] Acute ingestion of alcohol in combination with sulfonylureas can produce severe hypoglycemia. (*See also* Insulins, Drug Interactions.)

Parameters to Monitor. Monitor clinical symptoms of hyperglycemia (mainly polyphagia, polyuria, polydipsia, or numbing or tingling of feet) or hypoglycemia (hunger, nervousness, warmth, sweating, palpitations, headaches, confusion, drowsiness, anxiety, blurred vision, or paresthesias of lips). Monitor fasting serum glucose levels frequently at the initiation of therapy to gauge the adequacy of the dosage. Self-monitoring of fasting and selected postprandial blood glucose levels by the patient is also helpful. (*See* Blood Glucose Monitors Comparison Chart.) Long-term diabetic control may best be monitored using hemoglobin A_{1c}.

Notes. Sulfonylureas are usually an appropriate choice for nonobese, new-onset type 2 diabetic patients, whereas **metformin** is more appropriate for obese type 2 patients.[30] Individualize the choice of sulfonylurea based on the patient's characteristics (e.g., renal function, hepatic function, likelihood of hypoglycemia) and the pharmacokinetics of the drugs. Glyburide, glipizide, glimepiride, and chlorpropamide are more effective at lowering blood glucose than acetohexamide, tolazamide, or tolbutamide.[11] Acetohexamide, tolazamide, and tolbutamide probably should be reserved for mild hyperglycemia or in those likely to develop hypoglycemia (e.g., the elderly). In patients who do not respond to sulfonylurea monotherapy, combination therapy with **insulin, metformin, rosiglitazone, pioglitazone,** or **acarbose** may be effective.[31] **Glimepiride** is the most potent sulfonylurea agent, has the lowest rate of hypoglycemia, and does not affect potassium channels in the heart.[32]

SULFONYLUREA AGENTS COMPARISON CHART

DRUG	DOSAGE FORMS	DAILY DOSAGE	FATE	DURATION (h)	COMMENTS
FIRST GENERATION					
Acetohexamide Dymelor Various	Tab 250, 500 mg	250 mg–1.5 g in 2 divided doses	65% converted to an active metabolite (hydroxyhexamide)	12–18	May be useful in the elderly and others prone to hypoglycemia but avoid in patients with renal dysfunction.
Chlorpropamide Diabinese Various	Tab 100, 250 mg	100–500 mg in a single dose	Metabolized and 20% excreted unchanged	24–72	Avoid in elderly and in patients with renal dysfunction. Causes disulfiram-like reaction in 30% of patients.
Tolazamide Tolinase Various	Tab 100, 250, 500 mg	100 mg–1 g in 1–2 divided doses	Converted to weakly active metabolites	16–24	Delayed onset of action (3–4 h); may be useful in the elderly and others prone to hypoglycemia.
Tolbutamide Orinase Various	Tab 500 mg	500 mg–3 g in 2–3 divided doses	Converted to inactive compounds	6–12	May be useful in the elderly and others prone to hypoglycemia.
SECOND GENERATION					
Glimepiride Amaryl	Tab 1, 2, 4 mg	1–8 mg in a single dose	Converted to inactive and active metabolites	24	Similar to glyburide; lowest rate of hypoglycemia and does not affect cardiac potassium channels.
Glipizide Glucotrol Glucotrol XL	Tab 5, 10 mg SR Tab 2.5, 5, 10 mg	Non-SR 5–40 mg in 1–2 divided doses SR 5–20 mg in a single dose	Converted to inactive metabolites	10–24 (non-SR) 18–24 (SR)	Take non-SR product on an empty stomach.

(continued)

SULFONYLUREA AGENTS COMPARISON CHART (*continued*)

DRUG	DOSAGE FORMS	DAILY DOSAGE	FATE	DURATION (h)	COMMENTS
Glyburide DiaBeta Glynase Micronase Various	Tab 1.25, 2.5, 5 mg Tab (micronized) 1.5, 3, 4.5, 6 mg	Nonmicronized 1.25–20 mg in 1–2 divided doses Micronized 0.75–12 mg in 1–2 divided doses	Converted to inactive and active metabolites	18–24	The micronized product (Glynase, various) offers no advantage over the nonmicronized products.
COMBINATION PRODUCT					
Glyburide and Metformin Glucovance	Tab 1.25 mg glyburide plus 250 mg metformin, 2.5 mg or 5 mg glyburide plus 500 mg metformin	1.25 mg/250 mg daily bid initially, to a maximum of 20 mg/ 2000 mg daily in 1–2 divided doses	(See individual agents)	18–24	
Glipizide and Metformin Metaglip	2.5/250, 2.5/5000, 5/500	2.5/250 initially	(See individual agents)	10–24	
Rosiglitazone and Glimepiride Avandaryl	4/1, 4/2, 4/4	4/1 initially Maximum 8/4 mg/d	(See individual agents)	24	
Pioglitazone and Glimepiride Duetact	30/2, 30/4	30/2	(See individual agents)	24	

From Refs. 27 and 28 and product information.

795

PIOGLITAZONE Actos

Pharmacology. Pioglitazone is a thiazolidinedione antihyperglycemic agent used to improve insulin sensitivity in patients with type 2 diabetes. Insulin-dependent glucose disposal in skeletal muscle is improved and hepatic glucose production is decreased; both actions contribute to pioglitazone's glucose-lowering effects. Pioglitazone is only effective in the presence of insulin; by itself it does not lead to hypoglycemia and does not increase insulin secretion. Because insulin is required for its action, pioglitazone should not be used in patients with type 1 diabetes. **Rosiglitazone** (Avandia) is another thiazolidinedione antidiabetic agent that acts similarly to pioglitazone.

Administration and Adult Dosage. **PO for type 2 diabetes—(monotherapy)** 15–30 mg once daily with food; after a 4-week trial dosage can be increased to a maximum of 45 mg/d. If no response occurs at the maximum dose of 45 mg/d, other therapeutic options should be considered; **(combination therapy with insulin, sulfonylurea, or metformin)** 15–30 mg once daily initially, increasing q4wk to a maximum of 45 mg/d. Dosages of insulin or sulfonylurea may need to be decreased based on the glucose-lowering response. For those on **insulin,** decrease the insulin dosage when fasting plasma glucose levels are < 100 mg/dL or if hypoglycemic symptoms occur.

Special Populations. *Pediatric Dosage.* Safety and efficacy not established.

Geriatric Dosage. (>65 years) no differences in efficacy or safety; dosage adjustments are not required.

Other Conditions. No dosage adjustment is required in renal impairment.

Dosage Forms. **Tab** 15, 30, 45 mg.

Patient Instructions. Take once daily without regard to meals. If you are taking insulin, a sulfonylurea, or other glucose-lowering agent, you should understand the signs and symptoms of hypoglycemia and its appropriate treatment. Report nausea, vomiting, abdominal pain, loss of appetite, or dark urine immediately to your health care provider. Because pioglitazone's effect on oral contraceptives has not been established, other means of contraception may be required.

Missed Doses. If you forget to take a dose, take your regular dose the next day. Do not double the dose on the next day.

Pharmacokinetics. *Fate.* Oral absorption is rapid, with the peak plasma concentration in 2 h. Steady-state serum levels are achieved in 7 days. Extensively bound to serum albumin (>99%). V_d is 10.5–26.5 L/kg. Metabolized extensively by hydroxylation and oxidation in the liver and principally by CYP2C8 and CYP3A4. Renal elimination is negligible (15%–30%), with most of the oral dose believed to be excreted into the bile unchanged or as metabolites and subsequently eliminated in the feces.

$t_{1/2}$. 16–24 h.

Adverse Reactions. Mild-to-moderate hypoglycemia when used concurrently with a sulfonylurea or insulin. Headache, anemia (mean hemoglobin value decrease of 2%–4%), edema, weight gain.[33]

Contraindications. Diabetic keotacidosis, jaundice, active liver disease or ALT levels exceeding 2.5 times the upper limit of normal. Black box warning—symptomatic heart disease, CHF NYAC (New York Heart Association) III or IV.

Precautions. Premenopausal anovulatory individuals might resume ovulation, placing them at risk for pregnancy. Risk of edema, weight gain, or CHF increases when higher doses are used in conjunction with insulin in patients at risk of heart failure.[34]

Drug Interactions. Ethinyl estradiol and norethindrone plasma concentrations might be reduced, resulting in possible loss of contraceptive efficacy. Ketoconazole and possibly other drugs that inhibit CYP3A4 might inhibit the metabolism of pioglitazone. Additionally, CYP3A4-metabolized drugs such as calcium channel blockers, corticosteroids, cyclosporine, and HMG-CoA reductase inhibitors have not been specifically studied but might affect the metabolism of pioglitazone.

Parameters to Monitor. Monitor serum ALT levels at the start of therapy, and then periodically thereafter. If ALT is elevated 1–2.5 times the upper limit of normal at any time (before initiation or during therapy), the cause of the enzyme elevation should be determined. If ALT levels exceed 3 times the upper limit of normal or if at any time the patient is jaundiced, pioglitazone should be discontinued. Monitor fasting blood sugars and A_{1c}. (*See* Sulfonylureas.)

Notes. In patients with type 2 diabetes on insulin therapy, pioglitazone often results in a decreased requirement for **insulin.** Patients on concomitant therapy with insulin or **sulfonylureas** should not alter the doses of the latter medications until positive changes in fasting plasma glucose levels are obtained (fasting blood sugars <100 mg/dL) or if symptoms of hypoglycemia are experienced. (*See* Thiazolidinedione Comparison Chart.)

THIAZOLIDINEDIONE COMPARISON CHART

DRUG	MONOTHERAPY INITIATION DOSE	COMBINATION INITIATION DOSE	MAXIMUM DOSE	COMMENTS
Pioglitazone Actos	15–30 mg once daily	15–30 mg once daily	45 mg once daily	Approved for use with insulin, a sulfonylurea, or metformin. Increased risk of edema, weight gain, CHF when higher doses used with insulin. Black box warning regarding HF. May improve lipid profile.
Rosiglitazone Avandia	2 mg bid or 4 mg once daily	2 mg bid or 4 mg once daily	4 mg bid or 8 mg once daily	Approved for use with a sulfonylurea or metformin. Maximum 4 mg/d when used with insulin. Black box warning regarding HF and myocardial ischemia. May increase LDL and HDL cholesterol.[33]

SITAGLIPTIN
Januvia

Pharmacology. Dipeptidyl peptidase-4 (DPP-4) degrades the incretin hormones glucagon-like peptide-1 (GLP-1) and glucose-dependent insulinotropic peptide (GIP). Sitagliptin is an FDA approved DPP-4 inhibitor. Sitagliptin is used as monotherapy or with other antidiabetic agents to treat type 2 diabetes mellitus. Use with insulin has not been studied. When used as monotherapy or in combination with metformin or pioglitazone, a significant reduction in A_{1c} is obtained in the range of 0.3–0.6.[35] Vildagliptin, another DPP-4 inhibitor is under clinical investigation.

Administration and Adult Dosage. PO for type 2 diabetes—(monotherapy or in combination with other antidiabetic agents) 100 mg PO once daily.

Special Populations. *Pediatric Dosage.* Safety and efficacy not established.

Geriatric Dosage. Same as adult dosage.

Other Conditions. $Cl_{Cr} \geq 50$ mL/min no dosage adjustment. Cl_{Cr} 30–50 mL/min: 50 mg once daily. Cl_{Cr} <30 mL/min: 25 mg once daily.

Dosage Forms. **Tab** 25, 50, 100 mg.

Patient Instructions. Take once daily with or without meals. When used with a sulfonylurea, the dose of the sulfonylurea may need to be decreased to lessen the risk of hypoglycemia.

Missed Dose. If a dose is missed, take as soon as possible unless near the time of the next scheduled dose.

Pharmacokinetics. *Fate.* Rapid absorption after oral administration; 87% bioavailable. Mean plasma AUC is 8.52 μM/h and C_{max} of 950 nM. Mean volume of distribution is 198 L; 38% bound to plasma albumin; minimal hepatic metabolism. Primarily renally eliminated with 79% unchanged in the urine.

$t_{1/2}$. 12.4 h with normal renal function.

Adverse Reactions. Most common are nasopharyngitis, upper respiratory tract infection, and headache. Not associated with hypoglycemia when used with metformin or pioglitazone. When used with a sulfonylurea, incidence of hypoglycemia is increased.

Contraindications. Diabetic ketoacidosis, type 1 diabetes.

Precautions. Patients with altered GI function such as that seen with diarrhea, gastroparesis, GI obstruction, ileus, or vomiting. Dosage adjustment needed in patients with moderate-to-severe renal insufficiency and patients with ESRD requiring dialysis. Use cautiously in elderly because of possible altered renal function.

Drug Interactions. There are no unique drug interactions to sitagliptin. (See also Insulins, Drug Interactions.)

Parameters to Monitor. Blood glucose, A_{1c}.

PRAMLINTIDE
Symlin

Pharmacology. Pramlintide is a synthetic amylin analogue used as an adjunct to insulin for patients with type 1 or type 2 diabetes. Amylin is effective in lowering blood glucose by 3 primary mechanisms: slowing gastric emptying, suppressing postprandial glucagon secretion, and by central modulation of appetite that results in reduced caloric intake.[36,37]

Administration and Adult Dosage. Type 1 diabetes amylin is administered 15 μg subcutaneously immediately prior to each meal, or with a snack that contains ≥ 250 kcal or 30 g of carbohydrates. Dose titrated by 15 μg only after a 3-day period devoid of nausea. Target dose is 60 μg prior to each meal. Type 2 diabetes amylin 60 μg is administered subcutaneously prior to each meal, or with a snack that contains ≥ 250 kcal or 30 g of carbohydrates, with a target dose of 120 μg. Titration from 60 μg to 120 μg should only occur after a 3–7 day nausea-free period.

Special Populations. *Adolescents and Children.* Safe and effective use has not been established.

Geriatric Dosage. Same as adult dosage.

Dosage Forms. Pramlintide acetate 0.6mg/1mL solution for injection, Symlin Pen 60 and Symlin Pen 120 (1000 μg/mL solution for injection).

Patient Instructions. Do not mix pramlintide and insulin in the same syringe. Inject pramlintide in a separate site from insulin. May be necessary to decrease insulin dose by 50% when starting pramlintide, consult your physician. When using a vial, use insulin syringe only (0.3-mL syringe recommended). Inject SQ into abdomen or thigh. Do not inject into the arm. Rotate injection sites. Store unopened vials or pen injectors in the refrigerator and protect from light. Do not freeze. Pen injectors once used or opened vials should be stored in the refrigerator at room temperature up to 86°F. Severe hypoglycemia occurs most frequently in the first 4 weeks of therapy and within 3 h of injection. Do not drive or operate heavy equipment until response to therapy is known.

Pharmacokinetics. *Fate.* 30%–40% bioavailable, with a C_{max} of 39–147 pmol/L (dose proportional) and T_{max} reached in approximately 20 min; 40% albumin bound, metabolized primarily in the kidney with renal elimination.

$t_{1/2}$. 48 min.

Adverse Reactions. Nausea, vomiting, and anorexia are most common and tend to abate with time. Severe hypoglycemia occurs most frequently in patients with type 1 diabetes.

Contraindications. Hypersensitivity to pramlintide, metacresol, D-mannitol, acetic acid or sodium acetate. Gastroparesis, hypoglycemia unawareness.

Precautions. Only prescribe to patients without visual or dexterity impairment. Pramlintide has not been studied in patients with hepatic impairment, however, hepatic dysfunction is not expected to alter the response to pramlintide. Systemic allergic reaction is possible. Black box warning regarding severe hypoglycemia with the risk being higher in patients with type 1 diabetes and occurring within 3 h of injection.

Drug Interactions. Use with drugs that alter GI motility (e.g., anticholinergics, metoclopramide) or with α-glucosidase inhibitors (acarbose, miglitol) is not recommended due to pramlintide's effect on gastric emptying. Drugs that require rapid absorption should be given 1 h prior or 2 h after administration of pramlintide. (*See also* Insulins, Drug Interactions.)

Parameters to Monitor. Blood glucose, A_{1c}.

EXENATIDE
Byetta

Pharmacology. Exenatide is an incretin mimetic GLP-1 analogue. Exenatide enhances glucose-dependent insulin secretion, slows gastric emptying, suppresses glucagon secretion, and decreases caloric intake.[38] The net result of these mechanisms is to reduce fasting and postprandial blood glucose concentrations. Exenatide when used with metformin and/or a sulfonylurea has demonstrated reductions in A_{1c} in the range of 0.4%–0.9%.[39–41] Weight reductions in the range of 0.9–2.8 kg are reported.

Administration and Adult Dosage. 5 µg SQ twice daily, and at least 6 h apart and within 60 min of the morning and evening meals; can titrate to 10 µg twice daily after 1 month.

Special Populations. Children and adolescents—safe and effective use has not been established. Geriatric—pharmacokinetics unaffected by age. Race—no significant pharmacokinetic differences based on race (Caucasian, Hispanic, black). Obesity—pharmacokinetics unaffected.

Geriatric Dosage. Same as adult dosage.

Dosage Forms. 5 and 10 µg pen injections.

Patient Instructions. Administer subcutaneously into the thigh, abdomen, or upper arm within 60 min of breakfast and dinner and at least 6 h apart. Rotate injection sites. Do not administer after a meal. Prime pen prior to first use. Unopened prefilled pens should be stored in a refrigerator and can be stored at a temperature not to exceed 77°F after initial use. Do not freeze.

Pharmacokinetics. *Fate.* Mean peak plasma exenatide concentration 211 pg/mL reached within 2 h. Mean apparent V_d 28.3L. Primarily eliminated via glomerular filtration. Clearance 9.1 L/h.

$t_{1/2}$. 2.4 h.

Adverse Reactions. Nausea, diarrhea, vomiting, dizziness, headache, dyspepsia.[40,41]

Contraindications. Colitis, cresol hypersensitivity, Crohn's disease, DKA, gastroparesis, GI disease (e.g., ileus, inflammatory bowel disease, pseudomembranous colitis, ulcerative colitis), bleeding, obstruction or perforation, renal failure.

Precautions. Exenatide is not a substitute for insulin and therefore should not be used to treat DKA. Acute pancreatitis associated with exenatide has been reported. If pancreatitis is suspected, the use of exenatide should be suspended until the underlying etiology has been identified. Treatment with exenatide is not recommended in patients developing pancreatitis unless an alternate etiology has been confirmed. As patients can develop exenatide antibodies patients should be observed for hypersensitivity reactions or worsening of glycemic control.

Drug Interactions. Because of exenatide's effect on gastric emptying, it should be administered at least 1 h after consuming drugs dependent on threshold concentrations (e.g., oral contraceptives, antibiotics). (*See also* Insulins, Drug Interactions).

Parameters to Monitor. Blood glucose, A_{1c}.

BLOOD GLUCOSE MONITORS COMPARISON CHART

NAME MANUFACTURER	TEST STRIP USED	RANGE (mg/dL)	TEST TIME (s)	FEATURES
Accu-Chek Advantage (Roche Diagnostics)	Advantage or Comfort Curve	10–600	40	No clearing, wiping, or timing; touchable test strips; time and date; large target area; 100-value memory; PC down loading
Accu-Chek Complete (Roche Diagnostics)	Advantage or Comfort Curve	10–600	40	2-step procedure; pushbutton selection: stores and analyzes up to 1000 values
Accu-Chek Voice Mate (Roche Diagnostics)	Comfort Curve	10–600	40	For visually impaired and the blind; voice guidance; no need to clean
Accu-Chek Active (Roche Diagnostics)	Accu-Chek Active	10–600	5–10	Alternate site testing capabilities; 200-test memory
Accu-Chek Aviva (Roche Diagnostics)	Accu-Chek Aviva	10–600	5	500-test memory; Arthritis Foundation Ease-of-Use Commendation
Accu-Chek Compact Plus (Roche Diagnostics)	Accu-Chek Compact	10–600	5	Built-in detachable lancet device; 17-test strip drum; 500-test memory
Advance Intuition (ARKRAY)	Advance Intuition	30–550	10	Large display; single button control; 10-test memory
Advance Micro-Draw (ARKRAY)	Advance Micro-Draw	20–600	15	Small sample size requirement (1.5 µL); 250-test memory
Advocate Talking Blood Glucose Meter Kit (Sun Coast)	Advocate	20–600	7	Bilingua—English and Spanish; no coding required; 450-test memory
Advocate Duo (Sun Coast)	Advocate Duo TD-3223	20–600	7	Blood glucose and blood pressure monitoring; 450-test memory
Breeze2 (Bayer Diabetes Care)	Breeze2 Test Disc	20–600	5	10-test strip disc; no coding required; 420-test memory; Ease-Of-Use Commendation from the Arthritis Foundation

(continued)

801

BLOOD GLUCOSE MONITORS COMPARISON CHART (*continued*)

NAME MANUFACTURER	TEST STRIP USED	RANGE (mg/dL)	TEST TIME (s)	FEATURES
Contour (Bayer Diabetes Care)	Ascensia Contour	10–600	5	Basic and advanced modes; no coding necessary
Control AST (U.S. Diagnostics, Inc.)	Control	10–600	5	Alternate site testing; 250-test memory
EasyGluco (U.S. Diagnostics, Inc.)	EasyGluco	10–600	9	Alternate site testing; 200-test memory
FreeStyle Flash (Abbott Diabetes Care)	FreeStyle	20–500	7	Compact design; alternate site testing
FreeStyle Freedom (Abbott Diabetes Care)	FreeStyle Lite	20–500	5	Compact design; alternate site testing; 400-test memory
FreeStyle Lite (Abbott Diabetes Care)	FreeStyle Lite	20–500	5	Compact design; alternate site testing; 400-test memory
Nova Max (Nova Biomedical)	NovaMax	20–600	5	No coding necessary; NovaMax Link version can communicate with Medtronic insulin pumps
One Touch UltraSmart (LifeScan)	OneTouch Ultra	20–600	5	Organizes readings automatically into 9 charts and graphs; alternate site testing; 3000-test memory
One Touch Ultra2 (LifeScan)	OneTouch Ultra	20–600	5	Tabulates before and after meal averages; 500-test memory
OneTouch UltraMini (LifeScan) (Home Diagnostics)	OneTouch Ultra	20–600	5	Compact design; 50-test memory

(continued)

BLOOD GLUCOSE MONITORS COMPARISON CHART (*continued*)

NAME MANUFACTURER	TEST STRIP USED	RANGE (mg/dL)	TEST TIME (s)	FEATURES
Prestige IQ (Home Diagnostics)	Prestige Smart System	25–600	10–50	365-test memory; 14 or 30 d morning average, large display; English and Spanish videos available
Prodigy AutoCode Talking (Diagnostic Devices, Inc.)	Prodigy	20–600	6	English and Spanish voice; no coding required; alternate site testing; 1 button navigation
Prodigy Voice (Diagnostic Devices, Inc.)	Prodigy	20–600	6	Totally audible; no coding required; alternate site testing
Prodigy AutoCode (Diagnostic Devices, Inc.)	Prodigy	20–600	6	English and Spanish voice; no coding required
Prodigy Duo (Diagnostic Devices, Inc.)	Prodigy	20–600	6	Combined glucose and blood pressure testing; built in audio result reporting 450-test memory; alternate site testing
Prodigy Eject (Diagnostic Devices, Inc.)	Prodigy	20–600	6	Eject button for test-strip removal; alternate site testing
QuickTek (ARKRAY)	QuickTek	20–600	10–30	Durable test strips; 250-test memory
ReliOn Ultima (Solartek Products, Inc.)	ReliOn Ultima	20–500	5	Forearm testing capabilities; 450-test memory
Sidekick (Home Diagnostics)	Sidekick	52–473	10	No coding necessary; compact design; forearm testing capabilities; disposable unit containing 50 test strips
TrueTrack Smart System (Home Diagnostics)	TrueTrack	25–600	10	Simple 2-step testing; alternate site testing; 365-test memory
WaveSense Keynote (Agamatrix)	WaveSense Keynote	20–600	4	Large back-lit display for visually impaired

Adapted from Ref. 42.

■ REFERENCES

1. Mooradian AD, Thurman JE. Drug therapy of postprandial hyperglycaemia. *Drugs.* 1999;57:19-29.

2. Lebovitz HE. Glucosidase inhibitors in the treatment of hyperglycemia. In: Lebovitz HE, ed. *Therapy for Diabetes Mellitus and Related Disorders.* 2nd ed. Alexandria, VA: American Diabetes Association; 1994.

3. Anonymous. Tests of glycemia in diabetes. *Diabetes Care.* 1999;22(suppl 1):S77-S79.

4. Steele JW et al. Epalrestat: a review of its pharmacology, and therapeutic potential in late-onset complications of diabetes mellitus. *Drugs Aging.* 1993;3:532-535.

5. Hamada Y, Nakamura J. Clinical potential of aldose reductase inhibitors in diabetic neuropathy. *Treat Endocrinol.* 2004;3(4):245-255.

6. White CM. A review of potential cardiovascular uses of intravenous glucagon administration. *J Clin Pharmacol.* 1999;39:442-447.

7. Skyler JS. Insulin treatment. In: Lebovitz HE, ed. *Therapy for Diabetes Mellitus and Related Disorders.* 3rd ed. Alexandria, VA: American Diabetes Association; 1998:186-203.

8. Genuth S. Diabetic ketoacidosis and hyperosmolar hyperglycemic nonketotic syndrome in adults. In: Lebovitz HE, ed. *Therapy for Diabetes Mellitus and Related Disorders.* 3rd ed. Alexandria, VA: American Diabetes Association; 1998:83-96.

9. Kahn SE et al. Insulin secretion in the normal and diabetic human. In: Alberti KGMM et al., eds. *International Textbook of Diabetes Mellitus.* 2nd ed. New York: John Wiley & Sons; 1997:337-353.

10. The Diabetes Control and Complications Trial Research Group. The effect of intensive treatment of diabetes on the development and progression of long-term complications in insulin-dependent diabetes mellitus. *N Engl J Med.* 1993;329:977-986.

11. White JR Jr, Campbell RK. Pharmacologic therapies in the management of diabetes mellitus. In: Haire-Joshu D, ed. *Management of Diabetes Mellitus. Perspectives of Care Across the Life Span.* St. Louis, MO: Mosby–Year Book; 1994:119-148.

12. Peterson L et al. Insulin adsorbance to polyvinylchloride surfaces with implications for constant-infusion therapy. *Diabetes.* 1976;25:72-74.

13. Setter SM et al. Insulin aspart: a new rapid-acting insulin analog. *Ann Pharmacother.* 2000;34:1423-1431.

14. Dailey G, et al. Insulin glulisine provides improved glycemic control in patients with type 2 diabetes. *Diabetes Care.* 2004;27:2363-2368.

15. Rosskamp RH, Park G. Long-acting insulin analogs. *Diabetes Care.* 1999;22(suppl 2):B109-B113.

16. Plank J et al. A double-blind, randomized, dose-response study investigating the pharmacodynamic and pharmacokinetic properties of the long-acting insulin analog detemir. *Diabetes Care.* 2005;28:1107-1112.

17. Iltz JL, Odegard PS, Setter SM, et al. Update in the pharmacologic treatment of diabetes focus on insulin detemir, insulin glulisine, and inhaled dry powdered insulin. *Diabetes Educ.* 2007;33(2):215-253.

18. Bailey CJ, Turner RC. Metformin. *N Engl J Med.* 1996;334:574-579.

19. Bauman WA et al. Increased intake of calcium reverses vitamin B_{12} malabsorption induced by metformin. *Diabetes Care.* 2000;23:1227-1231.

20. Somogyi A et al. Reduction of metformin tubular secretion by cimetidine in man. *Br J Clin Pharmacol.* 1987;23: 545-551.

21. Hermann LS et al. Therapeutic comparison of metformin and sulfonylurea, alone and in various combinations. *Diabetes Care.* 1994;17:1100-1108.

22. Choudhury S et al. Single-dose pharmacokinetics of nateglinide in subjects with hepatic cirrhosis. *J Clin Pharmacol.* 2000;40:634-640.

23. Hirschberg Y et al. Improved control of mealtime glucose excursions with coadministration of nateglinide and metformin. *Diabetes Care.* 2000;23:349-353.

24. Wolffenbuttel BHR, Landgraf R; Dutch and German Repaglinide Study Group. A 1-year multicenter randomized double-blind comparison of repaglinide and glyburide for the treatment of type 2 diabetes. *Diabetes Care.* 1999;22:463-467.

25. Levien TL, Baker DE. *Drug evaluation—repaglinide.* Dana Point, CA: The Formulary Monograph Service; April 1998.

26. Gossain VV et al. Management of diabetes in the elderly: a clinical perspective. *J Assoc Acad Minor Phys.* 1996; 5:22-31.

27. Davidson MB. Rational use of sulfonylureas. *Postgrad Med.* 1992;92:69-85.

28. Gerich JE. Oral hypoglycemic agents. *N Engl J Med.* 1989;321:1231-1245.

29. White JR Jr, Campbell RK. Drug/drug and drug/disease interactions and diabetes. *Diabetes Educ.* 1995;21:283-289.

30. White JR. The pharmacologic management of patients with type II diabetes mellitus in the era of oral agents and insulin analogs. *Diabetes Spectrum.* 1996;9:227-234.

31. DeFronzo RA. Pharmacologic therapy for type 2 diabetes mellitus. *Ann Intern Med.* 1999;131:281-303.

32. Campbell RK, White JR. Overview of medications used to treat type 2 diabetes. In: *Medications for the Treatment of Diabetes.* Alexandria, VA: American Diabetes Association; 2000:23-43.
33. Campbell RK, White JR, eds. Glitazones. In: *Medications for the Treatment of Diabetes.* Alexandria, VA: American Diabetes Association; 2000:71-86.
34. Nesto RW et al. Thiazolidinedione use, fluid retention, and congestive heart failure. A consensus statement from the American Heart Association (AHA) and the American Diabetes Association (ADA). *Circulation.* 2003;108: 2941-2948.
35. Miller SA, St. Onge EL. Sitagliptin: a dipeptidyl peptidase IV inhibitor for the treatment of type 2 diabetes. *Ann Pharmacother.* 2006;40:1336-1343.
36. Kleppinger EL, Vivian EM. Pramlintide for the treatment of diabetes mellitus. *Ann Pharmacother.* 2003;37: 1082-1089.
37. Ryan GJ et al. Pramlintide in the treatment of type 1 and type 2 diabetes mellitus. *Clin Ther.* 2005;27:1500-1512.
38. Joy SV et al. Incretin mimetics as emerging treatments for type 2 diabetes. *Ann Pharmacother.* 2005;39:110-118.
39. Defronzo RA et al. Effects of exenatide (exendin-4) on glycemic control and weight over 30 weeks in metformin treated patients with type 2 diabetes. *Diabetes Care.* 2005;28:1092-1100.
40. Kendall DM et al. Effects of exenatide (exendin-4) on glycemic control over 30 weeks in patients with type 2 diabetes treated with metformin and a sulfonylurea. *Diabetes Care.* 2005;28:1083-1091.
41. Fineman MS et al. Effect on glycemic control of exenatide (synthetic exendin-4) additive to existing metformin and/or sulfonylurea treatment in patients with type 2 diabetes. *Diabetes Care.* 2003;26:2370-2377.
42. Anon. Your complete blood glucose meters reference guide from Diabetes Health. http://www.diabeteshealth.com/media/pdfs/PRG1207/Blood-Glucose-Meter-Reference-Guide-1207.pdf. Accessed November 18, 2008.

Chapter 51

Contraceptives

Peggy Piascik and T. Joseph Mattingly

Class Instructions. *Oral Contraceptives.* Take this drug at approximately the same time each day for maximum efficacy. This drug may be taken with food, milk, or an antacid if stomach upset occurs. Use an additional form of contraception concurrently during the first 7 days of oral progestin-only products or if you do not start your oral contraceptives on day 1 of menses. If spotting occurs and no oral doses have been missed, continue to take tablets even if spotting continues. Report immediately if any of the following occur: new severe or persistent headache; blurred or loss of vision; shortness of breath; severe leg, chest, or abdominal pain; or any abnormal vaginal bleeding. Hormonal contraceptives do not protect against HIV infection or other sexually transmitted diseases.

COMBINATION ORAL CONTRACEPTIVES

Pharmacology. These products contain an estrogen, ethinyl estradiol or mestranol, and a progestin derived from either 19-nortestosterone or spironolactone which are taken in a cyclic fashion, usually 21 of 28 days. As contraceptives, estrogens suppress follicle-stimulating hormone (FSH) and luteinizing hormone (LH) to inhibit ovulation, cause edematous endometrial changes that are hostile to implantation of the fertilized ovum, accelerate ovum transport, and produce degeneration of the corpus luteum (luteolysis). Progestins inhibit ovulation by suppression of LH, inhibit sperm capacitation, slow down ovum transport, produce a thin endometrium that hampers implantation, and cause cervical mucus changes that are hostile to sperm migration. Induction of a pseudopregnancy state and anovulation improves symptoms of endometriosis. Anovulatory dysfunctional uterine bleeding caused by unopposed estrogen or estrogen withdrawal responds to progestins. (*See* Contraception Efficacy and Risks and Benefits of Oral Contraceptives Comparison charts.)

Administration and Adult Dosage. **PO for contraception, acne (norgestimate- and drospirenone-containing products) and premenstrual dysphoric disorder (Yaz)—** (monophasic combinations) 1 tablet daily beginning on the first day of menses and continue for 21 days; stop for 7 days and start the next cycle of 21 tablets. Combination 28-day products (21 active tablets followed by 7 inert or iron tablets) are taken daily on a continuous basis; (multiphasic combinations) 1 tablet daily beginning either on the first day of menses (Triphasil only) or the first Sunday after the beginning of menstruation (if menstruation begins on Sunday, take first tablet on that day). (Extended cycle products) 84 active tablets followed by 7 placebo or low-dose ethinyl estradiol tablets; 24 active tablets followed by 4 placebo or iron-containing tablets; 21 active tablets followed by 2 placebo tablets and 5 reduced ethinyl estradiol tablets; 365 active tablets with no placebo tablets; 1 tablet daily continuously.[1,2] **PO for contraception postpartum**— start 6 weeks postpartum if not breastfeeding; lactation prolongs period of infertility. **PO for contraception postabortion**—start immediately if gestation is terminated at 12 weeks or earlier; start in 1 week if gestation is terminated at 13–28 weeks. **PO for emergency post-coital contraception**—(Yuzpe regimen) two doses taken 12 h apart, each dose contains 100 μg of ethinyl estradiol plus 0.5 mg of levonorgestrel.[3] Start regimen within 72 h of unprotected coitus. **PO for dysfunctional uterine bleeding (anovulatory cycles)**—(any combination agent) 1 tablet daily to qid for 5–7 days for acute bleeding, then 1 tablet daily as for contraception; continue for 3 months to prevent further bleeding.[4] **PO for dysmenorrhea or endometriosis**—(any combination tablet) 1 tablet daily continuously for 15 weeks, followed by 1 drug-free week; repeat 16-week cycle for 6–12 months to induce a pseudopregnant state.[5] **Transdermal for contraception**—(OrthoEvra) Apply one patch each week for 3 weeks (21 total days); followed by one week that is patch-free. Apply the patch on the same day each week ("patch change day"). Only one patch should be worn at a time. No more than 7 days should pass during the patch-free interval. **Vaginal for contraception**—(NuvaRing) One ring, inserted vaginally and left in place for 3 con-secutive weeks, then removed for 1 week. A new ring is inserted 7 days after the last was removed (even if bleeding is not complete) and should be inserted at approxi-mately the same time of day the ring was removed the previous week.

Special Populations. *Geriatric Dosage.* Same as adult dosage. *Pediatric Dosage.* Not to be used prior to menarche. *Smokers.* The risk of cardiovascular side effects increases in smokers, especially those who are >35 years of age; women who use combination hormonal contraceptives should be strongly advised not to smoke.[6]

Other Conditions Discontinue oral contraceptives at least 2 weeks before elective major surgery and do not reinstitute until at least 2 weeks afterward. Stop imme-diately in patients undergoing emergency surgery or immobilization for long peri-ods; institute low-dose SQ heparin or other appropriate thromboembolitic prophy-laxis in the postoperative period and restart cycle 4 weeks after returning to normal activities.[7] Start with an agent containing at least 50 μg estradiol in women receiv-ing rifampin or any cytochrome P450-inducing anticonvulsant.[7–8]

Dosage Forms. (*See* Oral Contraceptive Agents Comparison Chart.)

Patient Instructions. (*See* Class Instructions: Contraceptives.) (Contraception) any menstrual irregularities and bothersome side effects should diminish after the first 3–4 cycles. Report if no menses occur for 2 months. (Acute anovulatory bleed-ing) expect heavy and severely cramping flow 2–4 days after stopping therapy, with normal periods thereafter. (Vaginal Ring) Wash hands and remove ring from protective pouch (keep pouch for later ring disposal). Press sides of ring together between thumb and index finger and insert folded ring into vagina. Insert ring far enough into the vagina to be comfortable. To remove, hook index finger around rim and pull out. If the ring falls out, it may be rinsed with cool or warm (not hot) water and replaced. However, it must be replaced within 3 h. Refer to dosing if ring is out of place for > 3 h. Tampons do not interfere with the effectiveness of the ring; caution should be used when removing tampon, not to remove ring. The ring may interfere with correct placement of diaphragms; diaphragms should not be used as a backup method of contraception. Ensure proper vaginal placement of the ring to avoid inadvertent urinary bladder insertion. Check package insert for instructions when switching to the vaginal ring from another form of hormonal contraception. A spermicide or barrier method of contraception should be used until the ring has been in place for 7 consecutive days.[10] (Transdermal Patch) Apply to a clean, dry area of intact skin on the buttock, abdomen, upper outer arm, or upper torso. Press system firmly in place with the palm of the hand for about 10 seconds; ensure good contact, especially around the edges. Do not apply to sites that are oily, damaged, or irritated. Do not apply transdermal system to the breasts or to areas where tight clothing may cause the system to be rubbed off. If the system inadvertently gets detached and is removed for less than one day, reapply the system or, if necessary, apply a new system; if the system is removed for longer than 1 day, apply a new system immediately and start a new 4-week cycle; use a back-up method of contraception (e.g., condoms, spermicides, diaphragm) for the first week of the new cycle.[11]

Missed Doses. If the patient misses one active dose, take it as soon as remembered and take the next tablet at the correct time even if the patient takes 2 tablets on the same day or at the same time. If the patient misses 2 active doses in week 1 or 2, take 2 tablets on the day she remembers and 2 tablets the next day. If the patient misses 2 active doses in week 3 or misses 3 or more active tablets, then (if she starts on day 1) start a new pack the same day, or (if she starts on Sunday) take 1 tablet daily until Sunday and then start a new pack that day. The patient should use an alternative form of contraception for the next 7 days after she misses 2 or more active doses in weeks 1, 2, or 3 or abstain from sex for the next 7 days.

Pharmacokinetics. *Onset and Duration.* Onset of contraception within one week of beginning oral regimen. Dysfunctional uterine bleeding should decrease within 12–24 h of starting the regimen.[4]

Serum Levels. No correlation of estradiol or mestranol serum levels with pharmacologic activity.

Fate. There are marked intra- and interpatient variabilities in the pharmacokinetics of these agents. All are concentrated in body fat and endometrium and penetrate poorly into breast milk.[12–15]

Ethinyl estradiol. is rapidly absorbed, with peak concentrations in 60 ± 30 min; bioavailability is $59 \pm 13\%$.[12,14] It undergoes extensive small intestine and hepatic first-pass metabolism and conjugation to sulfates and hydroxylation to active 2-hydroxylethinyl estradiol and other hydroxylated metabolites. Ethinyl estradiol is 98.5% bound to albumin and not bound to sex hormone–binding globulin (SHBG). V_d is 5 ± 2 L/kg; reported CL has ranged from 0.4 ± 0.2 to 1 ± 0.3 L/h/kg. About 23%–59% is excreted in urine; 30%–53% in feces as glucuronides and sulfates; and 28%–43% undergoes enterohepatic circulation with a rebound in estradiol levels 10–14 h after administration.[7,12,14] **Mestranol** is approximately 54% demethylated to ethinyl estradiol; serum levels of ethinyl estradiol after oral administration of 50 μg of mestranol are equivalent to those after 35 μg of ethinyl estradiol.[14,15]

Desogestrel. is a prodrug that undergoes extensive first-pass and possibly gut-wall metabolism to its active form, 3-ketodesogestrel. Bioavailability is $63 \pm 7\%$; 65% bound to albumin and 35% to SHBG; SHBG increases by about 200% during long-term use. About 45% is recovered in urine as glucuronides (38%–61%), sulfates (23%–29%), and unconjugated forms (14%–28%); 31% is recovered in feces.[12,13] **Drospirenone** Peak concentration 1–3 h; bioavailability is 76%; V_d is 4 L/kg; 97% bound to SHBG and corticosteroid-binding globulin. **Ethynodiol diacetate** undergoes rapid absorption and hydrolysis to norethindrone and its metabolites in vivo. (*See* Progestin-Only Contraceptives.) **Norelgestromin** (transdermal) Reaches plateau by 48 h; 97% bound to albumin. Undergoes hepatic metabolism to norgestrel. First pass effect is avoided by transdermal administration. Metabolite norelgestromin binds to SHBG. Serum levels decrease after 3 weeks of continuous use. **Norgestrel/levonorgestrel, norethindrone, and norethindrone acetate.** (*see* Progestin-Only Contraceptives). **Norethynodrel** is rapidly converted to norethindrone in vitro.[15] **Norgestimate** undergoes hepatic and gut metabolism to levonorgestrel (15.4 ± 5.4%), norgestrel acetate (9.5 ± 1.7%), norgestrel oxime (10.6 ± 1.8%), and 8.1 ± 4.5% as other conjugated metabolites. It is not bound to SHBG; 35%–49% is excreted in urine (57% conjugated sulfates and glucuronides and 12% unconjugated) and 16%–49% in feces.

Half-life (Desogestrel)[16] 24 ± 5 h; (ethinyl estradiol)[12] 15 ± 3 to 33 ± 10 h; (levonorgestrel)[5,15] 31.4 ± 18.5 h; (norelgestromin) 28 h, (norgestimate) 16 h, (norethindrone)[13,15] 7.6 ± 1.9 h; (drospirenone) 30 h.

Adverse Reactions. The risk of major congenital malformations is not increased if oral contraceptives are taken during pregnancy.[17] The risks of oral contraceptives are minimal with the lower dosages of estrogens and progestins currently available.[7,18] (*See* Risks and Benefits of Oral Contraceptives and Hormone Excess and Deficiency Symptomatology Comparison Charts.)

Contraindications. Hypersensitivity to ethinyl estradiol, norelgestromin, or any component of the formulation. Known or suspected pregnancy; presence or history of thrombophlebitis or thromboembolic disorders; presence or history of carcinoma of breast or genitals, or other estrogen-dependent tumors; cerebral vascular or coronary artery disease; uncontrolled hypertension; focal migraine; markedly impaired liver function; hepatic adenoma or carcinoma; cholestatic jaundice of pregnancy or jaundice with prior oral contraceptive use; undiagnosed abnormal genital bleeding; malabsorption syndrome; heavy smoking (>15 cigarettes/d) in women[6] ≥35 year; polycythemia vera because of greater tendency for deep vein thrombosis. (*See* Notes.)

Precautions. Use with caution in patients with hyperlipidemia; diabetes; conditions that might be aggravated by fluid retention (e.g., hypertension, convulsions, migraine and cardiac or renal dysfunction), or severe varicosities; in adolescents in whom regular menses are not established; and during lactation. **Ortho Evra** The risk of nonfatal venous thromboembolism associated with use of the patch is similar to the risk associated with oral contraceptive pills containing higher doses of ethinyl estradiol (>30 μg).[11] **Desogestrel** The risk of thromboembolism may be higher with the third generation progestins.[19]

Drug Interactions. Oral contraceptives might be less effective, resulting in increased breakthrough bleeding or pregnancy, when given with some antibiotics (e.g., ampicillin, griseofulvin, metronidazole, nitrofurantoin, neomycin, penicillin, rifampin, tetracycline), or anticonvulsants (e.g., barbiturates, carbamazepine, phenytoin). Administer doses of vitamin C ≥1 g/d at least 4 h before or after oral contraceptives to avoid increasing the bioavailability of ethinyl estradiol; use caution if long-term vitamin C intake is discontinued.[7,20] Acitretin may diminish the therapeutic effect of oral contraceptives causing contraceptive failure. Retinoic acid derivatives may decrease the therapeutic effect of oral contraceptives. Two forms of contraception are recommended in females of childbearing potential during retinoic acid derivative therapy. Drospirenone may enhance the hyperkalemic effects of potassium-sparing diuretics, potassium supplements and ACE inhibitors.[21]

Parameters to Monitor. Complete pretreatment physical examination with special reference to blood pressure, breasts, abdomen, pelvic organs, and Pap smear at least every 1–2 years.

Notes. The initial oral contraceptive prescribed should be a combination product containing the smallest effective dose of estrogen (≤35 g ethinyl estradiol) and progestin (≤0.15 mg desogestrel or levonorgestrel, ≤1 mg norethindrone, or ≤0.25 mg norgestimate) that provides an acceptable pregnancy rate and minimizes side effects.[7] Prescribing oral contraceptives to smokers ≥35 years requires adequate informed consent because of a doubled risk of cardiovascular disease.[6] The health risks of pregnancy in healthy, nonsmoking women in their forties is greater than the risks of taking contraceptives containing ≧50 μg estrogen or progestin-only.[18] (*See* Risks and Benefits of Oral Contraceptives Comparison Chart.) Combination hormonal contraceptives do not protect against HIV infection or other sexually transmitted diseases.

PROGESTIN-ONLY CONTRACEPTIVES:	
ETONOGESTREL	Implanon
LEVONORGESTREL/NORGESTREL	Ovrette, Mirena, Plan B
MEDROXYPROGESTERONE ACETATE	Depo-Provera
NORETHINDRONE	Micronor, Nor-Q.D.

Pharmacology. Etonogestrel, norgestrel, and norethindrone are 19-nortestosterone derivatives; only the L-isomer of norgestrel (levonorgestrel) is active. Medroxyprogesterone acetate is a 17-α-acetoxyprogesterone derivative with greater progestational activity and oral efficacy than native progesterone. These compounds share the actions of progestins, although progestin-only contraceptives suppress ovulation in only about 50% of cycles. (*See* Combination Oral Contraceptives.)

Administration and Adult Dosage. PO for contraception—(norethindrone) 0.35 mg/d or (norgestrel) 0.075 mg/d continuously at the same time each day, starting on the first day of menses or immediately postpartum. IM (medroxyprogesterone acetate) 150 mg q3mo, starting within 5 days of menses or immediately postabortion or postpartum (within 5 days to 6 weeks of delivery). In breast-feeding mothers, the first dose is recommended at 6 weeks postpartum, although some clinicians give it 3–6 weeks postpartum.[22,23] PO for emergency postcoital contraception—(Plan B) 0.75 mg taken within 72 h after coitus and 0.75 mg taken 12 h later,[3] or take 1.5 mg as 1 single dose within 72 h after coitus[3]; subdermal (etonogestrel) 68 mg (single Implanon implant) q3y; insert within 5 days of onset of menstruation with no previous hormonal contraceptive use, or within seven days after last active pill if switching from a combination OC. If switching from another progestin-only method, insert implant on any day of the cycle.[24] Intrauterine System (levonorgestrel) 52 mg q5y; inserted by a trained provider within 7 days of onset of menstruation, or immediately postabortion, and may be replaced by a new IUS at any time during the menstrual cycle.[25] (*See also* Progesterone.)

Dosage Forms. **Tab** (norethindrone) 0.35 mg (Micronor, Nor-Q.D.); (norgestrel) 0.075 mg (Ovrette); (levonorgestrel) 0.75 mg (Plan B). **Implant Rod** (etonogestrel) single sterile rod containing 68 mg (Implanon). **IntraUterineSystem** (levonorgestrel) T-shaped intrauterine device containing 52 mg. **Inj** (medroxyprogesterone acetate) use only the 150 mg/mL dosage form of Depo-Provera for contraception.

Patient Instructions. (*See* Class Instructions: Oral Contraceptives.) Spotting and breakthrough bleeding occur more frequently than with the combination oral contraceptives during the first few months of use; notify prescriber if this persists through the third month.[22,23] (Plan B) If you vomit within 1 h of taking a tablet, call your health care provider to discuss whether to repeat the dose. You might experience spotting during use of this medication, and your next menstrual period might be delayed. If it is delayed more than 7 days, you might be pregnant. (Depo-Provera) Use an alternative form of contraception for the first 2 weeks if your first injection is more than 5 days after the start of menses. Cessation of menses is common after 1–2 years. (Implanon) If deviating from recommended timing of insertion, rule out pregnancy and use backup nonhormonal contraception for 7 days after insertion.[24] (Mirena) If IUS is removed midcycle and not replaced immediately then patient will be at risk of pregnancy. If patient wants to switch methods, remove Mirena during the first 7 days of menstrual cycle and start new method.[25]

Missed Doses. (Oral contraceptives) If you miss a dose, even if it is taken only 3 h late, use an additional backup method for the next 48 h. Take the missed dose as soon as you remember. If menses do not occur within 45 days, discontinue the contraceptive, use an alternate nonhormonal method of contraception, and make sure you are not pregnant. Because of the higher risk of failure if 1 tablet is missed every 1–2 cycles, consider changing the time of tablet taking or using a different contraceptive.

Pharmacokinetics. *Onset and Duration.* (Oral contraceptives) onset after 1 week; duration 24 h. (Depo-Provera) onset is within 24 h if given within 5 days of menses; the drug prevents ovulation the first month of use; ovulation is inhibited for at least 14 weeks after 150 mg IM; mean interval before return of ovulation after last injection is 9 months; 70% of former users conceive within the first 12 months after stopping.[13,26] (Implanon) onset immediately with first cycle if implanted as recommended, peak serum concentrations seen after first few weeks and the duration is 3 years. Implanon effectiveness in overweight women was not studied, but serum concentrations of etonogestrel is inversely related and could be less effective in that population.[24] (Mirena) Following insertion, initial levonorgestrel release into uterine cavity is 0.02 mg/d, which decreases gradually to approximately half of that value after 5 years.[25]

Serum Levels. (Ovulation inhibition) levonorgestrel 0.2 g/L (0.64 nmol/L); medroxyprogesterone <0.1 g/L (0.25 nmol/L)[27]; norethindrone 0.4 g/L (1.34 nmol/L).[28]

Fate. **Etonogestrel** is completely absorbed and obtains peak serum levels in 200 h. It is 32% bound to SHBG and 66% to albumin. Etonogestrel is metabolized via CYP3A4; excretion via urine, bile, and feces.[24] **Levonorgestrel** is completely absorbed orally with no first-pass metabolism.[12,13] Peak serum levels occur in 1.1 ± 0.4 h, are dose dependent, and exhibit considerable inter individual variations. Oral administration of 30 g yields peak levels of 0.9 ± 0.7 g/L (2.9 ± 2.2 nmol/L); 150 μg yields 3.6 ± 0.5 µg/L (11.5 ± 1.6 nmol/L); 250 g yields 5 ± 0.5 µg/L (16 ± 1.6 nmol/L). Levonorgestrel is concentrated in body fat and endometrium, but penetrates poorly into breast milk (~10% of serum levels); it is bound 69.4% to SHBG and 30% to albumin. V_d is 1.5 ± 0.4 L/kg; CL is 0.05 ± 0.01 L/h/kg. Conjugated glucuronides, sulfates, and unconjugated levonorgestrel and its metabolites are excreted 45% in urine and 32% in feces.[12,13] (*See* Medroxyprogesterone Acetate and Norethindrone.)

t₁/₂. (Etonorgestrel)[25] 29 h; (levonorgestrel)[12,13] 31.4 ± 18.5 h; (medroxyprogesterone acetate)[12,13] about 50 days, reflecting slow IM absorption from depot.

Adverse Reactions. (Oral contraceptives) Menstrual irregularities, including spotting, breakthrough bleeding, prolonged cycles, and amenorrhea, are frequent. Because ovulation is suppressed in only about 50% of cycles, functional ovarian cysts might occur. Most resolve spontaneously within 4 weeks, and surgical intervention is usually not necessary. Ectopic pregnancy occurs in 6% of all pregnancies. Low doses of progestins have minimal effects on the following: serum glucose, insulin or lipid levels; coagulation; liver or thyroid function; blood pressure; or cardiovascular complications.[26,27] (Plan B) nausea, abdominal pain, fatigue, headache and menstrual changes occur frequently. (Depo-Provera) menstrual irregularities, spotting, and breakthrough bleeding are frequent in the first 12 months after IM injection; amenorrhea (after 1 year), infertility (up to 18 months), and weight gain of 1–1.5 kg also occur. Reversible reduced bone density changes occur with more than 5 years of use as contraceptive, but there is no clinical evidence of fractures. Long-term use (>5 years) does not increase the overall risk of ovarian, liver, breast, or cervical cancer but reduces the risk of endometrial cancer for at least 8 years after stopping.[26,27]

Contraindications. Thrombophlebitis or history of deep vein thrombophlebitis or thromboembolic disorders; known or suspected carcinoma of the breast or endometrium, or other estrogen-dependent tumors; undiagnosed abnormal genital bleeding. Known or suspected pregnancy is a contraindication, but the risk of congenital malformations is not increased when progestin-only contraceptives are taken during pregnancy.[26] Although acute liver disease; benign or malignant liver tumors; history of cholestatic jaundice of pregnancy; or jaundice with prior hormonal contraceptive use are listed as contraindications by manufacturers—liver disease is not considered by others to be a contraindication to progestin-only contraceptives.[26] Intrauterine system: Congenital or acquired uterine anomaly; acute pelvic inflammatory disease; history of pelvic inflammatory disease (unless there has been a subsequent intrauterine pregnancy); postpartum endometritis or infected abortion within past 3 months; known or suspected uterine or cervical neoplasia; unresolved/abnormal Pap smear; untreated acute cervicitis or vaginitis; conditions which increase susceptibility to pelvic infections; unremoved IUD; undiagnosed abnormal uterine bleeding; known or suspected carcinoma of the breast.[25]

Precautions. Use with caution in patients with histories of depression, diabetes, gestational diabetes, coronary artery disease, cerebrovascular disease, hyperlipidemia, liver disease, or hypertension. Although progestins are not harmful to the fetus during the first 4 months of pregnancy, confirm a negative pregnancy test before reinjecting women >2 weeks late for their IM injection.[26] Progestin-only contraceptives used during breast-feeding pose no risk to the infant,[26] and they usually do not decrease breastmilk production if begun ≥6 weeks postpartum.

Intrauterine system: Increased incidence of group A streptococcal sepsis and pelvic inflammatory disease (may be asymptomatic). May perforate uterus or cervix; risk of perforation is increased in lactating women. Pregnancy may result if perforation occurs; delayed detection of perforation may result in migration of IUD outside of uterine cavity. Partial penetration or embedment in the myometrium may decrease effectiveness and lead to difficult removal. Use caution in patients with coagulopathy or receiving anticoagulants and in patients with congenital heart disease or other heart conditions, which may increase the risk of infective endocarditis during insertion of the device (prophylactic antibiotics may be required at time of insertion).[25]

Drug Interactions. Rifampin and cytochrome P450-inducing anticonvulsants can decrease efficacy. Long-term use of griseofulvin can increase menstrual irregularities.[26,27]

Parameters to Monitor. Complete pretreatment physical examination with special reference to blood pressure, breasts, abdomen, pelvic organs, and Pap smear at least every 1–2 years.

Notes. Progestin-only contraceptives are the hormonal contraceptives of choice during breastfeeding or in patients with contraindications to estrogen therapy (e.g., hypertension, diabetes, hyperlipidemia, smokers).[26–28] Long-term noncontraceptive benefits of IM medroxyprogesterone acetate are decreases in menstrual blood loss, anemia, candidal vulvovaginitis, pelvic inflammatory disease, and endometrial cancer. A 30% reduction in seizure frequency was observed in a small group of women with uncontrolled seizures who became amenorrheic with medroxyprogesterone.[27]

CONTRACEPTIVE EFFICACY OF HORMONAL METHODS

Percentage of women experiencing an unintended pregnancy during the first year of typical use and the first year of perfect use of contraception and the percentage continuing use at the end of the first year in the United States.

METHOD	WOMEN EXPERIENCING AN UNINTENDED PREGNANCY WITHIN THE FIRST YEAR OF USE (%)		WOMEN CONTINUING USE AT 1 YEAR (%)
	Typical Use	*Perfect Use*	
Combined Pill and Progestin-only Pill	8	0.3	68
Ortho Evra Patch	8	0.3	68
NuvaRing	8	0.3	68
Depo-Provera	3	0.3	56
IUD–ParaGard (copper T)	0.8	0.6	78
IUD–Mirena (LNG-IUS)	0.2	0.2	80
Implanon	0.05	0.05	84
Female Sterilization	0.5	0.5	100
Male Sterilization	0.15	0.1	100

From Ref. 8.

ORAL CONTRACEPTIVE AGENTS COMPARISON CHART

				POTENCY			BREAKTHROUGH BLEEDING AND
PRODUCT	CYCLE	ESTROGEN[a]	PROGESTIN[b]	Estrogenic[c]	Progestational[d]	Androgenic[e]	SPOTTING (%)[f]

MONOPHASIC COMBINATION AGENTS CONTAINING <50 µg OF ESTROGEN

PRODUCT	CYCLE	ESTROGEN[a]	PROGESTIN[b]	Estrogenic[c]	Progestational[d]	Androgenic[e]	SPOTTING (%)[f]
Alesse, Aviane, Lessina, Levlite, Lutera, Sronyx	21, 28	Ethinyl estradiol 20 µg	Levonorgestrel 0.1 mg	+	+	+	8
Junel 21 1/20, Junel Fe 1/20, Loestrin 21 1/20, Loestrin Fe 1/20, Microgestin 1/20, Microgestin Fe 1/20	21, 28	Ethinyl estradiol 20 µg	Norethindrone acetate 1 mg	+	++	++	25
Apri, Desogen, Ortho-Cept, Reclipsen, Solia	21, 28	Ethinyl estradiol 30 µg	Desogestrel 0.15 mg	+	+	±	4
Junel 21 1.5/30, Junel Fe 1.5/30, Loestrin 21 1.5/30, Loestrin Fe 1.5/30, Microgestin 1.5/30, Microgestin Fe 1.5/30	21, 28	Ethinyl estradiol 30 µg	Norethindrone acetate 1.5 mg	+	+++	+++	31

(continued)

ORAL CONTRACEPTIVE AGENTS COMPARISON CHART (*continued*)

				POTENCY			BREAKTHROUGH BLEEDING AND SPOTTING (%)[f]
PRODUCT	CYCLE	ESTROGEN[a]	PROGESTIN[b]	Estrogenic[c]	Progestational[d]	Androgenic[e]	
Levlen, Levora, Nordette, Portia	21, 28	Ethinyl estradiol 30 μg	Levonorgestrel 0.15 mg	–	+	+ +	14
Cryselle, Lo/Ovral, Low-Ogestrel	21, 28	Ethinyl estradiol 30 μg	Norgestrel 0.3 mg	+	+	+ +	10
Ocella, Yasmin	28	Ethinyl estradiol 30 μg	Drospirenone 3 mg[g]	+	+	0	—
Brevicon, ModiCon, Necon 0.5/30, Nortrel 0.5/30	21, 28	Ethinyl estradiol 35 μg.	Norethindrone 0.5 mg	+ +	+	+	15
Balziva, Femcon Fe Chewable, Ovcon-35, Zenchent	21, 28	Ethinyl estradiol 35 μg	Norethindrone 0.4 mg	+ +	+	+	15
Demulen 1/35, Kelnor 1/35, Zovia 1/35E	21,28	Ethinyl estradiol 35 μg	Ethynodiol diacetate 1 mg	+	+ +	+	38
Necon 1/35, Norethin 1/35, Norinyl 1+35, Nortrel 1/35, Ortho-Novum 1/35	21, 28	Ethinyl estradiol 35 μg.	Norethindrone 1 mg.	+ +	+ +	+	15

(*continued*)

ORAL CONTRACEPTIVE AGENTS COMPARISON CHART (continued)

PRODUCT	CYCLE	ESTROGEN[a]	PROGESTIN[b]	POTENCY Estrogenic[c]	POTENCY Progestational[d]	POTENCY Androgenic[e]	BREAKTHROUGH BLEEDING AND SPOTTING (%)[f]
Ortho-Cyclen, Mononessa, Previfem, Sprintec	21, 28	Ethinyl estradiol 35 µg.	Norgestimate 0.25 mg	++	++	+	11
BIPHASIC COMBINATION PRODUCTS CONTAINING <50 µg OF ESTROGEN							
Kariva, Mircette	28	Ethinyl estradiol 20 µg (days 1–21); 10 µg (days 24–28)	Desogestrel 0.15 mg (days 1–21)	++	+	±	12
Necon 10/11, Ortho-Novum 10/11	21, 28	Ethinyl estradiol 35 µg (days 1–21)	Norethindrone 0.5 mg (days 1–10); 1 mg (days 11–21)	++	+	+	20
TRIPHASIC COMBINATION PRODUCTS CONTAINING <50 µg OF ESTROGEN							
Cesia, Cyclessa, Velivet	28	Ethinyl estradiol 25 µg (days 1–21)	Desogestrel 0.1 mg (days 1–7); 0.125 mg (days 8–14); 0.15 mg (days 15–21)	+	+	±	—
Ortho Tri-Cyclen Lo	21, 28	Ethinyl estradiol 25 µg (days 1–21)	Norgestimate 0.18 mg (days 1–7); 0.215 mg (days 8–14); 0.25 mg (days 15–21)	++	+	+	8

(continued)

ORAL CONTRACEPTIVE AGENTS COMPARISON CHART (continued)

				POTENCY			BREAKTHROUGH BLEEDING AND
PRODUCT	CYCLE	ESTROGEN[a]	PROGESTIN[b]	Estrogenic[c]	Progestational[d]	Androgenic[e]	SPOTTING (%)[f]
Estrostep Fe; Tilia Fe	21, 28	Ethinyl estradiol 20 μg (days 1–5); 30 μg (days 6–12); 35 μg (days 13–21)	Norethindrone acetate 1 mg (days 1–21)	+	+	+	—
Necon 7/7/7, Nortrel 7/7/7, Ortho-Novum 7/7/7	21, 28	Ethinyl estradiol 35 μg (days 1–21)	Norethindrone 0.5 mg (days 1–7); 0.75 mg (days 8–14); 1 mg (days 15–21)	++	+	+	12
Ortho Tri-Cyclen, Trinessa, Tri-Previfem, Tri-Sprintec	21, 28	Ethinyl estradiol 35 μg (days 1–21)	Norgestimate 0.18 mg (days 1–7); 0.215 mg (days 8–14); 0.25 mg (days 15–21)	++	+	±1	9
Aranelle, Leena, Tri-Norinyl	21, 28	Ethinyl estradiol 35 μg (days 1–21)	Norethindrone 0.5 mg (days 1–7); 1 mg (days 8–16); 0.5 mg (days 17–21)	++	+	+	15
Enpresse, Tri-Levlen, Triphasil, Trivora-28	21, 28	Ethinyl estradiol 30 μg (days 1–6); 40 μg (days 7–11); 30 μg (days 12–21)	Levonorgestrel 0.05 mg (days 1–6); 0.075 mg (days 7–11); 0.125 mg (days 12–21)	+	+	+	15

(continued)

817

ORAL CONTRACEPTIVE AGENTS COMPARISON CHART (*continued*)

PRODUCT	CYCLE	ESTROGEN[a]	PROGESTIN[b]	POTENCY Estrogenic[c]	POTENCY Progestational[d]	POTENCY Androgenic[e]	BREAKTHROUGH BLEEDING AND SPOTTING (%)[f]
MONOPHASIC COMBINATION AGENTS CONTAINING 50 μg OF ESTROGEN							
Necon 1/50, *Norinyl 1 + 50* *Ortho-Novum 1/50*	21, 28	Mestranol 50 μg	Norethindrone 1 mg	++	++	+	11
Demulen 1/50, *Zovia 1/50*	21, 28	Ethinyl estradiol 50 μg	Ethynodiol diacetate 1 mg	+	++	+	13
Ovcon-50	21,28	Ethinyl estradiol 50 μg	Norethindrone 1 mg	++	++	++	12
Ogestrel	21, 28	Ethinyl estradiol 50 μg	Norgestrel 0.5 mg	++	+++	+++	5
EXTENDED-CYCLE COMBINATION PRODUCTS[h]							
Loestrin-24 Fe	28	Ethinyl estradiol 20 μg	Norethindrone 1 mg	+	++	++	—
Jolessa, Quasense, *Seasonale*	91	Ethinyl estradiol 30 μg	Levonorgestrel 0.15 mg	+	+	++	65
Seasonique	91	Ethinyl estradiol 30 μg (days 1–84); 10 μg (days 85–91)	Levonorgestrel 0.15 mg	+	+	++	64
Yaz	28	Ethinyl estradiol 20 μg	Drospirenone[g] 3 mg	+	+	0	25

(continued)

ORAL CONTRACEPTIVE AGENTS COMPARISON CHART (*continued*)

PRODUCT	CYCLE	ESTROGEN[a]	PROGESTIN[b]	POTENCY Estrogenic[c]	Progestational[d]	Androgenic[e]	BREAKTHROUGH BLEEDING AND SPOTTING (%)[f]
CONTINUOUS-CYCLE COMBINATION PRODUCTS							
Lybrel	28	Ethinyl estradiol 20 µg (days 1–28)	Levonorgestrel 0.09 mg	+	+	+	60
PROGESTIN ONLY							
Camila, Errin, Jolivette, Ortho Micronor, Nora-BE, Nor-QD	Continuous	—	Norethindrone 0.35 mg	0	+++	+	42
POSTCOITAL							
Plan B	2 doses of 1 tablet each (see monograph)	—	Levonorgestrel 0.75 mg	—	—	—	—

+++ = high; ++ = moderate; + = low; ± = very low; 0 = none.
[a]Estrogen potency: ethinyl estradiol is 1.5 times as potent as mestranol. Ovulation inhibition requires 50 µg of ethinyl estradiol or 80 µg of mestranol.

ORAL CONTRACEPTIVE AGENTS COMPARISON CHART (continued)

[b]Norethindrone may be preferred over norgestrel due to adverse effects on lipid profile (decreased HDL, increased LDL). Only levonorgestrel is biologically active. Older preparations contain norgestrel. Desogestrel and norgestimate have positive effects on lipids.

[c]Relative estrogenic potency (measured by affinity for estrogen receptor); norethynodrel > ethynodiol diacetate > norethindrone acetate > norethindrone > levonorgestrel/norgestimate/desogestrel. Antiestrogenic potency: norethindrone acetate > levonorgestrel > norethindrone > ethynodiol diacetate > norethynodrel > norgestimate > desogestrel.

[d]Progestational potency (measured by delay of menses test). Relative progestogenic potency: norgestimate > desogestrel > levonorgestrel > norethindrone > norethindrone acetate > ethynodiol diacetate > norethynodrel.

[e]Relative androgenic potency: levonorgestrel > norethindrone > norethindrone acetate > ethynodiol diacetate > norethynodrel > norgestimate > desogestrel. Drospirenone is antiandrogenic.

[f]BTB can result from either estrogen or progestin deficiency. Bleeding decreases after the first 6 months of use regardless of the formulation used.

[g]Drospirenone is a spironolactone analogue that has antiandrogenic and antimineralocorticoid activity. As such, it can cause mild diuresis and potassium retention. Use with caution in patients predisposed to potassium retention (e.g., renal insufficiency, ACE inhibitors, angiotensin receptor blockers, potassium-sparing diuretics).

[h]Extended cycle products may have the following advantages due to elimination of the hormone free interval: decreased menstrual-related adverse effects, improved efficacy, patient preference to eliminate menstrual bleeding.

From Refs. 7–9, 17, and 30.

RISKS AND BENEFITS OF ORAL CONTRACEPTIVES COMPARISON CHART

CONDITION	CLINICAL INFORMATION	COMMENTS
RISKS		
Breast Cancer	Reanalysis of 90% of the reported epidemiologic data found a small increased risk (relative risk [RR] = 1.24) of breast cancer in women while they were using OCs, with a decline to baseline risk 10 years after discontinuation.	Both the estrogen and progestin component of oral contraceptives have been implicated in tumor initiation and promotion.
Cerebrovascular Accidents	Risk of hemorrhagic stroke is increased 2.5-fold compared to nonusers; age and smoking increase risk. Hypertension is the strongest risk factor. Relative risk for ischemic stroke increases 4-fold for hypertensives and 3-fold for smokers.	Incidence of stroke is rare in women <35 years old who take low-dose products and do not have risk factors for smoking and hypertension.
Cervical Cancer	Increased risk of cervical erosions, eversions, dysplasias, and conversion to cancer in situ. Relative risk is 1.8–2.1 times that of nonusers and increased with duration of use >5 years; other risk factors include multiple sexual partners and early sexual activity.	Oral contraceptives may increase risk of herpes or papillomavirus infection.
Gallbladder Disease	Relative risk of 1.36 for gallstones in users compared to nonusers only during the first 4 years of use, then risk returns to baseline.	Estrogens increase cholesterol saturation.
Hepatic Tumors	Both benign and malignant tumors reported. Relative risk is 2.6 for 8 years of contraceptive use. Risk is greater in smokers and those with a history of hepatitis B infection or diabetes.	Mestranol and higher-dosage formulations are implicated. Progestin-only contraceptives not implicated.
Hyperglycemia	Abnormal glucose tolerance found in predisposed individuals (e.g., subclinical or gestational diabetes) and rare cases of diabetic ketoacidosis reported. These effects are minimal with combinations containing ≤35 μg/d of ethinyl estradiol or newer progestins. Norgestrel has greatest insulin-antagonizing activity.	Hyperinsulinemia with relative insulin resistance caused by progestins with minimal effect from estrogens.

(continued)

RISKS AND BENEFITS OF ORAL CONTRACEPTIVES COMPARISON CHART (*continued*)

CONDITION	CLINICAL INFORMATION	COMMENTS
Hyperlipidemia	Elevated triglycerides; adverse effects on lipids are greatest with progestin-dominant products, especially levonorgestrel and ethynodiol diacetate, and lowest with norgestimate, drospirenone, and desogestrel; patch and ring appear to be neutral with respect to effect on lipids.	Estrogens increase triglycerides and HDL; progestins increase LDL and decrease HDL. Minimal effect with progestin-only products.
Hypertension	Mild BP elevations of 4 mm Hg systolic and 1 mm Hg diastolic, usually reversible upon drug discontinuation, occur in 1%–5% of users. Rare with low-dose products. More common in older women and in those with a family history of hypertension.	Related to both estrogen and progestin components. Consider progestin-only contraceptives.
Infertility	Little risk of permanent sterility. Conception rate after discontinuation may temporarily lag behind that of nonusers for a few months.	Risk concentrated in older women with a long history of contraceptive use.
Myocardial Infarction	No increased risk in young, healthy nonsmokers; risk for smokers is 30-fold higher. Hypertension increases risk 4-fold. Other risk factors include age and diabetes.	Smoking status combined with age >35 years is a contraindication for use of oral contraceptives.
Postpill Amenorrhea	Prevalence is 0.2%–2.6% after use; check for pituitary tumor in presence of galactorrhea.	Risk is increased if menses were irregular prior to starting. Unrelated to duration or dose.
Pulmonary Embolism	Risk of fatal pulmonary embolism is 9.6-fold that of nonusers.	Risk appears related to progestin. Cyproterone, desogestrel and gestodene carry a 2- to 3-fold greater risk than levonorgestrel.

(continued)

RISKS AND BENEFITS OF ORAL CONTRACEPTIVES COMPARISON CHART (*continued*)

CONDITION	CLINICAL INFORMATION	COMMENTS
Thromboembolism and Thrombophlebitis	Risk is increased 2.8-fold over nonuser; risk is greatest in smokers, sedentary females >50 years, those with hypertension, and duration of use >5 years. Desogestrel-containing products have a 2-fold risk compared with other progestins and 4- to 5-fold that of nonusers. Minimal risk with progestin-only products. Use of the Ortho Evra transdermal patch increases exposure to estrogen by 60% over a 1-month period. Risk of VTE is increased 2-fold over women taking an oral product containing 30–35 μg of ethinyl estradiol.	Related to desogestrel use, transdermal patch, and estrogen dose. Estrogens decrease antithrombin III and increase coagulation factors and platelet aggregation. A history of venous thrombosis might be a reason to avoid combination products. Factor V Leiden is also a risk factor.
Teratogenesis	No increased risk of congenital cardiac, limb, or other malformations if oral or progestin-only contraceptives taken during pregnancy. Reports of masculinization of female genitalia reported when high doses of progestin were used for threatened abortion.	Exhaustive review of 18 prospective studies and meta-analysis of 12 prospective cohorts show relative risk of 0.99–1.04.
BENEFITS[a]		
Acne	Combined oral contraceptives lower serum testosterone levels with improvement of acne. Least androgenic progestins provide greatest effect.	Products containing norgestimate, norethindrone and drospirenone have FDA approval for acne treatment.
Benign Breast Disease	A 50%–75% reduction in fibrocystic disease and fibroadenoma with >2 years of use.	Protection greatest with progestin-dominant products. Does not prevent breast cancer.
Bone Mineral Density	Nineteen studies indicate positive effect on bone related to length of therapy and estrogen dose.	Effect may extend to protection from hip fracture in postmenopausal years
Ectopic Pregnancy	A 90% risk reduction.	Due to suppression of ovulation.

(continued)

RISKS AND BENEFITS OF ORAL CONTRACEPTIVES COMPARISON CHART (*continued*)

CONDITION	CLINICAL INFORMATION	COMMENTS
Endometrial Cancer	Risk is reduced by 52% and 66% after 4 and 8 years of use, respectively. Benefit persists for as long as 15 years after drug discontinuation. Greatest effects in nulliparous women.	Progestin component protective against endometrial adenomatous hyperplasia (precursor to adeno cancer) by opposing estrogen effect.
Menstrual Cycle Effects	Improvement in dysmenorrhea and dysfunctional uterine bleeding and reduced risk of iron deficiency anemia extend to low dose as well as older combination pills. Reduction in premenstrual symptoms (anxiety, depression, and headache) is reported with drospirenone-containing products. Progestin-only implants, IUS, and injection provide relief of menstrual-related symptoms.	Decrease in menstrual flow and menstrual fluid prostaglandins. Premenstrual Dysphoric Disorder is an approved indication for use of drospirenone-containing products.
Ovarian Cancer	Risk of ovarian cancer is reduced by 40% and 51% with use of oral contraceptives for 4 and 8 years, respectively. Protection persists for 10 years after drug discontinuation.	Mechanism unknown.
Ovarian Cysts	An 80%–90% risk reduction. Low-dose products (<35 μg) do not appear to retain these properties.	High-dose products decrease ovulation and production of functional cysts.
Pelvic Inflammatory Disease	Risk reduction of 50%–80% up to 1 year after discontinuing use; reduction of ectopic pregnancy rate.	Does not protect against gonorrhea or chlamydial cervicitis.
Rheumatoid Arthritis	Controversial; benefit appears to exist during but not following therapy.	Progesterone attenuates immune response.

[a]Most risks and benefits have been documented with the higher-dose estrogen products (>50 μg/d).
From Refs. 7, 17, 18, and 29.

■ REFERENCES

1. Anderson FD, Hait H. A multicenter, randomized study of an extended cycle oral contraceptive. *Contraception.* 2003;68:89-96.

2. Anderson FD et al. Safety and efficacy of an extended-regimen oral contraceptive utilizing continuous low-dose ethinyl estradiol. *Contraception.* 2006;73:229-234.

3. Grimes DA, Raymond EG. Emergency contraception. *Ann Intern Med.* 2002;137:180-189.

4. Bayer SR, De Cherney AH. Clinical manifestations and treatment of dysfunctional uterine bleeding. *JAMA.* 1993;269:1823-1828.

5. Lu PY, Ory SJ. Endometriosis: current management. *Mayo Clin Proc.* 1995;70:453-463.

6. Schiff I et al. Oral contraceptives and smoking, current considerations: recommendations of a consensus panel. *Am J Obstet Gynecol.* 1999;180(6 pt 2):S383-S384.

7. Weisberg E. Prescribing oral contraceptives. *Drugs.* 1995;49:224-231.

8. Hatcher RA et al. *Contraceptive technology.* 19th ed. New York: Irvington; 2007.

9. Van Look PFA, von Hertzen H. Emergency contraception. *Br Med Bull.* 1993;49:158-170.

10. Product Information: NuvaRing etonogestrel/ethinyl estradiol vaginal ring. Organon USA Inc. Roseland NJ, 2008.

11. Product Information: Ortho Evra norelgestromin/ethinyl estradiol transdermal system. Ortho-McNeil Pharmaceutical, Raritan NJ, 2006.

12. Shenfield GM, Griffin JM. Clinical pharmacokinetics of contraceptive steroids: An update. *Clin Pharmacokinet.* 1991;20:15-37.

13. Kuhl H. Pharmacokinetics of oestrogens and progestogens. *Maturitas.* 1990;12:171-197.

14. Goldzieher JW. Selected aspects of the pharmacokinetics and metabolism of ethinyl estrogens and their clinical implications. *Am J Obstet Gynecol.* 1990;163:318-22.

15. Orme ML'E et al. Clinical pharmacokinetics of oral contraceptive steroids. *Clin Pharmacokinet.* 1983;8:95-136.

16. McClamrock HD, Adashi EY. Pharmacokinetics of desogestrel. *Am J Obstet Gynecol.* 1993;168:1021-1028.

17. Kubba A, Guillebaud J. Combined oral contraceptives: acceptability and effective use. *Br Med Bull.* 1993;49:140-157.

18. Burkman R, Schlesselman JJ, and Zieman M. Safety Concerns and Health Benefits Associated With Oral Contraception. *Am J Obstet Gynecol.* 2004;190(suppl 4):5-22.

19. Spitzer WO et al. Third generation oral contraceptives and risk of venous thromboembolic disorders: an international case-control study. Transnational Research Group on Oral Contraceptives and the Health of Young Women. *BMJ.* 1996;312(7023):83-88.

20. Shenfield GM. Oral contraceptives: are drug interactions of clinical significance. *Drug Saf.* 1993;9:21-37.

21. Pearlstein TB, Bachmann GA, Zacur HA, et al. Treatment of Premenstrual Dysphoric Disorder with a new drospirenone-containing oral contraceptive formulation. *Contraception.* 2005;72(6):414-421.

22. World Health Organization Task Force for Epidemiological Research on Reproductive Health; Special Programme of Research, Development and Research Training in Human Reproduction. Progestogen-only contraceptives during lactation: I: infant growth. *Contraception.* 1994;50:35-53.

23. World Health Organization Task Force for Epidemiological Research on Reproductive Health; Special Programme of Research, Development and Research Training in Human Reproduction. Progestogen-only contraceptives during lactation: II: infant development. *Contraception.* 1994;50:55-68.

24. Product Information: Implanon, etonogestrel implant. Organon, Roseland, NJ, 2006.

25. Product Information: Mirena, levonorgestrel-releasing intrauterine system. Bayer HealthCare Pharmaceuticals, Wayne, NJ, 2008.

26. McCann MF, Potter LS. Progestin-only oral contraception: a comprehensive review. *Contraception.* 1994;50:S138-S148.

27. Kaunitz AM. Long-acting injectable contraception with depot medroxyprogesterone acetate. *Am J Obstet Gynecol.* 1994;170:1543-1549.

28. Darney PD. Hormonal implants: contraception for a new century. *Am J Obstet Gynecol.* 1994;170:1536-1543.

29. WHO. Cardiovascular Disease and Steroid Hormone Contraception: report of a WHO Scientific Group. Geneva, Switzerland: WHO Scientific Group on Cardiovascular Disease and Steroid Hormone Contraception; 1998. WHO Technical Report No. 877.

30. Portman D. Altering the hormone-free interval with extended cycle contraception. *Female Patient.* 2006; (suppl):1-4.

Chapter 52

Female Sex Hormones

Peggy Piascik

ESTRADIOL AND ITS ESTERS   Alora, Climara, Delestrogen, Divigel, Elestrin, Esclim, Estrace, Estraderm, Estrasorb, Estring, EstroGel, Evamist, Femring, Femtrace, Gynodiol, Menostar, Vagifem, Vivelle, Various

Pharmacology. Estradiol (17-β-estradiol) is the most potent of the naturally occurring estrogens and the major estrogen secreted during the reproductive years. Estradiol and other estrogens produce characteristic effects on specific tissues (such as breast), cause proliferation of vaginal and uterine mucosa, increase calcium deposition in bone, and accelerate epiphyseal closure after initial growth stimulation. Addition of the ethinyl radical results in an orally active compound that is 200 times more potent than estradiol. (*See* Notes.)

Administration and Adult Dosage. For patients with an intact uterus, continuous daily or cyclic (at least 10–12 days) administration of a progestin is recommended in combination with estrogen in postmenopausal women to induce endometrial sloughing and decrease the risk of endometrial cancer. **PO for vasomotor symptoms associated with menopause**—administer continuous daily or cyclic regimen of 3 weeks on followed by 1 week off, using the smallest effective dosage; (micronized estradiol) 0.5–2 mg/d initially, adjusted as necessary to control symptoms; (ethinyl estradiol) 0.02 mg/d or every other day, to a maximum of 0.05 mg/d; severe cases may require 0.05 mg tid initially until improvement, then decrease to 0.05 mg/d; administer as with micronized estradiol; (micronized estradiol plus norgestimate) 1 tablet daily per packaging (*see* Dosage Forms) (Prefest); (ethinyl estradiol plus norethindrone) 1 tablet daily and reevaluate at 3–6 months (Femhrt 1/5). **Transdermal patch for postmenopausal symptoms or osteoporosis**—initiate with a 25 or 50 μg/d patch; patch is changed once (Climara) or twice (Estraderm, Vivelle) weekly and administered continuously or cyclically (e.g., for 3 weeks followed by 1 week without patch). Dosage can be increased if symptoms are not controlled. Combi Patch can be used continuously or sequentially, in which a 50 μg/d estradiol-only patch is used for the first 14 days and Combi Patch is used for the second 14 days of a 28-day cycle. Start either method with the 0.14 mg norethindrone patch and change the patch twice weekly. **Vag for atrophic vaginitis and urogenital atrophy**—(micronized estradiol cream) 200–400 μg/d for 1–2 weeks, then reduce to 100–200 μg/d for 1–2 wk, then to maintenance of 100 μg 1–3 times/wk; (estradiol hemihydrate vaginal tablet; Vagifem) 1 tablet vaginally daily for 2 weeks, then 1 tablet vaginally twice weekly; (topical gel) one actuation (0.87 g/d of Elestrin or 1.2 g/d of Estrogel) applied at the same time of day; (Estring) insert one 2 mg ring into the upper vagina q3mo. **PO for prevention of osteoporosis**—use minimum effective dosage of 0.5 mg/d micronized estradiol; 20 μg/d of ethinyl estradiol or equivalent; or ethinyl estradiol 5 μg/d plus 1 mg norethindrone acetate (femhrt 1/5). **PO for dysfunctional uterine bleeding**—0.05–0.1 mg/d of micronized estradiol or 10–20 μg/d of ethinyl estradiol for 10–20 days with addition of progestin the third week.[1] **PO for palliation of breast cancer in postmenopausal women**—(ethinyl estradiol) 1 mg tid, or (micronized estradiol) 10 mg tid for at least 3 months. **PO for palliation of advanced inoperable prostatic cancer**—(ethinyl estradiol) 0.15–2 mg/d, or (micronized estradiol) 1–2 mg tid. **IM for postmenopausal symptoms and prevention of osteoporosis**—when oral or vaginal therapy does not provide expected response, is poorly tolerated, or when noncompliance occurs (estradiol cypionate) 1–5 mg q3–4wk; (estradiol valerate) 10–20 mg q4wk. **IM for dysfunctional uterine bleeding**—(estradiol valerate) 20 mg initially, then 5 mg q2wk with addition of progestin. **IM for palliation of advanced inoperable prostatic cancer**—(polyestradiol phosphate) 40 mg q2–4wk; (estradiol valerate) 30 mg or more q1–2wk depending on patient response.

Special Populations. *Geriatric Dosage.* Same as adult dosage. *Surgical patients.* Because estrogens can increase the risk of postsurgery thromboembolic complications, discontinue estrogens at least 4 weeks before surgery, if feasible.

Dosage Forms. **Tab** (estradiol) 0.5, 1, 1.5, 2 mg; (estradiol acetate) 0.45, 0.9, and 1.8 mg; **Tab** (combination with progestin) estradiol 1 mg/norethindrone acetate 0.5 mg, estradiol 0.5 mg/norethindrone acetate 1 mg (Activella); estradiol 1 mg/drospirenone 0.5 mg (Angeliq); estradiol 1 mg 3 tablets followed by estradiol 1 mg plus norgestimate 90 μg 3 tablets in continuous cycles (Prefest); ethinyl estradiol 2.5 μg/norethindrone acetate 0.5 mg or ethinyl estradiol 5 μg/norethindrone acetate 1 mg (Femhrt 1/5); **Topical Emulsion** (estradiol) 2.5 mg/g 2 pouches deliver 0.05 mg/d (Estrasorb); **Topical Gel** (estradiol) 0.06% or 0.1% (1 g/packet = 1 mg estradiol); **Topical Spray** (estradiol) 1.53 mg/spray; **Transdermal Patch** (estradiol) 14, 25, 37.5, 50, 60, 75, and 100 μg/d; **Transdermal Patch Combination** (estradiol) 50 μg/d plus norethindrone acetate 140 or 250 μg/d (Combi Patch); estradiol 45 μg plus 150 μg levonorgestrel. (*See* Notes.); **Vag Crm** (estradiol) 100 μg/g; **Vag Ring** (estradiol) 7.5 μg/24 h (Estring) and 0.05 mg/d (Femring); (estradiol acetate) 50 or 100 μg/24 h; **Vag Tab** 25 μg **(estradiol hemihydrate)** 25 μg; **Inj** (estradiol cypionate in oil) 5 mg/mL; 2 mg/mL with testosterone cypionate 50 mg/mL (DepoTestadiol, various); (estradiol valerate in oil) 10, 20, and 40 mg/mL; 2 mg/mL with testosterone enanthate 90 mg/mL. (*See* Notes.)

Patient Instructions. Report immediately if any of the following occur: new severe or persistent headache or vomiting; blurred or lost vision; speech impairment; calf, chest, or abdominal pain; weakness or numbness of extremities; or any abnormal vaginal bleeding. This drug may be taken with food, milk, or an antacid to minimize stomach upset. (Patch) Discard the protective liner and apply the patch to a clean, dry, and intact area of skin, preferably on the abdomen. Avoid excessively hairy, oily, or irritated areas. Apply immediately after opening and press the patch firmly in place with the palm of your hand for about 10 s to ensure good contact, particularly around the edges. Do not apply to the breasts or the waistline. To minimize irritation, rotate sites with an interval of at least 1 week between applications to a particular site.[2]

Pharmacokinetics. *Onset and Duration.* (Menopausal symptoms) onset of therapeutic estradiol levels after oral or vaginal administration is 0.5–1 h, with peak levels at 5 h and progressive decline toward baseline by 12–24 h. Onset of relief of menopausal symptoms occurs within days of the first cycle of therapy. Reductions of LH and FSH levels occur within 3 and 6 h, respectively, with a duration of 24 h.[3] Peak estradiol levels after administration of IM products are (valerate) 2.2 days, (cypionate) 4 days. Duration of depot products is variable after IM injection; (valerate) 14–21 days, (cypionate) 14–28 days, (polyestradiol phosphate) 14–28 days.[3,4] (Cancer) response to estradiol therapy should be apparent within 3 months after initiation of oral therapy.

Serum Levels. (Relief of menopausal symptoms) estradiol levels: apparent at >40 ng/L (147 pmol/L); 80% relief with 68 ng/L (250 pmol/L); 100% relief with 112 ng/L (411 pmol/L).[5–7] (Prevention of osteoporosis) 60 ng/L (220 pmol/L).

Fate. (Ethinyl estradiol) PO administration of 20 g yields ethinyl estradiol levels of 25 ng/L (84 pmol/L); 30 g yields 60 ng/L (202 pmol/L). (*See* Combination Oral Contraceptives.)

(Estradiol) oral bioavailability of micronized estradiol is 4.9 ± 5% because of extensive and rapid first-pass metabolism.[4] Topical absorption is affected by skin thickness and site of patch application: 100% (abdomen) and 85% (thigh).[2] Oral or vaginal administration results in unphysiologic levels of estrone.[3–7] Steady-state level after PO administration of 1 mg estradiol is 35 ± 5 ng/L (128 ± 18 pmol/L) or an increase of 25 ng/L (92 pmol/L) over baseline.[3,5] (Vag) 0.2 mg estradiol yields 80 ± 19 ng/L (293 ± 7 pmol/L) of E_2.[3] (Patch) 25 g yields 25 ng/L (92 pmol/L) of estradiol.[7] (*See* Notes.)

Estradiol is about 60% bound to albumin, 38% to SHBG, and 3% unbound. It is widely distributed and concentrated in fat. V_d is 10.9 ± 2.9 L; CL is 24.2 ± 7 L/h/m² or 0.77 L/h/kg.[3–5] Estradiol and its esters are converted in the liver, endometrium, and intestine, 15% to estrone (active), 65% to estrone sulfate and its conjugates (primarily sulfates and glucuronides with reconversions of 5% estrone and 1.4% estrone sulfate back to estradiol). Estradiol is excreted 50% in urine and 10% in feces, with some enterohepatic circulation. Less than 1% is excreted unchanged in urine and 50%–80% as conjugates: estrone 20%, estriol 20%, estradiol glucuronide 7%.[3–5]

Half-life (Estradiol)[3–5] 1 h; (ethinyl estradiol)[8,9] 15 ± 3 to 33 ± 10 h.

Adverse Reactions. (*See* Postmenopausal Hormone Replacement Risks and Benefits Comparison Chart.) Nausea, vomiting, bloating, breast tenderness, and spotting occur frequently. (*See* Hormone Excess and Deficiency Symptomatology Comparison Chart.) Hypercalcemia occurs occasionally in patients with breast cancer. Thromboembolism, thrombophlebitis, diabetes, hypertension, and gallbladder disease are less likely to occur with hormone replacement dosages than with oral contraceptive dosages. Pain at injection site occurs frequently. Occasional redness and irritation at application site with patch; rash rarely.

Contraindications. Hypersensitivity to estrogens or any component of the formulation; pregnancy; history or presence of estrogen-dependent cancer (except in appropriate patients treated for metastatic disease); undiagnosed abnormal genital bleeding; history or presence of thromboembolism or severe thrombophlebitis; porphyria. A history of breast cancer might not be an absolute contraindication to estrogen therapy in women with severe menopausal symptoms.[10] Active or severe chronic liver disease is a contraindication for combinations with testosterone.

Precautions. Use with caution in patients with disease states that could be exacerbated by increased fluid retention (e.g., asthma; epilepsy; migraine; and cardiac, hepatic, or renal dysfunction); in women with strong family histories of breast cancer or presence of fibrocystic disease, fibroadenoma, or abnormal mammogram; estrogen use may cause severe hypercalcemia in patients with breast cancer and bone metastases; in women with fibromyomata, cardiovascular disease, diabetes, hypertriglyceridemia, severe liver disease, or history of jaundice during pregnancy; and in young patients in whom bone growth is not complete; patients with cholestatic jaundice, gallbladder disease, porphyria, and systemic lupus erythematosus.

Oral estrogen can increase thyroid-binding globulin and cause false elevations in total T_4 and T_3 and false depression of resin T_3 uptake while the thyroid index, thyroid-stimulating hormone, and the patient remain euthyroid. Retinal vascular thrombosis: Estrogens may cause retinal vascular thrombosis; discontinue permanently if papilledema or retinal vascular lesions are observed on examination. Estrace 2 mg and Estinyl 0.02 mg contain tartrazine, which may cause allergic reactions, including bronchospasm, in susceptible individuals.

Drug Interactions. Estrogens can reduce the effects of tricyclic antidepressants and warfarin and increase the effects of corticosteroids and ropinirole by increasing their half lives. Estrogens may decrease the therapeutic effect of somatropin requiring a change in therapy. Estrogens may increase the risk of skin rash associated with tipranavir requiring a modification in therapy. Tipranavir may decrease serum levels of estrogen. Inducers of cytochrome P450 enzymes (CYP3A4 and CYP1A2) including barbiturates, rifampin and St John's wort can decrease estrogen levels. Herbs with estrogenic properties may enhance the adverse effects of estrogens; examples include black cohosh, bloodroot, hops, licorice, red clover, soybean, and wild yam.[11]

Parameters to Monitor. Signs and symptoms of side effects, especially abnormal bleeding. Pretreatment and physical examination with reference to blood pressure, breasts, abdomen, pelvic organs, and Pap smear. Baseline laboratory tests should include glucose, triglycerides, cholesterol, LFTs, and calcium. Repeat physical examination annually; repeat laboratory tests only if abnormal at baseline.

Notes. Estradiol has been advocated as the estrogen replacement of choice; however, advantages over other estrogens have not been established. Synthetic 17-α-alkylated estrogens (e.g., ethinyl estradiol) are generally not recommended in menopausal replacement therapy because of their potent hepatic effects. The combination of an androgen with estrogen is indicated for moderate to severe vasomotor symptoms in patients not improved by estrogen alone. Potential benefits include increased libido and psychological well-being. Alternatives to estrogens for hot flashes include **megestrol acetate** 20 mg bid.[12]

Nonoral estradiol administration (e.g., patch, vaginal, implant, injection), avoids first-pass effect and theoretically results in a preferable premenopausal physiologic serum level ratio of estradiol to estrone compared to oral administration.[3–5,7] Avoiding the first-pass effect allows a smaller dosage to be used and prevents undesirable changes from liver stimulation (i.e., increases in renin substrate, SHBG, thyroxine-binding globulin, coagulation factors, transferrin, growth hormone levels, and cortisol-binding globulin and a reduction in insulin like growth factor) and their sequelae (i.e., gallbladder disease, hypertension, and hypercoagulable states in some women).[7,13–16] Hepatic stimulation varies with oral preparations, with ethinyl estradiol > conjugated estrogens > estradiol. Enhanced liver action is also responsible for the cardioprotective effects on lipids and occurs even with vaginal estrogens.[17] Transdermal administration appears to exert favorable effects on serum lipoproteins (i.e., elevation of HDLs and depression of LDLs) after >4 months of use and protects against bone loss and fractures similarly to oral estrogens.[7,18,19]

In women requiring therapy for the treatment or prevention of osteoporosis, and in whom estrogen replacement therapy is intolerable or contraindicated, oral bisphosphonates, calcitonin, slow release fluoride or teriparatide have increased bone mass and reduced vertebral fractures, vertebral deformities, and loss of height.[20]

Hormone replacement therapy should not be used for the prevention of chronic disease. Treatment should be at the lowest dose for the shortest time necessary to control symptoms.[16]

ESTROGENS, CONJUGATED	Cenestin, Premarin, Various
ESTROGENS, ESTERIFIED	Estratab, Menest, Various

Pharmacology. Conjugated estrogens contain a mixture of 50%–65% sodium estrone sulfate, 20%–35% sodium equilin sulfate, and other estrogenic substances obtained from the urine of pregnant mares. Esterified estrogens are a combination of 75%–85% sodium estrone sulfate and 6.5%–15% sodium equilin sulfate prepared from Mexican yams. (*See* Estradiol and Its Esters.)

Administration and Adult Dosage. For patients with intact uteri, continuous daily or monthly (for at least 10–12 days) administration of a progestin is recommended to induce endometrial sloughing and decrease the risk of endometrial cancer; administration of progestin quarterly (14 days of progestin every 3 months) also might be effective. Cyclic administration of estrogen is either 3 weeks on, 1 week off or 25 days on followed by 5 days off. **PO for moderate to severe vasomotor symptoms associated with menopause and atrophic vaginitis**—use smallest effective dosage beginning with 0.3 mg/d continuously or cyclically. **PO for female hypogonadism**—0.3–0.62 5 mg/d cyclically, may be titrated every 6–12 months, add progestin when skeletal maturity is achieved. **PO for castration or primary ovarian failure**—1.25 mg/d given cyclically according to severity of symptoms. **PO for prevention of postmenopausal osteoporosis**—use minimum effective dosage initially 0.3 mg/d continuously, or cyclically if uterus is present; adjust dose based on clinical response and bone mineral density.[15,16] **PO for acute heavy dysfunctional uterine bleeding (unlabeled use)**—1.25 mg repeated every 4 h for 24 h, followed by daily dose for 10 days.[1] **IV (preferred) or IM for rapid cessation of acute heavy dysfunctional uterine bleeding**—25 mg, may repeat in 6–12 h prn, to a maximum of 3 doses, followed by oral estrogen/progestin combination therapy.[21] **PO for nonacute dysfunctional uterine bleeding (unlabeled use)**—1.25 mg daily for 7–10 days.[1] **IV for bleeding from uremia (unlabeled use)**—0.6 mg/kg/d diluted in 50 mL of NS and infused over 30–40 min for 5 days; dosages as high as 60 mg/d IV have been used.[21] **PO for palliation of breast cancer**—(patients should be ≥5 y postmenopausal) 10 mg tid. **PO for palliation of androgen-dependent prostatic cancer**—1.25–2.5 mg 3 times/da. **Vag for dyspareunia and atrophic vaginitis**—0.5 mg ranging from 2 times/wk up to daily on a cyclic basis.

Special Populations. *Geriatric Dosage.* Same as adult dosage. Consider lower dose or less frequent administration with mild -to moderate hepatic impairment.

Dosage Forms. **Tab** (conjugated) 0.3, 0.45, 0.625, 0.9, and 1.25 mg (Cenestin, Premarin, various); 0.625 mg with medroxyprogesterone acetate 2.5 and 5 mg (Prempro); 0.625 mg with medroxyprogesterone acetate 5 mg (Premphase); (esterified) 0.3, 0.625, 1.25, and 2.5 mg; 0.625 mg with testosterone 1.25 mg (Estratest H.S.); 1.25 mg with testosterone 2.5 mg (Estratest); **Inj** (conjugated) 25 mg; **Vag Crm** (conjugated) 0.625 mg/g.

Patient Instructions. Report immediately if any of the following occur: new severe or persistent headache or vomiting; blurred or loss of vision; speech impairment; calf, chest, or abdominal pain; weakness or numbness of extremities; or any abnormal vaginal bleeding. Take at bedtime to minimize adverse effects. This (oral) drug may be taken with food, milk, or an antacid to minimize stomach upset. (Vaginal) To clean applicator, remove plunger from barrel. Wash with mild soap and warm water; do not boil or use hot water.

Pharmacokinetics. *Onset and Duration.* (Menopausal symptoms) PO peak onset of equilin sulfate is 4 h; onset of estrone is 3 h, with a peak at 5 h; duration is >24 h. After vaginal administration, onset of therapeutic estradiol levels is 3 h and peak occurs in 6 h, with decline over 24 h to baseline values. Gonadotropin suppression occurs within 1 month of therapy, although suppression to premenopausal levels might not occur.[7] (Uremia) improvement in bleeding time occurs within 6 h after starting estrogens; maximum improvement occurs within 2 5 days after initiation of estrogens; effects last 3–10 days after drug discontinuation.[21]

Serum Levels. *See* Estradiol and Its Esters.

Fate. Conjugated equilin and estrone sulfate are rapidly absorbed and hydrolyzed to unconjugated forms when given orally or vaginally. Oral administration of 0.3 mg yields steady-state estradiol levels of 48 ± 12 ng/L (175 ± 45 pmol/L; Vaginal administration of 0.3 mg yields steady-state estradiol levels of 7 ± 22 ng/L (26 ± 81 pmol/L)[3–5]; (Estrone sulfate)[22,23] V_d is 38 ± 13 L; CL is 3.9 ± 1.2 L/h/m² Estrone sulfate is rapidly converted to estrone and estradiol. (Equilin sulfate) CL is 7.3 ± 4 L/h/m². Approximately 30% of equilin sulfate is metabolized to active 17-α-dihydroequilin sulfate and 2% to active 17-α-dihydroequilin.[22] Inactivation of estrogens occurs mainly in the liver, with degradation to less active estrogenic products (e.g., estrone). Metabolites are conjugated with sulfate and glucuronic acid; urinary recovery is 70%–88% within 5 days after oral administration. (*See* Estradiol and Its Esters.)

Half-life (Estrone sulfate) 4–5 h. (Equilin) 19–27 min. (Equilin sulfate) 190 min. (17 α-dihydroequilin) 45 ± 5 min. (17α-dihydroequilin sulfate) 2.5 ± 0.6 h.[22]

Adverse Reactions, Contraindications, Precautions, Drug Interactions, Parameters to Monitor. *See* Estradiol and Its Esters.

Notes. *See* Estradiol Notes, Postmenopausal Hormone Replacement Risks and Benefits Comparison Chart.

ESTROPIPATE	Ogen, Ortho-Est, Various

Pharmacology. Estropipate is estrone sulfate stabilized with inert piperazine. Estrone is the major estrogen produced in the postmenopausal period. It is one-half as potent as estradiol and shares the actions of other estrogens. (*See* Estradiol and Its Esters.)

Administration and Adult Dosage. For patients with intact uteri, continuous daily or monthly administration (minimum of 10–12 days) of progestin is recommended to induce endometrial sloughing and decrease the risk of endometrial cancer; administration of progestin quarterly (14 days of progestin every 3 months) also might be effective. **PO for postmenopausal symptoms, atrophic vaginitis or kraurosis vulvae, and prevention of osteoporosis**—use the smallest effective dosage in the range of 0.75–6 mg estropipate/d continuously or in cycles; administer as with conjugated estrogens. **PO for female hypogonadism, castration or primary ovarian failure**—1.5–9 mg daily for 3 weeks followed by a rest period of 8–10 days. Use lowest dose and regimen that controls symptoms.

Special Populations. *Geriatric Dosage.* Same as adult dosage. Reduce dose in cases of mild to moderate liver impairment. Not recommended in cases of severe liver impairment.

Dosage Forms. **Tab** (as conjugated estrogens equivalent) 0.625, 1.25, and 2.5 mg.

Patient Instructions. *See* Estradiol and Its Esters.

Pharmacokinetics. Estrone is not orally active because of enzymatic degradation in the gut and liver. Addition of a piperazine moiety increases oral absorption such that estradiol levels are similar to those after administration of estradiol. Oral administration of 0.6 mg estropipate yields estradiol serum levels of 34 ng/L (124 pmol/L).[3–5] Estrone is hydroxylated to α-hydroxyestrone, estriol, and 2-α hydroxyestrone. The half-life of estrone is estimated to be 12 h in serum; however, this does not reflect events in peripheral tissues. The half-life of estrone sulfate is 4–5 h.[3–5] (*See* Estradiol and Its Esters.)

Adverse Reactions, Contraindications, Precautions, Drug Interactions, Parameters to Monitor, Notes. *See* Estradiol and Its Esters.

MEDROXYPROGESTERONE ACETATE	Depo-Provera, Provera, Various

Pharmacology. Medroxyprogesterone is a 17-α-acetoxyprogesterone derivative with greater progestational effects and oral efficacy than progesterone. Progesterone transforms an estrogen-primed proliferative endometrium into a secretory endometrium.

Administration and Adult Dosage. **PO for secondary amenorrhea, or abnormal uterine bleeding, or to induce withdrawal bleeding after postmenopausal estrogen replacement therapy**—5–10 mg/day for 5–10 days, depending on the degree of endometrial stimulation desired, beginning on the presumed 16th or 21st day of the cycle for abnormal uterine bleeding. In secondary amenorrhea, therapy can be started at any time. **PO for endometriosis**—(depo-subQ and subQ) 104 mg every 12–14 weeks. **PO for postmenopausal symptoms**—(combined with continuous estrogen) 2.5–5 mg/d. (*See* Notes.) **PO for relief of vasomotor symptoms**—20 mg/d. **IM for relief of vasomotor symptoms**—150 mg/d. **IM for endometrial or renal carcinoma**—400 mg to 1 g/wk initially for few weeks, then, if improvement occurs, reduce to maintenance dosage of 400 mg/mo. **Accompanying postmenopausal cyclic estrogen therapy**—Oral: 5–10 mg for 12–14 consecutive days each month, starting on either day 1 or day 16 of the cycle; lower doses may be used if given with estrogen continuously throughout the cycle. (*See also* Progestin-Only Contraceptives.)

Special Populations. *Geriatric Dosage.* (Oral) Use is contraindicated with severe hepatic impairment. Consider lower dose or less frequent administration with mild to moderate hepatic impairment. Use of the contraceptive injection has not been studied in patients with hepatic impairment.

Surgical Patients. Progestins in combination with estrogens should be discontinued at least 4 weeks prior to and for 2 weeks following elective surgery associated with an increased risk of thromboembolism or during periods of prolonged immobilization.

Dosage Forms. **Tab** progesterone 2.5, 5, and 10 mg (medroxyprogesterone is the acetate salt); **Inj** 150, 400 mg/mL.

Patient Instructions. Report immediately if any of the following occur: new severe or persistent headache; blurred vision; calf, chest, or abdominal pain; or any abnormal vaginal bleeding. Use sunblock, wear protective clothing and eyewear, and avoid extensive exposure to direct sunlight; use caution when driving or engaging in tasks that require alertness until response to drug is known; maintain adequate hydration (2–3 L/day of fluids) unless instructed to restrict fluid intake and diet; dress in cool clothes and maintain cool environment if hot flashes occur. May cause discoloration of stool (green). This (oral) drug may be taken with food, milk, or an antacid to minimize stomach upset. (Dysfunctional uterine bleeding) expect heavy and severely cramping flow 2–4 days after stopping therapy; expect a normal period after a few days.

Pharmacokinetics. *Onset and Duration.* Withdrawal bleeding (in estrogen-primed endometrium) occurs 3–7 days after the last dose.[24] Onset of symptomatic relief of hot flashes within 4–7 days; maximum relief after 1 month; duration 8–20 weeks after discontinuation.

Serum Levels. Inhibition of ovulation and tumor response occurs with medroxyprogesterone levels >0.1 μg/L (0.25 nmol/L).[24]

Fate. Medroxyprogesterone acetate (MPA) is rapidly absorbed orally with no first-pass metabolism; oral bioavailability is 5.7 ± 3.8%; IM bioavailability is 2.5 ± 1.7%, with a large interpatient variation in serum levels after oral or IM administration.[5] Higher concentration depot formulation is associated with lower serum concentrations but equivalent bioavailability.[25] Peak concentrations occur in 2–7 h and are 2–10 times higher after oral than after IM depot injection.[5,25] The drug is stored in fat; >90% is protein bound to albumin; 83% of a dose is present in serum as the parent drug and conjugated medroxyprogesterone; it is hydroxylated to 6-α-hydroxy-MPA and 21-hydroxy-MPA, which have unknown activities. From 15% to 20% of a dose is excreted in urine as glucuronide and sulfate conjugates; 45%–80% is excreted in feces.[26]

    $t_{1/2}$. Oral 12–17 h; IM 50 days, SubQ ~40 days.

Adverse Reactions. Dizziness, headache, nervousness, decreased libido, menstrual irregularities including bleeding or amenorrhea, abdominal pain/discomfort, weight changes and muscle weakness occur in more than 5% of patients (PI) (*See* *also* Progestin-Only Contraceptives, Postmenopausal Hormone Replacement Risks and Benefits Comparison Chart, and Hormone Excess and Deficiency Symptomatology Comparison Chart.)

Contraindications. Known or suspected pregnancy or as a diagnostic test for pregnancy, thrombophlebitis, history of deep vein thrombophlebitis, or thromboembolic disorders; known or suspected carcinoma of the breast or endometrium, or other estrogen-dependent tumors; undiagnosed abnormal genital bleeding.

Precautions. Prolonged use of medroxyprogesterone contraceptive injection may result in a loss of bone mineral density related to the duration of use, and may not be completely reversible on discontinuation of the drug.[27]

An increased risk of invasive breast cancer was observed in postmenopausal women using medroxyprogesterone acetate in combination with conjugated equine estrogens. An increase in abnormal mammograms has also been reported with estrogen/progestin therapy. The risk of dementia may be increased in postmenopausal women; increased incidence was observed in women ≥65 years of age taking medroxyprogesterone in combination with conjugated equine estrogens.[13,16,28]

Use with caution in patients with histories of depression, diabetes, gestational diabetes, coronary artery disease, cerebrovascular disease, hyperlipidemia, liver disease, or hypertension. Confirm a negative pregnancy test before reinjecting a woman >2 weeks late for her IM injection.[27] Progestin-only contraceptives used during breastfeeding pose no risk to the infant,[27] and they usually do not decrease breast milk production if begun after 6 weeks postpartum.

Drug/Food Interactions. Rifampin and cytochrome P450-inducing anticonvulsants can increase progestin metabolism. Long-term use of griseofulvin can increase menstrual irregularities.[11,24,29] Bioavailability of the oral tablet is increased when taken with food.[27]

Parameters to Monitor. Complete pretreatment physical examination with special reference to blood pressure, breasts, abdomen, pelvic organs, and Pap smear yearly.

Notes. Continuous administration of low-dose progestin and estrogen combinations in postmenopausal syndrome causes amenorrhea in >50% of women and does not appear to negatively influence blood lipids when compared with cyclic therapy.[30] Concurrent administration of estrogen with progestin for amenorrhea might be associated with less breakthrough bleeding than with progestin alone. There is no evidence that progestins are effective in preventing habitual abortion or treating threatened abortion. Patients should be started at the lowest effective dose.

Risks versus benefits must be weighed for each postmenopausal patient receiving estrogen/progestin replacement therapy. Progestins with or without estrogen should be used for the shortest duration possible consistent with treatment goals. Medroxyprogesterone used in combination with estrogen may increase the risks of hypertension, myocardial infarction, stroke, pulmonary emboli, and deep vein thrombosis; incidence of these effects was shown to be significantly increased in postmenopausal women using conjugated equine estrogen in combination with medroxyprogesterone. Medroxyprogesterone/estrogen should not be used to prevent coronary heart disease.[13-16]

MIFEPRISTONE

Pharmacology. Mifepristone (RU-486) is a synthetic steroid with antiprogestational effects. It antagonizes the endometrial and myometrial effects of progesterone resulting in termination of pregnancy. It also has antiglucocorticoid and weak antiandrogenic activity.[31]

Adult Dosage. PO for pregnancy termination through day 49 of pregnancy— 600 mg as a single dose, followed in 2 days by misoprostol 400 mg PO. Patients should return on day 14 to assess efficacy of the procedure and bleeding.

Dosage Forms. Tab 200 mg.

Pharmacokinetics. Oral bioavailability is 69% with a 20 mg dose. It is 98% bound to albumin and alpha$_1$-acid glycoprotein. It is metabolized primarily by CYP3A4 to three major metabolites. Most of the drug is eliminated in feces, with 9% of the drug and metabolites eliminated in urine. Clearance is dose dependent, with 50% eliminated between 12 and 72 h; the remaining drug is eliminated with a half-life of 18 hours.

Adverse Reactions. Vaginal bleeding and cramping are expected effects of the drug (plus misoprostol) and occur mostly on day 3. Bleeding is generally more than a heavy menstrual period. Other frequent effects are abdominal pain, nausea, vomiting, diarrhea, headache, dizziness, and fatigue.

Contraindications. Confirmed or suspected ectopic pregnancy or undiagnosed abdominal mass; IUD in place; chronic adrenal failure; concurrent long-term corticosteroid use; allergy to mifepristone, misoprostol or other prostaglandin; hemorrhagic disorder; anticoagulant therapy; inherited porphyria.

Drug Interactions. Drugs that affect CYP3A4 can alter mifepristone metabolism. The metabolism of drugs metabolized by CYP3A4 might be affected

Notes. Pregnancy termination should be conducted only in a setting where a qualified physician can assess the gestational age of the fetus, diagnose ectopic pregnancies, and provide surgical intervention in case of incomplete abortion or severe bleeding (or have made plans to provide such care through others). Patients must receive a medication guide and sign a patient agreement before treatment. Patient should be informed to seek medical attention immediately if they experience heavy prolonged bleeding (may signify incomplete abortion) or sustained fever, malaise or severe abdominal pain due to the risk of serious infection and sepsis.[31]

NORETHINDRONE ACETATE

Pharmacology. Norethindrone acetate is a 19-nortestosterone derivative that shares the actions of progestins. It has oral efficacy, greater progestational activity than progesterone, and less androgenic activity than androgens. (*See also* Medroxyprogesterone Acetate, Progesterone.)

Administration and Adult Dosage. PO for amenorrhea and abnormal uterine bleeding—2.5–10 mg/d for 5–10 days during the second half of the menstrual cycle.[1] (*See* Medroxyprogesterone Acetate Notes.) **PO for amenorrhea or abnormal uterine bleeding**—2.5–10 mg/d for 5–10 days during second half of menstrual cycle. In cases of secondary amenorrhea, therapy can be started at any time.[32] **PO for endometriosis**—5 mg/d for 2 weeks, increasing in 2.5 mg/d increments every 2 weeks until a maintenance dosage of 15 mg/d is reached; continue for 6–9 months.[32]

Special Populations. *Geriatric Dosage.* Same as adult dosage.

Dosage Forms. **Tab** 5 mg.

Patient Instructions. Take dose at same time each day. Report immediately if any of the following occur: new severe or persistent headache; blurred vision; calf, chest, or abdominal pain; or any abnormal vaginal bleeding. This (oral) drug may be taken with food, milk, or an antacid to minimize stomach upset. In patients with secondary amenorrhea or dysfunctional uterine bleeding, withdrawal bleeding usually occurs 3–7 days after hormone therapy is discontinued.

Pharmacokinetics. *Onset and Duration.* (Uterine bleeding) after oral administration, acute bleeding should decrease in 1–2 days and stop in 3–4 days. (Withdrawal bleeding) onset 3–7 days after last oral dose.[8] Time to peak effect is 1–2 h.

Fate. Norethindrone acetate is rapidly and completely absorbed, with a mean bioavailability of 64 ± 16% because of first-pass metabolism.[5,8,26] Norethindrone acetate is rapidly converted to norethindrone in vivo.[8,9,33] Norethindrone is 36% bound to SHBG and 61% bound to albumin. It is concentrated in body fat and endometrium; breast milk levels are 10% of maternal serum levels. V_d is 4.3 ± 9 L/kg; CL is 0.5 ±1.5 L/h/kg. Over 50% is eliminated in urine and 20%–40% in feces as conjugated glucuronides and sulfates; <5% of norethindrone acetate is excreted as unchanged norethindrone.[8,9,26,33] Elimination half-life is about 8 h.

$t_{1/2}$. (Norethindrone) 6.4 ± 3 h.[5,8,9,26,33]

Adverse Reactions. *See* Medroxyprogesterone Acetate, Postmenopausal Hormone Replacement Risks and Benefits Comparison Chart, and Hormone Excess and Deficiency Symptomatology Comparison Chart.

Contraindications. *See* Medroxyprogesterone Acetate, Postmenopausal Hormone Replacement Risks and Benefits Comparison Chart.

Precautions. *See* Medroxyprogesterone Acetate, Postmenopausal Hormone Replacement Risks and Benefits Comparison Chart, and Hormone Excess and Deficiency Symptomatology Comparison Chart.

Drug Interactions, Parameters to Monitor, Notes. *See* Medroxyprogesterone Acetate.

PROGESTERONE	Crinone, Prometrium, Various
HYDROXYPROGESTERONE CAPROATE	Duralutin, Various

Pharmacology. Progesterone is the natural hormone that induces secretory changes in the endometrium, relaxes uterine smooth muscle, and maintains pregnancy. It also supports embryo implantation, promotes mammary gland development, and blocks follicular maturation and ovulation. Hydroxyprogesterone is a natural progestin with minimal progestational activity; esterification with caproic acid produces a progestational compound more potent than progesterone with a prolonged duration of activity.

Administration and Adult Dosage. **PO to prevent endometrial hyperplasia during postmenopausal estrogen replacement therapy**—(micronized progesterone)

200 mg/d for 12 days of cycle. **IM for amenorrhea**—5–10 mg for 6–8 consecutive days. **Secondary amenorrhea**—45 mg of 4% gel every other day for 6 doses; may increase to 90 mg if response is inadequate; 400 mg PO HS for 10 days. **Dysfunctional uterine bleeding**—5–10 mg IM for 6–8 days (hydroxyprogesterone caproate) 375 mg, may repeat in 4 weeks prn. **IM for palliation of metastatic endometrial cancer**—(hydroxyprogesterone caproate) 500 mg to 1 g 2–3 times/wk. **Vag for progesterone supplementation in ART patients**—(progesterone) 90 mg intravaginal gel daily or 100 mg tablet 2–3 times daily when oocyte retrieval begins for up to 10 weeks; **patients with partial or complete ovarian failure**— 90 mg of 8% gel twice daily, continue 10–12 weeks if pregnancy occurs.

Special Populations. *Geriatric Dosage.* Same as adult dosage.

Dosage Forms. **Cap** (micronized progesterone) 100 and 200 mg (Prometrium); **Inj** (progesterone in oil) 50 mg/mL; (hydroxyprogesterone caproate in oil) 125, 250 mg/mL; **Vag Tab** (progesterone) 100 mg (Endometrin); **Vag Gel** (progesterone 4%, 8%) 45 mg/applicatorful (Prochieve) and 90 mg/applicatorful (Crinone).

Patient Instructions. Report immediately if any of the following occur: new severe or persistent headache; blurred vision; calf, chest, or abdominal pain; or any abnormal vaginal bleeding. (Dysfunctional uterine bleeding) expect heavy flow and severe cramping 2–4 days after injection; expect a normal period after a few days. (Vaginal gel) Remove applicator from wrapper; holding applicator by thickest end, shake down to move contents to thin end; while holding applicator by flat section of thick end, twist off tab; gently insert into vagina and squeeze thick end of applicator. (Vaginal tablet) Insert tablet in vagina using disposable applicator provided.

Pharmacokinetics. *Onset and Duration.* Time to peak effect: oral = 3 h; IM = approximately 8 h; vaginal = 17–24 h. (Vag gel) absorption half-life = 25–50 h; (Amenorrhea) onset of withdrawal bleeding occurs 48–72 h after last dose of IM progesterone and 2 weeks after IM hydroxyprogesterone caproate; (dysfunctional uterine bleeding) onset within 6 days of IM progesterone. Duration is 12–24 h with oral progesterone and 9–17 days with IM hydroxyprogesterone caproate.

Serum Levels. (Endometrial progestational activity [luteal phase]) 15 μg/L (48 nmol/L) of progesterone.

Fate. (Progesterone) Bioavailability of oral progesterone is incomplete because of first-pass metabolism, with wide interpatient variations; micronized forms are somewhat better absorbed.[5,34,35] Higher levels of progesterone and active metabolites occur after IM, vaginal, or rectal administration because first-pass effect is avoided. Progesterone circulates 50%–54% bound to albumin and 43%–48% to corticosteroid-binding globulin and distributes into fat. It undergoes rapid gut and hepatic metabolism, with formation of active metabolites: 20-α-dihydroprogesterone (25%–50% of the progestational activity of progesterone), 17-hydroxyprogesterone, and 11-deoxycorticosterone (a potent mineralocorticoid).[5] Hydroxyprogesterone caproate is cleaved to form 17-hydroxyprogesterone in the body; 17-hydroxyprogesterone, whether formed from progesterone or exogenously administered, is further metabolized to 11-deoxycortisol and then cortisol. Urinary excretion of progesterone is 50%–60% as 5-α-pregnanediol glucuronide and other conjugated glucuronic acid or sulfate metabolites; 5%–10% excreted in feces.

$t_{1/2}$. (Progesterone) 32.6 ± 9.3 h.[34] (Vag gel) elimination half-life 5–20 min.

Adverse Reactions. Local reactions and swelling at the site of progesterone injection. The beneficial effects of estrogen-increased HDL levels are not reversed by progesterone.[30] (*See* Postmenopausal Hormone Replacement Risks and Benefits Comparison Chart, Hormone Excess and Deficiency Symptomatology Comparison Chart.)

Contraindications. (*See* Medroxyprogesterone Acetate.) Capsules are also contraindicated for use during pregnancy.

Precautions. (*See* Medroxyprogesterone Acetate, Postmenopausal Hormone Replacement Risks and Benefits Comparison Chart, and Hormone Excess and Deficiency Symptomatology Comparison Chart.) Patients allergic to peanuts should not use Prometrium.[36]

Drug Interactions. *See* Medroxyprogesterone Acetate.

Parameters to Monitor. Complete pretreatment and annual physical examinations with special reference to blood pressure, breasts, abdomen, pelvic organs, and Pap smear.

Notes. Progesterone is widely used in the treatment of premenstrual syndrome; however, in double-blind, controlled trials, oral micronized and vaginal progesterone were no better than placebo.[37,38] Progestins with or without estrogen should be used for shortest duration possible consistent with treatment goals. Conduct periodic risk: benefit assessments. Women should be informed of the risks and benefits, as well as possible effects of estrogen when added to progestin therapy.

RALOXIFENE
Evista

Pharmacology. Raloxifene is a selective estrogen receptor modulator similar to tamoxifen. It acts like an estrogen in the bone and cardiovascular system and like an estrogen antagonist on the breast and uterus. Raloxifene increases bone mineral density and decreases serum LDL and overall cholesterol levels but does not stimulate endometrial growth or affect HDLs.[39,40]

Administration and Adult Dosage. **PO for prevention of postmenopausal osteoporosis**—60 mg once daily with supplemental calcium. Patients should receive supplemental calcium and vitamin D if their daily dietary intake is inadequate; **PO for invasive breast cancer risk reduction**—60 mg daily for 5 years.[41]

Dosage Forms. **Tab** 60 mg.

Pharmacokinetics. Oral bioavailability is 2% because of an extensive first-pass effect. It is highly bound to albumin and alpha$_1$-acid glycoprotein and has a V_d of 2348 L/kg. CL is 40–60 L/h/kg. The drug is metabolized to glucuronide metabolites, some of which undergo enterohepatic recycling, and can be converted back to the parent drug. Metabolites are excreted primarily in feces. The half-life is about 28 h.[40]

Adverse Reactions. Hot flashes occur in 25%–30% of women and vaginal dryness is common; leg cramps also are frequent. It increases the risk of venous thromboembolism including deep vein thrombosis, pulmonary emboli, and retinal venous thrombosis. Raloxifene is a teratogen.

Contraindications. Women who might become pregnant or are pregnant or nursing mothers; those with active or a history of venous thromboembolism.

Precautions. Raloxifene has been associated with an increased risk of fatal stroke in women with coronary heart disease or increased risk for coronary events. Benefit versus risk should be assessed in women at risk for stroke secondary to a history of stroke or transient ischemic attack, atrial fibrillation, hypertension, or smoking cigarettes. Risk for deep vein thrombosis or pulmonary embolus may be increased. Raloxifene should not be used for the primary or secondary prevention of cardiovascular disease. Serum triglyceride concentrations should be monitored carefully during raloxifene therapy in women with a history of elevated triglyceride concentrations during therapy with oral estrogens/progestins.

Drug Interactions. Cholestyramine (and presumably colestipol) binds raloxifene and reduces its absorption and enterohepatic recirculation. Drugs should not be coadministered. Raloxifene decreases the effect of warfarin, and INR should be monitored carefully when they are given together. Use with highly protein bound drugs such as diazepam should be monitored due to the high protein binding of raloxifene.

Notes. Raloxifene increases bone mineral density, decreases the risk of vertebral fracture,[39] and decreases the risk of invasive breast cancer.[41] It also favorably alters serum LDL and overall cholesterol. The risk-benefit ratio should be considered for women at risk of stroke due to increased risk of death in postmenopausal women with documented coronary heart disease.[39] Postmenopausal women receiving raloxifene for the treatment or prevention of osteoporosis should engage in other measures including adequate vitamin D and calcium intake, weight-bearing exercise and lifestyle modifications including discontinuance of cigarette smoking and moderation of alcohol consumption.

POSTMENOPAUSAL HORMONE REPLACEMENT (HRT) RISKS AND BENEFITS COMPARISON CHART

RISKS/BENEFITS	CLINICAL INFORMATION	COMMENTS
Cancer, Breast	4–6 cases of invasive cancer per 10,000 women per year of estrogen/progestin are expected after 3–5 years of therapy. Estrogen only use did not increase risk after an average use of 7.1 years suggesting that <5 years of estrogen therapy has no significant impact on breast cancer risk. Use of HRT in women with a breast cancer history is controversial as no long-term randomized controlled trials have been completed.	Estrogen/progestin increases breast cell proliferation, breast pain, and mammography density that may impede diagnostic interpretation. Consider limiting duration of treatment to <5 years if risks of cancer outweigh benefits.
Cancer, Colon	46% decrease in colon cancer risk; no effect on rectal cancer.	In slender women, risk is reduced by up to 75%.
Cancer, Endometrial	Unopposed estrogen use (0.625 mg) for >3 years increases risk up to 5-fold; 10 years of use increases risk to 10-fold. Risk persists for several years after discontinuation of estrogen therapy. Risk is related to both dose and duration of estrogen therapy.	Relative risk of 1 with the concurrent addition of a minimum of 10–14 days of progestin. No increased risk of estrogen hyperplasia or need for hysterectomy with concurrent progestin therapy.
Cardiovascular Effects	Risk of coronary heart disease does not appear to be elevated in women aged 50–59 years or within 10 years of menopause when treating typical symptoms of menopause. Inconclusive evidence that use >5 years may be cardioprotective. In the WHI, initiation more than 10 years postmenopause was associated with increased risk of coronary heart disease; may increase risk of hypertension.	HRT is not recommended for women of any age as a primary indication for cardioprotection. Risk of first stroke may be increased by HRT use.
Cognitive aging/dementia	Risk of dementia may be increased in patients who begin estrogen therapy at ≥65 years of age.	Increased incidence documented with combination of conjugated equine estrogens and medroxyprogesterone.
Lipids	Unopposed oral estrogens reduce LDL and increase HDL by 10%–15%; however, estrogens can increase triglyceride levels.	Progesterone antagonizes beneficial effects of estrogen less than medroxyprogesterone. Nonoral estrogens (e.g., patch, vaginal) produce less HDL beneficial effects.

(continued)

POSTMENOPAUSAL HORMONE REPLACEMENT (HRT) RISKS AND BENEFITS COMPARISON CHART (continued)

RISKS/BENEFITS	CLINICAL INFORMATION	COMMENTS
Osteoporosis/Fractures	15%–50% increase in bone density if begun within 3 years of menopause. Osteoporosis risk increases in Caucasian and Asian ethnic groups with the following lifestyle factors: sedentary lifestyle, smoking, low calcium and vitamin D intake, and excessive alcohol or thyroxine intake. Spine and hip fractures decrease by 50% with >5 years of use, 28% reduction with 10 years use, 40% with 15 years use and 55% with 20 years. Risk returns near baseline 6 years or more after cessation of therapy.	Bone densitometry can identify women at highest risk. Therapy with bisphosphonates, intranasal calcitonin (Miacalcin), and slow-release fluoride are also effective. (See Estradiol Notes.)
Urinary Symptoms	Local estrogen therapy may be effective when stress incontinence occurs with vaginal atrophy. Benefits in cases of urge incontinence or systemic use for stress incontinence is controversial. Vaginal administration may reduce risk of recurrent urinary tract infection.	Use of vaginal HRT to reduce risk of recurrent UTI is a non-FDA approved use.
Vaginal Symptoms	Unpredictable bleeding occurs in 35%–40% of non-hysterectomized women yearly. Estrogen is the most effective agent for treating moderate to severe symptoms of vulvar and vaginal atrophy. Relief of vaginal atrophy may also relieve dyspareunia.	Amenorrhea usually occurs after 6–8 months of estrogen/progestin therapy. Vaginal administration of estrogen is preferred when this is the sole indication for estrogen therapy.
Venous Thromboembolism	In the WHI, there were 4 additional VTEs per 10,000 women/y for estrogen alone and 7 additional VTEs for estrogen/progestin therapy in women aged 50–59 years.	Risk is greater for women older than 60 years. Magnitude of risk decreases over time. Lower estrogen doses may reduce risk.

Although use of HRT is reported to increase the risks for a number of disease states, the risks generally fall into the category of rare occurrences and depend on several factors including time of initiation, duration of therapy, dose and route of estrogen administration, choice of progestin, and individual patient benefit/risk ratio.
From Refs. 10, 13–16, 18, 19, 28, and 30.

ESTROGENS COMPARISON CHART

DRUG	DOSAGE FORMS	EQUIPOTENT PHYSIOLOGIC DOSE[a,b]	COMMENTS
Conjugated Estrogens Premarin (equine)	Tab 0.3, 0.625, 0.9, 1.25 mg Vag Crm 0.625 mg/g Inj (powder for reconstitution) 25 mg	0.625 mg	Equine product is a mixture of 50%–65% sodium estrone sulfate, 20%–35% equilin sulfate, and other estrogenic substances from the urine of pregnant mares.
Cenestin, Enjuvia (synthetic, plant derived)	0.3, 0.45, 0.625, 0.9, 1.25 mg		Synthetic product is a mixture of 9–10 estrogens from soy and yams
Esterified Estrogens Covaryx Menest	Tab 0.3, 0.625, 1.25, 2.5 mg	0.625 mg	Similar to conjugated estrogens. Mixture of 75%–85% sodium estrone sulfate and 6.5–15% sodium equilin sulfate obtained from Mexican yams or soy.
Estradiol, Micronized Estrace EstroGel	Tab 0.5, 1, 2 mg Vag Crm 100 µg/g Gel 0.06%	0.75 mg/metered dose	Estradiol is the major estrogen secreted during the reproductive years
Estradiol Alora Climara Esclim Estraderm Menostar Vivelle	Transdermal System µg/day 25, 50, 75, 100 25, 37.5, 50, 60, 75, 100 25, 37.5, 50, 75, 100 50, 100 14 25, 37.5, 50, 75, 100		Some products contain alcohol and may be irritating to the skin; aerosol topical steroids may be applied under the patch to reduce allergic reactions; do not apply to an area exposed to direct sunlight (Estraderm).

(continued)

842

ESTROGENS COMPARISON CHART (continued)

DRUG	DOSAGE FORMS	EQUIPOTENT PHYSIOLOGIC DOSE[a,b]	COMMENTS
Estradiol	Topical Products: Gel		Absorption of estradiol is increased by application of sunscreen within 1 h; spray solution and gel are flammable, avoid fire or heat until spray has dried.
Divigel	Emulsion, spray	1 g/packet = 1 mg estradiol	
Elestrin	0.1%	0.53 mg estradiol/metered dose	
Evamist	0.06%		
	1.53 mg/spray		
Estradiol	Oral Tab		
Femtrace	0.45, 0.9, 1.8 mg (estradiol acetate)		
Gynodiol	0.5, 1, 1.5, and 2 mg		
Innofem	0.5, 1, and 2 mg		
Estradiol	Vaginal ring or tab		
Vagifem	25 μg tab (estradiol hemihydrate)		
Estring			
Femring	0.0075 mg/24 h ring		
	0.05 and 0.1 mg/24 h ring		
Estropipate	Tab 0.625, 1.25, 2.5, 5 mg	0.625 mg	Ogen 0.625 mg = 0.75 mg estropipate.
Ogen	Vag Crm 1.5 mg/g		Ogen 1.25 mg = 1.5 mg estropipate.
Ortho-Est			Ogen 2.5 mg = 3 mg estropipate.
			Ogen 5 mg = 6 mg estropipate.

[a]Potency of estrogens: estradiol > estrone. Potency is based on the effects on the liver.
[b]See monographs or product information for exact dosage regimens for various uses.

843

■ REFERENCES

1. Casablanca Y. Management of dysfunctional uterine bleeding. *Obstet Gynecol Clin North Am.* 2008;35(2):219-234.

2. Product Information: Estraderm, estradiol transdermal system. Novartis, East Hanover, NJ, 2006.

3. Lobo RA, Cassidenti DL. Pharmacokinetics of oral 17 beta-estradiol. *J Reprod Med.* 1992;37:77-84.

4. Anderson F. Kinetics and pharmacology of estrogens in pre- and postmenopausal women. *Int J Fertil.* 1993;38(suppl 1):53-64.

5. Kuhl H. Pharmacokinetics of oestrogens and progestogens. *Maturitas.* 1990;12:171-197.

6. Handa VL et al. Vaginal administration of low-dose conjugated estrogens: systemic absorption and effects on the endometrium. *Obstet Gynecol.* 1994;84:215-218.

7. Pang SC et al. Long-term effects of transdermal estradiol with and without medroxyprogesterone acetate. *Fertil Steril.* 1993;59:76-82.

8. Shenfield GM, Griffin JM. Clinical pharmacokinetics of contraceptive steroids: An update. *Clin Pharmacokinet.* 1991;20:15-37.

9. Goldzieher JW. Selected aspects of the pharmacokinetics and metabolism of ethinyl estrogens and their clinical implications. *Am J Obstet Gynecol.* 1990;163:318-22.

10. Xydakis et al. Hormone replacement therapy in breast cancer survivors. *Ann NY Acad Sci.* 2006;1092:349-360.

11. Shader RI, Greenblatt DJ. More on oral contraceptives, drug interactions, herbal medicines, and hormone replacement therapy. *J Clin Psychopharmacol.* 2000: 20(4):397-398.

12. Loprinzi CL et al. Megestrol acetate for the prevention of hot flashes. *N Engl J Med.* 1994;331:347-352.

13. Rossouw JE et al; for Women's Health Initiative Investigators. Risks and benefits of estrogen plus progestin in healthy postmenopausal women: principal results From the Women's Health Initaitive randomized controlled trial. *JAMA.* 2002;288:321-333.

14. Heiss G et al; for Women's Health Initiative Investigators. Health risks and benefits 3 years after stopping randomized treatment with estrogen and progestin. *JAMA.* 2008;299:1036-1045.

15. Hodis HN, Mack WJ. Postmenopausal hormone therapy in clinical perspective. *Menopause.* 2007;14:944-957.

16. Estrogen and progestogen use in postmenopausal women: July 2008 position statement of The North American Menopause Society. *Menopause.* 2008;15(4):584-603.

17. Walsh BW et al. Effects of postmenopausal estrogen replacement on the concentrations and metabolism of plasma lipoproteins. *N Engl J Med.* 1991;325:1196-1204.

18. L'hermite M, et al. Could transdermal estradiol + progesterone be a safer postmenopausal HRT? A review. *Maturitas.* 2008;60(3-4):185-201.

19. Vrablik M et al. Oral but not transdermal estrogen replacement therapy changes the composition of plasma lipoproteins. *Metabolism.* 2008;57(8):1088-1092.

20. Jenkins MR and Sikon AL. Update on nonhormonal approaches to menopausal management. *Cleve Clin J Med.* 2008;75(suppl 4):S17-S24.

21. McCarthy ML, Stoukides CA. Estrogen therapy of uremic bleeding. *Ann Pharmacother.* 1994;28(1):60-62.

22. Bhavnani BR, Cecutti A. Pharmacokinetics of 17_-dihydroequilin sulfate and 17_-dihydroequilin in normal postmenopausal women. *J Clin Endocrinol Metab.* 1994;78:197-204.

23. Steinberg KK et al. A meta-analysis of the effect of estrogen replacement therapy on the risk of breast cancer. *JAMA.* 1991;265:1985-1990. {Erratum *JAMA.* 1991;266:1362.}

24. Kaunitz AM. Long-acting injectable contraception with depot medroxyprogesterone acetate. *Am J Obstet Gynecol.* 1994;170:1543-1549.

25. Wright CE et al. Effect of injection volume on the bioavailability of sterile medroxyprogesterone acetate suspension. *Clin Pharm.* 1983;2:435-438.

26. Fotherby K. Pharmacokinetics and metabolism of progestins in humans. In: Goldzieher JW, Fotherby K, eds. *Pharmacology of the Contraceptive Steroids.* New York: Raven Press; 1994:99-126.

27. Product Information: Depo-Provera, medroxyprogesterone acetate. Pharmacia & Upjohn, Kalamazoo, MI, 2004.

28. Anderson GL et al. Prior hormone therapy and breast cancer risk in the Women's Health Initiative randomized trial of estrogen plus progestin. *Maturitas.* 2006;55:103-115.

29. Darney PD. Hormonal implants: contraception for a new century. *Am J Obstet Gynecol.* 1994;170:1536-1543.

30. The Writing Group for the postmenopausal estrogen/progestin interventions (PEPI) trial. Effects of estrogen or estrogen/progestin regimens on heart disease risk factors in postmenopausal women. *JAMA.* 1995;273(3):199-208.

31. Product Information: Mifiprex, mifepristone. Danco Laboratories, New York, NY, 2005.

32. Product Information: Aygestin, norethindrone. Duramed Pharm, Pomona, NY, 2003.

33. Orme ML'E et al. Clinical pharmacokinetics of oral contraceptive steroids. *Clin Pharmacokinet.* 1983;8:95-136.

34. Norman TR et al. Comparative bioavailability of orally and vaginally administered progesterone. *Fertil Steril.* 1991;56:1034-1039.

35. Munk-Jensen N et al. Continuous combined and sequential estradiol and norethindrone acetate treatment of post-menopausal women: effect of plasma lipoproteins in a two-year placebo-controlled trial. *Am J Obstet Gynecol.* 1994;171:132-138.

36. Product Information: Prometrium, progesterone. Solway Pharm Inc, Marietta, Ga, 2004.

37. Freeman EW et al. A double-blind trial of oral progesterone, alprazolam, and placebo in treatment of severe premenstrual syndrome. *JAMA.* 1995;274:51-57.

38. Freeman E et al. Ineffectiveness of progesterone suppository treatment of premenstrual syndrome. *JAMA.* 1990;264:349-353.

39. Product Information: Evista, raloxifene hydrochloride. Lilly, Indianapolis, IN, 2007.

40. Morello K. Pharmacokinetics of selective estrogen receptor modulators. *Clinl Pharmacokine.* 2003;42(4):361-372.

41. Vogel VG et al. for National Surgical Adjuvant Breast and Bowel Project (NSABP). Effects of tamoxifen vs raloxifene on the risk of developing invasive breast cancer and other disease outcomes: the NSABP study of tamoxifen and raloxifene (STAR) P-2 trial. *JAMA.* 2006;295:2727-2741.

Chapter 53

Thyroid and Antithyroid Drugs

Betty J. Dong

IODIDES

Various

Pharmacology. Iodide inhibits the synthesis and release of thyroid hormone and preoperatively decreases the size and vascularity of the hyperplastic thyroid gland. Large doses block the uptake of radioactive iodine by the thyroid gland.

Administration and Adult Dosage. **PO for hyperthyroidism, as an adjunct to antithyroid agents or following radioactive iodine therapy, or for preoperative thyroidectomy preparation**—3–10 drops daily in 1–2 divided doses of saturated solution of potassium iodide [SSKI] or 3–5 drops 3 times daily of Lugol's solution diluted in a glass of water, milk, or juice.[1] Administration of smaller doses of 30–50 mg iodine and continued suppression with doses of 15–50 mg/d also may be effective in patients with mild disease.[1] Use for 3–10 days before surgery.[2] **IV for hyperthyroidism, as an adjunct to antithyroid agents or following radioactive iodine therapy, or for preoperative thyroidectomy preparation**—sodium iodide (compounded by pharmacy) 500 mg every 12 h.[1] **PO for thyroid storm**—10 drops daily in divided doses of SSKI administered 1 h after thioamide administration but should not be withheld when thioamides cannot be given.[1] **PO for prophylaxis in radiation emergency 1 dose immediately before or within 1–2 h after exposure**—130 mg iodine.[3] When continued radiation exposure, additional daily doses can be taken for 3–7 days, to a maximum of 10 days after exposure.[3]

Special Populations. *Pediatric Dosage.* **PO for for preoperative thyroidectomy preparation**—SSKI q8h diluted as above. **PO for hyperthyroidism and thyroid storm**—1–3 drops Lugol's solution administered 1 h after thioamide administration but should not be withheld when thioamides cannot be given. **PO for prophylaxis in a radiation emergency 1 dose immediately before or within 1–2 h after exposure**—(birth to 1 month) 16 mg iodine; (1 month to 3 years) 32 mg iodine; (12–18 years) 65 mg iodine; (> 18 years or ≥ 70 kg) 130 mg iodine.[3] Avoid repeat doses in neonates. See repeat dosing as above for adults.

Geriatric Dosage. Same as adult dose.

Pregnant and Breastfeeding. Same as adult dose.[3] Do not repeat doses.

Dosage Forms. **Soln** (SSKI) 50 mg/drop iodide (1 g/mL); (Lugol's or strong iodine) 8 mg/drop iodide (50 mg/mL iodine plus 100 mg/mL potassium iodide); **Tab** 65, 130 mg potassium iodide; **Soln** potassium iodide 65 mg/mL; **EC Tab** not recommended.

Patient Instructions. Dilute solution in a glass (8 fl oz) of liquid before taking; it may be taken with food, milk, or an antacid to minimize stomach upset. Do not use when solution turns brownish yellow. When crystals form in the solution, they can be dissolved by warming the closed container in warm water. Dissolve tablets in one-half glass of water or milk before taking. Inform your physician when you are pregnant or breastfeeding. Discontinue use and report when fever, skin rash, epigastric pain, or joint swellings occur.

Pharmacokinetics. *Onset and Duration.* Onset 24–48 h in hyperthyroidism; maximum effect in 10–15 days. (*See* Notes.) Duration of protection after radiation exposure is 24 h after a single dose.[3]

Fate. Iodide is well absorbed throughout the GI tract and concentrated in the thyroid, stomach, salivary glands, and breast milk. (Iodide) >50 g/L (0.4 mmol/L) inhibits thyroid iodide binding in hyperthyroidism; >200 g/L (1.6 mmol/L) inhibit iodide uptake by normal thyroid.[4]

Renal clearance is 1.8 L/h/kg; approximately 100 g of iodine is excreted in urine daily; fecal excretion of iodine is negligible.[4]

Adverse Reactions. Any adverse reaction warrants drug discontinuation. Goiter, hypothyroidism, and hyperthyroidism occur frequently in euthyroid patients with a history of untreated thyroid disorder.[5–7] Iodism occurs with prolonged use and is indicated by metallic taste, GI upset, soreness of teeth and gums, coryza, frontal headaches, painful swelling of salivary glands, diarrhea, acneiform skin eruptions, and erythema of face and chest. Rarely, hypersensitivity occurs and is manifested by angioedema, cutaneous hemorrhages, and symptoms resembling serum sickness. (*See* Precautions.)

Contraindications. Pulmonary tuberculosis; pulmonary edema; multinodular goiters.[5–7]

Precautions. Pregnancy because of increased risk of fetal goiter, asphyxiation, or death; lactation. Use with caution in patients with untreated Hashimoto's thyroiditis, in iodide-deficient patients, in children with cystic fibrosis, and in euthyroid patients with a history of postpartum thyroiditis, subacute thyroiditis, amiodarone or lithium-induced thyroid disease, or previously treated Graves' disease because they can be particularly sensitive to iodide-induced hypothyroidism.[5–7] Patients with nontoxic multinodular goiters might be prone to development of hyperthyroidism. Avoid iodides entirely in patients with toxic nodular goiter or toxic nodules because thyrotoxicosis can be further aggravated.[5–7] Iodides are not recommended for use as expectorants because of their potential to induce acneiform eruptions, exacerbate existing lesions, and adversely affect the thyroid. Small bowel lesions are associated with enteric-coated potassium-containing tablets, which can cause obstruction, hemorrhage, perforation, and possible death. This dosage form is not recommended.

Drug Interactions. Iodide prevents uptake of ^{131}I for several weeks and delays onset of thioamide action when given before the thioamide. Lithium can potentiate the antithyroid action of iodide. Serum iodine can be elevated when potassium-sparing diuretics are taken with potassium iodide.

Parameters to Monitor. Monitor for signs of iodism (*see* Adverse Reactions), hypothyroidism, hyperthyroidism, and parotitis occasionally during long-term use. Monitor thyroid function tests at least every 6–12 months during long-term use in patients with family histories of thyroid disease or goiter. Monitor serum potassium frequently in patients who are taking other drugs that might affect serum potassium (e.g., diuretics).

Notes. Iodide has the most rapid onset of any treatment for hyperthyroidism. The therapeutic effects of iodide are variable and transient, with "escape" occurring after 10–14 days; do not use iodide alone in the therapy of hyperthyroidism. Pharmacologic amounts of iodide can be present in serum from **radiographic contrast agents** and vaginal douches such as **povidone-iodine.**[5–7]

LEVOTHYROXINE SODIUM

Levoxyl, Levo-T, Levothroid, Levolet, Novothyrox, Synthroid, Unithroid Various

Pharmacology. Levothyroxine is a synthetic hormone identical to the thyroid hormone T_4. Thyroid hormones are responsible for normal growth, development, and energy metabolism.

Administration and Adult Dosage. **PO for replacement in patients <50 years old with hypothyroidism (TSH < 50 mU/L)** 1.7 μg/kg/d (lean body weight) initially, increasing when needed and tolerated in 12.5–25 μg/d increments at 6- to 8-week intervals until thyroid-stimulating hormone (TSH) normalizes.[8,9] **Usual maintenance dosages**—75–100 μg/d for women and 100–150 μg/d for men. **PO for replacement of severe hypothyroidism (TSH >50 mU/L)**—12.5–25 μg/d increasing when needed and tolerated in 25 μg/d increments at 2- to 4-week intervals until TSH normalizes. Once-weekly replacement therapy for hypothyroidism can be effective.[10] **PO for replacement of subclinical hypothyroidism**—1 μg/kg/d may be adequate; benefits are greatest in those with TSH >10 mU/L, hypercholesterolemia, and subtle symptoms of hypothyroidism.[11] **PO for suppression therapy of thyroid nodules**—treatment is controversial and individualized; >2 μg/kg/d dose to suppress TSH to 0.1–1 mU/L to prevent further thyroid growth. Dosages are usually higher than those required for replacement therapy and risks must be assessed, especially in patients with cardiac disease. When no improvement after 1 year, consider stopping therapy.[12,13] **PO for suppression therapy of thyroid cancer after thyroidectomy**—approximately 2 μg/kg/d initially, increasing, when needed and tolerated, in 25–50 μg/d increments at 6- to 8-week intervals to a dosage of 150–250 μg/d to suppress the TSH level to <0.1 mU/L in high risk cancer patients and to 0.1–0.5 mU/L in lower risk patients.[14] **IV for myxedema coma**—200-300 μg (4 μg/kg/dose lean body weight) initially, followed in 24 h by 100 μg/d, and then 50 μg/d until oral administration is possible; use smaller dosages in cardiovascular disease.[15] **IM** indicated only for replacement therapy when the patient cannot take oral medication; parenteral dosage is about 80% of the oral dosage because of bioavailability differences.

Special Populations. *Pediatric Dosage.* **PO for hypothyroidism**—(preterm infants and full-term neonates to 1 year of life) 10–15 μg/kg/d (37.5–50 μg/d) to normalize T_4 to 10–16 μg/dL (130–206 nmol/L), free T4 to 1.4–2.3 ng/dL (18–30 pmol/L) within the first 2 weeks, and TSH within 1 month of life.[16] Higher dosages of 50 μg/d preferred initially, especially in infants with T4 level <5 μg/dL (65 nmol/L); 6–8 μg/kg/d; (1–5 years) 5–6 μg/kg/d; (6–12 years) 4–5 μg/kg/d; (>12 years but growth and puberty incomplete) 2–3 μg/kg/d; (growth and puberty complete) 1.7 μg/kg/d. Adjust maintenance dosage on the basis of growth, development, clinical response, and T_4 and TSH values.

Geriatric Dosage. **PO for hypothyroidism**—(>50 years) start with 25–50 μg/d initially, then increase when tolerated in 12.2–25 μg/d increments at 6- to 8-week intervals to a maintenance dosage necessary to normalize TSH; (>65 years) <1 μg/kg/d may be required. Poorly compliant elderly patients (mean age 86 years) have been maintained on a twice-weekly dosing regimen; however, this regimen might be dangerous in cardiac patients.[17] **IV for myxedema coma** (>55 years) same as adult dosage.

Other Conditions. **PO in patients with cardiovascular disease or severe, long-standing hypothyroidism**—25–50 μg/d initially, increasing, when tolerated in 12.5–25 μg/d increments at 6- to 8-week intervals until TSH normalizes. **PO for hypothyroidism in elderly patients with cardiac disease**—12.5–25 μg/d initially, increasing, when tolerated in 12.5–25 μg/d increments at 4- to 6-week intervals until TSH normalizes. In patients with cardiovascular disease, particularly angina, dosage increments should be balanced between exacerbation of angina and maintenance of euthyroidism. In some patients with severe coronary disease, incomplete control of hypothyroidism might be necessary to prevent further exacerbation of angina. **PO for hypothyroidism in pregnancy**—a 30%–50% dosage increase during the first trimester may be required to maintain a normal TSH level.[18]

Dosage Forms. **Tab** 25, 50, 75, 88, 100, 112, 125, 137, 150, 175, 200, 300 g; **Inj** IV 200, 500 mcg.

Patient Instructions. Take this medication regularly to maintain proper hormone levels in the body. Take this medication on an empty stomach 1 h before or 2 h after a meal or at bedtime and separate by at least 4 h from interacting medications. In infants, tablets should be crushed and mixed with breast milk, formula, or water. Do not mix tablets with soy formulas or preparations containing iron or calcium, both of which reduce the absorption of T_4. Report immediately when chest pain (especially in elderly patients), palpitations, sweating, nervousness, or other signs of overactivity occur.

Missed Doses. Take any missed dose as soon as it is remembered, but if more than 1 dose is missed, do not double the dosage.

Pharmacokinetics. *Onset and Duration.* PO onset 3–5 days; peak effect 6–8 weeks; duration after cessation of therapy 7–10 days. IV onset in myxedema coma 6–8 h, maximum effect in 1 day.[15]

Serum Levels. (Physiologic and therapeutic during levothyroxine therapy) free T_4 0.7–1.86 ng/dL (9–24 pmol/L); total T_4 5–12 μg/dL (64–164 nmol/L). Many drugs and pathologic and physiologic states affect binding and hence can affect results of some serum level determinations.[5,8,9]

Fate. Oral bioavailability ranges from 74 ± 11% to 93 ± 25% and can be decreased by many factors (e.g., malabsorption, concurrent food, and drugs; (*see* Drug Interactions).[8,9] Significantly higher free T4 levels achieved when administered at bedtime compared to 30 min before breakfast.[19] Peak free T_4 levels can be 12.7 ± 2.6%, and total T_4 levels 8.1 ± 1.2% higher than trough levels or levels obtained 10 h after a dose.[20,21] A dose of 500 μg IV increases serum T_4 levels by 3–5 μg/dL (39–65 nmol/L).[22] Only 0.03% is unbound in plasma. V_d is (hypothyroid) 0.17 ± 0.22 L/kg; (euthyroid) 0.16 ± 0.09 L/kg; (hyperthyroid) 0.23 ± 0.44 L/kg.

Turnover is (hypothyroid) $9.2 \pm 1.7\%/d$; (euthyroid) $11.2 \pm 1.7\%/d$; (hyperthyroid) $21 \pm 4.9\%/d$. CL is (hypothyroid) 0.0008 ± 0.0033 L/h/kg; (euthyroid) 0.00074 ± 0.0017 L/h/kg; (hyperthyroid) 0.002 ± 0.0007 L/h/kg.[23] About 80% is deiodinated in the body; 35% is peripherally converted to the more active T_3 and 45% to inactive reverse T_3.[6] Another 15%–20% is conjugated in the liver to form glucuronides and sulfates, which undergo enterohepatic recirculation with reabsorption or excretion in the feces.

Half-life (Hypothyroid) 7.5 ± 7.1 d; (euthyroid) 6.2 ± 4.7 d; (hyperthyroid) 3.2 ± 1.7 d.[23] Protein binding affects half-life (increased binding retards elimination and decreased binding increases elimination).

Adverse Reactions. Most are dose related and can be avoided by increasing the initial dosage slowly to the minimum effective maintenance dosage. Signs of overdosage include headache, palpitations, chest pain, heat intolerance, sweating, leg cramps, weight loss, diarrhea, vomiting, nervousness, and other symptoms of hyperthyroidism. Long-term thyroid administration that results in TSH suppression can predispose to ventricular hypertrophy, atrial fibrillation, osteoporosis, and increased fracture risk by increasing bone resorption in postmenopausal women with a history of hyperthyroidism[8,9,11]

Contraindications. Untreated subclinical hyperthyroidism, overt thyrotoxicosis; acute myocardial infarction, uncorrected adrenal insufficiency. Physiologic dosages of thyroid hormones should not be used for weight reduction, obesity, or premenstrual tension in euthyroid patients; larger dosages might result in toxicity.

Precautions. Initiate and increase dosage with caution in patients with cardiovascular disease, the elderly, and in long-standing hypothyroidism. In myxedema coma, give a corticosteroid concurrently.[15] The status of other metabolic diseases, including diabetes, adrenal insufficiency, hyperadrenalism, and panhypopituitarism, can be affected by changes in thyroid status.

Drug Interactions. Bran, coffee, fiber, soybean flour, walnuts, cholesterol-binding resins (e.g. cholestyramine, colestipol), sodium polystyrene sulfonate, iron sulfate, aluminum- and magnesium-containing antacids, raloxifene, sucralfate, simethicone, sevelamer hydrochloride, chromium picolinate, and calcium carbonate can decrease oral absorption.[8,9,24,25] Phenytoin, carbamazepine, phenobarbital, rifampin, and other enzyme inducers; sertraline and possibly other serotonin reuptake inhibitors, and ritonavir can increase levothyroxine requirements.[8,9] The action of some drugs (e.g., digoxin, warfarin, insulin, antidiabetic agents, sympathomimetics, theophylline) can be altered by changing thyroid status.[8,9]

Parameters to Monitor. (Adults) TSH, free T_4 or free T_4 index, and clinical status of the patient every 6–8 weeks initially. Monitor trough levels or obtain levels at least 10 h after tablet ingestion to avoid transient peak effects.[20,21] After stabilization, monitor free T_4 or free T_4 index, TSH, and clinical status at 6- to 12-month intervals or after any product change. (Infants and children) Monitor the parameters above every 2 and 4 weeks initially; every 1–2 months during the first 6 months of life; every 3–4 months between 6 months and 3 years of age; every 6–12 months thereafter until growth is complete. In congenital hypothyroidism, normalization of the T_4 and FT4 levels for the first 3 years of life result in higher cognitive, attention, and achievement scores; monitor T_4 because TSH can remain elevated despite adequate replacement doses. TSH values should normalize after the first month and range between 0.5 and 2 mU/L during the first 3 years of life.[16] (>50 years) Evaluate the replacement dosage annually and adjust downward as necessary because dosage requirements decrease with age.[8,9]

Notes. Levothyroxine is the drug of choice for thyroid replacement because of purity, long half-life, and close simulation to normal physiologic hormone levels. Protect from light and moisture. The FDA permits generic substitution for branded preparations although some organizations disagree.[21,26] Use of adjunctive thyroid hormones for depression may be effective; T_3 is used instead of T_4 (*see* Liothyronine).[27,28] (*See* Thyroid Replacement Products Comparison Chart.)

LIOTHYRONINE SODIUM   Cytomel, Triostat, Various

Pharmacology. Liothyronine is a synthetic hormone identical to the thyroid hormone T_3, which is 4 times as potent by weight as T_4. (*See* Levothyroxine.)

Administration and Adult Dosage. **PO for replacement in mild hypothyroidism**—25 μg/d initially, increasing, when needed and tolerated, in 12.5–25 μg/d increments at 1- to 2-week intervals to a maintenance dosage of 25–75 μg/d to normalize TSH. **PO for severe hypothyroidism**—5 μg/d initially, increasing in 5–10 μg/d increments at 1- to 2-week intervals until 25 μg/d is reached, then increase in 5–25 μg/d increments at 1- to 2-week intervals until euthyroid. Dividing daily dosage into 2–3 doses can prevent wide serum level fluctuations. **PO for augmentation of tricyclic therapy for depression (controversial)**—25–50 μg daily.[28,29] No data is available in combination with serotonin reuptake inhibitors. **IV for myxedema coma**—25–50 μg initially, then 10–12.5 μg q4–6 h to a minimum of 10–15 μg q12h until PO administration is possible. When given in combination with T_4, 10 μg initially, then, 10 μg q8–12h until oral therapy is feasible.[15] Avoid IM or SQ administration. Some suggest that T_3 is preferable in myxedema coma when impairment of T_4 to T_3 conversion is suspected or in cardiac disease because adverse effects will dissipate faster.[15] Limited experience exists with IV dosages >100 μg/d. **PO for T_3 suppression test**—75–100 μg/d in 2–3 divided doses for 7 days, then repeat ^{131}I thyroid up-take test.

Special Populations. *Pediatric Dosage.* **PO for congenital hypothyroidism**—T_3 not recommended; levothyroxine is the drug of choice in congenital hypothyroidism.[16]

Geriatric Dosage. Not recommended because of greater potential for cardiotoxicity. **PO**—when used, start at PO 5 μg/d and increase in 5 μg/d increments at 2-week intervals, when tolerated, until desired response is obtained. (*See* Levothyroxine.)

Other Conditions. Not recommended in those with cardiovascular disease but, when used, start at PO 5 μg/d and increase in 5 μg/d increments at 2-week intervals, when tolerated until desired response is obtained. (*See* Levothyroxine.) IV for myxedema coma in cardiac disease 10–20 μg initially, then adjust dosage depending on clinical response, administer every 4–12 h until oral therapy started.

Dosage Forms. **Tab** 5, 25, 50 μg; **Inj** IV10 μg/mL.

Patient Instructions. This medication must be taken regularly to maintain proper hormone levels in the body. Report immediately when chest pain (especially in elderly patients), palpitations, sweating, nervousness, or other signs of overactivity occur.

Missed Doses. Take any missed dose as soon as it is remembered, but if more than 1 dose is missed, do not double dosage.

Pharmacokinetics. *Onset and Duration.* **PO**—onset- 2–3 days; duration after cessation of therapy 3–5 days.

Serum Levels. (Physiologic and therapeutic during triiodothyronine therapy) free T_3 145–348 pg/dL (202–504 pmol/L); total T_3 79–149 ng/dL (1.2–2.3 nmol/L). During T_3 replacement, T_4 is maintained at ≤10 μg/L (13 nmol/L).[29]

Fate. Oral absorption is usually complete, 95% in 4 h but can decrease in CHF. With a typical replacement dosage, T_3 has a peak of 4.5–7 μg/L (7–11 nmol/L) 1–2 h postdose, returning to 0.88–1.6 μg/L (1.4–2.5 nmol/L) before the next dose 24 h later.[29] V_d is (hypothyroid) 0.53 ± 0.04 L/kg; (euthyroid) 0.52 ± 0.03 L/kg; (hyperthyroid) 0.94 ± 0.07 L/kg. Turnover is (hypothyroid) 50 ± 5%/d; (euthyroid) 68 ± 11%/d; (hyperthyroid) 110 ± 22%/d. CL is (hypothyroid) 0.012 ± 0.002 L/h/kg; (euthyroid) 0.02 ± 0.003 L/h/kg; (hyperthyroid) 0.043 ± 0.013 L/h/kg.[23,30] Excreted in urine as deiodinated metabolites and their conjugates.

Half-life. (Hypothyroid) 38 ± 6 h; (euthyroid) 25 ± 3 h; (hyperthyroid) 17 ± 4.7 h

Adverse Reactions. (*See* Levothyroxine.) Dose-related adverse effects are more likely and appear more rapidly than with levothyroxine because regulation of dosage is more difficult. Liothyronine and its mixtures (e.g., desiccated thyroid, liotrix) cause "unphysiologic" toxic peaks in serum T_3 levels not found during levothyroxine replacement therapy.[22]

Contraindications. (*See* Levothyroxine.) Concomitant use of intravenous T_3 and artificial rewarming of patients

Precautions. *See* Levothyroxine.

Drug Interactions. Normal serum T_3 levels are age related and can be decreased by a wide variety of pharmacologic agents (e.g., amiodarone, iodinated contrast dyes, corticosteroids, propylthiouracil) or clinical circumstances (e.g., malnutrition; chronic renal, hepatic, pulmonary, or cardiac disease; or acute sepsis) that impair peripheral or pituitary T_4 to T_3 conversion.[4,22] (*See also* Levothyroxine Drug Interactions.)

Parameters to Monitor. Serum TSH and T_3 levels. (*See* Levothyroxine.)

Notes. Liothyronine is not considered the drug of choice for replacement therapy in hypothyroidism because of its shorter half-life (necessitating more frequent administration), greater potential for cardiotoxicity, greater difficulty of monitoring, and greater expense.[22] T_3 administration is not necessary because normal T_3 levels are achieved after T_4 replacement therapy.[31] For those with continued mood disturbances on sole T_4 therapy, the addition of T_3 to T_4 replacement has not been found to be beneficial.[8,9] **Liothyronine** is the preparation of choice when thyroid supplements must be stopped before isotope scanning. After scanning, maintenance therapy with **levothyroxine** is recommended. The use of prophylactic T_3 during cardiopulmonary bypass to improve postoperative recovery and cardiac function in adults, children, and infants is controversial.[32] (*See* Thyroid Replacement Products Comparison Chart.)

METHIMAZOLE
Tapazole

Pharmacology. Methimazole is a thioamide antithyroid drug that interferes with the synthesis of thyroid hormones by inhibiting iodide organification. Unlike propylthiouracil (PTU), methimazole does not block peripheral conversion of T_4 to T_3. Titers of thyroid receptor–stimulating antibody (TRab) decline during therapy, suggesting an immunosuppressive effect. Methimazole is 10 times more potent than PTU on a weight basis.

Administration and Adult Dosage. PO for hyperthyroidism—15–30 mg/d as a single initial dose until euthyroid (usually 6–8 weeks), then decrease by 33%–50% over several weeks to a maintenance dosage of 5–15 mg/d in a single dose for a total duration of 12–18 mo.[33] GI intolerance or severe disease might require 2 divided doses. Methimazole can be continued indefinitely when well tolerated. Methimazole rather than PTU may be preferred before radioactive iodine therapy because PTU increases the failure rate of radioactive iodine therapy.[33,34] The addition of levothyroxine is not recommended because remission rates have not shown improvement.[33] **PO for thyroid storm**—60–120 mg/d divided q6h until euthyroid. In thyroid storm, PTU is preferred.[33,34] **PR and IV**—methimazole can be formulated for administration.[33,34]

Special Populations. Pediatric Dosage. PO—0.4 mg/kg/d to a maximum of 30–40 mg/d given in 1 or 2 divided doses, with a maintenance dosage 50% of the initial dosage.

Geriatric Dosage. Same as adult dosage.

Other Conditions. In pregnancy, dosages should be as low as possible to maintain maternal T_4 levels at approximately the upper limits of normal (<10% higher).[35] Initially give a maximum of 20–30 mg/d orally in 1 or 2 divided doses for 4–6 weeks, then decrease to 5–15 mg/d in a single dose. The intellectual development and growth of children exposed to methimazole in uteri appear to be similar to unexposed siblings.[33]

Dosage Forms. Tab 5, 10 mg

Patient Instructions. Report sore throat, fever, or oral lesions immediately because they might be early signs of a rare, but severe, blood disorder. Also report any skin rashes, itching, or yellowing of eyes and skin. Be sure to take at prescribed dosage intervals.

Missed Doses. If you miss a dose, take it as soon as possible. When it is time for the next dose, take both doses.

Pharmacokinetics. Onset and Duration. PO onset about 2–3 weeks, that is consistent with the elimination of existing T_4 stores. Duration intrathyroidally 40 h.[33,36]

Serum Levels.

Fate. Well absorbed orally. Considerable interindividual variations in pharmacokinetic parameters. <0.2 mg/L (1.8 mol/L) inhibits iodide organification.[36] Peak serum levels occur at 2.3 ± 0.8 h; levels after 30 mg orally is 0.8 ± 0.2 mg/L (6.8 ± 1.9 μmol/L); after 60 mg orally, 1.5 ± 0.5 mg/L (14 ± 4 μmol/L); after 60 mg rectally, 1.1 ± 0.5 mg/L (10 ± 5 μmol/L).[36,37] The drug is actively concentrated in the thyroid gland, with peak intrathyroidal levels[37] of 0.11–1.1 mg/L (1–10 µmol/L) within 1 h; there is minimal plasma protein binding; it is distributed into breast milk 10 times greater than PTU.[36] V_d is 1.4 ± 0.6 L/kg; CL is 0.072 ± 0.018 L/h/kg. There are no active metabolites; 7%–12% is excreted unchanged in urine, 6% excreted as inorganic sulfate, 1.5% as sulfur metabolites, and 50% as unknown metabolites.[36]

Half-life α phase 3 ± 1.4 h; β phase 18.5 ± 13 h in normal and hyperthyroid patients, increased to 21 h in cirrhosis.[36] Intrathyroidal half-life is 20 h.

Adverse Reactions. Side effects are dose related.[33] Gastric distress, nausea, maculopapular skin rashes, and itching occur frequently and can disappear spontaneously with continued treatment; urticaria requires drug discontinuation.[33] Methimazole can be given to patients who develop only a nonurticarial maculopapular rash on PTU. Arthralgias occur frequently and require methimazole discontinuation because it may progress to more severe arthritis. Mild transient leukopenia occurs frequently in untreated Graves' disease, does not predispose to agranulocytosis, and is not an indication to discontinue the drug. Agranulocytosis occurs occasionally, usually within the first 3 months of therapy but can occur at any time. Risk is higher with dosages >40 mg/d and in patients >40 years old. Discontinue thioamides when granulocyte count is less than 1000/mm³; granulocyte colony–stimulating factors (e.g., **filgrastim**) can hasten recovery.[33] Rarely, fever, cholestatic or hepatocellular toxicity, vasculitis, lupus-like syndrome, hypoprothrombinemia, aplastic anemia, thrombocytopenia, nephrotic syndrome, loss of taste, spontaneous appearance of circulating antibodies to insulin or glucagon, and congenital defects (e.g., aplasia cutis, esophageal atresia, transesophageal fistula) occur.[33–35]

Contraindications. Manufacturer states that breast-feeding is a contraindication, but thioamides are approved for nursing mothers by the American Academy of Pediatrics. Normal thyroid function and intellectual development have been shown in breast-fed infants.[33]

Precautions. Although methimazole crosses the placenta at rates 4 times greater than PTU and has been rarely associated with congenital defects, it can be given to pregnant patients intolerant of PTU.[33,35] Use with caution in patients with severe allergic reactions to other thioamides. A low prevalence of cross-sensitivity occurs between thioamide compounds for nonurticarial skin rashes, so when these occur, another thioamide can be substituted. However, a 50% chance of cross-sensitivity exists for severe reactions (e.g., agranulocytosis, hepatitis), so substitution with another thioamide is not recommended.[33]

Drug Interactions. Iodides given before a thioamide delay the response to the thioamide, especially in thyroid storm. Changes in thyroid status can alter pharmacodynamics and pharmacokinetics of digoxin, warfarin, theophylline, β-blockers, and insulin. (*See* Levothyroxine.)

Parameters to Monitor. Monitor clinical status; serum free T_4 or T_4 index, and TSH every 4–6 weeks initially until euthyroid, then every 3–6 months. Obtain baseline LFTs and CBC with differential (but these are not recommended routinely because they are not predictive of toxicity and transient leukopenia and elevations in LFTs can occur). Obtain AST, ALT, total bilirubin, and alkaline phosphatase when the patient reports signs of hepatitis; WBC and differential counts when the patient reports signs of agranulocytosis such as fever, sore throat, or malaise.

Notes. Methimazole is the drug of choice for treatment of uncomplicated hyperthyroidism because fewer tablets can be given once daily, improving patient compliance.[33] Remission rates of 40%–50% are common after cessation of therapy. Favorable remission rates correlate with longer duration of therapy, higher dosages, mild disease, shrinkage of goiter size with therapy, disappearance of thyroid receptor–stimulating antibodies, and initial presentation with T_3 toxicosis.[33,34] Adjunctive therapy with **cholestyramine** 4 g tid can lower thyroid hormone levels more rapidly.[34]

PROPYLTHIOURACIL	Varlous

Pharmacology. Propylthiouracil (PTU) is a thioamide antithyroid drug that blocks the synthesis of thyroid hormones and, at dosages >450 mg/d, decreases the peripheral conversion of T_4 to T_3. Titers of thyroid receptor–stimulating antibody decline during therapy, consistent with an immunosuppressive effect.

Administration and Adult Dosage. PO for hyperthyroidism—200–300 mg/d (depending on the severity of hyperthyroidism) divided q8h initially until euthyroid (usually 6–8 weeks), then decrease by 33%–50% over several weeks to a maintenance dosage of 50–150 mg/d in a single dose for a total duration of 12–18 months.[33,34] Rarely, initial dosages of 1–1.2 g/d (maximum dosage) in 3 divided doses might be necessary. PTU can be continued indefinitely when well tolerated. Methimazole rather than PTU may be preferred before radioactive iodine therapy because PTU increases the failure rate of radioactive iodine therapy.[33,34] The addition of levothyroxine is not recommended because remission rates have not shown improvement.[33] **PO for thyroid storm**—200–400 mg q6–8 h until euthyroid; maintenance dosage is determined by patient response. **PR** PTU can be formulated for rectal administration.[33,34]

Special Populations. *Pediatric Dosage.* Give orally in 3 divided doses. PO 150–300 mg/m²/d. Alternatively, (6–10 years) 5–10 mg/kg/d or 50–150 mg/d initially; (≥10 years) 150–300 mg/d initially. Maintenance dosage is determined by patient response.

Geriatric Dosage. Same as adult dosage.

Other Conditions. In pregnancy initially 300 mg/d orally in 3 divided doses for 4–6 weeks, then decrease to 50–150 mg/d in a single dose. (*See* Methimazole.)

Dosage Forms. Tab 50 mg.

Patient Instructions. Report sore throat, fever, fatigue, malaise, nausea, anorexia, or oral lesions immediately because they may be an early sign of a severe, but rare, blood disorder. Also report any skin rashes, itching, or yellowing of eyes and skin. Be sure to take at prescribed dosage intervals.

Missed Doses. If you miss a dose, take it as soon as possible. When it is time for the next dose, take both doses.

Pharmacokinetics. *Onset and Duration.* PO—onset of therapeutic effect 2–3 weeks; consistent with the elimination of existing thyroxine stores.

Serum Levels. Peak PTU levels >4 mg/L (24 mol/L) produce antithyroid activity; 3 mg/L (18 μmol/L) reduces organification by 50%; 0.8 mg/L (5 μmol/L) reduces peripheral conversion activity by 50%.[38,39]

Fate. Oral bioavailability is 77 ± 13%. Peak levels occur 2 ± 0.3 h after oral administration and 4.7 ± 1 h after rectal administration. Peak serum level after an oral dose of 50 mg is 1 ± 0.2 mg/L (6 ± 1.2 mol/L); after 200 mg, 4.5 ± 0.7 mg/L (26 ± 4 mol/L); after 300 mg, 7 ± 0.8 mg/L (42 ± 5 mol/L); after 400 mg rectally, 3 ± 0.8 mg/L (18 ± 5 mol/L).[33] PTU is actively concentrated in the thyroid gland, 40% as unknown metabolite, 32% as sulfate, and 20% as unchanged PTU; peak intrathyroidal levels of 0.17 ± 1.7 mg/L (1–10 mol/L) occur within 1 h.[38,39] The drug is 80% plasma protein bound; it distributes poorly into breast milk.[33,35] V_d is 0.29 ± 0.06 L/kg; CL is 0.23 ± 0.04 L/h/kg. About 85% is excreted in 24 h, 61% as glucuronides, 8%–9% as inorganic sulfates, 8%–10% as unknown sulfur metabolites, and <10% excreted unchanged in urine.[38,39]

Half-life 1.3 ± 0.6 h.[38,39]

Adverse Reactions. (*See* Methimazole.) Adverse effects are not dose related. Agranulocytosis is not more prevalent at higher doses. Risk of hepatitis, including fatal liver failure, is higher in children than adults; hepatocellular toxicity is more frequent than cholestatic jaundice.[33,40,41] Transient transaminase elevations, which normalize within 3 months of continued drug administration, can occur in asymptomatic individuals.

Contraindications. Manufacturer states that breastfeeding is a contraindication, but it can be used with infant thyroid monitoring because of low milk levels and lack of effect on infants.[33,35] (*See* Methimazole.)

Precautions. (*See* Methimazole.) Although it crosses the placenta poorly (25% that of methimazole), it can cause fetal hypothyroidism and goiter.[33,35] Thyroid dysfunction can diminish as pregnancy progresses, allowing a reduction in dosage and, in some cases, a withdrawal of therapy 2–3 weeks before delivery. Use with caution before surgery or during treatment with anticoagulants because of a rare hypoprothrombinemic effect.[33] Propylthiouracil should not be used in pediatric patients unless the patients is allergic to or intolerant of methimazole, and there are no other treatment options available due to highter risk of fatal liver failure.[42]

Drug Interactions. *See* Methimazole.

Parameters to Monitor. (*See* Methimazole.) INR monitoring is advisable, particularly before surgery.

Notes. Because propylthiouracil decreases peripheral conversion of T_4 to T_3, it is considered the thioamide of choice in treating thyroid storm. Some prefer PTU rather than methimazole in pregnancy and breastfeeding, although either can be used.[33,35] Reports of PTU induced liver failure can be reduced by limiting PTU administration to the first trimester and then chaning to methimazole. Patients pretreated with PTU might require a 25% higher dosage of radioactive iodine for efficacy.[33]

THYROID REPLACEMENT PRODUCTS COMPARISON CHART

DRUG	DOSAGE FORMS	EQUIVALENT DOSAGE	CONTENTS	RELATIVE ONSET AND DURATION[a]	COMMENTS
Levothyroxine Levoxyl, Levo-T, Levothroid, Levolet, Novothyrox, Synthroid, Unithroid Various	Tab 25, 50, 75, 88, 100, 112, 125, 137, 150, 175, 200, 300 μg Inj 200, 500 μg	60 μg	T_4	Long	Preparation of choice. T_4 content is now standardized using HPLC, and bioequivalence among products is likely. Absorption impaired by food and many medications.
Liothyronine Cytomel Triostat Various	Tab 5, 25, 50 μg Inj 10 μg/mL	25 μg	T_3	Short	Administration of T_4 produces T_3. Not recommended due to higher cost, need for multiple daily doses, and difficulty monitoring.
Liotrix Thyrolar	Tab 1/4, 1/2, 1, 2, 3[b]	#1 Tab[c]	T_4 and T_3 in 4:1 ratio	Intermediate	No advantage over T_4 administration; more costly and suffers from T_3 content. (See Thyroid, Desiccated.)
Thyroid, Desiccated Armour Various	Tab 15, 30, 60, 90, 120, 180, 240, 300 mg	60 mg	T_4 and T_3 in variable ratio	Intermediate	Inexpensive; allergy to animal protein rarely occurs; supraphysiologic elevations in T_3 occur leading to T_3 toxicosis.

[a]With equivalent dosages.
[b]Numbers represent equivalent dosage of thyroid in grains (i.e., 15, 30, 60, 120, 180 mg, respectively).
[c]Thyrolar-1 contains T4 50 μg and T3 12.5 μg; other strengths are in the same proportion.
From Refs. 21 and 22.

■ REFERENCES

1. Ross DS. Iodine in the treatment of hyperthyroidism. http://www.uptodate.com Accessed Nov 13, 2008.
2. Nayak B, Hodak SP. Hyperthyroidism. *Endocrinol Metab Clin North Am.* 2007;36:617-656.
3. CDC Fact Sheet on Potassium iodide for radiation emergencies. October 2006. http://www.bt.cdc.gov/radiation/pdf/ki.pdf. Accessed Novermber 20, 2008.
4. Braverman LE, Utiger RD. *Werner & Ingbar's the Thyroid: a Fundamental and Clinical Text.* 9th ed. Philadelphia: Lippincott Williams & Wilkins; 2005.
5. Basaria S, Cooper DS. Amiodarone and the thyroid. *Am J Med.* 2005;118:706-714
6. Roti E, Uberti ED. Iodine excess and hyperthyroidism. *Thyroid.* 2001;11:493-500.
7. Markou K et al. Iodine-induced hypothyroidism. *Thyroid.* 2001;11:501-10.
8. Vaidya B, Pearce SH. Management of hypothyroidism in adults. *BMJ.* 2008;337:337:284-289.
9. Roberts CGP, Ladenson PW. Hypothyroidism. *Lancet.* 2004;363:a801.
10. Rangan S et al. Once weekly thyroxine treatment as a strategy to treat non-compliance. *Postgrad Med J.* 2007;83(984):e3.
11. Surks MI et al. Subclinical thyroid disease. Scientific review and guidelines for diagnosis and management. *JAMA.* 2004;291:228-238.
12. Gharib H, Papini E. Thyroid nodules: clinical importance, assessment, and treatment. *Endocrinol Metab Clin North Am.* 2007;36:707-735.
13. Moalem J et al. Treatment and prevention of recurrence of multinodular goiter: an evidence-based review of the literature. *World J Surg.* 2008;32:1301-1312.
14. American Thyroid Association Guidelines Taskforce. Management guidelines for patients with thyroid nodules and differentiated thyroid cancer. *Thyroid.* 2006;16: 109-141.
15. Wartofsky L. Myxedema coma. *Endocrinol Metab Clin North Am.* 2006;35:687-698.
16. Rose SR et al Update of newborn screening and therapy for congenital hypothyroidism. *Pediatrics.* 2006;117:2290-2303
17. Taylor J et al. Twice-weekly dosing for thyroxine replacement in elderly patients with primary hypothyroidism. *J Int Med Res.* 1994;22:273-277.
18. Alexander EK et al. Timing and magnitude of increases in levothyroxine requirements during pregnancy in women with hypothyroidism. *N Engl J Med.* 2004;351:241
19. Bolk N et al. Effects of evening vs morning thyroxine ingestion on serum thyroid hormone profiles in hypothyroid patients. *Clin Endocrinolol.* 2007;66:43-48.
20. Ain KA et al. Thyroid hormone levels affected by time of blood sampling in thyroxine-treated patients. *Thyroid.* 1993;3:81-85.
21. Dong BJ et al. Bioequivalence of generic and brand-name levothyroxine products in the treatment of hypothyroidism. *JAMA.* 1997;277:1205-1213.
22. Singer PA et al. Treatment guidelines for patients with hyperthyroidism and hypothyroidism. *JAMA.* 1995;273:808-812.
23. Nicoloff JT et al. Simultaneous measurement of thyroxine and triiodothyronine peripheral turnover kinetics in man. *J Clin Invest.* 1972;51:473-483.
24. Benvenga S et al. Altered intestinal absorption of L-thyroxine caused by coffee. *Thyroid.* 2008;18:293-301.
25. John-Kalarickal J et al. New medications which decrease levothyroxine absorption. *Thyroid.* 2007;8:763-765.
26. Joint Statement on the US Food and Drug Administration's decision regarding bioequivalence of levothyroxine sodium. *Thyroid.* 2004;14:486.
27. Aronson R et al. Triiodothyronine augmentation in the treatment of refractory depression. A meta-analysis. *Arch Gen Psychiatry.* 1996;53:842-848.
28. Posternak M et al. A pilot effectiveness study: placebo-controlled trial of adjunctive L-triiodothyronine (T3) used to accelerate and potentiate the antidepressant response. *Int J Neuropsychopharmacol.* 2008;11:15-25
29. Salter DR et al. Triiodothyronine (T3) and cardiovascular therapeutics: a review. *J Card Surg.* 1992;7:363-374.
30. Zaninovich AA et al. Multicompartmental analysis of triiodothyronine kinetics in hypothyroid patients treated orally or intravenously with triiodothyronine. *Thyroid.* 1994;4:285-293.
31. Jonklaas J et al. Triiodothyronine levels in athyreotic individuals during levothyroxine therapy. *JAMA.* 2008;299:769-777
32. Ronald A, Dunning J. Does perioperative thyroxine have a role during adult cardiac surgery? *Interact Cardiovasc Thorac Surg.* 2006;5:166-178.
33. Cooper D. Antithyroid drugs. *N Engl J Med.* 2005;352:905-917.
34. Nayak B; Burman K. Thyrotoxicosis and thyroid storm. *Endocrinol Metab Clin North Am.* 2006;35:663-686.
35. Chan SW, Mandel SJ. Therapy insight: management of Graves' disease during pregnancy. *Nat Clin Pract Endocrinol Metab.* 2007;3:470-478.

36. Cooper DS et al. Methimazole pharmacology in man: studies using a newly developed radioimmunoassay for methimazole. *J Clin Endocrinol Metab.* 1984,58.473-479.

37. Nabil N et al. Methimazole: an alternative route of administration. *J Clin Endocrinol Metab.* 1982;54:180-181.

38. Cooper DS et al. Acute effects of propylthiouracil (PTU) on a thyroidal iodide organification and peripheral iodothyronine deiodination: correlation with serum PTU levels measured by radioimmunoassay. *J Clin Endocrinol Metab.* 1982;54:101-107.

39. Kampmann JP, Hansen JM. Clinical pharmacokinetics of antithyroid drugs. *Clin Pharmacokinet.* 1981;6: 401-428.

40. Cooper DS, Rivkees SA. Putting propythiouracil in perspective. *J Clin Endocrinol Metab.* 2009;94:1881-1882.

41. FDA 2009 Medication Safety Alerts for PTU. http://www.fda.gov/Safety/MedWatch/SafetyInformation/ SafetyAlertsforHumanMedicalProducts/ucm164162.htm. Accessed October 30, 2009.

42. http://www.fda.gov/Safety/MedWatch/SafetyInformation/SafetyAlertsforHumanMedicalProducts/ucm164162.htm. Accessed October 30, 2009.

Renal and Electrolytes | 9

Daniel M. Riche

Chapter 54

Diuretics

Paul G. Cuddy

Class Instructions. *Diuretics.* If you are taking more than one dose a day, take the last dose in the afternoon or early evening to avoid having urinate during the night. Avoid heavily salted foods; however, rigid salt restriction is not necessary. Avoid excessive water intake. Report any dizziness or lightheadedness (especially when arising from sitting or lying), muscle cramps, weakness, lethargy, dry mouth, thirst, or low urine output.

Missed Doses. Take this drug at regular intervals. If you miss a dose, take it as soon as you remember. If it is about time for the next dose, take that dose only. Do not double the dose or take an extra dose.

AMILORIDE HYDROCHLORIDE · Midamor, Various

Pharmacology. Amiloride is a potassium-sparing diuretic with a mechanism and site of action resembling triamterene. It has mild antihypertensive activity and a longer duration of action than triamterene.[1-3]

Adult Dosage. PO for congestive heart failure (HF) and hypertension—5 mg, which may be increased to 10 mg in 1–2 doses, to a maximum of 20 mg/d, although a dosage >10 mg/d is seldom necessary. (*See* Diuretics of Choice Comparison Chart.)

Dosage Forms. **Tab** 5 mg; **Tab** 5 mg with hydrochlorothiazide 50 mg (Moduretic 5–50).

Pharmacokinetics. Onset of action occurs within 2 h with maximal effects occurring 6–10 h after oral dose. The duration of action is approximately 24 h. The drug is approximately 50% orally absorbed, decreasing to 30% when taken with food. Nearly half of the absorbed drug is excreted in the urine. **Half-life** 6–9 h in normal renal function, increasing up to 144 h in renal failure.

Adverse Reactions. Adverse reactions are generally similar to triamterene; however, in contrast to triamterene, renal stone formation has not been reported with amiloride.

Notes. Moduretic 5–50 is only indicated for treatment of diuresis.

BUMETANIDE   Bumex, Various

Pharmacology. Bumetanide is a loop diuretic with renal pharmacology similar to furosemide. Bumetanide is estimated to be approximately 40 times as potent as furosemide on a weight basis.[1-6]

Administration and Adult Dosage. PO for edema—0.5–2 mg as a single dose and repeat every 4–5 h as needed, to a maximum of 10 mg/d. **IV or IM dose** is 0.5–1 mg, IV given over 1–2 min. Repeat doses may be administered as needed every 2–3 h, to a maximum of 10 mg/d. **IV infusion**—1 mg IV bolus, followed by (Cl$_{Cr}$ >75 mL/min) 0.5 mg/h; (Cl$_{Cr}$ 25–75 mL/min) 0.5–1 mg/h; (Cl$_{Cr}$ <25 mL/min) 1–2 mg/h.[3] (*See* Diuretics of Choice Comparison Chart.)

Special Populations. *Pediatric Dosage.* 0.015–0.1 mg/kg/dose every 6–24 h, to a maximum of 10 mg/d.

Geriatric Dosage. Start with a low initial dose and titrate to response.

Other Conditions. No adjustment is necessary for renal impairment, hemodialysis, or chronic ambulatory peritoneal dialysis.

Dosage Forms. Tab 0.5, 1, 2 mg; **Inj** 0.25 mg/mL.

Patient Instructions. *See* Diuretics, Class Instructions.

Pharmacokinetics. *Onset and Duration.* Onset of diuresis is within 30–60 min after oral administration and within minutes after IV administration. Durations of diuresis are 4–6 h orally and 2–3 h IV.[5,6]

Serum Levels. Site of action is within the renal tubule and not the serum; therefore, serum concentrations do not reflect diuretic activity.

Fate. Bioavailability is 80%–96%.[5,6] V_{dss} is 0.16–0.24 L/kg in normal subjects. Protein binding to albumin is 94%–97%. Renal excretion of total drug is 80% with 50% eliminated renally as unchanged drug. Hepatic metabolism and biliary excretion account for the remainder of the elimination. The metabolites are inactive. **Half-life** 0.3–1.5 h; 1.9 ± 0.1 h in renal insufficiency; 2.3 ± 0.4 h in cirrhosis.[5,6]

Adverse Reactions. Hypokalemia, hyponatremia, and hyperuricemia occur frequently. Muscle cramps, dizziness, hypotension, headache, and nausea occur occasionally. The ototoxic potential of bumetanide is believed to be less than that of furosemide and most likely associated with rapid IV administration, high-dose therapy, or use in renal impairment.

Contraindications. Anuria; hepatic coma; coexisting severe electrolyte depletion.

Precautions. *See* Furosemide.

Drug Interactions. Aminoglycoside-related ototoxicity risk can be increased with concomitant bumetanide therapy. Cardiac glycoside toxicity is enhanced with diuretic-induced hypokalemia and hypomagnesemia. Concomitant use with other loop or thiazide diuretics enhances diuresis.

Parameters to Monitor. *See* Furosemide.

Notes. Only edema associated with HF and hepatic/renal disease, including nephrotic syndrome, are approved to be treated with bumetanide. For long-term control of edema, intermittent regimens are recommended as alternate daily doses or daily doses for 3–4 days with 1–2 day drug holidays. (*See* Loop Diuretics Comparison Chart.)

EPLERENONE

Pharmacology. Eplerenone is a selective, competitive antagonist that interferes with aldosterone binding at mineralocorticoid receptors in epithelial and nonepithelial tissues. Chronic administration leads to increases in plasma renin and serum aldosterone; however, these increases do not diminish the therapeutic drug effect. Eplerenone has been shown to decrease mortality following acute myocardial infarction in patients with impaired left ventricular dysfunction and who have clinical evidence of HF.[7,8]

Administration and Adult Dosage. **PO for HF post acute myocardial infarction—** 25 mg/d once daily initially, then increase dosage to 50 mg within 1 month of initiation. **PO for essential hypertension—**50 mg/d initially, adjusting dosage after 2–4 weeks, if necessary to 50 mg twice daily. Doses greater than 100 mg daily are not recommended due to lack of efficacy.

Special Populations. *Pediatric Dosage.* (<18 years) Safety and efficacy not established.

Geriatric Dosage. Exercise caution if used in setting of age-related declines in renal function; however, no dosage adjustment is routinely recommended in the elderly.

Dosage Forms. Tab 25, 50 mg.

Patient Instructions. (*See* Diuretics, Class Instructions.) Avoid excessive amounts of high-potassium foods or salt substitutes that contain potassium. Avoid concomitant use of strong CYP 3A4 inhibitors.

Pharmacokinetics. *Onset and Duration.* Blood pressure (BP) reductions should become apparent within 2 weeks with full effect apparent 1 month after initiation of therapy.

Serum Levels. Not established and not used clinically.

Fate. Bioavailability is ~69%. Eplerenone undergoes extensive hepatic metabolism via CYP3A4 yielding inactive metabolites. Less than 5% of the parent compound is renally cleared in unchanged form. Plasma protein binding is 50% primarily to alpha 1-acid glycoprotein. Volume of distribution ranges from 43 to 90 L. **Half-life** 4–6 h.

Adverse Reactions. Hyperkalemia occurs most often in patients with renal impairment and the risk is inversely related to Cl_{Cr}. The presence of proteinuria and diabetes also increases risk of hyperkalemia. Other common adverse effects include dizziness, diarrhea, coughing, fatigue, hypertriglyceridemia, and flu-like symptoms.

Contraindications. Serum potassium concentrations >5.5 mEq/L at initiation of therapy and/or creatinine clearance of ≤30 mL/min, or concomitant use of strong CYP3A4 inhibitors. For hypertensive patients with type 2 diabetes, eplerenone is contraindicated in presence of microalbuminuria, serum creatinine >2.0 mg/dL in males or >1.8 mg/dL in females, creatinine clearance <50 mL/min with concomitant administration of potassium supplements or potassium-sparing diuretics.

Precautions. Pregnancy category B.

Drug Interactions. Use with strong CYP3A4 inhibitors is associated with increased eplerenone AUC, and the starting dose of eplerenone should be reduced to 25 mg. Concomitant use with ACE inhibitors or angiotensin-receptor blockers may increase risk of hyperkalemia. Concomitant use with St. John's Wort is associated with reduced eplerenone AUC.

Parameters to Monitor. Monitor serum electrolytes, in particular potassium prior to initiation of therapy. Continue to monitor periodically, especially early in the course of therapy and in patients who initiate concomitant therapy with a moderate CYP3A4 inhibitor. Monitor BUN and/or serum creatinine periodically. With increases in serum potassium to 5.5 mEq/L, dosage reduction is indicated; and the drug should be withheld if serum potassium rises >6 mEq/L. Screen for dose-related increases in serum triglycerides and cholesterol.

FUROSEMIDE   Lasix, Various

Pharmacology. Furosemide is a loop diuretic that is actively secreted via the non-specific organic acid transport system into the lumen and acts at the thick ascending limb of loop of Henle, where it decreases sodium reabsorption by interfering with the function of the Na^+-K^+-$2Cl^-$ symporter.[1,2] Medullary hypertonicity is diminished, thereby decreasing the kidney's ability to reabsorb water. Excretion of sodium, chloride, potassium, hydrogen ion, calcium, magnesium, ammonium, bicarbonate, and possibly phosphate is enhanced. IV furosemide increases venous capacitance independent of diuretic effect, producing rapid improvement in pulmonary edema.[1]

Administration and Adult Dosage. **PO for edema**—20–80 mg as a single dose initially; subsequent doses are increased by 20–40 mg and may be administered at 6- to 8-h intervals until the desired response is achieved. The maintenance dose may be administered once daily or as 2–3 divided doses, and dosage depends upon the size of the dose to which the patient originally responded. The maximum single oral dose depends on the disease state: 80 mg for hepatic cirrhosis with preserved renal function,[3] 240 mg for nephrotic syndrome,[3] 80–160 mg for HF (with normal kidney function)[3]; however, dosages up to 2500 mg/d have been recommended in refractory HF.[9] **PO for hypertension**—40 mg twice daily with titration to desired BP. **IV**—Should be used only when oral administration is not feasible. IV doses may be given over 1–2 min, except the rate should not exceed 4 mg/min when large doses are given. **IM or IV for edema**—20–40 mg as a single dose increased in 20 mg increments and repeated every 2 h as needed. **IV for acute pulmonary edema**—40 mg initially over 1–2 min and may be repeated in 60 min with 80 mg, if necessary. For patients with renal impairment, the initial and subsequent doses must be adjusted based on renal function. For example, if Cl_{Cr} is 50 mL/min (approximately one-half normal), the dose must be doubled; if Cl_{Cr} is 25 mL/min, the dose must be quadrupled. **Continuous IV infusion for edema**—40 mg loading dose followed by (Cl_{Cr} 75 mL/min) 10 mg/h; (Cl_{Cr} 25–75 mL/min) 10–20 mg/h; (Cl_{Cr} <25 mL/min) 20–40 mg/h.[3] (*See* Diuretics of Choice Comparison Chart.)

Special Populations. *Pediatric Dosage.* **PO for edema**—2 mg/kg in 1 dose initially, increasing by 1–2 mg/kg in 6–8 h, if necessary, to a maximum of 6 mg/kg/d. **IM or IV**—1 mg/kg in 1 dose initially, increasing by 1 mg/kg every 2 h or more until desired response is obtained, to a maximum of 6 mg/kg/d. Maximum single dose depends on renal function. (*See* Notes.)

Geriatric Dosage. Start with a low initial dose and titrate to response.

Other Conditions. For Cl_{Cr} <20 mL/min, maximal response is attained with single IV doses of 200 mg (400 mg PO). Hence, there appears to be no need to administer larger single doses to such patients.[10] A diminished response can occur in severe decompensated HF, caused in part by alterations in oral absorption[11] and decreased renal blood flow (despite relatively normal GFR), resulting in decreased delivery of furosemide to the renal tubule; IV administration circumvents absorption problems. However, decompensated HF usually affects only the rate rather than the extent of oral furosemide absorption.[12] For patients with cirrhosis, dosage is based on renal function.

Dosage Forms. **Soln** 8, 10 mg/mL; **Tab** 20, 40, 80 mg; **Inj** 10 mg/mL.

Patient Instructions. *See* Diuretics, Class Instructions.

Pharmacokinetics. *Onset and Duration.* (Venous capacitance) IV onset of action occurs within 5 min, with a duration of >1 h. (Diuresis) PO onset of action occurs within 30–60 min, with a peak at 1–2 h, and a duration 6–8 h; IV onset of action occurs within 5 min, with a peak at 30–60 min, and a duration 1–2 h. Duration might be prolonged in severe renal impairment. (Hypertension) Maximum effect on BP might not occur for several days.

Serum Levels. Site of action is within the renal tubules and not the serum; therefore, serum concentrations do not reflect diuretic activity. High serum levels can be associated with ototoxicity.[13]

Fate. Pharmacokinetics are variable and absorption is erratic; bioavailability is 71 ± 35% (range 43%–73%) in normal subjects, 30%–100% in renal failure.[13,14] The rate, but not the extent, of absorption might be decreased in patients with edematous bowel caused by decompensated HF[12]; 96%–99% is plasma protein bound, which may be reduced in HF, renal disease, or cirrhosis.[14] V_d is 0.11 L/kg; clearance is 0.12 ± 0.24 L/h/kg. Renal clearance is primarily by active secretion; (IV) 50%–80% and (PO) 20%–55% are excreted unchanged in urine. Renal clearance is decreased in renal failure, consistent with decreased renal blood flow, a reduction of functioning nephrons, and the presence of competitive inhibitors for secretion.[14] **Half-life** 92 ± 7 (range 30–120) min in normal subjects, can be extended in cirrhosis to 81 ± 8 min OR in HF to 122 min, and markedly prolonged in end-stage renal disease to 9.7 h, and in multiorgan failure to 11–20 h. Mean residence time has been proposed as a more appropriate estimate of duration: (IV) 51.4 min; (PO) 135–195 min.[11,12]

Adverse Reactions. Dehydration, hypotension, hypochloremic alkalosis, and hypokalemia are frequent. Hyperglycemia and glucose intolerance occur as with thiazides. (*See* Hydrochlorothiazide.) With high-dose therapy (>250 mg/d), hyperuricemia occurs frequently. Tinnitus and hearing loss, occasionally permanent, occur frequently in association with rapid IV injection of large doses in patients with renal impairment.[10,14,15] Rarely, thrombocytopenia, neutropenia, jaundice, pancreatitis, and a variety of skin reactions occur.

Contraindications. Anuria (except for single dose in acute anuria).

Precautions. Use with caution in patients with severe or progressive renal disease; discontinue if renal function worsens. Use with caution in liver disease (can precipitate hepatic encephalopathy), history of diabetes mellitus or gout, and in patients allergic to other sulfonamide derivatives. Use with caution in patients with hypokalemia, hypomagnesemia, or hypocalcemia.

Drug Interactions. Cholestyramine and colestipol decrease furosemide absorption, and NSAIDs can decrease the diuretic effect of furosemide. Aminoglycoside ototoxicity can be enhanced in renally impaired patients. IV furosemide can produce flushing, sweating, and BP variations in patients taking chloral hydrate.

Parameters to Monitor. Monitor serum potassium closely, other electrolytes periodically, and serum glucose, uric acid, BUN, and serum creatinine occasionally. Observe for clinical signs of fluid or electrolyte depletion such as dry mouth, thirst, weakness, lethargy, muscle pains or cramps, hypotension, oliguria, tachycardia, and gastrointestinal (GI) upset.

Notes. Furosemide is light sensitive; oral solution should be stored at 15°C–30°C and protected from light. In severe proteinuria (>3.5 g/d), urinary albumin binds furosemide and reduces its effectiveness, explaining the higher dosage required to achieve adequate free drug concentrations.[16] In general, clinical nonresponders tend to have a decreased fraction of loop diuretics excreted in the urine. For these patients and those with HF and renal impairment, larger doses may force more drug into the tubule; however, the risk of ototoxicity must be considered. Alternatively, combined use with a thiazide or metolazone orally can be effective by blocking sodium reabsorption at multiple tubule sites; however, these agents (especially metolazone) have a slow onset of action. (*See* Loop Diuretics Comparison Chart.)

LOOP DIURETICS COMPARISON CHART

DRUG	DOSAGE FORMS	ADULT DOSAGE[a]	PEDIATRIC DOSAGE[a]	DOSAGE IN RENAL IMPAIRMENT	COMMENTS
Bumetanide Bumex Various	Tab 0.5, 1, 2 mg Inj 0.25 mg/mL	PO for edema 0.5–2 mg/d, to a maximum of 10 mg/d; IM or IV over 1–2 min 0.5–1 mg, to a maximum of 10 mg/d IV continuous infusion 1 mg, then 1–2 mg/h	PO, IM, or IV 0.01–0.22 mg/kg, to a maximum of 0.4 mg/kg or 10 mg total daily dosage	Doses up to 20 mg IV have been administered to patients with impaired renal function; for patients with Cl_{Cr} <5 mL/min, single-dose studies have shown that doses greater than 2 mg IV were required to obtain a response	1 mg PO or IV = 40 mg IV furosemide
Ethacrynic Acid Edecrin	Tab 25, 50 mg Inj 50 mg	PO minimal dose in the range of 50–200 mg/d initially, to a maximum of 200 mg twice daily IV 50 mg or 0.5–1 mg/kg, to a maximum of 100 mg	PO (infants) not established; (children) 25 mg or 1 mg/kg initially, increased in 25 mg increments to desired effect; IV not established; 1 mg/kg has been used	Not recommended with Cl_{Cr} <10 mL/min; for Cl_{Cr} of 10–50 mL/min, increase interval to every 8–12 h	Nonsulfonamide; reliable potency data not available; however, 50 mg IV is approximately equal to furosemide 35 mg IV
Furosemide Lasix Various	Tab 20, 40, 80 mg Soln 8, 10 mg/mL Inj 10 mg/mL	(See furosemide monograph)	(See furosemide monograph)	Maximum response occurs with 200 mg IV or an average of 400 mg PO, although quite variable	IV dose averages 50% of PO dose, with great variability
Torsemide Demadex Various	Tab 5, 10, 20, 100 mg Inj 10 mg/mL	(See torsemide monograph)	(See torsemide monograph)	Single doses >200 mg have not been studied	5 mg PO or IV = 20 mg IV furosemide

[a]Higher doses needed for patients with HF, liver cirrhosis, and nephrotic syndrome.
From Refs. 5–9, 13, and 16 and product information.

| **HYDROCHLOROTHIAZIDE** | HydroDIURIL, Microzide, Various |

Pharmacology. Thiazides increase sodium and chloride excretion by interfering with their reabsorption in the cortical diluting segment of the nephron; a mild diuresis of slightly concentrated urine results.[1,2] Excretion of potassium, bicarbonate, magnesium, phosphate, and iodide is increased; calcium excretion is decreased. The antihypertensive effect is associated with initial reductions in extracellular volume and cardiac output. Over time, cardiac output and extracellular volume approach their baseline; however, peripheral vascular resistance remains decreased. Urine output is paradoxically decreased in diabetes insipidus.[1]

Administration and Adult Dosage. **PO for edema**—25–100 mg/d in 1–3 doses initially; 25–100 mg/d or intermittently for maintenance, to a maximum of 100 mg/d. **PO for hypertension**—12.5–50 mg/d. Maintenance dosages >50 mg/d provide little additional benefit in controlling essential hypertension and can increase the frequency of dose-related biochemical abnormalities.[17] (*See* Diuretics of Choice Comparison Chart.)

Special Populations. *Pediatric Dosage.* **PO for hypertension and edema**— (<6 months) Up to 3 mg/kg/d in 2 divided doses; (6–12 months) 1–2 mg/kg/d in 2 divided doses. (<2 years) Maximum dose is 37.5 mg/d; (2–12 years) Maximum dose is 100 mg/d.

Geriatric Dosage. Start with a low initial dose (e.g., 12.5 mg) and titrate to response.

Other Conditions. At a Cl_{Cr} <30 mL/min, usual dosages of thiazides and most related drugs are not very effective as diuretics but may be used in conjunction with loop diuretics.[18]

Dosage Forms. **Tab** 12.5, 25, 50, 100 mg; **Cap** 12.5 mg.

Patient Instructions. (*See* Diuretics, Class Instructions.) If stomach upset occurs, take drug with meals. Report persistent anorexia, nausea, or vomiting.

Pharmacokinetics. *Onset and Duration.* Onset of diuresis occurs within 2 h; peak in 4–6 h; duration 6–12 h. Onset of hypotensive effect in 3–4 days; duration ≤1 week after discontinuing therapy.

Serum Levels. The site of diuretic action is within the renal tubules and not the serum; therefore, serum concentrations do not reflect diuretic activity.

Fate. Oral bioavailability is 71 ± 15% in healthy individuals. There are no differences in absorption among single-entity formulations. The drug is 58 ± 17% plasma protein bound; V_d is 0.83 ± 0.31 L/kg; clearance is 0.29 ± 0.07 L/h/kg. Up to 75% of drug appears within the urine and more than 95% is excreted unchanged by filtration and secretion. In severe renal impairment, renal clearance is prolonged 5-fold, with nonrenal clearance (mechanism as yet unidentified) playing a larger role in elimination.[13,19] **Half-life** 2.5 ± 0.2 h; prolonged in uncompensated HF or renal impairment.[13,19,20]

Adverse Reactions. Hypokalemia is frequent with high dosage; however, its treatment in otherwise healthy hypertensive patients is usually unnecessary. Potassium supplements or potassium-sparing diuretics (*see* Notes) may be indicated in patients with arrhythmias, MI, or severe ischemic heart disease; those with chronic liver disease; elderly persons eating poor diets; patients taking digoxin, a corticosteroid, or drugs that interfere with ventricular repolarization such as phenothiazines and heterocyclic antidepressants; and those whose serum potassium level falls below 3 mEq/L. Although less common, hyponatremia may be life-threatening and requires intervention. Hyperuricemia is reversible, and treatment is unnecessary unless the patient has renal impairment or a history of gout.[21] Hyperglycemia and alterations in glucose tolerance (usually reversible), loss of diabetic control, or umasking of latent diabetes mellitus occur occasionally. Decreased glucose tolerance might increase in prevalence after several years of therapy.[22,23] Thrombocytopenia and pancreatitis occur rarely. Elevation of serum total and low-density lipoprotein (LDL) cholesterol and triglycerides occurs; the clinical importance is unknown but can increase the risk of coronary heart disease.

Contraindications. Anuria; allergy to sulfonamide derivatives.

Precautions. Use with caution in patients with renal function impairment, liver disease (can precipitate hepatic encephalopathy), history of diabetes mellitus, or gout. Use with caution in patients with diabetes mellitus because thiazides might worsen glucose intolerance.[22,23]

Drug Interactions. Cholestyramine and colestipol decrease oral absorption of thiazides, and NSAIDs can decrease the diuretic effect of thiazides. Anticholinergics can increase oral bioavailability. Dosage of potent hypotensive agents might have to be reduced if a thiazide is added to the regimen. Concurrent calcium-containing antacids can cause hypercalcemia. Long-term thiazides can reduce lithium excretion. Thiazide-induced hypokalemia may increase the risk for quinidine-induced torsades de pointes.

Parameters to Monitor. BP should be monitored regularly in hypertensive patients receiving hydrochlorothiazide to achieve target endpoints. Monitor serum potassium initially; subsequent frequency of monitoring should be influenced by concomitant therapies and disease states. Monitor all electrolytes more closely when other losses occur (e.g., vomiting, diarrhea). Observe for clinical signs of fluid or electrolyte depletion such as dry mouth, thirst, weakness, lethargy, muscle pains or cramps, hypotension, oliguria, tachycardia, and GI upset. Monitor serum total and LDL cholesterol concentrations.

Notes. For the prevention of hypokalemia during thiazide therapy, a potassium-sparing diuretic may be preferred over potassium supplements in alkalotic patients because these agents decrease hydrogen ion loss, which can correct alkalosis and drive more potassium extracellularly.[24] Potassium-sparing diuretics also may be preferred for patients predisposed to hypomagnesemia and for those with serum potassium <3 mEq/L because potassium supplements alone rarely correct hypokalemia of this severity. (*See* Thiazides and Related Diuretics Comparison Chart.) The Seventh Report of the Joint National Committee on Prevention, Detection, Evaluation, and Treatment of High Blood Pressure recommends diuretics as monotherapy or as part of combination therapy for hypertensive patients without concurrent compelling indications. Hydrochlorothiazide is available in combination with amiloride, aliskiren, benazepril, bisoprolol fumarate, candesartan cilexetil, captopril, enalapril maleate, eprosartan mesylate, hydralazine, irbesartan, lisinopril, losartan, metoprolol succinate, metoprolol tartrate, olmesartan medoxomil, spironolactone, telmisartan, triamterene, and valsartan.

THIAZIDES AND RELATED DIURETICS COMPARISON CHART[a]

DRUG	DOSAGE FORMS	ORAL DIURETIC DOSAGE RANGE (mg/d)[b]	EQUIVALENT DIURETIC DOSAGE (mg)	PEAK EFFECT (h)	DURATION OF DIURESIS (h)
Bendroflumethiazide Naturetin	Tab 5, 10 mg	2.5–20	5	4	12–16
Benzthiazide Exna Various	Tab 50 mg	50–150	50	4–6	16–18
Chlorothiazide Diuril Various	Tab 250, 500 mg Susp 50 mg/mL Inj 500 mg[c]	500–2000	500	4 (PO) 0.5 (IV)	6–12 (PO) 2 (IV)
Chlorthalidone[d] Hygroton Thalitone Various	Tab (Thalitone)[e] 15, 25 mg Tab 25, 50, 100 mg	50–200	50	2–6	24–72
Hydrochlorothiazide Microzide Various	Cap 12.5 mg Tab 25, 50, 100 mg	25–100	50	4–6	6–12
Hydroflumethiazide Diucardin Saluron Various	Tab 50 mg	25–200	50	3–4	12–24
Indapamide[d] Lozol Various	Tab 1.25, 2.5 mg	2.5–5	2.5	2	Up to 36

(continued)

THIAZIDES AND RELATED DIURETICS COMPARISON CHART[a] (continued)

DRUG	DOSAGE FORMS	ORAL DIURETIC DOSAGE RANGE (mg/d)[b]	EQUIVALENT DIURETIC DOSAGE (mg)	PEAK EFFECT (h)	DURATION OF DIURESIS (h)
Methyclothiazide Aquatensen Enduron Various	Tab 2.5, 5 mg	2.5–10	5	6	24
Metolazone[d] Mykrox Zaroxolyn	Tab (Mykrox)[e] 0.5 mg Tab 2.5, 5, 10 mg	5–20 0.5–1 (Mykrox)	5 (Zaroxolyn)	2	12–24
Polythiazide Renese	Tab 1, 2, 4 mg	1–4	2	6	24–48
Quinethazone[d] Hydromox	Tab 50 mg	50–200	50	6	18–24
Trichlormethiazide Metahydrin Naqua Various	Tab 2, 4 mg	2–4	2	6	24

[a]From product information: patients unresponsive to maximal dosage of one agent are unlikely to respond to another agent.
[b]Dosages are for edema.
[c]There is no therapeutic advantage in giving the drug parenterally.
[d]Not a thiazide, but similar in structure and mechanism of action.
[e]Thalitone and Mykrox are more bioavailable than other formulations of the respective drugs.

MANNITOL Osmitrol, Resectisol, Various

Pharmacology. Mannitol is filtered across the glomerulus and exerts its primary action at the loop of Henle and the proximal tubule. Renal blood flow is increased and the associated increase in medullary blood flow leads to a reduction in medullary tonicity.[25] Excretion of sodium, potassium, calcium, magnesium, and phosphate is increased. Mannitol increases serum osmolality and shifts fluid out of the eye and from the brain, which underlies its use in reducing intraocular pressure and for reduction of cerebral edema.

Administration and Adult Dosage. Never administer IM, SQ, or add to whole blood for transfusion. **IV as diagnostic evaluation of acute oliguria**—(if BP and CVP are normal and *after* cardiac output is maximized) give test dose of 0.2 g/kg as a 15%–20% solution over 3–5 min (often given with **Furosemide** 80–120 mg IV), may repeat in 1 h if urine output is <50 mL/h. If there is no response after 2 doses, give no more mannitol and treat for acute tubular necrosis. If response occurs, look for underlying cause of oliguria (e.g., hypovolemia). **IV for prevention of acute renal failure**—Give test dose as above to a total dose of ≥50 g in 1 h as a loading dose, then maintain urine output at 50 mL/h with continuous infusion of 5% solution, plus 20 mEq/L sodium chloride and 1 g/L calcium gluconate. **IV for reduction of intracranial or intraocular pressure**—0.25–2 g/kg over 30–60 min as a 15%–25% solution. **IV to decrease nephrotoxicity of cisplatin**—12.5 g IV push just before cisplatin, then 10 g/h for 6 h as a 20% solution. Replace fluids with 0.45% sodium chloride with 20–30 mEq/L potassium chloride at 250 mL/h for 6 h. Maintain urine output >100 mL/h with mannitol infusion.[26,27] (*See* Notes.)

Special Populations. *Pediatric Dosage.* **IV for oliguria or anuria**—Give test dose of 0.2 g/kg as above; the therapeutic dose is 0.25–2 g/kg over 2–6 h as a 15%–20% solution. **IV for reduction of intracranial or intraocular pressure**—1–2 g/kg over 30–60 min as a 15%–20% solution. **IV for intoxications**—2 g/kg as 5%–10% solution as needed to maintain a high urinary output. (*See* Notes.)

Geriatric Dosage. Start with a low initial dose and titrate to response.

Dosage Forms. **Inj** 5, 10, 15, 20, 25%.

Pharmacokinetics. *Onset and Duration.* Diuresis onset within 15–30 min, duration depends on half-life, but ranges from 2 to 8 h. Decrease in intraocular pressure onset within 30–60 min, duration 4–8 h. Decrease in intracranial pressure onset within 15–30 min, peak 60–90 min, duration 3–8 h after stopping infusion.[28]

Serum Levels. The site of diuretic action is within the renal tubules and not the serum; therefore, serum concentrations do not reflect diuretic activity.

Fate. Only approximately 17% is absorbed orally. IV doses of 1 and 2 g/kg increase serum osmolality by 11 and 32 mOsm/kg, decrease serum sodium by 8.7 and 20.7 mEq/L, and decrease hemoglobin by 2.2 and 2.5 g/dL, respectively.[29] V_c is 0.074 L/kg; $V_{d\beta}$ is 0.23 L/kg; Clearance is 0.086 L/h/kg.[30] Mannitol is eliminated largely (75%) unchanged in urine. **Half-life** α phase 0.11 ± 0.12 h; β phase 2.2 ± 1.3 h.[30]

Adverse Reactions. Most serious and frequent reactions are fluid and electrolyte imbalance, in particular symptoms of fluid overload (e.g., pulmonary edema, hypertension, water intoxication, and HF). Acute renal failure has been reported occasionally with high doses, especially in patients with renal impairment.[31,32] Dermal necrosis can occur if solution extravasates. Anaphylaxis has been reported rarely.

Contraindications. Patients with well-established anuria caused by severe renal disease or impaired renal function who do not respond to test dose; severe pulmonary congestion, frank pulmonary edema, or severe HF; severe dehydration; edema not caused by renal, cardiac, or hepatic disease associated with abnormal capillary fragility or membrane permeability; active intracranial bleeding except during craniotomy.

Precautions. Pregnancy. Observe solution for crystals before administering. (*See* Notes.) Water intoxication can occur if fluid input exceeds urine output. Masking of inadequate hydration or hypovolemia can occur by drug-induced sustaining of diuresis. If extravasation occurs, aspirate any accessible extravasated solution, remove the IV catheter, and apply a cold compress to the area. Mannitol should not be added to whole blood for transfusion.

Drug Interactions. None known.

Parameters to Monitor. Monitor urine output closely and discontinue drug if output is low. Monitor serum electrolytes closely, taking care not to misinterpret low serum sodium as a sign of hypotonicity. (*See* Fate.) If serum sodium is low, measure serum osmolality. Observe for clinical signs of fluid or electrolyte depletion such as dry mouth, thirst, weakness, lethargy, muscle pains or cramps, hypotension, oliguria, tachycardia, and GI upset.

Notes. Mannitol can crystallize out of solution at concentrations >15%. The crystals can be redissolved by warming containers in hot water and shaking or by autoclaving; making sure to cool to body temperature before administration. Administer concentrated solutions through an inline filter. Addition of electrolytes (sodium chloride or potassium chloride) to solutions of ≥20% concentration can cause precipitation.

SPIRONOLACTONE   Aldactone, Various

Pharmacology. Spironolactone is a steroidal competitive aldosterone antagonist that acts from the interstitial side of the distal and collecting tubular epithelium to block sodium–potassium exchange, producing a delayed and mild diuresis. The diuretic effect is maximal in states of hyperaldosteronism. Excretion of sodium and chloride is increased; excretion of potassium and magnesium is decreased.[33–35] Spironolactone has mild antihypertensive activity and has demonstrated a beneficial effect in class III and IV HF.[36]

Administration and Adult Dosage. **PO for hypokalemia**—25–100 mg/d. **PO for hypertension**—50–100 mg/d initially, adjusting dosage after 2 weeks. **PO for primary aldosteronism**—100–400 mg/d. **PO for HF, ascites, and edema from nephrotic syndrome**—25 mg once daily, if serum potassium ≤5.0 mEq/L and serum creatinine is ≤ 2.5 mg/dL. If tolerated after 5 days, dosage may be increased to 50 mg once daily as clinically indicated, to a maximum of 200 mg/d. If 25 mg once daily is not tolerated, reduce dosage to 25 mg every other day. If response is inadequate, add a thiazide or loop diuretic to the regimen. (*See* Diuretics of Choice Comparison Chart.)

Special Populations. *Pediatric Dosage.* **PO**—(neonates) 1–3 mg/kg/d every 12–24 h; (older children) 1.5–3.3 mg/kg/d OR 60 mg/m²/d in divided doses every 6–24 h.[37]

Geriatric Dosage. Start with a low initial dose and titrate to response.

Dosage Forms. **Tab** 25, 50, 100 mg; **Tab** 25 mg with hydrochlorothiazide 25 mg (Aldactazide); **Tab** 50 mg with hydrochlorothiazide 50 mg (Aldactazide 50/50).

Patient Instructions. (*See* Diuretics, Class Instructions.) Avoid excessive amounts of high-potassium foods or salt substitutes.

Pharmacokinetics. *Onset and Duration.* Onset of action occurs within 1–2 days, with peak effects noted after 2–3 days with continued administration; onset can be hastened by giving a loading dose; effects persist for 2–3 days after cessation of therapy.

Serum Levels. Not established and not used clinically.

Fate. Bioavailability is ~90%[33]; food promotes absorption and possibly decreases first-pass effect.[38] Spironolactone undergoes rapid and extensive metabolism to canrenone (active metabolite), 7α-thiomethylspironolactone (major metabolite), and other sulfur-containing metabolites; together with the parent drug, these metabolites contribute to the overall antimineralocorticoid activity.[33,39] Metabolites are eliminated primarily renally, with minimal biliary excretion. Little or no parent drug is excreted unchanged in urine.[38,39] **Half-life** (spironolactone) 1.4 ± 0.5 h; (7α-thiomethylspironolactone) 13.8 ± 6.4 h; (canrenone) 16.5 ± 6.3 h.[39]

Adverse Reactions. Hyperkalemia can occur, most frequently in patients with renal function impairment (especially those with diabetes mellitus) and those receiving potassium supplements or concomitant ACE inhibitors. Dehydration and hyponatremia occur occasionally, especially when the drug is combined with other diuretics. In patients receiving high doses, frequent estrogen-like side effects such as gynecomastia, decreased libido, and impotence occur in males; menstrual irregularities and breast tenderness occur in females. These effects are reversible after drug discontinuation.[40,41]

Contraindications. Anuria; acute renal insufficiency; rapidly deteriorating renal function; severe renal failure; serum potassium >5.5 mEq/L or development of hyperkalemia while taking the drug; hypermagnesemia.

Precautions. Pregnancy. Patients with renal impairment, especially those with diabetes mellitus and/or those receiving an ACE inhibitor, are at risk for developing hyperkalemia. Use with caution in patients with hepatic disease. Do not use with triamterene or amiloride. Give potassium supplements only to patients with demonstrated hypokalemia who are taking a proximally acting diuretic and a corticosteroid concurrently with spironolactone, or only for very short periods in treating cirrhosis and ascites.

Drug Interactions. Use with ACE inhibitors increases risk of hyperkalemia, especially in renal impairment. Spironolactone increases serum concentrations of digoxin by reducing renal clearance. In addition, spironolactone and its metabolites cross-react with digoxin-binding antibody in some digoxin immunoassays.

Blood from blood bank, potassium supplements, or potassium-containing medications may increase risk of hyperkalemia. Concurrent administration of spironolactone may reduce renal clearance of lithium or amantadine.

Parameters to Monitor. Monitor serum electrolytes, in particular potassium, periodically, especially early in the course of therapy. Monitor BUN and/or serum creatinine periodically. In ascites, also obtain daily weight and urinary electrolytes and maintain weight loss at no greater than 0.5–1 kg/d and urinary Na^+/K^+ ratio at >1. Observe for clinical signs of fluid or electrolyte depletion such as dry mouth, thirst, weakness, lethargy, muscle pains or cramps, hypotension, oliguria, tachycardia, and GI upset. Monitor BP periodically to achieve therapeutic goals.

Notes. Spironolactone is used in the diagnosis of primary aldosteronism and may be useful in the management of this condition in patients unable to undergo surgery.

TORSEMIDE
Demadex, Various

Pharmacology. Torsemide is a loop diuretic similar to furosemide. Over the normal dosage range, its diuretic potency by weight is approximately 2–4 times that of furosemide. Onset of diuresis is similar but duration is longer (up to 8–12 h orally).[42–44]

Administration and Adult Dosage. PO for hypertension—5 mg once daily. If therapeutic response is not achieved after 4–6 weeks, increase to 10 mg/d. **Initial PO or IV for edema or chronic renal failure**—20 mg/d; dosage may be doubled until the desired response is obtained, to a maximum of 200 mg/d OR IV by continuous infusion, give 20-mg loading dose, then 10–20 mg/h. **PO or IV for edema due to disease of the liver**—5–10 mg/d initially with a potassium-sparing diuretic, to a maximum of 40 mg/d. **PO or IV for HF**—10–20 mg once daily with titration until desired response is achieved, to a maximum dose of 200 mg daily. (*See* Furosemide, Notes and Loop Diuretics Comparison Chart.)

Dosage Forms. Tab 5, 10, 20, and 100 mg.

Pharmacokinetics. Oral bioavailability is 79%–91% (median 80); V_d is 0.14–0.19 L/kg. **Half-life** dose dependent, ranging from 2.2 to 3.8 h. Nonrenal clearance remains essentially constant over a dosage range of 5–20 mg, but renal clearance and fraction excreted decrease, suggesting saturable renal clearance. Renal impairment (Cl_{Cr} <60 mL/min) does not appreciably alter total clearance; hemodialysis and hemofiltration do not markedly influence serum clearance.

Adverse Reactions. Although the potential for hypokalemia exists, torsemide's kaliuretic potency is less than that of furosemide, suggesting that it is less potassium wasting during long-term therapy; the clinical relevance of this observation is unknown. Precautions and monitoring parameters are the same as those for furosemide.

Notes. Demadex injection (10 mg/mL) has been discontinued by Roche as of 4/30/08 for business reasons. Though Bedford Laboratories has approval for the generic formulation, the company has not launched the product, nor have they announced an estimated launch date.

TRIAMTERENE
Dyrenium, Various

Pharmacology. Triamterene acts directly from the distal tubular lumen on active sodium exchange for potassium and hydrogen ions, producing a mild diuresis that is independent of aldosterone concentration. Excretion of sodium, chloride, calcium, and possibly bicarbonate is increased; excretion of potassium and possibly magnesium is decreased. Antihypertensive activity is inconsistent and less pronounced than with thiazides or spironolactone.[34,35]

Administration and Adult Dosage. **PO for edema**—(Dyrenium) 100 mg twice daily with or immediately after meals, reduce dosage if used with another diuretic. Adjust the maintenance dosage to the needs of the patient, which can range from 100 mg/d to 100 mg every other day, to a maximum of 300 mg/d, (Dyazide) 1–2 capsules daily. **PO for hypertension**—(Maxzide, Dyazide) 1 tablet or capsule daily titrated every 2–3 weeks, to a maximum of 50/75 mg daily. (*See* Diuretics of Choice Comparison Chart.)

Special Populations. *Pediatric Dosage.* **PO**—2–4 mg/kg/d initially, may increase to 6 mg/kg/d in 1–2 doses after meals, to a maximum of 300 mg/d. Decrease dosage if used with another diuretic.

Geriatric Dosage. Start with a low initial dose and titrate to response.

Dosage Forms. **Cap** 50, 100 mg; **Cap** (Dyazide) 50 mg with hydrochlorothiazide 25 mg, 37.5 mg with hydrochlorothiazide 25 mg; **Tab** (Maxzide) 75 mg with hydrochlorothiazide 50 mg.

Patient Instructions. (*See* Diuretics, Class Instructions.) This drug may be taken with food or milk to minimize stomach upset. Report persistent loss of appetite, nausea, or vomiting. Avoid eating excessive amounts of high-potassium foods or salt substitutes.

Pharmacokinetics. *Onset and Duration.* Onset 2–4 h; full therapeutic effect might not occur for several days; duration of 7–9 h.

Serum Levels. The site of diuretic action is within the renal tubules and not the serum; therefore, serum concentrations do not reflect diuretic activity.

Fate. Variable absorption with bioavailability estimated at $51 \pm 18\%$. Plasma protein binding is $61 \pm 2\%$. Hepatic degradation occurs with formation of an active metabolite, 4-hydroxytriamterene sulfate, which is comparable in activity to the parent. Approximately $52 \pm 10\%$ of drug is eliminated through the urine with the sulfate compound accounting for most of the excreted drug, which accumulates in the presence of renal impairment.[25] **Half-life** 4.2 ± 0.7 h. Half-life is prolonged in renal impairment and in the elderly.

Adverse Reactions. Nausea, vomiting, diarrhea, and dizziness occur occasionally. Dehydration and hyponatremia with an increase in BUN occur occasionally, especially when the drug is combined with other diuretics. Triamterene-induced renal stones occur occasionally. Hyperkalemia occurs occasionally, especially in diabetics and those with renal impairment; metabolic acidosis has been reported. Megaloblastic anemia can occur in alcoholic cirrhosis.

Contraindications. Severe or progressive renal disease or dysfunction (except possibly nephrosis); severe renal failure; severe hepatic disease;

seium potassium >5.5 mEq/L or development of hyperkalemia while taking the drug; hypermagnesemia.

Precautions. Pregnancy. Patients with renal impairment, especially those with diabetes mellitus and/or receiving an ACE inhibitor are at risk for developing hyperkalemia. Can elevate serum uric acid in patients predisposed to gout. Do not use with spironolactone or amiloride.

Drug Interactions. Use with ACE inhibitors increases risk of hyperkalemia, especially in renal impairment. Indomethacin (and probably other NSAIDs) can reduce renal function when combined with triamterene. Use with dietary salt substitutes can increase risk of triamterene-induced hyperkalemia. Concurrent therapy with triamterene may lead to reduced renal clearance of lithium or amantadine.

Parameters to Monitor. Monitor serum electrolytes, in particular potassium, periodically, especially early in the course of therapy. Monitor BUN and/or serum creatinine periodically. Observe for clinical signs of fluid or electrolyte depletion such as dry mouth, thirst, weakness, lethargy, muscle pains or cramps, hypotension, oliguria, tachycardia, and GI upset. Monitor BP in hypertensive patients to achieve therapeutic endpoints.

Notes. Triamterene without hydrochlorothiazide (Dyrenium) is not approved, but used for hypertension at 50–100 mg in 1–2 divided doses.

DIURETICS OF CHOICE COMPARISON CHART[a]

CONDITION	LOOP DIURETICS	OSMOTIC DIURETICS	THIAZIDES	POTASSIUM-SPARING AGENTS	COMMENTS
Relative potency	>15%	10%–15%	5%–10%	<5%	Values refer to maximum fraction of filtered sodium excreted after maximally effective dose of drug
Hypertension	A	—	A	D	Sustained antihypertensive effect of thiazides exhibits a flat dose-response curve and occurs at doses below the threshold for diuresis; Loop diuretics are preferred with Cl_{Cr} <30 mL/min
Heart failure	A	—	A	A (spironolactone) A (eplerenone)	Begin with thiazide with low dosage; if ineffective, substitute a loop diuretic; loop diuretics are preferred with Cl_{Cr} <30 mL/min; spironolactone as adjunctive therapy reduces morbidity and mortality in NYHA class III and IV HF; adjunctive eplerenone therapy improves survival of stable patients with systolic dysfunction and HF after an acute MI
Pulmonary edema	A (IV)	—	—	—	Prompt venodilation precedes diuretic effect
Hepatic ascites	B	—	—	A	Spironolactone is the agent of choice; urine Na:K ratio <1 indicates need for higher dosage (200–1000 mg/d); rate of diuresis should not exceed 750 mL/d (no peripheral edema), or up to 2 L/d (if edema is present)
Renal failure	A	C	—	—	A loop diuretic plus a thiazide (in a high dose) can evoke a clinically useful diuresis even when Cl_{Cr} is <15 mL/min; however, provocative diuretic challenges in oliguric patients can be potentially hazardous, especially if the cause of renal failure is uncertain

(continued)

DIURETICS OF CHOICE COMPARISON CHART[a] (*continued*)

CONDITION	LOOP DIURETICS	OSMOTIC DIURETICS	THIAZIDES	POTASSIUM-SPARING AGENTS	COMMENTS
Diabetes insipidus	—	—	A	C	Thiazides are most useful in the nephrogenic form; a long-acting agent is preferred, amiloride is useful for lithium-induced DI
Hypercalcemia	A	—	—	—	High-dose furosemide (IV 80–100 mg every 1–2 h) with IV saline for forced diuresis to promote calcium excretion
Hypercalciuria	—	—	A	—	Thiazides cause marked reduction in urinary calcium excretion; they also appear effective in preventing calcium stone formation irrespective of whether urinary calcium is abnormally elevated

A, diuretic of choice; B, diuretic of second choice if patient is unresponsive to first choice; C, useful in some circumstances; D, useful as an adjunct to a more potent diuretic to reduce potassium loss and possibly enhance therapeutic effect.
[a]This table is a guide to the selection of the most appropriate diuretic for the condition listed but is not an all-inclusive guide to therapy.
From Refs. 34 and 35.

■ REFERENCES

1. Brater DC. Pharmacology of diuretics. *Am J Med Sci*. 2000;319:38-50.
2. Hebert SC. Molecular mechanisms. *Semin Nephrol*. 1999;19:504-523.
3. Brater DC. Diuretic therapy. *N Engl J Med*. 1998;339:387-395.
4. Ellison DH. Diuretic drugs and the treatment of edema: from clinic to bench and back again. *Am J Kidney Dis* 1994;23:623-643.
5. Ward A, Heel RC. Bumetanide. A review of its pharmacodynamic and pharmacokinetics properties and therapeutic use. *Drugs*. 1984;28:426-464.
6. Brater DC. Disposition and response to bumetanide and furosemide. *Am J Cardiol*. 1986;57:20A-25A.
7. Barnes BJ, Howard PA. Eplerenone: a selective aldosterone receptor antagonist for patients with heart failure. *Ann Pharmacother*. 2005;39:68-76.
8. Keating GM, Plosker GL. Eplerenone: a review of its use in left ventricular systolic dysfunction and heart failure after acute myocardial infarction. *Drugs*. 2004;64:2689-2707.
9. Gerlag PG, van-Meijel JJ. High-dose furosemide in the treatment of refractory congestive heart failure. *Arch Intern Med*. 1988;148:286-291.
10. Brater DC. Resistance to diuretics: mechanisms and clinical implications. *Adv Nephrol Necker Hosp*. 1993;22:349-369.
11. Vasko MR et al. Furosemide absorption altered in decompensated congestive heart failure. *Ann Intern Med*. 1985;102:314-318.
12. Van Meyel JJ et al. Absorption of high dose furosemide (frusemide) in congestive heart failure. *Clin Pharmacokinet*. 1992;22:308-318.
13. Thummel KE et al. Design and optimization of dosage regimens; pharmacokinetic data. In: Brunton LL et al., eds. *Goodman and Gilman's the Pharmacological Basis of Therapeutics*. 10th ed. New York: McGraw-Hill; 2005:1787-1888.
14. Ponto LL, Schoenwald RD. Furosemide (frusemide): a pharmacokinetic/pharmacodynamic review (part I). *Clin Pharmacokinet*. 1990;18:381-408.
15. Ponto LL, Schoenwald RD. Furosemide (frusemide): a pharmacokinetic/pharmacodynamic review (part II). *Clin Pharmacokinet*. 1990;18:460-471.
16. Ellison DH. Diuretic resistance: physiology and therapeutics. *Semin Nephrol*. 1999;19:581-597.
17. Kaplan NM. Diuretics: correct use in hypertension. *Semin Nephrol*. 1999;19:569-574.
18. Aronoff GR et al. *Drug Prescribing in Renal Failure. Dosing Guidelines for Adults*. 5th ed. Philadelphia, PA: American College of Chest Physicians; 2007.
19. Beermann B, Groschinsky-Grind M. Clinical pharmacokinetics of diuretics. *Clin Pharmacokinet*. 1980;5:221-245.
20. Welling PG. Pharmacokinetics of the thiazide diuretics. *Biopharm Drug Dispos*. 1986;7:501-535.
21. Greenberg A. Diuretic complications. *Am J Med Sci*. 2000;319:10-24.
22. O'Bryne S, Feely J. Effects of drugs on glucose tolerance in non-insulin–dependent diabetes (part II). *Drugs*. 1990;40:203-219.
23. O'Bryne S, Feely J. Effects of drugs on glucose tolerance in non-insulin–dependent diabetes (part I). *Drugs*. 1990;40:6-18.
24. Womack PL, Hart LL. Potassium supplements vs. potassium-sparing diuretics. *DICP*. 1990;24:710-711.
25. Jackson EK. Diuretics. In: Brunton LL, Lazo JS, Parker KL, eds. *The Pharmacological Basis of Therapeutics*. 11th ed. New York, NY: McGraw-Hill Companies; 2006:737.
26. Hoffman DM, Grossano D. Use of mannitol diuresis to reduce cis-platinum nephrotoxicity. *Drug Intell Clin Pharm*. 1978;12:489-490.
27. Anand AJ, Bashey B. Newer insights into cisplatin nephrotoxicity. *Ann Pharmacother*. 1993;27:1519-1525.
28. Nissenson AR. Mannitol. *West J Med*. 1979;131:277-284.
29. Manninen PH et al. The effect of high-dose mannitol on serum and urine electrolytes and osmolality in neurosurgical patients. *Can J Anaesth*. 1987;34:442-446.
30. Anderson P et al. Use of mannitol during neurosurgery: interpatient variability in the plasma and CSF levels. *Eur J Clin Pharmacol*. 1988;35:643-649.
31. Dorman HR et al. Mannitol-induced acute renal failure. *Medicine (Baltimore)*. 1990;69:153-159.
32. Horgan KJ et al. Acute renal failure due to mannitol intoxication. *Am J Nephrol*. 1989;9:106-109.
33. Skluth HA, Gums JG. Spironolactone: a re-examination. *DICP*. 1990;24:52-59.
34. Lant A. Diuretics: clinical pharmacology and therapeutic use (part II). *Drugs*. 1985;29:162-188.
35. Lant A. Diuretics: clinical pharmacology and therapeutic use (part I). *Drugs*. 1985;29:57-87.
36. Pitt B et al. The effect of spironolactone on morbidity and mortality in patients with severe heart failure. *N Engl J Med*. 1999;341:709-717.
37. Taketomo CK et al. *Pediatric Dosage Handbook*. 15th ed. Hudson, OH: Lexi-Comp, Inc.; 2008.

38. Overdiek HW, Merkus FW. Influence of food on the bioavailability of spironolactone. *Clin Pharmacol Ther.* 1986;40:531-536.
39. Gardiner P et al. Spironolactone metabolism: steady-state serum levels of the sulfur-containing metabolites. *J Clin Pharmacol.* 1989;29:342-347.
40. Overdiek JW, Merkus FW. Spironolactone metabolism and gynaecomastia. *Lancet.* 1986;1:1103.
41. Jeunemaitre X et al. Efficacy and tolerance of spironolactone in essential hypertension. *Am J Cardiol.* 1987;60:820-825.
42. Friedel HA, Buckley MM. Torsemide: a review of its pharmacological properties and therapeutic potential. *Drugs.* 1991;41:81-103.
43. Brater DC et al. Clinical pharmacology of torsemide, a new loop diuretic. *Clin Pharmacol Ther.* 1987;42:187-192.
44. Gehr TW et al. The pharmacokinetics of intravenous and oral torsemide in patients with chronic renal insufficiency. *Clin Pharmacol Ther.* 1994;56:31-38.

Chapter 55

Electrolytes

Paul G. Cuddy

Class Instructions. *Oral Electrolytes.* Take oral products with (tablets) or diluted in (liquids and powders) 6–8 fl oz of water or juice to avoid gastrointestinal injury or laxative effect. However, if you are undergoing hemodialysis, you may need to limit the volume of water you take. This medication may be taken with food or after meals if upset stomach occurs.

CALCIUM SALTS — Various

Pharmacology. Calcium plays an important role in neuromuscular activity, pancreatic insulin release, gastric hydrogen secretion, blood coagulation, and platelet aggregation; as a cofactor for some enzyme reactions; and in bone and tooth metabolism.[1]

Administration and Adult Dosage. PO as dietary supplement—(elemental calcium) recommended daily allowance (RDA) is (9–18 years, males and females) 1300 mg/d, (19–50 years, including pregnant and lactating women) 1000 mg/d; (≥50 years) 1200 mg/d.[2] **PO to lower serum phosphate in end-stage renal disease (ESRD)**—(calcium carbonate) 650 mg with each meal initially, adjust dosage to decrease serum phosphate to <6 mg/dL[3]; (calcium acetate) 1334 mg with each meal initially, adjust dosage to decrease serum phosphate to <6 mg/dL. (*See* Notes.) **IV for emergency elevation of serum calcium**—(calcium gluconate) 15 mg/kg in NS or D5W infused over 8–10 h (typically raises serum calcium by 2–3 mg/dL),[4] may repeat every 1–3 days depending on response; (calcium glucceptate) 1.1–1.4 g infused at a rate not to exceed 36 mg/min of elemental calcium. **IV for hypocalcemic tetany**—10–20 mL calcium gluconate infused over 10 min, may repeat until tetany is controlled. Faster IV infusion rates can result in cardiac dysfunction.[5]

Special Populations. *Pediatric Dosage.* PO as dietary supplement—(elemental calcium) adequate intake is (0–6 months) 210 mg/d; (7–12 months) 270 mg/d; (1–3 years) 500 mg/d; (4–8 years) 800 mg/d; (9–18 years) 1300 mg/d.[2] **PO for hypocalcemia**—(elemental calcium) (neonates) 50–150 mg/kg/d in 4– 6 divided doses, to a maximum of 1 g/d; (children) 20–65 mg/kg/d in 4 divided doses. **IV for emergency elevation of serum calcium**—(infants) <1 mEq, may repeat every 1–3 days depending on response; (children) 1–7 mEq, may repeat every 1–3 days depending on response. **IV for hypocalcemic tetany**—(infants) 2.4 mEq/d in divided doses; (children) 0.5–0.7 mEq/kg 3–4 times daily, or more until tetany controlled.

Geriatric Dosage. Postmenopausal women have a requirement of 1200 mg/d, including those on estrogen replacement or a bisphosphonate.[2] Lower dosage might be required in some patients because of the age-related decrease in renal function; conversely, requirements might increase with advanced renal insufficiency.

Other Conditions. Adolescence, renal impairment, and pregnancy might increase requirements; base maintenance dosage on serum calcium, serum phosphate, and diet.[1,2]

Dosage Forms. (*See* Oral Calcium Products Comparison Chart.) **Inj** (chloride) 1 g/10 mL (contains 273 mg or 13.6 mEq calcium); (gluconate) 1 g/10 mL (contains 93 mg or 4.65 mEq calcium); (gluceptate) 1.1 g/5 mL (contains 90 mg or 4.5 mEq calcium).

Patient Instructions. (*See* Oral Electrolytes, Class Instructions.) Do not take within 2 h of taking oral tetracycline or fluoroquinolone products. Take calcium tablets with food to maximize absorption. If used as a phosphate binder, calcium must be taken with food. Allow effervescent tablets to degas in a glass of water (approximately 4 min) before taking.

Missed Doses. Take this drug at regular intervals. If you miss a dose, take it as soon as you remember and then return to your normal dosage schedule.

Pharmacokinetics. *Serum Levels.* Normal serum total calcium is 8.4–10.2 mg/dL (2.1–2.6 mmol/L) for an adult with a serum albumin of 4 g/dL. Because a smaller fraction of calcium is protein bound in hypoalbuminemia, the patient's value must be corrected based on serum albumin:

Corrected serum calcium = serum calcium in mg/dL
+ (0.8 × [4 − serum albumin in g/dL]).

Fate. Oral calcium absorption is approximately 30% and depends on vitamin D and parathyroid hormone. Absorption decreases with age, high intake, achlorhydria, and estrogen loss at menopause[1]; absorption increases when taken with food or in divided doses.[5,6] Bioavailability from various salt forms does not appear to differ substantially in normals[7]; however, differences in disintegration and dissolution among commercial formulations exist.[3,5] Approximately 99% of total body calcium is found in bone and teeth; of the 1% in extracellular fluid, 40%–45% is plasma protein bound (mostly to albumin); 8%–10% is complexed to citrate, phosphate, and other anions; and 45%–50% is diffusible and physiologically active. Approximately 135–155 mg/d are secreted into the GI tract, with 85% reabsorbed. Fecal loss of unabsorbed dietary calcium and endogenous excretion is 100–130 mg/d, urine loss is 150 mg/d, and sweat loss is 15 mg/d.[6]

Adverse Reactions. IV calcium solutions, especially calcium chloride, are extremely irritating to the veins.[4] Constipation or flatulence occurs frequently, especially with high dosages; the frequency probably does not differ markedly among salt forms.[8] Calcium overload caused by oral calcium supplements is rare; immobilization, dosages in excess of 3–4 g/d, vitamin D therapy, and renal impairment can contribute to hypercalcemia, hypercalciuria, or nephrolithiasis during oral supplementation. Symptoms of calcium intolerance include nausea, intestinal bloating, excess gas, vomiting, constipation, abdominal pain, dry mouth, and polyuria.

Contraindications. Hypercalcemia; sarcoidosis; severe cardiac disease; digitalis glycoside therapy; calcium nephrolithiasis; calcium-phosphate product > 60–70 mg/dL in the setting of uremia is associated with calcification in extraosseous tissues and should be avoided. To determine calcium phosphate product, multiply the serum phosphate value (in mg/dL) by the serum calcium value (in mg/dL).

Precautions. Avoid extravasation of parenteral calcium products. If extravasation occurs, aspirate any accessible extravasated solution, remove IV catheter, and apply a cold compress to the area.

Drug Interactions. Concomitant thiazide diuretic therapy and sodium depletion or metabolic acidosis can increase tubular reabsorption of calcium. Calcium reduces oral absorption of fluoroquinolones, tetracyclines, and iron salts. Concomitant use with sodium polystyrene sulfonate can lead to metabolic alkalosis and compromised activity of the binding resin.

Parameters to Monitor. Serum calcium regularly, with frequency determined by patient's condition; BUN and/or serum creatinine, serum phosphate, magnesium, and serum albumin (especially if low) periodically.

Notes. Calcium supplementation also can be achieved by dietary measures: skim milk provides 300 mg calcium/8 fl oz, 300 mg/8 fl oz of low-fat yogurt, 272 mg/oz of Swiss cheese, and 200 mg/6 fl oz of calcium-fortified orange juice.[8] Calcium carbonate is inexpensive and a good first-line agent. However, dissolution of calcium from phosphate and carbonate salts is pH dependent. These salts might not be optimal calcium sources for patients with elevated GI pH, such as the elderly or those with achlorhydria. Calcium carbonate as a chewable tablet or nougat, or the use of an alternative calcium salt have been recommended.[5] In ESRD, use calcium salts when serum phosphate is <8 mg/dL; when serum phosphate is >8 mg/dL, use sevelamer or lanthanum. Calcium acetate binds approximately twice the amount of phosphorus for the same quantity of calcium absorbed[3]; however, the frequency of hypercalcemia does not seem to be diminished. (*See* Oral Calcium Products Comparison Chart.)

ORAL CALCIUM PRODUCTS COMPARISON CHART

PRODUCT	PERCENTAGE CALCIUM (%)	ELEMENTAL CALCIUM CONTENT
Calcium Acetate Calphron PhosLo	25	667-mg tablet = 169 mg 667-mg tablet = 169 mg
Calcium Carbonate Caltrate 600 Os-Cal 500 Nephro-Calci Tums E-X	40	1500-mg tablet = 600 mg 1250-mg tablet = 500 mg 1500-mg tablet = 600 mg 750-mg tablet = 300 mg
Calcium Citrate Citracal Tablets Citracal Liquitabs	21.1	950-mg tablet = 200 mg 2376-mg tablet = 500 mg
Calcium Glubionate Neo-Calglucon	6.5	5-mL syrup = 115 mg
Calcium Gluconate Various	9.3	500-mg tablet = 45 mg 650-mg tablet = 60 mg 975-mg tablet = 90 mg 1000-mg tablet = 93 mg
Calcium Lactate Various	13	500-mg tablet = 96 mg 650-mg tablet = 84.5 mg

(continued)

ORAL CALCIUM PRODUCTS COMPARISON CHART (*continued*)

PRODUCT	PERCENTAGE CALCIUM (%)	ELEMENTAL CALCIUM CONTENT
Calcium Phosphate, Tribasic Posture	39	1565-mg tablet = 600 mg
Dairy Products	—	Cheese 28 g = 300–400 mg Skim milk 250 mL = 300 mg Yogurt 28 g = 43 mg

From Refs. 2–4 and product information.

MAGNESIUM SALTS   Various

Pharmacology. Magnesium is the second most abundant intracellular cation, with an essential role in neuromuscular function and protein and carbohydrate enzymatic systems; it functions as a cofactor for enzymes involved in transfer, storage, and utilization of intracellular energy. Magnesium also is an integral component of bone matrix.[9]

Administration and Adult Dosage. PO as dietary supplement—(elemental magnesium) RDA is ≥19 years) 400–420 mg/d for males and 310–320 mg for nonpregnant, nonlactating women ≥19 years.[2] **PO for symptomatic chronic deficiency**—(elemental magnesium) 12–24 mg/kg in divided doses.[10] A renal threshold for magnesium excretion exists, so replacement is best accomplished slowly, usually over 5 days. **IV for prevention of negative balance**—(elemental magnesium) 100–200 mg/d in parenteral nutrition solution.[10] **IM for mild deficiency**—1 g $MgSO_4$ every 4–6 h until serum magnesium is normalized or signs and symptoms abate.[10] **IM for severe hypomagnesemia**—2 g $MgSO_4$ as a 50% solution every 8 h until serum magnesium is normalized or signs and symptoms abate; because IM injections are painful, continuous IV infusions might be preferred.[11] **IV infusion for severe hypomagnesemia**—48 mEq/d (6 g $MgSO_4$) for 3–7 days by continuous infusion.[11] **IV for life-threatening hypomagnesemia (acute arrhythmias and seizures)**—8–16 mEq (1–2 g $MgSO_4$) over 5–10 min, followed by continuous infusion of 48 mEq magnesium/d.[9] **IV for preeclampsia or eclampsia**—4–6 g $MgSO_4$, then 1–2 g/h by continuous infusion to maintain target serum level. (*See* Notes.)

Special Populations. *Pediatric Dosage.* **IV for hypomagnesemia**—25 mg/kg $MgSO_4$ as a 25% solution over 3–5 min every 6 h for 3–4 doses. **IM for seizures**—20–40 mg/kg $MgSO_4$ as a 20% solution as needed. **IV for severe seizures**—100–200 mg/kg $MgSO_4$ as a 1%–3% solution infused slowly with close monitoring of blood pressure. Administer one-half the dose during the initial 15–20 min and the total dose within 1 h.

Geriatric Dosage. Lower dosage might be required in some patients because of the age-related decrease in renal function.

Other Conditions. Base maintenance dosage on serum magnesium and diet. Renal impairment decreases requirement. In severe renal failure, reduce dosage by at least 50% of the recommended amount and monitor serum magnesium after each dose.[12] Concomitant administration of potassium and calcium may be necessary because many causes of hypomagnesemia also lead to hypocalcemia and hypokalemia.[10]

Dosage Forms. *See* Magnesium Products Comparison Chart.

Patient Instructions. *See* Oral Electrolytes, Class Instructions.

Missed Doses. Take this drug at regular intervals. If you miss a dose, take it as soon as you remember. Do not double the dose or take an extra dose.

Pharmacokinetics. *Onset and Duration.* Peak levels are achieved immediately after IV, 1 h after IM. Duration (anticonvulsant) is 30 min with IV, 3–4 h postonset with IM.

Serum Levels. (Normal) 1.3–2.1 mEq/L (0.65–1.1 mmol/L); (preeclampsia or eclampsia) 4–6 mEq/L (2–3 mmol/L).[9] Intracellular and extracellular concentrations can vary independently; hence, serum magnesium levels might not be indicative of total body stores.

Fate. Oral absorption varies inversely with intake; in general, 24%–76% is absorbed,[13] principally in upper small intestine. Total body content is approximately 24 g,[9] 60% of which is in bone, 39% in tissues, and 1% in extracellular fluid; 30% is plasma protein bound. Elimination is primarily by the kidneys, with only 1%–2% in feces. Raising the serum concentration above normal exceeds the maximum tubular reabsorption capacity with subsequent excretion of excess.

Adverse Reactions. Serum concentration related—(3–5 mEq/L; 1.5–2.5 mmol/L) hypotension; (5–10 mEq/L; 2.5–5 mmol/L) PR interval changes, QRS prolongation, peaked T waves; (10 mEq/L; 5 mmol/L) areflexia; (15 mEq/L; 7.5 mmol/L) respiratory paralysis; (25 mEq/L; 12.5 mmol/L) cardiac arrest.[13] Pain on IM injection occurs very frequently.[12]

Contraindications. Hypermagnesemia; heart block; myocardial damage; severe renal failure.

Precautions. Use with caution in patients with renal impairment (Cl_{Cr} <30 mL/min) and those concurrently taking a digitalis glycoside. With bolus $MgSO_4$ administration, 1 g of 10% calcium gluconate IV should be available in case apnea or heart block occurs.[13]

Drug Interactions. IV magnesium can potentiate neuromuscular blocking agents.

Parameters to Monitor. Serum magnesium regularly, frequency determined by condition of patient; BUN and/or serum creatinine, serum potassium, and calcium periodically. Deep tendon reflexes, respiratory rate, BP, and ECG periodically.

Notes. For mild deficiencies, dietary supplementation may be sufficient to normalize magnesium stores; sources are cereals, nuts, green vegetables, meat, and fish.[9] Magnesium gluconate is preferred for oral replacement and supplementation because it is possibly better absorbed and potentially causes less diarrhea.[10] Patients on long-term diuretic therapy who are prone to hypomagnesemia may benefit from using the minimally effective dose of diuretic and 20–30 mEq/d of magnesium orally or changing to a magnesium-sparing agent (e.g., amiloride, spironolactone, or triamterene).[14] Drugs known to produce hypomagnesemia are aminoglycoside antibiotics, amphotericin B, diuretics, alcohol, and cisplatin.[11,14] Coadministration of 3 g $MgSO_4$ IV with high-dose **cisplatin** chemotherapy has been recommended.[14] Correction of refractory hypocalcemia and hypokalemia with concurrent hypomagnesemia requires magnesium replacement to restore mineral balance.[10] (*See* Magnesium Products Comparison Chart.)

MAGNESIUM PRODUCTS COMPARISON CHART

PRODUCT	MAGNESIUM CONTENT[a] (mEq/g)	DOSAGE FORMS[b]	COMMENTS
Magnesium, Chelated Chelated magnesium	8.3	Tab 500 mg = 100 mg Mg	Amino acid chelate; sodium free; oral use only
Magnesium Chloride Slo-Mag Various	9.8	SR Tab 535 mg = 64 mg Mg Inj 200 mg/mL = 23.6 mg/mL Mg	Alternative to parenteral $MgSO_4$
Magnesium Citrate Various	4.4	Soln 60 mg/mL = 3.2 mg/mL Mg	Oral use only
Magnesium Gluconate Almora Magtrate Magonate	4.5–4.8	Tab 500 mg = 27–29 mg Mg Soln 11 mg/mL = 0.63 mg/mL Mg	Very soluble; well absorbed; produces no diarrhea
Magnesium Hydroxide Milk of Magnesia	34	Susp 40 mg/mL = 13.3 mg/mL Mg Susp 80 mg/mL = 32.6 mg/mL Mg Tab 300 mg = 122 mg Mg Tab 600 mg = 244 mg Mg	Readily available in combination antacid formulations; start with 5 mL suspension or 1 tablet, increase as tolerated to 4 times daily; requires gastric acid for absorption; inexpensive
Magnesium Oxide	49.6	Cap 140 mg = 84 mg Mg Tab 400 mg = 238 mg Mg	Poorly soluble; net absorption low, especially in malabsorptive states
Magnesium Sulfate Epsom salt	8.1	Inj 10% = 9.6 mg/mL Mg Inj 12.5% = 12 mg/mL Mg Inj 50% = 48 mg/mL Mg Pwdr 1 g = 97.2 g Mg	Use IV, IM, or PO

[a] 1 mEq = 12 mg = 0.5 mmol Mg.
[b] Magnesium products exhibit variable oral absorption; increase dosage incrementally until no further rise in serum magnesium occurs or until diarrhea occurs.

887

PHOSPHATE SALTS   Various

Pharmacology. Phosphate is a structural element of bone and is involved in carbohydrate metabolism, energy transfer, muscle contraction, and as a buffer in the renal excretion of hydrogen ion.[3] Many of the factors that influence serum calcium concentration also influence serum phosphate directly or indirectly.

Administration and Adult Dosage. The RDA is 700 mg/d for males and females ≥19 years.[2] **PO for phosphate replacement**—250–500 mg (8–16 mmol) of phosphorus 3–4 times daily. **IV replacement (recent and uncomplicated hypophosphatemia)**—0.08 mmol/kg, to a maximum of 0.2 mmol/kg; (prolonged and multiple causes) 0.16 mmol/kg, to a maximum of 0.24 mmol/kg. Infuse doses over 6 h and additional dosage guided by serum concentrations.[15] **IV for symptomatic hypophosphatemia**—patients with phosphorus levels of 1.6–1.9 mg/dL have received 15 mmol over 2 h[16] and those with phosphorus <1.24 mg/dL have received 30 mmol over 3 h[17] with success (both without regard to weight). Reassess at completion of infusion to determine need for additional therapy. When serum concentration reaches 2 mg/dL (0.67 mmol/L) and the patient can eat a normal diet, change to oral administration and a phosphate-rich diet.[18,19] (*See* Phosphate Products Comparison Chart.)

Special Populations. *Pediatric Dosage.* The RDAs are (0–6 months) 100 mg/d; (7–12 months) 275 mg/d; (1–8 years) 460–500 mg/d; (9–18 years) 1250 mg/d.[2] **PO for replacement**—(<4 years) 250 mg (8 mmol) of phosphorus qid initially; (<4 years) same as adult dosage. **IV replacement**—(serum phosphate 0.5–1 mg/dL) 0.05–0.08 mg/kg (0.15–0.25 mmol/kg) per dose over 4–6 h; (serum phosphate <0.5 mg/dL) 0.08–0.12 mg/kg (0.25–0.35 mmol/kg) per dose over 6 h. Repeat doses as needed to achieve desired serum concentration. Actual dosage depends on signs, symptoms, and serum phosphate concentration.

Geriatric Dosage. Lower dosage might be required in some patients because of the age-related decrease in renal function.

Other Conditions. Renal impairment decreases requirement. Choose the appropriate salt form based on the patient's sodium and potassium requirements. Requirement is increased during alcohol withdrawal, diabetic ketoacidosis, respiratory alkalosis, aluminum antacid therapy, burns, postsurgical status, and nutritional repletion.

Dosage Forms. *See* Phosphate Products Comparison Chart.

Patient Instructions. (*See* Oral Electrolytes, Class Instructions.) Do not take capsules whole; instead, dissolve contents in three-fourth glass of water before taking. Powder in packets must be dissolved in 1 gallon of water before using. Chilling solution may improve palatability. Do not take with calcium-containing products.

Missed Doses. Take this drug at regular intervals. If you miss a dose, take it as soon as you remember. Do not double the dose or take an extra dose.

Pharmacokinetics. *Serum Levels.* (As phosphorus) adults 2.7–4.5 mg/dL (0.9–1.5 mmol/L); children 4.5–5.5 mg/dL (1.5–1.8 mmol/L). Normal serum phosphorus concentrations can differ by as much as 0.6 mg/dL throughout the day because of changes in transcellular distribution. Concentrations <1.5 mg/dL indicate severe hypophosphatemia and require replacement therapy.[20]

Fate. Normal adult dietary intake is 1–1.8 g/d, 60%–70% of which is absorbed, primarily in the duodenum and jejunum.[3] Most of the absorbed phosphorus is excreted in urine.[15]

Adverse Reactions. Diarrhea and stomach upset occur frequently with oral administration.[15,21] Dose-related hyperphosphatemia, metastatic calcium deposition, dehydration, hypotension, hypomagnesemia, and hyperkalemia or hypernatremia (depending on salt used) can occur.

Contraindications. Hyperphosphatemia; hypocalcemia; hyperkalemia (potassium salt); hypernatremia (sodium salt); severe renal failure.

Precautions. Use cautiously in patients with renal impairment and those with hypercalcemia. Dilute IV forms before use and administer slowly.

Drug Interactions. None known.

Parameters to Monitor. Serum phosphorus regularly, frequency determined by condition of patient; BUN and/or serum creatinine, serum calcium, and magnesium periodically.[22] Monitor serum sodium and/or potassium periodically, depending on salt form used.

Notes. Phosphate salts can precipitate in the presence of calcium salts in IV solutions; add no more than 40 mmol of phosphate and 5 mEq of calcium/L. Calcium supplementation may be necessary to prevent hypocalcemic tetany during phosphate repletion. IV calcium gluconate or calcium chloride may be given until tetany subsides. Inorganic phosphorus exists in the body as mono- and dibasic forms, the relative proportions of which are pH dependent. It is therefore preferable to report concentrations as mg/dL or mmol/L rather than mEq/L.[15] (*See* Phosphate Products Comparison Chart.)

PHOSPHATE PRODUCTS COMPARISON CHART

PRODUCT	DOSAGE FORMS[a]	PHOSPHORUS CONTENT[b]		CATION CONTENT
		(mg)	(mmol)	
POTASSIUM SALTS				
K-Phos Original	Tab	114	3.6	3.7 mEq K$^+$/tablet
Neutra-Phos K	Pwdr packet	250 (per packet)	8	14.3 mEq K$^+$/packet
Potassium Phosphate	Inj	94 (per mL)	3	4.4 mEq K$^+$/mL
SODIUM SALTS				
Fleet's Phospho-Soda	Soln	128 (per mL)	4.1	111 mg (4.8 mEq) Na$^+$/mL
Sodium Phosphate	Inj	94 (per mL)	3	93 mg (4 mEq) Na$^+$/mL
SODIUM–POTASSIUM SALTS				
K-Phos Neutral	Tab	250 (per tablet)	8	298 mg (13 mEq) Na$^+$ and 1.1 mEq K$^+$/tablet
Neutra-Phos Plain	Pwdr packet	250 (per packet)	8	164 mg (7 mEq) Na$^+$ and 7 mEq K$^+$/packet
Skim Milk	Liquid	931 (per qt)	30	510 mg (22 mEq) Na$^+$ and 37 mEq K$^+$/qt

[a]Contents of capsules, tablets, and powders must be diluted in water before administration.
[b]31.25 mg = 1 mmol.
From Refs. 15, 18, and 19 and product information.

POTASSIUM SALTS
Various

Pharmacology. Potassium is the major cation of the intracellular space, where its major role is regulating muscle and nerve excitability. Another role is controlling intracellular volume (similar to sodium's control of extracellular volume), protein synthesis, enzymatic reactions, and carbohydrate metabolism.[23] The chloride salt is preferred for most uses because concomitant chloride loss and metabolic alkalosis frequently accompany hypokalemia. Non-chloride salts are preferred in acidosis (e.g., secondary to amphotericin B or carbonic anhydrase inhibitor therapy and in chronic diarrhea with bicarbonate loss).[24,25]

Administration and Adult Dosage. Variable, must be adjusted to needs of patient. **PO for prophylaxis with diuretic therapy**—prevention of hypokalemia can generally be accomplished by giving 20 mmol/d of KCl, whereas treatment requires as much as 40–100 mmol/d.[26] For nonedematous, ambulatory patients with uncomplicated hypertension, the goal should be to achieve a serum potassium of ≥4 mmol/L, and concentrations ≤3.4 mmol/L should be treated.[26] For edematous patients (e.g., with heart failure), consider routine supplementation with KCl even if the potassium is normal (e.g., 4 mmol/L).[26] In those with mild potassium deficits, 40–80 mEq/d is recommended; with severe deficit, 100–120 mEq/d is indicated with careful monitoring of serum potassium.[27] **IV administration in peripheral vein**—(serum potassium >2.5 mEq/L) may be infused at 10–20 mEq/h[25]; reserve rates faster than 20 mEq/h for emergency situations; may repeat every 2–3 h as needed; do not exceed a maximum concentration of 40 mEq/L. **IV administration in central vein**—(serum potassium <2.5 mEq/L) 30–60 mEq/h may be administered[25]; do not exceed a maximum concentration of 80 mEq/L. Infusion into a central vein requires use of a volume control device. Potassium concentration should not exceed 60 mEq/L unless the infusion site is through a large vein distal to the heart (e.g., femoral vein) or more than one IV line is available, in which case the potassium dose may be delivered through 2 different ports; however, more concentrated solutions (200 mEq/L) infused at slow rates (20 mEq/h) have been used with relative safety.[28] (*See* Other Conditions, Special Populations.)

Special Populations. *Pediatric Dosage.* **PO**—1–2 mEq/kg/d during diuretic therapy.

Geriatric Dosage. Lower dosage might be required in some patients because of the age-related decrease in renal function.

Other Conditions. Base maintenance dosage on serum potassium; renal impairment decreases requirement. For patients with renal impairment or any form of heart block, decrease infusion rate by one-half and do not exceed 5–10 mEq/h.[25]

Dosage Forms. **PO**—(*see* Potassium Products Comparison Chart.) **Inj** (potassium chloride) 2 mEq/mL; (potassium acetate) 2, 4 mEq/mL; (potassium phosphate) 4.4 mEq/mL of potassium and 3 mmol/mL of phosphate. (*See* Potassium Products Comparison Chart.)

Patient Instructions. (*See* Oral Electrolytes, Class Instructions.) Do not chew or crush tablets. The expanded wax matrix of sustained-release forms may be found in the stool, but this does not imply a lack of absorption.

Missed Doses. Take this drug at regular intervals. If you miss a dose, take it as soon as you remember and then return to your normal dosage schedule. Do not double the dose or take extra.

Pharmacokinetics. *Onset and Duration.* Peak elevation of serum potassium concentrations after SR preparations is slightly delayed (median of 2 h) compared with the liquid form (median of 1 h). Effect on serum potassium is most pronounced in the first 3 h after administration.[29]

Serum Levels. Differs depending on laboratory. Normal serum levels are (newborn) 5–7.5 mEq/L, (child) 3.4–4.7 mEq/L, and (adult) 3.5–5.1 mEq/L. Total-body stores are approximately 50 mEq/kg or 3500 mEq. As a general rule, a decrease of 1 mEq/L in serum potassium reflects a 10%–20% total-body deficit; however, there is considerable variation[27]; signs of hypokalemia appear <2.5 mEq/L; concentrations >7 mEq/L or <2.5 mEq/mL are dangerous. Clinical signs of hypokalemia or hyperkalemia are not reliable indicators of serum concentrations. Alkalosis decreases potassium concentrations, and acidosis increases potassium concentrations. Any hypokalemia-induced change in ECG must be treated as a medical emergency with IV potassium. Likewise, hyperkalemia-induced changes in ECG must be treated as a medical emergency.

Fate. When initially administered, the rates of absorption and excretion are more rapid with the liquid than with the SR forms; however, bioavailability is the same (78%–90%) during long-term administration.[29,30] Approximately 10 mEq/d is eliminated in feces, 60–90 mEq/d in urine, and 7.5 mEq/L in sweat.

Adverse Reactions. Bad taste, nausea, vomiting, diarrhea, and abdominal discomfort occur frequently with oral liquids. Do not use enteric-coated tablets because they can cause small-bowel and occasionally gastric ulceration.[27] Local tissue necrosis can occur if IV solution extravasates. Hyperkalemia can occur occasionally. Patients with diabetic nephropathy are at increased risk for hyperkalemia.[31]

Contraindications. Severe renal impairment; untreated Addison's disease; adynamia episodica hereditaria; acute dehydration; heat cramps; hyperkalemia; concurrent ACE inhibitor or potassium-sparing diuretic in patients with renal impairment.[27] In addition, all solid dosage forms (including SR products) are contraindicated in patients in whom delay or arrest of the tablet through the GI tract can occur.

Precautions. Use with caution (if at all) in patients receiving potassium-sparing diuretics or ACE inhibitors and those with digitalis-induced atrioventricular conduction disturbances or renal failure. Avoid extravasation of parenteral potassium products. If extravasation occurs, aspirate any accessible extravasated solution, remove IV catheter, and apply a cold compress to the area.

Drug Interactions. Use with an ACE inhibitor or potassium-sparing diuretic can result in hyperkalemia.

Parameters to Monitor. Serum potassium weekly to monthly initially, every 3–6 months when stable, BUN and/or serum creatinine periodically. For supplementation in patients on long-term diuretic therapy, obtain pretreatment serum levels of potassium and magnesium and reassess after 2–3 weeks and then monthly to determine pattern of potassium loss. Once steady state or normokalemia is achieved, assess quarterly or as condition requires.[27]

Notes. A potassium-sparing diuretic may be preferable to potassium supplementation when large supplements are needed, aldosterone concentrations are elevated, enhanced diuretic response is desired, or magnesium loss is of concern. If large doses of potassium fail to correct hypokalemia, suspect hypomagnesemia because potassium balance is strongly dependent on magnesium homeostasis.[24,32] If a hypokalemic patient is also hypomagnesemic, as occurs with **amphotericin B** therapy, the patient might not respond to potassium replacement therapy unless magnesium balance is restored. (*See* Potassium Products Comparison Chart.)

POTASSIUM PRODUCTS COMPARISON CHART

PRODUCT	DOSAGE FORMS	COMMENTS
Potassium Acetate Various	Inj 2, 4 mEq/mL	Useful in metabolic acidosis; avoid in metabolic alkalosis
PotassiuAcetate/ Bicarbonate/Citrate Trikates Tri-K	Soln 3 mEq/mL[a]	Preferred form in patients with delayed GI transit time or metabolic acidosis; avoid non chloride salts in metabolic alkalosis
Potassium Chloride K-I yte/Cl Adolph's Morton No Salt NuSalt	Inj 2 mEq/mL Soln 20, 30, 40, 45 mEq/15 mL[a] Pwdr packet 20, 25, 50 mEq[b] SR Cap/Tab 6.7, 8, 10, 20 mEq[b] Salt substitutes 50–70 mEq/tsp	Ideal for hypochloremic metabolic alkalosis
Potassium Bicarbonate/Citrate K-Lyte	Effervescent Tab 25, 50 mEq	Preferred form in patients with delayed GI transit time or metabolic acidosis; avoid non-chloride salts in metabolic alkalosis
Potassium Gluconate Kaon	Soln 1.33 mEq/mL[a]	Acidosis; avoid non-chloride salts in metabolic alkalosis

[a]Liquids have rapid absorption, low frequency of GI ulceration, and unpleasant taste.
[b]Bioequivalent to liquid forms; avoid in patients with delayed GI transit time.
From Refs. 24, 25, 26 and product information.

LANTHANUM CARBONATE   Fosrenol

Pharmacology. Lanthanum is a non-calcium–non-aluminum product, which binds dietary phosphate in intestinal tract following dissociation in acidic environments and is used in patients with ESRD to lower serum phosphate.[33] Compared to calcium-containing products, lanthanum is more effective at binding phosphate at lower system pH.[33] Lanthanum phosphate is poorly absorbed and is absorbed across the intestinal wall, which underlies its use in hyperphosphatemic patients.

Administration and Adult Dosage. PO for hyperphosphatemia in ESRD— 1500–3000 mg/d with meals. The recommended starting dose is 250–500 mg with each meal. At 2- to 3-week intervals, the dosage may be by titrated upward by 750 mg

(250 mg with each meal) to achieve the target serum phosphate concentration. Phosphate is lowered within 1–2 weeks of initiation of therapy.[34]

Special Populations. *Pediatric Dosage.* Safety and efficacy not established.

Dosage Forms. **Chew Tab** 250, 500, 750 1000 mg.

Patient Instructions. Tablets must be thoroughly chewed before swallowing with each meal of the day. The medication should be taken with or immediately after each meal.

Pharmacokinetics. Following chronic oral administration the drug is very poorly absorbed with bioavailability less than 0.6%. The drug is not metabolized and the majority of drug is eliminated in the feces.

Adverse Reactions. Only occasional nausea, abdominal pain, vomiting are reported in >5% of patients.

Contraindications. None reported.

Precautions. Use with caution in patients with peptic ulcer disease, Crohn's disease, ulcerative colitis, or bowel obstruction.

Drug Interactions. Lanthanum might bind with concomitantly administered drugs and decrease their absorption; therefore, drugs likely to interact with antacids should be avoided for 2 h prior to or after lanthanum administration.

SEVELAMER HYDROCHLORIDE
Renagel, Renvela

Pharmacology. Sevelamer is a metal-free cationic hydrogel polymer that binds phosphate in the GI tract. It is used in dialysis patients with ESRD to lower serum phosphate.[35] In vitro, sevelamer binds 2.6 mmol/L of phosphate/g of administered drug at neutral pH. It appears to be at least as effective as calcium-based therapy without worsening calcium balance. Sevelamer is a nonspecific binder and it also complexes with bile acids, which leads to a compensatory increase in LDL clearance via expression of cell surface LDL receptors.[35]

Administration and Adult Dosage. **PO for hyperphosphatemia in ESRD**—If patients are not currently receiving a phosphate binder, dosage is based on serum phosphate: serum phosphate of (>5.5 and <7.5 mg/dL) 800 mg 3 times daily; (≥7.5 and <9 mg/dL) 1200 mg 3 times daily; (≥9 mg/dL) 1600 mg 3 times daily. Dosage adjustments are undertaken at 2-week intervals by 1 tablet with each meal as necessary depending upon serum phosphorus.

Special Populations. *Pediatric Dosage.* Safety and efficacy not established.

Dosage Forms. **Tab** 400, 800 mg (as HCl salt, Renagel), 800 mg (as carbonate salt, Renvela).

Patient Instructions. Take the whole dosage form with meals. Do not chew tablet or capsule or take capsule apart. Take any other medications 1 h or more before or 3 h after taking this medication.

Pharmacokinetics. Sevelamer is not absorbed from the GI tract because of its large particle size, which increases further within the gastrointestinal tract. It is entirely eliminated in the feces.

Adverse Reactions. Well tolerated. Occasional nausea, dyspepsia, diarrhea, flatulence, and constipation reported.

Contraindications. Hypophosphatemia; bowel obstruction.

Precautions. Use with caution in patients with dysphagia, swallowing disorders, GI motility disorders, or major GI tract surgery.

Drug Interactions. Sevelamer might bind with concomitantly administered drugs and decrease their absorption. Concomitant administration of ciprofloxacin was associated with a 50% reduction in ciprofloxacin availability. It has also been shown to reduce the absorption of mycophenolate mofetil.

SODIUM POLYSTYRENE SULFONATE Kayexalate, Various

Pharmacology. A cation exchange resin that exchanges potassium for sodium. Each gram of resin binds up to 1 mEq of potassium and liberates 1–2 mEq of sodium.[36] Sorbitol is present in some products to induce diarrhea and reduce the potential for fecal impaction. (*See* Notes.)

Administration and Adult Dosage. **PO for hyperkalemia**—the usual oral dose is 15 g administered 1–4 times daily. If suspension does not contain sorbitol, give powder with, or suspended in a sorbitol solution (e.g., 15 mL of 70% sorbitol to a total final volume of 20–100 mL). **Rectally as enema for hyperkalemia**— 50 g retained for 30 min, if possible, may repeat as often as every 45 min.[25] Follow enema by an irrigation of up to 2 L of non–sodium-containing fluid to remove resin from bowel.

Special Populations. *Pediatric Dosage.* For small children and infants, calculate dosage on the basis of 1 g of resin binding 1 mEq of potassium.

Geriatric Dosage. Dosage adjustments not usually necessary in elderly, renal, or hepatic impairment.

Dosage Forms. **Pwdr** 454 g; **Susp** (containing sorbitol) 15 g/60 mL.

Pharmacokinetics. *Onset and Duration.* PO—onset 1–2 h; rectally retention enema lowers potassium within 0.5–1 h.[25]

Fate. Not absorbed from GI tract; binds potassium and liberates sodium as it passes through the intestine.

Adverse Reactions. Anorexia, nausea, and vomiting occur frequently with large doses; gastric irritation, constipation, and fecal impaction (especially in the elderly) occur occasionally. These effects can be avoided with enema. However, intestinal necrosis caused by enema has been reported. Use of sorbitol in the enema and failure to follow it with a cleansing enema are believed by some to predispose uremic patients to potentially fatal intestinal necrosis.[36]

Precautions. Use with caution in patients who cannot tolerate any additional sodium load (e.g., severe heart failure, severe hypertension, marked edema). In addition to potassium, other cations (e.g., magnesium, calcium) can bind to the resin, causing electrolyte imbalances. If rapid potassium lowering is required, give **insulin** with or without glucose.

Drug Interactions. Aluminum- or magnesium-containing antacids should be used concomitantly with caution due to the risk of precipitating metabolic alkalosis.

Parameters to Monitor. Serum potassium at least daily and more frequently if indicated; serum magnesium and calcium periodically; ECG and patient signs and symptoms are useful in evaluating status. Patients should be observed carefully for signs of sodium overload.

Notes. On average, 50 g of resin will lower serum potassium by 0.5–1 mEq/L.[37,38] Although sodium polystyrene sulfonate is used because of its ability to bind potassium, it also exchanges sodium for other di- and trivalent ions (e.g., calcium, magnesium, iron). Rectal administration is less effective than oral use. Heating can alter the exchange properties of the resin. Sodium polystyrene sulfonate–induced constipation may be treated with 70% **sorbitol** in oral doses (e.g., 10–20 mL/2 h) sufficient to produce 1 or 2 watery stools/d.

■ REFERENCES

1. Weaver CM, Heaney RP. Calcium. In: Shils ME et al., eds. *Modern Nutrition in Health and Disease.* 10th ed. Baltimore, MD: Lippincott Williams & Wilkins; 2005:194-210.

2. Food and Nutrition Board, Institute of Medicine. *Dietary Reference Intakes for Calcium, Phosphorus, Magnesium, Vitamin D and Fluoride.* Washington, DC: National Academy Press; 1997.

3. Delmez JA, Slatopolsky E. Hyperphosphatemia: its consequences and treatment in patients with chronic renal disease. *Am J Kidney Dis.* 1992;19:303-317.

4. Tohme JF, Bilezikian JP. Hypocalcemic emergencies. *Endocrinol Metab Clin North Am.* 1993;22:363-375.

5. Carr CJ, Shangraw RF. Nutritional and pharmaceutical aspects of calcium supplementation. *Am Pharm.* 1987;2:49-50, 54-57.

6. Blanchard J, Aeschlimann JM. Calcium absorption in man: some dosing recommendations. *J Pharmacokinet Biopharm.* 1989;17:631-644.

7. Sheikh MS et al. Gastrointestinal absorption of calcium from milk and calcium salts. *N Engl J Med.* 1987;317:532-536.

8. Anonymous. Calcium supplements. *Med Lett Drugs Ther.* 2000;42:29-31.

9. Rude RK, Shils ME. Magnesium. In: Shils ME et al., eds. *Modern Nutrition in Health and Disease.* 10th ed. Baltimore, MD: LippincottWilliams & Wilkins; 2005:223-247.

10. Al-Ghandi SMG et al. Magnesium deficiency: pathophysiologic and clinical overview. *Am J Kidney Dis.* 1994;5:737-752.

11. Rude RK. Magnesium metabolism and deficiency. *Endocrinol Metab Clin North Am.* 1993; 22:377-395.

12. Montgomery P. Treatment of magnesium deficiency. *Clin Pharm.* 1987;6:834-835.

13. Reinhart RA. Magnesium metabolism: a review with special reference to the relationship between intracellular content and serum levels. *Arch Intern Med.* 1988;148:2415-2420.

14. Berkelhammer C, Bear RA. A clinical approach to common electrolyte problems: hypomagnesemia. *Can Med Assoc J.* 1985;132:360-368.

15. Lloyd CW, Johnson CE. Management of hypophosphatemia. *Clin Pharm.* 1988;7:123-128.

16. Rosen GH et al. Intravenous phosphate repletion regimen for critically ill patients with moderate hypophosphatemia. *Crit Care Med.* 1995;23:1204-1210.

17. Perreault MM et al. Efficacy and safety of intravenous phosphate replacement in critically ill patients. *Ann Pharmacother.* 1997;31:683-688.

18. Hodgson SF, Hurley DL. Acquired hypophosphatemia. *Endocrinol Metab Clin North Am.* 1993;22:397-409.

19. Rubin MF, Narins RG. Hypophosphatemia: pathophysiological and practical aspect of its therapy. *Semin Nephrol.* 1990;10:536-545.

20. Subramanian R et al. Severe hypophosphatemia. Pathophysiologic implications, clinical presentations, and treatment. *Medicine (Baltimore).* 2000;79:1-8.

21. Peppers MP et al. Endocrine crises: hypophosphatemia and hyperphosphatemia. *Crit Care Clin.* 1991;7:201-214.

22. Kingston M, Al-Siba'i MB. Treatment of severe hypophosphatemia. *Crit Care Med.* 1985;13:16-18.

23. Martin ML et al. Potassium. *Emerg Med Clin North Am.* 1986;4:131-144.

24. Krishna GG. Hypokalemic states: current clinical issues. *Semin Nephrol.* 1990;10:515-524.

25. Zull DN. Disorders of potassium metabolism. *Emerg Med Clin North Am.* 1989;7:771-794.

26. Cohn JN et al. New guidelines for potassium replacement in clinical practice: a contemporary review by the National Council on Potassium in Clinical Practice. *Arch Intern Med.* 2000;160:2429-2436.

27. Stanaszek WF, Romankiewicz JA. Current approaches to management of potassium deficiency. *Drug Intell Clin Pharm.* 1985;19:176-184.

28. Kruse JA, Carlson RW. Rapid correction of hypokalemia using concentrated intravenous potassium chloride infusions. *Arch Intern Med.* 1990;150:613-617.

29. Toner JM, Ramsay LE. Pharmacokinetics of potassium chloride in wax-based and syrup formulations. *Br J Clin Pharmacol*. 1985;19:489-494.
30. Skoutakis VA et al. The comparative bioavailability of liquid, wax-matrix, and microencapsulated preparations of potassium chloride. *J Clin Pharmacol*. 1985;25:619-621.
31. Breyer JA. Diabetic nephropathy in insulin-dependent patients. *Am J Kidney Dis*. 1992;20:533-547.
32. Freedman BI, Burkart JM. Endocrine crises: hypokalemia. *Crit Care Clin*. 1991;7:143-153.
33. Swainston H et al. Lanthanum carbonate. *Drugs*. 2004;64:985-996.
34. Joy MS et al. Lanthanum carbonate. *Ann Pharmacother*. 2006;40:234-240.
35. Goldsmith DR et al. Sevelamer hydrochloride: a review of its use for hyperphosphataemia in patients with end-stage renal disease on haemodialysis. *Drugs*. 2008;68:85-104.
36. Lillemoe KD et al. Intestinal necrosis due to sodium polystyrene (Kayexalate) in sorbitol enemas: clinical and experimental support for the hypothesis. *Surgery*. 1987;101:267-272.
37. Alvo M, Warnock DG. Hyperkalemia. *West J Med*. 1984;141:666-671.
38. Greenberg A. Hyperkalemia: treatment options. *Semin Nephrol*. 1998;18:46-57.

Chapter 56

Bisphosphonates

Paul G. Cuddy

ALENDRONATE SODIUM Fosamax, Fosamax PLUS D

Pharmacology. Bisphosphonates are cleared rapidly from the circulation and localized to hydroxyapatite bone mineral surfaces where they influence osteoclast function. Postulated cellular mechanisms of action include inhibition of osteoclast formation/recruitment, inhibition of osteoclast activation, inhibition of mature osteoclast activity, and induction of osteoclast apoptosis.[1] Alendronate's action on osteoclast function is hypothesized to be related to the inhibition of the intracellular mevalonate pathway.[2]

Administration and Adult Dosage. PO for prevention of osteoporosis in postmenopausal women—5 mg/d or 35 mg once weekly.[3,4] PO for treatment of osteoporosis in postmenopausal women—10 mg/d or 70 mg (tab or soln) once weekly.[4-7] PO to increased bone mass in men with osteoporosis—10 mg/d or 70 mg (tab or soln) once weekly.[8] PO for glucocorticoid-induced osteoporosis in men and women—5 mg/d, except for postmenopausal women not receiving estrogen, for whom the recommended dosage is 10 mg/d.[9] PO for Paget's disease of bone in men and women—40 mg/d for 6 mo.[10]

Special Populations. *Pediatric Dosage.* (<18 y) Safety and efficacy not established. *Geriatric Dosage.* Same as adult dosage.

Other Conditions. Dosage adjustment is unnecessary in patients with hepatic impairment or Cl_{Cr} >35 mL/min.

Dosage Forms. **Tab** (Fosamax) 5, 10, 35, 40, 70 mg; **Tab** (Fosamax PLUS D) 70 mg/2800 International Units (IU) cholecalciferol, 70 mg/5600 IU cholecalciferol; **Oral Soln** 70 mg/75 mL.

Patient Instructions. Take alendronate with 180–240 mL (6–8 fl oz) of water on an empty stomach in the morning at least 30 min before any food, beverage, or other medicines. Food and beverages, including mineral water, coffee, tea, or juice, decrease alendronate absorption. Antacids or calcium or vitamin supplements also decrease the absorption of alendronate. Do not lie down for 30 min after taking alendronate. Patients should not suck or chew the tablets. Patients should take supplemental vitamin D and calcium to achieve recommended intake if dietary sources are deemed insufficient.

Missed Doses. If you miss a dose of this medicine, resume your usual schedule the next morning. Do not double doses. If you are taking your dose once weekly and miss a scheduled dose, take your weekly dose the next day. Do not take two tablets on the same day.

Pharmacokinetics. *Fate.* Oral bioavailability is 0.7% in women and 0.59% in men. Plasma protein binding is 78%; V_d is 28 L exclusive of bone distribution. Roughly

50% of absorbed drug is eliminated unchanged in the kidney within 72 h of administration.[11] **Half-life** The terminal half-life in humans is estimated to exceed 10 y, reflecting skeletal release of alendronate.[11]

Adverse Reactions. Mild, transient falls in serum calcium and phosphate have been reported. Dose-related abdominal pain, dyspepsia, constipation, diarrhea, esophageal ulcer, dysphagia, and abdominal distention can occur. Postmarketing surveillance showed an increased risk of erosive esophagitis, some with ulcerations, primarily in patients who did not comply with recommended administration guidelines.[12–14] Ulcerations are occasionally severe, necessitating hospitalization.[12] Severe joint and muscle pain has occasionally been reported with highly variable onset (days to months after initiating therapy).

Contraindications. Abnormalities of the esophagus that delay esophageal emptying such as stricture or achalasia; inability to stand or sit upright for at least 30 min; hypocalcemia.

Precautions. Pregnancy category C; avoid use with Cl_{Cr} <35 mL/min; osteonecrosis.

Drug Interactions. Concomitant calcium-containing products interfere with alendronate absorption and should be administered no sooner than 30 min after a dose. Concomitant use with IV ranitidine results in a 2-fold increase in bioavailability. Avoid concomitant ingestion with food, orange juice, or caffeine.

Parameters to Monitor. Monitor serum calcium, phosphorus, and creatinine. In osteoporosis, monitor bone mineral density by dual X-ray absorptiometry and for radiologic evidence of fractures. For evidence of active Paget's disease, monitor urinary hydroxyproline and creatinine. Assess pain in patients with Paget's disease who present with pain. (*See* Bisphosphonates Comparison Chart.). All patients should have a routine oral exam prior to treatment, especially those patients believed to be at increased risk (e.g., cancer, chemotherapy, radiotherapy, preexisting dental disease, and concomitant corticosteroids) for osteonecrosis of the jaw. Patients should also notify their health care professional if they notice pain in bones, joints, or muscles and should also be alert for jaw problems.

IBANDRONATE SODIUM   Boniva

Pharmacology. Ibandronate is a potent nitrogen-containing bisphosphonate that acts to inhibit bone resorption via interference with osteoclast function.

Administration and Adult Dosage. **PO for the treatment and prevention of postmenopausal osteoporosis**—2.5 mg/d OR 150 mg monthly;[15] **IV for postmenopausal osteoporosis**—3 mg every 3mo administered over 15–30 s by a health professional.[16]

Special Populations. *Pediatric Dosage.* Safety and efficacy not established.

Geriatric Dosage. Same as adult dosage.

Other Conditions. *Renal Impairment.* Not recommended in patients with Cl_{Cr} <30 mL/min.

Dosage Forms. **Tab** 2.5, 150 mg; **Inj** 1 mg/mL.

Patient Instructions. Take oral ibandronate with 180–240 mL (6–8 fl oz) of water on an empty stomach in the morning at least 1 h before any food, beverage, or other medicines. Food and beverages, including mineral water, coffee, tea, or juice

decrease ibandronate absorption. Antacids or calcium or vitamin supplements also decrease the absorption of ibandronate. Do not lie down for at least 1 h after taking ibandronate. Patients should not suck or chew the tablets and should swallow the tablet whole. Patients should take supplemental vitamin D and calcium to achieve recommended intake if dietary sources are deemed insufficient.

Missed Doses. If you miss a dose of this medicine and you are taking the medicine once each day, resume your usual schedule the next morning. If you are taking your dose once monthly and miss a scheduled dose and your next scheduled dose is more than seven days away, take the missed dose the morning of the next day and then resume your normal schedule. If your next scheduled dose is less than seven days away, wait until the next monthly dose is scheduled. Do not take two tablets the same week.

Pharmacokinetics. *Fate.* Bioavailability following oral administration is 0.6%. Bioavailability is reduced if ibandronate is taken within 1 hour of a meal (~90% reduction in absorption). Within 3 h of intravenous administration (and within 8 h of oral administration), concentrations fall to 10% of peak concentrations. V_d is estimated at 90 L. Ibandronate does not undergo any hepatic metabolism. Plasma protein binding is 86% and appears to vary with concentration. There is no hepatic degradation of ibandronate. Both the intravenously administered drug and absorbed oral drug are 50%–60% eliminated by the kidney in unchanged form. It is not excreted through the kidney and appears to be sequestered within bone with subsequent slow redistribution to the systemic circulation. **Half-life** (IV) 4.6–25.5 h; (PO) 37–157 h.

Adverse Reactions. Mild and transient infusion-related reactions include fever and a flulike syndrome consisting of chills, bone pain, arthralgias, and myalgias that seldom require treatment. Local reactions at the injection site include redness and swelling. Elevation in serum creatinine and decreases in serum calcium, phosphate, and magnesium are reported. Severe joint and muscle pain has occasionally been reported with highly variable onset (days to months after initiating therapy). Gastrointestinal intolerance, hypertension, and upper respiratory tract infections may also occur.

Contraindications. Unable or unwilling to stand or sit upright for 60 min following administration; uncorrected hypocalcemia.

Precautions. Pregnancy category C; Severe renal impairment (Cl_{Cr} <30 mL/min or serum creatinine of >2.3 mg/dL). Parenteral ibandronate may only be administered IV; osteonecrosis; Barrett's esophagus; and bone and mineral metabolism disturbances.

Drug Interactions. None documented. Any multivalent or trivalent cation—containing products are expected to interfere with oral absorption of ibandronate.

Parameters to Monitor. Serum electrolyte concentrations (e.g., phosphate, magnesium, potassium) should be monitored regularly. In osteoporosis—monitor bone mineral density by dual X-ray absorptiometry and monitor for radiologic evidence of fractures. For evidence of active Paget's disease, monitor urinary hydroxyproline and creatinine. All patients should have a routine oral exam prior to treatment, especially those patients believed to be at increased risk for

osteonecrosis of the jaw (e.g., cancer, chemotherapy, radiotherapy, preexisting dental disease, concomitant corticosteroids). Patients should also notify their health care professional if they notice pain in bones, joints, or muscles and should also be alert for jaw problems.

PAMIDRONATE DISODIUM   Aredia

Pharmacology. Pamidronate is a nitrogen-containing bisphosphonate that is about 100 times as potent as etidronate in inhibiting bone resorption in the rat.[17] (*See* Alendronate.)

Administration and Adult Dosage. IV for hypercalcemia of malignancy— (moderate hypercalcemia: corrected serum calcium of 12–13.5 mg/dL) 60–90 mg over 2–24 h, repeat in 1 wk, if needed;[18] (severe hypercalcemia: corrected serum calcium >13.5 mg/dL) 90 mg is recommended as an infusion over 2–24 h.

Corrected serum calcium = serum calcium in mg/dL
+ (0.8 × [4 − serum albumin in g/dL]).

IV for Paget's disease— 30 mg/d as a 4-h infusion on 3 consecutive days for a total of 90 mg. **IV for osteolytic bone lesions of metastatic breast cancer OR multiple myeloma**—90 mg once monthly as a 4-h infusion,[19] OR 90 mg q3–4wk as a 2-h infusion.[20,21]

Special Populations. *Pediatric Dosage.* Safety and efficacy not established.

Geriatric Dosage. Same as adult dosage.

Other Conditions. Although pharmacokinetic data are lacking, dosage adjustment appears unnecessary in patients with hepatic impairment. Renal clearance is correlated with Cl_{Cr}, and patients with renal impairment excrete less unchanged drug.[22] In patients receiving intermittent therapy, dosage adjustment is probably unnecessary.

Dosage Forms. Inj (Pwd for Soln) 30, 90 mg; (Soln) 3 mg/mL, 6 mg/mL, 9 mg/mL.

Pharmacokinetics. *Fate.* Oral bioavailability is estimated to be 0.3%. Pamidronate is not metabolized and eliminated exclusively by renal excretion. 46 ± 16% of the drug is excreted unchanged in the urine within 120 h. **Half-life** 28 ± 7 h.

Adverse Reactions. Generalized malaise has occurred. Hypocalcemia has been reported in patients with hypercalcemia and Paget's disease. Anemia is reported approximately 40%–48% of treated patients (38%–42% in placebo-treated patients). Abdominal pain, anorexia, constipation, nausea, and vomiting have been reported in at least 15% of patients receiving pamidronate for hypercalcemia and 5% of patients with Paget's disease. Transient mild temperature elevation (1°C) has occurred. Redness, swelling/induration, and pain on palpation can occur at the IV insertion site. Osteonecrosis of the jaw has been reported in patients receiving IV bisphosphonates. Risk factors for osteonecrosis include neoplasm, concurrent chemotherapy, radiation therapy, corticosteroids and associated dental procedures. Bone, joint, and muscle pain have been observed with parenteral bisphosphonate therapy.

Precautions. (*See* Adverse Reactions.) Pregnancy category D; obtain laboratory tests at the start of therapy; (*See* Parameters to Monitor.) Limited data exists for use of pamidronate in patients with serum creatinine >3 mg/dL.

Parameters to Monitor. Monitor serum potassium, calcium, phosphate, magnesium, creatinine, albumin, and complete blood count and temperature in patients with hypercalcemia of malignancy. In Paget's disease, reductions in serum alkaline phosphatase and urinary hydroxyproline excretion are indicative of a therapeutic response. Assessment of pain in patients with Paget's disease who present with pain is useful. A dental examination is recommended prior to initiation of intravenous bisphosphonate and subsequently to screen for oral infections and to permit initiation of preventive therapies. Therapy may need to be delayed or interrupted depending upon findings observed during dental examinations.

Notes. Do not mix pamidronate with any calcium-containing products. (*See* Bisphosphonates Comparison Chart.)

RISEDRONATE SODIUM   Actonel, Actonel with CALCIUM

Pharmacology. Risedronate is a potent pyridinyl bisphosphonate analog which acts to inhibit bone resorption via interference with osteoclast function.

Administration and Adult Dosage. **PO for the treatment or prevention of postmenopausal osteoporosis**—(Actonel) 5 mg daily, 35 mg once weekly, 75 mg on two consecutive days once per month, and 150 mg once per month.[23,24] **PO for osteoporosis in males**—35 mg once weekly. **PO for the treatment and prevention of glucocorticoid-induced osteoporosis**—5 mg once daily. **PO for Paget's disease**—30 mg once daily for 2 mo, repeat after a minimum of 2 mo.[25] **PO for the treatment or for prevention of osteoporosis in postmenopausal women**—(Actonel with CALCIUM) 35 mg once per wk 30 min prior to the first meal or liquid (except water) of the day; followed by 1250 mg calcium carbonate with food on the remaining days of the week.

Special Populations. *Pediatric Dosage.* Safety and efficacy not established.

Geriatric Dosage. Same as adult dosage.

Other Conditions. **Renal impairment.** Not recommended if Cl_{Cr} <30 mL/min; No adjustment required if Cl_{Cr} ≥30 mL/min or in hepatic impairment.

Dosage Forms. **Tab** 5, 30, 35, 75, and 150 mg; **Tab** (Actonel with CALCIUM) copackaged as (#4) 35 mg risedronate tablets and (#24) 1250 mg calcium carbonate tablets.

Patient Instructions. Take risedronate with 180–240 mL (6–8 fl oz) of water on an empty stomach in the morning at least 30 min before any food, beverage, or other medicines. Food and beverages, including mineral water, coffee, tea, or juice decrease risedronate absorption. Antacids or calcium or vitamin supplements also decrease the absorption of risedronate. Do not lie down for 30 min after taking risedronate. Patients should not suck on or chew the tablets. Patients should take supplemental vitamin D and calcium to achieve recommended intake if dietary sources are deemed insufficient

Pharmacokinetics. *Fate.* Bioavailability following oral administration is 0.63%, and it is reduced or substantially decreased if taken sooner than 30 min (55% reduction) or 1 h (35% reduction) following meals. The V_d is 6.3 L/kg with the majority of drug distributed to bone. Risedronate does not undergo hepatic metabolism.

Plasma protein binding is limited at ~24%. There is no hepatic degradation of risedronate. Slightly more than 50% of absorbed drug is excreted in the unchanged form through the urine within 24 h. **Half-life** 480 h.

Adverse Reactions. Elevation in serum creatinine and decreases in serum calcium, phosphate, and magnesium are reported. Severe joint and muscle pain has occasionally been reported with highly variable onset (days to months after initiating therapy). GI intolerance, asthenia, arthralgia, and flulike symptoms may also occur.

Contraindications. Orally administered risedronate is contraindicated in patients unable or unwilling to stand or sit upright for 60 min following administration. Uncorrected hypocalcemia contraindicates use of risedronate.

Precautions. Pregnancy category C. Not recommended for patients with severe renal impairment; Vitamin D deficiency; osteonecrosis. (*See* Other Conditions.)

Drug Interactions. None documented. Any multivalent or trivalent cation-containing products are expected to interfere with oral absorption of risedronate.

Parameters to Monitor. Serum electrolyte concentrations (e.g., phosphate, magnesium, potassium) and serum creatinine should be monitored regularly. In osteoporosis, monitor bone mineral density by dual X-ray absorptiometry and monitor for radiologic evidence of fractures. For evidence of active Paget's disease, monitor urinary hydroxyproline and creatinine. All patients should have a routine oral exam prior to treatment, especially those patients believed to be at increased risk of osteonecrosis of the jaw (e.g., cancer, chemotherapy, radiotherapy, preexisting dental disease, concomitant corticosteroids). Patients should also notify their health care professional if they notice pain in bones, joints, or muscles and should also be alert for jaw-related problems.

ZOLEDRONIC ACID   Zometa, Reclast

Pharmacology. Zoledronic acid is a potent nitrogen-containing bisphosphonate, which acts to inhibit bone resorption.[26–28] Zoledronic acid is approved for hypercalcemia of malignancy and for multiple myeloma and bone metastases from solid tumors, in conjunction with standard antineoplastic therapy.[29–30]

Administration and Adult Dosage. (Zometa) **IV for the treatment of hypercalcemia of malignancy**—4 mg over no less than 15 min for patients with an albumin-corrected serum calcium of at least 12 mg/dL, may repeat in 1 wk if resistant hypercalcemia. **IV for multiple myeloma and bone metastases from solid tumor**—4-mg dose over no less than 15 min every 3–4wk with calcium and a multivitamin containing vitamin D. (Reclast) **IV for treatment of osteoporosis in men and postmenopausal women, prophylaxis in patients with recent low-trauma hip fracture, treatment and prophylaxis of glucocorticoid-induced osteoporosis in patients expected to be on glucocorticoids for at least 12 mo**—5 mg infusion administered once yearly over no less than 15 min. **IV for Paget's disease of bone**—5 mg IV single infusion.

Special Populations. *Pediatric Dosage.* Safety and efficacy not established.

Geriatric Dosage. Same as adult dosage, unless renal impairment is present.

Other Conditions. **Renal impairment.** Specific to indication. Use in patients with severe renal impairment (Cl_{Cr} <30 mL/min) is not recommended.

Dosage Forms. (Zometa) **Inj** 4 mg/5 mL; (Reclast) **Inj** 5 mg/100 mL.

Pharmacokinetics. *Fate.* Following IV infusion, concentrations decline rapidly within a 24-h period. Zoledronic acid does not undergo any hepatic metabolism. Plasma protein binding ranges from 28%–53% and is dependent upon concentration. Drug clearance is correlated with Cl_{Cr} and 39 ± 16 % of the administered dose appears unchanged within 24 h.[29] Drug not excreted through the kidney appears to be sequestered within bone with subsequent slow redistribution to the systemic circulation. **Half-life** 146 h.

Adverse Reactions. Specific to indication. The predominate adverse effects are GI intolerance, arthralgia, peripheral edema, dizziness, and headache. Insomnia, nephrotoxicity, and fatigue may also occur. Mild and transient infusion-related reactions include fever and a flulike syndrome consisting of fever, chills, bone pain, and myalgias, which seldom require treatment. Local reactions at the injection site include redness and swelling. Displays the highest risk of osteonecrosis of the jaw with most cases occurring in patients with cancer who have undergone dental procedures. Atrial fibrillation (1.3%–2.8%) and stroke (2.3%) have been reported rarely in postmenopausal osteoporosis patients and most instances were reported several weeks after infusion.[27] All-cause death (up to ~10% of patients) seems to be associated with use.

Contraindications. In patients with hypersensitivity to zoledronic acid or any of its excipients; hypocalcemia.

Precautions. Pregnancy category D; severe renal impairment; high risk for osteonecrosis of the jaw; urticaria or aspirin-sensitive asthma; thyroid or parathyroid surgery; malabsorption syndromes; excision of small intestine.

Drug Interactions. Concomitant administration with calcium-containing infusion solutions should be avoided and the drug should be administered in a separate infusion line. Concomitant administration with loop diuretics should only be considered after adequate hydration has been achieved. Concomitant administration of loop diuretics with aminoglycosides appears to increase the risk of hypocalcemia.

Parameters to Monitor. Serum creatinine should be measured prior to each dose and dosage adjustments may be required depending upon the magnitude of decline in Cl_{Cr}. Serum electrolyte concentrations (e.g., phosphate, magnesium, potassium) should be monitored regularly. If not administered immediately after dilution, the drug should be refrigerated for up to 24 h. All patients should have a routine oral exam prior to treatment, especially believed to be at increased risk (e.g., cancer, chemotherapy, radiotherapy, preexisting dental disease, concomitant corticosteroids).[31]

Notes. If the drug has been previously refrigerated, it should be allowed to reach room temperature prior to infusion. Prehydration therapy with IV saline is appropriate. In Paget's disease, Reclast should be administered in conjunction with daily 800–1000 IU vitamin D supplementation and 1200–1500 mg of elemental calcium.

BISPHOSPHONATES COMPARISON CHART

DRUG	DOSAGE FORMS	INDICATIONS	DOSAGE
Alendronate Sodium Fosamax Fosamax PLUS D	Tab (Fosamax) 5, 10, 35, 40, 70 mg; Tab (Fosamax PLUS D) 70 mg/2800 IU cholecalciferol; 70 mg/5600 IU cholecalciferol; Soln 70/75 mL	Osteoporosis treatment and prevention; corticosteroid-induced osteoporosis; Paget's disease	(See monograph.)
Etidronate Disodium Didronel	Tab 200, 400 mg; Inj 300 mg	Hypercalcemia of malignancy; Paget's disease; heterotropic ossification.	IV for hypercalcemia. 7.5 mg/kg/d over ≥2 h for 3 d, followed by PO 20 mg/kg/d for 30 d as needed PO for Paget's disease. 5–10 mg/kg/d for up to 6 mo OR 11–20 mg/kg/d for up to 3 mo PO for heterotropic ossification. 20 mg/kg/d for 1 mo before and 3 mo after hip replacement OR if caused by spinal cord injury, 20 mg/kg/d for 2 wk, then 10 mg/kg/d for 10 wk
Ibandronate Sodium Boniva	Tab 2.5, 150 mg; Inj 3 mg/3 mL	Prevention and treatment of postmenopausal osteoporosis	(See monograph.)
Pamidronate Disodium Aredia	Inj 30, 90 mg	Hypercalcemia of malignancy; Paget's disease; osteolytic bone lesions and metastases	(See monograph.)
Risedronate Sodium Actonel Actonel with CALCIUM	Tab (Actonel) 5, 30, 35, 75, 150 mg Tab (Actonel with CALCIUM) (#4) 35 mg risedronate and (#24) 1250 mg calcium carbonate	Treatment and prevention of osteoporosis; Paget's disease	(See monograph.)

(continued)

905

BISPHOSPHONATES COMPARISON CHART (*continued*)

DRUG	DOSAGE FORMS	INDICATIONS	DOSAGE
Tiludronate Skelid	Tab 240 mg (200 mg of free acid)	Paget's disease	PO for Paget's disease. 400 mg daily for 3 mo
Zoledronic Acid Zometa Reclast	Inj 4 mg/5 mL (Zometa) Inj 5 mg/100 mL (Reclast)	Zometa: Hypercalcemia of malignancy; osteolytic bone lesions of metastatic breast cancer, multiple myeloma, and bone metastases from solid tumors and multiple myeloma; Reclast: Paget's disease, and postmenopausal osteoporosis	(*See* monograph.)

From Refs. 4–10, 18–21, 23–30, 32–35, and product information.

■ REFERENCES

1. Rodan GA. Mechanisms of action of bisphosphonates. *Annu Rev Pharmacol Toxicol.* 1998;38:375-388.
2. Rogers MJ et al. Cellular and molecular mechanisms of action of bisphosphonates. *Cancer.* 2000;88: 2961-2978.
3. Hosking D et al. Prevention of bone loss with alendronate in postmenopausal women under 60 years of age. *N Engl J Med.* 1998;338:485-492.
4. Schnitzer T et al. Therapeutic equivalence of alendronate 70 mg once-weekly and alendronate 10 mg daily in the treatment of osteoporosis. *Aging Clin Exp Res.* 2000;12:1-12.
5. Cummings SR et al. Effect of alendronate on risk of fracture in women with low bone density but without vertebral fractures. Results from the Fracture Intervention Trial. *JAMA.* 1998;280:2077-2082.
6. Black DM et al. Randomised trial of effect of alendronate on risk of fracture in women with existing vertebral fractures. *Lancet.* 1996;348:1535-1541.
7. Liberman UA et al. Effect of oral alendronate on bone mineral density and the incidence of fractures in post-menopausal osteoporosis. *N Engl J Med.* 1995;333:1437-1443.
8. Orwoll E et al. Alendronate for the treatment of osteoporosis in men. *N Engl J Med.* 2000;343:604-610.
9. Saag KG et al. Alendronate for the prevention and treatment of glucocorticoid-induced osteoporosis. *N Engl J Med.* 1998;339:292-299.
10. Lombardi A. Treatment of Paget's disease of bone with alendronate. *Bone.* 1999;24:59S-61S.
11. Sharpe M et al. Alendronate: an update of its use in osteoporosis. *Drugs.* 2001;61:999-1039.
12. de Groen PC et al. Esophagitis associated with the use of alendronate. *N Engl J Med.* 1996;335:1016-1021.
13. Liberman UA, Hirsch LJ. Esophagitis and alendronate [Letter]. *N Engl J Med.* 1996;335:1069-1070.
14. Bauer DC et al. Upper gastrointestinal tract safety profile of alendronate. The Fracture Intervention Trial. *Arch Intern Med.* 2000;160:517-525.
15. Chesnut CH. Treating osteoporosis with bisphosphonates and addressing adherence: a review of oral iban-dronate. *Drugs.* 2006;66:1351-1359.
16. Croom KF, Scott LJ. Intravenous ibandronate: in the treatment of osteoporosis. *Drugs.* 2006;66:1593-1601
17. Fleisch H. Bisphosphonates: mechanisms of action. *Endocr Rev.* 1998;19:80-100.
18. Nussbaum SR et al. Single-dose intravenous therapy with pamidronate for the treatment of hypercalcemia of malignancy: comparison of 30-, 60-, and 90-mg dosages. *Am J Med.* 1993;95:297-304.
19. Berenson JR et al. Efficacy of pamidronate in reducing skeletal events in patients with advanced multiple myeloma. *N Engl J Med.* 1996;334:488-493.
20. Hillner BE et al. American Society of Clinical Oncology guideline on the role of bisphosphonates in breast cancer. *J Clin Oncol.* 2000;18:1378-1391.
21. Hortobagyi GN et al. Efficacy of pamidronate in reducing skeletal complications in patients with breast cancer and lytic bone metastases. *N Engl J Med.* 1996;335:1785-1791.
22. Berenson JR et al. Pharmacokinetics of pamidronate disodium in patients with cancer with normal or impaired renal function. *J Clin Pharmacol.* 1997;37:285-290.
23. Harris ST et al. Effects of risedronate treatment on vertebral and nonvertebral fractures in women with post-menopausal osteoporosis. A randomized controlled trial. *JAMA.* 1999;282:1344-1352.
24. Reginster J et al. Randomized trial of the effects of risedronate on vertebral fractures in women with established postmenopausal osteoporosis. Vertebral Efficacy with Risedronate Therapy (VERT) Study Group. *Osteoporos Int.* 2000;11:83-91.
25. Siris ES et al. Risedronate in the treatment of Paget's disease of bone: an open label, multicenter study. *J Bone Miner Res.* 1998;13:1032-1038.
26. Deeks ED, Perry CM. Zoledronic acid: a review of its use in the treatment of osteoporosis. *Drugs Aging.* 2008;25:963-986.
27. Black DM et al. Once-Yearly Zoledronic Acid for Treatment of Postmenopausal Osteoporosis. *N Engl J Med.* 2007;356:1809-1822.
28. Reid IR et al. Comparison of a single infusion of zoledronic acid with risedronate for Paget's disease. *New Engl J Med.* 2005;353:898-908.
29. Wellington K, Goa KL. Zoledronic acid: a review of its use in the management of bone metastases and hyper-calcaemia of malignancy. *Drugs.* 2003;63:417-437.
30. Dhillon S et al. Zoledronic acid: a review of its use in the management of bone metastases of malignancy. *Drugs.* 2008;68:507-534.
31. Kyle RA et al. American Society of Clinical Oncology 2007 Clinical Practice Guideline Update on the Role of Bisphosphonates in Multiple Myeloma. *J Clin Oncol.* 2007;25:2464-2472.
32. Singer FR et al. Treatment of hypercalcemia of malignancy with intravenous etidronate. A controlled, multicenter study. *Arch Intern Med.* 1991;151:471-476.

33. Khairi MR et al. Treatment of Paget disease of bone (osteitis deformans). Results of a one-year study with sodium etidronate. *JAMA*. 1974;230:562-567.
34. Fraser WD et al. A double-blind, multicentre, placebo-controlled study of tiludronate in Paget's disease of bone. *Postgrad Med J*. 1997;73:496-502.
35. McClung MR et al. Tiludronate therapy for Paget's disease of bone. *Bone*. 1995;17(suppl 5):493S-496S.

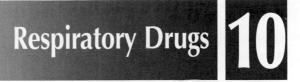

Respiratory Drugs 10

Nickole N. Henyan

Chapter 57

Antiasthmatics

Laura L. Sanders

Class Instructions. **Note:** The blue adapter supplied with albuterol inhalers should not be used with other product canisters, and adapters from other products should not be used with albuterol canisters. Do not cut, crush, or chew extended-release forms.

To use most metered-dose inhalers: Before using the inhaler for the first time, or if it has not been used for more than 4 weeks, "test spray" the inhaler by spraying 4 times into the air. To use the inhaler, remove the inhaler cap and hold the inhaler upright. Shake the inhaler immediately before using it. Tilt your head back and breathe out slowly through your mouth, exhaling as much air as possible. Place the mouthpiece fully in your mouth, holding the inhaler upright, and close your lips around it. As you breathe in deeply and slowly, fully depress the top of the metal canister with your index finger. Hold your breath as long as possible. Before breathing out, remove the inhaler from your mouth and release your finger from the canister. If more than one inhalation is prescribed, wait 1 min, shake the inhaler again, and repeat the steps for each inhalation. Discard the canister after you have used the labeled number of inhalations. Clean the inhaler daily by removing the metal canister and then rinsing the plastic cap and case in warm, running water. After thoroughly drying the case and cap, replace the canister and cap. Store inhalers away from heat and direct sunlight. Do not exceed the prescribed dosages of these medications. Report if symptoms do not completely clear or the inhaler is required more than prescribed. Bronchodilators can cause nervousness, tremors (especially with terbutaline or albuterol), or rapid heart rate. Report if these effects continue after dosage reduction; if chest pain, dizziness, or headache occur; or if asthmatic symptoms are not relieved.

Missed Doses. Take missed doses as soon as possible. However, if it is almost time for your next dose, skip the missed dose and go back to your regular schedule. Do not double your dose.

ALBUTEROL SULFATE   Proventil, Ventolin, ProAir, Accuneb, VoSpire ER, Various

Pharmacology. Albuterol is a short/intermediate acting, selective β$_2$-adrenergic agonist that produces bronchodilation, vasodilation, uterine relaxation, skeletal muscle stimulation, peripheral vasodilation, and tachycardia.[1] Short-acting β- adrenergic agonists are the therapy of choice for relief of acute symptoms and prevention of exercise-induced bronchospasm.[2]

Administration and Dosage. Inhalation aerosol for asthma (adults and children ≥4 years)—90–180 μg (1–2 inhalations) every 4–6 h prn. Inhalation powder (adults and children >4 years)—200–400 μg every 4–6 h. Inhalation for bronchospasm NEB (adults and children >12 years)—1.25–5 mg given over 5–15 min in 3 mL saline every 4–8 h prn.[2] Inhalation aerosol for prevention of exercise-induced bronchospasm (adults and children ≥4 years)—2 puffs 15–30 min before exercise, maximum 12 puffs/d; powder 200 μg 15 min before exercise. PO for asthma (adults)—2–4 mg every 6–8 h, increase as tolerated to a maximum of 32 mg/d; ER tablet 4–8 mg q12h, to a maximum of 32 mg/d. Do not crush or chew ER formulations.

Pediatric Dosage. Inhalation for asthma aerosol (children ≤4 years)—1–2 inhalations every 4–6 h prn. Powder dosage has not been established in children less than 4 years; NEB (children <5 years)—0.63–2.5 mg in 3 mL saline every 4–6 h prn; (children aged 5–11 years) 1.25–2.5 mg in 3 mL saline every 4–8 h prn.[2] Children weighing <15 kg who require <2.5 mg/dose should use 0.5% albuterol solution. PO for asthma—(children 2–6 years) 0.1–0.2 mg/kg/dose q8h, to a maximum of 4 mg q8h; (6–12 years) 2 mg every 6–8 h, to a maximum of 24 mg/d. ER tablet (6–12 years) 4 mg q12h; (>12 years) same as adult dosage—start with 4 mg if low body weight.

Geriatric Dosage. Inhalation for asthma—same as adult dosage. PO—2 mg tid–qid initially, increasing prn to a maximum of 8 mg tid–qid.

Dosage Forms. Inhal aerosol 90 μg/puff (200 puffs/inhaler); Inhal (HFA, does not contain chlorofluorocarbons [CFCs] as a propellant) (Proventil HFA, Ventolin HFA) 90 μg/puff (200 puffs/inhaler); Inhal Soln 0.63 (0.5% [5 mg/mL]), 0.083% (unit dose solution, 3 mL); Inhal Cap (Rotacap) 200 μg for use with powder inhaler; Tab 2, 4 mg; syrup 0.4 mg/mL; ER Tab 4, 8 mg. Inhal 90 μg plus ipratropium bromide 18 μg/puff (Combivent); Inhal Soln 3 mg plus ipratropium bromide 0.5 mg/3 mL (DuoNeb).

Patient Instructions. Refer to Class Instructions at the beginning of this chapter.

Pharmacokinetics. *Onset and Duration.* (Inhalation) 75% of maximal effect seen within 5 min, peak effect within 30–90 min. (PO)—onset 30–60 min, peak 2–3 h. Duration 4–6 h, depending on the dose, dosage form, and clinical condition. (*See* Sympathomimetic Bronchodilators Comparison Chart.)

Fate. Peak serum level after 0.15 mg/kg by inhalation is 5.6 μg/L (23 nmol/L). Following a 3-mg dose in adults (NEB), albuterol level at 0.5 h is 1.4–3.2 ng/mL. Oral bioavailability is 50% because of hepatic first-pass metabolism; peak after 4-mg tablet is 10 μg/L (42 nmol/L); 50% is excreted in urine as an inactive sulfate conjugate. The drug does not appear to be metabolized in the lung.[3]

$t_{1/2}$. (IV) 2–3 h; 5–6 h after oral and up to 7 h after inhalation because of prolonged absorption.[3]

Adverse Reactions. Paradoxical bronchospasm, dose-related reflex tachycardia from peripheral vasodilation and direct stimulation of cardiac β_2-receptors. Tremor, palpitations, and nausea are other dose-related effects that are markedly reduced with aerosol administration. All β_2-agonists lower serum potassium concentrations.

Precautions. Pregnancy; cardiac disorders including coronary insufficiency and cardiac arrhythmias and hypertension; diabetes; hyperthyroidism, convulsive disorders. Excessive or prolonged use may lead to tolerance.

Drug Interactions. Concurrent β-blockers may antagonize effects. Other short-acting sympathomimetic agents should not be used with albuterol. Digoxin levels are decreased. Tricyclic antidepressants and MAOI inhibitors may potentiate the action of albuterol on the vascular system.

Parameters to Monitor. Inhalation technique, asthma symptoms, frequency of use, pulmonary function, and heart rate.

Notes. A relationship between regular (i.e., not prn) use of inhaled β_2-agonists and death from asthma has been a concern.[4,5] However, the main short-acting β_2 agonists in use today (albuterol, levalbuterol, pirbuterol) are effective with few cardiovascular effects, contrasted with older less selective agents used at higher doses that were associated with severe and fatal asthma attacks.[6] Increasing use of short-acting β_2-agonists (>2 days/week or >1 canister/month for symptom relief, not prevention of exercise-induced bronchospasm) indicates inadequate control of asthma.[2] The FDA has phased out albuterol CFC inhalers effective December 2008. Only albuterol HFA inhalers are currently available.

CROMOLYN SODIUM   Gastrocrom, Intal, Nasalcrom, Opticrom, Various

Pharmacology. Cromolyn stabilizes the membranes of mast cells and other inflammatory cells (e.g., eosinophils), thereby inhibiting release and production of soluble mediators (e.g., histamine, leukotrienes) that produce inflammation and bronchospasm. The mechanism appears to be the inhibition of calcium ion influx through the cell membrane. Cromolyn inhibits the early and late responses to specific allergen and exercise challenges, and prevents the increase in nonspecific bronchial hyperreactivity that occurs during a specific allergen season in atopic asthmatics.[7] Cromolyn does not have immediate bronchodilating or antihistaminic activity.

Administration and Dosage. Inhalation for asthma (adults and children ≥5 years, MDI)—1.6 or 2 mg (2 puffs) qid at intervals of 4–6 h; maximum 16 puffs/d; (adults and children ≥2 years, NEB)—20 mg (1 ampule) qid at regular intervals of 4–6 h; maximum 160 mg/d. Inhalation for prevention of bronchospasm—(adults and children ≥5 years, MDI) 1.6–2 mg (2 puffs) a single dose 10–15 min (but not more than 60 min) before exercise or exposure to precipitating factor. Intranasal for prophylaxis of allergic rhinitis (adults and children ≥6 years)—5.2 mg/nostril (1 spray) in each nostril tid–qid at regular intervals. Dose may be increased to 6 times daily. Ophthalmic for allergic ocular

disorders—1–2 drops (1.6–3.2 mg) in each eye 4–6 times/d at regular intervals. For chronic conditions, the drug must be used continuously to be effective. **PO for mastocytosis**—200 mg qid, 30 min before meals and hs. **PO for food allergy**—200 mg qid 15–20 min before meals.

Pediatric Dosage. **Inhal (NEB, children <2 years)** dosage not established; **(MDI, <5 years)** dosage not established; **intranasal (>6 years)** dosage not established; **ophthalmic**—same as adult dosage. **PO for mastocytosis**—(term infants–2 years) 20 mg/kg/d in 4 divided doses, to a maximum of 30 mg/kg/d; (2–12 years) 100 mg qid, 30 min before meals and hs, increasing, if necessary, to a maximum of 40 mg/kg/d.

Geriatric Dosage. Same as adult dosage.

Other Conditions. The therapeutic effect is dose dependent, and patients with more severe disease may require more frequent administration initially. After a patient becomes symptom free, the frequency of administration may be reduced to bid–tid.

Dosage Forms. **Inhal Soln** 10 mg/mL (2-mL ampule); **Inhal** 800 μg/puff (112, 200 doses/inhaler); **nasal Inhal** 5.2 mg/spray (100, 200 doses/inhaler); **Ophth Drp** 4% (40 mg/mL, 250 drops/container); **PO Soln** 20 mg/mL.

Patient Instructions. See also Class Instructions at the beginning of this chapter.

Bronchospasm, NEB: Carefully follow directions for inhaler use included with the device. You may mix the nebulizer solution with any bronchodilator inhalant solution that does not contain benzalkonium chloride.

Allergies, nasal: Before using this medication, clear your nasal passages by blowing your nose. Wipe the nosepiece with a clean tissue and replace the dust cap after each use.

Mastocytosis, PO: Dissolve oral capsules in one-half glass (4 fl oz) of hot water, add an equal amount of cold water, and drink the entire amount. Do not mix with fruit juice, milk, or foods.

This medication must be used regularly and continuously to be effective.

Pharmacokinetics. *Onset and Duration.* (Bronchospasm) onset within 1 min for prevention of allergen-induced mast cell degranulation; duration dose dependent, 2–5 h.[7] It may require 4–6 weeks to achieve maximal response, although most asthmatics respond within 2 weeks.[8]

Fate. Oral bioavailability is 0.5%–1%. Amount absorbed after inhalation depends on the delivery system; approximately 10% of the dosage for a Spinhaler and <2% with the nebulizer solution.[7] Peak serum levels occur 15–20 min after inhalation. V_d is 0.2 ± 0.04 L/kg; Cl is 0.35 ± 0.1 L/h/kg. Rapidly excreted unchanged in equal portions in the bile and urine.[7]

$t_{1/2}$. 22.5 ± 1.6 min.[7]

Adverse Reactions. Mild burning or stinging can occur with ophthalmic solution. Occasionally, headache and diarrhea occur with oral capsules.

Precautions. Use with caution in patients with lactose sensitivity (capsules only). Watch for worsening of asthma in patients discontinuing the drug. The ophthalmic solution contains 0.01% benzalkonium chloride; therefore, do not wear soft contact lenses during therapy.

Drug Interactions. None known.

Parameters to Monitor. Monitor relief of asthmatic symptoms and the proper dosage and inhalation technique. Patient noncompliance or inappropriate inhalation technique often contributes to treatment failure. The measurement of peak expiratory flow rate with a peak flow meter is useful in severe chronic asthma. Periodic standard pulmonary function tests are indicated every 1–6 months.

Notes. Comparative studies have shown cromolyn and **theophylline** to be equally effective for the prophylaxis of chronic asthma, although cromolyn produces fewer side effects.[7,8] The inhalant solution is stable with all β_2-agonist and anticholinergic solutions for nebulization, although benzalkonium chloride-free solutions are preferred.[7] The nasal spray is most effective if started 1 week before the allergen season; however, patients receive benefit even if treatment is begun after symptoms occur.[8] Oral cromolyn has been used in the management of GI conditions such as food allergy and irritable bowel syndrome.[8] Cromolyn solution is incompatible with benzalkonium chloride.

IPRATROPIUM BROMIDE
Atrovent, Various

Pharmacology. Ipratropium is a competitive antagonist of acetylcholine at peripheral, but not central, muscarinic receptors because of its quaternary structure.[9] It is used primarily as a bronchodilator in COPD, emphysema, and bronchitis.

Administration and Dosage. Inhalation for bronchospasm of COPD including chronic bronchitis MDI (adults and children ≥12 years)—36–54 µg (2–3 puffs) qid by metered-dose inhaler, to a maximum of 204 µg (12 puffs)/d. **Inhalation for acute, severe asthma**—500 µg tid–qid with doses 6–8 h apart by nebulizer. Combivent or extemporaneous ipratropium/albuterol mixtures have the same dosage as above. **Nasal spray for rhinorrhea of perennial rhinitis**—2 sprays (21 µg/spray) in each nostril of 0.03% solution bid–tid; **Nasal spray for rhinorrhea of the common cold**—2 sprays of 0.06% solution (42 µg/spray)/nostril tid–qid for up to 4 days.

Pediatric Dosage. (<12 years) safety and efficacy not established. **Inhalation**—(**<2 years**) 125 µg/dose by nebulizer[10]; (**>2 years**) 125–250 µg every 6–8 h by nebulizer has been used.[11,12] **Nasal spray for rhinorrhea of perennial rhinitis**—(**<6 years**) safety and efficacy not established; (**6–11 years**) 2 sprays (21 µg/spray) in each nostril of 0.03% solution bid–tid; (**≥12 years**) same as adult dosage. **Nasal spray for rhinorrhea of the common cold (5–11 years)**—2 sprays 0.06% solution (42 µg/spray) per nostril tid for up to 4 days.

Geriatric Dosage. Same as adult dosage.

Dosage Forms. Inhal 17 µg/puff (200 doses/inhaler); **Inhal Soln** 0.02% in 2.5-mL vial; 200 µg/mL (500 µg/vial); **nasal spray** 0.03% 21 µg/spray, 345 sprays/bottle; 0.06% 42 µg/spray, 165 sprays/bottle. **Inhal** 18 µg plus 90 µg albuterol/puff (Combivent); 500 µg plus albuterol 3 mg/3 mL (DuoNeb).

Patient Instructions. Refer also to Class Instructions at the beginning of this chapter.

Inhalation for asthma (MDI). Atrovent HFA may taste and feel different when breathed compared to Atrovent CFC inhaler, but they contain the same medication.

Pharmacokinetics. *Onset and Duration.* Onset 3 min; peak 1–2 h[11]; duration 4–6 h, depending on intensity of response.[13]

Fate. Only ≤32% is orally absorbed and <1% of inhaled dose is absorbed.[11] Metabolized to 8 metabolites, which are excreted in urine and bile.

$t_{1/2}$. 1.5–4 h.[11]

Adverse Reactions. Dryness of the mouth. Because of the quaternary nature of the molecule, typical systemic anticholinergic side effects are absent.[11,13] With the nasal spray, epistaxis, nasal dryness, dry mouth, or throat and nasal congestion occur in 1%–10% of patients. During long-term use, headache, nausea, and upper respiratory tract infections also occur frequently.

Contraindications. Hypersensitivity to ipratropium; HFA is safe to use in patients with soy/nut allergies.

Precautions. Use with caution in narrow-angle glaucoma, prostatic hypertrophy, or bladder neck obstruction.

Drug Interactions. None known.

Parameters to Monitor. Inhalation technique, asthma symptoms, frequency of use, pulmonary function, and anticholinergic symptoms.

Notes. Anticholinergics appear to be as potent bronchodilators as β_2-adrenergic drugs in bronchitis and emphysema but less potent in asthma.[9,11] Anticholinergics produce an additive bronchodilation with β_2-adrenergic agents in severe asthma.[11,12] Ipratropium and albuterol nebulizer solutions can be mixed if the mixture is used within 1 h. Recent studies have evaluated the increased risk of cardiovascular death, myocardial infarction, and stroke in patients with COPD who used inhaled anticholinergic medications. Most of the excess risk appeared to come from studies in which ipratropium and tiotropium were taken for at least 6 months. The study concluded that decisions should be made by prescribers and patients regarding risk vs. benefits with these agents.[13]

| **LEVALBUTEROL** | Xopenex, Xopenex HFA |

Pharmacology. Levalbuterol is the active R-stereoisomer of albuterol, with greater affinity for the β_2-receptor than racemic albuterol and *S*-albuterol.[6] The mechanism of action is similar, relaxing smooth muscle and resulting in bronchodilation. Levalbuterol also inhibits the release of inflammatory mediators from airway mast cells.

Administration and Dosage. Inhalation for treatment or prevention of bronchospasm MDI (adults and children ≥4 years)—90 μg (2 puffs) every 4–6 h prn, up to 12 puffs/24 h; **NEB (adults and children ≥12 years)**—0.63–1.25 mg every 6–8 h, up to 1.25 mg tid.

Pediatric Dosage. MDI dose has not been established in children <4 years. **NEB (children 6–11 years)**—0.31 mg tid, not to exceed 0.63 mg tid.

Geriatric Dosage. (NEB)—in patients >65 years, initiate with 0.63-mg dose and increase as tolerated; **(MDI)**—initiate at lower end of dosing range.

Dosage Forms. Inhal MDI 45 μg/puff (200 puffs/inhaler); **NEB** 0.31, 0.63, 1.25 mg in 3-mL unit dose vials; 1.25 mg/0.5 mL unit dose vials.

Patient Instructions. Refer also to Class Instructions at the beginning of this chapter.

If you are using this medicine in a nebulizer, do not use it if the solution is cloudy.

This medication may cause a rapid heartbeat. Less common side effects are chest pain or tightness, dizziness, shortness of breath. Check with your health care professional if side effects are bothersome or worrying.

It is important to keep your appointments with your doctor to be sure your medicine is working properly. Do not start or stop taking this or any other asthma medications without checking with your doctor.

Pharmacokinetics. *Onset and duration.* (**Inhalation**) onset 10–17 min; duration 5–8 h.

Fate. Peak concentration (**NEB**) 0.2 h, (MDI, adults) 0.54 h, (MDI, children 4–11 years) 0.76 h; peak effect 1.5 h after 4 weeks of treatment; $t_{1/2}$ 3.3 h (single dose), 4.0 h (cumulative dosing); metabolized primarily by sulfotransferase enzymes; 80%–100% renal excretion of parent compound and primary metabolite; <20% in feces.

Adverse Reactions. Paradoxical bronchospasm, tachycardia, and other cardiovascular effects including hypertension, palpitations, chest pain; dyspnea, rhinitis, flu-like symptoms, viral infection, dry mouth, nervousness, tremor. Most adverse effects appear to be dose related.

Precautions. Use with caution in patients with cardiovascular disorders, especially cardiac insufficiency, hypertension, and cardiac arrhythmias. Large doses have been shown to exacerbate diabetes. All β_2-agonists may cause hypokalemia.

Drug Interactions. Concurrent use of β-blocking agents, especially propranolol, may inhibit therapeutic effects of both agents; serum digoxin levels may be decreased; tricyclic antidepressants and MAOIs may potentiate the effects of levalbuterol on the vascular system (do not use within 2 weeks of therapy with TCAs or MAOIs); concurrent use with methylxanthines may increase the risk of cardiac arrhythmias; short-acting epinephrine may increase cardiac adverse effects.

Monitoring Parameters. Inhalation technique, asthma symptoms, frequency of use; heart rate; serum potassium (especially when concomitant therapy with non–potassium-sparing diuretic agents).

Notes. It has been suggested that the use of racemic albuterol (mixture of *R*-albuterol and *S*-albuterol) increases proinflammatory effects and increases the risk of bronchial hyperreactivity. It has also been shown that levalbuterol 1.25 mg significantly improved lung function (as measured by forced expiratory volume (FEV_1)) compared to racemic albuterol 2.5 mg, and that *S*-albuterol may have an antagonist effect on bronchodilation and contribute to other adverse effects such as tachycardia. Other studies have found this not to be valid. Currently, the clinical significance of the differences between racemic albuterol and *R*-albuterol are unclear.[6,14,15]

MONTELUKAST SODIUM	Singulair

Pharmacology. Montelukast sodium is a selective and orally active leukotriene-receptor antagonist that inhibits the cysteinyl leukotriene ($CysLT_1$) receptor. Binding of leukotrienes to their receptors contributes to the pathophysiology of asthma, including airway edema, smooth muscle contraction, and other cellular activity associated with the inflammatory process. Montelukast inhibits this process and therefore inhibits bronchospasm due to antigen challenge.[16,17] Leukotriene-receptor antagonists are an alternative, not preferred, treatment option for mild persistent asthma, and can be used as adjunct therapy with inhaled corticosteroids.[2]

Administration and Dosage. **PO for asthma and seasonal allergic rhinitis (adults and children ≥15 years)**—10 mg/d qd. **PO for exercise-induced bronchospasm prophylaxis (adults and children >15 years)**—10 mg × 1 dose given >2 h before exercise. Do not give if on daily montelukast therapy.

Pediatric Dosage. **PO for asthma and seasonal allergic rhinitis**—(**infants <12 months**) safety and efficacy not established; (**infants 12–23 months**) oral granules 4 mg (1 packet) qd; (**children 2–5 years**) 4-mg chewable tablet or 4-mg oral granules (1 packet) qd; (**children 6–14 years**) 5-mg chewable tablet qd.

Geriatric Dosage. Same as adult dosage.

Dosage Forms. Oral granules 4 mg; Chew Tab 4, 5 mg; Tab 10 mg.

Patient Instructions. This drug is used for long-term control and prevention of mild persistent asthma symptoms and relief of the symptoms of seasonal allergic rhinitis. Take this medication daily, even when you are having no symptoms, and during periods of worsening asthma. This medication is not for the treatment of acute asthma attack management of exercise-induced bronchospasm. You should have appropriate short-acting β_2-agonist medication available to treat acute symptoms. Seek medical attention if short-acting inhaled bronchodilators are needed more often than usual, or if the maximum number of inhalations of short-acting bronchodilator treatment prescribed for a 24-h period is needed.

All montelukast oral forms can be administered without regard for meals. Chewable tablets contain aspartame. Oral granules may be administered directly into the mouth or mixed with a spoonful of cold or room temperature soft food.

Missed Doses. Take a missed dose as soon as possible. If it is almost time to take the next dose, skip the missed dose and go back to your regular dosage schedule. Do not double doses.

Pharmacokinetics. *Onset and Duration.* Treatment effect achieved after the first dose. Duration is 24 h.[16,17]

Fate. Montelukast is rapidly absorbed after oral administration. Mean oral bioavailabilities are 64% for the film-coated tablet and 73% for the chewable tablet in the fasted state, and 63% with a standard morning meal. The 4-mg oral granule dose is bioequivalent to the 4-mg chewable tablet. A high-fat meal decreased maximum concentration of the oral granules by 35%. Peak concentrations occur 3–4 h after administration of a 10-mg film-coated tablet, 2–2.5 h after the 5-mg chewable tablet, and 1.3–3.3 h after the oral granules in fasted adults. Montelukast is >99% protein bound; V_{dss} is 8–11 L; Cl is 2.7 L/h. CYP3A4 and 2C9 are involved in the metabolism of montelukast. Montelukast and its metabolites are excreted almost exclusively via the bile.

$t_{1/2}$ is 2.7–5.5 h in healthy young adults.

Adverse Reactions. Generally, well tolerated. Adverse events that occur with a frequency of ≥2% and more frequently in patients on montelukast than on placebo are headache, abdominal pain, dyspepsia, nausea, diarrhea, elevated ALT, cough, laryngitis, pharyngitis, otitis, sinusitis, flulike symptoms, and viral infection. Rare—systemic eosinophilia. Aggressive behavior and agitation have been observed in clinical practice, but the frequency cannot be determined. Other behavioral effects may include depression, anxiousness, tremor, and suicidal thoughts/behavior.

Contraindications. Patients with known aspirin sensitivity should continue to avoid aspirin or other NSAIDs while taking montelukast. Inform phenylketonuric patients that the chewable tablets contain phenylalanine (a component of aspartame) 0.824 mg/tablet. Patients with severe liver disease should be monitored.

Precautions. (*See* Patient Instructions.) Reduction in systemic corticosteroid dosage in patients on a leukotriene modifier has been followed rarely by eosinophilia, vasculitic rash, worsening pulmonary symptoms, cardiac complications, and/or neuropathy, sometimes presenting as Churg-Strauss syndrome. A causal relationship with leukotriene-receptor antagonists is not established.

Drug Interactions. Concurrent use with phenobarbital results in a reduction (40%) in the AUC of montelukast; no dosage adjustment is recommended.

Parameters to Monitor. Clinical symptoms of asthma. Appropriate monitoring recommended when systemic corticosteroid reduction is considered. Monitor patient for depression, anxiety, and other behavior changes.

Notes. The FDA is currently investigating a possible association between the use of Singulair and behavior/mood changes, suicidality (suicidal thinking and behavior) and suicide. The manufacturer (Merck) is reviewing Singulair study data for more information on suicidality and suicide and postmarketing reports of behavior/mood changes; suicidality and suicide are under review by the FDA. In April 2009, the FDA completed its review of neuropsychiatric events related to this class and advised that patients and healthcare providers should be aware of the potential for these events, that patients should report any occurrences to their healthcare providers and that if these symptoms develop, these medications should be discontinued. Since March 2007, Merck and Co., Inc., has updated prescribing and patient information to include the adverse effects of tremor, depression, suicidal thinking and behavior, and anxiousness. The FDA is also reviewing postmarketing reports it has received of behavior/mood changes and suicidality and suicide in patients receiving Zafirlukast (Accolate), Zileuton (Zyflo and Zyflo CR) and will assess whether further investigation is warranted.[18] According to a joint statement by ACAAI and AAAAI, there are no data from well-designed studies to indicate a link between Singulair and suicide and that the concern expressed by the FDA is based entirely on case reports with no indication that such effects apply to other leukotriene-modifying medications. These organizations recommend that patients taking Singulair should continue to take the medication as prescribed provided (1) the patient and physician feel the medication is effective and (2) the patient does not experience any suicidal behavior or thoughts.[19]

NEDOCROMIL SODIUM
Tilade (see Notes); Various

Pharmacology. Nedocromil sodium is the disodium salt of a pyranoquinolone dicarboxylic acid that is chemically dissimilar, but pharmacologically similar, to cromolyn sodium. Like cromolyn, nedocromil inhibits the activation of and mediator release from inflammatory cells important in asthma and allergy. Nedocromil appears to have more potent in vitro activity against allergic response than cromolyn.[20,21] The development of airway hyperresponsiveness to nonspecific bronchoconstrictors is also inhibited by nedocromil sodium.

Administration and Dosage. **Inhalation for asthma prevention MDI (adults and children ≥6 years)**—2 puffs qid at regular intervals. In patients under good control with qid administration (i.e., patients requiring inhaled or oral β-agonists not more than twice a week), a lower dosage can be tried. First reduce to a tid regimen, then, after several weeks of continued good control, attempt to reduce to a bid regimen. **Inhalation for exercise-induced bronchospasm prophylaxis MDI (adults and children ≥6 years)**—2 puffs up to 30 min before exercise or exposure to precipitating factors. **Ophthalmic for allergic conjunctivitis**—1–2 drops into each eye bid.

Pediatric Dosage. **(MDI) children up to 6 years**—dosage not established; **(ophthalmic)**—usual adult dose.

Geriatric Dosage. Usual adult dose.

Dosage Forms. **Inhal** 16.2 g canister, containing at least 104 actuations of 2-mg doses (1.75 mg reaches the patient); **Ophth Soln** 2%.

Patient Instructions. Before using the inhaler for the first time, or if it has not been used in more than 7 days, prime the inhaler before using. Remove the mouthpiece from the inhaler. Hold the canister away from you and press the top of the canister to spray the medication into the air. Repeat for a total of 3 sprays.

To use the inhaler, remove the cover from the inhaler, hold the inhaler upright with the mouthpiece toward you between your thumb and 1 or 2 fingers. Shake the inhaler 3–4 times. Breathe out slowly and completely. To use the open-mouth method, place the mouthpiece 1–2 in. (approximately 2 finger widths) in front of your mouth. Open your mouth widely and aim the inhaler so that the spray does not hit the roof of your mouth or your tongue. To use the closed-mouth method, place the mouthpiece in your mouth between your teeth and over your tongue and close your lips tightly around the mouthpiece, being sure that your tongue or teeth are not blocking the mouthpiece. Start to breathe in slowly through your mouth and at the same time, press the top of the canister once to expel 1 puff of medication. Continue to breathe in slowly for 5–10 s. Hold your breath as long as you can up to 10 s, then take the mouthpiece away from your mouth and breathe out slowly. If your doctor has prescribed more than 1 puff, shake the inhaler and take the second puff exactly as you did the first.

Clean the inhaler at least twice weekly and the mouthpiece daily. To clean the inhaler, remove the metal canister—do not get the metal canister wet. Rinse the mouthpiece and inhaler in hot water, shake off excess water, and allow to air dry completely before replacing the metal canister.

If your doctor has prescribed nedocromil to use every day, be sure and use it as ordered. It may take 2–4 weeks before you feel the full results of the medication.

Gargle or rinse your mouth after inhalation to relieve throat irritation and unpleasant taste.

Pharmacokinetics. *Onset and Duration.* Onset—shown to prevent bronchospasm when administered up to 30 min prior to exercise; when used as maintenance therapy, clinical improvement is usually seen within 2–4 weeks. Duration—12 h.

Fate. Absorption is 5%–6% from the respiratory tract; oral bioavailability is 2%–3% when absorbed from the GI tract after inhalation; $t_{1/2}$. is 1.5–3.3 h. Not metabolized and excreted as unchanged drug.

Adverse Reactions. *Frequent*—unpleasant taste; *less frequent, but indicate need for medical attention*—increased bronchospasm and abdominal pain; *less frequent and do not necessarily indicate need for medical attention*—cough, headache, rhinitis, sore throat.

Precautions. Nedocromil can decrease bronchial hyperreactivity but is only partly effective in steroid-dependent asthmatics. Nedocromil sodium is intended for regular maintenance treatment and should not be used in acute asthma attacks.

Drug Interactions. Nedocromil has been coadministered with inhaled and oral bronchodilators and inhaled corticosteroids with no evidence of increased adverse events. No formal drug–drug studies have been conducted.

Parameters to Monitor. Inhalation technique, asthma symptoms, pulmonary function.

Notes. Tilade inhalers containing CFCs were replaced by CFC-free inhalers beginning in January of 2006, thus Tilade inhaler will no longer be available as a branded product once current supplies are exhausted. The generic formulation is still available.[22]

OMALIZUMAB Xolair

Pharmacology. Omalizumab is a monoclonal antibody that prevents the binding of IgE to high-affinity receptors on basophils and mast cells. Decreasing the surface-bound IgE on these cells limits the release of mediators of the allergic response. Treatment with omalizumab also reduces the number of these high-affinity receptors. It is used as adjunctive therapy in patients ≥12 years who have allergies and persistent asthma. Omalizumab is defined as an immunomodulator whose addition to inhaled corticosteroid therapy produced a reduction in asthma exacerbations, improvement in lung function, and which appears to have a steroid-sparing effect.[2]

Dosage and Administration. **For asthma, persistent, moderate/severe prophylaxis SQ (adults and children ≥12 years)**—150–375 mg every 2–4 weeks.

Preparation of dosage form: Prepare SQ injection using sterile water for injection USP ONLY. Draw 1.4 mL SWFI, USP into a 3-mL syringe with a 1 in. 18-gauge needle. Place the vial upright on a flat surface using standard aseptic technique, insert the needle, and inject the SWFI onto the product. Keeping the vial upright, swirl the upright vial for 1 min to wet the powder. Do not shake. The lyophilized product takes 15–20 min to dissolve. Swirl the vial for 5–10 s every 5 min to dissolve any remaining solid product. If the contents do not dissolve in 40 min, do not use. The fully reconstituted product will be clear or slightly opalescent. Invert the vial for 15 sec to allow the solution to drain to the top of the vial. Using a new 3-mL needle with a 1 in. 18-gauge needle, insert the needle and position the tip at the bottom of the solution in the vial stopper. The reconstituted product is viscous; to obtain the full 1.2-mL dose, ALL of the product must be withdrawn from the vial before expelling air from the syringe.

Storage and stability: After reconstitution, the solution should be used within 8 h when stored in the refrigerator (36°F–46°F) or within 4 h if stored at room temperature. Protect reconstituted Xolair from light.

Administration: Replace the 18-gauge needle with a 25-gauge needle prior to injection. Expel air, bubbles, and any excess solution to obtain the 1.2-mL dose. (A thin layer of small bubbles may remain at the top of the solution.) Administer injection over 5–10 s. Doses and frequency are determined by serum total IgE level measured before the start of treatment and on body weight (kg). Doses of >150 mg should be given in more than 1 injection site; injection volume should not exceed 150 mg per site.

ADMINISTRATION EVERY 4 WEEKS

BASELINE SERUM IgE (IU/mL)	30–60 kg	>60–70 kg	>70–90 kg	>90–150 kg
≥30–100	150	150	150	300
>100–200	300	300	300	
>200–300	300		a	
>300		a		

[a]See table "Administration Every 2 Weeks."
Adapted from Xolair PI.

ADMINISTRATION EVERY 2 WEEKS

BASELINE SERUM IgE (IU/mL)	30–60 kg	>60–70 kg	>70–90 kg	>90–150 kg
≥30–100			a	
>100–200		a		225
>200–300	a	225	225	300
>300–400	225	225	300	Do not dose
>400–500	300	300	375	Do not dose
>500–600	300	375		Do not dose
>600–700	375			Do not dose

See table "Administration Every 4 Weeks."
Adapted from Xolair PI.

Pediatric Dosage. <12 years—dosing not established.

Geriatric Dosage. In patients ≥65 years—there were no apparent age-related differences seen in clinical studies, but the number of patients studied is insufficient to determine if response is significant enough to warrant dosage changes. Therefore, the usual adult dose is recommended.

Dosage Forms. SQ Inj—supplied as a lyophilized sterile powder in a single-use 5-mL vial designed to deliver 150 mg (1.2 mL) of drug upon reconstitution with 1.4 mL SWFI, USP. It contains no preservatives.

Patient Instructions. Omalizumab (Xolair) is used to treat moderate-to-severe persistent allergic asthma that works by blocking the effects of IgE, which is a substance that occurs in the body and plays a part in allergic reactions and asthma. Omalizumab is an injection given under the skin every 2 or 4 weeks. Your dose of medication will be determined by your IgE level, which will be measured with a blood test before you start treatment. Your health care provider will give your medication and will ask you to remain at the health care facility or clinic for a period of time after each injection to watch you for immediate side effects that can be serious.

Before using this medication, be sure and tell your doctor if you have had any unusual or allergic reaction to this or any other medication as well as other types of allergies, such as to foods, dyes, preservatives, or animals. It is important to know the signs of an allergic reaction to omalizumab and know what to do. If you have any symptoms such as a rash, itching, or swelling of your tongue and throat, get medical help immediately. Check with your doctor immediately also if you have a cough; difficulty swallowing; dizziness; a rapid heartbeat; hives; itching; puffiness of your eyelids or swelling around your eyes, face, lips, or tongue; shortness of breath; chest tightness; unusual tiredness; or wheezing. Other side effects that may occur include injection site reactions, bleeding, flulike symptoms, muscle aches, dry or sore throat, headache.

It is important that you continue all your asthma medications as prescribed by your doctor even though you are taking omalizumab.

Pharmacokinetics. Absorption is slow following SQ injection, with a bioavailability of 62%. Time to peak concentration is 7–8 days, with $t_{1/2}$ of 26 days. Clearance involves IgG clearance processes as well as clearance via complex formation with IgE. Of note, doubling body weight approximately doubles apparent clearance.

Adverse Reactions. Anaphylaxis, presenting as bronchospasm, hypotension, syncope, urticaria, and/or angioedema of the throat or tongue has been reported after administration of omalizumab. Anaphylaxis has occurred as early as after the first dose, but has also occurred after 1 year of dosing.

Other reactions include injection site reaction (45%), viral infection (23%), upper respiratory tract infection (20%), sinusitis (16%), headache (15%), pharyngitis (11%); musculoskeletal pain, malignant neoplasms (rare).

Precautions. Omalizumab should only be administered in a health care setting by providers prepared to manage life-threatening anaphylaxis. Patients should be monitored closely after administration for signs of anaphylaxis and should be informed of the signs and symptoms of anaphylaxis and instructed to seek immediate medical care should any of the symptoms occur.

Malignant neoplasms were observed in 0.5% of Xolair-treated patients (0.2% controls).

Do not discontinue corticosteroids upon initiation of Xolair therapy. In rare cases, patients on therapy with Xolair may present with systemic eosinophilia, which is usually associated with reduction of oral corticosteroid therapy.

Drug Interactions. No formal drug interaction studies have been performed.

Parameters to Monitor. Anaphylactic reactions; serum IgE prior to beginning therapy. (Note: Serum IgE levels remain elevated for up to 1 year following discontinuation of omalizumab. Therefore, IgE levels obtained less than 1 year following discontinuation should not be used to reassess dosing.) Monitor asthma symptoms, pulmonary function; monitor for presence of malignancy.

Notes. It is recommended that omalizumab be considered as adjunctive therapy for patients with allergies and severe persistent asthma that is inadequately controlled with the combination of high-dose inhaled corticosteroids and long-acting β-adrenergic agents.[2]

SALMETEROL XINAFOATE　　　　　　　　　　　　Serevent, Serevent Diskus

Pharmacology. Salmeterol is a β_2-agonist structurally and pharmacologically similar to albuterol. Salmeterol is a long-acting β_2-agonist intended for regular treatment of reversible airway obstruction and not for immediate symptomatic relief. By stimulating β_2-receptors in the lungs, salmeterol relaxes bronchial smooth muscle, relieving bronchospasm. β_2-receptors are also found in the heart and skeletal muscle, and stimulation of these areas can produce tachycardia and tremor. See **Precautions** and **Notes** sections for safety and other information.

Administration and Dosage. Inhalation for asthma prophylaxis powder (adults and children ≥4 years)—50 μg (1 inhalation) bid; MDI (adults and children ≥12 years)—42 μg (2 puffs) bid (12 h apart). Inhalation to prevent exercise-induced bronchospasm powder (adults and children ≥4 years)—50 μg (1 inhalation) at least 30 min before exercise. MDI (adults and children ≥12 years)—42 μg (2 puffs) 30–60 min before exercise. Inhalation for COPD-associated bronchospasm MDI (adults and children ≥12 years)—42 μg (2 puffs) bid (12 h apart).

Pediatric Dosage. **Inhalation MDI (children <12 years)** safety and efficacy not established; **powder (children ≥4 years)** same as adult dosage.

Geriatric Dosage. Usual adult dose.

Dosage Forms. **Inhal MDI** 21 μg/metered-dose puff, in 6.5 g (60 actuations) and 13 g (120 actuations) canisters; **Pwdr** 50 μg/blister. **Pwdr** 50 μg plus fluticasone 100, 250, or 500 μg/blister (Advair Diskus).

Patient Instructions. In patients with asthma, long-acting β-agonists, such as Serevent, may increase the chance of death from asthma problems. Talk with your health care provider about the risks and benefits of treating your asthma with Serevent. Serevent is not for adults and children who are well controlled with another asthma medication or only need short-acting β-agonists occasionally. Never use Serevent more often than prescribed and do not use other medications that contain a long-acting β-agonist for any reason. These included Advair, Foradil, Symbicort, Brovana, and Perforomist.

Powder Inhaler. To use the Serevent Diskus, take the Diskus out of the box and the foil pouch. Write the date the pouch was opened and the "Use By" date on the label on the top of the Diskus. The "Use By" date will be 6 weeks from the date you opened the pouch. The Diskus will be closed when you first open its pouch. The dose indicator on the top of the Diskus tells you how many doses are left and will decrease each time you use it.

　　　Hold the Diskus in one hand and put the thumb of your other hand on the thumb grip. Push your thumb away from you as far as it will go until the mouthpiece appears and snaps into position. Hold the Diskus in a flat, level position with the mouthpiece toward you. Slide the lever away from you as far as it will go until it clicks.

Exhale fully while holding the Diskus level and away from your mouth—never breathe out into the Diskus mouthpiece. Put the mouthpiece to your lips and breathe in quickly and deeply through your mouth (not your nose) through the Diskus. Remove the Diskus from your mouth and hold your breath for 10 sec or as long as is comfortable for you. Breathe out slowly. Close the Diskus when you are finished. Put your thumb and the thumb grip and slide it back toward you until the Diskus clicks shut and the lever returns to its original position.

The Diskus delivers your medication as a fine powder. Most people can feel or taste the powder. If you do not feel or taste the medicine, do not use another dose from the Diskus and contact your doctor.

Do not use the Diskus with a spacer device. Do not wash the mouthpiece or any part of the Diskus—it must be kept dry.

Metered-Dose Inhaler. Refer to Class Instructions at the beginning of this chapter.

Pharmacokinetics. *Onset and Duration.* **Onset**—approximately 10–20 min. Peak effect occurs within 3–4 h; 80% of maximal increase in FEV_1 occurs within 1 h of administration. **Duration**—approximately 12 h.

Fate. After inhalation, salmeterol is extensively metabolized by hydroxylation via CYP450 3A4, with the majority of a dose being eliminated within 72 h in the feces. (Approximately 25% of administered radioactivity was recovered in the urine and 60% in the feces after 7 days.); $t_{1/2}$. 5.5 h.

Adverse Reactions. **(Asthma)** increase in asthma-related deaths (see **Precautions**), headache, nasal/sinus congestion, rhinitis, flulike symptoms. **(COPD)** hypertension, throat irritation, cough, viral infection, musculoskeletal pain, headache. Observed in practice—laryngeal spasm, swelling, irritation; arrhythmias, atrial fibrillation, tachycardias; very rare anaphylactic reactions in patients with severe milk protein allergy.

Precautions. Long-acting β_2-adrenergic agents such as salmeterol may increase the risk of asthma-related death. When treating patients with asthma, Serevent (and other long-acting β_2-adrenergic agents) should only be used as additional therapy for patients not adequately controlled on other asthma controller medications such as inhaled corticosteroids or whose disease severity clearly warrants initiation of treatment with 2 maintenance therapies. Do not initiate Serevent in patients with significantly worsening or acutely deteriorating asthma. should not be stopped or reduced when Serevent is initiated.[2]

All sympathomimetic drugs can have cardiovascular and CNS effects such as hypertension, increased heart rate, and excitement. Use Serevent with caution in patients with cardiovascular disorders, especially coronary insufficiency, arrhythmias, and hypertension and in patients with convulsive disorders or hyperthyroidism. May exacerbate diabetes. May cause hypokalemia.

Drug Interactions. Concomitant administration with ketoconazole increased AUC of salmeterol 16-fold and C_{max} 1.4-fold. Therefore, concomitant use with CYP3A4 inhibitors is not recommended. Use with caution in patients receiving MAOIs and

TCAs. β-adrenergic antagonists may block the pulmonary effect of β-agonists. Hypokalemia may be exacerbated by the use of non–potassium-sparing diuretics.

Parameters to Monitor. Inhalation technique, asthma symptoms (with frequency of short-acting β_2-agonists), heart rate, pulmonary function.

Notes. The addition of a long-acting β-adrenergic agonist to therapy with inhaled corticosteroids leads to improved lung function and decreased need for short-acting β-adrenergic agents when compared with addition of a leukotriene-receptor antagonist or theophylline to inhaled corticosteroid therapy or to doubling the dose of inhaled corticosteroids. A large clinical trial comparing daily treatment with salmeterol added to usual asthma therapy resulted in an increased risk of asthma-related deaths in patients treated with salmeterol compared to placebo. In addition, increased numbers of asthma exacerbations were noted in the trials submitted to the FDA for formoterol approval. Thus the FDA determined that a black box warning was warranted on all preparations containing a long-acting β-adrenergic agent stating that these medications may increase the risk of severe asthma attacks and the risk of asthma-related death when these attacks occur.[23] Daily use of salmeterol should not exceed 100 μg.[2]

SYMPATHOMIMETIC BRONCHODILATORS COMPARISON CHART

		DOSAGE		RECEPTOR SELECTIVITY[a]		RELATIVE β₂ POTENCY[b]	DURATION OF ACTION BY INHALATION (h)[c]
DRUG	DOSAGE FORMS	Adult	Pediatric	β₁	β₂		

SINGLE-INGREDIENT PRODUCTS

Albuterol Accuneb Proventil Ventolin Volmax Various		Refer to albuterol monograph		+	+ + + +	5	4–6
Epinephrine Adrenalin Various	Inhal (Soln) 2.25% (racemic); Inj 0.1, 1 mg/mL	SQ 0.2–0.5 mL every 20 min–4 h prn; Inhal not recommended	SQ 0.01 mL/kg of 1:1000 every 15–20 min for 2 doses, then q4h prn; Inhal not recommended for asthma	+ + +	+ + +	5	0.5–2
Formoterol Foradil		Refer to formoterol monograph		+	+ + + +	70	12

(continued)

SYMPATHOMIMETIC BRONCHODILATORS COMPARISON CHART (*continued*)

DRUG	DOSAGE FORMS	DOSAGE Adult	DOSAGE Pediatric	RECEPTOR SELECTIVITY[a] β₁	RECEPTOR SELECTIVITY[a] β₂	RELATIVE β₂ POTENCY[b]	DURATION OF ACTION BY INHALATION (h)[c]
Isoetharine	Inhal (Soln) 1%	Inhal (Soln) 2.5–10 mg diluted 1:3 in NS every 2–4 h prn	Inhal (Soln) 0.1–0.2 mg/kg every 2–4 h prn	++	+++	1.7	0.5–2
Metaproterenol Alupent Various	Inhal (Soln) 0.4% (unit dose 10 mg), 0.6% (unit dose 15 mg), 5%; (metered-dose) 0.65 mg/puff Syrup 2 mg/mL Tab 10, 20 mg	Inhal (Soln) 5–15 mg every 2–4 h prn (every 1–2 h under medical supervision); (metered-dose) 1–3 puffs every 4–6 h and before exercise; PO 20 mg 3–4 times/d	Inhal (Soln) 0.25–0.5 mg/kg up to 15 mg every 2–4 h prn; (metered-dose) 1–2 puffs prn and before exercise; PO 0.5 mg/kg every 4–6 h, increase by 0.25 mg/kg as tolerated	++	++	1	3–4
Pirbuterol Maxair	Inhal (metered-dose) 0.2 mg/puff	Inhal 1–2 puffs every 4–6 h prn and before exercise	Inhal 1–2 puffs every 4–6 h prn and before exercise	+	++++	2.5	4–8

(continued)

SYMPATHOMIMETIC BRONCHODILATORS COMPARISON CHART (*continued*)

DRUG	DOSAGE FORMS	DOSAGE		RECEPTOR SELECTIVITY[a]		RELATIVE β_2 POTENCY[b]	DURATION OF ACTION BY INHALATION (h)[c]
		Adult	**Pediatric**	β_1	β_2		
Salmeterol Serevent	Inhal (metered-dose) 0.2 mg/puff;	Refer to salmeterol monograph		+	++++	20	12
Terbutaline Brethaire Brethine Bricanyl	Inj 1 mg/mL; Tab 2.5, 5 mg	Inhal 1–3 puffs every 4–6 h prn; 5–7 mg undiluted by nebulizer every 4–6 h prn; SQ 0.25–0.5 mg every 2–3 h prn; PO 5 mg every 6–8 h	Inhal 1–2 puffs every 4–6 h prn; 0.1– 0.3 mg/kg every 4–6 h (every 1–2 h under medical supervision; SQ 0.01 mg/kg up to 0.25 mg every 2–6 h prn; PO 0.075 mg/kg every 6–8 h	+	++++	2.5	4–8

COMBINATION PRODUCTS

Albuterol and Ipratropium Combivent DuoNeb	Inhal (metered-dose) albuterol 90 μg plus ipratropium 18 μg/ puff; Inhal Soln albuterol 3 mg plus ipratropium 0.5 mg/ 3 mL	Inhal 2 puffs qid to a maximum of 12 puffs/d	—	—	—	—	—

(continued)

SYMPATHOMIMETIC BRONCHODILATORS COMPARISON CHART (*continued*)

DRUG	DOSAGE FORMS	DOSAGE Adult	DOSAGE Pediatric	RECEPTOR SELECTIVITY[a] β_1	RECEPTOR SELECTIVITY[a] β_2	RELATIVE β_2 POTENCY[b]	DURATION OF ACTION BY INHALATION (h)[c]
Salmeterol and Fluticasone Advair Diskus	Inhal (dry Pwdr) salmeterol 50 mg plus fluticasone 100, 250 or 500 µg/Inhal	Inhal 1 puff bid	($\geq$12 y) same as adult dosage	—	—	—	—

+, minimal effect; +++, pronounced effect.

[a]β_2-selectivity does not equate to bronchoselectivity; β_2-stimulation produces reflex tachycardia from vasodilation as well as stimulation of cardiac β_2-receptors.

[b]Molar potency relative to metaproterenol; large numbers indicate more potent compounds.

[c]Onset and duration data apply to aerosol therapy only. Duration of bronchodilation only applies to otherwise stable asthmatics and is not applicable to acute severe asthma or protection from severe provocation (e.g., allergen, exercise, ozone). Duration may be shorter during acute exacerbation or with long-term therapy because of downregulation of β-receptors (tolerance). Oral tablets (especially SR tablets) and syrups are s7lower in onset but may be slightly longer acting than aerosols.

FORMOTEROL Foradil

Formoterol (Foradil) is a long-acting β_2-adrenergic agonist that is similar to salmeterol. Formoterol is indicated for long-term treatment of asthma in patients ≥ 5 years with reversible obstructive airway disease, including nocturnal asthma, who are receiving corticosteroid treatment.

Dosage: Inhalation for bronchoconstriction powder (adults and children ≥ 5 years)—12 μg bid approximately 12 h apart, not to exceed 24 μg/d. *Pediatric Dosage*—dosing not established for children <5 years. *Onset* 1–3 min; *duration* 12 h. *Fate*—metabolized by glucuronidation and demethylation/conjugation by CYP450 2D6, 2C19, 2C9 and 2A6 and excreted in the urine (59%–62%) and feces (32%–34%). Formoterol is available as a dry powder for inhalation. **Refer to Precautions, Patient Information, and Notes sections of Salmeterol.**

A fixed-dose combination with budesonide (Symbicort) is also available.

THEOPHYLLINE Theo-Dur, Slo-bid, Various

Pharmacology. Theophylline, the principally used methylxanthine, directly relaxes smooth muscles of bronchial airways and pulmonary blood vessels to act as a bronchodilator and pulmonary vasodilator. It is also a diuretic, coronary vasodilator, cardiac stimulant, and cerebral stimulant; it improves diaphragmatic contractility; and it lessens diaphragmatic fatigue. The exact cellular mechanism of smooth muscle relaxation is unknown, but intracellular calcium sequestration, inhibition of specific phosphodiesterase isozymes, adenosine-receptor antagonism, and stimulation of endogenous catecholamine release have been postulated to play a role.[17,24] **Aminophylline** is the ethylenediamine salt of theophylline.

Administration and Dosage. PO (theophylline) or IV (aminophylline) for acute asthma symptoms in the emergency department or in the hospital setting are no longer recommended because it appears to provide no additional benefit over optimal inhaled β_2-agonist therapy and might increase adverse effects; addition of IV theophylline to other therapies in hospitalized adults remains controversial. Sustained-release theophylline is used as alternative therapy with inhaled corticosteroids, not as preferred The following dosages have been used: 5 mg/kg (6 mg/kg aminophylline), if patient has taken no theophylline in previous 24 h. In emergencies, 2.5 mg/kg (3 mg/kg aminophylline) may be given if an immediate serum level cannot be obtained. Each 1 mg/kg (1.25 mg/kg aminophylline) results in approximately a 2 mg/L increase in serum theophylline. Infuse IV aminophylline no faster than 25 mg/min therapy.

Theophylline **(adults and children ≥ 12 years)**—starting dose 10 mg/kg/d, maximum 300 mg/dose. Maximum daily dose—800 mg.[2] **Maintenance dosage**—*see* Theophylline Dosage Adjustment Chart. **PO for chronic asthma (theophylline)**—(*see* Theophylline Dosage Adjustment Chart.) Adjust dosage to achieve serum concentration of 5–15 mg/L at steady state (at least 48 h of same dosage).[2,25,26] **IM, PR suppository**—not recommended.

Special Populations. All dosage recommendations are based on the average theophylline clearance for a given population group. There is a wide interpatient variability (often >2-fold) within all patient groups. Therefore, it is essential that serum concentrations be monitored in all patients. If no doses have been missed or extra doses have been taken during the previous 48 h, and if peak serum concentrations have been obtained (1–2 h after liquid or plain uncoated tablet and 4–6 h after most SR products), adjust dosage using the Theophylline Dosage Adjustment Chart.

Pediatric Dosage. **PO or IV for acute symptoms not recommended for children hospitalized for severe asthma. PO for chronic asthma (children 5–11 years)**—10 mg/kg/d starting dose, usual maximum 16 mg/kg/d; **(children ≤4 years)**—10 mg/kg/d. *Usual maximum (<1 year)*— 0.2 × (age in weeks) + 5 = mg/kg/d; *usual maximum (≥1 year)*—16 mg/kg/d.[2] **IM, PR suppository**—not recommended.

Geriatric Dosage. Not established, but the elderly as a group have slower hepatic clearance. Therefore, use lower initial doses and monitor closely for response and adverse reactions.

Other Conditions. Many factors can alter theophylline dosage requirements. (*See* Precautions and Factors Affecting Serum Theophylline Concentrations Chart.) Use IBW for dosage calculations in obese patients.

THEOPHYLLINE DOSAGE ADJUSTMENT CHART[a]

EVENT	DOSAGE	ACTION
Initial dosage	10 mg/kg/d to a maximum of 300 mg/d	If initial dosage is tolerated, increase dosage no sooner than 3 d to the first increment.
First increment	13 mg/kg/d to a maximum of 450 mg/d	If the first incremental increase is tolerated, increase dosage no sooner than 3 d to the second increment.
Second increment	16 mg/kg/d to a maximum of 600 mg/d	If the second incremental increase is tolerated, measure an estimate of the peak serum concentration after at least 3 d.

SERUM THEOPHYLLINE CONCENTRATION

<10 mg/L	—	Increase dosage by approximately 25%.
10–15.9 mg/L	—	Maintain dosage if tolerated.
16–19.9 mg/L	—	Consider a 10% dosage reduction.
20–25 mg/L	—	Hold next dose, then resume first incremental dosage.
>25 mg/L	—	Hold next 2 doses, then resume initial dosage.

[a]For children >1 years and adults with no risk factors for decreased clearance. These recommendations acknowledge interpatient variability in dosage requirements and are based on the principle of not exceeding two-thirds of mean dosage requirements initially and not reaching or exceeding mean dosage requirements without measurement of the serum theophylline concentration. The initial low dosage and spaced increases provide time for the tolerance to caffeine-like effects to occur.
From Refs. 27 and 28.

Dosage Forms. *See* Theophylline Products Comparison Chart.

Patient Instructions. Do not chew or crush sustained-release tablets or capsules. Take at equally spaced intervals around the clock. If you experience a fast heartbeat, nausea, vomiting, headache, excitement/restlessness, or seizures, stop your medication and contact your doctor.[2] Contents of sustained-release bead-filled capsules may be mixed with a vehicle (applesauce or jam) and swallowed without chewing for patients who have difficulty in swallowing capsules. Take Theo-24 and Uniphyl products at least 1 h before meals to avoid too rapid absorption of the drug.

Missed Doses. Take the missed dose as soon as possible. However, if it is almost time to take the next dose, skip the missed dose and go back to the regular dosage schedule. Do not double doses. Do not have your theophylline levels measured until you have missed no doses for 3 days.

Pharmacokinetics. *Onset and Duration.* IV onset within 15 min with loading dose.

Serum Levels. Well correlated with clinical effects—therapeutic is 10–15 mg/L (56–83 µmol/L); however, improvement in respiratory function can be observed with serum concentrations of 5 mg/L (28 µmol/L).[25,27] A serum concentration of 5–10 mg/L is often adequate for treatment of neonatal apnea. Toxicity increases at levels >20 mg/L. (*See* Adverse Reactions.)

Fate. Plain uncoated tablets and solution are well absorbed orally; enteric-coated tablets and some SR dosage forms might be unreliably absorbed. Food can affect the rate and extent of absorption of some SR formulations but has minimal effects on rapid-release forms. Food can increase the rate of absorption (Theo-24, Uniphyl), producing dose dumping, or impair absorption (Theo-Dur Sprinkle).[28] Rectal suppository absorption is slow and erratic, and suppositories (including aminophylline) are not recommended under any circumstances. Rectal solutions might result in serum concentrations comparable to oral solution. Approximately 60% is plasma protein bound (less in neonates); V_d is 0.5 ± 0.1 L/kg (greater in neonates). There can be marked intrapatient variability in clearance over time.[26] Cl also is affected by many factors. (*See* Precautions.) Smoking increases theophylline metabolism; this effect can last for 3 months–2 years after cessation of smoking. Clearance progressively increases in infants during the first year of life. Dose-dependent pharmacokinetics in the therapeutic range occur often in children and rarely in adults.[26] In the elderly, clearance declines with age to approximately 35 mL/h/kg.[29] Extensively metabolized in the liver to several inactive metabolites; 10% excreted unchanged in the urine.

$t_{1/2}$. 8 ± 2 h in adult nonsmokers, 4.4 ± 1 h in adult smokers (1–2 packs/d); 3.7 ± 1.1 h in children 1–9 years. In newborn infants, older patients with COPD or cor pulmonale, and patients with CHF or liver disease, the drug can have a half-life >24 h.

Adverse Reactions. Local GI irritation can occur. Reactions occur more frequently at serum concentrations >20 mg/L and include anorexia, nausea, vomiting, epigastric pain, diarrhea, restlessness, irritability, insomnia, and headache. Serious arrhythmias and convulsions (frequently leading to death or permanent brain damage) usually occur at levels >35 mg/L but have occurred at lower concentrations and might *not* be preceded by less serious toxicity; cardiovascular reactions include sinus tachycardia and life-threatening ventricular arrhythmias with PVCs. Rapid IV administration can cause hypotension, syncope, cardiac arrest (particularly if administered directly into central line), and death.[30] IM administration is painful and offers no advantage.

Contraindications. Active peptic ulcer disease; untreated seizure disorder. (Aminophylline) hypersensitivity to ethylenediamine.

Precautions. Use with caution in severe cardiac disease, hypoxemia, hepatic disease, acute myocardial injury, cor pulmonale, CHF, fever, viral illness, underlying seizure disorder, migraine, hepatic cirrhosis, and neonates. Do not give with other xanthine preparations. The alcohol in some oral liquid preparations might cause side effects in infants.

Drug Interactions. Numerous drugs and conditions can alter theophylline clearance and serum levels. Factors that can decrease serum levels are carbamazepine, charcoal-broiled beef, high-protein/low-carbohydrate diet, isoproterenol (IV), phenytoin, rifampin, and smoking. Factors that can increase serum levels are allopurinol (>600 mg/d), cimetidine, ciprofloxacin, cor pulmonale, macrolides (e.g., erythromycin, troleandomycin), oral contraceptives, and propranolol. (*See* Factors Affecting Serum Theophylline Concentrations Chart.)

Parameters to Monitor. (Inpatients) obtain serum theophylline concentrations before starting therapy (if patient previously took theophylline) and 1, 6, and 24 h after start of infusion; monitor daily during continuous infusion. (Outpatients) monitor serum concentrations q6mo, 3–5 days after any dosage change, and whenever there are symptoms of toxicity.[25,26]

Notes. The oral theophylline preparations of choice for long-term use, to achieve sustained therapeutic concentrations and improved compliance, are completely and slowly absorbed SR formulations that are minimally affected by food and pH.[28] (*See* Theophylline Products Comparison Chart.) Combination products containing **ephedrine** increase CNS toxicity and have no therapeutic advantage over adequate serum concentrations of theophylline alone. **Dyphylline** is chemically related to, but not a salt of, theophylline; the amount of dyphylline equivalent to theophylline is unknown. Because its potency is less than that of theophylline and it has a short half-life (2 h), its dosage is greater than that of theophylline and it must be given more frequently.

FACTORS AFFECTING SERUM THEOPHYLLINE CONCENTRATIONS CHART[a]

FACTOR	DECREASES IN THEOPHYLLINE CONCENTRATIONS	INCREASES IN THEOPHYLLINE CONCENTRATIONS	ACTION
Age	↑ Metabolism (1–9 y)	↓ Metabolism (<6 mo, elderly)	Adjust dosage according to serum concentration.
Diet	↑ Metabolism (high protein)	↓ Metabolism (high carbohydrate)	Inform patient that major changes in diet are not recommended while taking theophylline.
Food	↓ Or delays absorption of some SR preparations	↑ Rate of absorption (fatty food)	Select theophylline product that is not affected by food.
Hypoxia, cor pulmonale, decompensated CHF, cirrhosis	—	↓ Metabolism	Decrease dosage according to serum concentration.
Cimetidine	—	↓ Metabolism	Use alternative histamine H2-receptor antagonists (e.g., famotidine, nizatidine, ranitidine).
Macrolides: troleandomycin, erythromycin, clarithromycin	—	↓ Metabolism	Use alternative antibiotic or decrease theophylline dosage.
Phenobarbital, phenytoin, carbamazepine	↑ Metabolism	—	Increase dosage according to serum concentration.
Quinolones: ciprofloxacin, enoxacin	—	↓ Metabolism	Use alternative antibiotic or adjust theophylline dosage. Circumvent with levofloxacin if quinolone therapy is required.

(continued)

933

FACTORS AFFECTING SERUM THEOPHYLLINE CONCENTRATIONS CHART[a] (*continued*)

FACTOR	DECREASES IN THEOPHYLLINE CONCENTRATIONS	INCREASES IN THEOPHYLLINE CONCENTRATIONS	ACTION
Rifampin	↑ Metabolism	—	Increase dosage according to serum concentration.
Smoking	↑ Metabolism	—	Advise patient to stop smoking; increase dosage according to serum concentration.
Ticlopidine	—	↓ Metabolism	Decrease dosage according to serum concentration.
Viral illness, systemic febrile (e.g., influenza)	—	↓ Metabolism	Decrease theophylline dosage according to serum concentration. Decrease dosage by 50% if serum concentration is not available.

[a]This chart is not all inclusive; for other factors, see Chapter 79 of the section "Drug Interactions and Interferences" and product information.
From Ref. 2.

THEOPHYLLINE PRODUCTS COMPARISON CHART[a]

PRODUCT	ANHYDROUS THEOPHYLLINE CONTENT	MEASURABLE DOSE INCREMENT[b] (mg)	COMMENTS
RAPIDLY ABSORBED			
Plain Uncoated Tablets			
Various	Tab 100 mg scored	50	Serum level fluctuations are 459%/117%.[c]
	Tab 125 mg scored	62.5	
	Tab 200 mg scored	100	
	Tab 250 mg scored	125	
	Tab 300 mg scored	150	
Oral Liquids (Alcohol-Free)			
Aerolate	10 mg/mL	5	Sugar-free.
Slo-Phyllin 80 Syrup	5.3 mg/mL	5	Sugar-free.
Intravenous Solution			
Aminophylline[d]	20 mg/mL	5	Use rubber-stoppered vials to avoid glass particles from the breaking of ampules.
Theophylline	0.4, 0.8, 1.6, 2, 3.2, 4 mg/mL	—	Available in large volume solutions only.

(continued)

THEOPHYLLINE PRODUCTS COMPARISON CHART[a] (*continued*)

PRODUCT	ANHYDROUS THEOPHYLLINE CONTENT	MEASURABLE DOSE INCREMENT[b] (mg)	COMMENTS
SLOW-RELEASE PRODUCTS[e]			
Slo-bid Gyrocaps	Cap 50 mg Cap 75 mg Cap 100 mg Cap 125 mg Cap 200 mg Cap 300 mg	25	Excellent bioavailability in young infants; beads can be sprinkled on small amount of food; serum level fluctuations are 43%/18%.[c]
Theo-Dur	Tab 100 mg scored Tab 200 mg scored Tab 300 mg scored Tab 450 mg scored	25 100 150 225	Serum level fluctuations are 38%/16% for 200, 300, and 450 mg, and 87%/34% for 100-mg tablets[c]; some rapid metabolizers may require 8-h dosage intervals to avoid breakthrough of symptoms.
Uni-Dur	Tab 400 mg scored Tab 600 mg scored	200 300	The extent of absorption of Uni-Dur does not appear to be affected by food; however, large serum level fluctuations (78% in adults) may render this agent unreliable for once-daily administration.[26,31]

[a]Only products with documented bioavailability that are minimally affected by food and with dosage forms that permit incremental changes in dose are listed.

[b]Accuracy of measurement decreases below 0.5 mL with suspensions and syrups because of viscosity; smaller amounts cannot be accurately measured; measure all liquid dosage forms with a syringe.

[c]Predicted child/adult fluctuation between peak and trough (%) for 12-h dosage interval; average child $t_{1/2}$ = 3.7 h, average adult $t_{1/2}$ = 8.2 h.[23]

[d]The ethylenediamine portion of aminophylline may cause urticaria or exfoliative dermatitis rarely.

[e]Only Slo-bid Gyrocaps and Theo-Dur tablets have sufficiently slow and complete absorption to allow 12-h dosage intervals with minimal serum concentration fluctuations in most patients. Many products advertised for bid dosage do not maintain serum concentrations within the therapeutic range in many patients, especially children.[23] Some once-daily dosage products (e.g., Uniphyl) are affected by food and may be unreliable.[19,20]

TIOTROPIUM
Spiriva HandiHaler

Pharmacology. Tiotropium is a long-acting antimuscarinic agent with similar affinity for muscarinic receptors M_1–M_5. Its bronchodilating effects are due to its inhibition of the M_3 airway receptors. The bronchodilation produced by tiotropium is dose-dependent and lasts more than 24 h. Tiotropium has not received FDA approved labeling for use in asthma.[2]

Administration and Dosage. Adults: inhalation for bronchospasm—18 μg (1 capsule) qd.

Pediatric Dosage. Dosing not established.

Geriatric Dosage. Usual adult dosage.

Dosage Forms. Inhal Cap 18 μg.

Patient Instructions. Each capsule contains a dry powder blend of medication and lactose, but because the capsules contain only a small amount of medication, they appear almost empty. Once the capsule is used, you may notice a small amount of powder dusting in the capsule—this is normal. Each capsule is packaged in a blister, which can be separated from the blister card along the perforation. The capsules should be stored in the sealed blisters and only removed immediately before use. Do not store the capsules in the HandiHaler—once the capsule is removed from the blister it should be used immediately.

To take a dose of Spiriva, open the HandiHaler and the blister and remove the capsule from the blister pack by peeling back the corner of the blister— do not cut the foil or use sharp instruments to remove the capsule. Pull the dust cap up to expose the mouthpiece and open the mouthpiece. Insert the capsule in the center chamber of the HandiHaler device (it does not matter which end of the capsule is placed in the chamber). Close the mouthpiece until you hear a click. Hold the HandiHaler device with the mouthpiece pointed upward, press the green button until it is flush against the base, and release it—do not press the button more than once.

Breathe out completely. Hold the HandiHaler by the base, close your lips tightly around the mouthpiece, keeping your head in an upright position and the HandiHaler horizontal. Breathe in slowly and deeply until your lungs are full. You should breathe in quickly enough to hear or feel the capsule vibrate. Hold your breath as long as is comfortable and take the HandiHaler out of your mouth. Resume normal breathing. Repeat the above breathing steps again to be sure that you get a full dose of Spiriva. Do not press the green button again.

Once finished, open the mouthpiece, turn the HandiHaler upside down to tip out the used capsule and discard the used capsule. Close the mouthpiece and dust cap.

Clean the HandiHaler once monthly by opening the dust cap, mouthpiece, and base and rinse completely to remove any powder. Remove excess water and allow the HandiHaler to air dry for 24 h.

Missed Doses. Take Spiriva at regular intervals. If you miss a dose, take it as soon as you remember. If it almost time for the next dose, take that dose only (skip the missed dose) and then resume your regular schedule. Do not double the dose or take extra doses.

Pharmacokinetics. *Onset and Duration.* Time-to-peak concentration 5 min; time-to-peak effect 2–3 weeks; duration >24 h.

Fate. Dry powder administration results in the majority of the drug delivered into the GI tract and to a lesser extent to the lungs. The absolute bioavailability is 19.5%, indicating that the fraction reaching the lungs is highly bioavailable. Tiotropium is poorly absorbed from the gut. After dry powder inhalation, 14% is excreted via urinary tract, with the remainder eliminated via feces as unabsorbed drug.

$t_{1/2}$. is 5–6 days.

Adverse Reactions. Paradoxical bronchospasm, hypersensitivity reactions; angina, chest pain; dry mouth, dyspepsia, pharyngitis, rhinitis.

Precautions. May worsen signs and symptoms of narrow-angle glaucoma, benign prostatic hyperplasia or bladder neck obstruction. Patients with a creatinine clearance of <50 mL/min should be monitored closely, since tiotropium is predominantly renally eliminated.

Drug Interactions. Coadministration with other anticholinergic drugs such as ipratropium is not recommended, otherwise none known.

Parameters to Monitor. Hypersensitivity reactions; narrow-angle glaucoma (eye pain or discomfort, blurred vision, visual halos/colored images). Monitor renal function in patients with renal impairment. Also monitor administration technique, symptoms of bronchoconstriction.

Notes. Recent studies have evaluated the increased risk of cardiovascular death, myocardial infarction and stroke in patients with COPD who used inhaled anticholinergic medications. Most of the excess risk appeared to come from studies in which ipratropium and tiotropium were taken for at least 6 months. The study concluded that decisions should be made by prescribers and patients regarding risk vs. benefits of these agents.[13] The FDA has since received preliminary data from the UPLIFT trial as reported by the manufacturer of tiotropium demonstrating no increased risk of stroke with tiotropium bromide (Spiriva HandiHaler) compared to placebo.[32]

ZAFIRLUKAST	Accolate

Pharmacology. Zafirlukast is a selective competitive leukotriene-receptor antagonist (LTD_4 and LTE_4). Leukotrienes produce airway edema and smooth muscle constriction and are associated with the inflammatory process. Treatment with zafirlukast inhibits bronchoconstriction and bronchial hyperresponsiveness following allergen challenge. Leukotriene-receptor antagonists are an alternative, not preferred, treatment option for mild persistent asthma, and can be used as adjunct therapy with inhaled corticosteroids.[2]

Administration and Dosage. **PO for asthma (adults and children ≥12 years)**— 20 mg bid.

Administration with a high-fat or high-protein meal decreases bioavailability by 40%. Zafirlukast should be taken on an empty stomach, 1 h before or 2 h after a meal.

Pediatric Dosage. **PO for asthma (children 5–11 years)** 10 mg bid; **(children <5 years)** dosing not established.

Geriatric Dosage. Usual adult dose.

Dosage Forms. **Tab** 10 and 20 mg.

Patient Instructions. This medication is to help prevent the symptoms of your asthma. It is not for the quick reversal of an asthma attack. **Take this medication on an empty stomach, either 1 h before or 2 h after a meal.** Take it exactly as prescribed, even though you may not be having symptoms of your asthma. Be sure that your doctor knows all medications that you are taking, and contact your doctor if you begin taking any new prescription medicines, herbal or over-the-counter medicine. If you miss a dose of this medication, take it as soon as you remember; if it is almost time for your next dose, skip the missed dose and resume your regular schedule. Do not double doses.

A rare side effect of this medication is liver failure. Your doctor may test your blood to be sure that you do not develop this side effect. You should notify your doctor immediately if you have any of these symptoms: Pain in the upper right side of your abdomen, nausea, fatigue, itching, jaundice (yellowing of your skin or eyes), flulike symptoms, or if you have no appetite.

Pharmacokinetics. *Onset and Duration.* **Onset** 1 week; **peak** 3 h; **duration** $t_{1/2}$. 8–16 h. Accumulation in plasma following bid dosing is ~45%.

Fate. Absorption is rapid, but bioavailability is decreased after a high-fat or high-protein meal. Plasma protein binding is >99% (primarily albumin). Zafirlukast is extensively metabolized via CYP450 2C9 to metabolites that are less potent ($90\times$) than the parent drug. Elimination is 90% fecal and 10% renal.

Adverse Reactions. More common—headache, nausea, vomiting, diarrhea, abdominal pain, back pain, fever, infections (especially elderly patients). Rare—elevated serum transaminases (in particular ALT), systemic eosinophilia, usually associated with concomitant reduction in corticosteroid therapy, hypersensitivity reactions (including urticaria, angioedema, and rashes), agranulocytosis, bleeding/bruising.

Precautions. Use during breast-feeding is not recommended. In clinical trials (patients ≥55 years), the incidence of respiratory tract infections was greater than other age groups; the clinical significance is unknown.

Drug Interactions. **Warfarin:** Coadministration with zafirlukast results in a clinically significant increase in PT/INR; erythromycin (decrease zafirlukast levels by 40%); theophylline; aspirin. Zafirlukast is metabolized via the CYP450 2C9, but is also an inhibitor of CYP3A4 in vitro, so appropriate monitoring should be used when drugs affected by these pathways are coadministered, although no formal drug–drug interaction studies have been conducted.

Parameters to Monitor. Consider monitoring hepatic transaminases; watch for symptoms of liver dysfunction. Educate patient to self-monitor for liver dysfunction. Monitor asthma symptoms.

Notes. Refer to Notes of Montelukast (Singulair) regarding FDA review of behavioral/mood changes in patients receiving therapy with montelukast (Singulair), zafirlukast (Accolate), and zileuton (Zyflo).

ZILEUTON	Zyflo, Zyflo CR

Pharmacology. Zileuton inhibits the formation of leukotrienes LTC_4, LTD_4, LTE_4, and LTB_4. These leukotrienes augment the migration and aggregation of neutrophils, eosinophils, and monocytes, and increase leukocyte adhesion, capillary permeability, and smooth muscle contraction, all of which contribute to the inflammation, mucus secretion, edema, and bronchoconstriction in asthma. Because of more limited efficacy data and the need to monitor hepatic function, zileuton is a less desirable treatment option than the other leukotriene modifiers (leukotriene-receptor antagonists) montelukast and zafirlukast.[2]

Administration and Dosage. PO for asthma prophylaxis IR (adults and children ≥12 years)—600 mg qid with meals and at bedtime; CR (adults and children ≥12 years)—1200 mg bid with morning and evening meals. Do not chew, cut, or crush ER tabs. **Dosage** reduction may be necessary in hepatic dysfunction (see **Precautions**).

Pediatric Dosage. PO for asthma prophylaxis—(children <12 years) dosage not established.

Geriatric Dosage. PO for asthma prophylaxis—usual adult dose. However, females >65 years appear to be at increased risk for serum transaminase (ALT) elevations.

Hepatic Dysfunction. Contraindicated in patients with active liver disease or transaminase elevations ≥3× upper limits of normal.

Dosage Forms. Tab 600 mg; CR Tab 600 mg.

Patient Instructions. You should take Zyflo/Zyflo CR within 1 h after eating a meal. You should not take Zyflo/Zyflo CR if you have active liver disease or your liver enzymes are elevated. Inform your doctor before you take Zyflo/Zyflo CR if you have ever had liver disease, hepatitis, jaundice (yellowing of your skin or eyes), or dark colored urine. Also inform your doctor if you drink alcohol and about any prescription and nonprescription medications that you take (including over-the-counter medicines and herbal supplements). If you miss a dose of this medication, take it as soon as you remember; if it is almost time for your next dose, skip the missed dose and resume your regular schedule. Do not double doses.

Your doctor will evaluate your liver enzymes with a blood test before you start treatment with Zyflo/Zyflo CR, then once a month for the first 3 months that you are on this medication, and then every 2–3 months for the first year. After that, your liver enzymes will be checked periodically while you are on this therapy. Be sure and contact your health care provider if you have any of the following symptoms: Pain in the upper right side of your abdomen, nausea, fatigue, itching, jaundice (yellowing of your skin or eyes), flulike symptoms, or if you have no appetite.

Pharmacokinetics. *Onset* 2 h; *duration* 6–12 h.

Fate. Zileuton is well absorbed orally; absorption, peak plasma concentrations and half-life are increased in the presence of food. Time to peak concentration—1.7 h. It is 93% plasma protein bound (primarily albumin). It is metabolized by CYP1A2, 2C9, and 3A4. The mean plasma clearance in mild-to-moderate hepatic impairment was approximately half of that of healthy subjects. (**See Precautions.**)

$t_{1/2}$. IR 2.5h; ER 3.2h.

Adverse Reactions. Studies have shown that elevations of hepatic transaminases 2–5× ULN (particularly ALT) occurred in 1.9%–4.6% of patients treated with Zyflo. Females >65 years and patients with preexisting elevations of transaminases appeared to be at increased risk. See also **Precautions** for information regarding hepatic dysfunction.

The most common adverse reactions are headache, sinusitis, nausea, pharyngolaryngeal pain, and myalgia. GI effects such as upper abdominal pain, diarrhea, vomiting, and dyspepsia occur occasionally. Low WBC counts occur at rates greater than those in placebo-treated patients.

Precautions. Zileuton is contraindicated in patients with active liver disease or transaminase elevations $\geq 3\times$ upper limits of normal. Zileuton is not intended for use to reverse acute bronchospasm.

Drug Interactions. Zileuton increases the half-life and maximum concentration of theophylline and decreases clearance by $\sim 50\%$, which has resulted in an increase in theophylline-related adverse effects. Upon initiation of zileuton, theophylline dosage should be reduced by approximately one-half and theophylline levels monitored closely. Concomitant administration of zileuton and warfarin resulted in a decrease in warfarin clearance and a clinically significant increase in prothrombin time. Zileuton administration with propranolol decreases propranolol clearance and increases the C_{max}, AUC, and elimination half-life of propranolol, increasing β-blockade and resulting in decreased heart rate. Caution should be applied when administering zileuton concomitantly with other agents that share its metabolic pathways.

Parameters to Monitor. Obtain ALT at baseline and monthly for 3 months, then every 2–3 months for the remainder of the first year, then periodically. Monitor asthma symptoms and pulmonary function.

■ REFERENCES

1. Tashkin DP, Jenne JW. Beta adrenergic agonists. In: Weiss EB et al., eds. *Bronchial Asthma: Mechanisms and Therapeutics*. 3rd ed. Boston, MA: Little, Brown and Company; 1993:700-748.
2. National Heart, Lung and Blood Institute. *National Asthma Education and Prevention Program Expert Panel Report 3: Guidelines for the Diagnosis and Management of Asthma*. NIH Publication No. 08-5846. Bethesda, MD: National Heart, Lung and Blood Institute; 2007.
3. Spitzer OW et al. The use of β-agonists and the risk of death and near death from asthma. *N Engl J Med*. 1992;326:501-506.
4. Mullen M et al. The association between β-agonist use and death from asthma. A meta-analytic integration of case-control studies. *JAMA*. 1993;270:1842-1845.
5. Murphy S, Kelly HW. Cromolyn sodium: a review of its mechanisms and clinical use in asthma. *Drug Intell Clin Pharm*. 1987;21:22-35.
6. Berman BA. Cromolyn: past, present, and future. *Pediatr Clin North Am*. 1983;30:915-930.
7. Joseph JC. Compatibility of nebulized admixtures. *Ann Pharmacother*. 1997;31:487-489.
8. Edwards AM. Oral sodium cromoglycate: its use in the management of food allergy. *Clin Exp Allergy*. 1995; 25(suppl 1):31-33.
9. Milner AD. Ipratropium bromide in airways obstruction in childhood. *Postgrad Med J*. 1987;63(suppl 1): 53-56.
10. Gross NJ. Ipratropium bromide. *N Engl J Med*. 1988;319:486-494.
11. Shuk S et al. Efficacy of frequent nebulized ipratropium bromide added to frequent high-dose albuterol therapy in severe childhood asthma. *J Pediatr*. 1995;126:639-645.
12. Chung KF. Leukotriene receptor antagonists and biosynthesis inhibitors: potential breakthrough in asthma therapy. *Eur Respir J*. 1995;8:1203-1213.
13. Larsen JS et al. Antileukotriene therapy for asthma. *Am J Health Syst Pharm*. 1996;53:2821-2830.
14. Wasserman SI. A review of some recent clinical studies with nedocromil sodium. *J Allergy Clin Immunol*. 1993;92:210-215.
15. Brogden RN, Sorkin EM. Nedocromil sodium. An updated review of its pharmacological properties and therapeutic efficacy in asthma. *Drugs*. 1993;45:693-715.

16. Brogden RN, Faulds D. Salmeterol xinafoate. A review of its pharmacological properties and therapeutic potential in reversible obstructive airway disease. *Drugs*. 1991;42:895-912.

17. Jenne JW. Physiology and pharmacodynamics of the xanthines. In: Jenne JW, Murphy S, eds. *Drug Therapy for Asthma: Research and Clinical Practice*. New York: Marcel Dekker; 1987:297-334.

18. National Heart, Lung, and Blood Institute. *Expert Panel Report 2: Guidelines for the Diagnosis and Management of Asthma*. Publication No. 97-4051. Bethesda, MD: National Heart, Lung, and Blood Institute, National Asthma Education and Prevention Program, U.S. Department of Health and Human Services; 1997.

19. Weinberger MM et al. Theophylline in asthma. *N Engl J Med*. 1996;334:1380-1388.

20. Weinberger MM, Hendeles L. Theophylline. In: Middleton E et al., eds. *Allergy: Principles and Practice*. St. Louis, MO: Mosby; 1993:816-855.

21. Asmus MJ et al. Pharmacokinetics and drug disposition: apparent decrease in population clearance of theophylline: implications for dosage. *Clin Pharmacol Ther*. 1997;62:483-489.

22. Self TH et al. Reassessing the therapeutic range for theophylline on laboratory report forms: the importance of 5–15 μg/mL. *Pharmacotherapy*. 1993;13:590-594.

23. Hendeles L, Weinberger M. Selection of a slow-release theophylline product. *J Allergy Clin Immunol*. 1986;78:743-751.

24. Morris JF. Geriatric considerations. In: Weiss EB et al., eds. *Bronchial Asthma: Mechanisms and Therapeutics*. 3rd ed. Boston, MA: Little, Brown and Company; 1993:1017-1022.

25. Kelly HW. Theophylline toxicity. In: Jenne JW, Murphy S, eds. *Drug Therapy for Asthma: Research and Clinical Practice*. New York: Marcel Dekker; 1987:925-951.

26. González MA et al. Pharmacokinetic comparison of a once-daily and twice-daily theophylline delivery system. *Clin Ther*. 1994;16:686-692.

27. Campoli-Richards DM et al. Cetirizine. A review of its pharmacological properties and clinical potential in allergic rhinitis, pollen-induced asthma, and chronic urticaria. *Drugs*. 1990:40:762-781.

28. Mansmann HC et al. Efficacy and safety of cetirizine in perennial allergic rhinitis. *Ann Allergy*. 1992;68:348-353.

29. Spencer CM et al. Cetirizine. A reappraisal of its pharmacological properties and therapeutic use in selected allergic disorders. *Drugs*. 1993;46:1055-1080.

30. Barnes CL et al. Cetirizine: a new, nonsedating antihistamine. *Ann Pharmacother*. 1993;27:464-470.

31. González MA, Straughn AB. Effect of meals and dosage-form modification on theophylline bioavailability from a 24-hour sustained-release delivery system. *Clin Ther*. 1994;16:804-814.

32. Simons FER et al. Pharmacokinetics and efficacy of chlorpheniramine in children. *J Allergy Clin Immunol*. 1982;69:376-381.

Chapter 58

Antihistamines

Laura L. Sanders

Class Instructions. These medications can cause drowsiness, dry mouth, or occasional dizziness. The second-generation agents cetirizine, fexofenadine, loratadine, and desloratadine are preferred for initial management of allergic symptoms due to decreased sedation, performance impairment, and/or anticholinergic side effects compared to earlier agents.[1] Until the extent of drowsiness is known, caution should be used when driving, operating machinery, or performing other tasks requiring mental alertness or motor coordination while taking either first- or second-generation antihistamines. Excessive use of alcohol and other central nervous system depressants that cause drowsiness should be avoided while taking antihistamines. Consider risk–benefit ratio when using antihistamines (especially first generation agents) in patients with the following medical conditions: bladder neck obstruction, prostatic hypertrophy, urinary retention, and glaucoma. Intranasal antihistamines have demonstrated efficacy equal or superior to oral second-generation antihistamines for the treatment of allergic rhinitis, but are generally less effective than intranasal corticosteroids.[1] Antihistamines effectively suppress seasonal allergic rhinitis only when taken continuously. Extended-release (ER) formulations and capsules should be swallowed whole—do not cut, crush, or chew.

Missed Doses. Missed doses should be taken as soon as possible. However, if it is almost time for the next dose, skip the missed dose and go back to the regular dosage schedule. Do not double doses.

CETIRIZINE   Zyrtec OTC

Pharmacology. Cetirizine, a metabolite of hydroxyzine, is a low-sedating, long-acting peripheral H1 receptor antagonist. Cetirizine competitively inhibits the interaction of histamine with H1 receptors, thereby preventing the allergic response with low anticholinergic and antiserotonergic activity.

Administration and Dosage. PO for allergies tablet, chewable tablet, syrup (adults and children >6 years)— 5–10 mg/d depending on symptom severity.

Special Populations. *Pediatric Dosage.* PO for allergies (children 2–6 years)— syrup 2.5 mg (2.5 mL or half teaspoonful) qd–bid or 5 mg (5 mL or 1 teaspoonful) qd; do not exceed 5 mg (5 mL or 1 teaspoonful) in 24 h.

Geriatric Dosage. PO for allergies—reducing dosage in geriatric patients might be necessary because of a 50% increase in cetirizine's half-life and a 40% decrease in clearance. In patients >65 years, the recommended dosage is 5 mg qd.

Other Conditions. In patients with Cl_{Cr} of 11–31 mL/min, those on hemodialysis, and in hepatically impaired patients, give 5 mg/d.

Dosage Forms. Tab 5, 10 mg; Chew Tab 5, 10 mg; syrup 1 mg/mL.

Patient Instructions. *See* Class Information, Antihistamines.

Pharmacokinetics. *Onset and Duration.* Onset within 1 h. Duration is 24 h.

Fate. Cetirizine is rapidly absorbed after oral administration. Peak serum levels are reached within 1 h. Food does not affect the amount absorbed but might decrease the absorption rate. Protein binding averages 93%. Cl in normal adults is 0.04–0.05 L/kg/h. Cetirizine is oxidized to a small extent to inactive metabolites. After a 10-mg dose, 70% of the drug is excreted unchanged in the urine within 72 h and 10% is excreted in feces. Cetirizine is not appreciably dialyzable.[2–6]

$t_{1/2}$. (adults) 7–10 h; (children) 6–7 h; (elderly/renal insufficiency) 18–21 h.[2–6]

Adverse Reactions. The most frequent side effects are sedation, headache, dry mouth, fatigue, and nausea. Cetirizine 10 mg/d produces more sedation than loratadine 10 mg/d or placebo. Cetirizine has not been implicated in cardiac adverse events. Higher-than-recommended doses of cetirizine (up to 60 mg daily) did not prolong the QT interval in 25 healthy volunteers.

Contraindications/Precautions. Do not use cetirizine in patients who have a hypersensitivity to hydroxyzine or cetirizine. Sedative effects may be dose dependent.

Drug Interactions. Exercise caution when cetirizine is combined with anticholinergic agents, alcohol, or other CNS depressants. Because most of cetirizine is eliminated renally, cytochrome P450 interactions are not likely. Clinically important drug interactions have *not* been found with cetirizine and azithromycin, pseudoephedrine, ketoconazole, or erythromycin. Clearance of cetirizine was reduced slightly by a 400-mg dose of theophylline, but this reduction was not clinically important; however, larger doses might have a greater effect. Therefore, it seems appropriate to monitor patients for increased sedation or other CNS-related side effects when administering theophylline concomitantly with cetirizine.

Parameters to Monitor. (Allergic rhinitis) observe for sneezing, rhinorrhea, itchy nose, and conjunctivitis. Monitor for side effects such as sedation.

Notes. In 2008, Zyrtec became available without a prescription (OTC) and is no longer available by prescription. Children's Zyrtec Hives Relief Syrup contains 5 mg of cetiriaine/5 mL teaspoonful (1 mg/mL). The dosage for adults and children ≥6 years and adults ≥65 years is the same as children's Zyrtec syrup. A combination product, Zyrtec D, is available without a prescription, but is a "behind-the-counter" product. It is an antihistamine (cetirizine 5 mg) decongestant (pseudoephedrine HCl 120 mg) formulation. The dosage for adults and children ≥12 years is 1 tablet every 12 h (maximum 2 tablets/24 h).

CHLORPHENIRAMINE MALEATE	Chlor-Trimeton, Various

Pharmacology. Chlorpheniramine is a propylamine derivative that competitively antagonizes the activity of histamine at the H1-histamine receptor, preventing allergic responses mediated by histamine. It also has anticholinergic and transient sedative effects when used intermittently.

Administration and Dosage. **PO for seasonal allergic rhinitis tablets, chewable tablets, and syrup (adults and adolescents)**—4 mg every 4–6 h prn up to 24 mg/d; **ER tablets and capsules (adults and adolescents)**—8–12 mg every 8–12 h prn; do not cut, crush, or chew ER formulation. **IM, IV, SQ (adults and adolescents)**—5–40 mg once as needed, up to 40 mg/d. Effectiveness of PO dosing is maximized if given continuously, starting just before the pollen season.

Initiate dosing at 4 mg qhs initially, increasing gradually over 10 days as tolerated to 24 mg/d in 1–2 divided doses until the end of the season. **PO for acute allergic reactions**—12 mg in 1–2 divided doses. **ER**—(*See* Notes.)

Special Populations. *Pediatric Dosage.* **PO for seasonal allergic rhinitis (children <12 years)**— ER tablets and capsules not recommended; **(tablets, chewable tablets, syrup)**—87.5 μg (0.0875 mg)/kg body weight or 2.5 mg/m² q6h prn. **OR** 1 mg every 4–6 h up to 4 mg/d; **(children aged 6–12 years)**—2 mg every 4–6 h up to 12 mg/d. Initiate at 2 mg, increasing gradually over 10 days as tolerated to 12 mg/d in 1–2 divided doses until the end of the season.[7] (*See* Notes.)

Geriatric Dosage. **PO**—(≥60 years) 4 mg daily–bid.

Dosage Forms. **Chew Tab** 2 mg; **Tab** 4 mg; **syrup** 0.2 mg/mL, 0.4 mg/mL; **ER Cap** 8, 12 mg (*see* Notes); **ER Tab** 8, 12 mg (*see* Notes); **Cap** 4 mg; 10 mg with pseudoephedrine HCl 60 and 65 mg, respectively (various), and 8, 12 mg with pseudoephedrine HCl 120 mg (various); **IM, SQ, IV**—10 mg/mL.

Patient Instructions. *See* Class Information, Antihistamines.

Pharmacokinetics. *Onset and Duration.* Onset is 0.25–1 h; duration of suppression of wheal and flare response (IgE mediated) to skin tests with allergenic extract is 2 days.[8] Fast metabolizers have an earlier, greater, and more prolonged antihistaminic response than slow metabolizers because of rapid conversion to active metabolite.[9] Time to peak 2–6 h; duration is 4–8 h. In the elderly, duration of action can be ≥ 36 h, even when serum concentrations are low.[10]

Serum Levels. Serum chlorpheniramine levels do not correlate with histamine antagonist activity because of an unidentified active metabolite.[9] (Children) 2.3–12 μg/L (6–31 nmol/L) suppress allergic rhinitis symptoms; (children) 4–10 μg/L (11–26 nmol/L) suppress histamine-induced wheal and flare.[7]

Fate. Oral bioavailability is approximately 34%; 72% is plasma protein bound.[10] V_d is (adults) 3.2 ± 0.3 L/kg; (children) 7 ± 2.8 L/kg; Cl is (adults) 0.1 ± 0.006 L/h/kg; (children) 0.43 ± 0.19 L/h/kg.[7,11] Rapidly and extensively metabolized by CYP2D6 to mono- and didesmethylchlorpheniramine and unidentified metabolites, one or more of which are active. Metabolites and a small amount of parent drug are excreted in urine.[8,12]

$t_{1/2}$. (adults) 20 ± 5 h; (children) 13 ± 6 h; (chronic renal failure) 280–330 h.[7,11,12]

Adverse Reactions. Frequent drowsiness, dry mouth, dizziness, and irritability occur with intermittent therapy; however, most patients develop tolerance to these side effects during continuous therapy, particularly if the dosage is increased slowly.

Contraindications. Lactation; premature and newborn infants.

Precautions. Use chlorpheniramine with caution in patients ≥60 years. Dizziness, sedation, confusion, and hypotension may be more likely in geriatric patients, and geriatric patients may be more susceptible to anticholinergic side effects such as dry mouth and urinary retention. A paradoxical reaction of hyperexcitability may occur in older patients and in children. OTC labeling states to avoid in patients with narrow-angle glaucoma, symptomatic prostatic hypertrophy, asthma, emphysema, chronic pulmonary disease, shortness of breath, or breathing difficulties except under physician supervision; however, many studies have shown some bronchodilator effect of H1 receptor antagonists.[9]

Drug Interactions. MAOIs prolong and intensify the anticholinergic effects of antihistamines.[13] Alcohol or sedative-hypnotics can increase CNS depressant effects. Other medications with anticholinergic activity may potentiate the anticholinergic activity of antihistamines. Patients should report GI disturbances promptly due to risk of paralytic ileus with concurrent therapy.

Parameters to Monitor. In seasonal allergic rhinitis, observe for sneezing, rhinorrhea, itchy nose, and conjunctivitis.

Notes. Brompheniramine is a compound similar to chlorpheniramine (propylamine derivative). It is available in capsule, tablet, elixir and injectable forms. **PO antihistaminic: Adult and adolescent ($\geq$ 12 years)**—4 mg every 4–6 h prn with a maximum of 24 mg/d. **Children < 12 years (elixir)**—0.5 mg/kg or 15 mg/m^2 daily in 3–4 divided doses prn OR **children 2–6 years (elixir)**—1 mg every 4–6 h prn; **6–12 years (elixir)**—2 mg every 4–6 h prn.

CLEMASTINE FUMARATE
Tavist, Dayhist, Various

Pharmacology. Clemastine is an ethanolamine derivative H1 receptor antagonist used in the treatment of allergies that prevent allergen responses mediated by histamine. The anticholinergic action also provides a drying effect on the nasal mucosa. Ethanolamine derivatives show greater anticholinergic activity than other classes of antihistamines.

Dosage and Administration. PO for allergy: tablets (adults and children $\geq$12 years)—1 tab q12h, maximum 2 tablets/d; syrup 1.34 mg bid or 2.68 mg qd–tid prn. (Dermatological indications—2.68-mg dosage only).

Special Populations. *Pediatric Dosage.* PO for allergy: syrup, tablets (children 6–12 years)—0.67–1.34 mg bid, maximum 4.02 mg/d; (dermatological indications—1.34-mg dosage only). (Children <6 years)—dosage not established.
May be taken with food if causes GI distress.

Geriatric Dosage. Usual adult dosage. However geriatric patients may be more sensitive to effects; sedation, confusion, hypotension, and anticholinergic side effects may be more pronounced.

Dosage Forms. Tab 1.34, 2.68 mg; syrup 0.67 mg/5 mL.

Patient Information. Refer to Class Information at the beginning of this chapter.

Pharmacokinetics. *Onset and Duration.* Onset 15–60 min. Duration 12 h.

Fate. Absorption is rapid and complete, with time-to-peak plasma concentration 2–4 h; time to peak effect 5–7 h. Metabolized in the liver and excreted in the urine.

Adverse Reactions. Most common include drowsiness; dry mouth, nose, or throat; GI distress; headache. Clemastine has greater anticholinergic activity than other antihistamines, so these effects may be more numerous. Occasional paradoxical reactions of excitability are seen, particularly in the elderly.

Contraindications/Precautions. Refer to Class Information at the beginning of this chapter. Do not use concomitantly with MAOIs; do not use if breast-feeding or in infants.

Drug Interactions. Additive effects with CNS depressants; MAOIs may increase anticholinergic effects.

Parameters to Monitor. Allergy symptoms; dizziness, drowsiness, anticholinergic effects.

DESLORATADINE
Clarinex, Clarinex RediTabs

Pharmacology. Desloratadine, a major metabolite of loratadine, is a long-acting histamine antagonist with selective H1 receptor activity indicated for relief of seasonal and perennial allergic rhinitis and chronic idiopathic urticaria.

Administration and Dosage. PO for allergic rhinitis, chronic idiopathic urticaria (adults and children ≥ 12 years)—tablets 5 mg once daily; **syrup** 2 teaspoonfuls (5 mg in 10 mL) once daily.

Special Populations. *Pediatric Dosage.* **PO as antihistamine (children 6–11 years)— (syrup)** 1 teaspoonful (2.5 mg in 5 mL) once daily, **(RediTabs)** 2.5 mg once daily; **(children 12 months–5 years)—(syrup)** half teaspoonful (1.25 mg in 2.5 mL) once daily; **(children 6–11 months)—(syrup)** 2 mL (1.0 mg) once daily. Administer Clarinex syrup using a measuring dropper/syringe calibrated to deliver 2.0 and 2.5 mL. Place RediTabs on the tongue and allow to disintegrate before swallowing; administer with or without water.

Geriatric Dosage. See usual adult dosage.

Hepatic or Renal Impairment. (Adults) starting dose of one 5-mg tablet every other day is recommended. **(Children)** no dosing recommendations due to lack of pharmacokinetic data.

Dosage Forms. Tab 5 mg; **syrup** 0.5 mg/mL; **RediTabs** 2.5, 5 mg.

Patient Instructions. Clarinex may be taken without regard to meals. Use only as directed—do not increase dose or dosing frequency, as this does not increase effectiveness, but may increase drowsiness.

Pharmacokinetics. *Onset and Duration.* Onset within 1 h; duration up to 24 h.

Fate. Time to maximum plasma concentrations following sequential dosing (5 mg qd for 10 days) was 3 h. Desloratadine (a major metabolite of loratadine) is extensively metabolized to 3-hydroxydesloratadine. (The enzymes responsible have not been identified.) Approximately 6% of subjects in pharmacokinetic studies were poor metabolizers, resulting in increased exposure to desloratadine, which could result in an increased risk of adverse effects. Protein binding for desloratadine and its metabolite 3-hydroxydesloratadine is 82%–89%; $t_{1/2}$ is 27 h.

Adverse Reactions. There were no serious adverse events in patients receiving desloratadine in placebo-controlled trials. Adverse reactions reported by > 2% of patients that were more common than placebo included pharyngitis (4%), dry mouth (3%), myalgia, fatigue, somnolence, dysmenorrhea (all 2.1%).

Contraindications. Hypersensitivity to loratadine.

Precautions. Clarinex RediTabs contain phenylalanine (1.4 mg/2.5 mg or 2.9 mg/5 mg).

Drug Interactions. No significant interactions.

Parameters to Monitor. Symptoms of allergic rhinitis, urticaria.

Notes. Desloratadine is available in an ER formulation with pseudoephedrine as 2.5 mg desloratadine/120 mg pseudoephedrine (Clarinex-D 12 h ER) and desloratadine 5 mg/240 mg pseudoephedrine (Clarinex-D 24 h ER). Dosage for adults and children ≥12 years is 1 tablet once daily (Clarinex-D 24 h ER) or 1 tablet every 12 h (Clarinex-D 12 h ER). This formulation should be used with caution in patients with hypertension, diabetes, heart disease, increased intraocular pressure, hyperthyroidism, or prostatic hypertrophy. Clarinex-D ER is contraindicated in patients with narrow-angle glaucoma or urinary retention, and should be avoided in patients with renal or hepatic impairment. It should not be given within 14 days of MAOIs. Adverse reactions to Clarinex-D ER include insomnia, headache, dry mouth, fatigue, pharyngitis, dizziness, nausea, and anorexia. Clarinex-D ER tablets should be swallowed whole; do not break or chew.

DIPHENHYDRAMINE HYDROCHLORIDE
Benadryl, Various

Pharmacology. (*See* Chlorpheniramine.) Diphenhydramine is an ethanolamine derivative histamine antagonist. In addition to its antihistaminic uses, diphenhydramine is also indicated as an antidyskinetic, antiemetic, antitussive (syrup), antivertigo agent and a sedative-hypnotic. Diphenhydramine has strong sedating and anticholinergic properties.

Administration and Dosage. (**Adult and adolescent dose**): **PO as an antihistamine**—25–50 mg every 4–6 h prn; **PO for parkinsonism**—25 mg tid; may increase dose gradually prn to 50 mg qid; **PO for motion sickness/vertigo**—50 mg 30 min before exposure, then every 4–6 h prn; **PO as a nighttime sleep aid**—25–50 mg 20–30 min before bed; **PO as an antitussive**—25 mg every 4–6 h. **Maximum dose/d—300 mg PO.** **Deep IM or IV as an antihistamine or for allergic reactions to blood or plasma, adjunctive treatment of anaphylaxis, or parkinsonism**—10–50 mg/dose, up to 100 mg/dose if required, to a maximum of 400 mg/d. Do not exceed 25 mg/min IV. **Deep IM or IV as an antiemetic or antivertigo agent**—10 mg initially, then may increase to 20–50 mg every 2–3 h.

Special Populations. *Pediatric Dosage.* **PO as an antihistamine: capsules, tablets (children <6 years)**—6.25–12.5 mg every 4–6 h up to 37.5 mg/d; (**children 6–12 years**)—12.5–25 mg every 4–6 h up to 150 mg/d. **PO as an antiemetic or antivertigo agent**—1–1.5 mg/kg every 4–6 h up to 300 mg/d. (**Syrup) PO as an antihistamine**—(**elixir**) 1.25 mg/kg or 37.5 mg/m^2 every 4–6 h up to 300 mg/d; OR weight < 9.1 kg—6.25–12.5 mg every 4–6 h; weight ≥9.1 kg—12.5–25 mg every 4–6 h. **PO as an antiemetic or antivertigo agent (elixir)**—1–1.5 mg/kg every 4–6h prn up to 300 mg/d. **PO as an antitussive (elixir) (children < 2 years)**—dosage not available—use not recommended in premature and full-term neonates; (**children 2–6 years**)—6.25 mg every 4–6 h prn up to 25 mg/d; (**children 6–12 years**)—12.5 mg every 4–6 h prn up to 75 mg/d. **Deep IM or IV** (do not exceed 25 mg/min) 5 mg/kg/d or 150 mg/m^2/d in 4 divided doses, to a maximum of 300 mg/d.

Geriatric Dosage. **PO as an antihistamine**—25 mg bid–tid initially, then increase as needed.[14] (*See* Notes.)

Other Conditions. In renal impairment, increase dosage interval as follows: (Cl_{Cr} 10–50 mL/min), increase to 6–12 h; (Cl_{Cr} < 10 mL/min), increase to 12–18 h.[14]

Dosage Forms. **Cap** 25, 50 mg; **Chew Tab** 12.5 mg—this product has been discontinued—may be used until the expiration date; **Elxr** 2.5 mg/mL; **syrup** 1.25, 2.5 mg/mL; **prefilled spoons** 2.5 mg/mL (5-mL prefilled dose), **Tab** 25, 50 mg; **Inj** 10, 50 mg/mL.

Patient Instructions. *See* Class Information, Antihistamines.

Pharmacokinetics. *Onset and Duration.* Onset is 15 min after single oral dose; duration of suppression of wheal and flare is up to 2 days.[9,15] Duration of effect does not appear to be related to serum levels.

Serum Levels. (Antihistaminic effect) >25 μg/L (0.09 μmol/L); (sedation) 30–50 μg/L (0.1–0.17 μmol/L); (mental impairment) >60 μg/L (0.2 μmol/L).[11,15]

Fate. As a result of first-pass metabolism, oral bioavailability is variable, 61 ± 25%.[11,16] A single 50-mg oral dose in adults usually produces serum concentrations of 25–50 μg/L.[15] Approximately 85% is plasma protein bound and lower in Asians and those with cirrhosis.[17,18] V_d is 17.4 ± 4.8 L/kg in adults and larger in Asians and those with cirrhosis. Cl is 1.4 ± 0.6 L/h/kg in adults and higher in Asians and 0.7 ± 0.2 L/h/kg in the elderly.[11,14,16,17] Metabolized to N-dealkylated and acidic metabolites.[16,19] Less than 4% is excreted unchanged in urine.[20]

$t_{1/2}$. (adults) 9.2 ± 2.5 h; (elderly >65 years) 13.5 ± 4.2 h; (children 8–12 years) 5.4 ± 1.8 h[11,16]; (cirrhosis) 15 h.[18]

Adverse Reactions. Most common are sedation, dizziness, incoordination, gastric distress, thickening of bronchial secretions.

Contraindications. *See* Chlorpheniramine.

Precautions. Overdose in pediatric patients may cause hallucinations, convulsions or death. In the young pediatric patient, antihistamines may produce excitation. In the elderly, antihistamines are more likely to cause hypotension, sedation, and dizziness. Diphenhydramine possesses atropine-like effects and should be used with caution in patients with a history of asthma, increased intraocular pressure, cardiovascular disease, and hypertension.

Drug Interactions. Additive effects with alcohol and other CNS depressants. MAOIs may prolong the anticholinergic effects of antihistamines.

Parameters to Monitor. *See* Chlorpheniramine.

Notes. Because of its low degree of efficacy for pruritus, weak suppression of IgE-mediated skin tests, and high sedative potential, diphenhydramine is not the antihistamine of choice for most conditions. In the elderly, diphenhydramine is discouraged as a nighttime sleep aid because of its high anticholinergic potential. **Dimenhydrinate** (Dramamine), used for motion sickness, is the 8-chlorotheophyllinate salt of diphenhydramine; 100 mg dimenhydrinate is approximately equal to 50 mg diphenhydramine.

FEXOFENADINE   Allegra

Pharmacology. Fexofenadine is a histamine H1 receptor antagonist that is a metabolite of terfenadine. It causes little sedation and has little anticholinergic activity. (*See* Antihistamines Comparison Chart.)

Dosage and Administration. **PO for allergic rhinitis and chronic idiopathic urticaria tablet (adults and children ≥12 years)**—180 mg once daily or 60 mg bid; in renal impairment, reduce initial dosage to 60 mg/d. Administer with water.

Special Populations. *Pediatric Dosage.* **PO—tablets, capsules (<6 years)** safety and efficacy not established; **(6–11 years)** 30 mg bid with water; in pediatric patients with renal impairment, reduce initial dosage to 30 mg/d; **(≥12 years)** same as adult dosage. **(ODT)** only intended for use in patients 6–11 years; same dosage as tablet form. ODT should be allowed to disintegrate on the tongue and then swallowed, with or without water. It should be taken on an empty stomach and should not be chewed. **(Oral suspension) PO for seasonal allergic rhinitis and chronic idiopathic urticaria (children 2–11 years)**—30 mg (5 mL) bid; in decreased renal function, initial dose is 30 mg (5 mL) once daily. **Chronic idiopathic urticaria (children 6 months to <2 years)**—15 mg (2.5 mL) bid; in decreased renal function, 15 mg (2.5 mL) once daily. Shake bottle well before each use.

Dosage Forms. **Cap** 60 mg; **Tab** 30, 60, 180 mg; **ODT** 30 mg; **Oral Susp** 6 mg/mL; **ER Tab** 60 mg with pseudoephedrine 120 mg (Allegra-D 12 h) and 180 mg with pseudoephedrine 240 mg (Allegra-D 24 h).

Patient Instructions. Take with water; do not take with juices such as grapefruit, orange, apple, etc. Wait at least 15 min after taking fexofenadine to take an antacid containing aluminum or magnesium hydroxide. ER formulations (Allegra-D) should be taken on an empty stomach 1h before or 2 h after a meal; take with a full glass of water (no juice, milk, or antacids); do not crush or chew.

Pharmacokinetics. *Onset and Duration.* Onset is rapid; peak serum levels occur at 2.6 h (tablets, capsules), 2.0 h (ODT), 1 h (oral suspension). Food decreases oral absorption.

Fate. It is 60%–70% plasma protein bound and excreted unchanged in urine and feces. $t_{1/2}$ approximately 14 h in normal renal function and increases to approximately 19 h in severe renal impairment.

Adverse Reactions. Headache, back pain, cough, dysmenorrhea, somnolence/fatigue, fever, GI disturbances.

Precautions. Allegra ODT 30 mg contains 5.3 mg phenylalanine. Safety and efficacy of Allegra-D has not been established in children younger than 12 years.

Drug/Food Interactions. Antacids decrease AUC and C_{max} of fexofenadine; do not take closely in time. Erythromycin and ketoconazole increases plasma concentrations of fexofenadine; fruit juices (grapefruit, orange, apple) may reduce bioavailability of fexofenadine—take with water.

HYDROXYZINE HYDROCHLORIDE	Atarax, Vistaril, Various
HYDROXYZINE PAMOATE	Vistaril, Various

Pharmacology. Hydroxyzine is a piperazine derivative that is a competitive antagonist of histamine at the H1-histamine receptor. It also has antiemetic and sedative effects, thought to be a result of CNS subcortical suppression. Its bronchodilator, antihistaminic, and analgesic effects have been demonstrated experimentally and clinically, but claims of long-term antianxiety properties have not been substantiated by well-designed studies.

Administration and Adult Dosage. **PO for pruritus**—25 mg tid–qid. **PO for seasonal allergic rhinitis**—(effectiveness is maximized if given continuously just before the pollen season) 25 mg initially qhs until no sedation in the morning, then increase dosage every 2–3 days, to a maximum of 150 mg/d in 1–2 divided doses and maintain until the end of the season. Reduce dosage by one-third or more if sedation persists. Dosage may be increased, if tolerated, for symptoms during the peak of pollen season.[21] **PO for psychoneurosis-associated anxiety**—50–100 mg qid. **PO**

for sedation—50–100 mg. **IM for sedation before and after general anesthesia**—50–100 mg. **IM for nausea and vomiting and pre- and postoperative adjunctive medication**—25–100 mg. Preferred IM injection site is upper outer quadrant of gluteus maximus or midlateral thigh. **Not for SQ or intra-arterial use.**

Special Populations. *Pediatric Dosage.* **PO for pruritus**—(**<6 years**) 50 mg/d in 2–3 divided doses; (**≥6 years**) 50–100 mg/d in divided doses. **PO for seasonal allergic rhinitis**—10 mg initially qhs until no sedation in the morning, then increase dosage every 2–3 days, to a maximum of 75 mg/d in 1–2 divided doses and maintain until the end of the season. Reduce dosage by one-third or more if sedation persists. Dosage may be increased, if tolerated, for symptoms during the peak of pollen season.[21] **PO for psychoneurosis associated anxiety**—(**<6 years**) 50 mg daily in divided doses; (**>6 years**) 50–100 mg daily in divided doses. **IM for pre- and postoperative sedation**—0.5 mg/lb (HCl). **IM for nausea and vomiting and pre- and postoperative adjunctive medication**—1.1 mg/kg. Preferred site in children is midlateral muscles of the thigh.

Geriatric Dosage. **PO for pruritus**—10 mg tid–qid, increasing to 25 mg tid–qid if necessary.[22] In general, dosing should be initiated at the low end of the dosage range.

Dosage Forms. **Cap** (as pamoate equivalent of HCl salt) 25, 50, 100 mg; **Susp** (as pamoate equivalent of HCl salt) 5 mg/mL, **syrup** (as HCl) 2 mg/mL; **Tab** (as HCl) 10, 25, 50, 100 mg; **Inj** (as HCl) 25, 50 mg/mL (IM only).

Patient Instructions. (*See* Class Information, Antihistamines.) Shake suspension vigorously.

Pharmacokinetics. *Onset and Duration.* Onset 15–30 min after oral administration. Duration of suppression of wheal and flare response to allergenic extract skin test is 4 days.[9,22]

Serum Levels. (Pruritus) 6–42 μg/L (14–102 nmol/L) suppress pruritus in children.[23]

Fate. Peak serum level of 73 ± 11 μg/L occurs 2 ± 0.1 h after a 0.7 mg/kg dose in healthy adults, 117 ± 61 μg/L at 2.3 ± 0.7 h in primary biliary cirrhosis (mean dose 44 mg).[24,25] V_d is (healthy adults) 16 ± 3 L/kg,[24] (elderly) 23 ± 6 L/kg, (children) 19 ± 9 L/kg,[23] and (primary biliary cirrhosis) 23 ± 13 L/kg.[25] Cl is (healthy young and elderly adults) 0.6 ± 0.2 L/h/kg,[24,26] (children) 1.9 L/h/kg,[23] (primary biliary cirrhosis) 0.5 ± 0.4 L/h/kg.[25]

$t_{1/2}$. (healthy adults) 20 ± 4 h[24]; (elderly) 29 ± 10 h[26]; (children) 7 h, increasing with age[24]; (primary biliary cirrhosis) 37 ± 13 h.[25]

Adverse Reactions. Transient drowsiness and dry mouth occur frequently when the drug is taken intermittently. Most patients develop tolerance to these effects when the drug is taken continuously, particularly if the dosage is slowly increased over 7–10 days. IM injection can be painful and has caused sterile abscess. Hemolysis has been associated with IV administration and tissue necrosis with SQ or intra-arterial administration.

Contraindications. Early pregnancy, breast-feeding; SQ or intra-arterial use of injectable solution.

Precautions. Use with caution in the elderly.

Drug Interactions. MAOIs prolong and intensify the anticholinergic effects of antihistamines. Alcohol or sedative-hypnotics can increase CNS depressant effects.

When CNS depressants such as narcotics, nonnarcotic analgesics and barbiturates are administered concomitantly with hydroxyzine, their dosage should be reduced.

Parameters to Monitor. In seasonal allergic rhinitis, observe for sneezing, rhinorrhea, itchy nose, and conjunctivitis.

Notes. Hydroxyzine suppresses wheal and flare response to the greatest degree and for the longest duration of all antihistamines,[9] including the newer nonsedating antihistamines.[22]

LORATADINE
Claritin, Claritin RediTabs, Alavert, Various

Pharmacology. Loratadine is a long-acting piperidine antihistamine with selective peripheral H1 receptor antagonist activity. It is structurally similar to azatadine, with little or no action α-adrenergic or cholinergic receptors.[27] (*See* Antihistamines Comparison Chart.)

Dosage and Administration. PO for allergic rhinitis or urticaria (adults and children ≥6 years)—tablets and RediTabs 10 mg/d on an empty stomach; **(syrup)** 2 teaspoonfuls (10 mg).

Special Populations. *Pediatric Dosage.* PO (syrup)—**(<2 years)** safety and efficacy not established; **(2–5 years)** 1 teaspoonful (5 mg/d).

Geriatric Dosage. Usual adult dose.

Hepatic or Renal Failure. (GFR *<30 mL/min)*—**(adults and children ≥6 years)** start with dose of 10 mg every other day. **(Children 2–5 years)** start with dose of 5 mg every other day.

Dosage Forms. Tab 10 mg (conventional and rapidly dissolving); **Chew Tab** 5 mg; **syrup** 1 mg/mL; **Tab** 5 mg with pseudoephedrine 120 mg (Claritin-D); **Tab** 10 mg with pseudoephedrine 240 mg (Claritin-D 24 h).

Pharmacokinetics. The drug is rapidly absorbed; bioavailability and peak serum levels are increased by approximately 50% in the elderly (66–78 years) or when taken with food. It is 97% bound to plasma proteins and extensively metabolized to an active metabolite, descarboethoxyloratadine. Approximately 80% of a dose is excreted equally in urine and feces as metabolites after 10 days. The half-lives in healthy adults are 8.4 h (range 3–20) for loratadine and 28 h (range 8.8–92) for descarboethoxyloratadine.[27,28]

Adverse Reactions. Headache, somnolence, fatigue, dry mouth.

Notes. In 2002, the FDA approved loratadine as an over-the-counter (OTC) allergy drug product. It is available in tablet, rapidly disintegrating tablet and syrup forms for adults, and as flavored syrups, rapidly disintegrating tablets, and flavored chewables. Claritin-D is also available "behind-the-counter" as 12 h and 24 h formulations. The dosage of Claritin-D is 1 tablet bid on an empty stomach; Claritin-D 24 h is given once daily. This formulation should be used with caution in patients with hypertension, diabetes, heart disease, increased intraocular pressure, hyperthyroidism, narrow-angle glaucoma, urinary retention, or prostatic hypertrophy.

There have been postmarketing reports of upper GI tract obstruction in patients taking Claritin-D 24 h. In most cases, patients had a history of dysphagia. Patients with a known history of dysphagia should not use Claritin-D 24 h, but instead should be prescribed the 12-h formulation. The manufacturer has also redesigned the tablet shape.

ANTIHISTAMINES COMPARISON CHART

DRUG	DOSAGE FORMS	ADULT DOSAGE	PEDIATRIC DOSAGE	HALF-LIFE (h)	SIDE EFFECTS	
					Sedation[a]	Anticholinergic
Acrivastine	Tab 8 mg with pseudoephedrine 60 mg (Semprex-D)	PO 1 Tab every 4–6 h, to a maximum of 4/d	PO (>12 y) same as adult dosage	1.5–3	+	±
Azatadine Maleate Optimine	Tab 1 mg	PO 1–2 mg tid	(<12 y) safety and efficacy not established	12	+ +	+ +
Azelastine HCl Astelin	Nasal spray 125 μg/spray	2 sprays/nostril bid	(5–11 y) 1 spray/nostril bid; (≥12 y) same as adult dosage	22 (metabolite: 54)	+ +	+ +
Brompheniramine Maleate Dimetapp Allergy Various	Cap 4 mg Inj 10 mg/mL	PO 4 mg every 4–6 h, to a maximum of 24 mg/d SQ, IM, or slow IV 5–20 mg q12h, a maximum of 40 mg/d	PO (<12 y) 0.5 mg/kg/d In 3–4 doses SQ, IM, or slow IV 0.5 mg/kg/d in 3–4 divided doses	25	+	+ +

(continued)

953

ANTIHISTAMINES COMPARISON CHART (continued)

DRUG	DOSAGE FORMS	ADULT DOSAGE	PEDIATRIC DOSAGE	HALF-LIFE (h)	SIDE EFFECTS	
					Sedation[a]	Anticholinergic
Carbinoxamine Maleate Various	Drp 2 mg with pseudoephedrine 25 mg/mL Soln 0.4 mg/mL Syrup 0.4, 0.8 mg with pseudoephedrine 6, 12 mg/mL, respectively Tab 4 mg with pseudoephedrine 60 mg (Carbodec, Rondec) SR Tab 8 mg with pseudoephedrine 90 mg (Palgic-D)	PO 1 Tab qid	PO 0.2–0.4 mg/kg/d; (1–3 y) 2 mg tid–qid; (3–6 y) 2–4 mg tid–qid; (>6 y) 4–6 mg tid–qid (dosage refers to carbinoxamine component)	10–20	++	+++
Cetirizine HCl Zyrtec	Refer to cetirizine monograph			7–10	+	±
Chlorpheniramine Maleate Chlor-Trimeton Various	Refer to chlorpheniramine monograph			15–25	+	++
Clemastine Fumarate Tavist Various	Refer to clemastine monograph			21	++	+++

(continued)

ANTIHISTAMINES COMPARISON CHART (continued)

DRUG	DOSAGE FORMS	ADULT DOSAGE	PEDIATRIC DOSAGE	HALF-LIFE (h)	SIDE EFFECTS	
					Sedation[a]	Anticholinergic
Cyproheptadine HCl Periactin Various	Tab 4 mg Syrup 0.4 mg/mL	PO 4–20 mg/d, usually 4 mg tid–qid, to a maximum of 0.5 mg/kg/d	PO (2–6 y) 2 mg bid–tid, to a maximum of 12 mg/d; (7–14 y) 4 mg bid–tid, to a maximum of 16 mg/d	—	+	++
Desloratadine Clarinex	Refer to desloratadine monograph			28	±	±
Dexchlorpheniramine Maleate Polaramine Various	Syrup 0.4 mg/mL Tab 2 mg SR Tab 4, 6 mg	PO 2 mg every 4–6 h, to a maximum of 12 mg/d or SR 4–6 mg hs or every 8–10 h during the day	PO (2–5 y) 0.5 mg every 4–6 h, to a maximum of 3 mg/d, SR not recommended; (6–12 y) 1 mg every 4–6 h or SR 4 mg hs	15–25	+	++
Diphenhydramine HCl Benadryl Various	Refer to diphenhydramine monograph			9	+++	+++
Ebastine Kestine (Investigational–RPR)	—	PO 10–20 mg/d	—	15 (metabolite)	±	±
Fexofenadine HCl Allegra	Refer to fexofenadine monograph			14	±	±
Hydroxyzine HCl/Pamoate Atarax Vistaril Various	Refer to hydroxyzine monograph					

(continued)

955

ANTIHISTAMINES COMPARISON CHART (continued)

					SIDE EFFECTS	
DRUG	DOSAGE FORMS	ADULT DOSAGE	PEDIATRIC DOSAGE	HALF-LIFE (h)	Sedation[a]	Anticholinergic
Levocabastine HCl Livostin	Ophth Susp 0.05% Nasal Spray (investigational)	Ophth 1 drop qid	(>12 y) same as adult dosage	35–40	+	+
Loratadine Claritin	Refer to loratadine monograph			8 (metabolite: 28)	±	±
Phenindamine Tartrate Nolahist	Tab 25 mg	PO 25 mg every 4–6 h, to a maximum of 150 mg/d	PO (6–11 y) 12.5 mg every 4–6 h, to a maximum of 75 mg/d	—	+	++
Promethazine HCl Phenergan Various	Syrup 1.25, 5 mg/mL Tab 12.5, 25, 50 mg Inj 25, 50 mg/mL Supp 12.5, 25, 50 mg	PO (allergy) 25 mg hs or 12.5 mg ac and hs; (nausea and vomiting) 25 mg initial dose, then 12.5–25 mg every 4–6 h prn; (adjunctive preoperative use) 25–50 mg/dose IM, IV (IV maximum concentration 25 mg/mL, maximum rate 25 mg/ min) or PR (allergy) 25 mg, may repeat in 2 h; (nausea and vomiting) 12.5–25 mg q4h prn; (adjunctive pre- and postoperative use) 25–50 mg/dose	PO (allergy) 6.25–12.5 mg qid; (motion sickness or sedation) 12.5–25 mg/bid; IM, IV, or PR (PR not recommended <2 y); (allergy) 0.5 mg/kg/d in 4 divided doses; adjunctive preoperative use) 1 mg/kg/ dose, maximum dosage not to exceed one-half of adult dosage	12	++++	++++

(continued)

ANTIHISTAMINES COMPARISON CHART (continued)

DRUG	DOSAGE FORMS	ADULT DOSAGE	PEDIATRIC DOSAGE	HALF-LIFE (h)	Sedation[a]	Anticholinergic
Tripelennamine HCl PBZ Various	Tab 25, 50 mg SR Tab 100 mg	PO 25–50 mg every 4–6 h, to a maximum of 600 mg/d	PO 5 mg/kg/d in 4–6 divided doses, to a maximum of 300 mg/d; SR not recommended	2–4	++	±
Triprolidine HCl	Syrup 0.25 mg with pseudoephedrine 6 mg/mL Tab 2.5 mg with pseudoephedrine 60 mg (Actifed)	PO 2.5 mg every 4–6 h, to a maximum of 10 mg/d	PO (4 mo–2 y) 0.3 mg tid– qid; (2–5 y) 0.625 mg tid–qid; (6–12 y) 1.25 mg every 4–6 h, to a maximum of 4 doses/d	3	++	++

+ + +, very high; + + +, high; + + = moderate; +, low; ±, low to none; −, not known.
[a]Tolerance usually develops during long-term therapy.
From Refs. 27–32.

■ REFERENCES

1. Cook TJ et al. Degree and duration of skin test suppression and side effects with antihistamines. *J Allergy Clin Immunol.* 1973;51:71-77.
2. Usdin Yasuda S et al. Chlorpheniramine plasma concentration and histamine H1 receptor occupancy. *Clin Pharmacol Ther.* 1995;58:210-220.
3. Huang SM et al. Pharmacokinetics of chlorpheniramine after intravenous and oral administration in normal adults. *Eur J Clin Pharmacol.* 1982;22:359-365.
4. Benet LZ et al. Design and optimization of dosage regimens; pharmacokinetic data. In: Hardman JG et al., eds. *Goodman and Gilman's the Pharmacological Basis of Therapeutics.* 9th ed. New York: McGraw-Hill; 1996:1707-1792.
5. Paton DM, Webster DR. Clinical pharmacokinetics of H1 receptor antagonists (the antihistamines). *Clin Pharmacokinet.* 1985;10:477-497.
6. Simons FER. H1 receptor antagonists: clinical pharmacology and therapeutics. *J Allergy Clin Immunol.* 1989;84:845-861.
7. Simons KJ et al. Diphenhydramine: pharmacokinetics and pharmacodynamics in elderly adults, young adults, and children. *J Clin Pharmacol.* 1990;30:665-671.
8. Carruthers SG et al. Correlation between plasma diphenhydramine level and sedative and antihistamine effects. *Clin Pharmacol Ther.* 1978;23:375-382.
9. Blyden GT et al. Pharmacokinetics of diphenhydramine and a demethylated metabolite following intravenous and oral administration. *J Clin Pharmacol.* 1986;26:529-533.
10. Spector R et al. Diphenhydramine in Orientals and Caucasians. *Clin Pharmacol Ther.* 1980;28:229-234.
11. Meredith CG et al. Diphenhydramine disposition in chronic liver disease. *Clin Pharmacol Ther.* 1984;35:474-479.
12. Glazko AJ et al. Metabolic disposition of diphenhydramine. *Clin Pharmacol Ther.* 1974;16:1066-1076.
13. Albert KS et al. Pharmacokinetics of diphenhydramine in man. *J Pharmacokinet Biopharm.* 1975;3:159-170.
14. Schaaf L et al. Suppression of seasonal allergic rhinitis symptoms with daily hydroxyzine. *J Allergy Clin Immunol.* 1979;63:129-133.
15. Gendreau-Reid L et al. Comparison of the suppressive effect of astemizole, terfenadine, and hydroxyzine on histamine-induced wheals and flares in humans. *J Allergy Clin Immunol.* 1986;77:335-340.
16. Simons KJ et al. Pharmacokinetic and pharmacodynamic studies of the H1 receptor antagonist hydroxyzine in the elderly. *Clin Pharmacol Ther.* 1989;45:9-14.
17. Simons FER et al. Pharmacokinetics and antipruritic effects of hydroxyzine in children with atopic dermatitis. *J Pediatr.* 1984;104:123-127.
18. Simons FE et al. The pharmacokinetics and antihistaminic of the H1 receptor antagonist hydroxyzine. *J Allergy Clin Immunol.* 1984;73(1, pt 1):69-75.
19. Simons FER et al. The pharmacokinetics and pharmacodynamics of hydroxyzine in patients with primary biliary cirrhosis. *J Clin Pharmacol.* 1989;29:809-815.
20. Simons FER, Simons KJ. Antihistamines. In: Middleton E et al., eds. *Allergy. Principles and Practice.* St. Louis, MO: Mosby; 1993:856-879.
21. Gonzalez MA, Estes KS. Pharmacokinetic overview of oral second-generation H1-antihistamines. *Int J Clin Pharmacol Ther.* 1998;36:292-300.
22. Corey JP. Advances in the pharmacotherapy of allergic rhinitis: second-generation H1 receptor antagonists. *Otolaryngol Head Neck Surg.* 1993;109:584-592.
23. Korenblat PE, Wedner HJ. *Allergy. Theory and Practice.* 2nd ed. Philadelphia, PA: WB Saunders; 1992:300-333.
24. Desager J-P, Horsmans Y. Pharmacokinetic-pharmacodynamic relationships of H1-antihistamines. *Clin Pharmacokinet.* 1995;28:419-432.
25. Kobayaski RH et al. Beclomethasone dipropionate aqueous nasal spray for seasonal allergic rhinitis in children. *Ann Allergy.* 1989;62:205-208.
26. Krause HF. Antihistamines and decongestants. *Otolaryngol Head Neck Surg.* 1992;107:835-840.
27. Fauci AS et al. Glucocorticoid therapy: mechanisms of action and clinical considerations. *Ann Intern Med.* 1976;84:304-315.
28. Azarnoff DL, ed. *Steroid Therapy.* Philadelphia, PA: WB Saunders; 1975.
29. Barnes PJ. Inhaled glucocorticoids for asthma. *N Engl J Med.* 1995;332:868-875.
30. Barnes PJ, Pederson S. Efficacy and safety of inhaled corticosteroid in asthma. *Am Rev Respir Dis.* 1993;149:S1-S26.
31. Szefler SJ. A comparison of aerosol glucocorticoids in the treatment of chronic bronchial asthma. *Pediatr Asthma Allergy Immunol.* 1991;5:227-235.
32. Kamada AK. Therapeutic controversies in the treatment of asthma. *Ann Pharmacother.* 1994;28:904-914.

Chapter 59

Inhaled Corticosteroids

Laura L. Sanders

Pharmacology. Inhaled corticosteroids (ICS) are classified as long-term control medications for asthma and allergic rhinitis used to achieve and maintain control of persistent symptoms. Steroid nasal sprays are also used for prophylaxis/treatment of nasal polyps. Corticosteroids block late-phase reaction to allergens and reduce airway hyperresponsiveness. ICS inhibit the migration and activation of inflammatory cells (e.g., mast cells, eosinophils, neutrophils, macrophages, lymphocytes) and mediators (e.g., histamine, eicosanoids, leukotrienes, and cytokines). Anti-inflammatory corticosteroids exhibit potent glucocorticoid activity and weak mineralocorticoid activity. They are the most potent and effective anti-inflammatory medications currently available, and studies demonstrate that ICS improve asthma control more effectively in both children and adults than leukotriene-receptor antagonists or any other single long-term control medication. Dosages vary depending on the specific product and delivery devices and are in general well tolerated and safe at the recommended dosages.[1]

Dosage. (*See* Inhaled Corticosteroids Comparison Chart and Intranasal Corticosteroids Comparison Chart beginning page 965.) With all ICS, prescribers are advised to select the dosages appropriate for the patients' disease severity and titrate the dosage downward over time to the lowest level that maintains proper symptom control.

Patient Information. ICS will not relieve an acute asthma attack; be sure to keep your bronchodilator medication ready to relieve an acute attack.[2] In order for this medication to work, it must be used every day in regularly spaced doses as prescribed. It may take up to 4–6 weeks before you notice improvement in your symptoms. Gargle and rinse your mouth with water, spitting out the water (do not swallow the water after rinsing) after each dose to help prevent hoarseness, throat irritation, and mouth infections.

Be sure your doctor knows if you have an injury, infection, or surgery while taking this medicine; if you have an asthma attack that does not improve after you use your bronchodilator medication; if you are exposed to viral infections such as chickenpox or measles; if you have signs of infection (especially in your mouth, throat, and lungs); and if your symptoms do not improve or worsen.

If you take oral corticosteroid therapy, do not stop taking that medication without your doctor's advice, even if your asthma seems better.

Side effects of this medication may include cold-like symptoms, cough, dry mouth/throat, headache, hoarseness, voice changes, and trouble sleeping. Nasal sprays may cause sneezing, nasal stuffiness, runny nose, tearing eyes, or minor nosebleeds. Contact your health care provider immediately if any of the following side effects occur just after you use this medicine: shortness of breath; chest tightness; wheezing; swelling of your eyes, lips, or face. Let your doctor know as soon as possible if you have excessive bruising, pain on urination or blood in your urine, white patches in your mouth/throat or pain on eating/swallowing, fast heartbeat, weight gain/swelling.

If you miss a dose of this medication, take it as soon as possible, then use any remaining doses for that day at regularly spaced intervals.

Do not increase your dose of inhaled steroids unless your health care provider tells you to do so.

To prime most inhalers with removable canisters: When you use the inhaler for the first time, or if you haven't used it in a while, you must first prime the inhaler. To prime the inhaler, insert the metal canister into the mouthpiece, take the cover off the mouthpiece, and shake the inhaler 3–4 times. Hold the inhaler well away from you and press the top of the canister, spraying the medicine into the air 2 times. The inhaler is now ready to use.

To use most inhalers with removable canisters: Using your thumb and 1–2 fingers, hold the inhaler upright with the mouthpiece end down and pointing toward you. Take the cover off the mouthpiece, check it, and remove any foreign objects. Shake the inhaler gently 3–4 times. Hold the mouthpiece away from your mouth and breathe out slowly to the end of a normal breath. Use the inhalation method recommended by your doctor, open-mouth or closed-mouth.

To use the open-mouth method, place the mouthpiece approximately 1–2 in. (2 finger widths) in front of your widely opened mouth, making sure that the inhaler is aimed into your mouth so that the spray does not hit the roof of your mouth or tongue. To use the closed-mouth method, place the mouthpiece in your mouth between your teeth and over your tongue with your lips closed tightly around it. Do not block the mouthpiece with your teeth or tongue.

Begin to breathe in slowly through your mouth and at the same time, press the top of the canister once to get out 1 puff of medicine. Continue to breathe in for 3–5 s. Hold your breath as long as you can up to 10 s and then take the mouthpiece away from your mouth and breathe out slowly. If you are to inhale more than 1 puff, shake the inhaler again and repeat the steps.

If your health care provider has instructed you to use a spacer with your inhaler, attach the spacer to the inhaler according to the spacer's directions, gently shake the inhaler/spacer 3–4 times, hold the mouthpiece away from your mouth and breath out slowly and completely, and then place the mouthpiece of the spacer into your mouth between your teeth and over your tongue with your lips closed around it. Press down on the canister once to release 1 puff of medication into the spacer and within 1–2 s, breathe in slowly through your mouth for 3–5 s. Hold your breath as long as you can for up to 10 s and then breathe out slowly. Repeat the steps as needed for a second puff.

Clean the inhaler mouthpiece and spacer at least once a week by removing the canister from the inhaler (set the canister aside) and washing the mouthpiece and spacer with warm, soapy water. Rinse the mouthpiece and spacer under warm, running water, shake off the excess water, and let the parts air dry before putting the inhaler back together.

To use most nasal inhalers: Before removing the cover, shake the container prior to use and prime the pump by spraying 6–8 times into the air. If used daily, the pump does not need to be reprimed. If not used for 2 consecutive days, reprime with 1 spray or until a fine mist appears. If not used for > 14 days, rinse the applicator and reprime with 2 sprays or until a fine mist appears. Blow your nose before using. Remove the protective cap, insert the tip into your nostril, close the other nostril with your finger, and tilt your head forward slightly. Spray the medication into your nostril and breathe in gently. After spraying, lean your head back for a few seconds. Avoid blowing your nose for 15 min after using the spray. Wipe the nasal applicator and replace the cover.

To use Diskus: Take the Diskus out of the box and the foil pouch. Write the date the pouch was opened and the "Use By" date on the label on the top of the Diskus. The "Use By" date will be 4–6 weeks from the date you opened the pouch. The Diskus will be closed when you first open its pouch. The dose indicator on the top of the Diskus tells you how many doses are left and will decrease each time you use it. Hold the Diskus in one hand and put the thumb of your other hand on the thumb grip. Push your thumb away from you as far as it will go until the mouthpiece appears and snaps into position. Hold the Diskus in a flat, level position with the mouthpiece toward you. Slide the lever away from you as far as it will go until it clicks. Exhale fully while holding the Diskus level and away from your mouth—never breathe out into the Diskus mouthpiece. Put the mouthpiece to your lips and breathe in quickly and deeply through your mouth (not your nose) through the Diskus. Remove the Diskus from your mouth and hold your breath for 10 s or as long as it is comfortable for you. Breathe out slowly. Close the Diskus when you are finished. Put your thumb and the thumb grip and slide it back toward you until the Diskus clicks shut and the lever returns to its original position. The Diskus delivers your medication as a fine powder. Most people can feel or taste the powder. If you do not feel or taste the medicine, do not use another dose from the Diskus and contact your doctor. Do not use the Diskus with a spacer device. Do not wash the mouthpiece or any part of the Diskus—it must be kept dry.

To use most inhalers (nonremovable canister): (Flexhaler/Turbuhaler) Prime the inhaler before first use by holding the unit upright and removing the cover. Hold the inhaler in the middle (do not hold at the top of the mouthpiece). Twist the brown grip as far as it will go in one direction and then fully back again in the other direction until it stops. You will hear a click during one of the twisting movements. Repeat this step; the inhaler is now primed. You do not need to prime this inhaler again, even if it is not used for a long time. To use the inhaler to take a dose, hold the inhaler in the upright position, remove the cover and twist the brown grip fully in one direction as far as it will go, and then fully back in the other direction. You will hear a click. A dose is now loaded. **(Twisthaler)** Hold the inhaler upright with the colored base on the bottom. Hold the colored base and twist the cap once in a counterclockwise direction. As you remove the cap, the medicine is loaded into the Twisthaler.

Do not shake the inhaler once a dose is loaded. Turn your head away from the inhaler and breathe out. Place the mouthpiece in your mouth, close your lips around the mouthpiece, and inhale deeply and forcefully through the inhaler. Do not bite the mouthpiece. Remove the inhaler from your mouth and exhale. Be sure NOT to exhale into the mouthpiece. If more than one dose is prescribed, repeat the steps above. Place the cover back on the inhaler and twist it shut. Rinse your mouth with water after each use, but do not swallow. Do not immerse your inhaler in water. Wipe the outside of the mouthpiece once weekly with a dry tissue—do not use water. Do not use a spacer with the Flexhaler/Turbuhaler/Twisthaler. The Flexhaler/Turbuhaler/Twisthaler delivers your medicine as a fine powder, which you may not feel entering your lungs. This does not mean that you did not get the medication. So you should not repeat the inhalations even if you did not feel the medication.

Pharmacokinetics. *Onset.* Usually improvement in the control of asthma symptoms is seen within 2–8 days, but maximum improvement may take 4–6 weeks.

Corticosteroids are metabolized via CYP450 3A4.

Adverse Reactions. Local adverse reactions with ICS therapy include oral candidiasis, headache, cough nasopharyngitis, nasal congestion, pharyngitis, rhinitis, upper respiratory tract infection, wheezing, nausea, vomiting, diarrhea, unpleasant taste, and dysphonia. Nasal spray's use may cause rhinorrhea, epistaxis, sneezing, nasopharyngeal irritation. Rare adverse events reported include hypersensitivity reactions (including rash, angioedema, and bronchospasm), GI bleeding, edema/weight gain, tachycardia, palpitations, depression, anxiety, irritability, aggression, and psychosis. Steroid therapy including ICS may also lead to systemic effects as ICS may be absorbed into systemic circulation via the lungs or the GI tract. These adverse systemic effects may include adrenal suppression, decreased bone density, skin thinning/bruising, cataracts, and ocular hypertension. However, these systemic effects are often dose related and occur less frequently than with oral corticosteroid use.[3–5]

To reduce the potential for adverse effects, the following measures are recommended: use of spacers or holding chambers with non–breath-activated MDIs, rinsing the mouth and spitting after inhalation, use of the lowest effective dose, monitoring of growth in children, use of calcium supplements (1,000–1500 mg/d) and vitamin D (400–800 units/d) in adult patient.[1]

Contraindications/Precautions. Contraindicated in status asthmaticus. Cirrhosis/hepatic insufficiency may increase the effects of corticosteroids; ICS may increase intraocular pressure in glaucoma patients. Use with caution in hypothyroidism, untreated systemic infections (except upper respiratory viral infections), osteoporosis, and tuberculosis.

Use caution when transferring patients from oral steroid therapy to ICS because of risk of suppression of hypothalamic–pituitary–adrenal function. Patients maintained on 20 mg or more of prednisone (or equivalent) may be most susceptible. Patients on corticosteroid therapy may be more susceptible to infections such as chickenpox and measles. For patients receiving oral corticosteroids, taper oral therapy no faster than 2.5–5 mg/d on a weekly basis, beginning after at least 1 week of therapy with ICS. Monitor for symptoms of withdrawal such as fatigue, weakness, nausea, vomiting, and hypertension.

Drug Interactions. Ritonavir can significantly increase plasma fluticasone propionate exposure, resulting in reduced serum cortisol levels; reports during postmarketing have indicated clinically significant results of Cushing syndrome and adrenal suppression. Therefore, coadministration of fluticasone propionate and ritonavir is not recommended. Although extensive drug interactions have not been defined for ICS, consider that if ICS are used in high doses for extended periods, they may be absorbed systemically and have the potential for interactions seen with systemic corticosteroids (primarily with other drugs metabolized via the CYP450 3A4 pathway, or with drugs that are CYP450 3A4 inducers or 3A4 inhibitors). Steroid therapy may also decrease the efficacy of antidiabetic medications and increase hypokalemia associated with non–potassium-sparing diuretics or amphotericin B.

Parameters to Monitor. Periodic adrenal function assessment, especially when transferring a patient from systemic to ICS; growth in children (periodic stadiometry); inhalation technique; intraocular pressure in patients at risk for glaucoma, cataracts, vision changes; pulmonary function, asthma symptoms; signs of systemic absorption (patients on high doses); serum potassium, glucose as appropriate.

BECLOMETHASONE DIPROPIONATE	Beclovent, Beconase, Beconase AQ, QVAR, Vancenase, Vanceril, Vanceril DS

Dosage and Administration. Oral inhalation aerosol for asthma *Beclovent, Vanceril, Vanceril DS* (adults and children >12 years)—*42 or 50 μg per spray product* 84–100 μg (2 inhalations) tid–qid or 4 puffs bid, maximum 840–1000 μg (20 inhalations)/d; *84 μg/spray product* 168 μg (2 inhalations) bid, maximum 840 μg (10 puffs)/d. For severe asthma, may begin with 12–16 inhalations/d (*42–50 μg/ spray product*) or with 6–8 inhalations/d (*84 μg/spray product*), then decrease as possible.

40 or 80 μg/spray product *QVAR* (adults and children ≥ 12 years)—previous therapy with bronchodilators alone, 40–80 μg bid (1–2 inhalations), maximum 320 μg bid; previous therapy with ICS, 40–160 μg bid (1–4 inhalations), maximum 320 μg bid.

Intranasal for nasal congestion *Beconase AQ*—42–84 μg/nostril (1–2 sprays) bid (168–336 μg/d total dosage) for several days, then decrease dosage (if symptoms do not recur) to minimum amount necessary to control stuffiness.

Special Populations. *Pediatric Dosage.* Oral inhalation aerosol for asthma *Beclovent, Vanceril, Vanceril DS* (children 6–12 years)—*42 or 50 μg/spray product* 1–2 inhalations tid–qid or 4 inhalations bid, maximum 420 or 500 μg/d (10 inhalations); *84 μg/spray product* 2 inhalations bid, maximum 420 μg/d (5 inhalations). (**Children <6 years**)—dosage not established. Titrate dosage to the lowest effective dosage.

40 or 80 μg/spray product *QVAR* (children 5–11 years)—previous therapy with bronchodilators alone or with ICS: 40 μg bid, maximum 80 μg bid.

Intranasal for nasal congestion *Beconase AQ* (<6 years)—not recommended; (**6–12 years**) start with 42 μg (1 spray)/nostril bid; if no response or severe symptoms, may increase to 2 sprays/nostril (336 μg). Once control is achieved, decrease to 84 μg bid. Do not exceed 336 μg/d.

Geriatric Dosage. Same as adult dosage.

Other Conditions. Ineffective during a severe asthma attack.

Dosage Forms. **Inhal** (Beclovent, Vanceril) 42, 84 μg/puff (80 and 200 doses/inhaler, and 40 and 120 doses/inhaler, respectively); (QVAR) 40, 80 μg/puff (*see* Notes). **Nasal Inhal** (Beconase, Vancenase) 42 μg/spray (80, 200 doses/inhaler). **Aq Susp** (Beconase AQ, Vancenase AQ) 42, 84 μg/spray (200 and 120 doses/ bottle, respectively).

Pharmacokinetics. *Onset.* **(Beconase AQ)** improvement of symptoms of rhinitis usually becomes apparent within a few days. However, relief may not occur for up to 2 weeks. If symptom improvement is not significant after 3 weeks, discontinue therapy.

Fate. Only ≤10% of an inhaled dose is deposited in the lung; 80% is deposited in the mouth and swallowed. Oral absorption is slow and incomplete (61%–90%), and the drug undergoes extensive first-pass metabolism, resulting in oral bioavailability of less than 5%.[6] Well absorbed from the lung and extensively metabolized, with 65% excreted in the bile and <10% of unchanged drug and metabolites excreted in urine.[6]

$t_{1/2}$. 15 h.

Adverse Reactions, Contraindications, Precautions, Drug Interactions, Parameters to Monitor. Refer to Class Information at the beginning of this chapter.

INHALED CORTICOSTEROIDS COMPARISON CHART

DRUG	DOSAGE FORMS[a]	DAILY DOSAGE[a]			RECEPTOR HALF-LIFE	TOPICAL POTENCY[c]	ORAL BIOAVAILABILITY[d]
		Low (Step 2)	Medium (Step 3)	High (Step 4)			
SINGLE-INGREDIENT PRODUCTS							
Beclomethasone Dipropionate Beclovent Vanceril	MDI: 42, 84 μg/puff	Adult: 163–504 μg Child: 84–336 μg	504–840 μg 336–672 μg	>840 μg >672 μg	7.5 h	600	20%
Beclomethasone Dipropionate HFA QVAR	MDI: 40, 80 μg/puff	Adult: 80–160 μg	160–320 mg	>320 μg	7.5 h	600	20%
Budesonide Pulmicort	DPI: 200 μg/inhal NEB Susp: 125, 250 μg/mL	Adult: 200–400 μg Child: 100–200 μg	400–600 μg 200–400 μg	>600 μg >400 μg	5.1 h	980	11%
Flunisolide AeroBid AeroBid-M	MDI: 250 μg/puff	Adult: 500–1000 μg Child: 500–750 μg	1000–2000 μg 750–1250 μg	>2000 μg >1250 μg	3.5 h	330	21%
Fluticasone Propionate Flovent	MDI: 44, 110, 220 μg/puff DPI: 50, 100, 250 μg/inhal	Adult: 88–264 μg Child: 88–176 μg	264–660 μg 176–440 μg	>660 μg >440 μg	10.5 h	1200	1%

(continued)

INHALED CORTICOSTEROIDS COMPARISON CHART (continued)[a]

| DRUG | DOSAGE FORMS[b] | DAILY DOSAGE[a] | | | RECEPTOR HALF-LIFE | TOPICAL POTENCY[c] | ORAL BIOAVAILABILITY[d] |
		Low (Step 2)	Medium (Step 3)	High (Step 4)			
Triamcinolone Acetonide Azmacort	MDI: 100 µg/puff	Adult: 400–1000 µg Child: 400–800 µg	1000–2000 µg 800–1200 µg	>2000 µg >1200 µg	3.9 h	330	11%
COMBINATION PRODUCTS							
Fluticasone Propionate and Salmeterol Advair Diskus	DPI: fluticasone 100 µg, salmeterol 50 µg/Inhal; fluticasone 250 µg, salmeterol 50 µg/Inhal; fluticasone 500 µg, salmeterol 50 µg/Inhal	Adult: 100–50 bid	250–50 bid	500–50 bid	—	—	—

DPI, dry powder inhaler; MDI, metered-dose inhaler; NEB, nebulizer.

[a]Dosage ranges correspond to recommended treatment intensities for steps 2–4 of the NIH guidelines for diagnosis and management of asthma: step 1 = mild intermittent; step 2 = mild persistent; step 3 = moderate persistent; step 4 = severe persistent.[1] The most important determinant of appropriate dosage is the clinician's judgment of the patient's response to therapy; the clinician must monitor the patient's response on several clinical parameters and adjust the dosage accordingly. The stepwise approach to therapy emphasizes that once control of symptoms is achieved, the dosage of medication should be carefully titrated to the minimum dosage required to maintain control, thereby reducing the potential for adverse effects.

[b]MDI dosages are expressed as the actuator dose (the amount of drug leaving the actuator and delivered to the patient), which is the labeling required in the United States. This is different from the dosage expressed as the valve dose (the amount of drug leaving the valve, not all of which is available to the patient), which is used in many European countries and in some of the scientific literature. DPI doses are expressed as the amount of drug in the inhaler following activation.

[c]Potency determined from skin blanching; dexamethasone is the reference drug and has a value of 1 in this assay.

[d]Oral bioavailability of the swallowed portion of the dose received by the patient. Approximately 80% of the dose from an MDI without a spacer is swallowed. Nearly all of the drug delivered to the lungs is bioavailable. From 10% to 30% of an MDI dose is delivered to the lungs, depending on the product and device. Both the relative potency and the total bioavailability (inhaled + swallowed) determine the systemic activity of the product.

From Refs. 7–9.

INTRANASAL CORTICOSTEROIDS COMPARISON CHART

DRUG	DOSAGE FORMS	ADULT DOSAGE	PEDIATRIC DOSAGE[a]
Beclomethasone Dipropionate Beconase Vancenase	Aerosol, metered-dose 42 μg/spray Spray, aqueous 42, 84 μg/spray	1–2 sprays into each nostril bid–qid	1 spray into each nostril bid–tid
Budesonide Rhinocort	Aerosol, metered-dose 32 μg/spray	2 sprays into each nostril bid or 4 sprays into each nostril every morning, to a maximum of 800 μg/d	2 sprays into each nostril bid or 4 sprays into each nostril every morning, to a maximum of 400 μg/d
Flunisolide Nasalide Nasarel	Spray, aqueous 25 μg/spray	2 sprays into each nostril bid, to a maximum of 8 sprays/d into each nostril	1 spray into each nostril tid–qid
Fluticasone Propionate Flonase	Spray, aqueous 50 μg/spray	2 sprays into each nostril daily or 1 spray into each nostril bid; maintenance 1 spray into each nostril daily, to a maximum of 200 μg/d	(≥4 y) 1 spray in each nostril daily (100 μg/d); for nonresponders, 2 sprays in each nostril daily or 1 spray in each nostril bid, decrease to 100 μg/d once a response is achieved
Mometasone Furoate Nasonex	Spray, aqueous 50 μg/spray	2 sprays into each nostril once daily	(≤12 y) not established
Triamcinolone Acetonide Nasacort Nasarel	Spray, aqueous 55 μg/spray	2 sprays into each nostril daily; adjust to a maximum of 4 sprays/d in 1–4 divided doses; maintenance as low as 1 spray/d	Same as adult dosage

[a]Unless otherwise stated, pediatric dosage is for patients 6–12 years; dosages for patients <6 years have generally not been established.
From Refs. 3, 4, and 10.

BUDESONIDE	Pulmicort Flexhaler/ Turbuhaler, Respules; Rhinocort Aqua; Symbicort (budesonide/formoterol); Various

Refer to Class Information at the beginning of this chapter.

Administration and Dosage. Powder inhalation for asthma *Pulmicort Flexhaler* **(adults ≥ 18 years)**—360 μg bid, maximum 720 μg bid. In adult patients who are well controlled, consider 180 μg bid. *Turbuhaler* **(adults)**—previous therapy with bronchodilators alone 200–400 μg bid, maximum 400 μg daily; previous ICS therapy 200–400 μg bid, maximum 800 μg bid; previous therapy with oral corticosteroids 400–800 μg bid, maximum 800 μg bid. Inhalation suspension nebulizer for asthma *Pulmicort Respules* **(adults and adolescents)**—1–2 mg diluted with sterile NaCl inhalation solution to a volume of 2–4 mL via nebulizer over 10–15 min bid. Administer only via jet nebulizer. *Nasal Inhalation* **(adults and children ≥ 6 years)**—64 μg/d (1 spray/nostril) qd; maximum **(adults and children ≥ 12 years)**—256 μg/d (4 sprays/nostril) qd. Maximum dose (children <12 years)—128 μg (2 sprays/nostril) qd.

Pediatric Dosage. Powder inhalation for asthma *Pulmicort Flexhaler* **(children and adolescents 6–17 years)**—starting dosage is 180 μg bid; titrate as needed to a maximum of 360 μg bid. **(Children <6 years)**—dosing not established. *Turbuhaler* **(children)**—previous therapy with bronchodilator therapy alone 200 μg bid, maximum 400 μg bid; previous therapy with ICS 200 μg bid, maximum 400 μg bid. Inhalation suspension nebulizer for asthma *Pulmicort Respules* **(children 12 months–8 years)**—previous therapy with bronchodilators alone 0.5 mg qd or bid in divided doses, maximum 0.5-mg total daily dose; previous therapy with ICS 0.5 mg qd or bid in divided doses, maximum 1-mg total daily dose; previous therapy with oral corticosteroids 1 mg qd or 0.5 mg bid, maximum 1 mg total daily dose. **(Children < 12 months)**—dosage not established. Administer only via jet nebulizer. **Nasal inhalation (children < 6 years)**—dosage not established. **(Children ≥ 6 years)**—*See* adult dosage.

Geriatric Dosage. Usual adult dose; begin at lower end of dosage range.

Dosage Forms. **Pwdr for Inhal**—Pulmicort Flexhaler 90 μg/dose (60 doses), 180 μg/dose (120 doses); Pulmicort Turbuhaler 200 μg/dose (200 doses); combination product with formoterol (see Notes). **Inhal Susp Pulmicort Respules**—0.25 mg/2 mL, 0.5 mg/2 mL, 1 mg/2 mL supplied in single-dose ampules. **Nasal spray**—32 μg/pump spray bottle, 120 sprays/bottle.

Patient Instructions. Refer also to Class Information.

To use Pulmicort Respules: Use only with a jet nebulizer (not ultrasonic). Assemble the nebulizer according to the manufacturer's instructions. Open the sealed foil envelope along the dotted line and record the date you opened the foil on the back of the envelope. Put the unused ampules back into the foil envelope for storage. Gently shake the Respules in a circular motion. Hold the ampule upright without squeezing it and twist off the top. Place the open end into the nebulizer cup and slowly squeeze out all the medicine. If you are using a facemask, be sure that it fits so that the mist from the nebulizer does not get into the eyes. Turn on the compressor and continue the treatment until mist no longer comes out of the mouthpiece (approximately 5–10 min). Rinse mouth with water (do not swallow the water—spit it out) and wash face after each dose.

To use Rhinocort Aqua nasal spray: *See* Class Information at the beginning of this chapter.

Pharmacokinetics. *Onset.* **(Flexhaler/Turbuhaler)** Improvement in symptoms can occur within 24 h, but maximum benefit may not be seen for 1–2 weeks. **(Respules)** improvement may be seen in 2–8 days, but may take up to 4–6 weeks.

Fate. **(Powder for inhalation)** peak plasma concentrations are achieved in 1–2 h, and systemic bioavailability is 6%–13% following oral administration; 34% of a dose is delivered to the lungs, with 39% systemic bioavailability. Plasma protein binding is 85%–90%. Metabolism is rapid and extensive via CYP450 3A4. Half-life is 2–3 h, with excretion/elimination via urine (60%) and feces in the form of metabolites. (Inhalation suspension) in children aged 4–6 years, bioavailability ~6%, with peak plasma concentrations at ~20 min. Rapid and extensive metabolism via CYP450 3A4 with primary clearance by the liver and excretion/elimination in the urine (60%) and feces in the form of metabolites. The $t_{1/2}$ is 2.3 h.

Adverse Reactions, Contraindications, Precautions, Drug Interactions, Parameters to Monitor. Refer to Class Information at the beginning of this chapter.

Notes. A definite comparative therapeutic ratio has not been established between Pulmicort Flexhaler and Turbuhaler. The clinical response of Pulmicort Flexhaler tends to be lower compared with Pulmicort Turbuhaler. A patient who switches from one to the other should be dosed according to the specific product's dosing recommendations, with titration dictated by the clinical response. Flexhaler contains lactose.

In 2008, the FDA approved a generic formulation of Pulmicort Respules (0.25 mg/2 mL and 0.5 mg/2 mL).

A combination inhalation aerosol (MDI) product (Symbicort) is available as budesonide 80 μg/formoterol 4.5 μg and budesonide 160 μg/formoterol 4.5 μg.

FLUTICASONE PROPIONATE,	Flovent HFA/Diskus, Flonase, Veramyst,
FLUTICASONE FUROATE	Advair HFA/Diskus, Various

Refer to Class Information at the beginning of this chapter.

Administration and Dosage. **Inhalation aerosol for asthma (adults and children ≥12 years)**—previous therapy with bronchodilators alone 88 μg bid, maximum 440 μg bid; previous therapy with ICS 88–220 μg bid, maximum 440 μg bid; previous therapy with oral corticosteroids 440 μg bid, maximum 880 μg bid. **Inhalation powder for asthma (adults and children ≥12 years)**—previous therapy with bronchodilators alone 100 μg bid, maximum 500 μg bid; previous therapy with ICS 100–250 μg bid, maximum 500 μg bid; previous therapy with oral corticosteroids 500–1000 μg bid, maximum 1000 μg bid. **Nasal spray propionate/Flonase (adults)**—2 sprays (50 μg/spray; total 100 μg) in each nostril qd or 2 sprays (50 μg/spray; total 200 μg) in each nostril bid q12h. After a few days of 200 μg/d, dosage may be reduced to 100 μg daily (1 spray in each nostril qd). **Nasal spray furoate/Veramyst (adults and children ≥12 years)**—110 μg (2 sprays/nostril) qd.

Pediatric Dosage. **Inhalation aerosol for asthma (children 4–11 years)**—88 μg bid, maximum 88 μg bid. **(Children <4 years)**—dosage not established. **Inhalation powder for asthma (children 4–11 years)**—previous therapy with bronchodilators alone 50 μg bid, maximum 100 μg bid; previous therapy with ICS 50 μg bid, maximum 100 μg bid. **Nasal spray propionate/Flonase (adolescents and children ≥4 years)**—1 spray (50 μg/spray; total 100 μg) in each nostril qd up to

2 sprays (50 μg/spray; total 200 μg) each nostril, maximum 200 μg/d. **(Children <4 years)**—not recommended. **Nasal spray furoate/Veramyst (children 2–11 years)**—55 μg (1 spray/nostril) qd.

Geriatric Dosage. Usual adult dose.

Dosage Forms. Inhal aerosol (Flovent HFA) MDI 44 μg/Inhal, 120 Inhal/canister; 110 μg/Inhal, 120 Inhal/canister; 220 μg/Inhal, 120 Inhal/canister. **Inhal Pwdr (Flovent Diskus)** 50 μg, 100 μg, 250 μg. **Nasal spray (Flonase/various)** 50 μg/spray; 120 sprays/bottle. **(Veramyst)** 27.5 μg/spray; 120 sprays/bottle. Fluticasone propionate also available in combination with salmeterol as inhalation aerosol and powder for inhalation (**Advair HFA** 45/115/230 μg fluticasone propionate/21 μg salmeterol and **Advair Diskus** 100/250/500 μg fluticasone propionate/50 μg salmeterol).

Patient Instructions. Refer to Class Information at the beginning of this chapter.

Discard Flovent Diskus 50 μg 6 weeks after it has been removed from its foil pouch; discard the 100 μg or 250 μg strength Diskus 8 weeks after removed from the foil pouch.

Pharmacokinetics. *Fate.* Oral bioavailability negligible; the majority of fluticasone propionate delivered to the lung is systemically absorbed. Maximum plasma concentrations occurred in ~1 h with metabolism via the CYP450 3A4 pathway. Excretion of parent drug and metabolites is primarily via the feces. $t_{1/2}$. 7.8 h.

Adverse Reactions, Contraindications, Precautions, Drug Interactions, Parameters to Monitor. Refer to Class Information at the beginning of this chapter.

FLUNISOLIDE   AeroBid, AeroBid-M, Nasarel, Various

Refer to Class Information at the beginning of this chapter.

Administration and Dosage. Inhalation for asthma (adults and children ≥ 15 years)—500 μg (2 sprays) bid, morning and evening (total daily dose of 1 mg), maximum 4 inhalations bid (total daily dose of 2 mg). **Nasal spray (adults and children ≥ 15 years)**—2 sprays (50 μg) each nostril bid. May increase to 2 sprays each nostril tid, maximum 8 sprays/nostril/d (400 μg).

Pediatric Dosage. (Adolescents and children 6–14 years)—2 inhalations bid for a total daily dose of 1 mg. **(Children <6 years)**—dosage not available. **Nasal spray (adolescents and children 6–14 years)**—1 spray (25 μg) each nostril tid or 2 sprays (50 μg) each nostril bid, maximum 4 sprays/nostril/d (200 μg). **(Children <6 years)**—not recommended.

Dosage Forms. Inhal aerosol MDI 250 μg/Inhal, 100 Inhal/canister. AeroBid-M contains menthol. **Nasal spray** 25 μg/spray.

Patient Instructions. Refer to Class Information at the beginning of this chapter.

Pharmacokinetics. *Fate.* Following oral inhalation, total systemic bioavailability is 40%. Swallowed flunisolide is converted to the 6 β-OH metabolite during hepatic first-pass metabolism. $t_{1/2}$. 1.8 h.

Adverse Reactions, Contraindications, Precautions, Drug Interactions. Refer to Class Information at the beginning of this chapter.

Parameters to Monitor. When AeroBid and AeroBid-M are used chronically at 2 mg/d (adults) or 1 mg/d (pediatrics), monitor for effects on HPA axis.

Notes. Evidence suggests higher levels of systemic absorption with flunisolide than with other ICS. However, aerosol administration of 2 mg daily for 1 week in healthy volunteers did not reveal suppression of adrenal function nor the HPA axis.

MOMETASONE FUROATE
Asmanex Twisthaler, Nasonex

Refer to Class Information at the beginning of this chapter.

Administration and Dosage. In patients with known seasonal allergens, prophylaxis is recommended 2–4 weeks prior to the start of the pollen season.

Inhalation powder for asthma (adults and children ≥ 12 years)—previous therapy with bronchodilators alone or with ICS 220 μg qd in the evening, maximum 440 μg (may be administered qd or bid); previous therapy with oral corticosteroids 440 μg bid, maximum 880 μg. **Nasal inhalation for allergic rhinitis (adults and children ≥ 12 years)**—2 sprays (50 μg/spray) each nostril qd for a total dose of 200 μg/d **Nasal inhalation for polyps (adults ≥ 18 years)**—2 sprays (50 μg/spray)/nostril bid for a total daily dose of 400 μg/d. May be effective qd.

Pediatric Dosage. Inhalation powder for asthma (children 4–11 years)—110 μg qd in the evening (regardless of previous therapy), maximum 110 μg/d. **Nasal inhalation for allergic rhinitis (children 2–11 years)**— 1 spray (50 μg/spray)/ nostril for a total dose of 100 μg/d.

Geriatric Dosage. Usual adult dosage.

Dosage Forms. Inhal Pwdr 110 μg (100 μg/Inhal) available as 7, 30 inhalation units; 220 μg (200 μg/Inhal) available as 14, 30, 60, 120 inhalation units. **Nasal spray** 50 μg/spray, 120 sprays/bottle.

Patient Information. Refer to Class Information at the beginning of this chapter.

Pharmacokinetics. *Fate.* Mean absolute systemic bioavailability is < 1%, with mean time to peak concentration of 1–2.5 h. Metabolism is primarily and extensively hepatic via the CYP450 3A4 isoenzyme, with no major metabolites identified. Excretion is primarily via the feces (74%) and urine (8%).

$t_{1/2}$. 5h.

Adverse Reactions, Contraindications, Precautions, Drug Interactions, Parameters to Monitor. Refer to Class Information at the beginning of this chapter.

TRIAMCINOLONE ACETONIDE
Azmacort, Nasacort AQ

Refer to Class Information at the beginning of this chapter.

Dosage and Administration. Inhalation for asthma (adults and children ≥ 12 years)—2 inhalations (75 μg/inhalation) tid–qid or 4 inhalations bid, maximum 16 inhalations (1200 μg total dose)/d. Consider initial dosage of 12–16 inhalations/d in patients with severe asthma and titrate to lowest effective dose once stability is achieved. **Nasal spray for allergic rhinitis (adults and children ≥12 years)**—2 sprays (55 μg/spray) each nostril qd for a total and maximum dose of 220 μg/d.

Pediatric Dosage. Inhalation for asthma (children 6–12 years)—1–2 inhalations (75–150 μg) tid–qid or 2–4 inhalations (150–300 μg) bid, maximum 12 inhalations (900 μg)/d. **(Children <6 years)**—dosage not established. **Nasal spray for allergic rhinitis (children 6–12 years)**—1 spray each nostril qd for a total dose of 110 μg, maximum 220 μg (2 sprays each nostril qd).

Geriatric Dosage. Usual adult dose; initiate at lower end of dosing range.

Dosage Forms. **Inhal aerosol** 75 µg/Inhal, 240 actuations/canister. **Nasal spray** 55 µg/spray, 30 actuations/6.5 g bottle, 120 actuations/16.5 g bottle.

Patient Information. Refer also to Class Information at beginning of this chapter.

To use the Azmacort delivery system, begin by lining up the arrows on the inhaler and gently pulling each end of the inhaler until it is fully extended (you should see the small hole where the medication will come out). Adjust the inhaler into an "L" shape—it is hinged to swing in one direction only. The ridge on the top part of the inhaler should fit into the notch on the bottom part of the inhaler. Remove the mouthpiece cap. If using your inhaler for the first time, or if it has not been used in 3 or more days, prime the inhaler by holding it upright with the mouthpiece facing away from you. Shake the inhaler gently and press the canister firmly so that 2 puffs are released. If you don't need to prime your inhaler, simply open it and shake it before use. Breathe out to empty your lungs completely, place the mouthpiece in your mouth, close your lips tightly around it and press down firmly on the metal canister while breathing in slowly and deeply through your mouth only. Do not remove the inhaler from your mouth after breathing in the medication. Instead, hold your breath for 10 s and THEN remove the inhaler. Breathe out slowly. If you take more than 1 puff, wait 60 s between each puff and then repeat as your health care provider has instructed. After you have taken the prescribed number of puffs, thoroughly rinse your mouth with water. Do not swallow the water after rinsing—spit it out.

Pharmacokinetics. *Onset.* Relief of symptoms may be seen within a week, or may not occur for 2 or more weeks.

Fate. Triamcinolone acetonide is the more potent metabolite of triamcinolone; approximately 8 times more potent than prednisone in animal models of inflammation. It is rapidly absorbed following oral administration with peak plasma concentrations occurring at 1.5–2 h. Plasma protein binding is relatively low (~68%). Metabolism and excretion are rapid, with 3 metabolites identified and substantially less active than the parent compound. $t_{1/2}$. ~88 min.

Adverse Reactions, Contraindications, Precautions, Drug Interactions, Parameters to Monitor. Refer to Class Information at the beginning of this chapter.

■ REFERENCES

1. National Heart, Lung and Blood Institute. *National Asthma Education and Prevention Program Expert Panel Report 3: Guidelines for the Diagnosis and Management of Asthma.* NIH Publication No. 08-5846. Bethesda, MD; 2007.
2. Barnes PJ. Inhaled glucocorticoids for asthma. *N Engl J Med.* 1995;332:868-875.
3. McCubbin MM et al. A bioassay for topical and systemic effect of three inhaled steroids. *Clin Pharmacol Ther.* 1995;57:455-460.
4. Holliday SM et al. Inhaled fluticasone propionate. A review of its pharmacodynamic and pharmacokinetic properties, and therapeutic use in asthma. *Drugs.* 1994;47:318-331.
5. Matthys H et al. Dextromethorphan and codeine: objective assessment of antitussive activity in patients with chronic cough. *J Int Med Res.* 1983;11:92-100.
6. Kamada AK. Therapeutic controversies in the treatment of asthma. *Ann Pharmacother.* 1994;28:904-914.
7. Jacqz-Aigrain E et al. CYP2D6- and CYP3A-dependent metabolism of dextromethorphan in humans. *Pharmacogenetics.* 1993;3:197-204.
8. Woodworth JR et al. The polymorphic metabolism of dextromethorphan. *J Clin Pharmacol.* 1987;27:139-143.
9. Bryant BG, Lombardi TP. Cold, cough, and allergy products. In: Covington TR, ed. *Handbook of Nonprescription Drugs.* 10th ed. Washington, DC: American Pharmaceutical Association; 1993:89-115.
10. Toogood JH et al. Aerosol corticosteroid. In: Weiss EB et al., eds. *Bronchial Asthma: Mechanisms and Therapeutics.* 3rd ed. Boston, MA: Little, Brown and Company; 1993:818-841.

Chapter 60

Cough and Cold

Laura L. Sanders

| **DEXTROMETHORPHAN** | Delsym, Robitussin, Vicks 44, |
| **HYDROBROMIDE, POLISTIREX** | multiple branded products, Various |

Pharmacology. Dextromethorphan is the nonanalgesic, nonaddictive D-isomer of the codeine analogue of levorphanol. With usual antitussive doses, the cough threshold is elevated centrally with little effect on the respiratory, cardiovascular, or GI systems; it does not inhibit ciliary activity.

Dosage and Administration. (**Adults and children ≥ 12 years**)—(**PO as cough suppressant**) 10–20 mg q4h or 30 mg every 6–8 h; **ER** 60 mg q12h. Maximum 120 mg/d.

Special Populations. *Pediatric Dosage.* **PO as cough suppressant**—(**children < 4 years**) not recommended; (**children 4–6 years**) 2.5–5 mg q4h or 7.5 mg every 6–8 h, to a maximum of 30 mg/d; (**children 6–12 years**) 5–10 mg every 4h or 15 mg every 6–8 h, to a maximum of 60 mg/d. **ER**—(**children 4–6 years**) 15 mg q12h; (**children 6–12 years**) 30 mg q12h. (*See* Notes.)

Geriatric Dosage. Same as adult dosage.

Dosage Forms. **Cap** 30 mg; **Gel Cap** 15 mg; **lozenge** 2.5, 5, 7.5, 15 mg; **oral strips** 7.5 mg; **syrup** 0.67, 0.7, 1, 1.5, 2, 3 mg/mL; **ER Susp** 6 mg/mL; (available in many combination products in different concentrations).

Patient Instructions. Do not use this drug to suppress productive cough or chronic cough that occurs with smoking, asthma, or emphysema. Report if your cough persists. Some preparations contain alcohol. May cause drowsiness; alcohol and other CNS depressants may increase drowsiness.

Pharmacokinetics. *Onset and Duration.* PO—onset 15–30 min; duration up to 6 h with non-ER, 12 h for ER suspension.[1]

Fate. Rapidly absorbed from the GI tract and extensively metabolized, including appreciable first-pass effect, mainly to the active metabolite dextrorphan. Genetically determined polymorphic metabolism primarily by CYP2D6 with extensive (93%) and poor (7%) metabolizers. Peak plasma concentration in ~2.5 h. Excretion is primarily in the urine. (*See* Notes.)

$t_{1/2}$. (extensive metabolizers) 3–4 h to approximately 9 h; (poor metabolizers) 17–138 h.[2]

Adverse Reactions. Occasional mild drowsiness and GI upset. Intoxication, bizarre behavior, CNS depression, and respiratory depression can occur with extremely high dosages. Naloxone might be effective in reversing these effects.[3–6] Reports of dextromethorphan abuse have increased, especially among teenagers.[7,8]

Contraindications. MAOI therapy.[9]

Precautions. Generally, do not use in patients with chronic cough or cough associated with excessive secretions.

Drug Interactions. Concurrent MAOIs can cause hypotension, hyperpyrexia, nausea, and coma. Drugs that inhibit CYP2D6 (e.g., SSRIs) can inhibit dextromethorphan metabolism, but serious effects have not been reported.

Parameters to Monitor. Observe for relief of cough and CNS side effects.

Notes. Approximately equipotent with **codeine** in antitussive effectiveness in adults.[1,3] For cough associated with the common cold, first-generation antihistamine decongestants are recommended instead of newer, nonsedating antihistamines. Medications that alter the characteristics of mucus, peripheral cough suppressants, central cough suppressants, and zinc are not recommended to improve cough, nor are OTC combination cold medicines.[10] In patients with chronic bronchitis, codeine and dextromethorphan are recommended for short-term symptomatic relief of cough.[11]

One trial of dextromethorphan and codeine for night cough in children found not superior to placebo, and their efficacies have been questioned for this or any other use in children.[4,12] In October 2008, FDA completed its review of information about the safety of over-the-counter (OTC) cough and cold medicines in infants and children younger than 2 years. FDA is recommending that these drugs should not be used to treat infants and children younger than 2 years, because serious and potentially life-threatening side effects can occur. The FDA supports the Consumer Healthcare Products Association (CHPA), an association that represents most of the makers of nonprescription OTC cough and cold medicines for children, announcement that its members are voluntarily modifying the product labels for consumers of OTC cough and cold medicines to state "Do Not Use" in children younger than 4 years. Additionally, the manufacturers are introducing new child-resistant packaging and new measuring devices for use with the products.[13]

Used commonly for CYP2D6 phenotyping.[14] Dextromethorphan is currently being investigated for its analgesic-sparing effect.[15] Oral dextromethorphan in patients undergoing surgery with epidural lidocaine or general anesthesia reduces morphine and diclofenac use by approximately 50% in the immediate and late postoperative period compared with placebo, and improved subjectively scored levels of pain, sedation, and well-being.[16]

GUAIFENESIN	Guiatuss, Mucinex, Robitussin, Organidin NR, multiple branded products, Various

Pharmacology. Guaifenesin is proposed to have an expectorant action through an increased output of respiratory tract fluid, enhancing the flow of less viscid secretions, promoting ciliary action, and facilitating the removal of thickened or dried mucus. Evidence of the effectiveness of guaifenesin is largely subjective and not well established clinically.[3,10,17–20]

Administration and Dosage. PO as an expectorant: capsules, tablets, oral solution, syrup (adults and children ≥ 12 years)—200–400 mg q4h, maximum 2400 mg/d; ER capsules, tablets 600–1200 mg q12h, to a maximum of 2400 mg/d.[18]

Special Populations. *Pediatric Dosage.* **PO as an expectorant: capsules, tablets**—(children 4–6 years) liquid or ER capsule preferable for use in this age group; (children 6–12 years) 100–200 mg q4h, maximum 1200 mg/d. **ER capsules,**

tablets (children 4–6 years) 300 mg q12h; (children 6–12 years) 600 mg q12h, maximum 1200 mg/d. Oral solution, syrup (children 6–12 years) 100–200 mg q4h, maximum 1200 mg/d; (children 4–6 years) 50–100 mg q4h, maximum 600 mg/d.

Geriatric Dosage. Usual adult dosage.

Dosage Forms. Cap 200 mg; syrup 20, 40 mg/mL; Tab 100, 200, 1200 mg; SR Cap 300 mg; ER Tab 600, 1200 mg. Multiple combination products with pseudoephedrine, phenylephrine, and dextromethorphan.

Pharmacokinetics. Rapidly absorbed from the GI tract and eliminated renally; $t_{1/2}$. 1 h.

Patient Instructions. Take this drug with a large quantity of water to ensure proper drug action. Report if your cough persists for more than 1 week, recurs, or is accompanied by high fever, rash, or persistent headache. Excessive dosage can cause nausea and vomiting.

Adverse Reactions. Occasional nausea and vomiting, especially with excessive dosage; dizziness; headache.

Precautions. Generally, do not use in patients with chronic cough or cough associated with excessive secretions.

Drug Interactions. None known.

Notes. May interfere with certain laboratory determinations of 5-hydroxyindoleacetic acid and vanillylmandelic acid but does not cause a positive stool guaiac reaction in normal subjects.[19] *See* also Notes section of dextromethorphan monograph regarding administration of cough and cold preparations to children <4 years.

PSEUDOEPHEDRINE HYDROCHLORIDE	Sudafed, Various
PSEUDOEPHEDRINE SULFATE	Chlor-Trimeton Non-Drowsy, Drixoral

Pharmacology. Pseudoephedrine is an indirect-acting agent that stimulates α- and β-adrenergic receptors via release of endogenous adrenergic amines producing vasoconstriction (via α-stimulation) and bronchial relaxation (via β-stimulation). It is used primarily for decongestion of nasal mucosa through its action of shrinking swollen nasal mucous membranes, reducing tissue edema, and increasing nasal airway patency.

Administration and Dosage. Give with water or milk to decrease GI distress. Do not crush ER formulations.

PO as a decongestant: Capsules, tablets, oral solution, syrup (adults and children ≥ 12 years)—60 mg every 4–6 h, to a maximum of 240 mg/d. PO—ER capsules, tablets 120 mg q12h; 240 mg q24h, maximum 240 mg/d.

Special Populations. *Pediatric Dosage.* PO as a decongestant: oral solution, syrup. Note: For children up to 2 years, dosage should be individualized; 4 mg/kg body weight or 125 mg/m² BSA per day administered in 4 divided doses q6h. OR (children 4–12 months) 7.5 mg every 4–6 h, maximum 4 doses (30 mg)/24 h; (children 12–23 months) 11.25 mg every 4–6 h, maximum 4 doses (45 mg)/24 h; (children 2–5 years) 15 mg every 4–6 h, maximum 60 mg/24 h; (children 6–12 years) 30 mg every 4–6 h, maximum 120 mg/24 h. Do not give ER capsule/tablet 120 or 240 mg to patients <12 years.

Geriatric Dosage. Usual adult dosage. However, elderly patients are more likely to have prostatic hypertrophy and may require a dosage adjustment. Demonstrate safe use of short-acting formulation before using an ER product.

Dosage Forms. **(HCl) Cap** 30, 60 mg; **oral Soln** 9.4 mg/mL, 3 mg/mL, 6 mg/mL; **syrup** 3, 6 mg/mL; **Tab** 30, 60 mg; **ER Tab** (12 h) 120 mg; (24 h) 240 mg. **(Sulfate) Tab** 60 mg, **ER Tab** 120 mg.

Patient Instructions. Take the last dose of the day several hours before bedtime if you have difficulty sleeping. Do not crush or chew sustained-release preparations. Take with water or milk to decrease stomach upset.

Pharmacokinetics. *Onset and Duration.* Onset within 30 min on an empty stomach, within 1 h for ER forms; duration 3–4 h for immediate-release forms, 8–12 h for most ER forms.

Fate. Solution and immediate-release tablets are rapidly and completely absorbed orally. SR dosage forms attain peak serum levels in (12-h product) 4–6 h or (24-h product) 12 h. Food appears to delay absorption of non-ER forms, but not the ER forms.[21,22] V_d is 2.7 ± 0.2 L/kg; Cl averages 0.44 L/h/kg. Partly metabolized to inactive metabolite(s), and 6% metabolized to active metabolite, norpseudoephedrine; 45%–90% excreted unchanged in urine depending on urinary pH and flow.[23,24]

$t_{1/2}$. urinary flow and pH dependent; 13 ± 3 h at pH 8; 6.9 ± 1.2 h at pH 5.5–6; 4.7 ± 1.4 h at pH 5.[23,24]

Adverse Reactions. Frequent mild transient nervousness, insomnia, irritability, or headache. Usually negligible pressor effect in normotensive patients.[25,26]

Contraindications. Severe hypertension; coronary artery disease; MAOI therapy.

Precautions. Use with caution in patients with renal failure,[21] hypertension, diabetes mellitus, ischemic heart disease, increased intraocular pressure, prostatic hypertrophy, urinary retention, or thyroid disease. Elderly patients might be particularly sensitive to CNS effects. If use is necessary in infants with phenylketonuria, reduce dosage to avoid possible increased agitation.[22]

Drug Interactions. Concurrent MAOIs can increase pressor response. Urinary alkalinizers can decrease pseudoephedrine clearance; β-adrenergic agents may inhibit effect.

Parameters to Monitor. Nasal stuffiness, CNS stimulation, blood pressure in hypertensive patients.

Notes. Combination with an antihistamine can provide additive benefit in seasonal allergic rhinitis because antihistamines do not relieve nasal stuffiness.[23,24] Neither these combinations nor decongestants alone provide consistent long-term benefit for reduction of middle ear effusion in children with otitis media and are not recommended for this use.[25,26] *See* also Notes section of dextromethorphan monograph regarding administration of cough and cold preparations to children <4 years.

■ REFERENCES

1. American Academy of Pediatrics. Committee on Drugs. Use of codeine- and dextromethorphan-containing cough syrups in pediatrics. *Pediatrics.* 1997;99:918-920.
2. Katona B, Wason S. Dextromethorphan danger. *N Engl J Med.* 1986;314:993. Letter.
3. Bem JL, Peck R. Dextromethorphan. An overview of safety issues. *Drug Saf.* 1992;190-199.

4. Cranston JW, Yoast R. Abuse of dextromethorphan. *Arch Fam Med.* 1999;8:99-100.

5. Nierenberg DW, Semprebon M. The central nervous system serotonin syndrome. *Clin Pharmacol Ther.* 1993;53:84-88.

6. Taylor JA et al. Efficacy of cough suppressants in children. *J Pediatr.* 1993;122:799-802.

7. Streetman DS et al. Dose dependency of dextromethorphan for cytochrome P450 2D6 (CYP2D6) phenotyping. *Clin Pharmacol Ther.* 1999;66:535-541.

8. Henderson DJ et al. Perioperative dextromethorphan reduces postoperative pain after hysterectomy. *Anesth Analg.* 1999;89:399-402.

9. Anonymous. Guaiphenesin and iodide. *Drug Ther Bull.* 1985;23:62-64.

10. Anonymous. Cold, cough, allergy, bronchodilator, and antiasthmatic drug products for over-the-counter human use; expectorant drug products for over-the-counter human use; final monograph. *Fed Regist.* 1989;54:8494-8509.

11. Ziment I. Drugs modifying the sol-layer and the hydration of mucus. In: Braga PC, Allegra L, eds. *Drugs in Bronchial Mucology.* New York: Raven Press; 1989:293-322.

12. Sisson JH et al. Effects of guaifenesin on nasal mucociliary clearance and ciliary beat frequency in healthy volunteers. *Chest.* 1995;107:747-751.

13. Roth RP et al. Nasal decongestant activity of pseudoephedrine. *Ann Otol Rhinol Laryngol.* 1977;86:235-242.

14. Hamilton LH et al. A study of sustained action pseudoephedrine in allergic rhinitis. *Ann Allergy.* 1982;48:87-92.

15. Hwang SS et al. In vitro and in vivo evaluation of a once-daily controlled-release pseudoephedrine product. *J Clin Pharmacol.* 1995;35:259-267.

16. Kanfer I et al. Pharmacokinetics of oral decongestants. *Pharmacotherapy.* 1993;13(6, pt 2):116S-128S.

17. Brater DC et al. Renal excretion of pseudoephedrine. *Clin Pharmacol Ther.* 1980;28:690-694.

18. Kuntzman RG et al. The influence of urinary pH on the plasma half-life of pseudoephedrine in man and dog and a sensitive assay for its determination in human plasma. *Clin Pharmacol Ther.* 1971;12:62-67.

19. Chua SS, Benrimoj SI. Non-prescription sympathomimetic agents and hypertension. *Med Toxicol.* 1988;3:387-417.

20. Beck RA et al. Cardiovascular effects of pseudoephedrine in medically controlled hypertensive patients. *Arch Intern Med.* 1992;152:1242-1245.

21. Sica DA, Comstock TJ. Case report: pseudoephedrine accumulation in renal failure. *Am J Med Sci.* 1989;298:261-263.

22. Spielberg SP, Schulman JD. A possible reaction to pseudoephedrine in a patient with phenylketonuria. *J Pediatr.* 1977;90:1026.

23. Hendeles L. Selecting a decongestant. *Pharmacotherapy.* 1993;13(6, pt 2):129S-134S.

24. Bryant BG, Lombardi TP. Cold, cough, and allergy products. In: Covington TR, ed. *Handbook of Nonprescription Drugs.* 10th ed. Washington, DC: American Pharmaceutical Association; 1993:89-115.

25. Thoene DE, Johnson CE. Pharmacotherapy of otitis media. *Pharmacotherapy.* 1991;11:212-221.

26. Bahal N, Nahata MC. Recent advances in the treatment of otitis media. *J Clin Pharm Ther.* 1992;17:201-215.

27. Shaul WL et al. Dextromethorphan toxicity: reversal by naloxone. *Pediatrics.* 1977;59:117-119.

PART II

Clinical Information

Principal Editor: Kelly M. Smith

Drug-Induced Diseases

Kelly M. Smith

Chapter 61

Drug-Induced Blood Dyscrasias

Stephanie D. Sutphin

This table does not include all drugs capable of causing the specified dyscrasias and excludes cancer chemotherapeutic agents, which are known for producing dose-related bone marrow suppression. Five major types of blood dyscrasias have been selected for inclusion in this table; the following abbreviations indicate specific blood dyscrasias:

AA	—	Aplastic Anemia
AGN	—	Agranulocytosis, Granulocytopenia, or Neutropenia
APRCA	—	Acquired Pure Red Cell Aplasia
HA	—	Hemolytic Anemia
MA	—	Macrocytic Anemia
Th	—	Thrombocytopenia

DRUG AND DYSCRASIA	NATURE OF DYSCRASIA
Abciximab	
Th	The combination of abciximab and heparin presents twice the risk of mild and severe thrombocytopenia as the combination of placebo and heparin. (See also Heparin.)[1]
Acetaminophen	
Th	Scattered reports only; observed in 6 of 174 overdose patients in one report; might be an immune reaction.[1–3]

(continued)

DRUG AND DYSCRASIA	NATURE OF DYSCRASIA
Acetazolamide	
AGN	Eleven cases of acetazolamide-associated aplastic anemia were reported in Sweden during a 17-y period. The estimated incidence of reported acetazolamide-associated aplastic anemia is approximately 1 in 18,000 patient y.[4]
Th	Limited case reports.[5–7]
Alcohol	
HA	Most commonly encountered in chronic alcoholism.[8]
MA	Results from malnutrition and decreased folate absorption and/or utilization. Responds rapidly to folic acid administration.[8]
Th	Transient in many drinkers; persistent thrombocytopenia can accompany advanced alcoholic liver disease.[8]
Amphotericin B	
Th	Scattered reports only.[9]
Antidepressants, Heterocyclic	
AGN	Multiple case reports.[10] Idiosyncratic reaction, probably resulting from a direct toxic effect rather than allergy. Most commonly occurs between the 2nd and 8th wk of the therapy.[11]
Ascorbic Acid	
HA	In G-6-PD deficiency with large doses.[12,13]
Aspirin	
HA	Almost always encountered in patients with G-6-PD deficiency, usually in conjunction with infection, or other complicating factors.[13,14]
Th	Can occur in addition to the drug's effects on platelet adhesiveness. Some evidence for an immune reaction.[15]
Azathioprine	
AGN	WBC counts <2500/μL occur in about 3% of rheumatoid arthritis patients treated with azathioprine; an additional 15% develop some lesser degree of leukopenia.[16]
Captopril	
AGN	Neutropenia, once thought to be prevalent, now appears to be so only in patients with autoimmune or collagen-vascular disease; the majority of patients outside these groups are at low risk.[10,17]
Carbamazepine	
AA	27 cases reported from 1964 to1988; onset can be delayed until weeks or months after the initiation of therapy.[18]
AGN	Numerous case reports.[10] Leukopenia develops slowly, occurring in approximately 12% of children and 7% of adults. Its onset is typically within the first 3 mo of treatment, with patients at risk having a low or low-normal pretreatment white blood cell (WBC) count. Leukopenia often reverses, even if CBZ is continued.[19,20]
Th	Prevalence estimated at 2%.[1,19,20]

(continued)

DRUG AND DYSCRASIA	NATURE OF DYSCRASIA
Cephalosporins	
AGN	Rare; possibly the result of an immune reaction but occurs most often with high dosages and parenteral therapy lasting >2 wk.[10,21–23]
HA	Positive direct Coombs' test occurs frequently and can persist for up to 2 mo after discontinuation of therapy. Hemolysis is rare.[21–23]
Th	Rare; possibly the result of an immune reaction. Usually occurs late in the course of therapy.[21–23]
Chloramphenicol	
AA	Drug most commonly associated with marrow aplasia.[24]
HA	In G-6-PD deficiency.[13]
Chloroquine	
HA	Only a few cases have been reported; some association with G-6-PD deficiency is suspected.[13]
Chlorpromazine	
AGN	Several case reports, some fatal. Monitor blood counts if sore throat, or fever develop.[10,21]
Cimetidine	
AA	Scattered reports only; however, at least two fatalities with cimetidine reported (one fatality also was receiving chloramphenicol).[25]
AGN	Usually occurs in patients with systemic disease or other drug therapy that might have contributed to the dyscrasia.[10,25]
Th	Reversible upon discontinuation. Can occur with other H-2 antagonists.[1,26]
Ciprofloxacin	
Th	Rare case reports.[27,28]
Clopidogrel	
Th	At least 11 cases of clopidogrel-associated thrombotic thrombocytopenic purpura have been reported. Most cases occurred during the first 2 wk of treatment.[29]
Clozapine	
AGN	Frequency of granulocytopenia is calculated to be 0.4%–0.8% in closely monitored patients. Mild to moderate neutropenia occurs in 3%–20%. Most cases occur in the first 4 mo. Asians are more than twice as susceptible as whites. Recovery usually occurs 2–3 wk after drug withdrawal. Frequent WBC counts are mandated.[10,30–32]
Cocaine	
Th	Reported with IV and inhalational use.[33]
Dapsone	
AGN	Multiple case reports, some resulting in death.[10]
HA	In G-6-PD deficiency; might have other mechanism(s). Might be dose related; uncommon at 100 mg/d but frequent at 200–300 mg/d.[8]

(continued)

DRUG AND DYSCRASIA	NATURE OF DYSCRASIA
Digoxin	
Th	Scattered reports only; evidence of an immune mechanism.[34]
Dimercaprol	
HA	In G-6-PD deficiency.[8]
Doxepin	
Th	Rare.[35,36]
Dipyridamole	
Th	Relative risk of thrombocytopenia calculated to be 14 times higher than in untreated individuals, but needs confirmation.[34]
Diuretics, Thiazide	
HA	Exact mechanism is unclear; might be an immune reaction.[8,37]
Th	Mild thrombocytopenia occurs frequently, but severe cases are rare. Might be caused by an immune reaction.[1]
Eflornithine	
AA	Deaths caused by aplastic anemia have been reported.[38]
AGN	Leukopenia is reported in 18%–37% of patients.[38]
MA	Megaloblastic anemia is frequently reported.[38]
Erythropoetin	
APRCA	Cases of pure red cell aplasia and of severe anemia, with or without other cytopenias, associated with neutralizing antibodies to erythropoietin have been reported.[39]
Eptifibatide	
Th	Platelet inhibitor. Implicated in 5 or more reports.[1]
Etanercept	
AA	Although the causal relationship is unclear, some cases of aplastic anemia, including fatalities, have been associated with etanercept.[40]
Felbamate	
AA	More than 30 cases were reported shortly after the introduction of felbamate, resulting in the manufacturer and FDA urging withdrawal of patients from therapy. When a strict definition of aplastic anemia is applied and confounding factors are accounted for, the risk of aplastic anemia from felbamate might not be markedly different from the risk posed by carbamazepine. Most cases developed 2–6 mo after initiation of therapy. Monitoring has not been effective for early identification of cases.[41,42]
Fluconazole	
Th	Scattered reports only.[43]
Flucytosine	
AGN	Dose-related; usually requires plasma concentrations ≥100–125 mg/L.[44]
Th	Dose-related; usually requires plasma concentrations ≥100–125 mg/L.[44]

(continued)

DRUG AND DYSCRASIA	NATURE OF DYSCRASIA
Foscarnet	
AGN	Neutropenia occurs in 14% of patients treated for cytomegalovirus retinitis.[45]
Furosemide	
Th	Uncommon, mild, and asymptomatic.[46]
Ganciclovir	
AGN	Granulocytopenia occurs in about 40% of patients; it is usually reversible with drug discontinuation, but irreversible neutropenia and deaths have occurred.[45,47]
Th	Thrombocytopenia occurs in about 20% of patients.[47]
Gold Salts	
AA	Not dose-dependent; although this reaction is not common, numerous fatalities have been reported.[16,48]
AGN	Often brief and self-limiting; usually responds to withdrawal of therapy.[49,50]
Th	Not dose- or duration-dependent; prevalence estimated at 1%–3%; onset usually during the loading phase (first 1000 mg) but can be delayed until after the drug has been discontinued. Mechanism is unclear, but it often appears to be immunologically mediated. Up to 85% of patients with gold-induced thrombocytopenia have HLA-DR3 phenotype compared with 30% of all rheumatoid arthritis patients.[1,2,8,51,52]
Heparin	
Th	Many patients demonstrate a mild to moderate transient decrease in platelets after only a few days of heparin therapy. Up to 3% experience immune-mediated, persistent thrombocytopenia, which is associated with increased thrombin generation and development of serious thrombotic complications in 30%–60%. Intermittent, continuous infusion and "minidose" regimens have been implicated; this is uncommon with SQ administration. Prompt cessation of heparin minimizes serious complications; platelet count usually returns to normal within 7–10 d. Low-molecular-weight heparins (e.g., **dalteparin, enoxaparin, tinzaparin**) are much less likely than unfractionated heparin to stimulate the formation of immune complexes, leading to thrombocytopenia. Low-molecular-weight heparins offer very little protection from thrombocytopenia in patients who have already formed heparin-associated antibodies.[1,53–55]
Immune Globulin	
AGN	Transient neutropenia frequently accompanies IV use.[52]
HA	Acute Coombs' positive hemolysis has been reported in patients receiving high-dose therapy.[56]
Inamrinone	
Th	Prevalence during parenteral therapy has been estimated at 2.4%, although 8 of 16 children receiving parenteral inamrinone developed thrombocytopenia in one report. Thrombocytopenia might be caused by nonimmune peripheral platelet destruction.[57,58]

(*continued*)

DRUG AND DYSCRASIA	NATURE OF DYSCRASIA
Interferon Alfa	
AGN	Neutropenia may be observed at all dose levels. May be dose-limiting at higher dose ranges.[59]
AA	Rare cases.[59]
HA	<5% incidence.[59]
PRCA	Identified in postapproval use (rare).[59]
Th	Common, dose-limiting at higher ranges.[59,60]
Isoniazid	
AGN	Scattered reports only; some evidence of an immune reaction.[8,60]
Th	Scattered reports only; some evidence of an immune reaction.[8,60,61]
Isotretinoin	
AGN	Case reports; can be life-threatening.[10]
Lamotrigine	
AGN	Scattered reports only.[10,62]
Levamisole	
AGN	Multiple literature references.[10]
Th	Scattered reports only.[63]
Levodopa	
HA	Autoimmune reaction; positive direct and indirect Coombs' tests are frequent, but hemolysis is rare. **Carbidopa–levodopa** combinations also have produced hemolysis.[8]
Linezolid	
Th	Implicated in 5 or more reports.[1]
Methimazole	
AA	Scattered reports only, but some increased risk is present. Most cases occur during the first 3 mo of therapy.[64,65]
AGN	Prevalence estimated at 0.31%. Encountered overwhelmingly in women and appears to increase with age. Most cases occur in the first 3 mo of therapy; monitoring during this time might detect agranulocytosis before it is clinically apparent.[8,10,65,66]
Methyldopa	
AGN	Rare cases.[10]
HA	Autoimmune reaction; positive direct Coombs' test occurs in 5%–25% of patients, depending on dosage; hemolysis occurs in <1%, and its onset is gradual after ≥4 mo of therapy. Recovery is rapid after discontinuation of the drug.[8,67]
Th	Rare; might be caused by an immune reaction.[8,68]
Methylene Blue	
HA	In G-6-PD deficiency.[8]

(*continued*)

DRUG AND DYSCRASIA	NATURE OF DYSCRASIA
Nalidixic Acid	
HA	In G-6-PD deficiency; might have other mechanisms.[8]
Th	Scattered reports only; possibly associated with renal impairment in one series.[69]
Nifedipine	
AA	Increased risk identified in one long-term case surveillance study (absolute risk of 1.2 per 100,000 patient y).[70]
Nitrofurantoin	
HA	In G-6-PD deficiency; also encountered with enolase deficiency (mechanism unknown).[8]
NSAIDs	
AA	Although rare, indomethacin has been associated with a risk 12.7 times higher than in untreated individuals, especially when used regularly and for a long duration.[71]
HA	Thought to be autoimmune.[8,14]
AGN	Although rare, risk can be 8.9 times higher in patient receiving Indomethacin than in untreated individuals.[53]
Th	Commonly implicated.[1]
Penicillamine	
AA	Rare; develops after several months of therapy; due to direct marrow toxicity.[72,73]
AGN	Rare; most cases occur during the first month of therapy.[8,10,73]
HA	Scattered reports only; might be caused by G-6-PD deficiency or fluctuations in copper levels during therapy of Wilson's disease.[73,74]
Th	Prevalence estimated at 10%; some decrease in platelet counts occurs in 75% of penicillamine-treated patients. Might be the result of an immune reaction; most commonly occurs during the first 6 mo of therapy.[8,73,75]
Penicillins	
AA	Prevalence very low when extent of use is considered.[8]
AGN	Uncommon with most penicillins but frequent with **methicillin**; in one report, neutropenia developed in 23 of 68 methicillin-treated patients; resolution occurred within 3–7 d after drug withdrawal. The risk of penicillin-induced neutropenia is increased with parenteral treatment lasting >2 wk.[4,10,23,76]
HA	Positive direct Coombs' test occurs with large IV doses; hemolysis is rare.[8,14]
Th	Very rare.[1]
Phenazopyridine	
HA	Prevalence and mechanism unknown; renal insufficiency and overdose might be contributing factors. Often accompanied by methemoglobinemia.[8,77]
Phenobarbital	
MA	More than 100 cases reported; usually responds to folic acid.[8]

(continued)

DRUG AND DYSCRASIA	NATURE OF DYSCRASIA
Phenothiazines	
AGN	Most common during the first 2 mo of therapy and in older patients (>85% are >40 y). Rapid onset and general lack of dose dependence suggest an idiosyncratic mechanism. Prevalence estimated as high as 1/1200.[8,10,78,79]
Phenytoin	
AA	Fewer than 25 reported cases, but the association with phenytoin is strong.[8]
AGN	Scattered reports only; onset after days to years of therapy.[8,10]
MA	Caused by impaired absorption and/or utilization of folate and responds to folic acid therapy (although folate replacement can lower phenytoin levels). Mild macrocytosis is very common (>25%); onset is unpredictable but usually appears after >6 mo of therapy.[8]
Th	Scattered reports only; might be the result of an immune reaction.[1,8]
Primaquine	
HA	In G-6-PD deficiency.[8]
Primidone	
MA	Similar to phenobarbital, but prevalence might be lower; onset is unpredictable and can be delayed for several years during therapy. Some cases have responded to folic acid.[8]
Procainamide	
AGN	Prevalence usually estimated at <1%, but with a 25% fatal outcome. Occurs with conventional and sustained-release products; usually occurs within the first 90 d of use. No relationship with daily or total dosage.[8,10,80]
Propylthiouracil	
AA	Scattered reports only, but some increased risk is present. Most cases occur within the first 3 mo of therapy.[64,65]
AGN	Prevalence estimated at 0.55%. Occurs overwhelmingly in women and appears to increase with age. Most cases occur in the first 3 mo of therapy, and monitoring during this time might detect agranulocytosis before it becomes clinically apparent. Some evidence for an immune reaction.[8,10]
Quinidine	
AGN	Scattered reports only; an immune mechanism has been described.[10,81]
HA	In G-6-PD deficiency (but not in blacks).[8,14]
Th	Caused by quinidine-specific antibodies; little or no cross-reactivity with quinine. Accounts for a large portion of drug-induced thrombocytopenia.[1]
Quinine	
AGN	Scattered reports only.[8,10]
HA	In G-6-PD deficiency (but not in blacks). An immune mechanism is also suspected because quinine-dependent antibodies to RBCs have been demonstrated in cases of quinine-induced hemolytic-uremic syndrome.[8,82]
Th	Caused by quinine-specific antibodies; little or no cross-reactivity with quinidine. Fatalities have been reported. It has occurred in people drinking quinine-containing tonic water.[1]

(continued)

DRUG AND DYSCRASIA	NATURE OF DYSCRASIA
Rho Immune Globulin	
HA	Rare cases of intravascular hemolysis, usually within 4 h of administration.[83]
Rifabutin	
AGN	In a study of the pharmacokinetic interactions between rifabutin and azithromycin or clarithromycin, rifabutin, alone or in combination with either of those drugs, produced neutropenia in most of the patients. Neutropenia was not seen when either of the other drugs was used without rifabutin.[84]
Rifampin	
HA	Rare but many patients develop a positive Coombs' test; onset in h in some sensitized patients.[8,61,85]
Th	Peripheral destruction of platelets appears to result from an immune reaction; difficult to separate rifampin contribution from that of other drugs because it is usually used in combination therapy.[1]
Sulfasalazine	
AGN	Leukopenia reported in 5.6% of patients receiving the drug for rheumatoid arthritis and agranulocytosis/neutropenia in 4/1000 patients; prevalence of agranulocytosis/neutropenia among inflammatory bowel disease patients is considerably lower (0.3/1000 patients). Onset is usually during the first 3 mo of therapy; recovery takes 2 wk after drug discontinuation.[10,16,86,87]
HA	In G-6-PD deficiency but also occurs in nondeficient patients. Hemolysis might be more common in slow acetylators.[8,87–89]
MA	One series of 130 arthritis patients reported macrocytosis in 21% and macrocytic anemia in 3%.[90]
Sulfonamides	
AA	Historically an important cause of aplastic anemia, but most cases were reported after use of older sulfonamides; rarely occurs with products currently in use.[8]
AGN	Occurs mostly with older products; rarely occurs with products currently in use. Most current cases are in combined use with **trimethoprim**; also reported with **silver sulfadiazine**. Onset is usually rapid.[8,10,14,91,92]
HA	In G-6-PD deficiency but also occurs in nondeficient patients.[8,93]
Th	Scattered reports; probably an immune reaction. (See also Trimethoprim.)[1]
Ticlopidine	
AA	The growing number of cases of aplastic anemia associated with ticlopidine is disturbing; the incidence cannot be estimated.[94]
AGN	Incidence of neutropenia estimated at 2.4% of treated patients with severe neutropenia or agranulocytosis in 0.85%. Obtain CBC every 2 wk during the first 3 mo of treatment. Discontinue ticlopidine if the ANC is $<1200/\mu L$.[10,94]
Th	Thrombotic thrombocytopenia purpura occurs in 1 of every 1600–5000 exposed. Mean time to onset is 22 d. Plasmapheresis reduces the death rate from 60% to 21%.[95,96]

(*continued*)

DRUG AND DYSCRASIA	NATURE OF DYSCRASIA
Tirofiban	
Th	Platelet inhibitor. Implicated in 5 or more reports.[1]
Tocainide	
AGN	Prevalence estimated at 0.07%–0.18% of patients.[97,98]
Triamterene	
MA	Few cases reported, but it is a potent inhibitor of dihydrofolate reductase; greatest risk in those with folate deficiency before therapy (e.g., alcoholics).[8]
Trimethoprim	
AGN	Rare; occurs when used alone and in combination with **sulfonamides**, with the latter numerically more common.[8,10,92,99]
MA	Most cases occur after 1–2 wk of therapy; this drug can have weak antifolate action in humans that becomes important only in those with folate deficiency before therapy (e.g., alcoholics).[8]
Th	Thrombocytopenia is common, but severe cases are rare. Most commonly occurs in combination therapy with sulfonamides.[1]
Vaccines	
Th	A study of 9 million doses of measles, rubella, and mumps vaccines administered to children determined that the prevalence of thrombocytopenia was 0.17 cases/100,000 doses for measles vaccine and 0.23, 0.87, and 0.95 cases/100,000 doses for rubella, measles–rubella, and mumps–measles–rubella vaccines, respectively. These rates are similar to the rates of thrombocytopenia after the natural courses of the disease in unvaccinated children. Most of the cases had platelet counts >10,000/μL.[100]
Valproic Acid	
MA	Macrocytosis occurred in 11 of 60 patients in one report.[101]
Th	Thrombocytopenia occurred in 12 of 60 patients in one report. Immune and dose-dependent mechanisms have been suggested.[101]
Vancomycin	
AGN	Usually associated with therapy $\geq$12 d. Often resolves upon discontinuation of agent or with support of filgrastim therapy. Probable immune-mediated.[10,102]
Th	Multiple reports.[1]
Vitamin K	
HA	In G-6-PD deficiency; usually requires concurrent infection or other complicating factors. Hemolysis from high doses can contribute to jaundice in neonates; rarely toxic in older children and adults.[8]
Zidovudine	
AGN	Most patients experience at least a 25% reduction in neutrophil count; ANC of <500/μL occurs in 16% of patients. Usual onset is during the first 3 mo of therapy.[10,103,104]
MA	Macrocytosis develops in most patients, usually beginning during the first few weeks of therapy. Zidovudine is the leading cause of drug-induced macrocytosis.[103–105]

■ REFERENCES

1. Aster R, Bougie DW. Drug-induced immune thrombocytopenia. *N Engl J Med.* 2007;357:580-587.
2. Fischereder M, Jaffe JP. Thrombocytopenia following acute acetaminophen overdose. *Am J Hematol.* 1994;45:258-259.
3. Bougie D, Aster R. Immune thrombocytopenia resulting from sensitivity to metabolites of naproxen and acetaminophen. *Blood.* 2001;97:3846-3850.
4. Keisu M et al. Acetazolamide-associated aplastic anaemia *J Intern Med.* 1990;228(6):627-632.
5. Kodjikian L et al. Acetazolamide-induced thrombocytopenia. *Arch Ophthalmol.* 2004;122:1543-1544.
6. George JN et al. Drug-induced thrombocytopenia: a systematic review of published case reports. *Ann Intern Med.* 1998;129:886-890.
7. Fraunfelder FT et al. Hematologic reactions to carbonic anhydrase inhibitors. *Am J Ophthalmol.* 1985; 100:79-81.
8. Swanson M, Cook R. Drugs, chemicals and blood dyscrasias. Hamilton, IL: Drug Intelligence Publications; 1977.
9. Chan CSP et al. Amphotericin B—induced thrombocytopenia. *Ann Intern Med.* 1982;96:332-333.
10. Andersohn F et al. A systematic review: agranulocytosis induced by drugs other than chemotherapy. http://www.adverse effects.com. Accessed February 8, 2009.
11. Levin GM, DeVane CL. A review of cyclic antidepressant-induced blood dyscrasias. *Ann Pharmacother.* 1992;26:378-383.
12. Rees DC et al. Acute haemolysis induced by high dose ascorbic acid in glucose-6-phosphate dehydrogenase deficiency. *BMJ.* 1993;306:841-842.
13. Cappellini MD, Fiorelli G. Glucose-6-phosphate dehydrogenase deficiency. *Lancet.* 2008;371:64-74.
14. Sanford-Driscoll M, Knodel LC. Induction of haemolytic anemia by nonsteroidal anti-inflammatory drugs. *Drug Intell Clin Pharm.* 1986;20:925-934.
15. Garg SK, Sarker CR. Aspirin-induced thrombocytopenia on an immune basis. *Am J Med Sci.* 1974;267: 129-132.
16. George CS, Lichtin AE. Hematologic complications of rheumatic disease therapies. *Rheum Dis Clin North Am.* 1997;23:425-437.
17. Parish RC, Miller LJ. Adverse effects of angiotensin converting enzyme (ACE) inhibitors. An update. *Drug Saf.* 1992;7:14-31.
18. Handoko KB. Risk of aplastic anemia in patients using antiepileptic drugs. *Epilepsia.* 2006;47:1232-1236.
19. Sobotka JL et al. A review of carbamazepine's hematologic reactions and monitoring recommendations. *DICP.* 1990;24:1214-1219.
20. Tohen M et al. Blood dyscrasias with carbamazepine and valproate: a pharmacoepidemiological study of 2,228 patients at risk. *Am J Psychiatry.* 1995;132:413-418.
21. Andersohn F et al. Systematic review: agranulocytosis induced by nonchemotherapy drugs. *Ann Intern Med.* 2007;146:657-665.
22. Thompson JW, Jacobs RF. Adverse effects of newer cephalosporins. An update. *Drug Saf.* 1993;9:132-142.
23. Olaison L et al. Incidence of β-lactam—induced delayed hypersensitivity and neutropenia during treatment of infective endocarditis. *Arch Intern Med.* 1999;159:607-615.
24. Malkin D et al. Drug-induced aplastic anemia: pathogenesis and clinical aspects. *Am J Pediatr Hematol Oncol.* 1990;12:402-410.
25. Aymard J-P et al. Haematological adverse effects of histamine H2-receptor antagonists. *Med Toxicol Adverse Drug Exp.* 1988;3:430-448.
26. Wade E et al. H2 Antagonist-induced thrombocytopenia: is this a real phenomenon? *Intensive Care Med.* 2002;28:459-465.
27. Starr JA, Ragucci KR. Thrombocytopenia associated with intravenous ciprofloxacin. *Pharmacotherapy.* 2005;25:1030-1034.
28. Tuccori M et al. Severe thrombocytopenia and haemolytic anaemia associated with ciprofloxacin: a case report with fatal outcome. *Platelets.* 2008;19:384-387.
29. Bennett CL et al. Thrombotic thrombocytopenic purpura associated with clopidogrel. *N Engl J Med.* 2000;342:1773-1777.
30. Atkin K et al. Neutropenia and agranulocytosis in patients receiving clozapine in the UK and Ireland. *Br J Psychiatry.* 1996;169:483-488.
31. Honigfeld G. Effects of the Clozapine National Registry System on incidence of deaths related to agranulocytosis. *Psychiatr Serv.* 1996;47:52-56.
32. Munro J et al. Active monitoring of 12,760 clozapine recipients in the UK and Ireland. Beyond pharmacovigilance. *Br J Psychiatry.* 1999;175:576-580.

33. Leissinger CA. Severe thrombocytopenia associated with cocaine use. *Ann Intern Med.* 1990;112:708-710.

34. Kaufman DW et al. Acute thrombocytopenic purpura in relation to the use of drugs. *Blood.* 1993;82:2714-2718.

35. Nixon DD. Thrombocytopenia following doxepin treatment. *JAMA.* 1972;220:418.

36. Wolf B et al. A case of immune complex haemolytic anemia, thrombocytopenia and acute renal failure associated with doxepin use. *J Clin Psychiatry.* 1989;50:99-100.

37. Beck ML et al. Fatal intravascular immune hemolysis induced by hydrochlorothiazide. *Am J Clin Pathol.* 1984;81:791-794.

38. Sahai J, Berry AJ. Eflornithine for the treatment of *Pneumocystis carinii* pneumonia in patients with the acquired immunodeficiency syndrome: a preliminary review. *Pharmacotherapy.* 1989;9:29-33.

39. Product Information. Procrit®, epoetin alfa. Bridgewater, NJ: Ortho Biotech; 2008.

40. Food and Drug Administration. Important drug warning. http://www.fda.gov/medwatch/safety/2000/enbrel2.htm. Accessed October 12, 2000.

41. Pennell PB et al. Aplastic anemia in a patient receiving felbamate for complex partial seizures. *Neurology.* 1995;45:456-460.

42. Kaufman DW et al. Aplastic anemia among users of felbamate [Abstract]. *Pharmacoepidemiol Drug Saf.* 1996;5(suppl):S106.

43. Mercurio MG et al. Thrombocytopenia caused by fluconazole therapy. *J Am Acad Dermatol.* 1995;32:525-526.

44. Vermes A et al. Flucytosine: a review of its pharmacology, clinical indications, pharmacokinetics, toxicity, and drug interactions. *J Antimicrob Chemother.* 2000;46:171-179.

45. Morbidity and toxic effects associated with ganciclovir or foscarnet therapy in a randomized cytomegalovirus retinitis trial. Studies of Ocular Complications of AIDS Research Group, in collaboration with the AIDS Clinical Trials Group. *Intern Med.* 1995;155:65-74.

46. Offerhaus L. Diuretic drugs. In: Dukes MNG, ed. *Meyler's Side Effects of Drugs: An Encyclopedia of Adverse Reactions and Interactions.* 10th ed. Amsterdam, The Netherlands: Elsevier; 1984:368-385.

47. Cytovene product information. Palo Alto, CA: Syntex Laboratories; 1994.

48. Gibson J et al. Aplastic anemia in association with gold therapy for rheumatoid arthritis. *Aust N Z J Med.* 1983;13:130-134.

49. Gibbons RB. Complications of chrysotherapy. A review of recent studies. *Arch Intern Med.* 1979;139:343-346.

50. Gottlieb NL et al. The course of severe gold-associated granulocytopenia [Abstarct]. *Clin Res.* 1982;30:659A.

51. Coblyn JS et al. Gold-induced thrombocytopenia. A clinical and immunogenetic study of twenty-three patients. *Ann Intern Med.* 1981;95:178-181.

52. Adachi JD et al. Gold induced thrombocytopenia: platelet associated IgG and HLA typing in three patients. *J Rheumatol.* 1984;11:355-357.

53. Kelton, JG, Warkentin TE. Heparin-induced thrombocytopenia: a historical perspective. *Blood.* 2008;112: 2607-2616.

54. Warkentin TE et al. Heparin-induced thrombocytopenia in patients treated with low-molecular-weight heparin or unfractionated heparin. *N Engl J Med.* 1995;332:1330-1335.

55. Schmitt BP, Adelman B. Heparin-associated thrombocytopenia: a critical review and pooled analysis. *Am J Med Sci.* 1993;305:208-215.

56. Misbah SA, Chapel HM. Adverse effects of intravenous immunoglobulin. *Drug Saf.* 1993;9:254-262.

57. Treadway G. Clinical safety of intravenous amrinone — a review. *Am J Cardiol.* 1985;56:39B-40B.

58. Ross MP et al. Amrinone-associated thrombocytopenia: pharmacokinetic analysis. *Clin Pharmacol Ther.* 1993;53:661-667.

59. Product Information. Intron A® (interferon alfa 2-b). Kenilworth, NJ: Schering-Plough; 2008.

60. Murakami CS et al. Idiopathic thrombocytopenic purpura during interferon-α_{2B} treatment for chronic hepatitis. *Am J Gastroenterol.* 1994;89:2244-2245.

61. Holdiness MR. A review of blood dyscrasias induced by the antituberculosis drugs. *Tubercle.* 1987;68:301-309.

62. Nicholson RJ et al. Leucopenia associated with lamotrigine. *BMJ.* 1995;310:504.

63. El-Ghobarey AF, Capell HA. Levamisole-induced thrombocytopenia. *Br Med J.* 1977;2:555-556.

64. Anon. Risk of agranulocytosis and aplastic anemia in relation to use of antithyroid drugs. International Agranulocytosis and Aplastic Anaemia Study. *BMJ.* 1988;297:262-265.

65. Biswas N et al. Case report: aplastic anemia associated with antithyroid drugs. *Am J Med Sci.* 1991;301:190-194.

66. Thomas D et al. Antithyroid drug-induced aplastic anemia. *Thyroid.* 2008;18:1043-1048.

67. Kelton JG. Impaired reticuloendothelial function in patients treated with methyldopa. *N Engl J Med.* 1985;313:596-600.

68. Manohitharajah SM et al. Methyldopa and associated thrombocytopenia. *Br Med J.* 1971;1:494.

69. Meyboom RHB. Thrombocytopenia induced by nalidixic acid. *Br Med J.* 1984;289:962.

70. Laporte JR et al. Fatal aplastic anemia associated with nifedipine. *Lancet.* 1998;352:619-620.

71. Risks of agranulocytosis and aplastic anemia. A first report of their relation to drug use with special reference to analgesics. The International Agranulocytosis and Aplastic Anemia Study. *JAMA.* 1986;256:1749-1757.

72. Kay AGL. Myelotoxicity of D-penicillamine. *Ann Rheum Dis.* 1979;38:232-236.

73. Camp AV. Hematologic toxicity from penicillamine in rheumatoid arthritis. *J Rheumatol.* 1981;8(suppl 7):164-165.

74. Lyle WH. D-penicillamine and haemolytic anaemia [Letter]. *Lancet.* 1976;1:428.

75. Thomas D et al. A study of D-penicillamine induced thrombocytopenia in rheumatoid arthritis with Cr[51]-labelled autologous platelets [Abstract]. *Aust N Z J Med.* 1981;11:722.

76. Mallouh AA. Methicillin-induced neutropenia. *Pediatr Infect Dis J.* 1985;4:262-264.

77. Jeffery WH et al. Acquired methemoglobinemia and hemolytic anemia after usual doses of phenazopyridine. *Drug Intell Clin Pharm.* 1982;16:157-159.

78. Hollister LE. Allergic reactions to tranquilizing drugs. *Ann Intern Med.* 1958;49:17-29.

79. Pisciotta AV et al. Agranulocytosis following administration of phenothiazine derivatives. *Am J Med.* 1958;25:210-223.

80. Danielly J et al. Procainamide-associated blood dyscrasias. *Am J Cardiol.* 1994;74:1179-1180.

81. Alexander SJ, Gilmore RI et al. Quinidine-induced agranulocytosis. *Am J Hematol.* 1984;16:95-98.

82. Webb RF et al. Acute intravascular haemolysis due to quinine. *N Z Med J.* 1980;91:14-16.

83. Product Information. WinRho®, RhoD immune globulin intravenous (human). Winipeg, Manitoba: Cangene Corporation; 2005.

84. Apseloff G et al. Severe neutropenia caused by recommended prophylactic doses of rifabutin [Letter]. *Lancet.* 1996;348:685.

85. Tahan SR et al. Acute hemolysis and renal failure with rifampicin-dependent antibodies after discontinuous administration. *Transfusion.* 1985;25:124-127.

86. Marabani M et al. Leucopenia during sulfasalazine treatment for rheumatoid arthritis. *Ann Rheum Dis.* 1989;48:505-507.

87. Jick H et al. The risk of sulfasalazine- and mesalazine-associated blood disorders. *Pharmacotherapy.* 1995;13:170-181.

88. Cohen SM et al. Ulcerative colitis and erythrocyte G6PD deficiency. Salicylazosulfapyridine-provoked hemolysis. *JAMA.* 1968;205:528-530.

89. Das KM et al. Adverse reactions during salicylazosulfapyridine therapy and the relation with drug metabolism and acetylator phenotype. *N Engl J Med.* 1973;289:491-495.

90. Hopkinson ND et al. Haematological side-effects of sulphasalazine in inflammatory arthritis. *Br J Rheumatol.* 1989;28:414-417.

91. Jarrett F et al. Acute haemolytic during topical burn therapy with silver sulfadiazine. *Am J Surg.* 1978;135:818-819.

92. Anon. Anti-infective drug use in relation to the risk of agranulocytosis and aplastic anemia. The International Agranulocytosis and Aplastic Anemia Study. *Arch Intern Med.* 1989;149:1036-1040.

93. Zinkham WH. Unstable hemoglobins and the selective haemolytic action of sulfonamides. The International Agranulocytosis and Aplastic Anemia Study [Editorial]. *Arch Intern Med.* 1977;137:1365-1366.

94. Love BB et al. Adverse haematological effects of ticlopidine. Prevention, recognition and management. *Drug Saf.* 1998;19:89-98.

95. Steinhubl SR et al. Incidence and clinical course of thrombotic thrombocytopenic purpura due to ticlopidine following coronary stenting. *JAMA.* 1999;281:806-810.

96. Bennett CL et al. Thrombotic thrombocytopenic purpura associated with ticlopidine in the setting of coronary stents and stroke prevention. *Arch Intern Med.* 1999;159:2524-2528.

97. Volosin K et al. Tocainide associated agranulocytosis. *Am Heart J.* 1985;109:1392-1393.

98. Roden DM, Woosley RL. Tocainide. *N Engl J Med.* 1986;315:41-45.

99. Hawkins T et al. Severe trimethoprim induced neutropenia and thrombocytopenia. *N Z Med J.* 1993;106:251-252.

100. Jonville-Béra AP et al. Thrombocytopenic purpura after measles, mumps and rubella vaccination: a retrospective survey by the French Regional Pharmacovigilance Centres and Pasteur-Mérieux Sérums et Vaccins. *Pediatr Infect Dis J.* 1996;15:44-48.

101. May RB, Sunder TR. Hematologic manifestations of long-term valproate therapy. *Epilepsia.* 1993;34:1098-1101.

102. Segarra-Newnham M, Tagoff SS. Probable vancomycin-induced neutropenia. *Ann Pharmacother.* 2004;38:1855-1859.

103. Richman DD et al. The toxicity of azidothymidine (AZT) in the treatment of patients with AIDS and AIDS-related complex. A double-blind, placebo-controlled trial. *N Engl J Med.* 1987;317:192-197.

104. Rachlis A, Fanning MM. Zidovudine toxicity. Clinical features and management. *Drug Saf.* 1993;8:312-320.

105. Snower DP, Weil SC. Changing etiology of macrocytosis. Zidovudine as a frequent causative factor. *Am J Clin Pathol.* 1993;99:57-60.

Chapter 62

Drug-Induced Hepatotoxicity

Trenika R. Mitchell

This table includes only those drugs with well-established records of hepatotoxicity. Almost 1000 different medications have been associated with liver damage; therefore, if a drug is not listed in the table, it does not mean it cannot produce liver damage. Furthermore, combining drugs that have hepatotoxic potential commonly results in greater than additive liver damage. Patients with drug-induced liver injury can present with acute hepatitis, which is characterized by cellular necrosis and increased ALT and INR, cholestasis, which is characterized by canalicular and ductal injury and increased alkaline phosphatase, or a mixture of the two. In general, drug-induced hepatotoxicity is most prevalent in older patients, women, and those with preexisting hepatic impairment.[1,2]

ACE Inhibitors

Hepatic injury occurs occasionally with ACE inhibitors. **Captopril** and **enalapril** are implicated in most reported cases, but other ACE inhibitors have been shown to have hepatotoxic potential. Most cases show immune-mediated cholestatic injury, but mixed and hepatocellular damage also are reported.[1–3]

Acetaminophen

Centrilobular hepatic necrosis can follow acute overdose with ≥150 mg/kg in children or ≥7.5 g in adults. These doses saturate the normal metabolic pathways, producing large quantities of a hepatotoxic metabolite. Children appear to have a lower risk than adults of developing acetaminophen-induced hepatitis. Laboratory evidence of hepatotoxicity peaks 3–4 d after the acute exposure. Therapy with **acetylcysteine** to bind the metabolite is indicated when the 4h postingestion serum acetaminophen level is >150 mg/L. Even without acetylcysteine, fatalities are uncommon after acetaminophen overdose. Nonfatal cases usually recover fully in a few weeks. It is proposed that chronic alcohol ingestion and malnutrition may increase the risk of liver toxicity, but the supporting evidence remains controversial concerning these topics.[2,4–7]

Alcohol

Fatty infiltration of the liver occurs in 70%–100% of alcoholics. Fatty liver is generally without clinical manifestation, but 30% of alcoholics develop alcoholic hepatitis and about 10% develop cirrhosis. Malnutrition can potentiate alcoholic liver disease, and alcohol can enhance the hepatotoxicity of other drugs.[8]

Allopurinol

Hepatic granulomas, hepatitis, and hepatic necrosis can accompany other symptoms (especially rash, fever, eosinophilia, and vasculitis) of allopurinol hypersensitivity. Damage is usually focal, but widespread damage also is reported. This reaction is rare but serious when it occurs. Onset is usually after 3–6 wk of treatment. Renal impairment might be a predisposing factor for allopurinol-induced hepatitis. Cholestasis also has been attributed to allopurinol.[8,9]

(*continued*)

Aminosalicylic Acid

Up to 5% of patients develop a generalized hypersensitivity reaction. About 25% of these patients have evidence of mixed cholestatic and hepatocellular injuries as part of their hypersensitivity reactions. Fatalities have been reported.[8,10]

Amiodarone

Asymptomatic elevations of serum aminotransferases occur in 4%–25% of patients receiving oral amiodarone. Although most elevations are transient, cases of more severe hepatic injury, such as cirrhosis and fatal hepatocellular necrosis have been reported.[11]

Anticonvulsants

Several anticonvulsants are commonly associated with hepatic failure. **Carbamazepine** is associated with a dose-dependent liver toxicity in which hepatic necrosis, granulomas, and immunoallergic hepatitis have occurred, most often with the first 2 mo of therapy. During the first 6 wk of **phenytoin** therapy, patients may experience a hepatocellular necrosis accompanied by signs of hypersensitivity (e.g., eosinophilia, fever, rash, and lymphadenopathy). The most recent analysis of these patients revealed a mortality rate of 13%, although rates as high as 40% have been reported. Up to 44% of **valproic acid** patients have hepatic enzyme elevations, with clinically apparent liver disease characterized by fatigue, nausea, and prolonged vomiting in 1/15,000 cases. Severe hepatotoxic disease occurs most often in children ≤2 y of age and within the first 2–3 mo of therapy. Cases of **lamotrigine**-associated hepatotoxicity have been published in both pediatric and adult patients, include at least one case of severe hepatic failure with a fatal outcome, and are generally complicated by multiple-drug therapy. Although the prevalence of hepatocellular destruction is unclear, it, coupled with aplastic anemia toxicity, is of sufficient concern to limit the use of **felbamate** to carefully selected patients. At least 7 cases of hepatic failure can be attributed to felbamate use.[8,12–14]

Antidepressants

Hepatotoxic reactions have been observed with the majority of antidepressant agents. **Duloxetine** and **nefazodone** are the most commonly implicated antidepressant medications, with the former producing both hepatocellular and mixed-type hepatic injury and the latter demonstrating hepatocellular injury. In one analysis, approximately 1% of patients are receiving duloxetine developed ALT levels 3 times the ULN. The frequency of nefazodone-induced liver failure is estimated at 1 case of death or transplant per 250,000–300,000 patient years of nefazodone treatment.[15]

Antineoplastic Agents

Cisplatin and **carmustine** use have been connected with mild, transient elevations of hepatic enzymes in 15% and 26% of patients, respectively, and cholestatic changes are rapidly reversed upon **aldesleukin** discontinuation. 8%–12% of patients receiving **gefitinib** have been associated with grade 2 and 3 liver toxicity, while reversible grade 3 or 4 liver toxicity has been reported in patients ≥ 60 y of age receiving a generally well-tolerated chemotherapy agent, **gemtuzumab**. Minimal reports of liver necrosis and fatalities occur in **imatinib** patients, with 2%–6% developing grade 4 toxicity, and severe, but reversible hepatotoxicity has developed in patients administered the 5-d **clofarabine** regimen. An apparent dose-related, severe veno-occlusive disease of the liver has been reported in 10%–25% of bone marrow transplant patients receiving **busulfan** with rare cases of cholestatic hepatitis occurring in these patients. Due to **asparaginase's** influence on protein synthesis, 87% of patients develop a slowly reversible steatosis. Various types of liver toxicity including periportal fibrosis, cirrhosis, and liver atrophy are induced by **methotrexate**. While chronic low doses and cumulative doses >2 g of methotrexate are associated with potentially irreversible fibrosis and cirrhosis, increased liver enzymes more likely occur with transient high doses of the medication. Liver function tests may be normal in patients receiving methotrexate, so

(continued)

liver biopsy may be the most definitive indicator of liver toxicity. At least 20 reported deaths resulting from hepatic necrosis and possible cholestasis are reasonably attributed to **flutamide**-induced hepatotoxicity. The average latency period for hepatitis development is 3 mo, and therefore, baseline liver function tests followed by serial liver function testing are recommended for patients receiving flutamide. Hepatic arterial infusion of **floxuridine** results in elevated liver enzymes and bilirubin in up to 50% of patients, and biliary stricture or sclerosis in up to 16% of patients. Although the hepatitis generally improves after discontinuation of the medication, an irreversible sclerosing cholangitis can develop.[8,16,17]

Anti-Infectives, Antibacterial Agents

Occasional jaundice occurs in patients receiving macrolide antibiotics, **erythromycin** and **troleandomycin**. In erythromycin patients, reversible cholestasis likely due to hypersensitivity (60% have eosinophilia) appears in mainly adults after 5–20 d of initial therapy. Although most cases involve the estolate salt, hepatotoxicity has occurred with the ethylsuccinate, stearate, and propionate salts and with erythromycin base. The sulfonamides, such as **trimethoprim-sulfamethoxazole**, are associated with a probable immunoallergic form (characterized by eosinophilia and rash) of hepatitis that results in cholestatic or mixed hepatocellular–cholestatic injury, with the onset of symptoms occurring within weeks to the first 2 mo of therapy. Tetracycline antibiotics, such as **minocycline** and **tetracycline**, have been linked to various forms of hepatotoxicity. Autoimmune hepatitis associated with lupus-like symptoms (arthralgia, arthritis, fatigue, rash, and fever) with a median 1-y onset and hepatitis due to an apparent hypersensitivity mechanism, resulting in possible fulminant hepatic failure with a 1-mo onset, occurs with minocycline therapy. Hepatotoxicity caused by tetracycline is due to fatty infiltration of the liver with contributing factors including pregnancy, malnutrition, impaired renal function, and administering >2 g/d of the medication. At least 52 cases of **nitrofurantoin**-induced liver injury (likely due to hypersensitivity) resulting in acute cholestatic and hepatic injury have been reported, mainly in women receiving >6 mo of therapy. The penicillinase-resistant penicillins, such as **oxacillin** and **dicloxacillin**, are infrequently associated with cholestatic hepatitis, while **amoxicillin-clavulanic acid** is the antibiotic most frequently associated with hepatotoxicity (<1 case/100,000 persons exposed). Amoxicillin–clavulanic acid hepatic injury is cholestatic in nature, and patients with advancing age and repeated prescriptions have increased risk of developing toxic effects. Most reports of cephalosporin-induced hepatotoxicity occur in the first generation agents. However, **ceftriaxone** use is associated with development of "gallbladder sludge" in up to 25% of patients. 42 possible cases of **telithromycin**-associated acute liver injury have been assessed, with 5 cases resulting in death or the need for liver transplantation. Clinical features of this syndrome include jaundice, abdominal pain, and abrupt fever onset. The increased incidence of hepatotoxicity and lack of evidence of increased efficacy over existing acute bacterial sinusitis and acute exacerbation of chronic bronchitis therapies has resulted in an FDA advisory recommending restricted use of telithromycin.[8,18–26]

Anti-Infectives, Antifungal Agents

1%–5% of patients receiving **itraconazole** develop asymptomatic hepatitis; 15% of **ketoconazole**-treated patients develop elevated hepatic enzymes, with severe hepatocellular injury developing in 1/15,000 recipients. There have been at least 6 reports of acute drug-induced liver failure resulting in the need for liver transplantation and a few deaths in patients receiving ketoconazole. Although there have been a small number of reports of terbinafine-induced hepatotoxicity, severe cases requiring liver transplantation have occurred. Prolonged cholestasis involving liver test elevations up to 6 mo following cessation of therapy has been described.[18,19,24]

Anti-Infectives, Antitubercular Agents

Pyrazinamide-induced hepatitis appears to be dose-dependent and is more commonly noted in patients receiving doses >40 mg/kg, while **dapsone**-induced hepatitis occurs within the first

(*continued*)

2 wk of therapy. Dapsone-associated hepatitis is part of the "sulfone syndrome," a generalized hypersensitivity reaction that includes rash, fever, jaundice, and anemia in which fatalities have resulted. While 30% of **ethionamide** patients develop increased liver enzymes, 3%–5% of patients develop hepatitis after several months of therapy. Hepatotoxicity due to **isoniazid** use is associated with subclinical hepatitis that can resolve despite continued therapy. Elevated serum enzyme levels develop in 10%–30% of tuberculosis patients receiving isoniazid, and a syndrome resembling viral hepatitis with an onset usually during the first 2 mo of therapy occurs in 1% of patients. Despite the widespread assumption that patients <20 y of age are unlikely to develop isoniazid-induced fatal hepatotoxicity, reported deaths indicate otherwise.[8,18–19,27–29]

Chlorpropamide

Most hepatotoxic reactions are cholestatic and probably are caused by an immune mechanism. Prevalence is estimated at 0.5%–1.5%, with onset usually within the first 2 mo of therapy.[8]

Chlorzoxazone

Idiosyncratic hepatocellular damage occurs rarely, but fatalities have been reported. Discontinue the drug if elevated levels of transaminases or bilirubin are detected.[30]

Clozapine

Transient elevations of hepatic enzymes occur frequently during the first weeks to months of clozapine use. Although a case of fulminant hepatitis and at least 3 cases of icteric hepatitis have been reported, the risk of serious clozapine-induced hepatotoxicity remains small.[31]

Cocaine

Hepatic necrosis has been reported in cases of cocaine abuse; however, most of the cases occur in the setting of rhabdomyolysis and other conditions that can increase liver enzymes. Therefore, the prevalence of actual cocaine-induced hepatotoxicity is unknown.[8,32]

Contraceptives, Oral

Cholestasis, associated with mild transaminase and bilirubin elevations, occurs in 1/4,000–1/10,000 women receiving oral contraceptives. This adverse drug reaction generally occurs in the first 2–3 mo of therapy. An increased risk for contraceptive-induced cholestasis is noted in patients who previously developed cholestasis during pregnancy.[33]

Cyclosporine

Mild, and generally asymptomatic, cholestasis is associated with cyclosporine use. This is reversed upon dose reduction or drug withdrawal.[34]

Cyproterone

Cases of cyproterone acetate-induced fulminant hepatic failure and acute hepatitis have been assessed in the literature, and elevated liver enzymes were documented in 28.2% patients receiving cyproterone acetate in a retrospective study of 89 patients. Hepatocellular recovery is seen within 2–3 mo of medication withdrawal.[35]

Dantrolene

At least 1.8% of patients develop laboratory evidence of hepatic dysfunction, with symptomatic hepatitis in about 0.6%; the fatality rate among jaundiced patients is about 25%. Predisposing factors seem to include dosage (>300 mg/d), gender (women more than men), age (>30 y), and duration of therapy (≥2 mo).[8,36,37]

Disulfiram

Disulfiram use can produce a dose-dependent liver injury that has been previously confirmed with a rechallenge of the medication. An assessment of disulfiram-induced hepatotoxicity conducted in

(continued)

Sweden revealed a total of 82 reports of possible drug-associated liver injury, with increased morbidity and mortality in 16% of patients with jaundice. Signs and symptoms of disulfiram-induced hepatotoxicity include abdominal pain, fatigue, and nausea.[19,38]

Ezetimibe

Rare cases of severe cholestatic hepatitis and acute autoimmune hepatitis have been reported with ezetimibe use. The toxicity of ezetimibe may be related to an active metabolite that has considerable enterohepatic circulation.[39]

Ferrous Salts

Hepatic necrosis can appear within 1–3 d of an acute overdose. The fatality rate is high if the patient is not treated promptly.[8]

Gold Salts

Cholestasis occurs occasionally with normal doses of parenteral gold salts; hypersensitivity is the suspected mechanism. Onset is commonly within the first few weeks of therapy, and recovery usually occurs within 3 mo after drug discontinuation. Lipogranulomas are frequently found in liver biopsies of parenteral gold-treated patients. These can persist long after drug withdrawal but do not seem to impair liver function. Hepatic necrosis can result from overdose.[8,40,41]

Halothane

Halothane-associated acute hepatic necrosis is characterized by rash, fever, and pruritus that occurs 7–14 d following surgery. Despite extensive publicity, the actual frequency of severe halothane hepatitis is low, ranging from 1/10,000 to 1/35,000, with a reported case fatality rate of 50% for patients who develop fulminant hepatic failure. Although halothane is no longer available in the United States, other anesthetic agents, such as **methoxyflurane** and **enflurane**, produce similar hepatotoxic reactions, although less frequently.[8,19]

Histamine H2-Receptor Antagonists

Cimetidine and **ranitidine** are associated with transient, increased liver enzymes. The risk of acute liver injury with cimetidine is about once per every 300,000–600,000 prescriptions and once per every 75,000–150,000 ranitidine prescriptions.[42]

Methyldopa

Mild changes in liver function tests occur in up to 30% of patients taking methyldopa, but the prevalence of clinical acute hepatitis is probably <1%. Most cases occur during the first 3 mo of therapy. Most patients have rapid recovery after drug discontinuation; however, patient fatality due to massive hepatic necrosis has occurred.[19,43]

Nevirapine

Severe, life-threatening hepatotoxicity has been reported in patients taking nevirapine for HIV infection and health care workers taking the drug for postexposure prophylaxis. Coinfection with hepatitis B or hepatitis C and elevated CD4 counts associated with postexposure prophylaxis regimens are noted risk factors for developing hepatotoxicity. Hepatic failure and fatalities have occurred in HIV-infected patients.[2,4]

Niacin

Dose-related liver injury is associated with niacin use. The onset can be anywhere between 1 wk and 48 mo after the initiation of therapy, and this adverse event occurs much more commonly in patients receiving the sustained release formulation of the medication. Discontinuation of the medication alleviates symptoms, and recovery is seen within 2 mo.[39,44]

(continued)

Nonsteroidal Anti-Inflammatory Drugs

More than 91 cases of various types of liver injury have been reported with **sulindac**. Patients older than 50 y of age and of the female gender have a higher incidence of **sulindac**-induced hepatotoxicity. Over the past decade, **diclofenac** has also been indicated as a cause of severe hepatotoxicity. A population-based study conducted by de Abajo et al. estimated that serious hepatotoxicity occurs in 6.3 per 100,000 patients receiving the medication.[45]

Octreotide

Up to 63% of patients on long-term therapy develop cholelithiasis and/or gallbladder sludge. Some patients require cholecystectomy. The prevalence and speed of onset of symptoms might be dose-related.[33,46]

Papaverine

Numerous reports of hepatocellular injury and elevated liver enzymes in 27%–43% of patients indicate a marked hepatotoxic potential.[8,47]

Penicillamine

Rare cases of penicillamine-induced hepatotoxicity in patients with Wilson's disease have been reported.[48]

Phenothiazines

At least 20% of patients receiving phenothiazine therapy have asymptomatic, elevated liver function tests. Despite the dominance of **chlorpromazine** in the reported cases, other phenothiazines can produce similar hepatic damage. Jaundice proceeded by flu-like symptoms occur within the first month of therapy. Due to the early onset of symptoms and the presence of fever and eosinophilia in some cases, a hypersensitivity reaction has been projected as a possible cause of this toxicity.[19,32]

Propoxyphene

A small number of cases of propoxyphene-induced cholestasis have been reported; these are thought to be the result of hypersensitivity.[8,49]

Propylthiouracil

Although clinical hepatitis occurs rarely, at least 34 cases of severe hepatotoxicity have been reported. Symptoms occur within weeks to months of therapy initiation. Symptom reversal can occur; however, patients have developed fulminant hepatic failure.[19,50]

Riluzole

Elevated hepatic enzymes occur frequently; the prevalence appears to be dose-related.[51]

Ritonavir

Although several protease inhibitors have been associated with drug-induced hepatotoxicity, ritonavir is noted to have the highest incidence amongst the group. Patients receiving high-dose (600 mg PO bid) ritonavir have a projected 3%–9% incidence of severe hepatotoxicity.[24]

Quinidine

Hepatic damage is rare and usually accompanied by other signs of hypersensitivity, especially fever. Most reactions occur in the first 2 wk of therapy. The pathology is usually a mixture of hepatocellular necrosis and cholestasis; granulomas also have been reported. Symptoms cease with discontinuation of the medication.[52]

(*continued*)

Salicylates

The risk of developing salicylate-induced liver damage is greatest in patients with connective tissue disorders such as SLE or juvenile rheumatoid arthritis. Clinically apparent salicylate-induced hepatitis is uncommon, usually mild, and readily reversible. Hepatotoxicity most often occurs at serum salicylate concentrations >15 mg/dL.[19]

Steroids, C-17-α-Alkyl

Canalicular cholestasis occurs with a minimal amount of hepatic inflammation. The prevalence appears to be dose-related. Although laboratory changes are common (occurring in almost all patients taking anabolic steroids), jaundice is not. Jaundice may or may not be preceded by other clinical signs and usually follows 1–6 mo of therapy. Peliosis hepatitis also has been associated with these compounds, especially the anabolic steroids. Examples are **methyltestosterone, norethandrolone, methandrostenolone, fluoxymesterone, oxandrolone, oxymetholone,** and **stanozolol.** C-17-α-ethinyl steroids such as **ethinyl estradiol, mestranol, norethindrone,** and **norethynodrel** can produce similar reactions. An association between C-17-α-alkyl steroids and an increase in the prevalence of hepatocellular carcinoma is unclear.[8,53]

Sulfasalazine

Several cases of sulfasalazine-associated hepatic damage, including 9 fatalities, have been reported in children and adults. Hepatic necrosis is apparently part of a generalized hypersensitivity reaction that includes a morbilliform rash and fever with or without eosinophilia. Onset is usually within 6 wk of therapy.[54]

Tacrine

Tacrine induces a reversible hepatotoxicity in up to 50% of patients. Transaminase levels may reach up to 10 times the ULN. Liver function test elevation occurs within the first 6–12 wk of therapy. Due to the increased incidence of liver toxicity, the FDA requires weekly monitoring of ALT levels for the first 18 wk of therapy and every 3 mo after a stable dose is reached.[55,56]

Thiazolidinediones

There have been published case reports of hepatotoxicity development with **pioglitazone** and **rosiglitazone**. Manufacturers recommend liver function test monitoring for patients receiving these medications.[24]

Thiopurine Analogs

A study of 786 patients with inflammatory bowel disease reported a 7.1% incidence per patient year of abnormal liver enzymes and a 2.6% incidence per patient year of hepatotoxicity in patients receiving the thiopurine analogues, **azathioprine** and **mercaptopurine**. The use of both medications has been associated with the development of cholestasis and liver vascular disorder syndromes, such as peliosis hepatitis. Withdrawal of the medication or dose reduction may reverse the adverse conditions.[2,57,58]

Tolcapone

At least 22 cases of ALT level elevation to >3 times the ULN have been reported in tolcapone-treated patients. At least 3 deaths from fulminant hepatic failure have been reported, however, perilous increases in liver function tests were ignored in these patients. Therefore, the general consensus is that there is a low likelihood of developing hepatotoxicity when the medication is administered and monitored appropriately.[59]

Vitamin A

Hepatic disease, leading to ascites and portal hypertension, has occurred in patients receiving excessive doses (>40,000 IU per day) of vitamin A. Central vein sclerosis and perisinusoidal fibrosis, which can progress to cirrhosis, have been reported in cases of chronic intoxication.[60]

(continued)

Zafirlukast

Asymptomatic hepatic enzyme elevations occur frequently. At least 3 cases of severe hepatitis have been reported including one that resulted in liver transplantation.[61]

■ REFERENCES

1. Kaplowitz N. Drug-induced liver injury. *Clin Infect Dis.* 2004;38:S44-S48.
2. Abboud G, Kaplowitz N. Drug-induced liver injury. *Drug Saf.* 2007;30:277-294.
3. Nunes ACR et al. Fosinopril-induced prolonged cholestatic jaundice and pruritus: first case report. *Eur J Gastroenterol Hepatol.* 2001;13:271-282.
4. Murray KF et al. Drug-related hepatotoxicity and acute liver failure. *J Pediatr Gastroenterol Nutr.* 2008;47: 395-405.
5. Tan H et al. Acetaminophen hepatotoxicity: current management. *Mt Sinai J Med.* 2009;76:75-83.
6. Doyon S, Klein-Schwartz W. Hepatotoxicity despite early administration of intravenous *N*-acetylcysteine for acute acetaminophen overdose. *Acad Emerg Med.* 2009;16:34-39.
7. Larson AM et al. Acetaminophen-induced acute liver failure: results of a United States multicenter, prospective study. *Hepatology.* 2005;42:1364-1372.
8. Zimmerman HJ. *Hepatotoxicity: The Adverse Effects of Drugs and Other Chemicals on the Liver.* 2nd ed. Philadelphia, PA: Lippincott Williams & Wilkins; 1999.
9. Arellano F, Sacristán JA. Allopurinol hypersensitivity syndrome: a review. *Ann Pharmacother.* 1993;27: 337-343.
10. Simpson DG, Walker JH. Hypersensitivity to para-aminosalicylic acid. *Am J Med.* 1960;29:297-306.
11. Llanos L et al. Causality assessment of liver injury after chronic oral amiodarone intake. *Pharmacoepidemiol Drug Saf.* 2009;18:291-300.
12. Bjornsson E. Hepatotoxicity associated with antiepileptic drugs. *Acta Neurol Scand.* 2008;118:281-290.
13. Overstreet K et al. Fatal progressive hepatic necrosis associated with lamotrigine treatment: a case report and literature review. *Dig Dis Sci.* 2002;47:1921-1925.
14. Pellock JM. Felbamate in epilepsy therapy: evaluating the risks. *Drug Saf.* 1999;21:225-239.
15. Desanty KP, Amabile CM. Antidepressant-induced liver injury. *Ann Pharmacother.* 2007;41:1201-1211.
16. Field KM et al. Part I: liver function in oncology: biochemistry and beyond. *Lancet Oncol.* 2008;9:1092-1101.
17. Rodriguez-Frias EA, Lee WM. Cancer chemotherapy I: hepatocellular injury. *Clin Liver Dis.* 2007;11:641-662.
18. Thiim M, Friedman LS. Hepatotoxicity of antibiotics and antifungals. *Clin Liver Dis.* 2003;7:381-399.
19. Lewis JH. Drug-induced liver disease. *Med Clin North Am.* 2000;84:1-33.
20. Abusin S, Johnson S. Sulfamethoxazole/trimethoprim induced liver failure: a case report. *Cases J.* 2008;1:44.
21. Ford TJ, Dillon JF. Minocycline hepatitis. *Eur J Gastroenterol Hepatol.* 2008;20:796-799.
22. Lawrenson RA et al. Liver damage associated with minocycline use in acne. A systematic review of the published literature and pharmacovigilance data. *Drug Saf.* 2000;23:333-349.
23. Heaton PC et al. Association between tetracycline or doxycycline and hepatotoxicity: a population based case-control study. *J Clin Pharm Ther.* 2007;32:483-487.
24. Chang CY, Schiano TD. Review article: drug hepatotoxicity. *Aliment Pharmacol Ther.* 2007;25:1135-1151.
25. Polson JE. Hepatotoxicity due to antibiotics. *Clin Liver Dis.* 2007;11:549-561.
26. Brinker AD et al. Telithromycin-associated hepatotoxicity: clinical spectrum and causality assessment of 42 cases. *Hepatology.* 2009;49:250-257.
27. Tostmann A et al. Antituberculosis drug-induced hepatotoxicity: concise up-to-date review. *J Gastroenterol Hepatol.* 2008;23:192-202.
28. Shapiro MA, Lewis JH. Causality assessment of drug-induced hepatotoxicity: promises and pitfalls. *Clin Liver Dis.* 2007;11:477-505.
29. Conn HO et al. Ethionamide-induced hepatitis. A review with a report of an additional case. *Am Rev Resp Dis.* 1964;90:542-552.
30. Chou R et al. Comparative efficacy and safety of skeletal muscle relaxants for spasticity and musculoskeletal conditions: a systemic review. *J Pain Symptom Manage.* 2004;28:140-175.
31. Erdogan A et al. Management of marked liver enzyme increase during clozapine treatment: a case report and review of the literature. *Int J Psychiatry Med.* 2004;34:83-89.
32. Selim K, Kaplowitz N. Hepatotoxicity and psychotropic drugs. *Hepatology.* 1999;29:1347-1351.
33. Levy C, Lindor KD. Drug-induced cholestasis. *Clin Liver Dis.* 2003;7:311-330.
34. Corbani A, Burroughs AK. Intrahepatic cholestasis after liver transplantation. *Clin Liver Dis.* 2008;12:111-129.
35. Savidou I et al. Hepatotoxicity induced by cyproterone acetate: a report of three cases. *World J Gastroenterol.* 2006;12:7551-7555.
36. Utili R et al. Dantrolene-associated hepatic injury. Incidence and character. *Gastroenterology.* 1977;72:610-616.

37. Ward A et al. Dantrolene. A review of its pharmacodynamic and pharmacokinetic properties and therapeutic use in malignant hyperthermia, the neuroleptic malignant syndrome and an update of its use in muscle spasticity. *Drugs*. 1986;32:130-168.

38. Bjornsson E et al. Clinical characteristics and prognostic markers in disulfiram-induced liver injury. *J Hepatol*. 2006;44:791-797.

39. Bhardwaj SS, Chalasani N. Lipid lowering agents that cause drug-induced hepatotoxicity. *Clin Liver Dis*. 2007;11:597-613.

40. Howrie DL, Gartner JC. Gold-induced hepatotoxicity: case report and review of the literature. *J Rheumatol*. 1982;9:727-729.

41. Landas SK et al. Lipogranulomas and gold in the liver in rheumatoid arthritis. *Am J Surg Pathol*. 1992;16:171-174.

42. Fisher AA, Le Couteur DG. Nephrotoxicity and hepatotoxicity of histamine H2-receptor antagonists. *Drug Saf*. 2001;24:39-57.

43. Chitturi S, George J. Hepatotoxicity of commonly used drugs: nonsteroidal anti-inflammatory drugs, antihypertensives, antidiabetic agents, anticonvulsants, psychotropic drugs. *Semin Liver Dis*. 2002;22:169-183.

44. Gupta NK, Lewis JH. Review article: the use of potentially hepatotoxic drugs in patients with liver disease. *Aliment Pharmacol Ther*. 2008;28:1021-1041.

45. Aithal GP et al. Nonsteroidal anti-inflammatory drug-induced hepatotoxicity. *Clin Liver Dis*. 2007;11:563-575.

46. Trendle MC et al. Incidence and morbidity of cholestasis in patients receiving chronic octreotide for metastatic carcinoid and malignant islet cell tumors. *Cancer*. 1997;79:830-834.

47. Pathy MS, Reynolds AJ. Papaverine and hepatotoxicity. *Postgrad Med J*. 1980;56:488-490.

48. Deutscher J et al. Potential hepatotoxicity of penicillamine treatment in three patients with Wilson's disease. *J Pediatr Gastroenterol Nutr*. 1999;29:628.

49. Bassendine MF et al. Dextropropoxyphene induced hepatotoxicity mimicking biliary tract disease. *Gut*. 1986;27:444-449.

50. Aydemir S et al. Fulminant hepatic failure associated with propylthiouracil: a case report with treatment emphasis on the use of plasmapheresis. *J Clin Apher*. 2005;20:235-238.

51. Miller RG et al. Clinical trials of riluzole in patients with ALS. ALS/Riluzole Study Group—II. *Neurology*. 1996;47(suppl 2):S86-S92.

52. Farver DK, Lavin MN. Quinine-induced hepatotoxicity. *Ann Pharmcother*. 1999;33:32-34.

53. Haupt HA, Rovere GD. Anabolic steroids: a review of the literature. *Am J Sports Med*. 1984;12:469-484.

54. Jobanputra P et al. Hepatotoxicity associated with sulfasalazine in inflammatory arthritis: a case series from a local surveillance of serious adverse events. *BMC Musculoskelet Disord*. 2008;9:48.

55. Bonner LT, Peskind ER. Pharmacologic treatments of dementia. *Med Clin N Am*. 2002;86:657-674.

56. Schneider LS. Treatment of Alzheimer's disease with cholinesterase inhibitors. *Clin Geriatr Med*. 2001;17:337-358.

57. Gisbert JP et al. Liver injury in inflammatory bowel disease: long-term follow-up study of 786 patients. *Inflamm Bowel Dis*. 2007;13:1106-1114.

58. Shaye OA et al. Hepatotoxicity of 6-mercaptopurine (6-MP) and azathioprine (AZA) in adult IBD patients. *Am J Gastroenterol*. 2007;102:2488-2494.

59. Olanow CW, Watkins PB. Tolcapone: an efficacy and safety review. *Clin Neuropharmacol*. 2007;30:287-294.

60. Maddrey WC. Drug-induced hepatotoxicity: 2005. *J Clin Gastroenterol*. 2005;39:S83-S89.

61. Reinus JF et al. Severe liver injury after treatment with the leukotriene receptor antagonist zafirlukast. *Ann Intern Med*. 2000;133:964-968.

Chapter 63

Drug-Induced Nephrotoxicity

William R. Vincent III

This chapter includes agents that are associated with drug-induced nephrotoxicity but excludes drugs that produce nephrotoxicity as a result of damage to tissues other than the kidney (e.g., liver or skeletal muscle). The following abbreviations are used in the chapter:

Cl_{Cr}	— creatinine clearance
Cr_s	— serum creatinine
GFR	— glomerular filtration rate
mOsm	— milliosmole
NDI	— nephrogenic diabetes insipidus
ARF	— acute renal failure
AIN	— acute interstitial nephritis

Acetaminophen (APAP)

Tubular necrosis occurs in 1%–2% of acute overdoses and may occur in the absence of significant hepatotoxicity. The mechanisms of kidney injury are not clearly understood. In overdoses, glutathione and sulfate stores are depleted and metabolism shifts to CYP 2E1. The resultant *N*-acetyl-p-benzo-quinone imine (NAPQI) reactive intermediate forms adducts with cellular proteins, which leads to apoptosis in renal and hepatic tissues that contain CYP 2E1. Another proposed mechanism involves the direct nephrotoxicity of glutathione-APAP or glutathione-metabolite conjugates. Oliguria may accompany about 60% of cases of APAP nephrotoxicity and Cr_s peaks 7 d after overdose, on average. Although *N*-acetylcysteine prevents APAP-induced hepatotoxicity, it has not been shown to reduce APAP-induced nephropathy.[1,2]

ACE Inhibitors and Angiotensin II Receptor Blockers

Angiotensin II (AII) acts on angiotensin type I (AT1) receptors on the efferent arteriole and systemic vasculature to maintain GFR and renal blood flow, respectively. Inhibition of AII production or AT1 antagonism does not markedly affect renal function. However, in states of impaired renal blood flow, such as renal artery stenosis, diuretic therapy, vomiting, diarrhea, decompensated heart failure, cirrhosis, and nephrosclerosis, concomitant ACE inhibitor and angiotensin II receptor blocker therapy increases the risk of prerenal azotemia. Following a 30% or greater increase in Cr_s, the ACE inhibitor or ARB should be discontinued. Recovery of renal function usually follows discontinuation of the offending agent. Patients with impaired renal function were excluded from clinical trials of **aliskiren**, a direct renin inhibitor, and the manufacturer advises caution in this patient population.[3,4]

Acetazolamide

Glaucoma therapy with acetazolamide is associated with a 10-fold increase in the risk of renal stone formation. Calcium phosphate and calcium oxalate stones have been identified.[5,6]

(continued)

Acyclovir

Unchanged acyclovir is excreted in the urine, and accounts for 62%–91% of drug elimination. Due to its low urine solubility, precipitation in the collecting tubules with subsequent obstructive nephropathy occurs within 24–48 h of high-dose (500 mg/m^2) IV use with an estimated prevalence of 12%–48%. Oral and low-dose IV therapies are better tolerated. Aggressive hydration to achieve high urinary flow (100–150 mL/h) prior to acyclovir administration and administration over 1–2 h will prevent crystal formation. Normal renal function usually returns within 6 wk after drug withdrawal.[4,7–9]

Aldesleukin

Almost all patients receiving aldesleukin develop acute renal impairment marked by decreased Cl$_{Cr}$, oliguria or anuria, and fluid retention. It has been proposed that capillary leak syndrome caused by aldesleukin may lead to depletion of intravascular volume and acute renal failure. However, during therapy, normal renal blood flow is maintained. Most patients recover within 1 wk after drug discontinuation, but some require ≥1 mo.[10]

Allopurinol

Allopurinol hypersensitivity syndrome or drug rash with eosinophilia and systemic symptoms (DRESS) occurs in <1% of patients receiving allopurinol therapy, within 8 wk of drug initiation, and is characterized by rash, fever, enlarged lymph nodes, and organ involvement. Allopurinol-DRESS may be more common in patients with renal insufficiency, due to accumulation of a metabolite, oxypurinol, and immune-mediated glomerulonephritis may occur.[11]

Aminoglycosides

Proximal tubular necrosis occurs in up to 30% of patients treated with aminoglycosides for >7 d. Proximal tubular epithelial cells retain about 5% of an administered dose after glomerular filtration and because of slow clearance of these drugs from renal tissue, they still can be present in high concentrations in the kidney after serum levels are undetectable. This does not appear to be a good correlation between renal tissue concentrations of aminoglycosides and their nephrotoxic potential. Impaired organic acid, base, and water transport, protein synthesis, mitochondrial function, and other alterations contribute to tubular necrosis and mechanisms differ at low and high doses. Aminoglycoside-induced ARF is usually nonoliguric, which can delay its recognition. It is often first detected as an asymptomatic increase in Cr$_s$. Detectable changes in GFR usually occur at least 5 d after initiation of therapy and can progress after drug discontinuation. Aminoglycoside-induced renal damage is related to total dosage and duration of treatment. Administration of single daily doses may reduce the nephrotoxicity potential in children with cystic fibrosis but the data is less conclusive for adults. Partial to complete recovery of lost renal function can occur over several weeks after drug discontinuation. Monitoring of aminoglycoside plasma levels and serial renal function tests might be of value in recognizing nephrotoxicity. **Neomycin** has the greatest nephrotoxic potential. Renal failure has been reported following topical irrigation but oral neomycin administration is less likely to cause kidney damage because of its poor bioavailability. **Streptomycin** has the least nephrotoxic potential of the aminoglycosides. All other currently marketed aminoglycosides have intermediate nephrotoxic potentials. Concomitant therapy with other nephrotoxic drugs should be avoided.[12,13]

Amphotericin B

Mild or moderate renal impairment occurs in 50% of patients treated with conventional amphotericin B, with severe renal impairment in 8%. The drug causes a reduction in renal plasma flow as well as direct glomerular and tubular damage via pore formation in cellular membranes. Deoxycholate, a detergent used to solubilize conventional amphotericin B, may account for up to 50% of tubular toxicity. Most patients experience a rapid decline in GFR, which often stabilizes at

(continued)

20%–60% of normal and might not return to normal until several months after drug discontinuation. Distal tubular damage can lead to loss of concentrating ability, renal tubular acidosis, and electrolyte disturbances (most commonly hypokalemia but also hyponatremia and hypomagnesemia). These effects appear to be dosage related, and many patients respond favorably to temporary drug discontinuation or reduction in dosage. The prevalence of nephrotoxicity increases as the cumulative dose increases. Some investigators suggest that the total dosage of conventional amphotericin B should be kept below 3–5 g. Nephrotoxicity is increased by the coadministration of other nephrotoxic drugs, especially cyclosporine. Sodium loading (e.g., 1 L normal saline IV daily) reduces the frequency and severity of amphotericin B–induced nephrotoxicity. Newer lipid formulations appear to be less nephrotoxic, which may be partly due to the absence of deoxycholate. However, there is no consensus about differences in nephrotoxicity among the different products.[14–16]

Azacitidine

Proximal and distal tubular dysfunction may manifest as polyuria and glucosuria in 20%–30% and as a non-anion gap metabolic acidosis and hypophosphatemia in 60%–75% of patients receiving azacitidine therapy.[17]

Bisphosphonates

An increase in Cr_s by 0.5mg/dL or doubling from baseline may occur in 8%–24% of patients receiving intravenous **pamidronate** or **zoledronate**. The mechanisms of kidney injury are not well understood. Pamidronate may cause direct podocyte injury and focal segmental glomerulosclerosis, while zoledronate primarily causes tubular epithelial injury. On the other hand, **ibandronate** has not been associated with nephrotoxicity. Bisphosphonate nephrotoxicity is dose-dependent and infusion is time-dependent and Cr_s should be monitored prior to each dose. The drug should be held for unexplained increases in Cr_s. Oral bisphosphonates are not associated with nephrotoxicity but should be used cautiously in patients with $Cl_{Cr} < 30$ mL/min.[4,7,18,19]

Cephalosporins

The cephalosporin (and cephamycin) antibiotics are capable of producing rare interstitial nephritis similar to the penicillins. Increases in BUN and Cr_s occur occasionally. The nephrotoxicity of the newer cephalosporins is minimal compared with older drugs such as **cephalothin**.[20–22]

Cidofovir and Adefovir

Cidofovir uptake via organic anion transporters into proximal tubular epithelia leads to dose-dependent nephrotoxicity in 12%–25% of patients receiving cidofovir. Proteinuria and increased Cr_s occur in 50% and 12% of cases of cidofovir nephrotoxicity, respectively. **Probenecid** decreases the prevalence and magnitude of proteinuria and must be given with cidofovir. **Adefovir** nephrotoxicity may develop in 22%–50% of patient receiving doses greater than 30 mg/d. Cr_s elevations and hypophosphatemia may be predictive of adefovir nephrotoxicity.[4,7,8,23]

Contrast Media, Radiopaque

Contrast-induced nephropathy (CIN) is the third most common cause of ARF in hospitalized patients. CIN is defined by a 0.5 mg/dL or a 25% increase in Cr_s 48–72 h following exposure to contrast media and affects 1%–2% of the general population and up to 20% of select patient populations. The pathogenesis is not well understood but includes renal vasoconstriction and cytotoxicity to tubular epithelia. The most common pattern is acute oliguric renal failure developing within 24 h after the administration of the contrast agent and lasting 2–5 d; nonoliguric renal failure also has been reported. Most patients recover fully, but permanent renal impairment has been reported. Cr_s usually peaks 3–5 d after exposure and returns to baseline in 10–14 d. Patients with preexisting renal impairment are at much greater risk and constitute 60% of those experiencing nephrotoxicity. High-osmolality ionic contrast media might be more nephrotoxic than

(continued)

low-osmolality ionic or nonionic contrast media. Prevention strategies include hydration and bicarbonate therapy for patients at risk for developing CIN and *N*-acetylcysteine or ascorbic acid for high-risk patients. Dopamine, fenoldopam, loop diuretics, and mannitol may be harmful and should not be used for prevention.[24–27]

Cyclosporine

Dose-related nephrotoxicity occurs in 30%–50% of cyclosporine-treated patients and frequently limits the usefulness of the drug. Reduction in dosage usually reduces the renal toxicity. The drug produces decreased GFR, impaired tubular function, interstitial nephritis, hypertension, fluid retention, and hyperkalemia. Cyclosporine causes vasoconstriction in preglomerular arterioles, which can lead to chronic arteriopathy and tubular atrophy if the dosage is not reduced. Cyclosporine nephrotoxicity is usually reversible during the first 6 mo of therapy, but the risk of permanent renal impairment increases with time. **Calcium channel blockers** appear to reduce the prevalence of cyclosporine-induced nephrotoxicity in renal transplant patients.[28,29]

Demeclocycline

Dose-related, direct tubular toxicity of demeclocycline can lead to NDI. For this reason, it has been used in the management of the syndrome of inappropriate antidiuretic hormone secretion. Demeclocycline causes an inability to concentrate urine, which can lead to dehydration and renal ischemia, and may further promote kidney injury. Impaired hepatic metabolism of demeclocycline may result in increased serum drug concentrations and predispose to nephrotoxicity.[30,31] (*See* also Tetracyclines.)

Diuretics, Loop

Use of high-dose **furosemide** (5–10 mg/kg/d) in adults with refractory CHF is associated with a 40% decrease in Cl_{Cr}. Nephrocalcinosis and nephrolithiasis occur in up to 64% of low-birth-weight infants treated with **furosemide**. These effects usually resolve after drug discontinuation.[32,33]

Diuretics, Thiazide

Occasional cases of interstitial nephritis have been reported, which might be the result of hyper-sensitivity reactions. Long-term use of diuretics might increase the risk of renal cell carcinoma, especially in women.[34]

Fluoroquinolones

The incidence of Cr_s elevations with fluoroquinolones is 0.2%–1.3%. AIN is the most common mechanism; a hypersensitivity mechanism is suspected but remains to be confirmed. Urine alkalinity may promote crystal formation. Most patients reported to have fluoroquinolone-induced nephropathy are >50 y old.[35,36]

Foscarnet

Without intravenous hydration, renal failure may develop in up to 60% of patients receiving foscarnet. The primary pathogenic mechanism is direct tubular toxicity; increases in Cr_s typically occur after 6–15 d of therapy. Foscarnet also down regulates vasopressin-regulated aquaporin-2 channels in the collecting duct to cause polyuria and can lead to NDI. Electrolyte abnormalities are also common. Foscarnet–calcium and foscarnet-sodium crystal formation can occur and may result in hypocalcemia and glomerulopathy. The risk of nephrotoxicity is reduced to about 10%–20% when administered concomitantly with normal saline to promote urinary flow.[8,37]

Gallium Nitrate

Nephrotoxicity is the most frequent adverse effect of gallium, and elevations in BUN and Cr_s can occur after only 1 dose. At least 1 death has been associated with gallium-induced nephrotoxicity.[38]

(*continued*)

Gold Salts

A lesion resembling membranous glomerulonephritis with proteinuria can occur in 3%–10% of patients receiving parenteral gold therapy. Microhematuria and nephrotic syndrome are less frequent. One-half of the cases of proteinuria develop in the first 6 mo of therapy. Occasionally, acute tubular necrosis and interstitial nephritis are reported. Although recovery can take up to 18 mo, permanent renal impairment after drug withdrawal is uncommon. There is evidence for immune and direct toxic mechanisms for gold nephrotoxicity. Oral **auranofin** appears to be less nephrotoxic than parenteral gold products.[39,40]

Histamine H2-Receptor Antagonists

Cimetidine competes with Cr_s for tubular secretion and may produce transient elevations in Cr_s, an effect not seen with other drugs in the class. There are at least 25 case reports with fever and fatigue occurring in 85% and 67% of cases, respectively. Sterile pyuria and proteinuria are common findings on urinalysis. The immunomodulatory effects of H2RAs may contribute to AIN.[41]

Hydroxyethyl Starch

Hydroxyethyl starch (HES) is not degraded after uptake into proximal tubular cells, which can lead to osmotic nephrosis. Use of high-molecular weight HES products with high C2–C6 molar substitution ratios and exceeding the daily dose limit of 33 mL/kg/d may increase the risk for HES nephrotoxicity. However, use of a low-molecular weight HES product for fluid resuscitation in severe sepsis was recently associated with higher rates of ARF and renal replacement therapy in a dose-dependent manner than ringers lactate.[4,7,42]

Ifosfamide

Reversible, subclinical nephrotoxicity occurs in almost all ifosfamide-treated patients. Age and cumulative dose >45 g/m^2 are predictive of ifosfamide nephrotoxicity, which is typically mediated by proximal tubular dysfunction. Fanconi syndrome–like symptoms including renal loss of glucose, electrolytes, and small proteins occur in 4%. Mesna does not protect against ifosfamide nephrotoxicity.[17]

Immune Globulin

Intravenous administration of immune globulin can produce reversible ARF after first or repeated exposures. Osmotic nephrosis is caused by large amounts of sucrose used in some immune globulin products to reduce the formation of immunoglobulin aggregates. Maltose- and dextrose-stabilized products may have a lower propensity to cause kidney injury because they are metabolized by renal epithelial cells while sucrose is not.[4,43,44]

Indinavir

About 20% of indinavir is eliminated renally and may cause crystal nephropathy and nephrolithiasis related to the drug's pH-dependent insolubility in urine. Crystalluria occurs in most indinavir-treated patients and 8% of patients may experience urologic symptoms including back pain, dysuria, hematuria, and flank pain. Daily fluid intake of 2–3 L reduces crystal formation.[4,7–9,45]

Lithium

Lithium accumulates in the collecting duct and alters the response to antidiuretic hormone, resulting in the inability to concentrate urine, and may lead to NDI. This typically mild effect is usually reversible with drug withdrawal. Long-term therapy (10–15 y) is associated with an increased prevalence of reduced Cl_{Cr} and renal concentrating ability that are frequently not reversible, despite withdrawal of lithium. Interstitial nephritis and nephrotic syndrome also have been reported.[7,46–48]

(continued)

Mannitol

High doses (>200 g/d or >400 g/2 d) are associated with acute oliguric renal failure. The pathogenesis is unclear. Osmotic nephrosis is the predominant mechanism and with increased exposure, the profound diuresis caused by mannitol can lead to hypovolemia and prerenal azotemia. The osmolal gap should be maintained at less than 55 mOsm/kg to minimize the risk. ARF might require 7–10 d for recovery; dialysis shortens the recovery period to 1–2 d.[49,50]

Methotrexate

Acute renal impairment occurs in 30%–50% of patients treated with high-dose MTX and leucovorin rescue. Most cases are reversible within 3 wk. Approximately 20% of deaths associated with MTX are caused by ARF. Methotrexate (MTX) is excreted unchanged in the urine through glomerular filtration and tubular secretion. pH-Dependent urine solubility leads to crystal formation with high-dose (1–33 g/m^2) therapy. Mechanisms of kidney injury include crystal-induced obstructive nephropathy, direct tubular toxicity, and impaired renal blood flow due to afferent arteriole vasoconstriction. Close monitoring of MTX serum concentrations and adjustment of dosage might minimize the risk of nephrotoxicity, as do vigorous hydration and alkalinization during drug administration. Following carboxypeptidase-G2 administration, a >95% decrease in serum MTX concentrations occurs within minutes and, if given early, may prevent MTX nephrotoxicity. However, the enzyme is only currently available for investigational use.[9,17,51]

Methoxyflurane

NDI, proximal tubular damage, and interstitial nephritis have been reported. The nephrotoxicity of methoxyflurane appears to be dose-related and might be caused by increased circulating fluoride ion concentrations. Fluoride causes distal tubular dysfunction by inhibiting sodium and chloride transport in the ascending loop of Henle and reducing the response to antidiuretic hormone. Urinary oxalate crystallization also has been reported after methoxyflurane anesthesia.[52,53]

Mitomycin

ARF secondary to hemolytic uremic syndrome (HUS) may occur in more than 10% of patients receiving mitomycin. Cumulative doses >60 mg/m^2 may increase the risk of developing mitomycin nephrotoxicity and HUS may persist or worsen following drug discontinuation. Onset typically occurs within 5–12 mo following initial therapy. Plasmapheresis may reverse renal dysfunction.[17,54,55]

Nitrosoureas

The nitrosoureas, **carmustine, lomustine, semustine,** and **streptozocin**, can produce insidious nephrotoxicity in patients on long-term therapy. The pathogenic mechanism may be alkylation of renal tubular cell components. **Lomustine** seems to have the greatest nephrotoxic potential. Some cases of permanent renal function impairment have been reported.[17,56]

Nonsteroidal Anti-Inflammatory Drugs

NSAIDs, including **COX-2 inhibitors,** can reduce Cl$_{Cr}$ and produce renal insufficiency as a result of renal circulatory changes caused by inhibition of prostaglandin synthesis. These effects tend to be relatively minor and usually reversible. The prevalence is usually low (0.5%–1% of patients), but some patients are at increased risk; predisposing factors are advanced age, preexisting renal impairment, and states of renal hypoperfusion (e.g., sodium depletion, hypotension, diuretic use, hepatic cirrhosis, and CHF). Reversible AIN and necrosis occur occasionally. It is not possible at this time to accurately categorize the prevalence associated with each NSAID. **Fenoprofen** is the NSAID most commonly associated with interstitial nephritis and nephrotic syndrome. The removal of **phenacetin** from nonprescription analgesics has resulted in a marked decline in the incidence of analgesic nephropathy, a syndrome characterized by papillary necrosis, interstitial nephritis, and

(continued)

progressive renal medullary impairment that occurs in persons with long-term consumption of large quantities of oral, combination analgesic products.[4,7,57–59]

Pemetrexed

About 70%–90% of parent drug is eliminated unchanged in the urine. In phase III trials only patients with $Cl_{Cr} > 60$ mL/min were included and 2.4% developed renal failure and 0.6% required dialysis. NDI and renal tubular acidosis have also been reported. After uptake into tumor cells, pemetrexed undergoes polyglutamation and is retained in cells to disrupt folate-dependent metabolic processes involved in cell replication. A similar process may occur in renal tubular cells.[60]

Penicillamine

Slight to moderate proteinuria occurs in 7%–30% of patients on long-term (≥ 6 mo) therapy with penicillamine for rheumatoid arthritis. Most cases develop in the first year. Proteinuria is usually benign and slowly reversible over 6–12 mo, but nephrotic syndrome is occasionally encountered. The lesions appear to be perimembranous glomerulonephritis resulting from the deposition of antigen–antibody complexes on the renal basement membrane.[61]

Penicillins

Interstitial nephritis has been reported with most penicillins. **Methicillin** is by far the most frequently implicated penicillin (frequency 10%–16%); the reason for its dominance is unknown. Penicillin-induced interstitial nephritis is an immune reaction that most commonly occurs during a long course of therapy. The reaction is usually accompanied by other signs of hypersensitivity such as fever, rash, and eosinophilia; hematuria also can occur. The reduction of renal function might not be oliguric, so urine volume is not a reliable parameter to monitor. Recovery usually occurs within weeks to months after drug discontinuation.[62]

Pentamidine

Prospective trials of IV pentamidine for the treatment of *Pneumocystis jiroveci* pneumonia show nephrotoxicity in 4%–66% of patients. Onset is usually 8–12 d after the start of therapy and likely related to direct tubular toxicity. Similar to potassium-sparing diuretics, pentamidine acts on the collecting tubules to decrease sodium reabsorption, which reduces potassium excretion, and can cause life-threatening hyperkalemia. Hypomagnesemia and hypocalcemia are also common.[63]

Platinums

Dosage-related proximal tubular impairment is the major limiting factor in **cisplatin** therapy and can occur in 50%–75% of patients. Cl_{Cr} is typically reduced to 60%–80% of baseline with repeated courses of therapy. The greatest damage occurs in the first month of therapy, and it appears to be more likely when the drug is administered repetitively at close intervals. Forced hydration and mannitol diuresis can reduce renal toxicity, at least for the first cycle of therapy. Magnesium and calcium losses are common manifestations of cisplatin-induced nephrotoxicity. Cisplatin-induced renal effects can be detected as long as 6 mos after the end of therapy.

Although apparently less nephrotoxic than cisplatin, **carboplatin** therapy is frequently associated with reductions in GFR and increased electrolyte losses (especially calcium and magnesium). Patients with preexisting renal impairment and those who receive inadequate hydration during drug administration are at greatest risk. **Oxaliplatin** nephrotoxicity has not been reported.[17,64–66]

Polymyxins

Nephrotoxicity may occur in 10%–36% of patients receiving **colistimethate** or **polymyxin B** parenterally. Tubular necrosis most frequently occurs due to increased tubular cell permeability leading to cell swelling and lysis. High dosage, long duration of therapy, and renal impairment are predisposing factors. Polymyxin-induced renal damage is usually reversible, but some patients may continue to deteriorate after drug withdrawal.[67]

(continued)

Proton Pump Inhibitors

Interstitial nephritis occurs rarely during proton pump inhibitor (PPI) therapy. However, due to widespread use, PPI-induced nephrotoxicity is being reported with increasing frequency and may be one of the most common causes of drug-induced interstitial nephritis. Onset occurs typically after 10–11 wk of PPI therapy. Although initial reports implicated **omeprazole**, a class effect has been demonstrated.[68,69]

Rifampin

Rifampin nephrotoxicity is characterized by tubular necrosis, glomerulonephritis, interstitial nephritis, and proteinuria. It is mediated by a type II or III hypersensitivity reaction and most often occurs with intermittent or interrupted dosage regimens but also has been observed with continuous therapy.[70,71]

Sodium Phosphate, Oral

Acute phosphate nephropathy has been described in patients receiving oral sodium phosphate products (OSPs) for bowel cleansing. Transient elevations and reductions in serum phosphate and calcium occur, respectively, following OSP ingestion. Calcium phosphate crystals deposit in renal tubules and result in tubule injury. Achieving euvolemia and maintaining normal renal blood flow may prevent nephrotoxicity. OSPs now carry a boxed warning to warn of the risks of acute phosphate nephropathy and over-the-counter use is no longer recommended.[7]

Sulfonamides, Antibacterial

Crystalluria occurs in 8%–29% of **sulfadiazine**-treated patients because the drug is a weak acid and tends to precipitate at urinary pH <5.5. ARF is typically oliguric and asymptomatic. Crystallization occurs less frequently in patients receiving **sulfamethoxazole**. Interstitial nephritis, glomerulonephritis, and tubular necrosis are reported rarely and may be allergic in origin.[4,7,9]

Tacrolimus

Acute nephrotoxicity occurs with prevalence similar to that of cyclosporine. Progressive nephrotoxicity is reported with long-term (>1 y) therapy. The risk of nephrotoxicity can be greatly limited by keeping the tacrolimus whole blood concentration <20 μg/L.[28,29,72,73]

Tenofovir

Mild reductions in GFR may occur in 5%–7% patients receiving tenofovir and typically occur after 5–11 mo of therapy. Like **adefovir** and **cidofovir**, tenofovir is a substrate for tubular organic anion transporters and may cause tubular dysfunction at higher concentrations. Combination therapy with ritonavir may increase the risk of nephrotoxicity by inhibiting tenofovir efflux from renal tubules. Fanconi syndrome has also been reported in rare cases.[4,7,8,45,74]

Topiramate

Nephrolithiasis occurs in 1.5% of topiramate-treated patients during the first year of therapy. Topiramate promotes bicarbonate urinary excretion via carbonic anhydrase inhibition in proximal and distal tubules, which can lead to systemic metabolic acidosis. The increase in urinary pH decreases calcium phosphate solubility and results in crystal formation.[75]

Triamterene

Triamterene may precipitate in acidic urine and cause crystal nephropathy. The drug is also associated with an increase in urinary sediment, and can be incorporated into existing renal calculi. One report suggests that 1/1500 users of the drug will develop triamterene-associated calculi during the course of 1 y. Triamterene also might be associated with the development of interstitial nephritis. As a precaution, the drug probably should not be used in patients with a history of renal calculi and concomitant NSAID therapy is not advised.[9]

(continued)

Vancomycin

Nephrotoxicity from vancomycin was commonly reported early in its history. Currently, the prevalence of vancomycin-induced renal impairment (usually mild) is 5%–17% and the mechanism of injury may be tubular necrosis or interstitial nephritis. It is usually reversible after discontinuation of the drug. Concomitant administration of **aminoglycosides** and other nephrotoxins results in at least additive nephrotoxicity. Additionally, prolonged therapy and serum concentrations >15 mg/L have been associated with reductions in Cl_{Cr}.[76–78]

Vorinostat

Transient increases in Cr_s and proteinuria occurred in 46%–51% of patients, respectively, receiving the histone deacetylase inhibitor, vorinostat, for cutaneous T-cell lymphoma in phase II trials. Blocking histone deacetylation in renal tubular cells may lead to mitochondrial injury and apotosis.[79]

■ REFERENCES

1. Mazer M, Perrone J. Acetaminophen-induced nephrotoxicity: pathophysiology, clinical manifestations, and management. *J Med Toxicol.* 2008;4(1):2-6.
2. Eguia L, Materson BJ. Acetaminophen-related acute renal failure without fulminant liver failure. *Pharmacotherapy,* 1997;17(2):363-370.
3. Textor SC. Renal failure related to angiotensin-converting enzyme inhibitors. *Semin Nephrol.* 1997;17:67-76.
4. Perazella MA. Drug-induced acute renal failure: update on new medications and unique mechanisms of nephrotoxicity. *Am J Med Sci.* 2003;325(6):349-362.
5. Kass MA et al. Acetazolamide and urolithiasis. *Ophthalmology,* 1981;88:261-265
6. Tawil R et al. Acetazolamide-induced nephrolithiasis: implications for treatment of neuromuscular disorders. *Neurology,* 1993;43:1105-1106.
7. Markowitz GS, Perazella MA. Drug-induced renal failure: a focus on tubulointerstitial disease. *Clinica Chimica Acta.* 2005;351:31-47.
8. Izzedine J et al. Antiviral drug-induced nephrotoxicity. *Am J Kidney Dis.* 2005;45(5):804-817.
9. Perazella MA. Crystal-induced acute renal failure *Am J Med.* 1999;106:459-465.
10. Vial T, Descotes J. Clinical toxicity of interleukin-2. *Drug Saf.* 1992;7:417-433.
11. Markel A. Allopurinol-induced DRESS syndrome. *Isr Med Assoc J.* 2005;7(10):656-660.
12. Mingeot-Leclercq MP Tulkens PM. Aminoglycosides: nephrotoxicity. *Antimicrob Agents Chemother.* 1999;43(5):1003-1012.
13. Smyth AR et al. Once-daily versus multiple-daily dosing with intravenous aminoglycosides for cystic fibrosis. *Cochrane Database Syst Rev.* 2006;(3). Art. No.: CD002009. DOI: 10.1002/14651858.CD002009.pub2.
14. Deray G. Amphotericin B nephrotoxicity. *J Antimicrob Chemother.* 2002;49(suppl 1):37-41.
15. Johansen HK, Gøtzsche PC. Amphotericin B lipid soluble formulations versus amphotericin B in cancer patients with neutropenia. *Cochrane Database Syst Rev.* 2000;(3). Art. No.: CD000969. DOI: 10.1002/14651858. CD000969.
16. Barrett JP et al. A systematic review of the antifungal effectiveness and tolerability of amphotericin B formulations. *Clin Ther.* 2003;25(5):1295-1320.
17. Kintzel PE. Anticancer drug-induced kidney disorders: incidence, prevention and management. *Drug Saf.* 2001;24(1):19-38.
18. Perazella MA, Markowitz GS. Bisphosphonate nephrotoxicity. *Kidney Int.* 2008;74(11):1385-1393.
19. Henrich WL. Nephrotoxicity of several newer agents. *Kidney Int.* 2005;67(suppl 94):S107-S109.
20. Quin JD. The nephrotoxicity of cephalosporins. *Adverse Drug React Acute Poison Rev.* 1989;8:63-72.
21. Zhanel GG. Cephalosporin-induced nephrotoxicity: does it exist? *DICP.* 1990;24:262-265.
22. Thompson JW, Jacobs RF. Adverse effects of newer cephalosporins. An update. *Drug Saf.* 1993;9:132-142.
23. Dando TM, Plosker GL. Adefovir dipivoxil: a review of its use in chronic hepatitis B. *Drugs.* 2003;63(20):2215-2234.
24. Mehran R, Nikolsky E. Contrast-induced nephropathy: definition, epidemiology, and patients at risk. *Kidney Int.* 2006;69:S11-S15.
25. Persson PB, Tepel M. Contrast medium-induced nephropathy: the pathophysiology. *Kidney Int.* 2006;69:S8-S10.
26. Briguori C, Marenzi G. Contrast-induced nephropathy: pharmacologic prophylaxis. *Kidney Int.* 2006;69: S30-S38.
27. Pannu N et al. Prophylaxis strategies for contrast-induced nephropathy. *JAMA.* 2006;295:2765-2779.

28. Andoh TF et al. Nephrotoxicity of immunosuppressive drugs: experimental and clinical observations. *Semin Nephrol.* 1997;17:34-45.

29. Rossi SJ et al. Prevention and management of the adverse effects associated with immunosuppressive therapy. *Drug Saf.* 1993;9:104-131.

30. Forrest JN et al. Superiority of demeclocycline over lithium in the treatment of chronic syndrome of inappropriate secretion of antidiuretic hormone. *N Engl J Med.* 1978;298:173-177.

31. Curtis NJ et al. Irreversible nephrotoxicity from demeclocycline in the treatment of hyponatremia. *Age Ageing.* 2002;31(2):151-152.

32. Alon US et al. Nephrocalcinosis and nephrolithiasis in infants with congestive heart failure treated with furosemide. *J Pediatr.* 1994;125:149-151.

33. Cotter G et al. Increased toxicity of high-dose furosemide versus low-dose dopamine in the treatment of refractory congestive heart failure. *Clin Pharmacol Ther.* 1997;62:187-193.

34. Grossman E et al. Does diuretic therapy increase the risk of renal cell carcinoma? *Am J Cardiol.* 1999;83:1090-1093.

35. Lomaestro BM. Fluoroquinolone-induced renal failure. *Drug Saf.* 2000;22:479-485.

36. Lipsky BA, Baker CA. Fluoroquinolone toxicity profiles: a review focusing on newer agents. *Clin Infect Dis.* 1999;28:352-364.

37. Deray G et al. Foscarnet nephrotoxicity: mechanism, incidence and prevention. *Am J Nephrol.* 1989;9:316-321.

38. Chitambar CR. Gallium nitrate revisited. *Semin Oncol.* 2003;30(2 suppl 5):1-4.

39. Hall CL. Gold nephropathy. *Nephron.* 1988;50:265-272.

40. Newton P et al. Proteinuria with gold therapy: when should gold be permanently stopped? *Br J Rheumatol.* 1983;22:11-17.

41. Fisher AA, LeCouteur DG. Nephrotoxicity and hepatotoxicity of histamine H2-receptor antagonists. *Drug Saf.* 2001;24(1):39-57.

42. Brunkhorst FM et al. Intensive insulin therapy and pentastarch resuscitation in severe sepsis. *N Engl J Med.* 2008;358:125-139.

43. Anon. Renal insufficiency and failure associated with immune globulin intravenous therapy—United States, 1985-1998. *MMWR Morb Mortal Wkly Rep.* 1999;48:518-521.

44. Winward DB, Brophy MT. Acute renal failure after administration of intravenous immunoglobulin: review of the literature and case report. *Pharmacotherapy.* 1995;15:765-772.

45. Roling J et al. HIV-associated renal diseases and highly active antiretroviral therapy-induced nephropathy. *Clin Infect Dis.* 2006;42:1488-1495.

46. Gitlin M. Lithium and the kidney. An updated review. *Drug Saf.* 1999;20:231-243.

47. Bendz H et al. Kidney damage in long-term lithium patients: a cross-sectional study of patients with 15 years or more on lithium. *Nephrol Dial Transplant.* 1994;9:1250-1254.

48. Walker RG. Lithium nephrotoxicity. *Kidney Int.* 1993;44(suppl 42):S93-S98.

49. Visweswaran P et al. Mannitol-induced acute renal failure. *J Am Soc Nephrol.* 1997;8:1028-1033.

50. Dickenmann M et al. Osmotic nephrosis: acute kidney injury with accumulation of proximal tubular lysosomes due to administration of exogenous solutes. *Am J Kidney Dis.* 2008;51:491-503.

51. Widemann BC, Adamson PC. Understanding and managing methotrexate nephrotoxicity. *Oncologist.* 2006; 11:694-703.

52. Cousins MJ, Mazze RI. Methoxyflurane nephrotoxicity. A study of dose response in man. *JAMA.* 1973;225:1611-1616.

53. Desmond JW. Methoxyflurane nephrotoxicity. *Can Anaesth Soc J.* 1974;21:294-307.

54. Valavaara R, Nordman E. Renal complications of mitomycin C therapy with special reference to the total dose. *Cancer.* 1985;55:47-50.

55. Verwey J et al. Mitomycin C–induced renal toxicity, a dose-dependent side effect? *Eur J Cancer Clin Oncol.* 1987;23:195-199.

56. Weiss RB et al. Nephrotoxicity of semustine. *Cancer Treat Rep.* 1983;67:1105-1112.

57. Gambaro G, Perazella MA. Adverse renal effects of anti-inflammatory agents: evaluation of selective and nonselective cyclooxygenase inhibitors. *J Intern Med.* 2003;253:643-652.

58. De Broe ME, Elseviers MM. Analgesic nephropathy. *N Engl J Med.* 1998;338:446-452.

59. Mihatsch MJ et al. Obituary to analgesic nephropathy—an autopsy study. *Nephrol Dial Transplant.* 2006;21:3139-3145.

60. Vootukuru V et al. Pemetrexed-induced acute renal failure, nephrogenic diabetes insipidus, and renal tubular acidosis in a patient with non-small cell lung cancer. *Med Oncol.* 2006;23(3):419-422.

61. Hall CL et al. Natural course of penicillamine nephropathy: a long term study of 33 patients. *Br Med J.* 1988;296:1083-1086.

62. Appel GB. A decade of penicillin related acute interstitial nephritis—more questions than answers. *Clin Nephrol.* 1980;13:151-154.

63. O'Brien JG et al. A 5-year retrospective review of adverse drug reactions and their risk factors in human immunodeficiency virus–infected patients who are receiving intravenous pentamidine therapy for *Pneumocystis carinii* pneumonia. *Clin Infect Dis.* 1997;24:854-859.

64. Cornelison TL, Reed E. Nephrotoxicity and hydration management for cisplatin, carboplatin, and ormaplatin. *Gynecol Oncol.* 1993;50:147-158.

65. Yao X, Panichpisal K, Kurtzman N. Cisplatin nephrotoxicity: a review. *Am J Med Sci.* 2007;334(2):115-124.

66. Cassidy J, Misset JL. Oxaliplatin-related side effects: characteristics and management. *Semin Oncol.* 2002;29(5 suppl 15):11-20.

67. Falagas ME, Kasiakou SK. Toxicity of polymyxins: a systematic review of the evidence from old and recent studies. *Crit Care.* 2006;10(4):R123.

68. Brewster UC, Perazella MA. Proton pump inhibitors and the kidney: a critical review. *Clin Nephrol.* 2007;68(2):65-72.

69. Brewster UC, Perazella MA. Acute kidney injury following proton pump inhibitor therapy. *Kidney Int.* 2007;71:589-593.

70. De Vriese AS et al. Rifampicin-associated acute renal failure: pathophysiologic, immunologic, and clinical features. *Am J Kidney Dis.* 1998;31:108-115.

71. Munoz ME et al. Rifampin-related acute renal failure, thrombocytopenia, and leukocytoclastic vasculitis. *Ann Pharmacother.* 2008;42:727-728.

72. Porayko MK et al. Nephrotoxicity of FK 506 and cyclosporine when used as primary immunosuppression in liver transplant recipients. *Transplant Proc.* 1993;25:665-668.

73. Böttiger Y et al. Tacrolimus whole blood concentrations correlate closely to side-effects in renal transplant recipients. *Br J Clin Pharmacol.* 1999;48:445-448.

74. James CW et al. Tenofovir-related nephrotoxicity: case report and review of the literature. *Pharmacotherapy.* 2004;24(3):415-418.

75. Welch BJ, Graybeal D, Moe OW. Biochemical and stone-risk profiles with topiramate treatment. *Am J Kidney Dis.* 2006;48:555-563.

76. Bailie GR, Neal D. Vancomycin ototoxicity and nephrotoxicity. A review. *Med Toxicol Adverse Drug Exp.* 1988;3:376-386.

77. Rybak MJ et al. Nephrotoxicity of vancomycin, alone and with an aminoglycoside. *J Antimicrob Chemother.* 1990;25:679-687.

78. Jeffries MN et al. A retrospective analysis of possible renal toxicity associated with vancomycin in patients with health care-associated methicillin-resistant *Staphylococcus aureus. Clin Ther.* 2007;29(6):1107-1115.

79. Dong G et al. Induction of apoptosis in renal tubular cells by histone deacetylase inhibitors, a family of anticancer agents. *J Pharmacol Exper Ther.* 2008;325(3):978-984.

Chapter 64

Drug-Induced Oculotoxicity

Melanie Mabins

Occasionally, nonspecific blurred vision occurs with almost all drugs. The agents in this table are associated with a specific pattern of drug-induced oculotoxicity when administered *systemically*. Class-related effects are reported when applicable.

Acetaminophen

It can cause erythema multiforme.[1]

Allopurinol

Despite the discovery of allopurinol in cataractous lenses taken from patients on long-term (>2 y) therapy, there is no clinical evidence for an increased risk of cataracts in allopurinol-treated patients. Allopurinol can also cause erythema multiforme.[1-3]

Alpha-1 Blocking Agents

Patients treated with nonspecific α-1 blockers who undergo cataract surgery are at risk of intraoperative floppy iris syndrome. This is well documented with **tamsulosin** and was seen after 4 mo of therapy and 1 y after drug discontinuation in one case study. This does not affect vision or eye health.[1,2]

Amiodarone

Most patients treated with amiodarone develop bilateral corneal microdeposits (75% after 1 y of therapy) that may be clinically irrelevant as they rarely cause significant visual impairment. Visual symptoms occur in 6%–14%. Halo vision at night is most commonly reported, but patients also might complain of photophobia and blurred vision. The deposits are apparently dose related and reversible, appearing within 1–4 mo and disappearing 3–7 mo after drug discontinuation. Minute lens opacities occurred in 7 of 14 amiodarone-treated patients in one study. Amiodarone has also been found to cause erythema multiforme. It is probable this agent could also cause bilateral optic neuropathy upon initiation and may improve or disappear upon discontinuation.[3-8]

Anticancer (Antineoplastic) Agents

Docetaxel and **paclitaxel** can cause or exacerbate open-angle glaucoma. In several case reports, epidermal growth factor receptor pathway inhibitors such as **cetuximab, erlotinib,** and **gefitinib** appeared to cause external ocular changes and ocular side effects such as meibomitis, periocular cutaneous toxicity and cicatricial ectropion. Multiple reports indicate **vascular endothelial growth factor–modulating therapy** is associated with retinal pigment epithelium tears, commonly presenting as abrupt and significant vision loss. Adverse effects are easily treatable and reversible with drug discontinuation. Various ocular disorders occur frequently with the **vinca alkaloids.** Most (ptosis, blurred vision, night blindness) are thought to be the result of cranial nerve impairment. Ptosis occurs in up to 50% of vincristine-treated patients. Time to onset ranges widely (2–44 wk) as does resolution after drug discontinuation (2–24 wk). **Vincristine** might be more oculotoxic than **vinblastine.** Long-term therapy (usually ≥1 y) with **busulfan** is associated with the development of posterior subcapsular cataracts in approximately 10% of patients. Blurred vision and altered color perception are frequently associated with high-dose **cisplatin.** Blurred vision gradually improves after drug discontinuation, although altered color vision can persist.

(continued)

Pigmentary retinopathy is also reported with this agent. Keratoconjunctivitis occurs in up to 50% of patients on **cyclophosphamide**. One report showed a 17% prevalence of transient reversible blurred vision during high-dose cyclophosphamide therapy. Recovery took from 1 h to 14 d. Keratoconjunctivitis, corneal damage, ocular pain, and photophobia are frequent, dose-related side effects of **cytarabine**. These symptoms usually resolve 1–2 wk after drug discontinuation. Pretreatment with corticosteroid eye drops can be beneficial but should be used with caution in patients with corneal damage. **Doxorubicin** stimulates excessive lacrimation shortly after administration in approximately 25% of patients. Conjunctivitis also has been reported with this agent. Adverse ocular effects occur in 25%–50% of patients receiving **fluorouracil** systemically. Blurred vision, ocular irritation and pain, conjunctivitis, keratitis, and excessive lacrimation occur frequently. These effects resolve in 1–2 wk after drug discontinuation. Some patients can develop eversion of the eyelid margin (cicatricial ectropion) or potentially irreversible fibrosis of the tear duct (dacryostenosis) with prolonged therapy. Adverse ocular effects associated with systemic **methotrexate** occur in up to 25% and include conjunctivitis, increased or decreased lacrimation, photophobia, and eye pain. Onset is during the first week of therapy, and resolution usually occurs 1–2 wk after drug discontinuation. Scintillating scotomas or photopsia occur frequently during **paclitaxel** infusions. The onset of these short-lived effects is usually during the last hour of the infusion. They do not always recur during subsequent infusions. With **tamoxifen**, fine, refractile retinal opacities and retinopathy occur frequently; corneal opacities also are reported. The prevalence of retinopathy has been rare, 1.5%–11.8%, in prospective studies. Although these lesions can occur with any dosage, they occur most often with daily dosages >180 mg or cumulative dosages >100 g. Perhaps due to estrogenic properties, this manifests as loss of vision, retinal edema, hemorrhage, and optic disc swelling after a few weeks. These can result in retinal changes, reduced visual acuity, and decreased color vision and are slowly reversible after drug discontinuation. Tamoxifen can also induce cataracts and macular edema. Ocular toxicity (in the cornea, lens, retina, and optic nerve) can be caused at standard and high doses. Also, the long-term, standard dosage of tamoxifen can cause ocular toxicity and a level of loss of color vision. Retinopathy and keratopathy from low doses of tamoxifen are well defined. There is little reporting on visual function impairment with limitations to color vision defects. Some level of color vision loss and ocular toxic effects were found in one study.[3,4,7,9,27]

Anticholinergic Agents

Blurring of vision can result from paralysis of accommodation (cycloplegia). These drugs also dilate the pupil (mydriasis), which can produce photophobia and precipitate narrow-angle (or acute angle-closure) glaucoma. With systemic administration, large doses are usually required to produce mydriasis, which is most commonly associated with potent anticholinergics such as **atropine, scopolamine,** or **benztropine.** Photophobia and impaired vision because of pupil dilation and paralysis of accommodation can occur from scopolamine skin patches due to its anticholinergic properties. Patients being treated for narrow-angle glaucoma can usually tolerate systemic anticholinergic therapy but nevertheless should avoid these drugs unless absolutely necessary. Patients with open-angle glaucoma, particularly if treated, can receive anticholinergic medications without much risk. Patients receiving nebulized **ipratropium** by facemask are at risk for developing increased intraocular pressure and precipitation of narrow-angle glaucoma, probably from the drug escaping from beneath the ill-fitting masks and directly affecting the eyes. All of the ocular effects of anticholinergics are dose related and reversible.[4,7,28–31]

Anticonvulsants

Diplopia and nystagmus occur frequently. Blurred vision can be caused by mydriasis (**phenytoin**) or cycloplegia (**carbamazepine**). All of these effects are dose related. Visual field defects have been frequently reported with **vigabatrin** and infrequently with long-term **valproic acid** (bilateral

(continued)

concentric) therapy. Sulfa-based drugs such as **topiramate** can cause ocular adverse effects like refractive changes and swelling of the ciliary body, which leads to acute angle-closure glaucoma. The acute increase in intraocular pressure commonly occurs within the first few weeks of therapy. The most common clinical presentation is blurred vision. Over 100 cases have been documented. Visual field loss (concentric or bilateral nasal) occurs to some degree in 30%–50% of **vigabatrin**-treated patients and is severe in 9%. Males are more susceptible than females. This specifically presents as visual field constriction and alterations in the full-field electroretinogram. A high maximum dose is most likely to cause the visual field defects versus high cumulative doses or a long duration of therapy. These adverse effects may remain years after discontinuing vigabatrin therapy, suggesting permanent retinal damage by the drug.[7,32–40]

Antidepressants

SSRIs such as **fluoxetine, paroxetine, fluvoxamine,** and **venlafaxine** have anticholinergic properties that cause pupillary dilation and can precipitate narrow-angle glaucoma and cycloplegia at usual doses. (*See* Anticholinergic Agents.) There is a 10%–30% prevalence of blurred vision resulting from cycloplegia, but it is rarely troublesome and is reversible with drug discontinuation. Blurred vision usually resolves despite continued antidepressant use as the eye becomes tolerant to the drug's effects. Reports of angle closure have been made with the tricyclic antidepressants (**amitriptyline** and **imipramine**) in addition to SSRIs (**citalopram**). Another case report indicates that **escitalopram** may be the cause of choroidal effusions and secondary angle closure.[4,9,33,41]

Antihistamine Drugs (H1 Blockers)

With the exception of **loratadine** and **fexofenadine,** these drugs have some anticholinergic properties and can precipitate narrow-angle glaucoma and cycloplegia. (*See* Anticholinergic Agents.) These effects are minor and reversible with drug discontinuation. Antihistamines (most notably **diphenhydramine**) can reduce night vision.[4,30,42]

Anti-infectives

Several anti-infectives have been known to cause an ocular presentation of Stevens-Johnson syndrome such as mucopurulent conjunctivitis or pseudomembrane formation (erythema multiforme of the eyelids). Some of these agents include **ampicillin, cefazolin, clindamycin, doxycycline, isoniazid, penicillin, sulfadiazine, sulfonamides,** and **vancomycin**. Sulfonamides are also reported to be a frequent cause of acute myopia. Other complications include conjunctival shrinkage, misdirection of eyelashes, and dry eye. There have been 12 reported cases of optic neuropathy with long-term **linezolid** use. The optic neuropathy presented in an average of 5–11 mo. This clinically presents as decreased vision and color vision, visual field defects, and swollen or pale optic disc. Vision improves after discontinuation of linezolid. **Ethambutol** has over 50 reported cases of optic neuropathy that is dose dependent. Some studies report an incidence of 18% after a few months of a 35 mg/kg/d dose; severe loss of vision in both eyes is also reported. Overall, at recommended doses, the incidence is only 1%. Specific symptoms are loss of visual acuity, loss of color vision, and visual field defect. Optic neuritis, papilledema, and visual field defects are occasionally reported with chloramphenicol. These effects can occur after weeks or years of therapy but are most common after several months of **chloramphenicol** use. Most cases are reported in children with cystic fibrosis, but the association with this disorder is unclear and might only reflect the types of patients who received long-term chloramphenicol therapy. Permanent visual impairment and recovery are reported after drug discontinuation. There are anecdotal reports that large doses of vitamins B_6 and B_{12} have beneficial effects on these adverse ocular effects. Dark blue discoloration of the sclera has been reported with **minocycline**. Although the prevalence cannot be accurately estimated, the growing use of minocycline as an antiarthritic drug should increase the number of cases. It is not known if the discoloration is reversible. Uveitis occurs frequently during **rifabutin** treatment and prophylaxis of *Mycobacterium avium* complex infection in

(*continued*)

AIDS patients. Its onset is variable (2 wk to 7 mo after starting treatment). Uveitis can be unilateral or bilateral and responds to topical corticosteroid therapy.[4,7,12,43–51]

Antimalarials

Loss of visual acuity and reduction of the visual field to the point of blindness can occur with **quinine** therapy or (especially) overdose. Other reported ocular effects are impaired color vision and night blindness. These effects are usually reversible, but permanent constriction of the visual field and blindness are reported. The ocular effects of quinine might be the result of changes in the retinal vasculature. The oculotoxicity of **chloroquine** and **hydroxychloroquine** limits their usefulness; two general types of ocular change occur: corneal deposits and retinopathy. Approximately 50% of patients demonstrate corneal deposits, less than one-half of whom have visual impairment resulting from these deposits. Opacities present as punctate or whirling patterns. They can appear after 2 mo, usually do not interfere with vision, and are commonly reversible in 6–8 wk after drug discontinuation. Early changes in the retina (deposition of pigment in the macula) are usually asymptomatic and reversible. However, both chloroquine and hydroxychloroquine can cause an irreversible retinal degeneration. More advanced damage includes hyperpigmentation of the macula surrounded by a depigmented ring and hyperpigmented retina ("bull's eye" retinopathy). Patients complain of reading difficulty, blurred vision, visual field defects, and photophobia; some also report defective color vision and light flashes. The prevalence ranges from 3% to 45% in various reports. The drug should be discontinued if these symptoms develop. Limiting the chloroquine daily dosage to 4 mg/kg up to a maximum of 250 mg in adults minimizes the risk. Corneal deposits occur only with high daily doses of hydroxychloroquine. Limiting the daily dosage to 6.5 mg/kg up to a maximum of 400 mg of hydroxychloroquine in adults minimizes the risk of retinopathy. Weekly use of chloroquine for malarial prophylaxis does not seem to cause retinopathy. More recent data suggest that the toxic effects of these agents appear to be dependent on the total dose, duration of use, and patient age. Patients at risk include those with renal disease; those who are small, thin, and elderly; and those who receive a large baseline dose, especially those who are obese. Though commonly reversible, toxic maculopathy must be detected in its early phases for successful treatment. Patients receiving long-term therapy with chloroquine 3 mg/kg/d should have ophthalmologic examinations at least every 6 mo initially and then annually if their vision remains stable. Those receiving >3 mg/kg/d should be examined every 6 mo.[1,4,15,23–27,52–61]

Antitubercular Agents

Retrobulbar neuritis is the primary ocular complication with the agent **ethambutol**. Symptoms include blurred vision, scotoma, and reduction of the visual field. Color vision defects also occur, usually presenting as a reduction in green perception. Retrobulbar neuritis is dose related, occurring most frequently with dosages ≥25 mg/kg/d of ethambutol. Its onset is usually after 3–6 mo of therapy, and it is slowly reversible after drug discontinuation. Dosages ≤15 mg/kg/d appear relatively free of ocular side effects. Optic neuritis occurs occasionally with use of **isoniazid**, most commonly in malnourished or alcoholic patients, and often manifests itself as impaired red-green perception. It responds to pyridoxine therapy. Exudative conjunctivitis, ocular pain, and orange staining of tears (and consequent staining of soft contact lenses) are occasionally reported with **rifampin**. These effects are rapidly reversible when the drug is withdrawn.[4,62–64]

Antivirals

At least 9 cases of diffuse, white, subendothelial corneal opacities have been reported with **amantadine,** which usually resolved within a few weeks after drug discontinuation. Anterior uveitis occurs in approximately one-third of AIDS patients receiving **cidofovir** intravenously for the treatment of cytomegalovirus retinitis. The onset is usually after 4–5 d of treatment. Uveitis usually responds to topical cycloplegics and corticosteroids and does not require discontinuation of cidofovir.[47,65]

(continued)

β-Adrenergic Blocking Agents

A reduction in tear production occurs, which can produce a hot, dry, gritty sensation in the eyes. This is rapidly reversible with drug discontinuation.

Bromocriptine

Myopia is a frequent complication of long-term bromocriptine therapy and often goes unappreciated until the patient complains of blurred vision. The cause is not fully determined but might be due to lens swelling. Myopia is reversible within 1–2 wk after drug discontinuation.[4,66,67]

Clomiphene

Visual disturbances, most commonly blurred vision, occur frequently with clomiphene. These disturbances usually disappear after the drug is withdrawn, but one report of 3 patients describes prolonged afterimages, shimmering of the peripheral visual field, and photophobia.[68]

Contraceptives, Oral

A variety of retinal vascular disorders have been attributed to oral contraceptives, but the association remains unproved. It is purported that some oral contraceptive users cannot tolerate contact lenses, possibly because of ocular edema or dryness; however, a prospective study failed to show any differences in lens tolerance between oral contraceptive users and nonusers.[69,70]

Corticosteroids

Topical, periocular, local (nasal and inhalation), and systemic corticosteroid administration, including intravitreal injection (**triamcinolone**), of these drugs can produce a variety of ocular disorders when used for extensive periods at reasonably high doses with long-term therapy. The most notable ocular disorders caused are glaucoma and cataracts. Corticosteroid-induced increases in intraocular pressure occur in approximately 30% of long-term users and appear to be dose related. Glaucoma can persist for several months after drug discontinuation. Corticosteroid-induced cataracts (usually 5%–15% posterior subcapsular) are found in 10%–40% of patients on long-term, systemic therapy and are correlated with total dosage and duration of therapy. Corticosteroid-induced cataracts occur in both adults and children. Outcome is variable, ranging from improvement despite continued therapy to rare loss of sight. Most patients have no vision impairment. Although they most commonly occur with large oral doses, increased intraocular pressure and cataracts are reported in patients receiving corticosteroids by the topical ophthalmic, inhalation, and intranasal routes. Children develop cataracts more frequently than adults; Hispanics might be affected more often than blacks or non-Hispanic whites. Central serous chorioretinopathy is a complication with corticosteroids that specifically presents as bilateral and multifocal retinal pigment epithelium detachment.[2–4,7,11,12,71–81]

Cyclosporine

Retinopathy occurs frequently with cyclosporine and severe visual disturbances, including cortical blindness, occur occasionally. Oculotoxicity appears to be dose related and resolves after drug discontinuation.[12,82]

Deferoxamine

Oculotoxicity, including severe, acute visual impairment, blurred vision, impaired color vision, night blindness, and retinal deposits, occurs in 4%–11% of patients receiving deferoxamine for chronic iron overload. Retinal pigment epithelial changes can also occur. These effects are commonly reported in the literature and appear to be dose related and might be caused by the chelation of trace minerals.[83–88]

Digitalis Glycosides

The most unique ocular effect is the frosted or snowy appearance of objects or colored halos around them. These effects are most noticeable in bright light. Color vision might be affected such that objects appear yellow (green or other colors are reported, but far less frequently). With **digoxin,**

(*continued*)

color changes usually occur when the plasma level exceeds 1.5 μg/L. Digitalis glycosides also are reported to produce photophobia, blurred vision, central scotomas, and flickering or light flashes before the eyes. Reversible ocular side effects occur in up to 25% of patients with digitalis intoxication.[4,89,90]

Disopyramide

The anticholinergic effects of disopyramide frequently produce blurred vision.[91]

Disulfiram

A few cases of retrobulbar neuritis have occurred, manifested by a dramatic decline in visual acuity and impairment of color vision. In most patients, vision returns to normal after drug discontinuation.[4,92]

Fenoldopam

Treatment of hypertensive emergencies with fenoldopam results in dose-dependent, mild increases in intraocular pressure during the infusion. Increases in intraocular pressure occur in patients with and without ocular hypertension. The importance of these findings is not established.[93,94]

Gold Salts

Parenteral gold can produce microscopic crystalline deposits in the cornea, most commonly in the superficial layers. These deposits are dose related and rarely occur until the total dosage of parenteral gold exceeds 1 g. The deposits slowly resolve after drug discontinuation, do not appear to affect vision, and are not a reason to stop gold therapy. **Auranofin** does not seem to produce these ocular effects.[4,95,96]

Histamine-2 Receptor Antagonists

Cimetidine and **ranitidine** have weak anticholinergic properties that can cause pupillary dilation and angle-closure **glaucoma**.[7]

Interferons

Although the prevalence cannot be accurately determined, retinal vascular complications have been reported with **interferon alfa**. Onset is usually after 2–3 mo of treatment. These effects appear to be reversible after drug discontinuation. Though retinopathy with interferon alfa is well documented, there appears to be only one case report of retinopathy with **interferon beta-1a**.[97,98]

Iodine, Radioactive (I^{131})

Ophthalmopathy, including diplopia and changes in visual acuity, occurred or worsened in 15% of patients with Graves' hyperthyroidism treated with I^{131} after a 3–4 mo course of methimazole. Patients treated with a combination of I^{131} and prednisone or continued methimazole did not show any increased ophthalmopathy. All changes occurred during the first 6 mo after I^{131} treatment. Ophthalmic changes persisted for 2–3 mo in 65% of those affected, longer in the other 35%.[99]

Monoclonal Antibodies

Cetuximab is reported to cause accelerated growth of eyelashes and impairment of corneal wound healing. Severe and sustained ocular hypertension (increased ocular pressure) occurred in 4 cases following intravitreal **ranibizumab**. Retinal pigment epithelial tears that can cause vision loss occurred in 1.6% of 920 eyes treated with intravitreal **bevacizumab** in a retrospective study.[100–102]

Muromonab-CD3

Conjunctivitis and photophobia occur frequently.[103]

Niacin

There is a case report that intraocular pressure is increased during use. The intraocular pressure decreased to original levels each time niacin was ceased.[104]

(continued)

Nilutamide

Delayed dark adaptation is a dose-dependent adverse effect reported with an incidence of 12.9%–90%. One patient in a case report experienced impaired dark adaptation following use.[105]

Oprelvekin

Transient blurred vision and conjunctival injection occur frequently during oprelvekin therapy. Papilledema occurs in 1.5%.

Oxygen

Retrolental fibroplasia is an important complication of oxygen therapy in neonates, in particular premature or other low-birthweight neonates. The risk of retrolental fibroplasia in these patients increases whenever the concentration of inspired oxygen exceeds normal.[106–108]

Pamidronate

Reversible anterior uveitis and conjunctivitis are occasional complications of pamidronate therapy. Onset is usually 24–48 h after IV infusion.[47,109]

Pentostatin

Conjunctivitis and keratitis frequently occur during pentostatin therapy. Whereas conjunctivitis is usually mild, keratitis can be severe.[3]

Phenothiazines

The most common agents in this class that cause cataracts in a dose and drug-dependent manner are **chlorpromazine** and **thioridazine**. Case reports observe corneal deposits from chlorpromazine therapy. When administered systemically, fine, white to yellowish brown granules in the anterior cortex begin to build up. Over time, the granules develop a pattern that becomes a cataract. These lesions of the lens, cornea, and retina are the most important features of phenothiazine-induced oculotoxicity. The deposits in the lens most frequently occur with long-term, high total dose (>600 g) of **chlorpromazine** therapy. Epithelial keratopathy, possibly resulting from a drug-induced photosensitivity reaction, can occur after only a few months of high-dose therapy. It is characterized by diffuse opacification of the corneal epithelium. The consistent use of sunglasses can reduce the risk of keratopathy. Lens and corneal deposits usually do not interfere with vision, and all of these effects might be slowly reversible. **Thioridazine** is most noted for producing pigmentary retinopathy. As with most phenothiazine-induced ocular effects, pigmentary retinopathy is dose related. It can occur within a few weeks or months of high-dose usage. Patients might complain of blurred vision, decreased night vision, loss of visual field, brown discoloration of vision, and central scotoma. Vision might improve if the drug is withdrawn soon enough; however, some cases continue to deteriorate despite drug discontinuation. Other phenothiazines can cause pigmentary retinopathy, but the supporting data are limited to case reports. Phenothiazines (especially thioridazine) have anticholinergic effects and might precipitate narrow-angle glaucoma. Corneal edema is a rare, but dangerous, complication of phenothiazine use, requiring immediate discontinuation of therapy.[4,41,110–112]

Phosphodiesterase-5 Inhibitors

Sildenafil, tadalafil, and **vardenafil** can cause ocular side effects such as changes in color perception, blurred vision, and sensitivity to light (photosensitivity). These uncommon side effects are dose dependent and fully reversible. Over 40 case reports suspect optic neuropathy with the use of these agents where approximately 14 case reports specifically demonstrate a common optic neuropathy, nonarteritic anterior ischemic optic neuropathy (NAION). This is an ischemic disorder of the optic disc that may follow transient visual symptoms. Decreased visual field/loss attributed to NAION is reported to be dose dependent in one particular case of a patient who took an unusual, doubled dose. This oculotoxicity is only probable as candidates for such agents already have predisposing risk factors of optic neuropathy.[4,113,114]

(continued)

Psoralens

The combination of psoralens and long-wave ultraviolet light (PUVA therapy) radiation is associated with the development of conjunctivitis, photophobia, and other signs of ocular irritation. The use of UVA protective lenses during therapy greatly reduces the prevalence. An experimentally demonstrated connection between PUVA therapy and cataracts has not been confirmed clinically.[4,115,116]

Retinoids

Ocular adverse effects such as dry eyes, blurred vision, cataracts, color and night blindness, abnormal dark-adaptation curves, abnormal Meibomian gland atrophy, myopia, ocular discomfort, sicca syndrome, increased tear osmolarity, papilledema, photophobia, teratogenic ocular abnormalities, and blepharoconjunctivitis are all reported with **isotretinoin**. Blepharoconjunctivitis occurs in >50% of patients receiving isotretinoin. This painful condition appears to be dose related, and its onset is usually during the first 2 mo of therapy. Dry eyes can occur with or without blepharoconjunctivitis. Other effects associated with retinoid therapy include corneal opacities (which clear in 6–7 wk after drug discontinuation) and elevated intracranial pressure. There are numerous reports of ocular adverse effects with one case report indicating corneal steepening (drop in visual acuity) after systemic treatment that subsided with discontinuation. Resolution usually occurs within a week after retinoid discontinuation. Similar effects were reported with **etretinate**.[4,7,12,117–123]

Sympathomimetic Agents

These drugs can dilate the pupil and precipitate narrow-angle glaucoma. Sympathomimetics with marked α-adrenergic activity (e.g., **ephedrine, phenylpropanolamine, tetrahydrozoline**) should be avoided. The risk of this reaction is slight unless large doses are taken orally or the drugs are applied topically.[30]

TNF-α Antagonists

Infliximab, etanercept, and **adalimumab** have been associated with optic neuropathy.[124]

■ REFERENCES

1. Lerman S et al. Further studies on allopurinol therapy and human cataractogenesis. *Am J Ophthalmol.* 1984;97:205-209.
2. Clair WK et al. Allopurinol use and the risk of cataract formation. *Br J Ophthalmol.* 1989;73:173-176.
3. Burns LJ. Ocular toxicities of chemotherapy. *Semin Oncol.* 1992;19:492-500.
4. Davidson SI, Rennie IG. Ocular toxicity from systemic drug therapy. An overview of clinically important adverse reactions. *Med Toxicol.* 1986;1:217-224.
5. Flach AJ et al. Amiodarone-induced lens opacities. *Arch Ophthalmol.* 1983;101:1554-1556.
6. Naccarelli GV et al. Adverse effects of amiodarone. Pathogenesis, incidence and management. *Med Toxicol Adverse Drug Exp.* 1989;4:246-253.
7. Li J et al. Drug-induced ocular disorders. *Drug Saf.* 2008;31:127-141.
8. Erdurmus M et al. Amiodarone-induced keratopathy: full-thickness corneal involvement. *Eye Contact Lens.* 2008;34:131-132.
9. Ritch R et al. Oral imipramine and acute angle closure glaucoma. *Arch Ophthalmol.* 1994;112:67-68.
10. Podos SM, Canellos GP. Lens changes in chronic granulocytic leukemia. Possible relationship to chemotherapy. *Am J Ophthalmol.* 1969;68:500-504.
11. Imperia PS et al. Ocular complications of systemic cancer chemotherapy. *Surv Ophthalmol.* 1989;34:209-230.
12. Al-Tweigeri T et al. Ocular toxicity and cancer chemotherapy. A review. *Cancer.* 1996;78:1359-1373.
13. Kende G et al. Blurring of vision. A previously undescribed complication of cyclophosphamide therapy. *Cancer.* 1979;44:69-71.
14. Lass JH et al. Topical corticosteroid therapy for corneal toxicity from systemically administered cytarabine. *Am J Ophthalmol.* 1982;94:617-121.
15. Herzig RH et al. High-dose cytosine arabinoside therapy for refractory leukemia. *Blood.* 1983;62:361-369.
16. Curran CF, Luce JK. Ocular adverse reactions associated with Adriamycin (doxorubicin). *Am J Ophthalmol.* 1989;108:709-711.
17. Straus DJ et al. Cicatricial ectropion secondary to 5-fluorouracil therapy. *Med Pediatr Oncol.* 1977;3:15-19.
18. Haidak DJ et al. Tear-duct fibrosis (dacryostenosis) due to 5-fluorouracil. *Ann Intern Med.* 1978;88:657.

19. Capri G et al. Optic nerve disturbances: a new form of paclitaxel neurotoxicity. *J Natl Cancer Inst.* 1994;86:1099-1101.
20. Seidman AD, Barrett S. Photopsia during 3-hour paclitaxel administration at doses ≥250 mg/m^2 [letter]. *J Clin Oncol.* 1994;12:1741-1742.
21. Nayfield SG, Gorin MB. Tamoxifen-associated eye disease: a review. *J Clin Oncol.* 1996;14:1018-1026.
22. Albert DM et al. Ocular complications of vincristine therapy. *Arch Ophthalmol.* 1967;78:709-713.
23. Chang LK, Sarraf D. Tears of the retinal pigment epithelium: an old problem in a new era. *Retina.* 2007;27:523-534.
24. Frankfort BJ, Garibaldi DC. Periocular cutaneous toxicity and cicatricial ectropion: a potential class effect of antineoplastic agents that inhibit EGFR signaling. *Ophthal Plast Reconstr Surg.* 2007;23:496-497.
25. Zhang G et al. Acquired trichomegaly and symptomatic external ocular changes in patients receiving epidermal growth factor receptor inhibitors: case reports and a review of literature. *Cornea.* 2007;26:858-860.
26. Bourla DH et al. Intravitreous vascular endothelial growth factor (VEGF) inhibitor therapy for tamoxifen-induced macular edema. *Semin Ophthalmol.* 2007;22:87-88.
27. Salomao SR et al. Multifocal electroretinography, color discrimination and ocular toxicity in tamoxifen use. *Curr Eye Res.* 2007;32:345-352.
28. Saeed M et al. Hyoscine skin patches for drooling dilate pupils and impair accommodation: spectacle correction for photophobia and blurred vision may be warranted. *Dev Med Child Neurol.* 2007;49:426-428.
29. Hiatt RL et al. Systemically administered anticholinergic drugs and intraocular pressure. *Arch Ophthalmol.* 1970;84:735-740.
30. Durkee DP, Bryant BG. Drug therapy reviews: drug therapy of glaucoma. *Am J Hosp Pharm.* 1978;35:682-690.
31. Singh J et al. Nebulized bronchodilator therapy causes acute angle closure glaucoma in predisposed individuals [letter]. *Respir Med.* 1993;87:559-561.
32. Tilz C. et al. Visual field defect during therapy with valproic acid. *Eur J Neurol.* 2007;14:929-932.
33. Massaoutis P et al. Bilateral symptomatic angle closure associated with a regular dose of citalopram, an SSRI antidepressant. *Br J Ophthalmol.* 2007;91:1086-1087.
34. Giuliari GP et al. Closed-angle glaucoma after topiramate therapy for migraine in a patient with undiagnosed pseudotumor cerebri. *Can J Ophthalmol.* 2008;43:371.
35. Guier CP. Elevated intraocular pressure and myopic shift linked to topiramate use. *Optom Vis Sci.* 2007;84:1070-1073.
36. Tsui I et al. Electronegative electroretinogram associated with topiramate toxicity and vitelliform maculopathy. *Doc Ophthalmol.* 2008;116:57-60.
37. Kjellstrom U et al. Full-field ERG and visual fields in patients 5 years after discontinuing vigabatrin therapy. *Doc Ophthalmol.* 2008;117:93-101.
38. Conway M et al. Visual field severity indices demonstrate dose-dependent visual loss from vigabatrin therapy. *Epilepsia.* 2008;49:108-116.
39. Wild JM et al. Vigabatrin and epilepsy: lessons learned. *Epilepsia.* 2007;48:1318-1327.
40. Goldman MJ, Schultz-Ross RA. Adverse ocular effects of anticonvulsants. *Psychosomatics.* 1993;34:154-158.
41. Oshika T. Ocular adverse effects of neuropsychiatric agents. Incidence and management. *Drug Saf.* 1995;12:256-263.
42. Luria SM et al. Effects of aspirin and dimenhydrinate (Dramamine) on visual processes. *Br J Clin Pharmacol.* 1979;7:585-593.
43. Cocke JG et al. Optic neuritis with prolonged use of chloramphenicol. Case report and relationship to fundus changes in cystic fibrosis. *J Pediatr.* 1966;68:27-31.
44. Huang NN et al. Visual disturbances in cystic fibrosis following chloramphenicol administration. *J Pediatr.* 1966;68:32-44.
45. Cocke JG. Chloramphenicol optic neuritis. Apparent protective effects of very high daily doses of pyridoxine and cyanocobalamin. *Am J Dis Child.* 1967;114:424-426.
46. Fraunfelder FW, Randall JA. Minocycline-induced scleral pigmentation. *Ophthalmology.* 1997;104:936-938.
47. Fraunfelder FW, Rosenbaum JT. Drug-induced uveitis. Incidence, prevention and treatment. *Drug Saf.* 1997;17:197-207.
48. Saran BR et al. Hypopyon uveitis in patients with acquired immunodeficiency syndrome treated for systemic *Mycobacterium avium* complex infection with rifabutin. *Arch Ophthalmol.* 1994;112:1159-1165.
49. Karbassi M, Nikou S. Acute uveitis in patients with acquired immunodeficiency syndrome receiving prophylactic rifabutin. *Arch Ophthalmol.* 1995;113:699-701.
50. Mahesh G et al. Drug-induced acute myopia following chlorthalidone treatment. *Indian J Ophthalmol.* 2007;55:386-388.
51. Zoumalan CI, Saun AA. Optical coherence tomography can monitor reversible nerve-fibre layer changes in a patient with ethambutol-induced optic neuropathy. *Br J Ophthalmol.* 2007;91:839-840.

52. Easterbrook MA, Bernstein H. Ophthalmological monitoring of patients taking antimalarials: preferred practice patterns. *J Rheumatol*. 1997;24:1390-1392.
53. Ritenhour RJ et al. Chloroquine-related myasthenic syndrome with severe retinopathy [abstract]. *Can J Ophthalmol*. 2008;43:241-243.
54. Kellner U et al. Chloroquine retinopathy: lipofuscin- and melanin-related fundus autofluorescence, optical coherence tomography and multifocal electroretinography. *Doc Ophthalmol*. 2008;116:119-127.
55. Easterbrook M. Ocular effects and safety of antimalarial agents. *Am J Med*. 1988;85(suppl 4A):23-29.
56. Kerdel F et al. Antimalarial agents and the eye. *Dermatol Clin*. 1992;10:513-519.
57. Easterbrook M. The ocular safety of hydroxychloroquine. *Semin Arthritis Rheum*. 1993;23(suppl 1):62-67.
58. Bernstein HN. Ocular safety of hydroxychloroquine sulfate (Plaquenil). *South Med J*. 1992;85:274-279.
59. Gangitano JL, Keltner JL. Abnormalities of the pupil and visual-evoked potential in quinine amblyopia. *Am J Ophthalmol*. 1980;89:425-430.
60. Dyson EH et al. Death and blindness due to overdose of quinine. *Br Med J*. 1985;291:31-33.
61. Hanna B et al. Retinal toxicity secondary to Plaquenil therapy. *Optometry*. 2008;79:90-94.
62. Cayley FE, Majumdar SK. Ocular toxicity due to rifampicin. *Br Med J*. 1976;1:199-200.
63. Lyons RW. Orange contact lenses from rifampin [letter]. *N Engl J Med*. 1979;300:372-373.
64. Harris J, Jenkins P. Discoloration of soft contact lenses by rifampicin [letter]. *Lancet*. 1985;2:1133.
65. Fraunfelder FT, Meyer SM. Amantadine and corneal deposits [letter]. *Am J Ophthalmol*. 1990;110:96-97.
66. Calne DB et al. Long-term treatment of parkinsonism with bromocriptine. *Lancet*. 1978;1:735-738.
67. Manor RS et al. Myopia during bromocriptine treatment [letter]. *Lancet*. 1981;1:102.
68. Purvin VA. Visual disturbance secondary to clomiphene citrate. *Arch Ophthalmol*. 1995;113:482-484.
69. De Vries Reilingh A et al. Contact lens tolerance and oral contraceptives. *Ann Ophthalmol*. 1978;10:947-952.
70. Petursson GJ et al. Oral contraceptives. *Ophthalmology*. 1981;88:368-371.
71. Renfro L, Snow JS. Ocular effects of topical and systemic steroids. *Dermatol Clin*. 1992,10.505-512.
72. Toogood JH et al. Association of ocular cataracts with inhaled and oral steroid therapy during long-term treatment of asthma. *J Allergy Clin Immunol*. 1993;91:571-579.
73. Opatowsky I et al. Intraocular pressure elevation associated with inhalation and nasal corticosteroids. *Ophthalmology*. 1995;102:177-179.
74. Cumming RG et al. Use of inhaled corticosteroids and the risk of cataracts. *N Engl J Med*. 1997;8:8-14.
75. Mendrinos E et al. Bilateral multifocal retinal pigment epithelium detachments associated with systemic corticosteroids [abstract]. *Eur J Ophthalmol*. 2008;118:649-651.
76. Yildirim N et al. The relationship between plasma MMP-9 and TIMP-2 levels and intraocular pressure elevation in diabetic patients after intravitreal triamcinolone injection. *J Glaucoma*. 2008,17:253-256.
77. James ER. The etiology of steroid cataract. *J Ocul Pharm Ther*. 2007;23:403-420.
78. Lau LI et al. Intraocular pressure elevation after intravitreal triamcinolone acetonide injection in a Chinese population. *Am J Ophthalmol*. 2008;146:573-578.
79. Vasconcelos-Santos DV et al. Secondary ocular hypertension after intravitreal injection of 4 mg of triamcinolone acetonide: incidence and risk factors. *Retina*. 2008;28:573-580.
80. Ideta S et al. Ptosis after sub-Tenon's capsule triamcinolone. *Ophthalmology*. 2008;115:410.
81. Inatani M et al. Intraocular pressure elevation after injection of triamcinolone acetonide: a multicenter retrospective case-control study. *Am J Ophthalmol*. 2008;145:676-681.
82. Memon M et al. Reversible cyclosporine-induced cortical blindness in allogenic bone marrow transplant recipients. *Bone Marrow Transplant*. 1995;15:283-286.
83. Baath JS et al. Deferoxamine-related ocular toxicity: incidence and outcome in a pediatric population. *Retina*. 2008;28:894-899.
84. Lu M et al. Effects of deferoxamine on retinal and visual function. *Arch Ophthalmol*. 2007;125:1581-1582.
85. Olivieri NF et al. Visual and auditory neurotoxicity in patients receiving subcutaneous deferoxamine infusions. *N Engl J Med*. 1986;314:869-873.
86. De Virgiliis S et al. Depletion of trace elements and acute ocular toxicity induced by desferrioxamine in patients with thalassemia. *Arch Dis Child*. 1988;63:250-255.
87. Cases A et al. Acute visual and auditory neurotoxicity in patients with end-stage renal disease receiving desferrioxamine. *Clin Nephrol*. 1988;29:176-178.
88. Cases A et al. Ocular and auditory toxicity in hemodialyzed patients receiving desferrioxamine. *Nephron*. 1990;56:19-23.
89. Robertson DM et al. Ocular manifestations of digitalis toxicity. Discussion and report of three cases of central scotomas. *Arch Ophthalmol*. 1966;76:640-645.
90. Aronson JK, Ford AR. The use of colour vision measurement in the diagnosis of digoxin toxicity. *Q J Med*. 1980;49:273-282.
91. Bauman JL. Long-term therapy with disopyramide phosphate: side effects and effectiveness. *Am Heart J*. 1986;111:654-660.

92. Norton AL, Walsh FB. Disulfiram-induced optic neuritis. *Trans Am Acad Ophthalmol Otolaryngol.* 1972;76:1263-1265.

93. Everitt DE et al. Effect of intravenous fenoldopam on intraocular pressure in ocular hypertension. *J Clin Pharmacol.* 1997;37:312-320.

94. Elliott WJ et al. Intraocular pressure increases with fenoldopam, but not nitroprusside, in hypertensive humans. *Clin Pharmacol Ther.* 1991;49:285-293.

95. Bron AJ et al. Epithelial deposition of gold in the cornea in patients receiving systemic therapy. *Am J Ophthalmol.* 1979;88:354-360.

96. Kincaid MC et al. Ocular chrysiasis. *Arch Ophthalmol.* 1982;100:1791-1794.

97. Folden DV et al. Interferon beta-associated retinopathy in patients treated for multiple sclerosis. *Neurology.* 2008;70:1153-1155.

98. Guyer DR et al. Interferon-associated retinopathy. *Arch Ophthalmol.* 1993;111:350-356.

99. Bartalena L et al. Relation between therapy for hyperthyroidism and the course of Graves' ophthalmopathy. *N Engl J Med.* 1998;338:73-78.

100. Bakri SJ et al. Persistent ocular hypertension following intravitreal ranibizumab. *Graefes Arch Clin Exp Ophthalmol.* 2008;246:955-958.

101. Foerster CG et al. Persisting corneal erosion under cetuximab (Erbitux) treatment (epidermal growth factor receptor antibody). *Cornea.* 2008;27:612-614.

102. Garg S et al. Retinal pigment epithelial tears after intravitreal bevacizumab injection for exudative age-related macular degeneration. *Clin Experiment Ophthalmol.* 2008;36:252-256.

103. Dukar O, Barr CC. Visual loss complicating OKT3 monoclonal antibody therapy. *Am J Ophthalmol.* 1993;115:781-785.

104. Tittler EH et al. Oral niacin can increase intraocular pressure. *Ophthalmic Surg Lasers Imaging.* 2008;39:341-342.

105. Chan P, Odel JG. Delayed dark adaptation caused by nilutamide. *J Neuroophthalmol.* 2008;28:158-159.

106. Committee on Fetus and Newborn, American Academy of Pediatrics. History of oxygen therapy and retrolental fibroplasia. *Pediatrics.* 1976;57(suppl):591-642.

107. Betts EK et al. Retrolental fibroplasia and oxygen administration during general anesthesia. *Anesthesiology.* 1977;47:518-520.

108. Naiman J et al. Retrolental fibroplasia in hypoxic newborn. *Am J Ophthalmol.* 1979;88:55-58.

109. Macarol V, Fraunfelder FT. Pamidronate disodium and possible ocular adverse drug reactions. *Am J Ophthalmol.* 1994;118:220-224.

110. Toshida H et al. In vivo observations of a case of chlorpromazine deposits in the cornea using an HRT II Rostock corneal module. *Cornea.* 2007;26:1141-1143.

111. Bond WS, Yee GC. Ocular and cutaneous effects of chronic phenothiazine therapy. *Am J Hosp Pharm.* 1980;37:74-78.

112. Ngen CC, Singh P. Long-term phenothiazine administration and the eye in 100 Malaysians. *Br J Psychiatry.* 1988;152:278-280.

113. Carter JE. Anterior ischemic optic neuropathy and stroke with use of PDE-5 inhibitors for erectile dysfunction: cause or coincidence? *J Neurol Sci.* 2007;262:89-97.

114. Pepin S, Pitha-Rowe I. Stepwise decline in visual field after serial sildenafil use. *J Neuroophthalmol.* 2008;28:76-77.

115. Farber EM et al. Current status of oral PUVA therapy for psoriasis. Eye protection revisions. *J Am Acad Dermatol.* 1982;6:851-855.

116. Stern RS. Ocular lens findings in patients treated with PUVA. Photochemotherapy follow-up-study. *J Invest Dermatol.* 1994;103:534-538.

117. Fraunfelder FT et al. Adverse ocular reactions possibly associated with isotretinoin. *Am J Ophthalmol.* 1985;100:534-537.

118. Lebowitz MA, Berson DS. Ocular effects of oral retinoids. *J Am Acad Dermatol.* 1988;19:209-211.

119. Gold JA et al. Ocular side effects of the retinoids. *Intern J Dermatol.* 1989;28:218-225.

120. Gross EG, Helfgott MA. Retinoids and the eye. *Dermatol Clin.* 1992;10:521-531.

121. Santodomingo-Rubido J et al. Drug-induced ocular side-effects with isotretinoin. *Ophthalmic Physiol Opt.* 2008;28:497-501.

122. Burkhart CG. Another threat to the availability of isotretinoin: ocular side effects have aviation authorities considering restricting use from (even potential) pilots [abstract]. *Dermatol Online J.* 2008;14:2.

123. Finsterer J. Enhanced ocular isotretinoin toxicity in mitochondrial disorder [letter]. *South Med J.* 2008;101: 664-665.

124. von Jagow B, Kohnen T. Anterior optic neuropathy associated with adalimumab. *Ophthalmologica.* 2008;222:292-294.

Chapter 65

Drug-Induced Ototoxicity

William R. Vincent III

Drug-induced ototoxicity can affect hearing (auditory or cochlear function), balance (vestibular function), or both, depending on the drug. Drugs of almost every class have been reported to produce tinnitus, as have placebos. The agents in this section are associated with measurable changes in hearing or vestibular defect when administered *systemically*.

Aminoglycosides

Aminoglycoside antibiotics chelate metal ions that promote the production of reactive oxygen species and can cause cochlear and vestibular toxicities. Cochlear toxicity presents as progressive hearing loss, starting with the highest tones and advancing to lower tones. Thus, considerable damage can occur before the patient is cognizant of it. Vestibular damage presents as dizziness, vertigo, or ataxia. Both forms of ototoxicity are usually bilateral and potentially reversible, but permanent damage is common and can progress after aminoglycoside discontinuation. Estimates of the prevalence of aminoglycoside-induced ototoxicity vary widely depending on the criteria applied. Clinically detectable ototoxicity probably occurs in as many as 5% of patients, with a much higher percentage demonstrating audiometrically detectable damage. Most aminoglycoside-induced ototoxicity is associated with parenteral therapy, but it has followed topical, oral, and irrigation use of these drugs, especially **neomycin**. A patient should receive dosages by these routes that are no greater than the dosages given by injection. Possible predisposing factors for ototoxicity are decreased renal function, long duration of therapy, large total dosage, plasma levels exceeding the therapeutic range, previous aminoglycoside use, concurrent use of other ototoxic drugs, dehydration, and old age. Up to one-third of patients who develop ototoxicity may carry an inherited mutation in a mitochondrial RNA gene that predisposes to aminoglycoside-induced ototoxicity. Hearing impairment is less common in neonates and children. Once daily and multiple daily dosing of aminoglycosides seem to have similar effects on hearing. The comparative effects on vestibular function have not been adequately investigated. Serial audiometry might be useful in early detection of ototoxicity. Each aminoglycoside has a slightly different spectrum of ototoxicity; the table below serves as a general guide to their relative ototoxic potentials.[1–10]

RELATIVE OTOTOXIC POTENTIAL		
DRUG	**COCHLEAR**	**VESTIBULAR**
Amikacin	+++	++
Gentamicin	++	+++
Kanamycin	+++	++
Neomycin	++++	++
Netilmicin	+	+
Streptomycin	++	++++
Tobramycin	++	++

(*continued*)

Antidepressants, Tricyclic

The prevalence of tricyclic antidepressant–associated tinnitus is estimated to be 1%. Tinnitus can subside despite continued therapy. Although **imipramine** and **amitriptyline** may cause tinnitus, they have also been used to treat tinnitus.[2,4,11]

Bortezomib

Peripheral neuropathies may occur in over 30% of patients receiving bortezomib. Hearing impairment and vertigo have been reported in clinical trials and a case report described irreversible, unilateral deafness that occurred after the second cycle of bortezomib and persisted despite immediate drug discontinuation.[12]

Carbamazepine

Carbamazepine (CBZ) inhibits auditory nerve conduction and can cause reversible, transient pitch perception deficits. A case series described deficits that occurred in mostly Japanese patients aged 4–42 y, developed 2 h to 2 wk following initiation, and occurred at serum CBZ concentrations within the therapeutic range. Symptoms resolved despite continued therapy in some cases. Reversible sensorineural hearing loss has also been described following ingestion of 36 g of the drug.[13,14]

Deferoxamine

Dosage-related hearing impairment occurs during long-term deferoxamine therapy. The prevalence reported varies among studies from 6% to 57%. High-frequency hearing is affected first; reversible and irreversible hearing losses have been reported. The mechanism of ototoxicity is unclear although it may be related to direct toxicity to retinal cells or indirectly via trace metal chelation.[4,15]

Diuretics, Loop

Rapid-onset hearing loss is a frequent feature of high-dose, rapid IV administration of **furosemide.** Hearing loss and tinnitus are less common with furosemide administration via IV continuous infusion. The onset might be more gradual with **ethacrynic acid.** Renal failure is usually listed as a predisposing factor, but only renal failure patients are likely to receive large IV doses. Coadministration with **aminoglycoside antibiotics** is often said to result in increased ototoxicity, but one study did not confirm this. The hearing loss is usually transient, but permanent loss has been reported, more often with ethacrynic acid than with furosemide. Hearing loss and vestibular toxicity after oral therapy have been reported. **Bumetanide** or **torsemide** produce less ototoxicity than ethacrynic acid or furosemide.[1–5,16–18]

Efalizumab

Immune- or inflammatory-mediated reactions requiring hospitalization occurred in 0.4% of patients receiving efalizumab in clinical trials. In one case, this led to sensorineural hearing loss.[19]

Eflornithine

High- and low-frequency hearing impairments are reported frequently and dizziness occurs occasionally.[20]

Hydrocodone

Rapidly progressing bilateral hearing loss has been reported in at least 3 case series of a total of 17 patients receiving hydrocodone/acetaminophen. Prolonged use or high doses over a short period of time were common among reported cases. Ototoxicity is likely cochlear in origin and vestibular symptoms are typically absent.[21,22]

Interferons

Tinnitus and hearing impairment may occur in up to 44% of patients receiving parenteral interferon or pegylated interferon therapy. Interferon may be directly toxic to auditory nerves and

(*continued*)

autoimmune inner ear disease may lead to sudden hearing loss. These effects seem to be related to cumulative exposure and usually resolve 1–2 wk after drug discontinuation. Interferon beta may be more ototoxic than interferon alfa.[4,20,23,24]

Macrolides

In elderly patients or patients with AIDS treated with **azithromycin** at doses of 600 mg/d for *Mycobacterium avium* complex or toxoplasmosis, hearing loss occurs in 15%–25%. Hearing loss occurs at all frequencies, but lower frequencies, including the speech range, are affected most often. Drug withdrawal or reduction of the dose to 300 mg/d resolves the hearing loss. Tinnitus and vestibular disturbances also occur frequently.

Hearing loss has occasionally followed parenteral or oral high-dose **erythromycin** (>4 g/d) therapy and does not seem to be caused by any particular salt form. Impaired hepatic or renal function and advanced age can increase the risk. The loss occurs at speech frequencies and is usually reversible, but irreversible hearing loss has also been reported. Recovery usually begins within 24 h of drug discontinuation. Hearing impairment and tinnitus have also been reported with **clarithromycin** therapy.[1,3–5,25–31]

Minocycline

Reversible vestibular toxicity, manifested primarily by dizziness, loss of balance, and lightheadedness, is a frequent occurrence. This adverse effect was noted in an average of 76% of patients in 6 studies and required 12%–52% of affected patients to discontinue the drug or to cease employment. Other studies have found lower, but still large, percentages of patients with vestibular toxicity. Women are more susceptible than men. Onset is often during the first 2 d of therapy, and recovery begins soon after minocycline discontinuation.[1,4,32–34]

Nonsteroidal Anti-Inflammatory Drugs

Tinnitus, high-frequency hearing loss, and occasional vertigo are common features of salicylate intoxication. Hearing loss appears to be related to the unbound plasma salicylate level, explaining the marked interpatient variability in the total salicylate serum level at which it is first detected. Most patients demonstrating ototoxicity from salicylates are receiving long-term, high-dose therapy, such as for rheumatoid arthritis. Salicylate ototoxicity, even if severe, is almost always reversible in 48–72 h, but permanent hearing loss has been reported. Although not as common as with salicylates, other NSAIDs have been associated with hearing impairment and deafness, including some cases of permanent damage. Tinnitus and vestibular dysfunction also have been reported.[1–5,35,36]

Nucleoside Reverse Transcriptase Inhibitors (NRTIs)

Audiometry determined that hearing loss occurred in 29% of 99 patients receiving antiretroviral drugs, with most cases associated with **zidovudine**. The prevalence of hearing loss was marked for patients >35 y. NRTI combinations with **didanosine**, **stavudine**, **lamivudine**, and zidovudine have been implicated in cases of hearing impairment, which is likely caused by mitochondrial toxicity.[37,38]

Ototopicals

The incidence of ototoxicity with ototopical aminoglycoside drops has been estimated to be <1% although vestibular toxicity may be underreported. More than 1 million patients in the United States require tympanostomy tube (TT) placement for otitis media with effusion. Otic solutions may pass through TTs into the middle ear and reach the inner ear by passive and active transport across the round window membrane (RWM). The ototopical aminoglycosides neomycin and **gentamicin** may cause ototoxicity by this mechanism. Additionally, systemic **absorption** may occur with topical gentamicin administration. However, there are no reports of ototoxicity in patients with an intact

(*continued*)

tympanic membrane. Topical antiseptics like **chlorhexidine** and **ethanol** may also be ototoxic. Conversely, **ciprofloxacin-** and **ofloxacin**-containing otic drops are not ototoxic.[39,40]

Phenytoin

Cerebellar toxicity caused by phenytoin is concentration-dependent and manifests as nystagmus at total serum concentrations >20 μg/ml and ataxia at >30 μg/ml. Hearing is not affected by phenytoin.[41]

Platinums

Cisplatin causes cochlear toxicity via the formation of reactive oxygen species. Tinnitus occurs frequently and usually subsides within 1 wk of cisplatin discontinuation. It cannot be relied on to predict further ototoxicity. Hearing loss occurs frequently in patients receiving cisplatin and can be dose limiting. Audiometric abnormalities can be detected in most patients and appear within a few days after the drug is started, although a delay of several months is common. High frequencies are lost first. If therapy continues despite early hearing loss, most patients experience hearing loss in the speech frequencies. Effects are cumulative, dose-related, and probably irreversible. Prolonged, low-dose therapy might produce less ototoxicity than short-term, high-dose treatment. Ototoxicity occurs more frequently in children and the elderly, and those with preexisting hearing loss appear to be at increased risk. Routine use of **amifostine** to prevent cisplatin ototoxicity is not recommended. **Carboplatin** is less ototoxic than cisplatin but can contribute to hearing loss when used in high-dose regimens or as consolidation-phase treatment after cisplatin-containing induction. Carboplatin ototoxicity is dependent on cumulative AUC and in a case series of 9 patients with an AUC of 24, all developed hearing impairment. **Sodium thiosulfate** 16–20 g/m^2 IV given 2 h after carboplatin may protect against hearing loss in patients with CNS malignancies. There is a lower risk for **oxaliplatin** ototoxicity than with cisplatin or carboplatin.[1–5,42–50]

Quinoline Derivatives

Tinnitus and high-frequency hearing impairment occur frequently with **quinine** therapy. Although these effects are usually reversible, permanent hearing impairment has occurred with long-term therapy. Vestibular effects also have been described.

Nerve deafness is a rare but consistent feature of **chloroquine** therapy. Its onset is usually delayed, irreversible, and associated with long-term therapy. However, a partially reversible case and a case resulting from only 1 g of chloroquine have been reported. **Hydroxychloroquine** hearing impairment has also been reported and **artemether/lumefantrine** may have a lower risk of ototoxicity than other quinoline derivatives.[1–5,51–53]

Sildenafil

Irreversible hearing loss has been reported in a case report after 15 d of sildenafil therapy.[54]

Tyrosine Kinase Inhibitors

Bilateral irreversible hearing loss has been reported during **imatinib** and **erlotinib** therapy and may be related to mitochondrial toxic effects.[55,56]

Valproic Acid

Hearing loss and tinnitus have been reported with valproic acid (VPA) therapy. Although VPA ototoxicity was not reported in a recent study of pediatric patients with epilepsy, routine audiometric monitoring during therapy may be warranted.[57,58]

Vigabatrin

Vigabatrin is an antiepileptic that increases γ-aminobutyric acid concentrations in the brain and may cause reversible hearing impairment.[59]

(continued)

Vancomycin

Transient and permanent hearing loss, tinnitus, and dizziness have occurred. Hearing impairment is rare with plasma levels <30 mg/L (21 μmol/L). In many of the reported cases, the patients also had been exposed to other ototoxic drugs, especially **aminoglycoside antibiotics.** In a recent retrospective study, the prevalence of vancomycin-induced ototoxicity, after an average of 27 d of therapy with serum concentrations <20 mg/L, was 12%. Ototoxicity may be more common with advanced age.[1,4,5,60,61]

Vinca Alkaloids

Hearing loss and tinnitus have been reported with **vincristine, vinblastine,** and **vinorelbine.** Vincristine is the most toxic to cochlear cells and has been implicated in more case reports than other vincas.[62,63]

■ REFERENCES

1. Huang MY, Schacht J. Drug-induced ototoxicity. Pathogenesis and prevention. *Med Toxicol Adverse Drug Exp.* 1989;4:452 467.
2. Griffin JP. Drug-induced ototoxicity. *Br J Audiol.* 1988;22:195-210.
3. Norris CH. Drugs affecting the inner ear. A review of their clinical efficacy, mechanisms of action, toxicity, and place in therapy. *Drugs.* 1988;36:754-772.
4. Seligmann H et al. Drug-induced tinnitus and other hearing disorders. *Drug Saf.* 1996;14:198-212.
5. Tange RA. Ototoxicity. *Adverse Drug React Toxicol Rev.* 1998;17:75-89.
6. Brummett RE, Fox KE. Aminoglycoside induced hearing loss in humans. *Antimicrob Agents Chemother.* 1989;33:797-800.
7. Rizzi MD, Hirose K. Aminoglycoside ototoxicity. *Curr Opin Otolaryngol Head Neck Surg.* 2007;15:352-357
8. Guthrie OW. Aminoglycoside induced ototoxicity. *Toxicol.* 2006;249:91-96.
9. Smyth AR et al. Once-daily versus multiple daily dosing with intravenous aminoglycosides for cystic fibrosis. *Cochrane Database Syst Rev.* 2006;(3): CD002009. doi: 10.1002/14651858.CD002009.
10. Fischel-Ghodsian N. Genetic factors in aminoglycoside toxicity. *Pharmacogenomics.* 2005;6:27-36.
11. Mendis D, Johnston M. An unusual case of prolonged tinnitus following low-dose amitriptyline. *J Psychopharmacol.* 2008;22:574-576.
12. Chim CS, Wong LG. Deafness associated with the use of bortezomib in multiple myeloma. *Acta Oncol.* 2008;47:323-324.
13. Taieno A et al. Carbamazepine-induced transient auditory pitch perception deficit. *Pediatr Neurol.* 2006;35:131-134.
14. de la Cruz M, Bance M. Carbamazepine-induced sensorineural hearing loss. *Arch Otolaryngol Head Neck Surg.* 1999;125:225-227.
15. Kanno H et al. The ototoxicity of deferoxamine mesylate. *Am J Otolaryngol.* 1995;16:148-152.
16. Rybak LP. Ototoxicity of loop diuretics. *Otolaryngol Clin North Am.* 1993;26:829-844.
17. Smith CR, Lietman PS. Effect of furosemide on aminoglycoside-induced nephrotoxicity and auditory toxicity in humans. *Antimicrob Agents Chemother.* 1983;23:133-137.
18. Salvador DRK et al. Continuous infusion versus bolus injection of loop diuretics in congestive heart failure. *Cochrane Database Syst Rev.* 2005(3): CD003178. doi: 10.1002/14651858.CD003178.
19. Scheinfeld N. Efalizumab: a review of events reported during clinical trials and side effects. *Expert Opin Drug Saf.* 2006;5:197-209.
20. Formann E et al. Sudden hearing loss in patients with chronic hepatitis C treated with pegylated interferon/ribavirin. *Am J Gastroenterol.* 2004;99:873-877.
21. Friedman RA et al. Profound hearing loss associated with hydrocodone/acetaminophen abuse. *Am J Otol.* 2000;21:188-191.
22. Ho T et al. Hydrocodone use and sensorineural hearing loss. *Pain Physician.* 2007;10:467-472.
23. Kanda Y et al. Sudden hearing loss associated with interferon. *Lancet.* 1994;343:1134-1135.
24. Elloumi H et al. Sudden hearing loss associated with peginterferon and ribavirin combination therapy during hepatitis C treatment. *World J Gastroenterol.* 2007;13:5411-5412.
25. Tseng AL et al. Azithromycin-related ototoxicity in patients infected with human immunodeficiency virus. *Clin Infect Dis.* 1997;24:76-77.
26. Brown BA et al. Relationship of adverse events to serum drug levels in patients receiving high-dose azithromycin for mycobacterial lung disease. *Clin Infect Dis.* 1997;24:958-964.
27. Lo SE et al. Azithromycin-induced hearing loss. *Am J Health Syst Pharm.* 1999;56:380-383.
28. Brummett RE. Ototoxic liability of erythromycin and analogues. *Otolaryngol Clin North Am.* 1993;26:811-819.

29. Sacristán JA et al. Erythromycin-induced hypoacusis: 11 new cases and literature review. *Ann Pharmacother.* 1993;27:950-955.
30. Uzun C. Tinnitus due to clarithromycin. *J Laryngol Otol.* 2003;117:1006-1007.
31. Coulston J, Balaratnam N. Irreversible sensorineural hearing loss due to clarithromycin. *Postgrad Med J.* 2005;81:58-59.
32. Schofield CBS, Masterton G. Vestibular reactions to minocycline. *MMWR Morb Mortal Wkly Rep.* 1976;25:31.
33. Gump DW et al. Side effects of minocycline: different dosage regimens. *Antimicrob Agents Chemother.* 1977;12:642-646.
34. Greco TP et al. Minocycline toxicity: experience with an altered dosage regimen. *Curr Ther Res.* 1979;25:193-201.
35. Jung TTK et al. Ototoxicity of salicylate, nonsteroidal anti-inflammatory drugs, and quinine. *Otolaryngol Clin North Am.* 1993;26:791-810.
36. Brien J. Ototoxicity associated with salicylates. A brief review. *Drug Saf.* 1993;9:143-148.
37. Marra CM et al. Hearing loss and antiretroviral therapy in patients infected with HIV-1. *Arch Neurol.* 1997;54:407-410.
38. Simdon J et al. Ototoxicity associated with use of nucleoside analog reverse transcriptase inhibitors: a report of 3 possible cases and review of the literature. *Clin Infect Dis.* 2001;32:1623-1627.
39. Haynes DS et al. Ototoxicity of ototopical drops—an update. *Otolaryngol Clin North Am.* 2007;40:669-683.
40. Matz G et al. Ototoxicity of ototopical antibiotic drops in humans. *Otolaryngol Head Neck Surg.* 2004;130:S79-S82.
41. De Diego JI et al. Vestibular and hearing manifestations of phenytoin toxicity: a retrospective series. *Ear Nose Throat J.* 2001;80:404,407-409.
42. Blakley BW, Myers SF. Patterns of hearing loss resulting from cis-platinum therapy. *Otolaryngol Head Neck Surg.* 1993;109:385-391.
43. Li Y et al. Predicting cisplatin ototoxicity in children: the influence of age and the cumulative dose. *Eur J Cancer.* 2004;40:2445-2451.
44. Bokemeyer C et al. Analysis of risk factors for cisplatin-induced ototoxicity in patients with testicular cancer. *Br J Cancer.* 1998;77:1355-1362.
45. Dubs A et al. Ototoxicity in patients with dose-intensive therapy for cisplatin-resistant germ cell tumors. *J Clin Oncol.* 2004;22:1158.
46. Hensley ML et al. American Society of Clinical Oncology 2008 clinical practice guidelines update: use of chemotherapy and radiation therapy protectants. *J Clin Oncol.* 2008;26:1-22.
47. Freilich RJ et al. Hearing loss in children with brain tumors treated with cisplatin and carboplatin-based high dose chemotherapy with autologous bone marrow rescue. *Med Pediatr Oncol.* 1996;26:95-100.
48. van der Hulst RJ et al. High frequency audiometry in prospective clinical research of ototoxicity due to platinum derivatives. *Ann Otol Rhinol Laryngol.* 1988;97:133-137.
49. Neuwelt EA et al. First evidence of otoprotection against carboplatin-induced hearing loss with a two compartment system in patients with central nervous system malignancy using sodium thiosulfate. *J Pharmacol Exp Ther.* 1998;286:77-84.
50. Pasetto LM et al. Oxaliplatin-related neurotoxicity: how and why? *Crit Rev Oncol Hematol.* 2006;59:159-168.
51. Bortoli R, Santiago M. Chloroquine ototoxicity. *Clin Rheumatol.* 2007;26:1809-1810.
52. Seckin U et al. Hydroxychloroquine ototoxicity in a patient with rheumatoid arthritis. *Rheumatol Int.* 2000;19:203-204.
53. Gurkov R et al. Ototoxicity of artemether/lumefantrine in the treatment of falciparum malaria: a randomized trial. *Malar J.* 2008;7:179.
54. Mukherjee B, Shivakumar T. A case of sensorineural deafness following ingestion of sildenafil. *J Laryngol Otol.* 2007;121:395-397.
55. Attili VSS et al. Irreversible sensorineural hearing loss due to imatinib. *Leuk Res.* 2008;32:991-992.
56. Koutras AK et al. Irreversible ototoxicity with the use of erlotinib in a patient with pancreatic cancer. *Acta Oncol.* 2008;47:1171-1173.
57. Armon C et al. Sensorineural hearing loss: a reversible effect of valproic acid. *Neurology.* 1990;40:1896-1898.
58. Incecik F et al. Effects of valproic acid on hearing in epileptic patients. *Int J Pediatr Otorhinolaryngol.* 2007;71:611-614.
59. Papadeas E et al. Sensorineural hearing loss: a reversible effect of vigabatrin. *Neurology.* 2003;61:1020-1021.
60. Forouzesh A et al. Vancomycin ototoxicity: a re-evaluation in an era of increasing doses. *Antimicrob Agents Chemother.* 2009;53:483-486.
61. Gendeh BS et al. Vancomycin administration in continuous ambulatory peritoneal dialysis: the risk of ototoxicity. *Otolaryngol Head Neck Surg.* 1998;118:551-558.
62. Moss PE et al. Ototoxicity associated with vinblastine. *Ann Pharmacother.* 1999;33:423-425.
63. Tibaldi C et al. A case of ototoxicity in a patient with metastatic carcinoma of the breast treated with paclitaxel and vinorelbine. *Eur J Cancer.* 1998;34:1133-1134.

Chapter 66

Drug-Induced Pancreatitis

Trenika R. Mitchell

Drug-induced pancreatitis is rare with an estimated overall incidence of 0.1%–2%. Although pancreatitis can be an acute or chronic condition, most drug-induced cases are acute. The diagnosis of acute drug-induced pancreatitis requires laboratory (elevated serum amylase and lipase levels) and clinical (abdominal pain) evidence, as well as characteristic findings of acute pancreatitis via a CT scan. Because acute pancreatitis has so many possible etiologies, the strongest associations of drug-induced acute pancreatitis are made when re-administration of the drug results in a recurrence of pancreatitis (i.e., a positive rechallenge). Pancreatitis development has been associated with the administration of many drugs; however, the drugs included in the following table are those that present sufficient evidence to establish themselves as probable causes of pancreatitis.

ACE Inhibitors and Angiotensin Receptor Antagonists

There are numerous cases of ACE inhibitor–induced pancreatitis in the literature and the files of manufacturers. **Captopril, enalapril, ramipril,** and **lisinopril** have been implicated. In addition, there have been case reports of pancreatitis development with the angiotensin receptor antagonist, **losartan.** It is not possible to estimate a prevalence of ACE inhibitor and angiotensin receptor antagonist-induced pancreatitis. However, cases have been confirmed by rechallenge with agents in both drug classes.[1,2]

Alcohol

Alcohol is the greatest cause of drug-induced pancreatitis. It is projected that about one-third of acute pancreatitis cases in the United States are induced by alcohol use. Acute pancreatitis occurs in about 5%–10% of alcoholics and usually develops after several years of alcohol abuse.[3,4]

Asparaginase

The estimated prevalence of asparaginase-induced acute pancreatitis is 0.7%–18%. Many patients who develop pancreatitis during asparaginase therapy are in poor condition and receiving other chemotherapeutic agents. Pancreatitis has developed in patients receiving all formulations of asparaginase.[1,4]

Azathioprine

There are many published cases of azathioprine-induced pancreatitis. The majority of the cases have been reported in patients with inflammatory bowel disease; however, azathioprine-induced pancreatitis has also been noted in the renal transplant patient population.[1,5]

Contrast Media

Up to 14% of patients receiving contrast media through endoscopic retrograde cholangiopancreatography develop pancreatitis. Use of lower-osmolarity agents reduces the prevalence of pancreatitis.[4,7]

(continued)

Cyclosporine

Cyclosporine-induced pancreatitis was identified in 5 of 143 heart and heart–lung transplant recipients in one study. In another study, 4 of 105 cyclosporine-treated renal transplant recipients developed pancreatitis, compared with only 2 of 180 **azathioprine**-treated patients. All cases occurred within 4 mo of the start of cyclosporine therapy.[8,9]

Diuretics, Thiazide and Loop

Although there are at least 25 published case reports of thiazide-associated pancreatitis and several cases of loop-associated pancreatitis, the quality of the evidence is poor. A recent study of antihypertensive agents and their subsequent risk for pancreatitis development revealed no increased risk for the adverse effect in patients receiving these medications.[2,10]

Enfuvirtide

Three percent of patients (corresponding to a rate of 3.6 events per 100 patient years) receiving enfuvirtide, a fusion inhibitor, versus 2.5 events per 100 patient years in the background regimen group developed pancreatitis during Phase 3 clinical trials of the medication. There are currently no published post-marketing reports of enfuvirtide-induced pancreatitis.[11]

Estrogens

Estrogen therapy increases the risk of pancreatitis in patients with pre-existing hyperlipidemia, especially hypertriglyceridemia. Hypertriglyceridemia is a known cause of pancreatitis, and estrogen therapy raises serum triglyceride levels. An increased incidence of estrogen-induced hypertriglyceridemia has been noted in women older than 40 y of age and those receiving higher doses of estrogen.[1]

Exenatide

Exenatide is a glucagon-like peptide 1 analogue that is indicated for the adjunctive management of type 2 diabetes. Since exenatide's release, the FDA has received more than 30 reports of possible exenatide-induced pancreatitis, which include two fatalities. Due to these reports, the FDA has released two special alerts concerning exenatide's link with pancreatitis, and it is currently working with Amylin Pharmaceuticals to strengthen warnings of this risk in the prescribing information. The risk of developing pancreatitis is currently included in the "Precaution" section of the package insert.[12,13]

HMG-CoA Reductase Inhibitors

There are more than 53 case reports of pancreatitis following the use of HMG-CoA reductase inhibitors, commonly known as statins. Statin-induced pancreatitis generally occurs after patients have had long-term exposures (e.g., months to years) to the medication. The pancreatitis is not dose-related, as pancreatitis has developed in statin users receiving a wide range of doses.[1,14]

Interferon Alfa

Although few cases have been reported, the association with the administration of interferon alfa is strong.[15]

Mercaptopurine

Inflammatory bowel disease is associated with pancreatitis. In one study of patients with inflammatory bowel disease, 3% of patients developed pancreatitis while receiving mercaptopurine (50–100 mg/d). Seven of the cases were rechallenged and all developed recurrent pancreatitis, thereby establishing a strong cause-and-effect relationship. Pancreatitis developed during the first month of initial treatment in all patients.[1]

(continued)

Mesalamine Derivatives

Inflammatory bowel disease is associated with pancreatitis, but **mesalamine, sulfasalazine,** and **olsalazine** have been implicated in cases of acute pancreatitis confirmed by rechallenge. Positive rechallenge can occur after rectal administration.[1]

Metronidazole

Pancreatitis occurs occasionally with metronidazole. One study of 6485 HMO patients found a rate of pancreatitis requiring hospitalization of 4.6/10,000 in patients receiving metronidazole. The study did not report on nonhospitalized cases.[1]

Nonsteroidal Anti-Inflammatory Drugs

There are isolated case reports of pancreatitis associated with most NSAIDs, but **sulindac** is clearly the most commonly reported. Several cases have positive rechallenges. The onset of symptoms is from 3 wk to 5 y after initiation of therapy.[1]

Nucleoside Reverse Transcriptase Inhibitors

Nucleoside reverse transcriptase inhibitors (NRTI), such as **didanosine** and **stavudine**, have been associated with an increased risk for developing drug-induced pancreatitis. One longitudinal study conducted at the Johns Hopkins HIV Clinic with 2613 patients receiving at least one NRTI-containing regimens showed a relative risk of 1.26 for patients receiving stavudine alone and 2.08 when patients received stavudine in combination with didanosine. The highest relative risk (8.56) was noted in patients receiving didanosine and hydroxyurea in combination. The lowest relative risk was noted in patients receiving zidovudine therapy.[16]

Octreotide

There is conflicting evidence concerning the effect of octreotide on reducing endoscopic retrograde cholangiopancreatography-induced pancreatitis. Previous studies have found no significant reduction in pancreatitis development in patients receiving octreotide. However, a more recent study randomized 961 patients into placebo and octreotide treatment groups, which resulted in a statistically significant decrease in the incidence of pancreatitis in the treatment group versus the placebo group.[17]

Pentamidine

Investigators at Johns Hopkins Hospital's HIV clinic conducted a 10-y analysis of the incidence and associated risk factors for the development of pancreatitis in their HIV patient population. As confirmed in previous studies, the use of aerosolized pentamidine for the prevention of various opportunistic infections resulted in an increased risk of pancreatitis. This study demonstrated an increased incidence of pancreatitis development that was independent of the patient's CD4 count.[18]

Propofol

Multiple cases of pancreatitis associated with propofol have been reported. Pancreatitis can most likely be attributed to the development of hypertriglyceridemia in patients receiving propofol. In a study conducted with 159 intensive care unit patients receiving propofol, 29 (18%) patients developed hypertriglyceridemia with 3 of those cases resulting in pancreatitis.[19]

Valproic Acid

There are at least 80 published cases of valproic acid–induced pancreatitis, including three case reports providing rechallenge data. Pediatric patients have an increased likelihood of developing valproic acid–induced pancreatitis and currently account for 75% of reported cases. There is no obvious connection with dosage or duration of therapy, although cases generally occur within the first 3–17 mo of therapy.[1,20]

(continued)

■ REFERENCES

1. Balani AR, Grendell JH. Drug-induced pancreatitis. *Drug Saf*. 2008;31:823-837.
2. Eland IA et al. Antihypertensive medication and the risk of acute pancreatitis: the European case-control study on drug-induced acute pancreatitis. *Scand J Gastroenterol*. 2006;41:1484-1490.
3. Chodhury P, Gupta P. Pathophysiology of alcoholic pancreatitis: an overview. *World J Gastroenterol*. 2006;12:7421-7427.
4. Cappell MS. Acute pancreatitis: etiology, clinical presentation, diagnosis, and therapy. *Med Clin North Am*. 2008;92:889-923.
5. Knoderer H et al. Predicting asparaginase-associated pancreatitis. *Pediatr Blood Cancer*. 2007;49:634-639.
6. Bermejo F et al. Acute pancreatitis in inflammatory bowel disease, with special reference to azathioprine-induced pancreatitis. *Aliment Pharmacol Ther*. 2008;28:623-628.
7. Pezzilli R et al. Mechanisms involved in the onset of post-ERCP pancreatitis. *JOP*. 2002;3:162-168.
8. Steed DL et al. General surgical complications in heart and heart-lung transplantation. *Surgery*. 1985;98:739-745.
9. Yoshimura N et al. Effect of cyclosporine on the endocrine and exocrine pancreas in kidney transplant recipients. *Am J Kidney Dis*. 1988;12:11-17.
10. Greenberg A. Diuretic complications. *Am J Med Sci*. 2000;319:10-24.
11. Product Information. Fuzeon (R), enfuvirtide. Nutley, NJ: Roche; 2007.
12. Product Information. Byetta (R), exenatide. San Diego, CA: Amylin Pharmaceuticals, Inc.; 2008.
13. U.S. Food and Drug Administration. Information for healthcare professionals: exenatide (marketed as Byetta) 2008 update. http://www.fda.gov/cder/drug/InfoSheets/HCP/exenatide2008HCP.htm. Accessed December 1, 2008.
14. Signh S, Loke YK. Statins and pancreatitis: a systemic review of observational studies and spontaneous case reports. *Drug Saf*. 2006;29:1123-1132.
15. Eland IA et al. Acute pancreatitis attributed to the use of interferon alfa-2b. *Gastroenterology*. 2000;119:230-233.
16. Moore RD et al. Incidence of pancreatitis in HIV-infected patients receiving nucleoside reverse transcriptase inhibitor drugs. *AIDS*. 2001;15:617-620.
17. Copper ST, Slivka A. Incidence, risk factors, and prevention of post-ERCP pancreatitis. *Gastroenterol Clin North Am*. 2007;36:259-276.
18. Riedel DJ et al. A ten-year analysis of the incidence and risk factors for acute pancreatitis requiring hospitalization in an urban HIV clinical cohort. *AIDS Patient Care STDS*. 2008;22:113-121.
19. Devlin JW et al. Propofol-associated hypertriglyceridemia and pancreatitis in the intensive care unit: an analysis of frequency and risk factors. *Pharmacotherapy*. 2005;25:1348-1352.
20. Gerstner T et al. Valproic acid-induced pancreatitis: 16 new cases and a review of the literature. *J Gastroenterol*. 2007;42:39-48.

Chapter 67

Drug-Induced Sexual Dysfunction

Melanie Mabins

The large subjective component of human sexual response makes the evaluation of drug-induced sexual dysfunction difficult. Variations in study design have produced widely divergent reported rates of sexual dysfunction in the "normal" or control populations. In addition, most of the literature indicates there is great reluctance of self-reporting of sexual dysfunction during clinical interviews and even more if not directly asked or aggressively sought by clinicians. Common drug-induced sexual dysfunctions are decreased libido or sexual drive, impotence (failure to achieve or maintain an erection in men), priapism (persistent and often painful erection), delayed ejaculation or failure of ejaculation, retrograde ejaculation (into the urinary bladder), and, in women, failure to achieve orgasm and decreased vaginal lubrication. Gynecomastia (enlargement of the male breast) has been included in this table. Although not life-threatening, drug-induced sexual dysfunction has a negative effect on quality of life and is an important contributor to noncompliance with prescribed drug regimens. Class-related effects are reported when applicable.

ACE-Inhibitors

Studies have shown ACE-inhibitor therapy contributes to the prevalence of erectile dysfunction.[1]

Alcohol

Low doses result in behavioral disinhibition and can increase libido. With higher doses libido is decreased, and sexual response is impaired, frequently resulting in failure of erection in men and reduced vaginal vasodilation and delayed orgasm in women. In chronic alcoholics, sexual dysfunction frequently persists long after alcohol withdrawal and is permanent in some. Chronic alcoholism has an 8%–54% rate of impotency. The long-term effects are probably neurologic and endocrine in origin; alcohol reduces testosterone levels and increases luteinizing hormone levels. Long-term effects are independent of liver disease.[2–10]

α-Adrenergic Blocking Agents

Unspecified sexual dysfunction has been reported in 9% of the population receiving α-blockers. **Prazosin** and **terazosin** have been reported as the cause of priapism and impotence in some case reports. Gynecomastia occurs in 0.4% of **finasteride**-treated men. Onset is usually delayed until after 5–6 mo of treatment. In a meta-analysis of 3 double-blind studies including 2511 patients randomized to finasteride, Permixon (phytotherapy), or **tamsulosin** therapy, ejaculation disorders were the most frequently reported. Decreased libido, impotence, and ejaculation disorders were reported in 0.8%–9% of patients treated with finasteride or tamsulosin; 4%–6% reported retrograde ejaculation with tamsulosin. Other reports also indicate that tamsulosin causes retrograde ejaculation (4%–11% of patients treated with 0.4 mg in one trial and 4.2% of 354 men randomized to tamsulosin reported ejaculation disorder in another trial) while finasteride has a higher incidence of decreased libido and erectile dysfunction slightly more than placebo (still low, less than 10%). Finasteride and tamsulosin have a slight impact on sexual function (per MSF-4

(continued)

questionnaire that assesses interest in sexuality, quality of erection, and achievement of ejaculation and orgasm), especially on ejaculation. These effects are rare, but in line with previous reports. **Phenoxybenzamine** is associated with dosage-related failure of ejaculation but not interference with orgasm. This effect was present in all 19 patients in one study and reversed 24–48 h after drug discontinuation.[2–5,11–14]

Alprostadil

Intracavernous injection of alprostadil produces penile pain in 44% of patients, prolonged erection in 8%, and priapism in 1%. Fibrotic nodules or scarring occur frequently. Intraurethral administration does not appear to cause priapism or fibrosis, but 36% experience penile pain.[15–17]

Aminocaproic Acid

This drug can inhibit ejaculation without affecting libido and has produced "dry" ejaculation. Effects are rapidly reversible with drug discontinuation.[3,4,18,19]

Amphetamines

Low doses can increase libido and delay male orgasm. High doses have been associated with failure to achieve an erection in men and loss of orgasm in both sexes.[4,20–22]

Anabolic Steroids

Impotence and gynecomastia occur frequently in men and might be the result of reduction in the circulating levels of natural testosterone.[3,5,23]

Anti-Cancer Agents

Gynecomastia results from the antiandrogen effects of **cyproterone** and **flutamide**. The use of **tamoxifen** increases the prevalence of vaginal dryness and painful intercourse. Sexual dysfunction has been reported with **methotrexate**, along with several other chemotherapeutic agents likely due to gonadal suppression.[2,23,24]

Anticonvulsants

Because patients with epilepsy already experience various forms of sexual dysfunction, it is generally difficult to isolate drug-induced sexual dysfunction from the underlying disease state. Female and male libido can be reduced. Self-reported sexual dysfunction has been described in a widely varying percentage of patients. Social and psychological aspects of epilepsy probably play important roles in these findings. Some effects might be caused by a reduction in the level of free testosterone, resulting from hepatic enzyme induction and higher concentrations of sex hormone–binding globulins. Increased metabolism of androgens caused by the induction of the cytochrome P450 pathway has been reported with **carbamazepine, phenobarbital, phenytoin,** and **primidone**. Sexual dysfunction is more common in women receiving phenytoin and carbamazepine vs **lamotrigine** or **valproate**. Severely decreased libido and anorgasmia have been reported in women treating bipolar disorder with valproate. There are case reports of anorgasmia in epileptic women receiving **gabapentin**.[2,3,6,25–28]

Antidepressants

Most antidepressants cause sexual dysfunction with anorgasmia and delayed ejaculation being the most common. As demonstrated by large observational studies of women, agents such as **venlafaxine** and **SSRIs** are widely reported (one-third to one-half) to cause anorgasmia due to their serotonin agonist activity. **Mirtazapine** and **nefazodone** have minimal to no sexual dysfunction reported in these studies due to their additional mechanism of postsynaptic blockade of the 5-HT-2 receptor, which in turn blocks orgasmic dysfunction. Numerous cases of priapism have been reported with **trazodone** therapy, usually during the first month. **Desipramine,** nefazodone, and **bupropion** may produce the lowest incidence of sexual side effects in this class as a whole.

(continued)

Decreased libido and impaired ejaculation is associated with selective and nonselective serotonin reuptake inhibitors. The number of self-reports of complete erectile dysfunction among men who used SSRIs has increased and arousal disturbance (i.e., decreased vaginal lubrication) has been reported among women. However, anorgasmia and delay of orgasm are the most well-known adverse effects of SSRIs, affecting the majority of patients in some studies. **Fluvoxamine, fluoxetine, paroxetine,** and **sertraline** are the most frequently mentioned. These effects have been confirmed in patients without depression. Some patients have benefited from a dosage reduction. Bupropion, mirtazapine, and nefazodone should be considered in patients with SSRI-induced dysfunction.

The effect of tricyclic antidepressants on sexual dysfunction is reported to be common; however, due to their less frequent use, the reports have somewhat diminished. With **imipramine** at doses ranging from 200 to 300 mg, orgasmic delay was reported in 27% vs 11% of women in a 6-wk placebo-controlled trial. There appears to be a significant increase in self-reports of complete erectile dysfunction among men who used tricyclics.

With use of heterocyclic antidepressants, impotence, delayed ejaculation, and painful ejaculation have been reported in men. Women and men have reported delayed orgasm, anorgasmia, increased and, more commonly, decreased libido. **Clomipramine** is the worst offender. The frequency of these effects varies considerably among published reports, perhaps reflecting the influence of the underlying depressive illness.

Also highly variable are reported adverse sexual effects of MAOIs. Impotence, spontaneous erections, and ejaculatory delay in men and orgasmic failure in men and women have all been described. The true prevalence of these effects cannot be determined from available data, but MAOIs might be associated with more sexual dysfunction than heterocyclic antidepressants. With **phenelzine** at doses ranging from 60 to 90 mg, orgasmic delay was reported in 36% vs 11% of women in a 6-wk placebo-controlled trial.[2–6,18,22,25,29–40]

Antipsychotics

These drugs have been implicated in producing a wide variety of adverse sexual effects such as impotence and priapism, absent and spontaneous ejaculation, painful ejaculation, retrograde ejaculation, menstrual irregularities, and decreased libido. Decreased libido has been the most commonly reported sexual adverse effect in this class, especially with the agents **thioriduzine** and **fluphenazine.** The incidence of decreased libido overall can be up to 25%. These effects result from the complex actions of the drugs on the patient's hormonal balance and central sympathetic and parasympathetic pathways. With the exception of priapism, these effects are usually benign and respond to drug discontinuation. **Thioridazine** is the most commonly implicated drug.

Erectile and ejaculatory dysfunction are reported with **chlorpromazine**, thioridazine, **fluphenazine,** and **trifluoperazine**. Priapism is reported with most neuroleptic agents, including haloperidol. In a small study, quetiapine was reported to cause diminished libido and erectile dysfunction at week 4. In a much larger study consisting of 4,783 patients, at 12 mo and in patients prescribed only one antipsychotic at baseline, sexual dysfunction was reported with **olanzapine** (55.7%), **quetiapine** (60.2%), **risperidone** (67.8%), and **haloperidol** (71.1%). The possible contribution of the underlying disease state cannot be overlooked.[2–6,22,41–44]

β-Adrenergic Blocking Agents

These drugs are associated with a variety of sexual problems, most commonly impotence. It is reported that impotence is frequent at 160 mg or greater doses of **propranolol**. However, decreased libido and ejaculatory dysfunction is frequent (1–4% and 28%, respectively) at doses higher than 320 mg. In a study of 46 men, 7 experienced "complete" impotence, 13 noted reduced potency, and 2 complained of reduced libido. In a larger trial, the frequencies of impotence during propranolol therapy were 13.8% and 13.2% after 12 wk and 2 y, respectively.

(continued)

However, these figures did not differ significantly from placebo. Most of the published reports implicate propranolol; other more cardioselective β-blockers are less frequently associated with complaints of adverse sexual effects. In addition to impotence, studies show beta-blocker therapy contributes to the prevalence of erectile dysfunction. In general, there has been a decrease in the reporting of sexual adverse effects with β-blockers, which is attributed to a trend toward the use of lower drug doses. A study including 10,088 hypertensive patients had no reports of sexual dysfunction while treated with metoprolol and only 30 unspecified reports occurred in another study including 9837 hypertensive patients. There have been at least 25 reported patients who complained of sexual dysfunction (18 impotence, 9 decreased libido) while receiving topical ophthalmic treatment with **timolol**. Some of these patients were rechallenged, with positive results.[1–3,6,18,29,41,45–50]

Benzodiazepines

Studies show therapy significantly contributes to the prevalence of erectile dysfunction.[1]

Calcium Channel Blockers

Verapamil is the most commonly implicated calcium channel blocker, but **nifedipine** and **diltiazem** also can produce gynecomastia. Other calcium channel blockers seem less likely to cause gynecomastia. Studies show that calcium channel blocker therapy contributes to the prevalence of erectile dysfunction.[1,3,51]

Carbonic Anhydrase Inhibitors

Many patients receiving carbonic anhydrase inhibitors (e.g., **acetazolamide, methazolamide**) develop a syndrome of malaise, fatigue, weight loss, and depression, which often includes loss of libido. These patients appear to be more acidotic than those without the syndrome and some respond to therapy with sodium bicarbonate. Decreased libido has occurred in men and women and usually requires 2 wk of carbonic anhydrase inhibitor therapy to develop.[3,4]

Danazol

Most women treated with danazol for endometriosis experience reversible decreased libido.[52]

Digoxin

Studies show that digoxin can contribute to the prevalence of erectile dysfunction. Digitalis glycosides have some estrogen-like activity, and digoxin has been associated with decreased libido, impotence, and gynecomastia in men. In one study, digoxin use was associated with a 60% decrease in testosterone and a similar increase in estrogen in men. **Disopyramide**, another antiarrhythmic agent, is also linked to erectile dysfunction.[1–6,18,53]

Diuretics, Thiazide

The data propose that sexual dysfunction occurring with diuretics is infrequent. In a few studies, patients receiving thiazide therapy experienced an increased incidence of impotence. The frequency of impotence with furosemide and ethacrynic acid is approximately 5%, while spironolactone is considered a more common offender compared to all. Studies show that thiazide therapy significantly contributes to the prevalence of erectile dysfunction. In one large study, the prevalence of impotence was reported to be significantly higher with **bendroflumethiazide** than with placebo (23% after 2 y compared with 10% for placebo), and in another, **hydrochlorothiazide** was reported to produce more impotence and loss of libido than propranolol. In a well-designed study, 14% of men taking **chlorothiazide** complained of impotence, as did 14% of placebo-treated men. In 3 studies, **chlorthalidone** therapy resulted in more impotence than placebo (17% vs 8% in one).[1,2–6,18,29,46–48,50,54–57]

(*continued*)

Ephedrine

Few case reports associate priapism with nonprescription weight loss products containing ephedrine.[58]

Estrogens

Impotence and gynecomastia occur frequently in men taking estrogens for prostate cancer. Estrogens have been used to reduce libido and sexual activity of male sex offenders.[3–6,59]

Gonadotropin-Releasing Hormone Analogues

Most men and women treated with **goserelin** experience reversible decreased libido. **Leuprolide**-treated patients likely react similarly.[52]

Guanethidine

Up to 54% of men have reported impotence and up to 71% have reported ejaculatory impairment. Sexual dysfunction occurs often with guanethidine, but does not affect parasympathetic function and would not be expected to produce impotence, leading some to suggest that the impotence is secondary to the inhibition of ejaculation. Retrograde ejaculation occurs as a result of the failure of the internal urethral sphincter to close; this action is sympathetically mediated. Although not well characterized, decreased libido in women taking guanethidine has been reported. Guanethidine effects are reversible with drug discontinuation and can be alleviated by a reduction in dosage.[2–6,18,55]

Histamine-2 Receptor Antagonists

Sexual dysfunction, including impotence and painful erections is associated with cimetidine, famotidine, and ranitidine. **Cimetidine** is understood to cause an antiandrogen effect, therefore producing sexual dysfunction. Studies show that therapy contributes to the prevalence of erectile dysfunction. In a group of 22 men treated with high dosages of cimetidine for hypersecretory states, 11 developed gynecomastia and 9 experienced impotence. These effects appear to be dose-related and readily reversible and are not an important problem at dosages used for peptic ulcers. Cimetidine has some antiandrogenic effects, possibly the result of hyperprolactinemia, which are thought to be responsible for sexual dysfunction. Displacement of androgens from breast androgen receptors might contribute to the development of gynecomastia. **Ranitidine** does not appear to be associated with as high a prevalence of sexual dysfunction, and **famotidine** is not antiandrogenic.[1–6,18,23,51,60]

Lipid-Lowering Agents

Lipid-lowering agents are related to diminished libido and impotence. Erectile dysfunction is correlated with statins and fibrates, which affect the substrates of sex hormones, according to a systematic review article. At least 47 cases of **simvastatin**-associated impotence have been reported, including some with positive rechallenge. There are scattered reports of impotence with **lovastatin** and **pravastatin.** In large multicenter trials with the agent clofibrate, impotence has been reported more frequently than with placebo.[2–6,18,61–64]

Ketoconazole

Gynecomastia has been reported, apparently the result of the inhibition of testosterone synthesis.[3,23,51]

Marijuana

Positive and negative effects on sexual function are possible. Low doses can have a disinhibiting effect, whereas large doses have been associated with decreased libido and impotence. Long-term use also can result in gynecomastia.[4,51,65]

(*continued*)

Metoclopramide

Gynecomastia and galactorrhea have been reported in adults and children receiving metoclopramide. Diminished libido and erectile function can also be caused. These effects are probably due to metoclopramide-induced hyperprolactinemia.[2,66]

Narcotics

Long-term narcotic use (especially abuse) is frequently associated with decreased libido and orgasmic failure in both sexes and impotence in men. These effects are dose-related, with the highest frequency of impotence reported in narcotic addicts (80%–90% in some series), and are reversible with drug discontinuation. Although **cocaine** is often perceived as a sexual stimulant, its use is associated with difficulty in establishing an erection and delayed ejaculation. Priapism has been discovered in case reports.[4,22,59,67–71]

Nitrates and Nitrites

These vasodilators have been used (primarily by inhalation) to enhance the perception of orgasm. However, when they are used too soon before orgasm, the vasodilation rapidly produces loss of erection. This effect has been used therapeutically to reduce spontaneous erections in men undergoing urologic procedures. Studies show that nitrate therapy contributes to the prevalence of erectile dysfunction.[1,4,72,73]

Omeprazole

Although the prevalence is unclear, impotence and gynecomastia in men and breast enlargement in women have been described. Sexual dysfunction, including impotence and painful erections is associated with omeprazole.[2,3,74]

Peripheral Vasodilators

Intracavernous injection of **papaverine** resulted in priapism (defined as an erection lasting >3 h) in 17% of 400 patients. Those with psychogenic or neurogenic impotence were more likely to experience priapism than those with vasculogenic impotence. Rare cases of priapism are reported with the agent **hydralazine**.[2,15,34]

Progestins

Impotence has been reported in 25%–70% of men receiving progestins for prostatic hypertrophy. Progestins have been used to reduce libido and sexual activity of male sex offenders.[4,58,75]

Reserpine

Sexual dysfunction such as impotence (33%) and failure of ejaculation (14%) in men and reduced libido in both sexes occur frequently.[2–4,6,18,55]

Sedative-Hypnotic Drugs

In a manner similar to alcohol, low doses can produce some disinhibition, whereas large doses can reduce sexual performance.[3–6]

Somatropin

Benign gynecomastia can occur in prepubertal and adult males receiving somatropin. Onset might not occur until after months or years of treatment.[76]

Spironolactone

Gynecomastia in men and painful breast enlargement or menstrual irregularities in women are frequent with large dosages. Less frequently reported effects are impotence, inhibition of vaginal

(continued)

lubrication, and loss of libido. The structural similarity of the drug to estrogens and progestins is thought to be a key factor in the genesis of adverse sexual effects. Spironolactone might inhibit the formation of testosterone and its breast receptor binding. It also might increase the metabolic clearance of testosterone and its rate of peripheral conversion to estradiol. These effects appear to be dose-related. Studies show that spironolactone therapy significantly contributes to the prevalence of erectile dysfunction.[3,4,6,18,23,29,51,55]

Sympatholytics

Centrally acting sympatholytic agents can cause sexual dysfunction with an average frequency of 20%–30%. There is a high frequency with **α-methyldopa, clonidine, guanabenz,** and **guanfacine.** Although some reports have indicated no sexual problems, others have indicated problems in up to 24% of patients taking clonidine. Impotence is the most frequently noted effect with this agent, but delayed or retrograde ejaculation in men and failure of arousal and orgasm in women have been described. Studies show that clonidine therapy significantly contributes to the prevalence of erectile dysfunction. Impotence and ejaculatory failure in men and reduced libido in both sexes have been described with methyldopa. The frequency of sexual dysfunction varies from quite low in some reports to >50% in response to direct questioning. These effects are dose-related and reversible. They might be the result of drug-induced sympathetic inhibition and mild CNS depression. Gynecomastia in men and painful breast enlargement in women have also occurred with methyldopa. In addition, studies show that methyldopa therapy contributes to the prevalence of erectile dysfunction.[2–6,18,26,29,48,55,77]

■ REFERENCES

1. Derby CA et al. Drug therapy and prevalence of erectile dysfunction in the Massachusetts Male Aging Study cohort. *Pharmacotherapy.* 2001;21:676 683.
2. Thomas DR et al. Medications and sexual function. *Clin Geriatr Med.* 2003;19:553-562.
3. Forman R et al. *Drug-Induced Infertility and Sexual Dysfunction.* Cambridge, UK: Cambridge University; 1996.
4. Buffum J. Pharmacosexology: the effects of drugs on sexual function. A review. *J Psychoactive Drugs.* 1982;14:5-44.
5. Brock GB, Lue TF. Drug-induced male sexual dysfunction. An update. *Drug Saf.* 1993;8:414-426.
6. McWaine DE, Procci WR. Drug-induced sexual dysfunction. *Med Toxicol Adverse Drug Exp.* 1988;3:289-306.
7. Lemere F, Smith JW. Alcohol-induced sexual impotence. *Am J Psychiatry.* 1973;130:212-213.
8. Wilson GT, Lawson DM. Effects of alcohol on sexual arousal in women. *J Abnorm Psychol.* 1976;85:489-497.
9. Gordon GG et al. Effect of alcohol (ethanol) administration on sex-hormone metabolism in normal men. *N Engl J Med.* 1976;295:793-797.
10. Dudek FA, Turner DS. Alcoholism and sexual functioning. *J Psychoactive Drugs.* 1982;14:47-54.
11. Zlotta AR et al. Evaluation of male sexual function in patients with lower urinary tract symptoms (LUTS) associated with benign prostatic hyperplasia (BPH) treated with a phytotherapeutic agent (permixon), tamsulosin or finasteride. *Eur Urol.* 2005;48:269-276.
12. Debruyne F et al. Comparison of a phytotherapeutic agent (permixon) with an α-blocker (tamsulosin) in the treatment of benign prostatic hyperplasia: a 1-year randomized international study. *Eur Urol.* 2002;41:497-506.
13. Wilton L et al. The safety of finasteride used in benign prostatic hypertrophy: a non-interventional observational cohort study in 14,772 patients. *Br J Urol.* 1996;78:379-384.
14. Kedia KR, Persky L. Effect of phenoxybenzamine (dibenzyline) on sexual function in man. *Urology.* 1981;18:620-622.
15. The European Alprostadil Study Group. The long-term safety of alprostadil (prostaglandin-E1) in patients with erectile dysfunction. *Br J Urol.* 1998;82:538-543.
16. Chen RN et al. Penile scarring with intracavernous injection therapy using prostaglandin E1: a risk factor analysis. *J Urol.* 1996;155:138-140.
17. Padma-Nathan H et al. Treatment of men with erectile dysfunction with transurethral alprostadil. *N Engl J Med.* 1997;336:1-7.
18. Buffum J. Pharmacosexology update: prescription drugs and sexual function. *J Psychoactive Drugs.* 1986;18:97-106.
19. Evans BE, Aledort LM. Inhibition of ejaculation due to epsilon aminocaproic acid [Letter]. *N Engl J Med.* 1978;298:166-167.

20. Greaves G. Sexual disturbances among chronic amphetamine users. *J Nerv Ment Dis*. 1972;155:363-365.

21. Smith DE et al. Amphetamine abuse and sexual dysfunction: clinical and research considerations. In: Smith DE et al, eds. *Amphetamine Use, Misuse, and Abuse: Proceedings of the National Amphetamine Conference, 1978*. Boston, MA: GK Hall; 1979:228-248.

22. Segraves RT. Effects of psychotropic drugs on human erection and ejaculation. *Arch Gen Psychiatry*. 1989;46:275-284.

23. Braunstein GD. Gynecomastia. *N Engl J Med*. 1993;328:490-495.

24. Mortimer JE et al. Effect of tamoxifen on sexual functioning in patients with breast cancer. *J Clin Oncol*. 1999;17:1488-1492.

25. Gutierrez MA et al. Sexual dysfunction in women with epilepsy: role of antiepileptic drugs and psychotropic medications. *Int Rev Neurobiol*. 2008;83:157-167.

26. Toone BK et al. Sex hormone changes in male epileptics. *Clin Endocrinol*. 1980;12:391-395.

27. Dana-Haeri J et al. Reduction of free testosterone by antiepileptic drugs. *Br Med J*. 1982;284:85-86.

28. Morrell MJ. Sexual dysfunction in epilepsy. *Epilepsia*. 1991;32(suppl 6):S38-S45.

29. Francis ME et al. The contribution of common medical conditions and drug exposures to erectile dysfunction in adult males. *J Urol*. 2007;178:591-596.

30. Harrison WM et al. Effects of antidepressant medication on sexual function: a controlled study. *J Clin Psychopharmacol*. 1986;6:144-149.

31. Shen WW, Sata LS. Inhibited female orgasm resulting from psychotropic drugs. A five-year, updated, clinical review. *J Reprod Med*. 1990;35:11-14.

32. Balon R et al. Sexual dysfunction during antidepressant treatment. *J Clin Psychiatry*. 1993;54:209-212.

33. Segraves RT. Antidepressant-induced sexual dysfunction. *J Clin Psychiatry*. 1998;59(suppl 4):48-54.

34. Lomas GM, Jarow JP. Risk factors for papaverine-induced priapism. *J Urol*. 1992;147:1280-1281.

35. Warner MD et al. Trazodone and priapism. *J Clin Psychiatry*. 1987;48:244-245.

36. Labbate LA et al. Antidepressant-related erectile dysfunction: management via avoidance, switching antidepressants, antidotes, and adaptation. *J Clin Psychiatry*. 2003;64:11-19.

37. Williams VS et al. Estimating the prevalence and impact of antidepressant-induced sexual dysfunction in 2 European countries: a cross-sectional patient survey. *J Clin Psychiatry*. 2006;67:204-210.

38. Piazza LA et al. Sexual functioning in chronically depressed patients treated with SSRI antidepressants: a pilot study. *Am J Psychiatry*. 1997;154:1757-1759.

39. Modell JG et al. Comparative sexual side effects of bupropion, fluoxetine, paroxetine, and sertraline. *Clin Pharmacol Ther*. 1997;61:476-487.

40. Nafziger AN et al. Incidence of sexual dysfunction in healthy volunteers on fluvoxamine therapy. *J Clin Psychiatry*. 1999;60:187-190.

41. Pollack MH et al. Genitourinary and sexual adverse effects of psychotropic medication. *Int J Psychiatry Med*. 1992;22:305-327.

42. Thompson JW et al. Psychotropic medication and priapism: a comprehensive review. *J Clin Psychiatry*. 1990;51:430-433.

43. Mir A et al. Change in sexual dysfunction with aripiprazole: a switching or add-on study. *J Psychopharmacol*. 2008;22:244-253.

44. Atmaca M et al. A new atypical antipsychotic: quetiapine-induced sexual dysfunctions. *Int J Impot Res*. 2005;17:201-203.

45. Fraunfelder FT, Meyer SM. Sexual dysfunction secondary to topical ophthalmic timolol [Letter]. *JAMA*. 1985;253:3092-3093.

46. Medical Research Council Working Party on Mild to Moderate Hypertension. Adverse reactions to bendrofluazide and propranolol for the treatment of mild hypertension. *Lancet*. 1981;2:539-542.

47. Veterans Administration Cooperative Study Group on Antihypertensive Agents. Comparison of propranolol and hydrochlorothiazide for the initial treatment of hypertension. II. Results of long-term therapy. *JAMA*. 1982;248:2004-2011.

48. Bansal S. Sexual dysfunction in hypertensive men. A critical review of the literature. *Hypertension*. 1988;12:1-10.

49. Prisant LM et al. Sexual dysfunction with antihypertensive drugs. *Arch Intern Med*. 1994;154:730-736.

50. Grimm RH Jr. et al. Long-term effects on sexual function of five antihypertensive drugs and nutritional hygienic treatment in hypertensive men and women. Treatment of Mild Hypertension Study (TOMHS). *Hypertension*. 1997;29:8-14.

51. Thompson DF, Carter JR. Drug-induced gynecomastia. *Pharmacotherapy*. 1993;13:37-45.

52. Shaw RW. An open randomized comparative study of the effect of goserelin depot and danazol in the treatment of endometriosis. Zoladex Endometriosis Study Team. *Fertil Steril*. 1992;58:265-272.

53. Neri A et al. Subjective assessment of sexual dysfunction of patients on long-term administration of digoxin. *Arch Sex Behav*. 1980;9:343-347.

54. Buranakitjaroen P et al. Prevalence of erectile dysfunction among treated hypertensive males. *J Med Assoc Thai.* 2006;89:S28-S36.
55. Duncan L, Bateman DN. Sexual function in women. Do antihypertensive drugs have an impact? *Drug Saf.* 1993;8:225-234.
56. Wassertheil-Smoller S et al. Effect of antihypertensives on sexual function and quality of life: the TAIM study. *Ann Intern Med.* 1991;114:613-620.
57. Chang SW et al. The impact of diuretic therapy on reported sexual function. *Arch Intern Med.* 1991;151:2402-2408.
58. Munarriz R et al. Cocaine and ephedrine-induced priapism: case reports and investigation of potential adrenergic mechanisms. *Urology.* 2003;62:187-192.
59. Bancroft J et al. The control of deviant sexual behavior by drugs: I. Behavioural changes following oestrogens and anti-androgens. *Br J Psychiatry.* 1974;125:310-315.
60. Jensen RT et al. Cimetidine-induced impotence and breast changes in patients with gastric hypersecretory states. *N Engl J Med.* 1983;308:883-887.
61. The Coronary Drug Project Research Group. Clofibrate and niacin in coronary heart disease. *JAMA.* 1975;231:360-381.
62. Oliver MF et al. A co-operative trial in the primary prevention of ischaemic heart disease using clofibrate. Report from the Committee of Principal Investigators. *Br Heart J.* 1978;40:1069-1118.
63. Boyd IW. HMG-CoA reductase inhibitor-induced impotence [Letter]. *Ann Pharmacother.* 1996;30:1199.
64. Jackson G. Simvastatin and impotence. *Br Med J.* 1997;315:31.
65. Halikas J et al. Effects of regular marijuana use on sexual performance. *J Psychoactive Drugs.* 1982;14:59-70.
66. Madani S, Tolia V. Gynecomastia with metoclopramide use in pediatric patients. *J Clin Gastroenterol.* 1997;24:79-81.
67. Cushman P. Sexual behavior in heroin addiction and methadone maintenance. Correlation with plasma luteinizing hormone. *N Y State J Med.* 1972;72:1261-1265.
68. Langrod J et al. Methadone treatment and physical complaints: a clinical analysis. *Int J Addict.* 1981;16:947-952.
69. Rosenbaum M. When drugs come into the picture, love flies out the window: women addicts' love relationships. *Int J Addict.* 1981;16:1197-1206.
70. Siegel RK. Cocaine and sexual dysfunction: the curse of mama coca. *J Psychoactive Drugs.* 1982;14:71-74
71. Wesson DR. Cocaine use by masseuses. *J Psychoactive Drugs.* 1982;14:75-76.
72. Sigell LT et al. Popping and snorting volatile nitrites: a current fad for getting high. *Am J Psychiatry.* 1978;135:1216-1218.
73. Welti RS, Brodsky JB. Treatment of intraoperative penile tumescence. *J Urol.* 1980;124:925-926.
74. Lindquist M, Edwards IR. Endocrine adverse effects of omeprazole. *Br Med J.* 1992;305:451-452.
75. Meiraz D et al. Treatment of benign prostatic hyperplasia with hydroxyprogesterone-caproate: placebo-controlled study. *Urology.* 1977;9:144-148.
76. Malozowski S, Stadel BV. Prepubertal gynecomastia during growth hormone therapy. *J Pediatr.* 1995;126:659-661.
77. Meston CM. Inhibition of subjective and physiological sexual arousal in women by clonidine. *Psychosom Med.* 1997;59:399-407.

Chapter 68

Drug-Induced Skin Disorders

Katherine D. Mieure

Drug-induced skin disorders frequently occur.[1] The mechanisms involved in the pathogenesis of these reactions are immunologic and nonimmunologic, with non-immunologic accounting for 75% of the reactions.[2] It has been reported that many commonly used drugs have dermatologic reaction rates above 1%.[1] However, esti-mating the frequency of occurrence of these reactions are limited by the difficulty of determining a correct diagnosis of a skin disorder and the complexity of estab-lishing a causal relationship with drug therapy. Fortunately, most reactions are not severe, and few are fatal.[3]

The following table includes a list of drugs and associated skin disorders. Drugs believed to be among the most common causes of a particular drug-induced skin disorder are designated by "XX" in the table. Only skin disorders resulting from *systemic* administration of drugs are represented in this table. The following abbreviations are used to indicate the specific skin disorders listed:

AE	—	Acneiforms Eruptions
AL	—	Alopecia
ED	—	Exfoliative Dermatitis
FE	—	Fixed Drug Eruptions
LE	—	Lupus Erythematosus-Like Reactions
ME	—	Maculopapular Exanthems
PE	—	Palmoplantar Erythrodysesthesia
PH	—	Photosensitivity and Phototoxicity Reactions
SJ/TN	—	Stevens–Johnson Syndrome/Toxic Epidermal Necrolysis
UT	—	Urticaria

Note that in the above list Stevens–Johnson syndrome and toxic epidermal necrol-ysis have been combined into a single column because of their similarity in histopathology and because they are usually caused by the same drugs.

DRUG	AE	AL	ED	FE	LE	ME	PE	PH	SJ/TN	UT	REFERENCES
Abacavir						X			X	X	4
Acetaminophen			X			X				X	5, 6
Acetazolamide									X		7
Allopurinol		X	X			X			XX		2, 5, 7–9
Amikacin									X		7

(continued)

DRUG	AE	AL	ED	FE	LE	ME	PE	PH	SJ/TN	UT	REFERENCES
Aminosalicylic Acid			X								9
Amiodarone		X						X			2, 5, 8, 10, 11
Amphetamines		X									12
Androgens	XX	X									2, 5, 8, 9
Anti-TNFα Agents					X						13
Anticoagulants		X									2, 5, 8, 9
Antidepressants, Heterocyclic	X							X		X	5, 8, 10, 14
Atazanavir						X			X		4
Auranofin		X									5
Azathioprine		X									5
Barbiturates	X		X	X		X			XX		2, 5, 7–9, 15, 16
Bleomycin		XX									5
Bromocriptine		X									5, 8, 12
Capecitabine		X					X				7, 17
Captopril		X	X		X	X					2, 5, 7, 13
Carbamazepine			X	X	X			X	X		2, 3, 5, 7, 9, 13, 15, 16
Carboplatin		X									5, 7
Cephalosporins			X	X					X	X	2, 3, 16, 17
Chlorambucil		X								X	7
Chlordiazepoxide			X								6, 10
Chloroquine			X	X				X	X		2, 8, 10
Chlorpromazine				X				X			2, 7, 11, 13
Cimetidine		X	X						X		2, 8, 12
Cisplatin		X					X				7, 19
Clindamycin					X						6
Clofibrate		X									9
Colchicine		XX							X		2, 5, 9
Contraceptives, Oral	X	X		X	X			X			2, 5, 7–10, 12
Corticosteroids	XX										2, 5, 8, 9
Cyclophosphamide		XX					X		X	X	2, 5, 7, 19
Cyclosporine	X	X									5
Cytarabine		XX					X				5, 7, 17
Dacarbazine		X						X			5, 10, 7
Dactinomycin	XX	X							X		5, 7

(continued)

DRUG	AE	AL	ED	FE	LE	ME	PE	PH	SJ/TN	UT	REFERENCES
Dapsone	X		X	X		X		X	X	X	3, 5, 10, 20
Darunavir						X			X		4
Daunorubicin		X					X			X	5, 7, 17
Demeclocycline								X			2, 11
Dextran										X	7
Diflunisal						X					2
Disulfiram	X										5
Docetaxel							X				19
Doxorubicin		XX					X				2, 5, 7, 19
Efavirenz						X		X	X		4
Emtricitabine						X				X	4
Epirubicin							X				19
Ethionamide	X										5
Etoposide		XX					X				5, 19
Fluoroquinolones								XX	X		5, 7, 10, 15, 16, 21
Fluorouracil		XX					X	X			2, 5, 7, 8, 10, 17
Fosamprenavir						X			X		4
Furosemide								X			2, 11
Gentamicin						X					2
Gold Salts		X	XX	X		X		X	X		2, 5, 7, 9, 10
Griseofulvin				X	X			X			2, 7, 8, 10
Hydralazine					XX			X			2, 5, 7, 9, 13
Hydroxychloroquine									X		22
Hydroxyurea		X					X				7, 19
Ifosfamide		XX									5, 7
Indinavir		X									4
Indomethicin		X									2
Interferon Alfa (2a, 2b)		XX									5
Iodides	X										2
Isoniazid	X	X	X	X	X	X		X	X	X	2, 5, 7–9, 13
Ketoconazole		X									5
L-asparaginase										X	7
Lamotrigine									XX		23, 24
Leflunomide									X		25
Levodopa		X									2, 9, 12
Lithium	XX	X	X			X					2, 5, 8, 9, 12

(*continued*)

DRUG	AE	AL	ED	FE	LE	ME	PE	PH	SJ/TN	UT	REFERENCES
Lopinavir/ritonavir		X				X					4
Melphalan		X								X	7
Meprobamate				X		X					5, 7
Mercaptopurine		X					X				7, 19
Methotrexate		XX					X	X	X	X	2, 5, 7, 8, 10, 19
Methyldopa					X						2, 5, 7, 9, 13
Metronidazole			X								5
Minocycline				X	X						10, 13, 26
Mitomycin		X									5
Mitotane							X				2, 19
Multitargeted Kinase Inhibitors							X				27
Nalidixic Acid					X			X			2, 7, 10, 11
Nitrofurantoin		X		X					X		7, 8
NSAIDs		X		X	X			X	X	X	2, 3, 5, 8, 10, 12, 13, 16
Opiates										X	7
Paclitaxel		XX					X				5, 19
Penicillamine		X		X	X						2, 5, 7, 8, 13
Penicillins			XX	X		X			X	X	2, 5, 7–9, 15
Pentazocine								X			7
Phenolphthalein				X				X			2, 5, 7–9
Phenothiazines	X	X	X	X	X	X		XX	X		2, 5, 7–9, 10
Phenytoin	X		X	X	X	X			X		2, 3, 5, 7–9, 15, 16
Piroxicam								X			2, 11
Procainamide					XX			X			2, 5, 7, 9, 13
Promethazine								X			7
Propranolol		X		X	X						2, 7–9
Propylthiouracil		X			X						2, 5, 9, 13
Psoralens	X				X			XX			2, 5, 7, 11
Pyrazinamide	X							X			28
Quinacrine		X									2, 9
Quinidine	X		X	X	X	X		X	X	X	2, 7, 9, 10, 13
Quinine	X			X		X		X			2, 5, 7
Radiocontrast dye					X					X	7
Retinoids		XX						X			2, 5, 8, 10, 12

(continued)

DRUG	AE	AL	ED	FE	LE	ME	PE	PH	SJ/TN	UT	REFERENCES
Rifampin	X								X		5, 15
Salicylates		X		X					X	X	2, 3, 5, 7, 8, 12
Streptomycin			XX	X					X		5, 8, 28
Sulfonamides			XX	X	X	X		XX	XX	X	2, 3, 5, 7–11, 13, 15, 16
Sulfonylureas		X						X	X		2, 5, 8–10
Sulindac									X		2
Tenofovir					X					X	4
Tetracyclines				X				XX	X	X	2, 3, 5, 7–11
Thiazides					X	X		XX			2, 5, 7–11
Thiouracil					X						2
Tipranavir					X			X		X	4
Tolbutamide								X			2
Trimethadione	X	X			X						5, 7, 9
Troxacitabine							X				19
Valproic Acid		X							X		5, 9, 12, 16
Vancomycin					X						29
Vinblastine		XX						X			5, 8, 10
Vincristine		XX									5
Vinorelbine							X				17
Vitamin A		X									2, 30
Voriconazole								X	X		31

■ REFERENCES

1. Bigby M et al. Drug-induced cutaneous reactions: a report from the Boston Collaborative Drug Surveillance Program on 15,438 consecutive inpatients, 1975 to 1982. *JAMA*. 1986;256:3358-3363.
2. Habif TP. Exanthems and drug eruptions. In: *Clinic Dermatology: A Color Guide to Diagnosis and Therapy*. 4th ed. Edinburgh: Mosby, Inc; 2003:457-496.
3. Raksha MP, Marfatia YS. Clinical study of cutaneous drug eruptions in 200 patients. *Indian J Dermatol Venereol Leprol*. 2008;74:80-84.
4. Borras-Blasco J. Adverse cutaneous reactions associated with the newest antiretroviral drugs in patients with human immunodeficiency virus infection. *J Antimicrob Chemother*. 2008;62:879-888.
5. Zürcher K, Krebs A. *Cutaneous Drug Reactions*. 2nd ed. Basel, Switzerland: Karger; 1992.
6. Rallis E et al. Drug eruptions in children with ENT infections. *Int J Pediatr Otorhinolaryngol*. 2006;70:53-57.
7. Duvic M. Urticaria, drug hypersensitivity rashes, nodules and tumors, and atrophic diseases. In: Goldman L, Ausiello D, eds. *Cecil Medicine*. 23rd ed. Philadelphia, PA: WB Saunders; 2008:2957-2969.
8. Blacker KL et al. Cutaneous reactions to drugs. In: Fitzpatrick TB et al., eds. *Dermatology in General Medicine*. 4th ed. New York, NY: McGraw-Hill; 1993:1783-1806.
9. Millikan LE. Drug eruptions (dermatitis medicamentosa). In: Moschella SL, Hurley HJ, eds. *Dermatology*. 3rd ed. Philadelphia, PA: WB Saunders; 1992:535-573.
10. Anon. Drugs that cause photosensitivity. *Med Lett Drugs Ther*. 1995;37:35-36.
11. Habif TP. Light-related diseases and disorders of pigmentation. In: *Clinic Dermatology: A Color Guide to Diagnosis and Therapy*. 4th ed. Edinburgh: Mosby, Inc; 2003:661-697.
12. Llau ME et al. Drug-induced alopecia: review of the literature. *Therapie*. 1995;50:145-150.
13. Vedove CD et al. Drug-induced lupus erythematosus. [published online ahead of print September 17, 2008]. *Arch Dermatol Res*. 2009;301:99-105.

14. Milionis HJ et al. Hypersensitivity syndrome caused by amitriptyline administration. *Postgrad Med J.* 2000;76:361-363.

15. Roujeau JC, Stern RS. Severe adverse cutaneous reactions to drugs. *N Engl J Med.* 1994;331:1272-1285.

16. Sharma VK et al. Stevens Johnson syndrome (SJS), toxic epidermal necrolysis (TEN) and SJS-TEN overlap: a retrospective study of causative drugs and clinical outcome. *Indian J Dermatol Venereol Leprol.* 2008;74:238-240.

17. Ozkaya E et al. Ceftriaxone-induced fixed drug eruption: first report. *Am J Clin Dermatol.* 2008;9:345-347.

18. Sakai H et al. A case of fixed drug eruption presenting with a butterfly rash-like exanthema in a patient with Sjogren's syndrome. *Int J Dermatol.* 2005;44:260-262.

19. Gilbar P. Palmar-plantar erythrodysesthesia. *J Oncol Pharm Pract.* 2003;9:137-150.

20. De D et al. Dapsone induced acute photosensitivity dermatitis; a case report and review of literature. *Lepr Rev.* 2007;78:401-404.

21. Mehlhorn AJ, Brown DA. Safety concerns with fluoroquinolones. *Ann Pharmacother.* 2007;41:1859-1866.

22. Callaly EL et al. Hydroxychloroquine-associated, photo-induced toxic epidermal necrolysis. *Clin Exp Dermatol.* 2008;33:527-524.

23. Mackay FJ et al. Safety of long-term lamotrigine in epilepsy. *Epilepsia.* 1997;38:881-886.

24. Sahin S et al. Cutaneous drug eruptions by current antiepileptics: case reports and alternative treatment options. *Clin Neuropharmacol.* 2008;31:93-96.

25. Hassikou H et al. Leflunomide-induced toxic epidermal necrolysis in a patient with rheumatoid arthritis. *Joint Bone Spine.* 2008;75:597-599.

26. Shapiro LE et al. Comparative safety of tetracycline, minocycline, and doxycycline. *Arch Dermatol.* 1997;133:1224-1230.

27. Lacouture ME et al. Evolving strategies for the management of hand-foot skin reaction associated with multitargeted kinase inhibitors sorafenib and sunitinib. *Oncologist.* 2008;13:1001-1011.

28. Tan WC et al. Two years review of cutaneous adverse drug reaction from first line anti-tuberculous drugs. *Med J Malaysia.* 2007;62:143-146.

29. Prey S et al. Cutaneous drug reactions induced by glycopeptides. *Med Mal Infect.* 2007;37:270-274.

30. Cetaruk EW. Vitamins. In: Ford MD et al, eds. *Clinical Toxicology.* 1st ed. Philadelphia, PA: WB Saunders; 2001:296-304.

31. Malani AN, Aronoff DM. Voriconazole-induced photosensitivity. *Clin Med Res.* 2008;6:83-85.

Drug Use in Special Populations

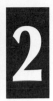

2

Kelly M. Smith

Chapter 69

Drugs and Pregnancy

Kristina E. Ward

In the United States, fetal malformations occur in 3%–6% of pregnancies. These include major and minor malformations from any cause, be it drug, infection, maternal disease state, genetic defect, or pollutant.[1,2] Drug use during pregnancy can be associated with risk to the developing fetus and the pregnant woman. Drugs are probably responsible for only approximately 1%–5% of fetal malformations; 60%–70% of malformations have unknown causes.[2-4]

The genetic makeup of the fetus and the mother influence the extent to which an agent affects the developing fetus. For example, the rates of absorption, metabolism, and elimination of an agent by the mother; its rate of placental transfer; or the way it interacts with cells and tissues of the embryo are genetically determined factors. Thus, human teratogenicity cannot be predicted based only on animal data or extrapolated from one pregnancy to another.

■ PHYSIOLOGIC AND DEVELOPMENTAL FACTORS

Teratogenic substances rarely cause a single defect. Most often, a spectrum of defects occur that corresponds with the systems undergoing major development at the time of exposure. Major malformations are usually the result of first-trimester exposure during critical periods of organogenesis. Exposures during the second and third trimesters can result in alterations or damage in fine structure and function. Intrauterine growth retardation is perhaps the most reliable indicator that a teratogen was present during the second and third trimesters of fetal development. Several organs and systems continue to develop after birth. Therefore, exposure to agents late in pregnancy carries some risk and can result in debilitating alterations in development such as mental retardation. Figure 69–1 shows the stages of human structural development in relation to teratogenic potential.[5]

1051

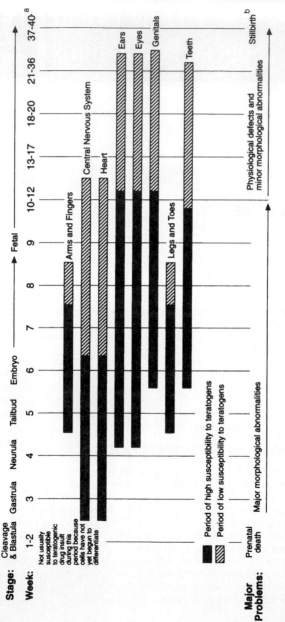

Figure 69–1. Variation in teratogenic susceptibility of organ systems during stages of human intrauterine development. "a" indicates average time for fertilization to parturition is 38 wk. "b" indicates drugs administered during this period can cause neonatal depression at birth (or other effects directly related to the pharmacologic effect of the administered drug). *Reproduced with permission from Ref. 5.*

■ DRUG FACTORS

Most chemicals in the maternal bloodstream cross the placenta. Movement of compounds across the placenta is generally bidirectional, although the net transfer occurs from mother to fetus in most instances.[6,7] Although active and facilitated transport of some substances across the placenta have been demonstrated, the transplacental passage of most agents occurs primarily by simple diffusion.[6,8,9] Only the unbound (free) fraction of a drug is subject to placental transfer; therefore, the greater the degree of protein binding of a drug, the less that is transferred to the fetus.[6,8,9] Early in pregnancy, the placental membrane is relatively thick, and this characteristic tends to reduce permeability.[6] The thickness of the trophoblastic epithelium decreases and surface area increases in the last trimester. The passage of drugs is increased during this stage of pregnancy.[6,10]

The rate-limiting factors in placental transfer of drugs are the same as those that govern membrane diffusion by molecules in general. Thus, the rate of diffusion across the placental barrier is directly proportional to the maternal–fetal concentration gradient and the surface area of the placenta.[6,8,9] Higher concentrations are generally attained in fetal serum and amniotic fluid after bolus injection than after continuous infusion of drug into the mother and by multiple-dose rather than single-dose therapy.[6] Certain physicochemical properties of drugs or chemicals favor transport to the fetus, including low molecular weight, lipid solubility, and nonionization at pH 7.4.[7,9,10]

Each drug has a threshold above which fetal defects can occur and below which no effects are discernible. Whether an agent reaches a "threshold concentration" in the fetus depends on maternal factors (e.g., rates of absorption and clearance) and the chemical nature of the agent.

Administration of drugs near term poses another potential threat to the fetus. Before birth, the fetus relies on maternal systems for drug elimination. After birth, the neonate must rely on its own metabolic and excretory capabilities, which have not yet fully developed. Drugs given near term or during birth, especially those with long half-lives, can have an even more prolonged action in the neonate. Drugs that cause maternal addiction also are known to cause fetal addiction. Neonatal withdrawal symptoms can occur when mothers have been addicted to drugs during pregnancy or when they have taken addicting drugs near term, even though the mothers themselves are not addicted.

■ EFFECTS OF PREGNANCY ON THE MOTHER

Maternal physiology changes as pregnancy progresses and can have an effect on drug disposition and clearance. Maternal plasma volume increases by approximately 20% at midgestation and 50% at term[9] and then falls toward prepregnancy levels postpartum. The volume of distribution for many drugs increases as the fetal compartment enlarges, causing changes in maternal serum drug concentrations. Drugs with narrow therapeutic ranges require careful monitoring during pregnancy and possibly dosage increases. As postpartum maternal plasma volume returns to normal, dosages of many drugs require reduction. Changes in plasma protein concentrations during pregnancy can affect the degree of binding and thus the amount of unbound drug.[8,9] Despite an increase in production of serum albumin, the increased intracellular and intravascular volumes cause serum albumin concentrations to decline.[11] A decrease in total plasma protein concentrations of approximately 10 g/L occurs during pregnancy.[8] Body fat increases by 3–4 kg during pregnancy and can act as a depot for fat-soluble drugs, thereby increasing their volume of distribution.[9] Renal blood flow and glomerular filtration rate increase by almost 50% during pregnancy because of increased cardiac output. Renally excreted drugs, therefore, can have increased rates of clearance.[9]

■ INTERPRETATION OF STUDIES

There are few controlled, prospective studies of drug use in pregnancy. Most of the available information comes from case reports or case-control studies. Cause-and-effect relationships between drugs and teratogenicity are difficult to establish retrospectively because of the numerous variables in each report. These include maternal drug dosage, time of ingestion relative to the date of conception, duration of therapy, concomitant exposure to other potential teratogens, and questionable study design or methodology. Because studies cannot disprove that a slight teratogenic risk might occur with in utero exposure to drugs, drugs should be used during pregnancy only when absolutely necessary. The following table provides information concerning the effects of drugs used during pregnancy on the pregnant woman and on pregnancy outcome. For a more thorough discussion of the principles of teratology, the reader should consult Reference 1.

The following abbreviation is used in the table:

IUGR—intrauterine growth retardation, less than the 10th percentile (of an appropriate standard) birth weight for gestational age.[12]

DRUGS AND PREGNANCY

ANALGESIC AND ANTI-INFLAMMATORY DRUGS

ANTIMIGRAINE DRUGS

Ergot Derivatives

Ergotamine and dihydroergotamine are contraindicated during pregnancy.[13] Both can stimulate uterine contraction through effects at 5-HT$_2$ receptors,[14] and potentially cause abortion.[15] Exposure during pregnancy can also cause neural tube defects, preterm birth, and low birth weight.[16]

Triptans

Evidence collected through the Swedish Medical Birth Registry (658 pregnancies) and the Sumatriptan and Naratriptan Pregnancy Registry (507 pregnancies) indicates no increased risk of birth defects with sumatriptan exposure.[17] Data on other triptans (e.g., almotriptan, eletriptan, frovatriptan, naratriptan, rizatriptan, and zolmitriptan) are sparse.

(continued)

ANALGESIC AND ANTI-INFLAMMATORY DRUGS

NONSTEROIDAL ANTI-INFLAMMATORY DRUGS

Acetaminophen

Acetaminophen does not cause congenital malformations and is the analgesic-antipyretic of choice for use near term because it does not affect platelet function or peripheral prostaglandin synthesis.[18–20] In maternal acetaminophen overdose, most infants are normal at birth,[21] but neonatal liver toxicity can occur.[22] Treat overdose as usual with acetylcysteine. Acetaminophen might prevent fetal distress in laboring women with chorioamnionitis and fever.[23]

Nonsteroidal Anti-inflammatory Drugs (NSAIDs)

Large population-based studies and case-control studies have not shown the NSAIDs, as a class, to be teratogens.[24–28] However, links to cardiac defects have been reported.[29,30] **Naproxen** has been linked to orofacial clefts; however, this link needs to be confirmed through further study.[29] Although controversial, NSAIDs have been reported to increase the risk of spontaneous abortion if used early in pregnancy.[26,28] Most commonly reported with **indomethacin**, NSAID use in the third-trimester can cause constriction or early closure of the ductus arteriosus leading to pulmonary hypertension.[24,26,31] Oligohydramnios resulting from decreased fetal urine output has been reported with indomethacin, **ibuprofen**, naproxen, **ketoprofen, diclofenac, celecoxib,** and **piroxicam**.[24,26,32] Fatal anuria has also been reported with indomethacin.[24] Indomethacin inhibits uterine contractions and has been used as a tocolytic agent.[33] Echocardiographic surveillance of the fetus might be indicated to monitor effects on the ductus arteriosus.

   Aspirin use during pregnancy has been extensively studied. First-trimester aspirin use does not increase the risk of congenital malformations, stillbirth, or decreased birthweight.[24,34] Repeated third-trimester administration of aspirin 325 mg can result in prolonged constriction of the ductus arteriosus and pulmonary hypertension.[18] Maternal ingestion of aspirin 325 mg during the third trimester can interfere with uterine contractility and prolong gestation and labor.[35] Maternal and neonatal platelet function can be affected, resulting in increased maternal blood loss at delivery and abnormal platelet function tests and clinical bleeding in newborns, including intracranial hemorrhage.[24] Although used in low doses to prevent hypertension, preeclampsia, IUGR, and perinatal death, aspirin treatment has not consistently shown efficacy.[24]

OPIOIDS

Narcotics

Narcotic analgesics do not cause fetal malformations, but narcotic abuse during pregnancy or use near term can lead to fetal tolerance and neonatal withdrawal. Meconium might be present in the amniotic fluid, caused most likely by increased bowel activity during periods of fetal withdrawal and/or hypoxia, putting the fetus at risk for meconium aspiration.[36] Withdrawal symptoms such as irritability, increased muscle tone, sleep disturbances, vague autonomic nervous system symptoms, tremulousness, high-pitched crying, frantic and uncoordinated sucking, and seizures can occur in neonates born to narcotic-addicted women and nonaddicted women using narcotics near term.[37] Use of opioids during labor can decrease the pain of labor and allow the patient to rest although fetal heart rate tracings may be more difficult to interpret. Epidural anesthesia is effective and early concerns about increased risk of cesarean delivery and longer duration of labor have not materialized.[38] Neonatal respiratory depression can occur when narcotic analgesics are given during labor and is dependent on the drug, dose, dosing interval, and route of administration (IV > IM).[18] Higher doses of intrathecal **sufentanil** cause more fetal bradycardia and decelerations than low doses or epidural administration.[39] **Meperidine** crosses the placenta rapidly and can cause a sinusoidal fetal heart rate pattern.[40] It is eliminated by the fetus at a rate

(continued)

ANALGESIC AND ANTI-INFLAMMATORY DRUGS

much slower than the mother's; its metabolite, normeperidine, is long acting.[18] Meperidine given during delivery can interfere with the early establishment of breast-feeding because of infant sedation; **morphine** interferes less.[41,42] Infants born to narcotic-dependent women maintained on **methadone** during pregnancy are reported to have lower birth weights, jaundice, thrombocytosis, and withdrawal. Divided doses of methadone better stabilize the fetal activity pattern (which might indicate fetal withdrawal) before and after drug administration than do single daily doses.[43] Methadone clearance increases with each trimester.[44] It is not known if opioids can cause alterations in the neurobehavioral function of infants exposed in utero.

Narcotic Partial Agonists

All narcotics, including the partial agonists and agonist-antagonists, can cause respiratory depression and possibly some behavioral abnormalities in the newborn if used at the time of delivery. Long-term use may cause withdrawal symptoms similar to those reported in offspring of heroin and methadone addicts. **Butorphanol** and **nalbuphine** during labor can cause a sinusoidal fetal heart rate pattern. Nalbuphine offers no advantage over pure narcotics and can cause severe fetal bradycardia possibly resulting in neurological damage.[45] Small for gestational age infants, prematurity, and fetal distress also have been observed.[18] **Tramadol** can cause neonatal seizures, withdrawal, fetal death, and stillbirth when used during pregnancy.

OTHER ANTI-INFLAMMATORY DRUGS

Gold Salts

Although teratogenic in animals, a few reports describe normal children born to women using gold salts during pregnancy.[46,47]

Penicillamine

Data on the teratogenicity of penicillamine are contradictory. Most pregnant women taking penicillamine deliver normal healthy babies, even at the high dosages used in treating Wilson's disease.[18] However, there have been cases of fetal connective tissue abnormalities.[18] Penicillamine is best avoided during pregnancy.[47]

ANTIMICROBIAL DRUGS

AMINOGLYCOSIDES

There is no evidence that aminoglycosides are teratogenic.[48,49] **Streptomycin** and kanamycin can cause congenital hearing loss, ranging from minor high-frequency loss to total deafness, when given to pregnant women for the treatment of tuberculosis. Prevalence is low, especially with careful dosage calculation and limited duration of therapy.[18,48] There is a theoretical risk of nephrotoxicity and ototoxicity for all aminoglycosides.[18,48]

ANTIFUNGAL DRUGS

Amphotericin

Use of amphotericin throughout pregnancy is considered safe.[18]

Azoles

Fluconazole is teratogenic at doses above 400 mg/d given during the first trimester.[18,50] Reported congenital anomalies include craniofacial abnormalities, cleft palate, skeletal defects, and cardiovascular defects. More data is available on the safety of lower fluconazole doses. A population-based cohort study of 1079 women who received fluconazole any time during pregnancy found no increased risk of teratogenicity. The majority (n = 1032; 96%) received ≤300 mg in total.[51] A small study reported the outcomes of 165 women who took fluconazole

(continued)

ANTIMICROBIAL DRUGS

150 mg for vaginal candidiasis during pregnancy. Rates of preterm delivery, low birth weight, and congenital malformations were not different compared to controls.[52] There are no reports of **voriconazole** use in pregnant women, but it is teratogenic in rats and rabbits; avoid use. In 229 women exposed to **itraconazole** during pregnancy (198 first-trimester exposures), the rate of malformations was similar to the control group; however, pregnancy loss was greater and birth weight was lower in itraconazole-exposed pregnancies.[53] Topical use of azole antifungals is probably safe.[18,54,55] However, a recent case-control study found a potential association between azole antifungal use for vaginal candidiasis and hypoplastic left heart syndrome.[56]

Echinocandins

No data are available regarding the use of **anidulafungin, caspofungin,** or **micafungin** during pregnancy. Preclinical studies suggest a fetal risk.

ANTIMALARIAL DRUGS

Chloroquine is the drug of choice for prophylaxis and treatment of malaria during pregnancy in areas with no reports of chloroquine-resistant *Plasmodium falciparum*.[18,57] Chloroquine or **hydroxychloroquine** malaria prophylaxis does not cause adverse fetal effects; however, larger anti-inflammatory doses have resulted in spontaneous abortion.[26,57,58] For chloroquine-resistant *P. falciparum*, **mefloquine** prophylaxis is recommended because it does not appear to be teratogenic although data on its use in the first trimester are limited.[18,57] **Proguanil** does not appear to cause fetal defects, but is only available in combination with atovaquone.[18,59] Folic acid or leucovorin supplementation is necessary because of proguanil's folate antagonism.[18] There are no reports of **primaquine** teratogenicity. There is a risk of hemolysis in fetuses that are G-6-PD deficient; its use would require mother and fetal testing for G-6-PD.[57,60] **Pyrimethamine** is a microbial folate antagonist. Although methotrexate, a mammalian folate antagonist, is teratogenic, pyrimethamine use in pregnancy does not appear to be teratogenic.[18,60] **Quinine** has been used as a folk medicine abortifacient, despite its poor efficacy. Fetal anomalies include blindness, optic nerve hypoplasia, deafness, and hearing impairment.[18,59]

ANTIMYCOBACTERIAL DRUGS

Antituberculars

The treatment of choice for tuberculosis during pregnancy is **isoniazid, rifampin** and **ethambutol** for 9 mo.[61] Also include **pyridoxine** to prevent isoniazid-induced neurologic toxicity.[62,63] Isoniazid is the safest antitubercular used during pregnancy with the occurrence of malformations similar to the expected frequency in nonexposed pregnancies, although there is an increased risk of hepatotoxicity in pregnant women.[62] Rifampin was not associated with an increased risk of fetal malformations in 204 pregnancies as compared to the expected rate of malformations in the general population.[18,62] In most reports, rifampin was taken with isoniazid or ethambutol. Neonatal hypoprothrombinemia has been reported and raises some concern about the use of rifampin, especially near term.[18,62,64] If rifampin is given during pregnancy, maternal oral prophylaxis with vitamin K 20 mg/d for 2 wk before delivery is recommended.[65] Infants should receive 0.5–1 mg of vitamin K IM or SQ within 1 h after delivery.[66,67] Experience using rifabutin and rifapentine during pregnancy is limited. Ethambutol appears safe and did not increase miscarriages, premature births, stillbirths, or malformations in 655 reported exposures.[18,62,63] Some advocate including **pyrazinamide** in the treatment regimen to decrease the risk of treatment failure.[62,68]

Sulfones

Dapsone does not appear to increase the risk of fetal abnormalities.[18,69] There are, however, some reports of hemolytic anemia in mothers and their infants after dapsone use.[69] Because

(continued)

ANTIMICROBIAL DRUGS

dapsone is similar to sulfonamides, it might displace bilirubin from albumin-binding sites and increase the risk of kernicterus in the infant caused by hyperbilirubinemia.[69] This risk is minimized if the drug is discontinued 1 mo before the expected date of delivery.[18,70] (*See* Sulfonamides.)

Thalidomide

Thalidomide is a well-known human teratogen that causes a myriad of congenital malformations including (but not limited to) bilateral limb reduction defects and other skeletal defects; craniofacial defects such as refractive eye errors, deafness, cataracts, glaucoma, and hypoplastic nasal bridge; CNS effects including hydrocephalus, meningomyelocele, and facial palsies; esophageal and duodenal atresia; and anomalies of the kidneys and heart. The time of greatest risk is 34–50 d after the last menstrual period (LMP; correlates to gestational days 20–36). If exposure occurs between days 38 and 43 after the LMP, the arms are most often affected; with exposure between days 40 and 47, the legs and arms are affected.[18] There are no reports documenting the use of lenalidomide during pregnancy. Use in women of childbearing age requires either abstention from **intercourse** or the use of 2 forms of contraception during treatment and for 4 wk thereafter.[71]

ANTIRETROVIRAL DRUGS

Nucleoside Reverse Transcriptase Inhibitors (NRTI)

No evidence of teratogenicity exists for **lamivudine, zidovudine, stavudine, emtricitabine** and **abacavir**.[18,72] Defects with first-trimester use of **didanosine** (5.8%; n = 259) are higher than with use in later trimesters (1%; n = 195).[72] All, including didanosine, are recommended as part of highly active antiretroviral therapy (HAART), with zidovudine and lamivudine preferred.[72] Zidovudine administration with nevirapine (see below) during the intrapartum and postpartum period substantially reduces vertical transmission of HIV from mother to fetus and is the standard of care for HIV-infected pregnant women.[72] Avoid concurrent use of stavudine and didanosine; fatal lactic acidosis may occur.[72,73]

Nonnucleoside Reverse Transcriptase Inhibitors (NNRTI)

Nevirapine is not teratogenic.[18,72] **Efavirenz** caused major malformations in monkeys and there are 3 cases of neural tube defects after first-trimester exposure.[72,74,75] Use is not recommended during pregnancy.[72] Limited experience with **delavirdine** during pregnancy limits its use.[18,72]

Protease Inhibitors

Protease inhibitors can cause hyperglycemia and new onset diabetes mellitus; theoretically, pregnancy may contribute. **Lopinavir** (combined with low-dose ritonavir) does not appear to cause abnormalities.[18,72] **Indinavir** causes hyperbilirubinemia in adults and may contribute to neonatal hyperbilirubinemia; no cases have been reported.[18,72] The prevalence rate of birth defects associated with **nelfinavir** is similar to the expected background rate in the general population.[18,76] **Ritonavir** is used to boost concentrations of other protease inhibitors; low doses are recommended.[18,72] Limited data suggest that **saquinavir** is not associated with abnormalities.[18,72] **Amprenavir, atazanavir, darunavir, fosamprenavir,** and **tipranavir** are not recommended; limited data exist regarding their safety in pregnancy.[72]

Miscellaneous Antiretrovirals

No data exist for **raltegravir** or **maraviroc** use during pregnancy. Five cases of exposure to **enfuvirtide** did not result in birth defects.[18] **Tenofovir** decreased fetal growth and bone porosity in animals. Similar effects in human pregnancies have not been reported.[18,72]

ANTIVIRAL DRUGS

Maternal **acyclovir** has not been shown to cause malformations[18,77,78] and is recommended for various infections during pregnancy. **Valacyclovir** use after the 36 wk of gestation for treatment of recurrent genital herpes has yielded some data suggesting safety.[79,80] Some suggest valacyclovir

(continued)

ANTIMICROBIAL DRUGS

use for primary and recurrent genital herpes during pregnancy.[81,82] There are limited data concerning **famciclovir** use during pregnancy.

β-LACTAMS

Cephalosporins and **penicillins** are thought to be without teratogenic risk.[18,83,84] Treatment of early syphilis with penicillin (or other drugs) during pregnancy might produce the Jarisch-Herxheimer reaction, resulting in uterine cramping, decreased fetal movement, and, in some cases, fetal death.[85]

FLUOROQUINOLONES

Fluoroquinolones (e.g., **ciprofloxacin, norfloxacin, ofloxacin, levofloxacin, gemifloxacin, moxifloxacin**) cause cartilage erosion in weight-bearing joints of immature animals.[18,84] Data have not shown this effect in humans.[18,84] The rate of malformations documented with ciprofloxacin, ofloxacin, and norfloxacin is similar to the expected background rate.[18,84] No pattern of defects is apparent, but hypospadias, skeletal dysplasias, cardiac anomalies, and other defects have been repoted.[18] There are no data on the use of gemifloxacin, levofloxacin, or moxifloxacin during pregnancy.

MACROLIDES

There is no evidence that **erythromycin** is harmful to the fetus.[18,84] Approximately 10% of women treated with **erythromycin estolate** in the second-trimester develop elevated serum AST levels that normalize when therapy is discontinued[18]; other derivatives are preferred. Preliminary studies of women exposed to **clarithromycin** during pregnancy show no increased risk of anomalies despite evidence of teratogenicity and risk in animals.[18,84,86] A prospective study in 157 pregnant women exposed to clarithromycin (122 in first trimester) found no differences in the rate of major malformations when compared to matched controls.[87] A retrospective surveillance study of 149 infants with first-trimester exposure to clarithromycin found no difference in rate of major malformation compared to the expected background rate.[88] In 123 pregnant women exposed to **azithromycin** (88 in first-trimester), the rate of major malformations and spontaneous abortions was not different from matched controls.[89]

SULFONAMIDES

There are occasional reports of abnormalities, but no malformation pattern has emerged. Evidence associating sulfonamide use near term with neonatal kernicterus is lacking, despite sulfonamide displacement of bilirubin from albumin-binding sites.[18,84] There is a theoretical risk for hemolysis in the fetus or neonate because of its relative deficiencies in G-6-PD and glutathione.[18,84]

TETRACYCLINES

Tetracyclines can cause permanent yellow-brown staining of the teeth when taken after 4–5 mo of gestation when calcification of the teeth begins.[18,84,90] **Doxycycline** might be less likely to discolor enamel.[84] Early reports of depressed fetal bone growth have not been confirmed in larger surveillance studies. Pregnant women with pyelonephritis or underlying renal disease or receiving high doses are at risk for developing acute fatty necrosis of the liver and azotemia, putting the fetus at risk for still or premature birth.[18,90] First-trimester use of **oxytetracycline** caused neural tube defects, cleft palate, and cardiovascular defects in a recent retrospective study.[18,84] Avoid use of tetracycline antibiotics in pregnant women.

MISCELLANEOUS ANTIMICROBIALS

Chloramphenicol

Although reports of fetal abnormality or toxicity from maternal chloramphenicol are lacking, there is a theoretical risk of blood dyscrasias. Particular caution should be exercised near term because

(continued)

ANTIMICROBIAL DRUGS

of the "gray baby" syndrome, the result of toxic accumulation of chloramphenicol in neonates caused by their slow elimination of the drug.[18,91]

Clindamycin

Available data do not support a link between clindamycin and birth defects after administration during the first-trimester.[18,84] Although it has been used during the second trimester to prevent preterm birth resulting from bacterial vaginosis, recent studies have not found a benefit.[92,93]

Daptomycin

Two cases of daptomycin use in pregnancy are published. In the first, a woman of 27 wk gestation received daptomycin for 14 d. The patient delivered prematurely at 35 wk; no adverse neonatal effects were observed.[94] A 1-wk course of daptomycin was given to a woman in her third-trimester; no neonatal outcomes were reported.[95]

Linezolid

No data are available regarding the use of linezolid during pregnancy. Reserve for use when maternal benefit outweighs fetal risk.

Metronidazole

Almost 40 y of experience and several studies demonstrate no definitive association of metronidazole with congenital malformations, abortions, or stillbirths.[18,84] However, a few cases of facial clefting have been reported.[84]

Nitrofurantoin

No fetal abnormalities or neonatal hemolytic anemia have been observed with nitrofurantoin use during pregnancy.[18,84] A theoretical risk for the development of hemolysis in neonates exists if the drug is taken by mothers near term because of infants' relative G-6-PD and glutathione deficiencies.[18,84]

Quinupristin/Dalfopristin

No data are available regarding the use of quinupristin/dalfopristin during pregnancy. Reserve for use when maternal benefit exceeds fetal risk.

Trimethoprim

Because it is a folate antagonist, caution is advised with trimethoprim use in pregnancy.[18,96] (*See* Methotrexate and Pyrimethamine.) While some data suggest a lack of teratogenicity, recent evidence links trimethoprim use in the first trimester to neural tube defects, oral clefts, and congenital heart defects.[18,96–99] Supplementation with folic acid may reduce the risk.

Vancomycin

There is a theoretical risk for auditory and renal toxicity in the fetus. However, in one small prospective trial, IV vancomycin during the second or third trimester produced no cases of fetal renal toxicity or hearing impairment.[18,84]

ANTINEOPLASTICS AND IMMUNOSUPPRESSANTS

ANTINEOPLASTICS

Antineoplastic agents have teratogenic and mutagenic potential, and reports of infertility and congenital defects exist. Male and female fertility is affected by antineoplastic agents. The extent depends on the type and cumulative dose received.[100] Although aggressive treatment of malignancy is necessary on occasion, avoidance or minimum use of these drugs, especially during the first-trimester, is recommended because of minimal reports of teratogenicity and spontaneous abortion.[101,102] However, normal pregnancy outcome has occurred, particularly if exposure is early

(*continued*)

ANTINEOPLASTICS AND IMMUNOSUPPRESSANTS

in gestation (first 2 wk after conception).[102] Chemotherapeutic exposure during the second and third trimester generally produces a decrease in birth weight and increases the risk of IUGR.[102] Use of antineoplastics after 35 wk might cause spontaneous delivery to occur before recovery of neonatal bone marrow suppression because the drugs might not have been eliminated before delivery.[102] Chemotherapy-induced tumors in the infant are a theoretical possibility.

ALKYLATING AGENTS

Busulfan

Use during pregnancy has been associated with IUGR and multiple malformations, although no specific pattern is evident.

Chlorambucil

Treatment in the first and second trimesters can cause spontaneous abortion, cleft palate, renal agenesis, or skeletal abnormalities.[18,25,103] There also have been reports of normal pregnancy.[104]

Cyclophosphamide, Ifosfamide

Use in the first-trimester has resulted in fetal malformations, particularly of the toes, syndactyly, cleft palate, facial anomalies, IUGR, and possible developmental delay. The overall risk of malformation is estimated to be 16%–22%.[25,102] No malformations have been reported with second- or third-trimester use, but pancytopenia occurred in neonates exposed late in pregnancy.[18] A report of malignancies in a child that occurred 10 and 14 y after exposure in utero raises the question of whether intrauterine exposure to cyclophosphamide can cause iatrogenic or secondary cancers.[102] Second-trimester exposure to ifosfamide resulted in fetal growth cessation, absence of amniotic fluid, and intraventricular hemorrhage. Seven days after emergency cesarian section, the infant died.[10] Another report of ifosfamide exposure beginning in the second trimester resulted in mild IUGR.[105] Exposure to 3 courses of ifosfamide in the third trimester resulted in an infant with mild IUGR, that otherwise healthy.[106] Cyclophosphamide and ifosfamide should be avoided in pregnancy.

Procarbazine, Dacarbazine

Use in pregnancy is limited, but several fetal abnormalities have occurred, all with first-trimester exposure. There is one report of procarbazine administration for 30 d starting in the 12th wk of pregnancy; a healthy infant was delivered at term.[18] There is little experience with dacarbazine during pregnancy. A total of 19 patients exposed to dacarbazine resulted in one case of IUGR and one case of syndactyly.[102]

ANTIMETABOLITES

Cytarabine

Cytarabine can cause IUGR, intrauterine fetal death (IUFD), chromosomal abnormalities, and congenital anomalies including limb and auditory canal defects.[18,102] Reports of normal infants exposed to cytarabine in utero exist.[18]

Fluorouracil

Use can cause malformations consistent with inhibition of cell division and cell growth as well as IUGR and IUFD.[18,102] Inadvertent first-trimester topical administration of 5% fluorouracil to the lower genital tract resulted in normal-appearing infants in 12 pregnancies.[107–109] However, cleft palate, ventricular septal defect, and spontaneous abortions have been reported with topical and mucous membrane application.[18]

Methotrexate

Use in the first trimester at doses above 10 mg/wk causes methotrexate embryopathy which consists of IUGR, cranial anomalies, limb abnormalities, growth retardation, and developmental

(*continued*)

ANTINEOPLASTICS AND IMMUNOSUPPRESSANTS

abnormalities.[18,25,26,102] Spontaneous abortions may occur, but normal pregnancy outcome has occurred after second- and third-trimester use.[25,26] Methotrexate should be discontinued for 3–4 mo before conception and the mother should be taking folic acid.[25,110,111]

Thioguanine

Use in the first and second trimesters has been associated with chromosomal and congenital abnormalities.[18]

DNA INTERCALATING DRUGS

Anthracycline-induced cardiomyopathy in the fetus may occur, although infants without cardiomyopathy have been delivered.[112] **Daunorubicin** and **doxorubicin** have been given without resultant fetal malformation, although some spontaneous abortions, IUGR, and IUFD have occurred.[102] Premature delivery and transient bone marrow suppression have been reported. **Dactinomycin** use during the second- or third-trimester in 6 pregnancies resulted in normal infants.[18] Data regarding the use of **idarubicin** and epirubicin during pregnancy are limited; **doxorubicin** is preferred if considered equally effective.[102]

VINCA ALKALOIDS

Most case reports of **vinblastine** and **vincristine** use during pregnancy describe a lack of congenital malformations.[18,103] However, secundum atrial septal defect resulting in neonatal death, IUGR, and spontaneous abortion have occurred.[18,102] **Vinorelbine** use in a limited number of patients did not result in malformations.[18,113]

IMMUNOSUPPRESSANTS

Azathioprine

Azathioprine (and 6-mercaptopurine) are not converted to active metabolites because the fetal liver lacks the required enzyme.[111] Normal pregnancy outcome has occurred with azathioprine taken for immunosuppression for transplantation, inflammatory bowel disease, and systemic lupus erythematosus.[18,110,114] However, IUGR, neonatal lymphopenia, hypogammaglobulinemia, thymic hypoplasia, fetal bone marrow suppression, leukopenia, and thrombocytopenia have occurred.[114] Older studies showed some chromosomal aberrations; however, there is no evidence of permanent genomal or gonadal damage.

Cyclosporine

Use of cyclosporine throughout pregnancy after renal or hepatic transplant does not appear to cause malformations, although experience is limited.[111] IUGR has occurred; however, normal size for gestational age infants are often delivered.[18,115] No neonatal distress or increased mortality has been reported.

Mycophenolate

Mycophenolate is teratogenic and has caused cleft lip and palate, facial abnormalities, limb defects, and defects of the heart, kidneys, and esophagus.[18,111] Many patients are switched to azathioprine if pregnancy is detected.[115]

Sirolimus

Experience with sirolimus use during pregnancy is limited. A few cases of normal pregnancies exist.[18,116]

(continued)

ANTINEOPLASTICS AND IMMUNOSUPPRESSANTS

Tacrolimus

Registry data indicate that use in pregnancy causes miscarriage (22%), low birth weight (53%), prematurity (55%), and stillbirth (3%); all of which are higher than background rates.[117] The risk for congenital malformations appears low.[18]

CARDIOVASCULAR DRUGS

ANTIARRHYTHMIC DRUGS

Amiodarone

Neonatal hypothyroidism with and without goiter and hyperthyroidism have occurred with amiodarone use.[18,118] Neonatal hypothyroidism appears more common than hyperthyroidism, affecting 23% (16/69) infants compared to 2.8% (2/69).[118] Neurodevelopmental delays have been reported anecdotally.[118]

Digoxin

Digoxin is not a teratogen. Maternal digitalis toxicity can cause fetal toxicity, miscarriage, and infant death.[18,119] As pregnancy progresses, renal clearance of digoxin increases lowering serum concentrations by 50%.[119] Therefore, maternal serum concentrations might fluctuate and should be monitored.

Disopyramide

Use during pregnancy has not been well studied, but in one report, uterine contractions precipitated by disopyramide subsided when the drug was discontinued.[18,110]

Lidocaine

Lidocaine does not appear to cause congenital malformations, but can cause fetal bradycardia, decrease placental blood flow, and increase myometrial tone.[18,119]

Procainamide

Even when used during the first-trimester, procainamide does not appear teratogenic.[18,119] However, because of the potential for SLE, caution is advised.[119]

Quinidine

Quinidine is not teratogenic. It can cause uterine contractions; this effect is not usually observed at therapeutic doses. Neonatal thrombocytopenia has occurred after maternal use of quinidine.[18,119]

ANTIHYPERTENSIVE DRUGS

α_1-Adrenergic Antagonists

Prazosin and **phenoxybenzamine** are used during pregnancy for hypertension associated with pheochromocytoma.[120] In a controlled trial, 153 women with hypertension were randomized to receive either prazosin or nifedipine in addition to methyldopa. A total of 71 women received prazosin. More pulmonary edema and intrauterine deaths occurred in the prazosin group.[121]

α_2-Adrenergic Agonists

Most clinicians consider **methyldopa** the drug of choice to treat hypertension in pregnancy.[120,122] Available data show no teratogenicity. Experience using **clonidine** during the first trimester is limited although no reports of congenital defects during any trimester are published. In a small study, 22 neonates exposed to clonidine developed sleep disturbance.[120]

ACE Inhibitors

Use of ACE inhibitors during the second and third trimesters causes oligohydramnios, IUGR, pulmonary hypoplasia, joint contractures, hypocalvaria (malformed skull dome), and neonatal anuric renal failure (some cases resulting in fetal death).[120,123] Renal dysgenesis can also

(*continued*)

CARDIOVASCULAR DRUGS

occur.[120,123] Evidence of first-trimester risk was found in an analysis of 29,507 pregnancies. Of those, 209 were exposed to ACE inhibitors, 202 were exposed to other antihypertensive agents, and 29,096 had no exposure. Risk of major congenital malformation was 2.71 (95% CI, 1.71–4.27) and 0.66 (0.25–1.75) for ACE inhibitor use and other antihypertensive used compared to no exposure, respectively. The increase in risk was attributed to effects in the cardiovascular and central nervous systems (e.g., atrial and ventricular septal defect, patent ductus arteriosus, spina bifida, microcephaly). Avoid use of ACE inhibitors during pregnancy.

Angiotensin II Receptor Blockers

Emerging evidence suggests a teratogenicity profile similar to the ACE inhibitors.[18,120,124] Out of 47 reports of ARB use in the first-trimester, 37 were normal infants while 2 fetal deaths, 5 spontaneous abortions, and 3 congenital anomalies (e.g., patent ductus arteriosus, anencephaly, IUGR, cleft palate, renal tubular dysplasia, craniofacial defects) occurred.[125] In 20 reported cases of second- and third-trimester use, oligohydramnios (n = 17), neonatal anuria (12 of 15 live births), renal dysgenesis (n = 9), and pulmonary hypoplasia (n = 3) occurred.[125] Renal failure leading to fetal death has also been reported.[120] Avoid use of ARBs during pregnancy.

β-ADRENERGIC BLOCKING DRUGS

β-Blockers such as **acebutolol, pindolol, metoprolol, labetalol**, and **propranolol** are not associated with congenital anomalies and are generally safe in pregnancy.[120,122] Maternal hypertension can cause IUGR, decreased placental size, neonatal respiratory depression, and hypoglycemia. IUGR and neonatal hypoglycemia and hypotension have occurred after taking β-blockers. Whether these effects are caused by the drugs or maternal disease is not known although evidence suggests an association between β-blocker use and IUGR.[126] Neonatal bradycardia might be caused by these agents, but is usually mild.[120] The association between **atenolol** and decreased IUGR and placental weight is stronger than for other antihypertensives, including other β-blockers.[120,122] No reports of carvedilol use in pregnancy exist. Increasingly, labetalol given intravenously is preferred over **hydralazine** for control of severe hypertension because of fewer adverse effects.[120]

CALCIUM CHANNEL BLOCKING DRUGS

No malformations have been associated with the use of **nifedipine** and **verapamil**.[120,122] Lesser evidence suggests a lack of teratogenicity with other agents (i.e., **amlodipine, diltiazem, felodipine, isradipine, nicardipine, nisoldipine**).[127,128] Nifedipine and nicardipine have been used as tocolytic agents.[129]

INOTROPIC DRUGS

The treatment of hypotension during pregnancy with sympathomimetic agents (e.g., **dopamine, dobutamine, norepinephrine**) is complicated by the fact that the uterine vasculature is supplied solely with α-adrenergic receptors and is maximally dilated under basal conditions. Pure α-adrenergic agents markedly constrict uterine vessels and decrease blood flow, thereby compromising the fetus; β-adrenergic agents cause peripheral vasodilation and tend to shunt blood away from the uterus and also can cause fetal compromise. Volume-expanding agents seem to be the most prudent treatment for sudden hypotension in pregnancy.

Vasodilators

Hydralazine is not associated with congenital anomalies.[120] Use in pregnancy can affect uteroplacental blood flow and fetal heart rate after acute administration. Neonatal thrombocytopenia and drug-induced lupus have also been reported.[18,120]

(continued)

CENTRAL NERVOUS SYSTEM DRUGS

ANTICONVULSANTS

Congenital malformations have been reported in children of women with epilepsy, and all anticonvulsants for which data are adequate have been implicated as possible causes of malformations. Mothers with epilepsy have an incidence of fetal malformation 2–3 times higher compared to mothers without epilepsy, and anticonvulsant drugs appear to increase these frequencies.[130] Major malformations are more common after combination therapy than with monotherapy.[131] Inherited fetal deficiency of epoxide hydrolase, a major enzyme in the metabolic pathway of many anticonvulsants (e.g., **carbamazepine, phenytoin,** and **valproic acid**) that helps eliminate toxic intermediates, might mediate teratogenic effects.[132] Total and free concentrations of carbamazepine, phenytoin, and *phenobarbital* decline as pregnancy progresses, caused by changes in plasma protein binding, metabolizing capacity, increased volume of distribution, and changes in absorption.[130] Free concentrations of valproic acid increase.[18] Measurement of free anticonvulsant drug concentrations allows for appropriate dosage adjustment. Decreased folic acid concentrations have been linked with neural tube defects in the general population and in women with epilepsy receiving antiepileptic drugs.[130] Folic acid supplementation (e.g., 4 mg/d) during pregnancy might decrease the risk of abnormal offspring.

Carbamazepine

Carbamazepine is associated with a 0.5%–1% risk of spina bifida.[133] Malformations similar to those ascribed to other anticonvulsants also have been reported: specific facial features, nail hypoplasia, and small head circumference. Data concerning developmental delay or impairment require substantiation.[18,133] Mothers receiving carbamazepine should receive supplemental folic acid.

Gabapentin

There is little information about gabapentin in pregnancy. Rates of malformations and fetal and maternal adverse effects were similar to the expected background rates in 44 live births.[134] However, of 30 gabapentin exposures, one resulted in a major malformation (bilateral abnormally positioned fifth digit and prominent eyelid folds), 2 had anticonvulsant facies, and 2 had neurologic abnormalities.[135]

Lamotrigine

In the manufacturer's registry, congenital malformations occurred in 2.9% (26/908) infants whose mothers took lamotrigine during pregnancy.[18,130] Reported rates of malformation range from 0% to 4.4%.[130,136] Lamotrigine may have a lower risk of teratogenicity compared with other anticonvulsants; however, a recent association with oral clefts is concerning.[137]

Levetiracetam

Reports of levetiracetam use during pregnancy are limited. No malformations were reported in 39 monotherapy exposures.[130,133] Of 11 women who took the drug during pregnancy, 9 infants were born without defects; however, birth weight was low to very low in 3 infants.[138] One spontaneous and one elective abortion accounted for the remaining two pregnancies. A larger report of 117 pregnancies exposed to levetiracetam found an abnormality in 8 infants, with a major congenital malformation occurring in 3 (2.7%) infants (2 spina bifida, 1 pyloric stenosis; all occurred with polytherapy).[139]

Oxcarbazepine

Oxcarbazepine is structurally similar to carbamazepine. A review of 248 pregnancies exposed to oxcarbazepine monotherapy and 61 to polytherapy with other antiepileptic drugs found 6 malformations (2.4%) with monotherapy and 4 (6.6%) with polytherapy.[130,133] Folic acid supplementation should be given with oxcarbazepine.

(continued)

CENTRAL NERVOUS SYSTEM DRUGS

Phenobarbital

Although causality was previously questioned, it is now accepted that phenobarbital use during pregnancy increases the risk for oral clefts and cardiovascular malformations.[136] It can also cause reduced birth weight, decreased head circumference and impaired cognitive abilities.[18,136] Craniofacial abnormalities have also been reported.[18,136] Phenobarbital can lead to decreased folic acid levels; mothers should receive folic acid supplementation.[18] Barbiturates can cause a decrease in vitamin K–dependent clotting factors, leading to bleeding in the newborn.[18] Neonatal withdrawal can occur after phenobarbital use during pregnancy.

Phenytoin

Phenytoin is a teratogen that causes a number of anomalies such as heart defects and facial clefts. It also can cause a cluster of anomalies called the fetal hydantoin syndrome (FHS), the principal features of which are craniofacial anomalies (e.g., bowed upper lip, ocular hypertelorism, broad nasal bridge, short nose, epicanthal folds), digital hypoplasia with small or absent nails, and pre- and postnatal growth deficiency.[18,136] The risk of developing FHS is approximately 10% when phenytoin is taken throughout pregnancy.[136] Maternal phenytoin use also can result in developmental delay and intellectual impairment.[136] Phenytoin can cause a decrease in vitamin K–dependent clotting factors, leading to bleeding in the newborn as well as decreases in folic acid levels.[18] Mothers taking phenytoin should receive folic acid supplementation.

Valproic Acid

Of the antiepileptic agents, valproic acid and its derivatives appear the most teratogenic. Major congenital anomalies are 4 times more likely to occur with valproic acid monotherapy than with any other antiepileptic agent.[136,140] Neural tube defects (e.g., spina bifida) occur in 1%–2% of valproic acid–exposed fetuses.[136] The risk for neural tube defects might be 10- to 20-fold higher with valproic acid compared with the background frequency.[136] Risk appears to increase with increasing serum levels; therefore, serum concentrations should be kept as low as possible during pregnancy and the mother should be given supplemental folic acid.[18] Fetal valproate syndrome has been described and involves craniofacial anomalies, digital anomalies, urogenital defects (e.g., hypospadias), and developmental delay.[18,140] Multiple other defects have been reported, including cardiovascular abnormalities. Mothers taking valproic acid should receive folic acid supplementation. Valproic acid has also been associated with autism and autistic spectrum disorders.[18,136,140]

ANTIDEPRESSANTS

Serotonin Norepinephrine Reuptake Inhibitors

No evidence suggests that **venlafaxine** is a teratogen.[18,141,142] A prospective, controlled study compared pregnancy outcomes of women exposed to venlafaxine, other selective serotonin reuptake inhibitors (SSRIs), or other nonteratogenic agents (150 outcomes evaluated in each group).[18,141,142] No difference was observed in spontaneous abortions, live births, birth weight, gestational age, or congenital malformations. Use of venlafaxine in the third-trimester can cause postnatal complications such as respiratory distress, cyanosis, apnea, symptoms of withdrawal, or potentially serotonin syndrome. Data on **duloxetine** use in pregnancy are limited. One case described poor neonatal adaptation after duloxetine use at least during the third trimester with symptoms similar to those seen with venlafaxine.[143] Respiration at birth was minimal, requiring transfer to intensive care. On day 3, the infant began having jerky movements and twitching. EEG on day 7 suggested subclinical seizures. By week 7 the infant had no seizure activity. At 2 y, the child was developing normally.

(continued)

CENTRAL NERVOUS SYSTEM DRUGS

Selective Serotonin Reuptake Inhibitors

With the exception of paroxetine, the SSRIs do not appear teratogenic.[141,142] First-trimester use of **paroxetine** increases the risk of congenital malformations by almost 2 times. Cardiac malformations, most often atrial or ventricular septal defect, are increased with paroxetine by 1.5- to 2-fold.[18,141,142] SSRI use during pregnancy is linked to increases in premature birth, low birth weight, spontaneous abortion, and persistent pulmonary hypertension of the newborn.[18,142] Neonatal adaptation syndrome has been reported with third-trimester use of SSRIs. Symptoms are respiratory distress, restlessness, irritability, crying, tremors, increased muscle tone, poor feeding, and sleep disturbance.[18,142] On the basis of limited data, neurodevelopment does not appear substantially affected.[142]

Tricyclic Antidepressants

Although there are several case reports of different fetal anomalies after maternal use of tricyclic antidepressants (TCAs) during pregnancy, no consistent pattern of malformation has been observed and they are not considered to pose a teratogenic risk. Maternal use of TCAs during pregnancy occasionally has produced neonatal symptoms of breathlessness, respiratory distress, and hypertonia with tremor, clonus, spasm, cyanosis, tachypnea, irritability, and feeding difficulties. Neurodevelopmental assessments of offspring exposed in utero do not show abnormalities.[144]

ANTIPSYCHOTIC DRUGS

There is some evidence that women with psychoses can have preterm delivery, low-birth-weight infants, and small for gestational age infants.[145] An increased risk of cardiac malformations[146] and occurrence of fetal malformation twice that seen in the general population[147] has been documented.

Atypical Antipsychotics

In general, there are little data regarding the use of atypical antipsychotics during pregnancy. Folic acid supplementation (e.g., 4 mg/d) should be considered. Limited evidence suggests that **clozapine** does not cause congenital malformations.[147] However, spontaneous abortion, floppy infant syndrome, and low birth weight have been reported.[145,148] Data from 144 pregnancies in the **olanzapine** pregnancy registry found no increases in the risk of spontaneous abortions, stillbirths, or premature deliveries compared to background risk; however, malformations occurred in 6 (4.2%) cases.[147] Cases of major fetal malformations, gestational metabolic complications, and neurodevelopmental impairment have been reported.[148] A report generated from pregnancy registry data found that of 53 prospectively followed pregnancies exposed to **risperidone** with known outcomes, organ malformations and spontaneous abortions occurred in 2 (3.8%) and 9 (15.9%), respectively, both within expected background rates.[149]

Typical Antipsychotics

Most data do not implicate **phenothiazines** or **haloperidol** as teratogens.[18,145,147,148] Phenothiazine use near term can result in extrapyramidal effects and withdrawal reactions in the neonate. If drug therapy is necessary during pregnancy, high-potency agents (e.g., **haloperidol, fluphenazine**) are preferred to low-potency agents (e.g., **chlorpromazine, thioridazine**) because the latter can cause maternal hypotension.[18,147]

ANXIOLYTICS, SEDATIVES, AND HYPNOTICS

High dosages of any sedative-hypnotic close to or during delivery can result in neonatal CNS and respiratory depression.

Barbiturates

First-trimester use of **butalbital, pentobarbital,** or **secobarbital** has not been associated with defects.[18] Barbiturate addiction during pregnancy can result in neonatal withdrawal. (*See* Anticonvulsants and Phenobarbital.)

(*continued*)

CENTRAL NERVOUS SYSTEM DRUGS

Benzodiazepines

Recent data do not support a previously reported association between **diazepam** or **chlordiazepoxide** and oral clefting.[150,151] Benzodiazepines can cause preterm birth and low birth weight after early and late exposure, but do not appear strongly correlated with teratogenicity.[18,150,152] Infants of mothers using benzodiazepines near term might exhibit withdrawal symptoms (including tremors, irritability, and hypertonicity) and cardiovascular, respiratory, and CNS effects consistent with benzodiazepine pharmacology. Many exhibit the "floppy baby syndrome" characterized by muscular relaxation, poor sucking, disturbances in thermoregulation, and regurgitation.[18,153] **Oxazepam, lorazepam,** and **temazepam** are short acting and predominantly metabolized into inactive glucuronides and subsequently excreted by the kidneys; therefore, they might be preferred to diazepam, although irritability, feeding difficulties, respiratory depression, and muscle tone disorders have been reported with lorazepam, and temazepam is rated pregnancy category X by the manufacturer.[18,153] It is not known if benzodiazepines cause behavioral abnormalities after prolonged intrauterine exposure.

LITHIUM

Lithium use during the first-trimester of pregnancy increases the risk of cardiovascular abnormalities, including Ebstein's anomaly.[154–156] Although the relative risk of Ebstein's anomaly compared to the general population is elevated (1:20,000 vs. 1–2:1000), the absolute risk is small.[155] Of 225 infants included in the lithium registry, 18 (8%) had cardiac malformations, 6 with Ebstein's anomaly.[154] Other anomalies as well as macrosomia have been reported.[18,155] Lithium has also caused fetal loss and premature delivery.[156] Symptoms of lithium toxicity, including lethargy, hypotonia, poor sucking reflex, respiratory distress, cyanosis, arrhythmias, and thyroid depression with goiter and hypothermia, have been reported in newborns of women receiving lithium therapy near term.[18,155,156] Monitor maternal serum concentrations frequently during pregnancy because lithium clearance changes as pregnancy progresses.[155,156]

GASTROINTESTINAL DRUGS

ACID–PEPTIC THERAPY

Antacids

Available data do not suggest teratogenicity for commonly used antacids (aluminum, magnesium, calcium salts).[157,158] Long-term administration, however, is not recommended because of the potential toxicity.[157] Sodium bicarbonate should be avoided because of the potential for fluid overload and metabolic alkalosis.[159]

Histamine H2-Receptor Antagonists

No reports link **cimetidine, famotidine,** or **ranitidine** to adverse pregnancy outcome.[18,157,158] Less data are available for **nizatidine**, although increased risk is not expected.[18] Cimetidine possesses antiandrogenic properties in animals and adults; some recommend avoiding cimetidine during pregnancy.[18,158]

Proton Pump Inhibitors

The majority of safety data available for proton pump inhibitors concerns omeprazole. **Omeprazole** does not appear teratogenic.[18,159,160] Of 534 patients exposed to omeprazole compared to nonexposed controls, the relative risk for malformations was 1.05 (95% CI, 0.59–1.85).[161] In 62 pregnancies exposed to **lansoprazole,** the rate of major congenital malformations was not different than in controls (3.9% [2/51] vs. 3.8% [30/792], respectively).[160,162] The same study evaluated 53 pregnancies exposed to **pantoprazole**. Major congenital

(continued)

GASTROINTESTINAL DRUGS

malformations were 2.1% (1/48) with pantoprazole, which was not different compared to the control rate of 3.8%.[160,162]

Sucralfate

No adequate studies exist on the use of sucralfate in pregnant women. Because little drug is absorbed, little risk is expected.[18,159]

ANTIEMETICS

Studies of women with nausea and vomiting of pregnancy (NVP) treated with **metoclopramide** or **prochlorperazine** demonstrate no increased risk for malformations or neonatal problems.[18,163,164] Of the selective serotonin subtype 3 (5-HT$_3$) receptor antagonists, only **ondansetron** has published data on use during pregnancy. A study evaluating 176 pregnancies exposed to ondansetron found no differences between ondansetron or other antiemetics and controls for live births, miscarriage, stillbirth, major malformations, birth weight, or gestational age.[165] Compared with other drugs used in NVP, there is relatively little experience with ondansetron. Antihistamines used for pregnancy-induced emesis **(dimenhydrinate, diphenhydramine, doxylamine, meclizine)** are not considered teratogens; however, use during the last 2 wk of pregnancy has been associated with retinopathy of prematurity.[18,163,164,166] Uterine stimulation and fetal distress resulting from the oxytocic effects of dimenhydrinate have been reported.[18] (*See* Antihistamines.)

MISCELLANEOUS GASTROINTESTINAL DRUGS

Mesalamine Derivatives

Mesalamine derivatives including **sulfasalazine** have not been associated with teratogenic risk.[18,167] Compared to women without inflammatory bowel disease, women with inflammatory bowel disease are at an increased risk of premature delivery, having low birth weight infants and requiring cesarean section.[167] It is not clear, however, if the drugs or the disease for which they are used contribute adverse effects such as low birth weight. (*See also* Antimicrobial Drugs, Sulfonamides.)

HEMATOLOGIC DRUGS

COAGULANTS AND ANTICOAGULANTS

Heparin

Heparin does not cross the placenta because of its large molecular weight and has not been associated with an increased risk for structural or functional defects, IUGR, or fetal bleeding.[18,168] However, maternal thrombocytopenia and hemorrhage can occur.

Low-Molecular-Weight Heparins

Low-molecular-weight heparins do not cross the placenta and do not pose a teratogenic risk.[18,168] Maternal thrombocytopenia and hemorrhage can occur.

Other Anticoagulants

Danaparoid does not appear to cross the placenta, as demonstrated by a lack of detectable anti-Xa activity in fetal cord plasma. It has been used successfully in cases of heparin-induced thrombocytopenia (HIT), although the evidence supporting its use is limited.[18,168] Although **fondaparinux** does not appear to cross the placenta, it has been found in fetal cord plasma.[18,168] Its use should be reserved for women with HIT who cannot tolerate danaparoid.

(continued)

HEMATOLOGIC DRUGS

Warfarin

Warfarin and related anticoagulants can produce the fetal warfarin syndrome or warfarin embryopathy. The critical period of risk appears to be between 6 and 12 wk of gestation. Features include nasal hypoplasia, neonatal respiratory distress from upper airway obstruction, stippled epiphyses, IUGR, and different degrees of hypoplasia of the extremities. Eye abnormalities, including blindness, have also been reported. Approximately one-third of exposed cases result in adverse pregnancy outcomes.[18,168] CNS defects appear to occur independent of the fetal warfarin syndrome. Critical periods of risk for CNS effects appear to be during the second and third trimesters.[168] Warfarin also increases the risk for fetal and maternal hemorrhage, especially when used near term.

HORMONAL DRUGS

ADRENAL HORMONES

Although corticosteroids do not represent a major teratogenic risk, an increased risk of oral clefts, consistent with animal studies, has been demonstrated after first-trimester use of corticosteroids.[18,169,170] Some studies show decreased birth weight and increased rates of prematurity, although these effects might have been due to underlying maternal disease.[169] Women who had status asthmaticus during pregnancy were more likely to have infants with low birth weight or IUGR.[169] Use of corticosteroids during pregnancy does not appear to increase the risk of adverse events, except in women with gestational diabetes and endometritis.[170] A placental enzyme (11-β-OH-dehydrogenase) inactivates certain corticosteroids, leading to low fetal concentrations. This inactivation is greater with **hydrocortisone, prednisone, prednisolone,** and **methylprednisolone** than with **betamethasone, beclomethasone,** or **dexamethasone**.[18,171] The fetal liver is relatively ineffective in converting prednisone into the active prednisolone, even at term. Therefore, prednisone or hydrocortisone might be preferred during pregnancy. Neonates born to women taking long-term corticosteroids should be monitored for adrenal insufficiency, although this rarely occurs. Corticosteroids (e.g., betamethasone, dexamethasone) are used to prevent respiratory distress in infants born between 28 and 34 wk of gestation, with no apparent adverse effects.[172]

ANTIDIABETIC DRUGS

Poor glucose control in women with diabetes increases the rate of congenital malformations. Poorly controlled diabetes causes macrosomia, perinatal death, and increased trauma during birth.[173–175] Oral antidiabetic agents are typically avoided during pregnancy because of the risk for fetal and neonatal hypoglycemia.[173] **Glipizide** does not cross the placenta as readily as first-generation sulfonylureas, and **glyburide** does not cross in appreciable amounts.[18,174] A meta-analysis of 745 women treated with glyburide and 637 treated with insulin for diabetes during pregnancy found no differences in macrosomia, low birth weight, prematurity, neonatal hypoglycemia, or ICU admission.[173] However, one study found an increased risk of preeclampsia and neonatal need for phototherapy with glyburide compared to insulin.[176] An analysis comparing sulfonylureas and metformin found no difference in the rate of major malformation after first-trimester use compared to controls.[175] First-trimester use of **metformin** does not appear to cause major malformations or cause neonatal hypoglycemia, respiratory distress, or prematurity.[18,177,178] Avoid use of **thiazolidinediones** during pregnancy as experience is limited. Pregnant women with diabetes should be treated with **insulin** since it does not cross the placenta.[18,174]

(continued)

HORMONAL DRUGS

FEMALE SEX HORMONES

Estrogens

Although considered contraindicated during pregnancy,[18] there is some epidemiologic evidence that estrogens do not increase the risk of congenital anomalies or external genital effects.[18,179] However, estrogens can feminize male fetuses. Diethylstilbestrol (DES), well known to cause genital tract anomalies and vaginal adenocarcinoma, is no longer marketed.[18,179]

Progestins

Progesterone is routinely used as part of in vitro fertilization protocols for luteal support.[179] Progestins do not appear to cause nongenital malformations.[180] Hypospadias have occurred in males, most likely occurring during the period of external genitalia development (8–12 wk postconception).[18,179] High doses of progestins (e.g., **medroxyprogesterone, norethindrone**) during pregnancy can cause masculinization of female external genitalia because of weakly androgenic effects. Inadvertent exposure to normal doses used for contraception does not appear to cause major malformations.[18]

THYROID AND ANTITHYROID DRUGS

Propylthiouracil (PTU) and **methimazole** are not considered major human teratogens.[18] Both drugs have been associated with aplasia cutis (a fetal scalp defect) and neonatal goiter.[18,181,182] Although it was earlier thought that PTU crossed the placenta to a lesser extent than methimazole, this has been disproven.[181,183] Transient neonatal hypothyroidism and neonatal thyrotoxicosis can occur. Hypothyroidism can be prevented by discontinuing the drug at 36–37 wk gestation if the mother has remained euthyroid.[182] Uncontrolled hyperthyroidism in pregnancy can cause preterm labor, preeclampsia, IUGR, and increased maternal and perinatal mortality.[182] No adverse effects have been reported after inadvertent exposure to I^{131} before 10 wk of gestation.[182] After 10 wk of gestation, the fetal thyroid actively concentrates iodine; any radioactive iodine ingested by the mother will cross the placenta and destroy fetal thyroid tissue.[18]

Untreated hypothyroidism increases the risk for miscarriage, preeclampsia, IUGR, placental abruption, perinatal mortality, and neonatal morbidity.[182] Thyroid hormones (**levothyroxine, liothyronine**) may be used during pregnancy for the treatment of hypothyroidism.[18]

MISCELLANEOUS HORMONAL AGENTS

Oxytocin

Oxytocin given for induction of labor can cause tetanic uterine contractions, resulting in decreased uterine blood flow and fetal distress. Oxytocin may increase the risk of neonatal hyperbilirubinemia and jaundice.[184]

Prostaglandins

Misoprostol is a teratogen and has uterotonic effects; it should not be used during pregnancy. Anomalies reported include paralysis of cranial nerves VI and VII and limb, orofacial, and musculoskeletal defects.[18,185] A meta-analysis comparing 4899 cases and 5742 controls found increased risks for any congenital anomaly (OR 3.56; 95% CI, 0.98–12.98), Möbius sequence (congenital palsy of the sixth and seventh cranial nerves; OR 25.31; 95% CI, 11.11–57.66), and terminal transverse limb defects (OR 11.86; 95% CI, 4.86–28.9).[185] Misoprostol has been used off-label for cervical ripening.[18] Endocervical and vaginal administration of **dinoprostone** (prostaglandin E_2) is used for cervical ripening. Dinoprostone probably shortens labor more than oxytocin.[186]

(continued)

RENAL AND ELECTROLYTES

DIURETICS

Diuretics should be used cautiously during pregnancy because they can decrease maternal intravascular volume and consequently diminish uteroplacental perfusion, thereby compromising fetal oxygenation and growth.[122] This effect is most rapid and severe with loop diuretics (e.g., **bumetanide, furosemide,** and **torsemide**). Neonatal hyperbilirubinemia may occur with loop diuretic use.[122] IV furosemide administration to the pregnant woman has enabled ultrasonic imaging of the fetal bladder because of increased fetal urine output.[18] **Thiazide** diuretic use is not associated with birth defects; however, use during late pregnancy can produce neonatal hypoglycemia, hyponatremia, hypokalemia, and thrombocytopenia.[122]

ELECTROLYTES

Long-term infusion of **magnesium sulfate** during the second-trimester occasionally causes bone abnormalities and dental enamel hypoplasia.[18] However, infusions between 24 and 34 wk of gestation in women with preterm labor generally do not cause adverse neonatal outcomes. Use of magnesium sulfate as a tocolytic agent near term can cause dosage-related neonatal hypotonia, hyporeflexia, respiratory distress, hypocalcemia, and hypermagnesemia.[18,187]

RESPIRATORY DRUGS

ANTIALLERGICS

Cromolyn sodium use during pregnancy is not known to have any teratogenic effects.[188,189] Experience with **nedocromil** use in pregnancy is limited, but teratogenic risk is expected to be low.[18] Nedocromil use in 35 pregnancies resulted in 8 elective abortions, 1 spontaneous abortion, 1 birth defect (congenital heart disease), and 22 live births with 3 lost to follow-up.[190]

ANTIASTHMATICS

β-Adrenergic Agonists

Aerosol inhalation of **metaproterenol** and **albuterol** is considered safe during pregnancy. In one study, **salmeterol** was taken during the first trimester in 65 pregnancies. The 65 pregnancies resulted in 4 elective abortions, 7 spontaneous abortions, 2 ectopic pregnancies, and 47 live births with 5 outcomes unknown.[190] The small number of fetuses exposed to salmeterol during this study precludes any definitive conclusions about its safety. **Terbutaline** and **ritodrine** have been given for tocolysis during the third-trimester without permanent harm to the fetus, although hypertension, hypoglycemia, hypokalemia, and hypocalcemia have been reported.[18,191]

Inhaled Corticosteroids

This route is preferred during pregnancy to minimize fetal exposure. (*See* Corticosteroids.)

Theophylline

Maternal theophylline pharmacokinetics change during pregnancy. Reports of increased and decreased serum theophylline concentrations exist based on either decreased clearance or increased volume of distribution.[18,189] Pregnant women should have serum theophylline concentrations monitored frequently for dosage adjustments. No adverse fetal effects from long-term theophylline use during pregnancy are known.[189,192] Theophylline withdrawal has been reported in neonates of mothers receiving theophylline.[18]

ANTIHISTAMINES

The relative risk of malformations for first-generation antihistamines (e.g., **chlorpheniramine, doxylamine, diphenhydramine**) is not statistically significant.[18,188] **Hydroxyzine** and **cetirizine** have not shown a significant teratogenic risk.[18,188] In one large study, **loratadine** was associated

(*continued*)

RESPIRATORY DRUGS

with a greater risk of hypospadias; this finding was not confirmed in 2 later studies.[188] Use of antihistamines during the last 2 wk of pregnancy has been associated with retinopathy of prematurity. **Dimenhydrinate** might have an oxytocic effect on the term uterus, causing shortened labor.[18] (*See* Antiemetics.)

COUGH AND COLD

Use of **sympathomimetics** (e.g., **phenylephrine, pseudoephedrine**) for treatment of nasal congestion can cause increased fetal activity and fetal tachycardia. Some studies link first-trimester use of decongestants to gastroschisis, small intestine atresia, and hemifacial microsomia, which may be caused in part by the vasoconstrictive action of decongestants.[166,193] Intranasal decongestant use (e.g., oxymetazoline) may have lower systemic concentrations resulting in fewer fetal effects.[193]

MISCELLANEOUS DRUGS

ANESTHETICS, LOCAL

Most data available for local anesthetics are derived from use during labor and delivery. Even though all local anesthetics cross the placenta, epidural administration of **bupivacaine, ropivacaine, levobupivacaine,** or **lidocaine** might be the safest for obstetric analgesia.[194] However, local anesthetics have resulted in fetal and neonatal CNS depression and fetal bradycardia after maternal use during labor.[18,195] Epidural lidocaine was shown to decrease neonatal neurobehavioral performance, but the effects were not duplicated in further studies.[18]

RETINOIDS

Isotretinoin

Isotretinoin is a known teratogen. Use during pregnancy causes defects of the CNS, heart, external ear, and thymus. Other reported malformations include cleft palate, microphthalmia, micrognathia, facial dysmorphia, and limb reduction defects. Infants might exhibit hearing and visual impairments and mental retardation. The risk for malformations with isotretinoin is estimated at almost 30% compared to the baseline risk of 3%–5%.[196] The risk for spontaneous abortion is also increased.[18,196] An effective form of contraception must be used for at least 1 mo before starting and 1 mo after discontinuation of isotretinoin.

Tretinoin

Topical application of tretinoin results in absorption of vitamin A with equivalent activity less than that of a prenatal vitamin. Therefore, the risk of teratogenicity, although theoretically possible, is low when used topically without occlusive dressing as directed.[18] While case reports of retinoic acid embryopathy with topical tretinoin exist, studies of first-trimester exposure do not implicate topical retinoids in malformations.[18,197]

Vitamin A

Retinol or retinyl esters (but not beta-carotene) in toxic doses are teratogenic in animals, producing defects in almost all organ systems. Doses of vitamin A contained in prenatal vitamin supplements (<8000 IU, the RDA) do not appear to increase the risk of fetal malformation.[18,198] Defects observed when mothers ingested ≥ 25,000 IU/d of vitamin A during pregnancy include craniofacial, CNS, cardiac, urinary, vertebral, and other skeletal malformations.[18,198]

VACCINES

See section "Immunization", page 1141, for information regarding vaccination during pregnancy.

■ REFERENCES

1. Wilson JG, Fraser RC, eds. *Handbook of Teratology.* Vol I. *General Principles and Etiology.* New York: Plenum Press; 1977.
2. Beckman DA et al. Mechanism of known environmental teratogens: drugs and chemicals. *Clin Perinatol.* 1986;13:649-687.
3. Brent RL. The complexities of solving the problem of human malformations. *Clin Perinatol.* 1986;13:491-503.
4. Friedman JM et al. Potential human teratogenicity of frequently prescribed drugs. *Obstet Gynecol.* 1990;75: 594-599.
5. Pagliaro LA, Pagliaro AM, eds. *Problems in Pediatric Drug Therapy.* 3rd ed. Hamilton, IL: Drug Intelligence Publications; 1995.
6. Chow AW et al. Pharmacokinetics and safety of antimicrobial agents during pregnancy. *Rev Infect Dis.* 1985;7:287-313.
7. Berlin CM. Effects of drugs on the fetus. *Pediatr Rev.* 1991;12:282-287.
8. Landers DV et al. Antibiotic use during pregnancy and the postpartum period. *Clin Obstet Gynecol.* 1983;26:391-406.
9. Murray L et al. Drug therapy during pregnancy and lactation. *Emerg Med Clin North Am.* 1994;12:129-149.
10. Pacifici GM et al. Placental transfer of drugs administered to the mother. *Clin Pharmacokinet.* 1995;28:235-269.
11. Frey BM et al. Drug therapy in pregnancy and lactation. *J Pharm Pract.* 1989;2:2-12.
12. Kramer MS. Intrauterine growth and gestational duration determinants. *Pediatrics.* 1987;80:502-511.
13. Goadsby PJ et al. Migraine in pregnancy. *BMJ.* 2008;336:1502-1504.
14. Schiff PL. Ergot and its alkaloids. *Am J Pharm Educ.* 2006;70:98.
15. Sanders-Bush E et al. 5-hydroxytryptamine (serotonin): receptor agonists and antagonists. In: Brunton LL Lazo JS, Parker KL, eds. *Goodman & Gilman's the Pharmacological Basis of Therapeutics.* 11th ed. New York: McGraw-Hill Medical Publishing Division; 2006:297-315.
16. Banhidy F et al. Ergotamine treatment during pregnancy and a higher rate of low birthweight and preterm birth. *Br J Clin Pharmacol.* 2007;64:510-516.
17. Evans EW et al. Use of 5-HT1 agonists in pregnancy. *Ann Pharmacother.* 2008;42:543-549.
18. Briggs GG, Freeman RK, Yaffe SJ. *Drugs in Pregnancy and Lactation: A Reference Guide to Fetal and Neonatal Risk.* 8th ed. Philadelphia, PA: Lippincott Williams & Wilkins; 2008.
19. Rebordosa C et al. Acetaminophen use during pregnancy: effects on risk for congenital abnormalities. *Am J Obstet Gynecol.* 2008;198:178,e1-e7.
20. Czeizel AE et al. Short-term paracetamol therapy during pregnancy and a lower rate of preterm birth. *Paediatr Perinat Epidemiol.* 2005;19:106-111.
21. McElhatton PR et al. Paracetamol overdose in pregnancy analysis of the outcomes of 300 cases referred to the Teratology Information Service. *Reprod Toxicol.* 1997;11:85-94.
22. Wilkes JM et al. Acetaminophen overdose in pregnancy. *South Med J.* 2005;98:1118-1122.
23. Kirshon B et al. Effect of acetaminophen on fetal acid-base balance in chorioamnionitis. *J Reprod Med.* 1989;34:955-959.
24. Ostensen ME et al. Anti-inflammatory pharmacotherapy during pregnancy. *Expert Opin Pharmacother.* 2004;5:571-580.
25. Ostensen M et al. Treatment of inflammatory rheumatic disorders in pregnancy: what are the safest treatment options? *Drug Saf.* 1998;19:389-410.
26. Chambers CD et al. Human pregnancy safety for agents used to treat rheumatoid arthritis: adequacy of available information and strategies for developing post-marketing data. *Arthritis Res Ther.* 2006;8:215. doi:10.1186/ar1977.
27. Tassinari MS et al. NSAIDs and developmental toxicity. *Birth Defects Res B Dev Reprod Toxicol.* 2003;68:3-4.
28. Nielsen GL et al. Risk of adverse birth outcome and miscarriage in pregnant users of non-steroidal anti-inflammatory drugs: population based observational study and case-control study. *BMJ.* 2001;322:266-270.
29. Ericson A et al. Nonsteroidal anti-inflammatory drugs in early pregnancy. *Reprod Toxicol.* 2001;15:371-375.
30. Ofori B et al. Risk of congenital anomalies in pregnant users of non-steroidal anti-inflammatory drugs: A nested case-control study. *Birth Defects Res B Dev Reprod Toxicol.* 2006;77:268-279.
31. Koren G et al. Nonsteroidal antiinflammatory drugs during third trimester and the risk of premature closure of the ductus arteriosus: a meta-analysis. *Ann Pharmacother.* 2006;40:824-829.
32. Benini D et al. In utero exposure to nonsteroidal anti-inflammatory drugs: neonatal renal failure. *Pediatr Nephrol.* 2004;19:232-234.
33. Loe SM et al. Assessing the neonatal safety of indomethacin tocolysis: a systematic review with meta-analysis. *Obstet Gynecol.* 2005;106:173-179.
34. Kozer E et al. Aspirin consumption during the first trimester of pregnancy and congenital anomalies: a meta-analysis. *Am J Obstet Gynecol.* 2002;187:1623-1630.

35. Kozer E et al. Effects of aspirin consumption during pregnancy on pregnancy outcomes: meta-analysis. *Birth Defects Res B Dev Reprod Toxicol.* 2003;68:70-84.

36. Minozzi S et al. Maintenance agonist treatments for opiate dependent pregnant women. *Cochrane Database Syst Rev.* 2008;(2):CD006318.

37. Ebner N et al. Management of neonatal abstinence syndrome in neonates born to opioid maintained women. *Drug Alcohol Depend.* 2007;87:131-138.

38. Lockwood CJ et al, eds. *Guidelines for Perinatal Care.* 6th ed. Elk Grove Village, IL; American Academy of Pediatrics [and] the American College of Obstetricians and Gynecologists. 2007.

39. Van de Velde M et al. Intrathecal sufentanil and fetal heart rate abnormalities: a double-blind, double placebo-controlled trial comparing two forms of combined spinal epidural analgesia with epidural analgesia in labor. *Anesth Analg.* 2004;98:1153-1159.

40. Cunningham FG et al. Intrapartum assessment. In: Cunningham FG, Leveno KJ, Bloom SL et al, eds. *Williams Obstetrics.* 22nd ed. New York: McGraw-Hill Medical Publishing Division; 2005:443-472.

41. Wittels B et al. Postcesarean analgesia with both epidural morphine and intravenous patient-controlled analgesia: neurobehavioral outcomes among nursing neonates. *Anesth Analg.* 1997;85:600-606.

42. Ransjo-Arvidson AB et al. Maternal analgesia during labor disturbs newborn behavior: effects on breastfeeding, temperature, and crying. *Birth.* 2001;28:5-12.

43. Wittman BK et al. A comparison of the effects of single- and split-dose methadone administration on the fetus: ultrasound evaluation. *Int J Addict.* 1991;26:213-218.

44. Wolff K et al. Changes to methadone clearance during pregnancy. *Eur J Clin Pharmacol.* 2005;61:763-768.

45. Rathmell JP et al. Management of nonobstetric pain during pregnancy and lactation. *Anesth Analg.* 1997; 85:1074-1087.

46. Almarzouqi M et al. Gold therapy in women planning pregnancy: outcomes in one center. *J Rheumatol.* 2007;34:1827-1831.

47. Janssen NM et al. The effects of immunosuppressive and anti-inflammatory medications on fertility, pregnancy, and lactation. *Arch Intern Med.* 2000;160:610-619.

48. Czeizel AE et al. A teratological study of aminoglycoside antibiotic treatment during pregnancy. *Scand J Infect Dis.* 2000;32:309-313.

49. Nahum GG et al. Antibiotic use in pregnancy and lactation: what is and is not known about teratogenic and toxic risks. *Obstet Gynecol.* 2006;107:1120-1138.

50. Abramowicz M, ed. *Handbook of Antimicrobial Therapy.* New Rochelle, NY: The Medical Letter, Inc; 2005.

51. Norgaard M et al. Maternal use of fluconazole and risk of congenital malformations: a Danish population-based cohort study. *J Antimicrob Chemother.* 2008;62:172-176.

52. Sorensen HT et al. Risk of malformations and other outcomes in children exposed to fluconazole in utero. *Br J Clin Pharmacol.* 1999;48:234-238.

53. Bar-Oz B et al. Pregnancy outcome after in utero exposure to itraconazole: a prospective cohort study. *Am J Obstet Gynecol.* 2000;183:617-620.

54. Czeizel AE et al. Preterm birth reduction after clotrimazole treatment during pregnancy. *Eur J Obstet Gynecol Reprod Biol.* 2004;116:157-163.

55. Czeizel AE et al. Population-based case-control teratologic study of topical miconazole. *Congenit Anom (Kyoto).* 2004;44:41-45.

56. Carter TC et al. Antifungal drugs and the risk of selected birth defects. *Am J Obstet Gynecol.* 2008;198:191,e1-e7.

57. Brunette GW, Kozarsky PE, Magill AJ, Shlim DR. *CDC Health Information for International Travel 2010.* St. Louis MO: Mosby Ltd. 2009.

58. Chambers C et al. Are new agents used to treat rheumatoid arthritis safe to take during pregnancy? Organization of Teratology Information Specialists (OTIS) Study. *Can Fam Physician.* 2007;53:409-412.

59. Taylor WR et al. Antimalarial drug toxicity: a review. *Drug Saf.* 2004;27:25-61.

60. Schlagenhauf P et al. Malaria chemoprophylaxis: strategies for risk groups. *Clin Microbiol Rev.* 2008;21:466-472.

61. American Thoracic Society, CDC, Infectious Diseases Society of America. Treatment of tuberculosis. *MMWR Recomm Rep.* 2003;52(RR-11):1-77.

62. Bothamley G. Drug treatment for tuberculosis during pregnancy: safety considerations. *Drug Saf.* 2001;24:553-565.

63. Efferen LS. Tuberculosis and pregnancy. *Curr Opin Pulm Med.* 2007;13:205-211.

64. Sutor AH et al. Vitamin K deficiency bleeding (VKDB) in infancy. ISTH Pediatric/Perinatal Subcommittee. International Society on Thrombosis and Haemostasis. *Thromb Haemost.* 1999;81:456-461.

65. Autret-Leca E et al. Vitamin K in neonates: how to administer, when and to whom. *Paediatr Drugs.* 2001;3:1-8.

66. American Academy of Pediatrics Committee on Fetus and Newborn. Controversies concerning vitamin K and the newborn. *Pediatrics.* 2003;112(1, pt 1):191-192.

67. *Physicians' Desk Reference.* Montvale, NJ: Medical Economics Company; 2002.

68. Joint Tuberculosis Committee of the British Thoracic Society. Chemotherapy and management of tuberculosis in the United Kingdom: recommendations 1998. *Joint Tuberculosis Committee of the British Thoracic Society. Thorax.* 1998;53:536-548.

69. Brabin BJ et al. Dapsone therapy for malaria during pregnancy: maternal and fetal outcomes. *Drug Saf.* 2004;27:633-648.

70. Thornton YS et al. Neonatal hyperbilirubinemia after treatment of maternal leprosy. *South Med J.* 1989;82:668.

71. Revlimid (lenalidomide)[package insert]. Summit, NJ: Celgene Corporation; 2007.

72. Perinatal HIV Guidelines Working Group. *Public Health Service Task Force Recommendations for Use of Anti-retroviral Drugs in Pregnant HIV-Infected Women for Maternal Health Interventions to Reduce Perinatal HIV Transmission in the United States.* April 29, 2009:1-90. http://aidsinfo.nih.gov/contentfiles/perinatalgl.pdf. Accessed October 23, 2009.

73. Sarner L et al. Acute onset lactic acidosis and pancreatitis in the third trimester of pregnancy in HIV-1 positive women taking antiretroviral medication. *Sex Transm Infect.* 2002;78:58-59.

74. De Santis M et al. Periconceptional exposure to efavirenz and neural tube defects. *Arch Intern Med.* 2002;162:355.

75. Fundaro C et al. Myelomeningocele in a child with intrauterine exposure to efavirenz. *AIDS.* 2002;16:299-300.

76. Covington DL et al. Risk of birth defects associated with nelfinavir exposure during pregnancy. *Obstet Gynecol.* 2004;103:1181-1189.

77. Brown ZA et al. Genital herpes complicating pregnancy. *Obstet Gynecol.* 2005;106:845-856.

78. Sheffield JS et al. Acyclovir prophylaxis to prevent herpes simplex virus recurrence at delivery: a systematic review. *Obstet Gynecol.* 2003;102:1396-1403.

79. Andrews WW et al. Valacyclovir therapy to reduce recurrent genital herpes in pregnant women. *Am J Obstet Gynecol.* 2006;194:774-781.

80. Sheffield JS et al. Valacyclovir prophylaxis to prevent recurrent herpes at delivery: a randomized clinical trial. *Obstet Gynecol.* 2006;108:141-147.

81. Majeroni BA et al. Screening and treatment for sexually transmitted infections in pregnancy. *Am Fam Physician.* 2007;76:265-270.

82. ACOG Committee on Practice Bulletins. ACOG Practice Bulletin. Clinical management guidelines for obstetrician-gynecologists: No. 82, June 2007. Management of herpes in pregnancy. *Obstet Gynecol.* 2007;109:1489-1498.

83. Czeizel AE et al. Use of cephalosporins during pregnancy and in the presence of congenital abnormalities: a population-based, case-control study. *Am J Obstet Gynecol.* 2001;184:1289-1296.

84. Einarson A et al. Effects of antibacterials on the unborn child: what is known and how should this influence prescribing. *Paediatr Drugs.* 2001;3:803-816.

85. Myles TD et al. The Jarisch-Herxheimer reaction and fetal monitoring changes in pregnant women treated for syphilis. *Obstet Gynecol.* 1998;92:859-864.

86. Schick B et al. Pregnancy outcome following exposure to clarithromycin [abstract of the Ninth International Conference of the Organization of Teratology Information Services; May 2–4, 1996; Salt Lake City, UT.] *Reprod Toxicol.* 1996;10:162.

87. Einarson A et al. A prospective controlled multicentre study of clarithromycin in pregnancy. *Am J Perinatol.* 1998;15:523-525.

88. Drinkard CR et al. Postmarketing surveillance of medications and pregnancy outcomes: clarithromycin and birth malformations. *Pharmacoepidemiol Drug Saf.* 2000;9:549-556.

89. Sarkar M et al. Pregnancy outcome following gestational exposure to azithromycin. *BMC Pregnancy Childbirth.* 2006;6:18. doi:10.1186/1471-2393-6-18.

90. Macejko AM et al. Asymptomatic bacteriuria and symptomatic urinary tract infections during pregnancy. *Urol Clin North Am.* 2007;34:35-42.

91. Bentov Y et al. Mediterranean spotted fever during pregnancy: case presentation and literature review. *Eur J Obstet Gynecol Reprod Biol.* 2003;107:214-216.

92. McDonald HM et al. Antibiotics for treating bacterial vaginosis in pregnancy. *Cochrane Database Syst Rev.* 2007;(1):CD000262.

93. Simcox R et al. Prophylactic antibiotics for the prevention of preterm birth in women at risk: a meta-analysis. *Aust N Z J Obstet Gynaecol.* 2007;47:368-377.

94. Shea K et al. Successful treatment of vancomycin-resistant *Enterococcus faecium* pyelonephritis with daptomycin during pregnancy. *Ann Pharmacother.* 2008;42:722-725.

95. Cunha BA et al. Daptomycin cure after cefazolin treatment failure of methicillin-sensitive *Staphylococcus aureus* (MSSA) tricuspid valve acute bacterial endocarditis from a peripherally inserted central catheter (PICC) line. *Heart Lung.* 2005;34:442-447.

96. Shepard TH et al. Update on new developments in the study of human teratogens. *Teratology.* 2002;65:153-161.

97. Hernandez-Diaz S et al. Folic acid antagonists during pregnancy and the risk of birth defects. *N Engl J Med.* 2000;343:1608-1614.

98. Hernandez-Diaz S et al. Neural tube defects in relation to use of folic acid antagonists during pregnancy. *Am J Epidemiol.* 2001;153:961-968.

99. Czeizel AE et al. The teratogenic risk of trimethoprim-sulfonamides: a population based case-control study. *Reprod Toxicol.* 2001;15:637-646.

100. Roberts JE et al. Fertility preservation: a comprehensive approach to the young woman with cancer. *J Natl Cancer Inst Monogr*. 2005:57-59.

101. Gwyn K. Children exposed to chemotherapy in utero. *J Natl Cancer Inst Monogr*. 2005:69-71.

102. Cardonick E et al. Use of chemotherapy during human pregnancy. *Lancet Oncol*. 2004;5:283-291.

103. Sorosky JI et al. The use of chemotherapeutic agents during pregnancy. *Obstet Gynecol Clin North Am*. 1997;24:591-599.

104. Ali R et al. Pregnancy in chronic lymphocytic leukemia: Experience with fetal exposure to chlorambucil. *Leuk Res*. 2009;33:e26-28.

105. Nakajima W et al. Good outcome for infant of mother treated with chemotherapy for Ewing sarcoma at 25 to 30 weeks' gestation. *J Pediatr Hematol Oncol*. 2004;26:308-311.

106. Merimsky O et al. Management of cancer in pregnancy: a case of Ewing's sarcoma of the pelvis in the third trimester. *Ann Oncol*. 1999;10:345-350.

107. Odom LD et al. 5-fluorouracil exposure during the period of conception: report on two cases. *Am J Obstet Gynecol*. 1990;163(1 pt 1):76-77.

108. Kopelman JN et al. Inadvertent 5-fluorouracil treatment in early pregnancy: a report of three cases. *Reprod Toxicol*. 1990;4:233-235.

109. Van Le L et al. Accidental use of low-dose 5-fluorouracil in pregnancy. *J Reprod Med*. 1991;36:872-874.

110. Khamashta MA. Systemic lupus erythematosus and pregnancy. *Best Pract Res Clin Rheumatol*. 2006;20:685-694.

111. Temprano KK et al. Antirheumatic drugs in pregnancy and lactation. *Semin Arthritis Rheum*. 2005;35:112-121.

112. Pereg D et al. The treatment of Hodgkin's and non-Hodgkin's lymphoma in pregnancy. *Haematologica*. 2007;92:1230-1237.

113. Mir O et al. Emerging therapeutic options for breast cancer chemotherapy during pregnancy. *Ann Oncol*. 2008;19:607-613.

114. Ferrero S et al. Inflammatory bowel disease: management issues during pregnancy. *Arch Gynecol Obstet*. 2004;270:79-85.

115. Petri M. Immunosuppressive drug use in pregnancy. *Autoimmunity*. 2003;36:51-56.

116. Chu SH et al. Sirolimus used during pregnancy in a living related renal transplant recipient: a case report. *Transplant Proc*. 2008;40:2446-2448.

117. Grimer M. The CARI guidelines. Calcineurin inhibitors in renal transplantation: pregnancy, lactation and calcineurin inhibitors. *Nephrology*. 2007;12(suppl 1):S98-S105.

118. Lomenick JP et al. Amiodarone-induced neonatal hypothyroidism: a unique form of transient early-onset hypothyroidism. *J Perinatol*. 2004;24:397-399.

119. Ferrero S et al. Maternal arrhythmias during pregnancy. *Arch Gynecol Obstet*. 2004;269:244-253.

120. Podymow T et al. Update on the use of antihypertensive drugs in pregnancy. *Hypertension*. 2008;51:960-969.

121. Hall DR et al. Nifedipine or prazosin as a second agent to control early severe hypertension in pregnancy: a randomised controlled trial. *BJOG*. 2000;107:759-765.

122. Ghanem FA et al. Use of antihypertensive drugs during pregnancy and lactation. *Cardiovasc Ther*. 2008;26:38-49.

123. Cooper WO et al. Major congenital malformations after first-trimester exposure to ACE inhibitors. *N Engl J Med*. 2006;354:2443-2451.

124. Alwan S et al. Angiotensin II receptor antagonist treatment during pregnancy. *Birth Defects Res A Clin Mol Teratol*. 2005;73:123-130.

125. Alwan S et al. Addendum: sartan treatment during pregnancy. *Birth Defects Res A Clin Mol Teratol*. 2005;73:904-905.

126. Magee LA et al. Oral beta-blockers for mild to moderate hypertension during pregnancy. *Cochrane Database Syst Rev*. 2003(3):CD002863.

127. Weber-Schoendorfer C et al. The safety of calcium channel blockers during pregnancy: a prospective, multicenter, observational study. *Reprod Toxicol*. 2008;26:24-30.

128. Fletcher H et al. An open trial comparing isradipine with hydralazine and methyldopa in the treatment of patients with severe pre-eclampsia. *J Obstet Gynaecol*. 1999;19:235-238.

129. Oei SG. Calcium channel blockers for tocolysis: a review of their role and safety following reports of serious adverse events. *Eur J Obstet Gynecol Reprod Biol*. 2006;126:137-145.

130. Battino D et al. Management of epilepsy during pregnancy. *Drugs*. 2007;67:2727-2746.

131. Holmes LB et al. The teratogenicity of anticonvulsant drugs. *N Engl J Med*. 2001;344:1132-1138.

132. Sankar R. Teratogenicity of antiepileptic drugs: role of drug metabolism and pharmacogenomics. *Acta Neurol Scand*. 2007;116:65-71.

133. Perucca E. Birth defects after prenatal exposure to antiepileptic drugs. *Lancet Neurol*. 2005;4:781-786.

134. Montouris G. Gabapentin exposure in human pregnancy: results from the Gabapentin Pregnancy Registry. *Epilepsy Behav*. 2003;4:310-317.

135. Chambers CD et al. Pregnancy outcome in infants prenatally exposed to newer anticonvulsants [abstract]. *Birth Defects Res A Clin Mol Teratol*. 2005;73:316.

136. Ornoy A. Neuroteratogens in man: an overview with special emphasis on the teratogenicity of antiepileptic drugs in pregnancy. *Reprod Toxicol*. 2006;22:214-226.

137. Holmes LB et al. Increased risk for non-syndromic cleft palate among infants exposed to lamotrigine during pregnancy [abstract]. *Birth Defects Res A Clin Mol Teratol*. 2006;76:318.

138. ten Berg K et al. Levetiracetam use and pregnancy outcome. *Reprod Toxicol*. 2005;20:175-178.

139. Hunt S et al. Levetiracetam in pregnancy: preliminary experience from the UK Epilepsy and Pregnancy Register. *Neurology*. 2006;67:1876-1879.

140. Duncan S. Teratogenesis of sodium valproate. *Curr Opin Neurol*. 2007;20:175-180.

141. Bellantuono C et al. Serotonin reuptake inhibitors in pregnancy and the risk of major malformations: a systematic review. *Hum Psychopharmacol*. 2007;22:121-128.

142. Way CM. Safety of newer antidepressants in pregnancy. *Pharmacotherapy*. 2007;27:546-552.

143. Eyal R et al. Poor neonatal adaptation after in utero exposure to duloxetine. *Am J Psychiatry*. 2008;165:651.

144. Nulman I et al. Child development following exposure to tricyclic antidepressants or fluoxetine throughout fetal life: a prospective, controlled study. *Am J Psychiatry*. 2002;159:1889-1895.

145. ACOG Committee on Practice Bulletins—Obstetrics. ACOG Practice Bulletin: Clinical management guidelines for obstetrician-gynecologists: No. 92, April 2008 (replaces bulletin No. 87, November 2007). Use of psychiatric medications during pregnancy and lactation. *Obstet Gynecol*. 2008;111:1001-1020.

146. Jablensky AV et al. Pregnancy, delivery, and neonatal complications in a population cohort of women with schizophrenia and major affective disorders. *Am J Psychiatry*. 2005;162:79-91.

147. Trixler M et al. Use of antipsychotics in the management of schizophrenia during pregnancy. *Drugs*. 2005;65:1193-1206.

148. Gentile S. Antipsychotic therapy during early and late pregnancy. A systematic review. *Schizophr Bull*. 2008. doi:10.1093/schbul/sbn107.

149. Coppola D et al. Evaluating the postmarketing experience of risperidone use during pregnancy: pregnancy and neonatal outcomes. *Drug Saf*. 2007;30:247-264.

150. Wikner BN et al. Use of benzodiazepines and benzodiazepine receptor agonists during pregnancy: neonatal outcome and congenital malformations. *Pharmacoepidemiol Drug Saf*. 2007;16:1203-1210.

151. Czeizel AE et al. A population-based case-control study of oral chlordiazepoxide use during pregnancy and risk of congenital abnormalities. *Neurotoxicol Teratol*. 2004;26:593-598.

152. Eros E et al. A population-based case-control teratologic study of nitrazepam, medazepam, tofisopam, alprazolum and clonazepam treatment during pregnancy. *Eur J Obstet Gynecol Reprod Biol*. 2002;101(2):147-154.

153. Iqbal MM et al. Effects of commonly used benzodiazepines on the fetus, the neonate, and the nursing infant. *Psychiatr Serv*. 2002;53:39-49.

154. Giles JJ et al. Teratogenic and developmental effects of lithium. *Curr Pharm Des*. 2006;12:1531-1541.

155. Yonkers KA et al. Management of bipolar disorder during pregnancy and the postpartum period. *Am J Psychiatry*. 2004;161:608-620.

156. Eberhard-Gran M et al. Treating mood disorders during pregnancy: safety considerations. *Drug Saf*. 2005;28:695-706.

157. Black RA et al. Over-the-counter medications in pregnancy. *Am Fam Physician*. 2003;67:2517-2524.

158. Conover EA. Herbal agents and over-the-counter medications in pregnancy. *Best Pract Res Clin Endocrinol Metab*. 2003;17:237-251.

159. Ali RA et al. Gastroesophageal reflux disease in pregnancy. *Best Pract Res Clin Gastroenterol*. 2007;21:793-806.

160. Nava-Ocampo AA et al. Use of proton pump inhibitors during pregnancy and breastfeeding. *Can Fam Physician*. 2006;52:853-854.

161. Nikfar S et al. Use of proton pump inhibitors during pregnancy and rates of major malformations: a meta-analysis. *Dig Dis Sci*. 2002;47:1526-1529.

162. Diav-Citrin O et al. The safety of proton pump inhibitors in pregnancy: a multicentre prospective controlled study. *Aliment Pharmacol Ther*. 2005;21:269-275.

163. Magee LA et al. Evidence-based view of safety and effectiveness of pharmacologic therapy for nausea and vomiting of pregnancy (NVP). *Am J Obstet Gynecol*. 2002;186(suppl 5 Understanding):S256-S261.

164. Williamson C. Drugs in pregnancy. Gastrointestinal disease. *Best Pract Res Clin Obstet Gynaecol*. 2001;15:937-952.

165. Einarson A et al. The safety of ondansetron for nausea and vomiting of pregnancy: a prospective comparative study. *BJOG*. 2004;111:940-943.

166. Erebara A et al. Treating the common cold during pregnancy. *Can Fam Physician*. 2008;54:687-689.

167. Brar H et al. Effects and treatment of inflammatory bowel disease during pregnancy. *Can Fam Physician*. 2008;54:981-983.

168. Bates SM et al. Venous thromboembolism, thrombophilia, antithrombotic therapy, and pregnancy: American College of Chest Physicians Evidence-Based Clinical Practice Guidelines (8th Edition). *Chest*. 2008;133(suppl 6):844S-886S.

169. Lam J et al. Safety of dermatologic drugs used in pregnant patients with psoriasis and other inflammatory skin diseases. *J Am Acad Dermatol.* 2008;59:295-315.

170. Fardet L et al. Corticosteroid-induced adverse events in adults: frequency, screening and prevention. *Drug Saf.* 2007;30:861-881.

171. Mottet C et al. Pregnancy and breastfeeding in patients with Crohn's disease. *Digestion.* 2007;76:149-160.

172. Roberts D et al. Antenatal corticosteroids for accelerating fetal lung maturation for women at risk of preterm birth. *Cochrane Database Syst Rev.* 2006;3:CD004454.

173. Moretti ME et al. Safety of glyburide for gestational diabetes: a meta-analysis of pregnancy outcomes. *Ann Pharmacother.* 2008;42:483-490.

174. Klieger C et al. Treating the mother–protecting the unborn: the safety of hypoglycemic drugs in pregnancy. *J Matern Fetal Neonatal Med.* 2008;21:191-196.

175. Gutzin SJ et al. The safety of oral hypoglycemic agents in the first trimester of pregnancy: a meta-analysis. *Can J Clin Pharmacol.* 2003;10:179-183.

176. Jacobson GF et al. Comparison of glyburide and insulin for the management of gestational diabetes in a large managed care organization. *Am J Obstet Gynecol.* 2005;193:118-124.

177. Rowan JA et al. Metformin versus insulin for the treatment of gestational diabetes. *N Engl J Med.* 2008; 358:2003-2015.

178. Gilbert C et al. Pregnancy outcome after first-trimester exposure to metformin: a meta-analysis. *Fertil Steril.* 2006;86:658-663.

179. Elizur SE et al. Drugs in infertility and fetal safety. *Fertil Steril.* 2008;89:1595-1602.

180. Brent RL. Nongenital malformations following exposure to progestational drugs: the last chapter of an erroneous allegation. *Birth Defects Res A Clin Mol Teratol.* 2005;73:906-918.

181. Clark SM et al. Pharmacokinetics and pharmacotherapy of thionamides in pregnancy. *Ther Drug Monit.* 2006;28:477-483.

182. Lao TT. Thyroid disorders in pregnancy. *Curr Opin Obstet Gynecol.* 2005;17:123-127.

183. Koren G et al. Therapeutic drug monitoring of antithyroid drugs in pregnancy: the knowledge gaps. *Ther Drug Monit.* 2006;28:12-13.

184. Oral E et al. Oxytocin infusion in labor: the effect different indications and the use of different diluents on neonatal bilirubin levels. *Arch Gynecol Obstet.* 2003;267:117-120.

185. da Silva Dal Pizzol T et al. Prenatal exposure to misoprostol and congenital anomalies: systematic review and meta-analysis. *Reprod Toxicol.* 2006;22:666-671.

186. Keirse MJ. Natural prostaglandins for induction of labor and preinduction cervical ripening. *Clin Obstet Gynecol.* 2006;49:609-626.

187. Nassar AH et al. Adverse maternal and neonatal outcome of prolonged course of magnesium sulfate tocolysis. *Acta Obstet Gynecol Scand.* 2006;85:1099-1103.

188. Gilbert C et al. Fetal safety of drugs used in the treatment of allergic rhinitis: a critical review. *Drug Saf.* 2005;28:707-719.

189. Gluck JC et al. Asthma controller therapy during pregnancy. *Am J Obstet Gynecol.* 2005;192:369-380.

190. Wilton LV et al. The outcomes of pregnancy in women exposed to newly marketed drugs in general practice in England. *Br J Obstet Gynaecol.* 1998;105:882-889.

191. ACOG Committee on Practice Bulletins. ACOG Practice Bulletin. Clinical management guidelines for obstetrician-gynecologist, No. 43, May 2003. Management of preterm labor. *Obstet Gynecol.* 2003; 101(5 pt 1):1039-1047.

192. Chambers C. Safety of asthma and allergy medications in pregnancy. *Immunol Allergy Clin North Am.* 2006;26:13-28.

193. Werler MM. Teratogen update: pseudoephedrine. *Birth Defects Res A Clin Mol Teratol.* 2006;76:445-452.

194. Mattingly JE et al. Effects of obstetric analgesics and anesthetics on the neonate: a review. *Paediatr Drugs.* 2003;5:615-627.

195. Hill JB et al. A comparison of the effects of epidural and meperidine analgesia during labor on fetal heart rate. *Obstet Gynecol.* 2003;102:333-337.

196. Berard A et al. Isotretinoin, pregnancies, abortions and birth defects: a population-based perspective. *Br J Clin Pharmacol.* 2007;63:196-205.

197. Loureiro KD et al. Minor malformations characteristic of the retinoic acid embryopathy and other birth outcomes in children of women exposed to topical tretinoin during early pregnancy. *Am J Med Genet A.* 2005;136:117-121.

198. Tzimas G et al. The role of metabolism and toxicokinetics in retinoid teratogenesis. *Curr Pharm Des.* 2001;7:803-831.

Chapter 70

Drugs and Breast-Feeding

Philip O. Anderson

With the increasing recognition of the benefits of breast-feeding, clinicians must often weigh the benefits versus risks of drug therapy in lactating women. The physicochemical, pharmacokinetic, and clinical factors involved with drug use in nursing women can be summarized as follows.[1,2]

■ PHYSICOCHEMICAL FACTORS

Small water-soluble nonelectrolytes pass into breast milk by simple diffusion through pores in the mammary epithelial membrane that separates serum from milk. Equilibration between the two fluids is rapid, and breast milk concentrations of drugs approximate serum concentrations. For larger molecules, only the lipid-soluble, nonionized forms pass through the membrane by crossing the cell wall and diffusing across the interior of the cell to reach the milk. Because the pH of breast milk is generally lower than that of serum, breast milk can act as an "ion trap" for basic drugs. At equilibrium, these compounds can be concentrated in breast milk relative to serum. Conversely, acidic drugs are inhibited from entering milk. The pK_a of weak acids and bases is an important determinant of their equilibrium concentration in milk.

Protein binding is also an important determinant because serum proteins bind drugs much more avidly than do breast milk proteins. Highly protein-bound drugs do not pass into breast milk in high concentrations. Lipid solubility favors passage of some drugs into milk because the fat component of breast milk can concentrate lipid-soluble drugs. However, because breast milk contains only a small percentage of fat, its capacity for concentrating drugs is limited. Active transport of drugs into breast milk has been shown for a few drugs, but is the exception.

■ PHARMACOKINETIC FACTORS

Because the breast is periodically emptied by the breast-feeding infant and refilled with newly formed milk, equilibrium between serum and breast milk is rarely reached. Therefore, the rate of drug passage from serum into breast milk is important in determining the concentration of a drug in milk. Factors favoring rapid passage into breast milk are high lipid solubility and low molecular weight.

Passage of drugs between serum and breast milk occurs in both directions. When the concentration of nonionized, unbound drug is higher in breast milk than in serum, net transfer of drug from breast milk to serum occurs. Thus, the maneuver of pumping and discarding breast milk does not appreciably hasten the elimination of most drugs from milk nor does it have a marked effect on the overall clearance of the drug from the mother's body.

■ METHODS OF EXPRESSING THE EXTENT OF PASSAGE

The ratio of concentrations of a drug in breast milk and serum (the milk/serum or M/P ratio) has often been used as a measure of a drug's passage into breast milk. However, the M/P ratio has shortcomings that make it meaningless as a measure of drug safety during nursing. There is no standard method of calculating the value, and the value is not constant as often calculated but changes with the time after the dose and the number of doses given. It also does not take into account the safety or potential toxicity of the drug.

The percentage of the maternal dosage that is excreted into breast milk is also used to express the extent of passage. Usually a weight-adjusted (i.e., mg/kg) infant dosage <10% of the mother's is is considered safe; of 205 drugs studied, 87% of drugs fell into this category. The likelihood of an adverse effect in the infant increases markedly in those few drugs (about 3%) that have a dosage in breast milk that exceeds 25% of the maternal weight-adjusted dosage.[3]

Drug clearance can be a useful factor for identifying drugs that can accumulate in infants and thereby have a pharmacologic effect.[4] Drugs with an adult total body clearance of 0.3 L/h/kg or greater and that have no active metabolites are unlikely to have pharmacologic effects in a nursing infant because they are rapidly eliminated by the mother and infant.

All of the above methods fall short of providing a complete assessment of the safety of a drug during breast-feeding in a specific mother–infant pair. Several additional factors must be considered.

■ CLINICAL CONSIDERATIONS

Factors that should be considered when determining the advisability of using a particular drug in a nursing mother are the potential acute toxicity of the drug, dosage and duration of therapy, age of the infant (infants younger than 2 mo are the most susceptible)[5], quantity of breast milk consumed, experience with the drug in infants, oral absorption of the drug by the infant, potential long-term effects, and possible interference with lactation.

A stepwise approach to using medications in breast-feeding women can be followed to minimize infant exposure to medications in milk.[1] Starting from the strategies that are least disruptive to nursing and progressing to those that are most disruptive, the prescriber can consider the following steps: withhold the drug; delay drug therapy temporarily; choose drugs that pass poorly into milk; use alternative routes of administration (e.g., topical, inhalation); avoid nursing at times of peak breast milk concentrations; administer the drug before the infant's longest sleep period; withhold breast-feeding temporarily; and, infrequently, discontinue breast-feeding.

Another consideration is non–dose-related adverse effects such as allergic reactions and some hemolytic anemias; however, these reactions are uncommon. GI intolerance caused by antimicrobial agents in breast milk can occur whether or not the drugs are absorbed by the infant. Antimicrobial agents are among the most commonly used maternal medications during nursing, and although serious side effects are rare, diarrhea occurs in about 12% of infants.[6]

Although the above considerations are important, serious side effects in breast-fed infants from maternal medications are uncommon.[5,6] Nursing seldom needs to be completely discontinued because of concern of acute toxicity from maternal drug therapy.

The following section contains information on the use of specific drugs during nursing. The risks are assessed and alternatives are presented based on the principles discussed. Recent review articles are provided when available. More detailed information and a complete bibliography is available in the National Library of Medicine's LactMed database at http://lactmed.nlm.nih.gov.

DRUGS AND BREAST-FEEDING

ANALGESICS AND ANTI-INFLAMMATORY DRUGS

ANTIMIGRAINE DRUGS

Ergotamine

When given daily for 6 d postpartum ergotamine did not affect lactation or infant weight in 1 study; however, the excretion of ergotamine into breast milk during lactation has not been studied. Avoid its use during lactation, because older ergot preparations have produced toxicity in infants.[7]

Sumatriptan

Minimally excreted in milk, sumatriptan has poor oral absorption by the infant. It poses little risk during breast-feeding.[8]

NONSTEROIDAL ANTI-INFLAMMATORY DRUGS[9]

Acetaminophen

The amount of acetaminophen excreted into breast milk is small. Acetaminophen is a good analgesic choice during nursing.

Nonsteroidal Anti-inflammatory Drugs

Amounts of most NSAIDs in breast milk are low because they are weak acids that are extensively serum protein-bound. However, short-acting agents are preferred, particularly in the case of breast-fed neonates. Some agents have active metabolites (e.g., **sulindac**) or glucuronide metabolites (e.g., **salicylate, fenoprofen,** and **ketoprofen**) that can add to infant intake. Because of the increased likelihood of accumulation, avoid long-acting agents such as **diflunisal, naproxen, piroxicam,** and **sulindac** in mothers of neonates,[10] although amounts of piroxicam in breast milk are low. Naproxen caused prolonged bleeding time, thrombocytopenia, and acute anemia in one 7-d-old infant, and possibly drowsiness and vomiting in others. The more toxic NSAIDs such as **mefenamic acid** and **indomethacin** should also be avoided, although recent studies on indomethacin indicate that it might not be contraindicated. **Ketorolac** is contraindicated during nursing by an FDA boxed warning; its antiplatelet effects are much greater than other NSAIDs. **Diclofenac** was not detected in breast milk after a single dose of 50 mg IM, or 100 mg/d for 1 wk, and the amount of **tolmetin** in 1 woman's breast milk was low. **Ibuprofen** and **flurbiprofen** have the best documentation of safety during breast-feeding; the dose of ibuprofen that an infant receives in breast milk is less than 0.001% of the mother's dosage, and flurbiprofen concentrations are low to undetectable after dosages up to 50 mg tid. **Celecoxib** appears in milk in small amounts that are unlikely to affect breast-fed infants.[11,12]

(*continued*)

ANALGESICS AND ANTI-INFLAMMATORY DRUGS

Salicylates

Salicylate enters breast milk in a low concentration relative to that in serum, although its glucuronide metabolite increases the overall infant dosage. Doses >1 g yield markedly higher salicylate concentrations in breast milk and can result in high infant serum concentrations. One case of thrombocytopenic purpura from **aspirin** in breast milk (confirmed by rechallenge) was reported in a 5-mo-old infant. The risk of Reye's syndrome caused by salicylate in breast milk is unknown. If aspirin is taken occasionally, avoid breast-feeding for 1–2 h after a dose to minimize antiplatelet effects. NSAIDs such as ibuprofen are preferred to aspirin for long-term therapy.

OTHER ANTI-INFLAMMATORY DRUGS[13–15] *See also* Antimalarials

Anti-TNF drugs

These medications are generally large molecules that are poorly excreted into breast milk. They would also not be expected to be absorbed from the GI tract of an older infant, although some absorption might theoretically take place in the first month after birth, if possible. **Adalimumab** has been used during nursing and milk excretion was minimal. **Etanercept** excretion into breast milk is poor, but no safety data are available. It should probably be avoided during the first month postpartum. A few infants have been breast-fed during maternal **Infliximab** therapy without harm, but it should probably be avoided during the first month postpartum, if possible.

Gold

During maternal administration of **aurothioglucose** and **gold sodium thiomalate,** gold was detected in the blood and urine of some nursing infants. The weight-adjusted infant dosage might be greater than the maternal dosage, but the amount of gold that infants absorb orally is not known. Sufficient amounts are absorbed, however, to potentially cause adverse effects. Opinions vary, but gold therapy is a reason to very carefully monitor the breast-fed infant, and might be a reason for withholding breast-feeding.

Penicillamine

Penicillamine was used during 3 mo of breast-feeding in 2 women who nursed 3 infants without harm, but data are insufficient to judge its safety during lactation.[16,17]

OPIOIDS

Neonates are particularly susceptible to narcotics in breast milk. Postpartum maternal opioids (oral **codeine** or **propoxyphene** with or without prior IM **meperidine**) can be a causative factor in episodes of apnea, bradycardia, and cyanosis during the first week of life. Avoid maternal narcotics when the breast-fed neonate has experienced such an episode. Although single analgesic doses of most narcotics are excreted into breast milk in small amounts, infant drowsiness caused by repeated administration of postpartum oral narcotics in breast milk is more prevalent than commonly thought—about 20% in 1 study.[6] A newborn infant death occurred during breast-feeding by a mother who was an ultrarapid CYP2D6 metabolizer; she experienced excessive drowsiness and excreted large amounts of morphine in her breast milk.[18] Maternal and infant pharmacogenetic makeup appears to be an important factor in causing adverse reactions to codeine during breast-feeding.[19] **Hydrocodone** concentrations were found to be low in 2 nursing mothers,[20] but more data are needed to evaluate the safety of hydrocodone during breast-feeding. Drowsiness from narcotics in breast milk is dose related and can be severe with the maximum dosage. Limiting oral opioid dosage to 1 tablet (e.g., **codeine** 30 mg, **hydrocodone** 5 mg, or **oxycodone** 5 mg) q4h is advisable; analgesia can be

(*continued*)

ANALGESICS AND ANTI-INFLAMMATORY DRUGS

supplemented with additional acetaminophen or ibuprofen. With any opioid, if the infant shows signs of increased sleepiness, difficulty breast-feeding, breathing difficulties, or limpness, a physician should be contacted immediately.

Meperidine

Meperidine is particularly likely to interfere with infant nursing behavior when given during labor.[21,22] Furthermore, repeated postpartum meperidine doses, including patient-controlled analgesia, cause diminished alertness and orientation in breast-fed neonates compared with equivalent doses of **morphine**.[23] Meperidine should be avoided during labor and nursing, although a single small maternal dose for anesthesia or conscious sedation usually does not cause problems in older breast-fed infants.[24]

Methadone

Methadone has been relatively well studied in breast-feeding mothers who were taking the drug during pregnancy and postpartum for maintenance of narcotic abstinence. Breast-feeding may decrease neonatal withdrawal symptoms and reduce hospitalization time for infants exposed *in utero*. However, because methadone is transferred to breast milk in only small amounts, a breast-fed newborn or infant may require treatment for withdrawal.[25–30] The amount of methadone in breast milk is insufficient to warrant lowering the dosage of diluted tincture of opium given to the newborn to mitigate methadone withdrawal.[31] These observations do not apply to the situation in which methadone is begun *de novo* postpartum, because the infant would not be tolerant to methadone. Severe respiratory depression occurred in one infant in this setting.

Morphine

Morphine 10–15 mg in single parenteral doses produces only low concentrations in milk, but repeated doses can result in drug accumulation in infant serum to near therapeutic concentrations. Morphine glucuronides in breast milk contribute an additional 50%–100% to the infant. Epidural administration and patient-controlled analgesia cause fewer effects in infants than IV administration and are preferred.[9,23]

Fentanyl and related drugs

IV or epidural fentanyl and **sufentanil** produce low breast milk concentrations.[32,33] **Remifentanil** has not been studied, but it is unlikely to enter milk in large amounts. In addition, these drugs have poor oral bioavailability and have short half-lives, so they are good choices for maternal analgesia during nursing.

Narcotic Partial Agonists

IV narcotic agonist-antagonists given during labor can interfere with establishment of lactation.[21,22] Despite breast-feeding and relatively high infant serum drug concentrations, mild withdrawal occurred in the neonate of a mother taking **buprenorphine** during pregnancy and postpartum for heroin addiction.[34] Oral buprenorphine for narcotic abstinence appears to have little impact on the breast-fed infant because of low amounts of the drug and metabolite in breast milk.[35,36] **Butorphanol** and **nalbuphine** concentrations in breast milk are low, and oral bioavailability in the infant should be low.[9,37] Amounts of **tramadol** in milk are low and have little or no impact in breast-fed infants.[38] **Naltrexone** was used in 1 mother without adverse effects in her breast-fed infant.[39] Excretion of **naloxone** into breast milk has not been studied, but is unlikely to have an effect on the infant.

(continued)

ANTIMICROBIAL DRUGS

AMINOGLYCOSIDES

Systemic effects of **amikacin, gentamicin, streptomycin, tobramycin,** and other aminoglycosides are unlikely in infants because of the small amounts in breast milk and poor oral absorption; however, observe infants for disruptions of the GI flora, such as diarrhea and thrush.

ANTIFUNGAL DRUGS

Amphotericin B and **nystatin** are virtually unabsorbed orally, and the latter is frequently used orally for treating thrush in infants; therefore, both are safe for use in nursing mothers, including topical application to the nipples. Likewise, **clotrimazole** has poor oral bioavailability and has been used orally in infants with thrush, sometimes successfully after nystatin has failed.[40] **Miconazole** has efficacy and safety similar to clotrimazole.[41] These two imidazoles are preferred for topical or vaginal application during nursing. **Fluconazole** amounts in breast milk are much less than the dosage prescribed for infants and can be used for recalcitrant *Candida* infections,[42–44] given to the mother and infant simultaneously. **Ketoconazole** concentrations in breast milk are low,[45] but it is best avoided in nursing mothers orally or topically to the nipples because of its oral absorption, occasional hepatotoxicity, and the availability of safer alternatives. Other imidazole antifungals have not been studied. **Gentian violet** is potentially toxic (toxic to mucous membranes, potential tattooing of the skin, and carcinogenic and mutagenic in rodents) and is best avoided topically on the nipples or in the infant's mouth.[46]

ANTIMYCOBACTERIAL DRUGS

Clofazimine

Clofazimine is excreted into milk, reportedly coloring it bright pink. Infants receive about 15%–30% of the maternal mg/kg dose. Breast-fed infants can develop the typical skin discoloration. In 1 infant, the skin color returned to normal 5 mo after the end of maternal therapy.[47,48]

Antituberculars[49]

Antituberculars pass into breast milk in small quantities. Use caution in nursing mothers because many of these drugs can cause hepatic damage. However, inadequate maternal therapy poses a much greater risk to the infant than the drugs in milk. The Centers for Disease Control and Prevention and other professional organizations state that breast-feeding should not be discouraged in women taking the first-line antituberculars.[50] **Isoniazid** is excreted into breast milk in amounts that are less than those given to treat an infant.[51] Nursing mothers who are taking isoniazid should take 25 mg of oral pyridoxine daily.[50] **Pyrazinamide** concentrations in breast milk in 1 woman were low and would give the baby less than a therapeutic dosage. **Rifampin** has not been well studied, but amounts in breast milk are small. **Cycloserine** is excreted in small amounts and no adverse reactions have been reported in infants. **Ethambutol** has not been adequately studied.

Sulfones

Newborns and glucose-6-phosphate dehydrogenase (G-6-PD)—deficient infants are particularly susceptible to **dapsone** hemolysis; avoid the drug while nursing these infants. Older infants might tolerate the amounts of sulfones excreted into milk.

ANTIPARASITIC DRUGS

Anthelmintics

Mebendazole was undetectable in breast milk in one woman and is poorly absorbed orally; therefore, it is unlikely to cause adverse effects in an infant. Contrary to an early case report, it

(continued)

ANTIMICROBIAL DRUGS

does not inhibit lactation. **Albendazole** has not been adequately studied during breast-feeding. Only small amounts of **praziquantel** and **ivermectin** reach the infant, and these drugs appear safe during nursing.[52,53]

Antimalarials

Hydroxychloroquine used daily for rheumatoid arthritis has not adversely affected infants' vision.[54] Weekly prophylactic doses of **chloroquine** are unlikely to be harmful during breast-feeding because the amount of drug in breast milk is less than the infant prophylactic dose. Small amounts of **quinine** in breast milk are unlikely to harm the infant, although allergic reactions might occur. **Pyrimethamine** appears to be acceptable and can be excreted into breast milk in quantities sufficient to treat or protect infants younger than 6 mo of age against malaria; however, breast-feeding is not a reliable method of drug administration. **Atovaquone** and **proguanil** are not recommended when breast-feeding infants under 5 kg, but may be used in heavier infants. **Mefloquine** appears in breast milk in small amounts after a single dose, but has not been studied after repeated weekly administration for malaria prophylaxis.[55]

Scabicides and Pediculocides

Lindane was excreted into breast milk at up to 30 times the typical background concentration (from environmental pollution) after maternal topical application of a 0.3% emulsion daily for 3 d. Breast milk concentrations remained elevated over background concentrations for at least 7 d.[56] Lindane should be avoided in nursing mothers. Although not well studied, **permethrin** and **pyrethrins** are preferred for nursing mothers because of their low toxicity.[53]

ANTIVIRAL DRUGS

Acyclovir and related drugs

A breast-fed infant would receive only about 1% of the mother's weight-adjusted oral dosage of acyclovir. The low dosage in breast milk and its poor oral bioavailability indicate that it might be well tolerated by the nursing infant, even with large IV doses.[57,58] Likewise, the amounts of acyclovir in milk after **valacyclovir** are low.[59] **Famciclovir** has not been studied during breast-feeding. Topical acyclovir or **penciclovir** applied to small areas of the mother's body away from the breast should pose no risk to the infant.

Antiretrovirals

Breast-feeding is considered to be contraindicated in HIV-infected mothers living in developed countries where acceptable, feasible, and safe alternatives to breast milk are available and affordable. In developing countries, **lamivudine, nevirapine,** and **zidovudine** are commonly used in nursing mothers to prevent mother-to-child transmission of HIV infection. Because of the long half-life of nevirapine, subtherapeutic nevirapine concentrations can persist in breast milk and infant serum for relatively long periods, potentially increasing the risk of development of nevirapine-resistant HIV infections when it is used alone for prophylaxis.[60–62] **Efavirenz, indinavir,** and **nelfinavir** have been studied to a lesser extent. Breast-fed infants generally tolerate these drugs well, but the use of highly active antiretroviral therapy during breast-feeding might increase the risk of neutropenia in breast-fed infants.[63]

Drugs for influenza

Amantadine is a dopamine agonist that decreases serum prolactin and theoretically can decrease lactation, so it is best avoided during nursing. Limited data on **oseltamivir** indicate that it is acceptable to use during breast-feeding.[64]

(continued)

ANTIMICROBIAL DRUGS

BETA-LACTAMS

Cephalosporins

Cephalosporins appear in trace amounts in breast milk and can lead to disruption of the GI flora or, rarely, allergic sensitization. Breast-feeding is safe with first- and second-generation agents. The risk might be greater with the third-generation cephalosporins and similar agents (e.g., **aztreonam, imipenem**), which are more active against GI flora. Observe infants for diarrhea, thrush, and rash.

Penicillins

Penicillins appear in trace amounts in breast milk, which can occasionally lead to allergic sensitization, allergic reactions in previously sensitized infants, or disruption of the GI flora, especially with the broader-spectrum agents (e.g., **piperacillin, ticarcillin plus clavulanate**). Unless the infant is allergic to penicillin, breast-feeding is generally safe. Observe infants for diarrhea, rash, and thrush.

MACROLIDES

Erythromycin, clarithromycin, and **azithromycin** are excreted into the breast milk in amounts much smaller than a typical infant dosage and are usually harmless to the infant.

NITROFURANS

Avoid these drugs in infants younger than 1 mo of age and those with G-6-PD deficiency because of the risk of hemolysis. If the infant is older than 1 mo, **furazolidone**, which is poorly absorbed orally, can be used to treat maternal giardiasis; **nitrofurantoin** is excreted into breast milk in pharmacologically unimportant amounts.

QUINOLONES

Ciprofloxacin, fleroxacin, nalidixic acid, ofloxacin, and **pefloxacin** have been detected in milk.[65,66] Ciprofloxacin seems to have caused pseudomembranous colitis in an infant via breast milk exposure,[67] and nalidixic acid caused hemolytic anemia in a breast-fed neonate.[68] Although short courses of these agents are unlikely to be problematic for most infants, **norfloxacin** might be the best choice among quinolones for maternal UTI treatment because of its low breast milk excretion and poor oral bioavailability.[69]

SULFONAMIDES

Some sulfonamides can cause hemolysis in G-6-PD–deficient infants; theoretically, sulfonamides in milk might increase the risk of kernicterus in neonates although documentation is lacking. **Sulfamethoxazole,** with or without **trimethoprim,** and **sulfisoxazole** can be used by mothers of healthy, full-term infants older than 2 mo old.[70]

TETRACYCLINES

Tooth staining from a tetracycline in breast milk has never been reported. Breast milk calcium apparently inhibits absorption of the small amounts of **tetracycline** in milk. Infant absorption and serum concentrations have not been reported with other tetracyclines, but infants would only receive a few milligrams per day of **demeclocycline, doxycycline,** or **minocycline** with usual maternal dosages. Minocycline has caused black milk.[71] Although other drugs are preferred for most infections, tetracyclines can be used for up to 2 wk during breast-feeding; avoid prolonged or repeat courses during nursing.[70]

(continued)

ANTIMICROBIAL DRUGS

MISCELLANEOUS ANTIMICROBIALS

Chloramphenicol

Breast-feeding is contraindicated during maternal chloramphenicol treatment. Breast milk concentrations are not sufficient to induce "gray baby" syndrome, but theoretically might be enough to cause the rare, idiosyncratic aplastic anemia. Adverse reactions in infants, including refusal of the breast, falling asleep during feeding, and vomiting after feeding, have occurred.[70]

Clindamycin

Clindamycin is excreted variably in small amounts into milk. It is not certain what effects these amounts might have on infants' GI flora (e.g., pseudomembranous colitis), but a single case of bloody stools in an infant with normal stool flora was reported during maternal clindamycin use. Clindamycin is best avoided if possible, but a few days of therapy with close monitoring of the infant is acceptable. Vaginal or topical clindamycin presents less infant risk than oral or IV use.

Metronidazole

Both metronidazole and its hydroxy metabolite are found in the serum of nursing infants in concentrations that are 10%–20% of maternal serum concentrations. Anecdotal cases of "spitting up" (possibly from a bad taste), diarrhea and isolation of *Candida* species in infants have been reported, but most infants do not have immediate reactions. Because of the carcinogenicity in animals, possible mutagenicity, and the relatively high infant serum concentrations achieved, metronidazole probably should be avoided in nursing mothers. When essential to treat trichomoniasis, metronidazole can be given as a single 2-g dose, and an alternative feeding method used for the next 24 h. After longer courses for anaerobic infections, nursing can resume 12–24 h after the final dose.[70]

Vancomycin

Because it is excreted into breast milk in only small amounts and is not orally absorbed, vancomycin can be used during nursing.[72]

ANTINEOPLASTICS AND IMMUNOSUPPRESSANTS

Few reports exist, but breast-feeding is generally considered to be contraindicated in women receiving antineoplastics because of the potential for immunosuppression and carcinogenicity.

ALKYLATING AGENTS

Busulfan

Busulfan in a dosage of 4 mg/d for 5 wk was taken by 1 woman while breast-feeding, with no apparent adverse effects on her infant's leukocytes or hemoglobin. This case is not conclusive and breast-feeding is not recommended.

Cisplatin

Platinum has been detected in the breast milk after maternal administration. Because the platinum might be in a reactive form, nursing is not recommended during cisplatin therapy.

Cyclophosphamide

Cyclophosphamide is detectable in milk and has caused bone marrow suppression in infants of women who nursed while receiving the drug. Breast-feeding is contraindicated during cyclophosphamide therapy.

(*continued*)

ANTIMICROBIAL DRUGS

ANTINEOPLASTICS AND IMMUNOSUPPRESSANTS

Methotrexate

Low amounts of methotrexate were found in breast milk in 1 patient; however, this case is not conclusive. Low weekly doses (e.g., 25 mg or less) for arthritis probably pose only a slight risk to the infant and are acceptable.

CYTOKINES

Interferons

IV **interferon alfa** results in only a slight increase over physiologic interferon breast milk concentrations.[73,74]

DNA INTERCALATING DRUGS

Doxorubicin

Doxorubicin and its primary active metabolite, **doxorubicinol**, appear in milk, with their highest breast milk concentrations occurring 24 h after a dose. Nursing is not recommended during doxorubicin therapy.

Mitoxantrone

Measurable concentrations of mitoxantrone occurred in breast milk for at least 28 d after 6 mg/kg was given daily for 3 d.[75] Nursing is not recommended during mitoxantrone therapy.

MITOTIC INHIBITORS

Etoposide

Etoposide is undetectable in breast milk 24 h after a dose.[75]

MISCELLANEOUS ANTINEOPLASTICS

Hydroxyurea

Only small amounts of hydroxyurea are found in milk, but breast-feeding is not advised.

Imatinib

Maternal doses of imatinib up to 400 mg daily result in low levels in milk. One breast-fed infant experienced no adverse effects during maternal use of imatinib, but no long-term data are available. Imatinib should be used only with careful monitoring during breast-feeding. Avoiding nursing for 8–9 h after a dose should considerably reduce the dose that the infant receives.[76–78]

IMMUNOSUPPRESSANTS[13,79]

Many infants reportedly were breast-fed safely during maternal **azathioprine** use (up to 200 mg/d) after renal transplantation and treatment of ulcerative colitis. Low concentrations of the azathioprine metabolite, **mercaptopurine,** are found in milk. Breast-feeding during azathioprine use is usually acceptable, but it may be desirable to monitor exclusively breast-fed infants with a complete blood count with differential, and liver function tests if azathioprine is used during lactation. Although probably not necessary, nursing the infant just before the dose and then pumping the breasts and discarding the milk 3–4 h after the dose would markedly reduce the dose received by the infant. Maternal **cyclosporine** therapy results in the infant receiving less than 2% of the mother's mg/kg dosage. **Tacrolimus** colostrum concentrations are about 50% of maternal serum concentrations. Numerous infants have been breast-fed during maternal cyclosporine or tacrolimus therapy after organ transplantation with no reported adverse effects.[80]

(continued)

CARDIOVASCULAR DRUGS

ANTIARRHYTHMIC DRUGS[81]

Some antiarrhythmics reach near-therapeutic concentrations in infants. **Amiodarone** is excreted in amounts that might pose a hazard to the infant and it should not be used during nursing. Data on **disopyramide** indicate that infants can receive relatively large amounts of the drug and its active metabolite, with infant serum concentrations near the therapeutic range. Disopyramide can be used cautiously while breast-feeding older infants when other alternatives are unacceptable. Observe the infant for anticholinergic symptoms, and monitor infant serum concentrations if there is a concern. The anticholinergic activity of disopyramide might also suppress lactation. (*See* Anticholinergics.) Sparse data from 1 patient indicate that **tocainide** should be used with caution during nursing. Infants receive trivial doses of **digoxin** via breast milk. Amounts of **flecainide** in breast milk are small and unlikely to affect the infant. **Lidocaine** concentrations in breast milk during continuous IV infusion, epidural administration, and with high doses as a local anesthetic are low and poorly absorbed by the infant, so it poses no hazard to the infant. Amounts of **mexiletine** in breast milk are too low to be detected in the serum of infants. **Procainamide** and its active metabolite, **N-acetylprocainamide,** are found in breast milk in fairly small amounts; procainamide can be used with careful monitoring in nursing mothers. **Propafenone** breast milk concentrations are very low, but no clinical experience has been reported. **Quinidine** excretion seems inconsequential.

ANTIHYPERTENSIVE DRUGS[82]

Certain antihypertensives are less desirable than others during nursing. Breast-fed infants have serum **clonidine** concentrations approaching those of the mother. Clonidine and **guanfacine** can also decrease maternal prolactin secretion. These drugs must be used with caution during breast-feeding and should be avoided if possible. The angiotensin-converting enzyme (ACE) inhibitors, **benazepril, captopril, enalapril,** and **quinapril,** are found in small amounts and no adverse effects have occurred in breast-fed infants. In addition, breast milk ACE activity was in the normal range after a dose of enalapril. These ACE inhibitors are good choices during lactation; others have not been studied. Limited data and extensive clinical experience indicate that low-dose, short-term use of **hydralazine** (i.e., a few days postpartum) is safe. There is limited information on oral **minoxidil** in milk, but amounts are small. However, use minoxidil with caution, particularly when therapy involves large dosages and long-term use. Several studies indicate that **methyldopa** is excreted in unimportant amounts.

BETA-ADRENERGIC ANTAGONISTS[82]

The excretion of β-blockers into breast milk has been studied extensively. The infant's dosage differs greatly among the different compounds, allowing a range of choices. The most water-soluble drugs reach the infant in the greatest amounts because of low serum protein binding. Water-soluble agents also have the longest half-lives, are renally eliminated, and therefore are more likely to accumulate in infants. Maternal therapy with **atenolol** and **acebutolol** has resulted in adverse effects (e.g., bradycardia, hypotension, tachypnea, and cyanosis) in infants. These two drugs, as well as **betaxolol, nadolol, sotalol,** and **timolol,** should be avoided in mothers of newborn infants or when high dosage is required. **Propranolol, metoprolol,** and **labetalol** are excreted in low enough quantities to allow nursing even in the neonatal period. However, labetalol apparently affected a 26-wk preterm infant who was given his mother's pumped milk.[83]

CALCIUM-CHANNEL ANTAGONISTS[82]

Case reports indicate that only small amounts of **diltiazem, nifedipine, nimodipine,** and **nitrendipine** are excreted into milk. Several case reports indicate that the amounts of **verapamil** and **norverapamil** in breast milk and infant serum are low. Verapamil also appears to be acceptable during nursing.

(*continued*)

CENTRAL NERVOUS SYSTEM DRUGS

ANTICONVULSANTS[84,85]

Breast-fed infants can achieve serum anticonvulsant concentrations that produce pharmacologic effects. Mild drowsiness, irritability, and feeding difficulties can occur in the infants of mothers taking sedating anticonvulsants, especially during the early neonatal period. Breast-feeding can mitigate withdrawal symptoms in infants whose mothers took sedating anticonvulsants during pregnancy and withdrawal symptoms have been observed after abrupt weaning. Serum concentration monitoring in infants might be indicated, particularly in infants who are excessively drowsy, feed poorly, or gain weight inadequately. Infants of mothers taking anticonvulsants might have more difficulty nursing and breast-feed for a shorter duration, possibly because of negative or equivocal safety advice given by health professionals.[86–88] Long-term effects of exposure are not well studied, but preliminary evidence indicates that breast-fed infants of mothers taking anticonvulsant monotherapy have better mental development than non–breast-fed infants.[89]

Carbamazepine

Both carbamazepine and its major active metabolite are excreted into breast milk and can be detected in nursing infants' serum; concentrations are usually low but near the therapeutic range in some infants. Two cases of hepatic dysfunction in neonates have been reported. Poor feeding and sedation have been reported occasionally, but most breast-fed infants tolerate the drug in milk well.[90] Carbamazepine can be used during lactation, but close observation of the infant for jaundice and other signs of possible adverse idiosyncratic effects is advisable. Measurement of the infant serum carbamazepine concentration might be indicated if symptoms occur.[85]

Clonazepam

Serum concentrations of clonazepam were low to unmeasurable in several nursing infants, and no effects were noted. In 1 infant, breast-feeding increased serum concentrations over those present at birth.[91] Clonazepam has been detected in the serum of a neonate whose mother was receiving the drug before and after delivery, but was undetectable in 4 others.[92] Observation of the infant for drowsiness and monitoring of the infant's serum concentration might be indicated.

Ethosuximide

Breast-fed infants can attain ethosuximide serum concentrations near the therapeutic range, and some infants might become drowsy or fussy. Breast-feed with caution, especially with neonates, and keep the mother's serum concentrations as low as possible while remaining in the therapeutic range. Infant serum drug concentration monitoring is indicated.

Gabapentin

Serum concentrations in breast-fed infants have been low in a small number of cases. Adverse effects are unlikely.[93]

Levetiracetam

Serum concentrations of levetiracetam in breast-fed infants are low and adverse effects are not expected, but infants should be monitored for sedation and other adverse effects.[94]

Lamotrigine

Lamotrigine serum concentrations in infants breast-fed during maternal lamotrigine therapy is variable, but can approach the maternal serum concentration. No adverse effects have been reported with these relatively high concentrations.[95] Infants can be allowed to nurse but close monitoring for side effects such as rash (which can be life-threatening), drowsiness, or poor sucking is essential. Obtain an infant serum concentration if adverse effects are suspected and discontinue breast-feeding if a rash occurs.

(continued)

CENTRAL NERVOUS SYSTEM DRUGS

Oxcarbazepine

Data from a few breast-fed infants indicate that serum concentrations are low.[96,97] Because of its similarity to carbamazepine, few adverse effects are expected during nursing. Follow precautions as for carbamazepine. (*See* Carbamazepine.)

Phenobarbital

The effect of phenobarbital is unpredictable: drowsiness leading to feeding difficulties can occur; however, breast-feeding can mitigate withdrawal symptoms in infants whose mothers took phenobarbital during pregnancy; and withdrawal symptoms have been observed after abrupt weaning. Phenobarbital can be used in low to moderate dosages, but monitor infant behavior, weight gain, and, if there is concern, serum concentrations. Sometimes breast-feeding must be discontinued because of excessive drowsiness and poor weight gain.

Phenytoin

Only small amounts of phenytoin are excreted into milk. Rarely, infants experience idiosyncratic reactions such as cyanosis and methemoglobinemia, but infants generally tolerate phenytoin in breast milk well.

Primidone

Primidone and its metabolites (**phenylethylmalonamide, phenobarbital,** and **parahydroxyphenobarbital**) appear in breast milk in large amounts. Considerations are the same as those for phenobarbital. (*See* Phenobarbital.)

Topiramate

Limited data indicate that serum topiramate concentrations in breast-fed infants are low to undetectable and breast-fed infants are not affected with maternal doses up to 200 mg/d.[98–100]

Valproic Acid

Milk concentrations of valproate are low, and usually no effects occur in infants.[101] One case of probable infant thrombocytopenic purpura from valproate in breast milk has been reported.[102] Observe infants for rare idiosyncratic effects such as thrombocytopenia and hepatotoxicity.[103]

Zonisamide

Limited data indicate that serum concentrations in breast-fed newborns are similar to maternal concentrations. No adverse effects have been reported, but standard anticonvulsant monitoring is advisable.[104]

ANTIDEPRESSANTS

Heterocyclic Antidepressants[105–109]

Although concern is often expressed about the use of antidepressants during breast-feeding, the consequences of untreated depression are also a great concern. When antidepressant therapy is required, **sertraline, paroxetine,** and **nortriptyline** are considered the drugs of choice because of their low concentrations in breast milk and usually undetectable serum concentrations in the breast-fed infants. Follow-up of infants up to 1 yr have found no adverse effects on growth and development with these drugs. Sedating TCAs and those with active metabolites (e.g., **amitriptyline, doxepin,** and **imipramine**) might be less desirable than other TCAs, but maternal dosages of **amitriptyline** up to 150 mg/d, **clomipramine** 150 mg/d, **desipramine** 300 mg/d, **imipramine** 200 mg/d, or **nortriptyline** 125 mg/d have not caused observable effects in the infants studied. Respiratory depression was reported in 1 infant whose mother was taking

(continued)

CENTRAL NERVOUS SYSTEM DRUGS

doxepin 25 mg tid, and another report found poor sucking and swallowing, muscle hypotonia and vomiting in a 9-d-old infant whose mother was taking doxepin 35 mg/d.[110,111] Doxepin should be avoided during breast-feeding.

Selective Serotonin Reuptake Inhibitors

As stated above, sertraline and paroxetine are generally considered to be the SSRIs of choice during breast-feeding, with sertraline probably used most frequently. The average daily dosages of **fluoxetine** and **norfluoxetine** in breast milk are about 7% of the mother's weight-adjusted dosage, but some mothers excrete as much as 12% of their dosage and the drugs' half-lives are very long.[112] One case of colic (increased crying, decreased sleep, watery stools, and vomiting) and unexplained high serum concentrations was reported in a 6-wk-old infant. The infant improved after switching to formula and colic reappeared upon rechallenge. Other case reports with fluoxetine include seizure-like activity, irritability, hyperglycemia and glycosuria, and withdrawal symptoms.[112] Norfluoxetine is often detectable in infants' serum.[92,112,113] Fluoxetine should be avoided during breast-feeding if possible, although older infants might be less susceptible to fluoxetine's effects than newborns. Monitor infants carefully for behavioral symptoms and adequate weight gain.

Citalopram reaches the infant in dosages of about 5% of the mother's mg/kg dosage.[114–116] The manufacturer states that drowsiness and weight loss in infants have occurred, and uneasy sleep occurred in the infant of a mother taking citalopram.[117] Higher serum concentrations of citalopram were found in 2 breast-fed infant twins whose mother was a poor metabolizer of citalopram and 5 infants who were heterozygous for the CYP2C19*1/*2 genotype had average serum levels that were 3.75 times higher than 5 other infants with the CYP2C19*1/*1 extensive metabolizer genotype.[35] These findings indicate that both maternal and infant genotypes can influence the serum concentration in breast-fed infants. Citalopram is not a good choice while breast-feeding a newborn; however, use of **escitalopram** in a dose of 25% that of citalopram reduces breast milk concentrations by about half and is a better alternative.[118,119]

Fluvoxamine has not been as well studied, but infants receive a weight-adjusted dose of <1% of the maternal dose. Several infants grow and developed normally with maternal fluvoxamine use.[120–122]

Monoamine Oxidase Inhibitors

There are no data on the amounts of older nonselective MAOIs excreted into milk. Because of their potential for toxicity and lactation inhibition, avoid MAOIs during nursing.

Other Antidepressants

Bupropion milk concentrations are low, but experience during nursing is limited.[123] One seizure was possibly caused by bupropion in breast milk.[124] Limited data indicate that **duloxetine** passes into milk poorly and does not adversely affect breast-fed infants.[125] **Mirtazapine** has not been studied well, but it appears that amounts excreted into breast milk are less than 5% of the maternal weight-adjusted dosage.[126,127] **Nefazodone** and **trazodone** dosages in the infant are <1% of the mother's mg/kg dosage, but only a few cases have been reported.[128] One case of drowsiness, lethargy, poor feeding, and inability to maintain normal body temperature was reported in a small preterm infant whose mother was taking nefazodone 300 mg/d.[129] Infants receive **venlafaxine** doses of up to 9.2% of the mother's mg/kg dosage and the active metabolite is detectable in the infant's serum. Although adverse effects have not been reported, caution should be used with venlafaxine until more experience is gained.[130–132]

(continued)

CENTRAL NERVOUS SYSTEM DRUGS

ANTIPSYCHOTIC DRUGS[108,133,134]

Data on the use of antipsychotics during lactation are sparse. **Phenothiazines** and **thioxanthenes** pass into breast milk somewhat unpredictably, but usually in small amounts. Drowsiness can occur with the more sedating agents, such as **chlorpromazine.** Limited follow-up, ranging from 15 mo to 6 yr, indicates no long-term effects on infant development in most infants. However, 3 infants whose mothers were taking large dosages of chlorpromazine (200–600 mg/d) and **haloperidol** (20–40 mg/d) in combination showed deterioration of mental and psychomotor developmental scores over the first 12–18 mo of life.[135] Nine other infants whose mothers were taking lower dosages of a single antipsychotic (including haloperidol up to 20 mg/d) showed normal development. It appears that maternal phenothiazines, thioxanthenes and haloperidol cause no problems for nursing infants unless dosage is at the high end of the range or combinations of drugs are used.[136–138] In 1 reported case, **aripiprazole** concentrations in milk were very low.[139] Breast-feeding during **clozapine** use in 4 infants resulted in sedation in 1 and agranulocytosis in another, which resolved upon discontinuation; nursing is not recommended during clozapine use. **Olanzapine** has been more thoroughly studied than some older antipsychotics. Amounts in milk are less than 1% of the maternal weight-adjusted dosage. Some unpublished reports received by the manufacturer indicate that the drug may be associated with extrapyramidal reactions and sedation in breast-fed infants.[140] **Quetiapine** breast milk dosages are low and the drug is low to undetectable in the serum of breast-fed infants.[141] Slight developmental delays occurred in 2 infants exposed to both quetiapine and paroxetine, but not to quetiapine alone. **Risperidone** dosages in milk are higher than those of olanzapine and similar to quetiapine's, but no adverse effects have been reported. One report found only small amounts of ziprasidone in breast milk, but other drugs are preferred.

ANXIOLYTICS, SEDATIVES, AND HYPNOTICS

Many sedatives and hypnotics pass into breast milk in measurable and potentially important amounts. Minimize sedative and hypnotic intake during lactation.

Anesthetics, General[32,33]

Compared with epidural anesthesia, general anesthesia used during cesarean delivery can decrease the frequency and duration of breast-feeding.[32] Excretion of most inhalation anesthetics in breast milk has not been well studied. Blood concentrations of anesthetic gases such as **desflurane, enflurane, halothane, isoflurane, nitrous oxide,** and **sevoflurane** drop rapidly after termination of anesthesia, are predicted to pass poorly into milk, and are probably poorly absorbed by the infant. **Etomidate** breast milk concentrations drop rapidly after a dose and should pose little risk to the infant. Amounts of **propofol** in breast milk are small and do not have good oral bioavailability in the infant.[142] Typical IV doses of **methohexital** or **thiopental** for induction of anesthesia produce low concentrations in breast milk that do not cause effects in the infant. Current opinion suggests that breast-feeding can be resumed as soon as the mother has recovered sufficiently from general anesthesia to nurse.

Barbiturates

Short-acting agents are preferable to long-acting agents, because smaller amounts are excreted into milk. Large single doses have more potential for causing infant drowsiness than multiple small doses. (*See also* Anesthetics, General; Anticonvulsants.)

(*continued*)

CENTRAL NERVOUS SYSTEM DRUGS

Benzodiazepines

Long-acting benzodiazepines and those with active metabolites (e.g., **diazepam**) can accumulate and cause adverse effects in infants, especially with repeated doses and in neonates, because of their immature excretory mechanisms. A single dose of diazepam for short dental, surgical, or diagnostic procedures is not likely to cause sedation in infants past the neonatal period.[24] **Bromazepam** taken by the mother might have contributed to the death of her 4-wk-old breast-fed infant with a 5-d history of apneic episodes.[143] Breast milk **alprazolam** concentrations are low,[144] but infant drowsiness and withdrawal symptoms have been reported with alprazolam use during nursing. When oral therapy is essential, the short-acting agents, **oxazepam** or **lorazepam,** are preferred; **temazepam** might also be acceptable.[138,145] **Midazolam** concentrations in breast milk are low and unlikely to affect the infant after a single dose or short course of therapy.[142]

Chloral Hydrate

Chloral hydrate and its active metabolite, **trichloroethanol,** appear in breast milk in dosages that approximate an infant sedative dosage and are detectable for up to 24 h after a single dose. Using another hypnotic is advisable during nursing.

Zaleplon

The dose in breast milk is very small and the drug disappears from breast milk rapidly.[146]

Zolpidem

Zolpidem breast milk concentrations are low for 3 h after a dose and undetectable thereafter.[147]

LITHIUM

Lithium in breast milk can adversely affect the infant when its elimination is impaired, as in dehydration or in neonates or premature infants. Neonates can also have transplacentally acquired serum lithium concentrations. The long-term effects of lithium on infants are not known; many investigators consider lithium therapy a contraindication to breast-feeding, but others do not. Lithium can be used cautiously in mothers who are carefully selected for their ability to monitor their full-term infants. Discontinue breast-feeding immediately if the infant appears restless or looks ill. Measurement of serum lithium concentrations in the infant can help rule out lithium toxicity.[148,149]

PARKINSONISM DRUGS

Dopamine Agonists

Some ergot alkaloids have dopaminergic activity that can suppress prolactin release and lactation. **Bromocriptine** was used therapeutically for this purpose, but has lost this indication in the United States because of potentially serious maternal toxicity (i.e., stroke, death). **Cabergoline** has also been used as a single dose to suppress lactation. Some mothers being treated with bromocriptine for other conditions have successfully breast-fed their infants.[150,151] No breast-feeding information is available on newer dopaminergic agents such as **pergolide, pramipexole,** and **ropinirole,** but they all might inhibit lactation.

Levodopa

Levodopa decreases serum prolactin in nonnursing women with hyperprolactinemia and galactorrhea in a dose-dependent fashion and inhibits lactation in animals at high dosages. One mother taking SR levodopa 200 mg-carbidopa 50 mg qid successfully breast-fed her infant whose development was normal at age 2 yr.[152]

(continued)

GASTROINTESTINAL DRUGS[153]

ACID-PEPTIC THERAPY[154]

Antacids

Although **aluminum, calcium,** and **magnesium** antacids are partially absorbed, they are unlikely to appreciably increase concentrations of these ions in breast milk and are safe to use.

Histamine H2-Receptor Antagonists

Cimetidine is concentrated in breast milk because of ion trapping and possibly by active secretion;[155] the dose of **ranitidine** that infants receive in breast milk is lower. **Famotidine** and **nizatidine** have the lowest doses in breast milk and are preferred during nursing.

Proton Pump Inhibitors

Proton pump inhibitors have not been well studied during breast-feeding, but since they are given safely to infants, it is unlikely they are harmful. In 1 mother, omeprazole breast milk concentrations were low and her newborn infant was breast-fed without harm.[156] Results were similar in another mother taking **pantoprazole**.[157] **Esomeprazole, lansoprazole,** and **rabeprazole** have not been studied during breast-feeding, but are probably similarly poorly excreted into milk.

Sucralfate

Because sucralfate is virtually nonabsorbable, it is unlikely to affect the breast-fed infant.

GASTROINTESTINAL MOTILITY

Antidiarrheals

The **loperamide** prodrug loperamide oxide results in only small amounts of loperamide in breast milk. **Diphenoxylate** excretion into breast milk has not been studied. One or two small doses of loperamide or diphenoxylate daily should pose little risk to the nursing infant. Avoid **bismuth subsalicylate** because salicylate is absorbable.

Cathartics and Laxatives

Some **anthraquinone** derivatives, such as **aloe** and **cascara,** and other stimulant cathartics (e.g., **phenolphthalein**) should be avoided during nursing because of a laxative effect in breast-fed infants. Laxatives that are nonabsorbable or poorly absorbed, such as bulk-forming (e.g., **psyllium**), osmotic (e.g., **magnesium** or **phosphate salts**), or stool-softening (e.g., **docusate**) types, are preferred during lactation. **Senna** in moderate dosages is acceptable if other measures fail. **Bisacodyl** is virtually unabsorbed from the GI tract and should be safe.

Gastrokinetic Agents

Metoclopramide elevates serum prolactin via central dopaminergic antagonism. It has been used in mothers who are producing insufficient quantities of milk, such as the mothers of premature or sick infants, or adoptive mothers, but clinical results are equivocal. Although infant dosages of metoclopramide from breast milk are low, the infant's serum prolactin concentrations are sometimes elevated. Metoclopramide can induce depression and tardive dyskinesia with long-term use, so limiting the duration of metoclopramide therapy is essential; it should not be used in mothers with a history of depression. **Domperidone** has been used to increase breast milk supply and results in lower breast milk drug concentrations than metoclopramide.[158,159] The use of antidopaminergic drugs as galactagogues should be seen as a last resort and not a substitute for good lactation management.[160]

(continued)

GASTROINTESTINAL DRUGS[153]

MISCELLANEOUS GASTROINTESTINAL DRUGS

Mesalamine Derivatives

Small amounts of **sulfasalazine** and **sulfapyridine** have been found in breast milk and infants' sera after oral sulfasalazine use. The small amount of sulfapyridine released should cause no bilirubin displacement. **Olsalazine** is not detectable in milk, but its metabolite N-acetyl-5-ASA is found in small amounts.[161] Small amounts of **mesalamine** and larger amounts of its metabolite are found in breast milk after oral administration.[162] Diarrhea has been reported in infants of mothers using mesalamine derivatives, but a controlled study found the frequency of diarrhea to be no greater than that in infants of untreated mothers.[163] Sulfasalazine and mesalamine and its derivatives are acceptable during nursing.

Ursodiol

Ursodiol was undetectable in the breast milk of 1 lactating mother, and her nursing infant developed normally during therapy.[164] Maternal ursodiol therapy decreased the bile acid concentration in colostrum and was found in trivial amounts in breast milk in 16 mothers with intrahepatic cholestasis of pregnancy. Their breast-fed infants showed no adverse effects.[165]

HEMATOLOGIC DRUGS

COAGULANTS AND ANTICOAGULANTS

Coumarins

Amounts of **warfarin** in milk are of no clinical consequence with a maternal dosage of 12 mg/d or less because of extensive protein binding. Higher dosages have not been studied. Other coumarin derivatives (e.g., **acenocoumarol, dicumarol,** and **phenprocoumon**) also appear to be safe.[166]

Direct Thrombin Inhibitors

Lepirudin is not detectable in milk.[167] **Ximelagatran** and **melagatran** are excreted into breast milk in low amounts unlikely to affect breast-fed infants.[168]

Heparins

Although minimal documentation exists, it is unlikely that **heparin** passes into breast milk or is absorbed orally by the infant. Low-molecular-weight heparins (e.g., **enoxaparin, dalteparin**) pass poorly into milk and do not affect the breast-fed infant.[169,170] **Danaparoid** likewise has no effect on the breast-fed infant.[171,172] **Fondaparinux** has not been studied in breast-feeding.

HORMONES AND SYNTHETIC SUBSTITUTES

ADRENAL HORMONES[13,153]

Corticosteroids

Excretion of **prednisone** and **prednisolone** into breast milk is minimal even with large oral doses.[173] The infant dosage can be reduced even further by using prednisolone rather than prednisone and avoiding nursing for 3–4 h after a dose. Three infants reportedly have been breast-fed during long-term maternal use of **methylprednisolone** 6–8 mg/d with apparent safety. Large IV doses of corticosteroids or use of long-acting agents such as **dexamethasone** have not been studied, and caution is warranted. Depot injections, inhaled corticosteroids (e.g., **beclomethasone, fluticasone**), nonabsorbable oral corticosteroids (e.g., **budesonide**) or topical corticosteroids should present little or no risk to the infant because of low maternal serum concentrations.[79,174] However, topical application to the nipple has caused adverse effects in the infant because of direct ingestion.[175]

(continued)

HORMONES AND SYNTHETIC SUBSTITUTES

ANTIDIABETIC DRUGS[176]

Insulin

Diabetic mothers using insulin may nurse their infants. However, the mother might need to reduce her insulin dosage to 55%–75% of the prepregnancy dosage. Close monitoring is required postpartum, because the return to prepregnancy insulin dosage has been variably reported to take 1–6 wk.[177,178] Exogenous insulin appears in milk in similar concentrations to endogenous insulin.[179]

Sulfonylureas

Tolbutamide is excreted in breast milk in small amounts that should cause no harm. The manufacturer reports that **chlorpropamide** concentrations in breast milk are low. **Glyburide** and **glipizide** also appear in milk in only low concentrations.[180]

Other Antidiabetic Agents

Acarbose and **miglitol** have not been studied during breast-feeding, but are unlikely to affect the infant because of their poor oral absorption. **Metformin** has been used widely in treating polycystic ovary syndrome during breast-feeding with no adverse effects in breast-fed infants.[181] The excretion of **pioglitazone, rosiglitazone, exenatide,** and **pramlintide** has not been studied during lactation.

FEMALE SEX HORMONES

Estrogen–Progestin Combination Oral Contraceptives

Although present in breast milk in small amounts, estrogens and progestins are readily metabolized by nursing infants. Combined oral contraceptives do not affect the composition of milk substantially in healthy, well-nourished mothers. They might transiently affect growth negatively during the first month after introduction, but an 8-yr follow-up of infants of mothers taking contraceptives containing **ethinyl estradiol** 50 μg found no adverse effects on the infants' development or behavior. Rare case reports of breast enlargement in infants have been attributed to older high-dose (>50 μg) estrogen-containing oral contraceptives. Estrogen-containing contraceptives can suppress lactation in a dose-dependent fashion, especially when administered immediately postpartum. Women taking these drugs introduce formula sooner than those not taking them.[182] Expert opinion holds that combination contraceptive products should not be started sooner than 6 wk postpartum. Between 6 wk and 6 mo postpartum, their potential suppression of lactation generally outweighs the advantages of this method during breast-feeding. After 6 mo postpartum, combination contraceptives (including oral tablets, transdermal patches, and vaginal rings) can be used, but progestin-only methods are preferred if breast-feeding will be continued.[183–185]

Progestin Only Contraceptives

Progestin-only contraceptives such as **levonorgestrel** intrauterine devices or implants, depot **medroxyprogesterone acetate,** or oral **norethindrone** or **norgestrel** are considered the hormonal contraceptives of choice during lactation. They appear not to affect the composition of milk, the growth and development of the infant or the milk supply. The timing of initiation of postpartum contraception with levonorgestrel is somewhat controversial. It is preferable to initiate progestin-only contraception no sooner than 6 wk postpartum. Starting sooner theoretically could affect the newborn infant adversely because of slower metabolism of the drug than older infants. Administration sooner than 3 d postpartum could inhibit lactogenesis and interfere with the

(*continued*)

HORMONES AND SYNTHETIC SUBSTITUTES

establishment of lactation, although 2 medium-quality studies found no adverse effects on breast-feeding. Use of 2 doses of 0.75 mg of levonorgestrel 12 h apart for postcoital contraception has not been studied, but data from a study on a single 1.5 mg dose indicate that nursing can be resumed after 8 h.[184,186,187]

Progesterone

Progesterone-releasing vaginal and intrauterine devices transfer little progesterone to the infant, and any drug in breast milk is minimally absorbed by the infant. Breast milk progesterone concentrations have not been measured after higher doses used to treat premenstrual syndrome.[188,189]

THYROID AND ANTITHYROID DRUGS

Iodides

Inorganic **iodide** is contraindicated during breast-feeding because of possible thyroid suppression and rash. Topical **povidone-iodine** use in nursing mothers can result in elevated breast milk iodine concentrations and occasionally causes thyroid suppression or abnormal thyroid function tests in nursing infants. Its use should be minimized. Maternal application vaginally or to open wounds has caused severe electrolyte abnormalities in breast-fed infants.[190–192]

Thioamides

Propylthiouracil is the antithyroid drug of choice during lactation because little passes into breast milk and infant thyroid suppression does not occur. Dosages as high as 750 mg/d have been given to nursing mothers with no adverse effects in their infants. **Methimazole** 20 mg/d or **carbimazole** (a methimazole prodrug) 15 mg/d can also be used, but these drugs pass into breast milk in greater quantities and have longer half-lives than propylthiouracil. Infants of mothers who took 20 mg/d of methimazole while nursing had no decrease in intellectual or physical development at age 1 yr. A potential for idiosyncratic reactions (e.g., agranulocytosis) and hypothyroidism exists, and measurement of the infant's serum thyroxine and TSH concentrations at 2 to 4 wk intervals might be prudent during maternal antithyroid drug use.[193,194]

Thyroid Hormones

Normal lactation requires thyroid hormones. **Levothyroxine** (T_4) passes into breast milk poorly, although **liothyronine** (T_3) might pass in more physiologically relevant amounts. Breast milk concentrations of thyroid hormones have not been measured after exogenous administration, but a physiologic replacement dosage of levothyroxine to a breast-feeding mother is not expected to result in excessive thyroid administration to the infant. Replacement therapy with liothyronine or supraphysiologic maternal levothyroxine dosage might transfer larger amounts of liothyronine to the infant.[195,196]

MISCELLANEOUS HORMONAL AGENTS

Calcitriol

Calcitriol requirements in hypoparathyroid women decrease during lactation. Failure to substantially decrease (up to two-thirds) the calcitriol dosage can result in maternal hypercalcemia.[197,198]

Desmopressin

Desmopressin is excreted in negligible amounts into breast milk and is poorly absorbed orally by the infant, so it appears acceptable to use.

(continued)

HORMONES AND SYNTHETIC SUBSTITUTES

Human Growth Hormone

Somatropin can increase milk production in mothers with an insufficient breast milk production.[199]

RENAL AND ELECTROLYTES

Diuretics

Large dosages of short-acting thiazide-type diuretics (e.g., **hydrochlorothiazide**), usual dosages of loop diuretics (e.g., **furosemide**), or long-acting thiazide-type diuretics (e.g., **chlorthalidone** and **bendroflumethiazide**) can suppress lactation and should be avoided. Long-acting agents can also accumulate in infants' serum. Low dosages of short-acting thiazide-type diuretics (e.g., 25 mg/d or less of hydrochlorothiazide) should pose no problems to the infant or suppress lactation. **Acetazolamide** appears in breast milk in small amounts that are unlikely to harm the infant. The amounts of **spironolactone** and its metabolites in breast milk are inconsequential.[200–203]

Bisphosphonates

Pamidronate was used successfully in 1 patient to treat bone loss associated with reflex sympathetic dystrophy. The drug was undetectable in breast milk.[204]

Fluoride

Fluoride supplementation is not recommended during the first 6 mo after birth; from 6 mo to 3 yr of age, fluoride supplementation of 0.25 mg/d is recommended only if the mother's water supply contains <0.3 ppm fluoride.[205]

Iron

Intravenous **iron sucrose** given to nursing mothers appears not to increase breast milk iron out of the normal range.[206]

Magnesium Sulfate

Infants exposed to magnesium sulfate transplacentally during delivery may be hypotonic and have lower APGAR scores postpartum. However, IV magnesium sulfate increases breast milk magnesium concentrations only slightly. Oral absorption of magnesium is poor, so maternal magnesium therapy is not a contraindication to breast-feeding.[207,208]

ANTIGOUT AGENTS

Allopurinol

This drug and its active metabolite, **oxypurinol,** are excreted into breast milk in nearly therapeutic amounts, and oxypurinol is detectable in the nursing infant's serum in near-therapeutic concentrations. Although 1 infant reportedly breast-fed without harm during maternal allopurinol therapy, observe infants for side effects, especially hypersensitivity reactions. If possible, give allopurinol to the mother in a single dose after the last nursing of the day.[209]

Colchicine

Several infants have been breast-fed safely during long-term, low-dose administration of colchicine to the mother for familial Mediterranean fever. The amount excreted in breast milk indicates that toxicity might occur with higher dosages. Use colchicine with great caution and in low dosages when breast-feeding, especially with a neonate.[210–212]

(continued)

RESPIRATORY DRUGS

ANTIASTHMATICS

Anticholinergics

Excretion of anticholinergics into breast milk has not been studied. Theoretical hazards of the orally absorbable compounds include anticholinergic effects such as drying of secretions, temperature elevations, and CNS disturbances in the infant. Theoretically, anticholinergics inhibit lactation by inhibiting growth hormone and oxytocin secretion.[213] Observe infants carefully for anticholinergic symptoms and signs of decreased lactation (e.g., insatiety, poor weight gain) when anticholinergics are given to the mother. It is unlikely that inhaled **ipratropium** affects the infant or breast milk production.

Terbutaline

Oral administration results in low breast milk terbutaline concentrations, causes no symptoms in infants, and is not expected to decrease breast milk supply. Other beta$_2$-receptor agonists (e.g., **albuterol**) appear safe to use orally, but inhaler products should transfer the lowest amount of drug to the infant and are preferred.[214]

Theophylline

Maternal theophylline use occasionally causes irritability and fretful sleep in infants. There is no need to avoid theophylline products; however, keep maternal serum concentrations in the lower part of the therapeutic range and measure infant serum concentrations if side effects occur. Newborn and preterm infants have much slower elimination of theophylline which can result in high serum concentrations.[215]

ANTIHISTAMINES

There are few studies on antihistamine use during lactation. One study found drowsiness or irritability occurred in 12% of infants whose mothers took antihistamines.[6] Avoid older, sedating (and more anticholinergic) antihistamines such as **diphenhydramine** in high dosages, in SR formulations, or in combinations with a sympathomimetic agent, because they affect the infant and might suppress lactation. (*See Anticholinergics.*) Nonsedating antihistamines are preferred agents for long-term therapy.[216,217] **Cetirizine** has not been studied, but is recommended as an alternative to older antihistamines.[216] **Clemastine** has caused drowsiness in a breast-fed infant.[218] **Cyproheptadine** lowers maternal serum prolactin and should be avoided during lactation.[219] Based on terfenadine experience, **fexofenadine** is likely to be well tolerated by breast-fed infants.[6,220] **Loratadine** is excreted into breast milk in seemingly unimportant amounts.[221] Only small amounts of **triprolidine** are found in breast milk.[222]

COUGH AND COLD

Alpha-adrenergic **sympathomimetics** decrease breast milk flow in animals by central inhibition of secretion and release of prolactin and oxytocin. **Norepinephrine** might decrease prolactin release. Lactation inhibition and infant irritability occurs with maternal **pseudoephedrine** use; therefore, sympathomimetic nasal sprays (e.g., **oxymetazoline**) are recommended over oral decongestant products. Pseudoephedrine also causes irritability in some breast-fed infants.[6,223] Furthermore, the FDA has recommended against cough and cold preparation use in infants and children under 2 yr of age.

MISCELLANEOUS DRUGS

Baclofen

Only small amounts of baclofen appear in milk, and it can be used in nursing mothers with caution.[224]

(*continued*)

MISCELLANEOUS DRUGS

Bupivacaine

Bupivacaine appears in breast milk in small amounts when administered to the mother by intrapleural or epidural routes but has no effect on the infant.[225] Epidural analgesia with bupivacaine post-cesarean section improved breast-feeding performance in 1 study.[226] (*See also* Lidocaine in Antiarrhythmics.)

Cholinergic Drugs

Six infants of mothers treated with **neostigmine** for myasthenia gravis were reportedly breast-fed successfully. Neostigmine was not found in milk, but 1 infant appeared to have abdominal cramps after each breast-feeding. **Pyridostigmine** has been used safely during breast-feeding in 3 patients with myasthenia gravis.[227,228]

Dantrolene

Several dantrolene doses totaling 720 mg IV over 2 d to a postpartum mother yielded peak breast milk concentrations of 12 mg/L. Dantrolene half-life in breast milk was 9.2 h. Data are insufficient to establish safety during breast-feeding.[229]

Ergot Alkaloids

Ergonovine can lower postpartum serum prolactin concentrations and reduce lactation rates, but **methylergonovine** apparently does not. Methylergonovine is not found in breast milk in important quantities.[230–233] Short-term, low-dose regimens of these agents immediately postpartum pose no hazard to the infant, but methylergonovine is preferred because it does not inhibit lactation. Courses of these drugs given several days postpartum might expose the infant to greater risk of ergot side effects because of the larger amount of breast milk consumed at this age.

Nicotine

With a 21 mg transdermal patch, nicotine passes into breast milk in amounts equivalent to smoking 17 cigarettes daily. Lower patch strengths of 7 and 14 mg provide proportionately lower amounts of nicotine to the breast-fed infant. No studies on nicotine spray or nicotine gum use in nursing mothers have been reported.[234]

Pyridoxine

In high doses (200–600 mg/d), pyridoxine has been used to suppress lactation, although it is often not effective. With usual dosages found in foods and low-dose vitamin supplements, pyridoxine has no effect on prolactin or lactation.[235,236]

Retinoids

Acitretin passes into breast milk in a quantity sufficient to merit avoidance of nursing while taking it.[237] Although there is no information on use during lactation, the manufacturers of oral **isotretinoin** and topical **tretinoin** state that they are not compatible with nursing. Based on the systemic bioavailability of tretinoin applied topically to a small area such as the face, it is unlikely that harmful amounts reach the infant via breast milk.[238] Avoid contact of the infant's skin with treated areas of the mother's skin.

Stimulants

In mothers taking **amphetamine** or **dextroamphetamine** 15–45 mg/d for narcolepsy or attention deficit disorder, amphetamine concentrations in breast milk were low and no adverse effects on the infant were noted.[239,240] This is consistent with an old report of mothers taking amphetamine for postpartum depression with no adverse infant effects.[241] Methamphetamine and its metabolite, amphetamine, are detectable in breastmilk and infant's serum after abuse of methamphetamine

(*continued*)

MISCELLANEOUS DRUGS

by nursing mothers. Four infants were breast-fed during maternal use of **methylphenidate** 15–80 mg/d for attention deficit disorder. None of the infants experienced adverse reactions.

Vaccines

Breast-feeding is not a contraindication to the use of most vaccines (live or inactivated) in the nursing mother. However, nursing mothers should generally not receive the smallpox or yellow fever vaccine.[242–244]

DIAGNOSTIC AGENTS

Iodinated Contrast Media

Although data are limited, the contrast agents **diatrizoate, iohexol,** and **metrizamide** are detectable in small amounts in breast milk after IV administration. Because the iodine is tightly bound in these compounds, the risk of iodine toxicity in the infant is minimal. Both the American College of Radiology and the European Society of Urogenital Radiology state that breast-feeding need not be interrupted after a nursing mother receives an iodine-containing contrast medium.[245,246]

Fluorescein

Fluorescein is detectable in breast milk after IV or topical administration. After IV administration, it had a breast milk half-life of 62 h in 1 mother. The drug might present a risk to neonates who are undergoing phototherapy.[247,248] Temporarily withholding nursing after IV fluorescein use seems appropriate.

Gadolinium

Gadodiamide and **gadopentetate,** used in magnetic resonance imaging (MRI), are detectable in milk in low concentrations, but have poor oral absorption and are rapidly excreted renally. Breast-feeding need not be interrupted after their use.[245,246,249] Other MRI contrast agents have not been studied during breast-feeding.

Radiopharmaceuticals

Exposure of the infant to excessive amounts of radioactivity is usually the primary concern raised by administration of radiopharmaceuticals to nursing mothers, rather than any pharmacologic toxicity of the agent. Some, but not all radiopharmaceuticals require discontinuation of breast-feeding, at least temporarily, after administration to a nursing mother. The period needed for breast milk radioactivity to decline (by means of both radioactive decay and maternal excretion) to a safe exposure concentration depends on several factors: dosage, biological half-life, radionuclide half-life, condition being treated, and "contamination" with other isotopes. The age of the infant, potential for oral absorption of the radionuclide from the infant's GI tract, and threshold concentration that is considered safe are also important factors. Measurement of breast milk radioactivity can aid in determining when breast-feeding can resume. **Radioactive iodine-131** is the most dangerous and usually requires complete cessation of breast-feeding. Agents that contain **technetium 99m** compounds require at most a few hours of withholding of breast-feeding. Consult specialty sources for more detailed information.[250,251]

■ REFERENCES

1. Anderson PO. Drug use during breast-feeding. *Clin Pharm.* 1991;10:594-624.
2. Anderson GD. Using pharmacokinetics to predict the effects of pregnancy and maternal-infant transfer of drugs during lactation. *Expert Opin Drug Metab Toxicol.* 2006;2:947-960.
3. Bennett PN, Notarianni LJ. Risk from drugs in breast milk: an analysis by relative dose [abstract]. *Br J Clin Pharmacol.* 1996;42:P673-P674.

4. Ito S, Koren G. A novel index for expressing exposure to the infant to drugs in breast milk. *Br J Clin Pharmacol.* 1994;38:99-102.

5. Anderson PO et al. Adverse drug reactions in breastfed infants: less than imagined. *Clin Pediatr (Phila).* 2003;42:325-340.

6. Ito S et al. Prospective follow-up of adverse reactions in breast-fed infants exposed to maternal medication. *Am J Obstet Gynecol.* 1993;168:1393-1399.

7. Jolivet A et al. Effect of ergot alkaloid derivatives on milk secretion in the immediate postpartum period. *J Gynecol Obstet Biol Reprod (Paris).* 1978;7:129-134.

8. Wojnar-Horton RE et al. Distribution and excretion of sumatriptan in human milk. *Br J Clin Pharmacol.* 1996;41:217-221.

9. Spigset O, Hagg S. Analgesics and breast-feeding: safety considerations. *Paediatr Drugs.* 2000;2:223-238.

10. Anderson PO. Medication use while breast feeding a neonate. *Neonatal Pharmacol Q.* 1993;2:3-14.

11. Gardiner SJ et al. Quantification of infant exposure to celecoxib through breast milk. *Br J Clin Pharmacol.* 2006;61:101-104.

12. Hale TW et al. Transfer of celecoxib into human milk. *J Hum Lact.* 2004;20:397-403.

13. Ostensen M, Motta M. Therapy insight: the use of antirheumatic drugs during nursing. *Nat Clin Pract Rheumatol.* 2007;3:400-406.

14. Rayburn WF. Connective tissue disorders and pregnancy. Recommendations for prescribing. *J Reprod Med.* 1998;43:341-349.

15. Skomsvoll JF et al. Drug insight: anti-tumor necrosis factor therapy for inflammatory arthropathies during reproduction, pregnancy and lactation. *Nature Clin Pract Rheumatol.* 2007;3:156-164.

16. Gregory MC, Mansell MA. Pregnancy and cystinuria. *Lancet.* 1983;2:1158-1160.

17. Messner U et al. Wilson disease and pregnancy. Review of the literature and case report. *Z Geburtshilfe Neonatol.* 1998;202:77-79.

18. Madadi P et al. Pharmacogenetics of neonatal opioid toxicity following maternal use of codeine during breast-feeding: a case-control study. *Clin Pharmacol Ther.* 2009;85:31-35.

19. Madadi P et al. Establishing causality of CNS depression in breastfed infants following maternal codeine use. *Paediatr Drugs.* 2008;10:399-404.

20. Anderson PO et al. Hydrocodone excretion into breastmilk: the first two reported cases. *Breastfeed Med.* 2007;2:10-14.

21. Rajan L. The impact of obstetric procedures and analgesia/anaesthesia during labour and delivery on breast feeding. *Midwifery.* 1994;10:87-103.

22. Nissen E et al. Effects of routinely given pethidine during labour on infants' developing breastfeeding behaviour. Effects of dose-delivery time interval and various concentrations of pethidine/norpethidine in cord plasma. *Acta Paediatr.* 1997;86:201-208.

23. Wittels B et al. Postcesarean analgesia with both epidural morphine and intravenous patient-controlled analgesia: neurobehavioral outcomes among nursing neonates. *Anesth Analg.* 1997;85:600-606.

24. Borgatta L et al. Clinical significance of methohexital, meperidine, and diazepam in breast milk. *J Clin Pharmacol.* 1997;37:186-192.

25. Philipp BL et al. Methadone and breastfeeding: new horizons. *Pediatrics.* 2003;111:1429-1430.

26. Fong G. High doses of methadone in breastfeeding. Presented at: *ASHP Annual Meeting;* 2000;57:pp INTL-3. IPA accession number 37-05332.

27. Malpas TJ et al. Breastfeeding reduces the severity of neonatal abstinence syndrome [abstract P20]. *J Paediatr Child Health.* 1997;33:A38.

28. Oei J, Lui K. Management of the newborn infant affected by maternal opiates and other drugs of dependency. *J Paediatr Child Health.* 2007;43:9-18.

29. Jansson LM et al. Concentrations of methadone in breast milk and plasma in the immediate perinatal period. *J Hum Lact.* 2007;23:184-190.

30. Lim S et al. High-dose methadone in pregnant women and its effect on duration of neonatal abstinence syndrome. *Am J Obstet Gynecol.* 2009;200:70.e1-e5.

31. Meites E . Opiate exposure in breastfeeding newborns [letter]. *J Hum Lact.* 2007;23:13.

32. Lee JJ, Rubin AP. Breast feeding and anaesthesia. *Anaesthesia.* 1993;48:616-625.

33. Hale TW. Anesthetic medications in breastfeeding mothers. *J Hum Lact.* 1999;15:185-194.

34. Marquet P et al. Buprenorphine withdrawal syndrome in a newborn. *Clin Pharmacol Ther.* 1997;62:569-571.

35. Jernite M et al. Buprenorphine excretion in breast milk [abstract]. *Anesthesiology.* 1999;91:A1095.

36. Lindemalm S et al. Transfer of buprenorphine into breast milk and calculation of infant drug dose. *J Hum Lact.* 2009;25:199-205.

37. Wischnik A et al. Elimination von nalbuphin in die muttermilch Elimination of nalbuphine in human milk. *Arzneimittelforschung.* 1988;38:1496-1498.

38. Ilett KF et al. Use of a sparse sampling study design to assess transfer of tramadol and its O-desmethyl metabolite into transitional breast milk. *Br J Clin Pharmacol.* 2008;65:661-666.

39. Chan CF et al. Transfer of naltrexone and its metabolite 6,beta-naltrexol into human milk. *J Hum Lact.* 2004;20:322-326.

40. Johnstone HA, Marcinak JF. Candidiasis in the breastfeeding mother and infant. *J Obstet Gynecol Neonatal Nurs.* 1990;19:171-173.

41. Amir LH, Pakula S. Nipple pain, mastalgia and candidiasis in the lactating breast. *Aust N Z J Obstet Gynaecol.* 1991;31:378-380.

42. Schilling CG et al. Excretion of fluconazole in human breast milk [abstract]. *Pharmacotherapy.* 1993;13:287.

43. Force RW. Fluconazole concentrations in breast milk. *Pediatr Infect Dis J.* 1995;14:235-236.

44. Wiener S. Diagnosis and management of Candida of the nipple and breast. *J Midwifery Womens Health.* 2006;51:125-128.

45. Moretti ME et al. Disposition of maternal ketoconazole in breast milk. *Am J Obstet Gynecol.* 1995;173:1625-1626.

46. Utter AR. Gentian violet treatment for thrush: can its use cause breastfeeding problems [letter]. *J Hum Lact.* 1990;6:178-180.

47. Venkatesan K et al. Excretion of clofazimine in human milk in leprosy patients. *Lepr Rev.* 1997;68:242-246.

48. Waters MFR. G 30 320 or B 663-Lampren (Geigy). A working party held at the Royal Garden Hotel London, September 1968. *Lepr Rev.* 1969;40:21-47.

49. Tran JH, Montankitikul P. The safety of antituberculosis medications during breastfeeding. *J Hum Lact.* 1998;14:337-340.

50. Blumberg HM et al. American Thoracic Society/Centers for Disease Control and Prevention/Infectious Diseases Society of America: treatment of tuberculosis. *Am J Respir Crit Care Med.* 2003;167:603-662.

51. Singh N et al. Transfer of isoniazid from circulation to breast milk in lactating women on chronic therapy for tuberculosis. *Br J Clin Pharmacol.* 2007;65:418-422.

52. Ogbuokiri JE et al. Ivermectin levels in human breast milk. *Eur J Clin Pharmacol.* 1994;46:89-90.

53. Porto I. Antiparasitic drugs and lactation: focus on anthelmintics, scabicides, and pediculicides. *J Hum Lact.* 2003;19:421-425.

54. Costedoat-Chalumeau N et al. Safety of hydroxychloroquine in pregnant patients with connective tissue diseases. Review of the literature. *Autoimmun Rev.* 2005;4:111-115.

55. Arguin P, Mali S. Prevention of Specific Infectious Diseases. In: Arguin PM, Kozarsky PE, Reed C, eds. Centers for Disease Control and Prevention. Health Information for International Travel 2008. Atlanta: US Department of Health and Human Services, Public Health Service; 2007:chap 4.

56. Senger VE et al. Therapy-induced lindane concentration in breast milk. *Derm Beruf Umwelt.* 1989;37:167-170.

57. Taddio A et al. Acyclovir excretion in human breast milk. *Ann Pharmacother.* 1994;28:585-587.

58. Bork K, Benes P. Concentration and kinetic studies of intravenous acyclovir in serum and breast milk of a patient with eczema herpeticum. *J Am Acad Dermatol.* 1995;32:1053-1055.

59. Sheffield JS et al. Acyclovir concentrations in human breast milk after valacyclovir administration. *Am J Obstet Gynecol.* 2002;186:100-102.

60. Arrive E et al. Prevalence of resistance to nevirapine in mothers and children after single-dose exposure to prevent vertical transmission of HIV-1: a meta-analysis. *Int J Epidemiol.* 2007;36:1009-1021.

61. Kunz A et al. Persistence of nevirapine in breast milk and plasma of mothers and their children after single-dose administration. *J Antimicrob Chemother.* 2009;63:170-177.

62. Moorthy A et al. Nevirapine resistance and breast-milk HIV transmission: effects of single and extended-dose nevirapine prophylaxis in subtype C HIV-infected infants. *PLoS One.* 2009;4:e4096.

63. Bae WH et al. Hematologic and hepatic toxicities associated with antenatal and postnatal exposure to maternal highly active antiretroviral therapy among infants. *AIDS.* 2008;22:1633-1640.

64. Wentges-van Holthe N et al. Oseltamivir and breastfeeding. *Int J Infect Dis.* 2008;12:451.

65. Dan M et al. Penetration of fleroxacin into breast milk and pharmacokinetics in lactating women. *Antimicrob Agents Chemother.* 1993;37:293-296.

66. Gardner DK et al. Simultaneous concentrations of ciprofloxacin in breast milk and in serum in mother and breast-fed infant. *Clin Pharm.* 1992;11:352-354.

67. Harmon T et al. Perforated pseudomembranous colitis in the breast-fed infant. *J Pediatr Surg.* 1992;27:744-746.

68. Belton EM, Jones RV. Haemolytic anaemia due to nalidixic acid [letter]. *Lancet.* 1965;286:691.

69. Takase Z et al. Basic and clinical studies on AM-715 in the field of obstetrics and gynecology. *Chemotherapy (Tokyo).* 1981;29(suppl 4):697-704.

70. Chin KG et al. Use of anti-infective agents during lactation: Part 2–Aminoglycosides, macrolides, quinolones, sulfonamides, trimethoprim, tetracyclines, chloramphenicol, clindamycin, and metronidazole. *J Hum Lact.* 2001;17:54-65.

71. Hunt MJ et al. Black breast milk due to minocycline therapy. *Br J Dermatol.* 1996;134:943-944.

72. Chin KG et al. Use of anti-infective agents during lactation: part 1 – beta-lactam antibiotics, vancomycin, quin-upristin-dalfopristin, and linezolid. *J Hum Lact.* 2000;16:351-358.

73. Kumar AR et al. Transfer of interferon alfa into human breast milk. *J Hum Lact.* 2000;16:226-228.

74. Haggstrom J et al. Two cases of CML treated with alpha-interferon during second and third trimester of pregnancy with analysis of the drug in the new-born immediately postpartum [letter]. *Eur J Haematol.* 1996;57:101-102.

75. Azuno Y et al. Mitoxantrone and etoposide in breast milk [letter]. *Am J Hematol.* 1995;48:131-132.

76. Ali R et al. Imatinib use during pregnancy and breast feeding: a case report and review of the literature. *Arch Gynecol Obstet.* 2009;280:169-175.

77. Russell MA et al. Imatinib mesylate and metabolite concentrations in maternal blood, umbilical cord blood, placenta and breast milk. *J Perinatol.* 2007;27:241-243.

78. Gambacorti-Passerini CB et al. Imatinib concentrations in human milk. *Blood.* 2007;109:1790.

79. Mottet C et al. Pregnancy and breastfeeding in patients with Crohn's disease. *Digestion.* 2007;76:149-160.

80. Coscia LA et al. Report from the National Transplantation Pregnancy Registry (NTPR): outcomes of pregnancy after transplantation. *Clin Transplant.* 2007;29-42.

81. Qasqas SA et al. Cardiovascular pharmacotherapeutic considerations during pregnancy and lactation. *Cardiol Rev.* 2004;12:201-221.

82. Beardmore KS et al. Excretion of antihypertensive medication into human breast milk: a systematic review. *Hypertens Pregnancy.* 2002;21:85-95.

83. Mirpuri J et al. What's mom on? A case of bradycardia in a premature infant on breast milk [abstract]. *J Invest Med.* 2008;56:409.

84. Tomson T, Battino D. Pharmacokinetics and therapeutic drug monitoring of newer antiepileptic drugs during pregnancy and the puerperium. *Clin Pharmacokinet.* 2007;46:209-219.

85. Hovinga CA, Pennell PB. Antiepileptic drug therapy in pregnancy II: fetal and neonatal exposure. *Int Rev Neurobiol.* 2008;83:241-258.

86. Meador K et al. Effects of breastfeeding in women taking antiepileptic drugs on their children's cognitive outcomes. *Neurology.* 2008;70:A400-A401.

87. Hartmann AM et al. Stillen, gewichtszunahme und verhalten bei neugeborenen epileptischer frauen. Breast feeding, weight gain and behaviour in newborns of epileptic women. *Monatsschr Kinderheilkd.* 1994;142:505-512.

88. Ito S et al. Initiation and duration of breast feeding in women receiving antiepileptics [abstract]. *Clin Pharmacol Ther.* 1994;55:177.

89. Lee A et al. Physicians' advice as an influential factor on the decision to breastfeed in a cohort of women on carbamazepine [abstract]. *Pediatr Res.* 2000;47:472A.

90. Merlob P et al. Transient hepatic dysfunction in an infant of an epileptic mother treated with carbamazepine during pregnancy and breast feeding. *Ann Pharmacother.* 1992;26:1563-1565.

91. Bossi L et al. Pharmacokinetics and clinical effects of antiepileptic drugs in newborns of chronically treated epileptic mothers. In: Janz D et al, eds. Epilepsy, Pregnancy and the Child. New York, NY. Raven Press; 1982:373-381.

92. Birnbaum CS et al. Serum concentrations of antidepressants and benzodiazepines in nursing infants: a case series. *Pediatrics.* 1999;104:e11.

93. Kristensen JH et al. Gabapentin and breastfeeding: a case report. *J Hum Lact.* 2006;22:426-428.

94. Tomson T et al. Pharmacokinetics of levetiracetam during pregnancy, delivery, in the neonatal period, and lactation. *Epilepsia.* 2007;48:1111-1116.

95. Newport DJ et al. Lamotrigine in breast milk and nursing infants: determination of exposure. *Pediatrics.* 2008;122:e223-e231.

96. Lutz UC et al. Oxcarbazepine treatment during breast-feeding: a case report. *J Clin Psychopharmacol.* 2007;27:730-732.

97. Bulau P et al. Pharmacokinetics of oxcarbazepine and 10-hydroxy-carbazepine in the newborn child of an oxcarbazepine-treated mother. *Eur J Clin Pharmacol.* 1988;34:311-313.

98. Ohman I et al. Topiramate kinetics during lactation. *Epilepsia.* 2007;48(suppl 7):156-157.

99. Froscher W, Jurges U. Topiramate used during breast feeding. *Aktuel Neurol.* 2006;33:215-217.

100. Gentile S. Topiramate in pregnancy and breastfeeding. *Clin Drug Investig.* 2009;29:139-141.

101. Piontek CM et al. Serum valproate levels in 6 breastfeeding mother-infant pairs. *J Clin Psychiatry.* 2000;61:170-172.

102. Stahl MMS et al. Thrombocytopenic purpura and anemia in a breast-fed infant whose mother was treated with valproic acid. *J Pediatr.* 1997;130:1001-1003.

103. Chaudron LH, Jefferson JW. Mood stabilizers during breastfeeding: a review. *J Clin Psychiatry.* 2000;61:79-90.

104. Kawada K et al. Pharmacokinetics of zonisamide in perinatal period. *Brain Dev.* 2002;24:95-97.

105. Field T. Breastfeeding and antidepressants. *Infant Behav Dev.* 2008;31:481-487.

106. The Academy of Breastfeeding Medicine Protocol Committee. ABM clinical protocol #18: use of antidepressants in nursing mothers. *Breastfeed Med.* 2008;3:44-52.

107. Weissman AM et al. Pooled analysis of antidepressant levels in lactating mothers, breast milk, and nursing infants. *Am J Psychiatry.* 2004;161:1066-1078.

108. ACOG Practice Bulletin No. 92: use of psychiatric medications during pregnancy and lactation. *Obstet Gynecol.* 2008;111:1001-1020.

109. Hendrick V et al. Weight gain in breastfed infants of mothers taking antidepressant medications. *J Clin Psychiatry.* 2003;64:410-412.

110. Matheson I et al. Respiratory depression caused by *N*-desmethyldoxepin in breast milk [letter]. *Lancet.* 1985;326:1124.

111. Frey OR et al. Adverse effects in a newborn infant breast-fed by a mother treated with doxepin. *Ann Pharmacother.* 1999;33:690-693.

112. Kristensen JH et al. Distribution and excretion of fluoxetine and norfluoxetine in human milk. *Br J Clin Pharmacol.* 1999;48:521-527.

113. Isenberg KE. Excretion of fluoxetine in human breast milk [letter]. *J Clin Psychiatry.* 1990;51:169.

114. Jensen PN et al. Citalopram and desmethylcitalopram concentrations in breast milk and in serum of mother and infant. *Ther Drug Monit.* 1997;19:236-239.

115. Spigset O et al. Excretion of citalopram in breast milk. *Br J Clin Pharmacol.* 1997;44:295-298.

116. Rampono J et al. Citalopram and demethylcitalopram in human milk; distribution, excretion and effects in breast fed infants. *Br J Clin Pharmacol.* 2000;50:263-268.

117. Schmidt K et al. Citalopram and breast-feeding: serum concentration and side effects in the infant. *Biol Psychiatry.* 2000;47:164-165.

118. Rampono J et al. Transfer of escitalopram and its metabolite demethylescitalopram into breastmilk. *Br J Clin Pharmacol.* 2006;3:316-322.

119. Castberg I, Spigset O. Excretion of escitalopram in breast milk. *J Clin Psychopharmacol.* 2006;26:536-538.

120. Hagg S et al. Excretion of fluvoxamine into breast milk [letter]. *Br J Clin Pharmacol.* 2000;49:286-287.

121. Piontek CM et al. Serum fluvoxamine levels in breastfed infants. *J Clin Psychiatry.* 2001;62:111-113.

122. Arnold LM et al. Fluvoxamine concentrations in breast milk and in maternal and infant sera. *J Clin Psychopharmacol.* 2000;20:491-492. Letter.

123. Haas JS et al. Bupropion in breast milk: an exposure assessment for potential treatment to prevent post partum tobacco use. *Tob Control.* 2004;13:52-56.

124. Chaudron LH, Schoenecker CJ. Bupropion and breastfeeding: a case of a possible infant seizure. *J Clin Psychiatry.* 2004;65:881-882.

125. Lobo ED et al. Pharmacokinetics of duloxetine in breast milk and plasma of healthy postpartum women. *Clin Pharmacokinet.* 2008;47:103-109.

126. Klier CM et al. Mirtazapine and breastfeeding: maternal and infant plasma levels. *Am J Psychiatry.* 2007;164:348-349.

127. Kristensen JH et al. Transfer of the antidepressant mirtazapine into breast milk. *Br J Clin Pharmacol.* 2007;63:322-327.

128. Dodd S et al. Nefazodone in the breast milk of nursing mothers: a report of two patients [letter]. *J Clin Psychopharmacol.* 2000;20:717-718.

129. Yapp P et al. Drowsiness and poor feeding in a breast fed infant: association with nefazodone and its metabolites. *Ann Pharmacother.* 2000;34:1269-1272.

130. Dodd S et al. Antidepressants and breast-feeding. A review of the literature. *Paediatr Drugs.* 2000;2:183-192.

131. Ilett KF et al. Distribution of venlafaxine and its O-desmethyl metabolite in human milk and their effects in breastfed infants. *Br J Clin Pharmacol.* 2002;53:17-22.

132. Hendrick V et al. Venlafaxine and breast-feeding [letter]. *Am J Psychiatry.* 2001;158:2089-2090.

133. Winans EA. Antipsychotics and breastfeeding. *J Hum Lact.* 2001;17:344-347.

134. Gentile S. Infant safety with antipsychotic therapy in breast-feeding: a systematic review. *J Clin Psychiatry.* 2008;69:666-673.

135. Yoshida K et al. Neuroleptic drugs in breast-milk: a study of pharmacokinetics and of possible adverse effects in breast-fed infants. *Psychol Med* 1998;28:81 91.

136. Yoshida K et al. Psychotropic drugs in mothers' milk: a comprehensive review of assay methods, pharmacokinetics and safety of breast feeding. *J Psychopharmacol.* 1999;13:64-80.

137. Tenyi T et al. Antipsychotics and breast-feeding. A review of the literature. *Paediatr Drugs.* 2000;2:23-28.

138. Pons G et al. Excretion of psychoactive drugs into breast milk. Pharmacokinetic principles and recommendations. *Clin Pharmacokinet.* 1994;27:270-289.

139. Schlotterbeck P et al. Aripiprazole in human milk. *Int J Neuropsychopharmacol.* 2007;10:433.

140. Goldstein DJ et al. Olanzapine use during breast-feeding [abstract]. *Schizophr Res.* 2002;53:185.

141. Rampono J et al. Quetiapine and breast feeding. *Ann Pharmacother.* 2007;41:711-714.

142. Nitsun M et al. Pharmacokinetics of midazolam, propofol, and fentanyl transfer to human breast milk. *Clin Pharmacol Ther.* 2006;79:549-557.

143. Martens PR. A sudden infant death like syndrome possibly induced by a benzodiazepine in breast-feeding. *Eur J Emerg Med.* 1994;1:86-87.

144. Oo CY et al. Pharmacokinetics in lactating women: prediction of alprazolam transfer into milk. *Br J Clin Pharmacol.* 1995;40:231-236.

145. Lebedevs TH et al. Excretion of temazepam in breast milk [letter]. *Br J Clin Pharmacol.* 1992;33:204-206.

146. Darwish M et al. Rapid disappearance of zaleplon from breast milk after oral administration to lactating women. *J Clin Pharmacol*. 1999;39:670-674.

147. Pons G et al. Zolpidem excretion in breast milk. *Eur J Clin Pharmacol*. 1989;37:245-248.

148. Moretti ME et al. Monitoring lithium in breast milk: an individualized approach for breast-feeding mothers. *Ther Drug Monit*. 2003;25:364-366.

149. Viguera AC et al. Lithium in breast milk and nursing infants: clinical implications. *Am J Psychiatry*. 2007;164:342-345.

150. Verma S et al. Breastfeeding a baby with mother on bromocriptine. *Indian J Pediatr*. 2006;73:435-436.

151. Cozzi R et al. Pregnancy in acromegaly: a one-center experience. *Eur J Endocrinol*. 2006;155:279-284.

152. Thulin PC et al. Levodopa in human breast milk: clinical implications. *Neurology*. 1998;50:1920-1921.

153. Mahadevan U, Kane S. American Gastroenterological Association Institute Technical Review on the Use of Gastrointestinal Medications in Pregnancy. *Gastroenterology*. 2006;131:283-311.

154. Ali RA, Egan LJ. Gastroesophageal reflux disease in pregnancy. *Best Pract Res Clin Gastroenterol*. 2007;21:793-806.

155. Oo CY et al. Active transport of cimetidine into human milk. *Clin Pharmacol Ther*. 1995;58:548-555.

156. Marshall JK et al. Omeprazole for refractory gastroesophageal reflux disease during pregnancy and lactation. *Can J Gastroenterol*. 1998;12:225-227.

157. Plante L et al. Excretion of pantoprazole in human breast. *J Reprod Med*. 2004;49:825-827.

158. Hofmeyr GJ et al. Domperidone: secretion in breast milk and effect on puerperal prolactin levels. *Br J Obstet Gynaecol*. 1985;92:141-144.

159. Knoppert DC et al. A randomized, double blind, placebo controlled trial of domperidone in lactating mothers of premature newborns [abstract OII-B-1]. *Clin Pharmacol Ther*. 1999;65:176.

160. Anderson PO, Valdes V. A critical review of pharmaceutical galactagogues. *Breastfeed Med*. 2007;2:229-242.

161. Miller LG et al. Disposition of olsalazine and metabolites in breast milk. *J Clin Pharmacol*. 1993;33:703-706.

162. Klotz U, Harings-Kaim A. Negligible excretion of 5-aminosalicylic acid in breast milk [letter]. *Lancet*. 1993;342:618-619.

163. Moretti ME et al. Prospective follow-up of infants exposed to 5-aminosalicylic acid containing drugs through maternal milk [abstract]. *J Clin Pharmacol*. 1998;38:867. Abstract.

164. Rudi J et al. Therapy with ursodeoxycholic acid in primary biliary cirrhosis in pregnancy. *Z Gastroenterol*. 1996;34:188-191.

165. Brites D, Rodrigues CMP. Elevated levels of bile acids in colostrum of patients with cholestasis of pregnancy are decreased following ursodeoxycholic acid therapy. *J Hepatol*. 1998;29:743-751.

166. Clark SL et al. Coumarin derivatives and breast-feeding. *Obstet Gynecol*. 2000;95:938-940.

167. Lindhoff-Last E et al. Hirudin treatment in a breastfeeding woman. *Lancet*. 2000;355:467-468.

168. Hellgren M et al. The oral direct thrombin inhibitor, ximelagatran, an alternative for anticoagulant treatment during the puerperium and lactation. *BJOG*. 2005;112:579-583.

169. Guillonneau M et al. L'allaitement est possible en cas de traitement maternel par l'enoxaprine. *Arch Pediatr (Paris)*. 1996;4:513-514.

170. Richter C et al. Excretion of low molecular weight heparin in human milk. *Br J Clin Pharmacol*. 2001;52:708-710.

171. Schindewolf M, Lindhoff-Last E. Alternative anticoagulation with danaparoid in two pregnancies in a patient with former heparin-induced thrombocytopenia (hit), homozygous factor v leiden mutation, a history of venous thrombosis and recurrent pregnancy losses. *Thromb Haemost*. 2008;99:776-778.

172. Lindhoff-Last E et al. Treatment of 51 pregnancies with danaparoid because of heparin intolerance. *Thromb Haemost*. 2005;93:63-69.

173. Greenberger PA et al. Pharmacokinetics of prednisolone transfer to breast milk. *Clin Pharmacol Ther*. 1993;53:324-328.

174. Falt A et al. Exposure of infants to budesonide through breast milk of asthmatic mothers. *J Allergy Clin Immunol*. 2007;120:798-802.

175. De Stefano B et al. Factitious hypertension with mineralocorticoid excess in an infant. *Helv Paediatr Acta*. 1983;38:185-189.

176. Merlob P et al. Oral antihyperglycemic agents during pregnancy and lactation. A review. *Paediatr Drugs*. 2002;4:755-760.

177. Alban Davies H et al. Insulin requirements of diabetic women who breast feed. *BMJ*. 1989;298:1357-1358.

178. Murtaugh MA et al. Energy intake and glycemia in lactating women with type 1 diabetes. *J Am Diet Assoc*. 1998;98:642-648.

179. Whitmore TJ et al. Insulin content of human milk [abstract]. *Breastfeed Med*. 2008;3:83-84.

180. Feig DS et al. Transfer of glyburide and glipizide into breast milk. *Diabetes Care*. 2005;28:1851-1855.

181. Goldenberg N, Glueck C. Medical therapy in women with polycystic ovarian syndrome before and during pregnancy and lactation. *Minerva Ginecol*. 2008;60:63-75.

182. van Wouwe JP et al. Breastfeeding duration related to practised contraception in the Netherlands. *Acta Paediatr*. 2009;98:86-90.

183. Truitt ST et al. Hormonal contraception during lactation: systematic review of randomized controlled trials. *Contraception*. 2003;68:233-238.
184. Queenan JT. Contraception and breastfeeding. *Clin Obstet Gynecol*. 2004;47:734-739.
185. Gaffield ME et al. Medical eligibility criteria for new contraceptive methods: combined hormonal patch, combined hormonal vaginal ring and the etonogestrel implant. *Contraception*. 2006;73:134-144.
186. World Health Organization. *Medical eligibility criteria for contraceptive use*. 3rd ed. Geneva: Reproductive Health and Research, World Health Organization; 2004.
187. Halderman LD, Nelson AL. Impact of early postpartum administration of progestin-only hormonal contraceptives compared with nonhormonal contraceptives on short-term breast-feeding patterns. *Am J Obstet Gynecol*. 2002;186:1250-1258.
188. Massai R et al. Extended use of a progesterone-releasing vaginal ring in nursing women: a phase II clinical trial. *Contraception*. 2005;72:352-357.
189. Chen JH et al. The comparative trial of TCu 380A IUD and progesterone-releasing vaginal ring used by lactating women. *Contraception*. 1998;57:371-379.
190. Casteels K et al. Transient neonatal hypothyroidism during breastfeeding after post-natal maternal topical iodine treatment. *Eur J Pediatr*. 2000;159:716-717.
191. Koga Y et al. Effect on neonatal thyroid function of povidone-iodine used on mothers during perinatal period. *J Obstet Gynaecol*. 1995;21:581-585.
192. Rakover Y, Adar H. Thyroid function disturbances in an infant following maternal topical use of Polydine. *Harefuah*. 1989;116:527-529.
193. Azizi F. Treatment of post-partum thyrotoxicosis. *J Endocrinol Invest*. 2006;29:244-247.
194. Abalovich M et al. Management of thyroid dysfunction during pregnancy and postpartum: an Endocrine Society clinical practice guideline. *J Clin Endocrinol Metab*. 2007;92:S1-S7.
195. van Wassenaer AG et al. The quantity of thyroid hormone in human milk is too low to influence plasma thyroid hormone levels in the very preterm infant. *Clin Endocrinol (Oxf)*. 2002;56:621-627.
196. Koldovsky O. Hormones in milk. *Vitam Horm*. 1995;50:77-149.
197. Caplan RH, Wickus GG. Reduced calcitriol requirements for treating hypoparathyroidism during lactation. A case report. *J Reprod Med*. 1993;38:914-918.
198. Cathebras P et al. Hypercalcemia induced by lactation in 2 patients with treated hypoparathyroidism. *Rev Med Interne*. 1996;17:675-676.
199. Milsom SR et al. Potential role for growth hormone in human lactation insufficiency. *Horm Res*. 1998;50:147-150.
200. Miller ME et al. Hydrochlorothiazide disposition in a mother and her breast-fed infant. *J Pediatr*. 1982;101:789-791.
201. Cominos DC et al. Suppression of postpartum lactation with furosemide. *S Afr Med J*. 1976;50:251 252.
202. Mulley BA et al. Placental transfer of chlorthalidone and its elimination in maternal milk. *Eur J Clin Pharmacol*. 1978;13:129-131.
203. Phelps DL, Karim A. Spironolactone: relationship between concentrations of dethioacetylated metabolite in human serum and milk. *J Pharm Sci*. 1977;66:1203.
204. Siminoski K et al. Intravenous pamidronate for treatment of reflex sympathetic dystrophy during breastfeeding. *J Bone Miner Res*. 2000;15:2052-2055.
205. Nainar SM, Mohummed S. Diet counseling during the infant oral health visit. *Pediatr Dent*. 2004;26:459-462.
206. Breymann C et al. Milk iron content in breast-feeding mothers after administration of intravenous iron sucrose complex. *J Perinat Med*. 2007;35:115-118.
207. Riaz M et al. The effects of maternal magnesium sulfate treatment on newborns: a prospective controlled study. *J Perinatol*. 1998;18:449-454.
208. Cruikshank DP et al. Breast milk magnesium and calcium concentrations following magnesium sulfate treatment. *Am J Obstet Gynecol*. 1982;143:685-688.
209. Kamilli I et al. Allopurinol in breast milk. *Adv Exp Med Biol*. 1991;309A:143-145.
210. Ben-Chetrit E et al. Colchicine in breast milk of patients with familial Mediterranean fever. *Arthritis Rheum*. 1996;39:1213-1217.
211. Guillonneau M et al. Colchicine is excreted at high concentrations in human breast milk [letter]. *Eur J Obstet Gynecol Reprod Biol*. 1995;61:177-178.
212. Milunsky JM, Milunsky A. Breast-feeding during colchicine therapy for familial Mediterranean fever [letter]. *J Pediatr*. 1991;119 (1 Pt 1):164.
213. Daniel JA et al. Methscopolamine bromide blocks hypothalmic-stimulated release of growth hormone in ewes. *J Anim Sci*. 1997;75:1359-1362.
214. Lindberg C et al. Transfer of terbutaline into breast milk. *Eur J Respir Dis Suppl*. 1984;134:87-91.
215. McNamara PJ, Abbassi M. Neonatal exposure to drugs in breast milk. *Pharm Res*. 2004;21:555-566.
216. Powell RJ et al. BSACI guidelines for the management of chronic urticaria and angio-oedema. *Clin Exp Allergy*. 2007;37:631-650.
217. Incaudo GA, Takach P. The diagnosis and treatment of allergic rhinitis during pregnancy and lactation. *Immunol Allergy Clin North Am*. 2006;26:137-154.

218. Kok THHG et al. Drowsiness due to clemastine transmitted in breast milk [letter]. *Lancet.* 1982;319:914-915.

219. Wortsman J et al. Cyproheptadine in the management of the galactorrhea-amenorrhea syndrome. *Ann Intern Med.* 1979;90:923-925.

220. Lucas BD Jr. et al. Terfenadine pharmacokinetics in breast milk in lactating women. *Clin Pharmacol Ther.* 1995;57:398-402.

221. Hilbert J et al. Excretion of loratadine in human breast milk. *J Clin Pharmacol.* 1988;28:234-239.

222. Findlay JWA et al. Pseudoephedrine and triprolidine in plasma and breast milk of nursing mothers. *Br J Clin Pharmacol.* 1984;18:901-906.

223. Aljazaf K et al. Pseudoephedrine: effects on milk production in women and estimation of infant exposure via breastmilk. *Br J Clin Pharmacol.* 2003;56:18-24.

224. Eriksson G, Swahn CG. Concentration of baclofen in serum and breast milk from a lactating woman. *Scand J Clin Lab Invest.* 1981;41:185-187.

225. Ortega D et al. Excretion of lidocaine and bupivacaine in breast milk following epidural anesthesia for cesarean delivery. *Acta Anaesthesiol Scand.* 1999;43:394-397.

226. Hirose M et al. The effect of postoperative analgesia with continuous epidural bupivacaine after cesarean section on the amount of breast feeding and infant weight gain. *Anesth Analg.* 1996;82:1166-1169.

227. Fraser D, Turner JWA. Myasthenia gravis and pregnancy. *Proc R Soc Med.* 1963;56:379-381.

228. Hardell LI et al. Pyridostigmine in human breast milk. *Br J Clin Pharmacol.* 1982;14:565-567.

229. Fricker RM et al. Secretion of dantrolene into breast milk after acute therapy of a suspected malignant hyperthermia crisis during cesarean section. *Anesthesiology.* 1998;89:1023-1025.

230. Begley CM. The effect of ergometrine on breast feeding. *Midwifery.* 1990;6:60-72.

231. Symes JB. A study on the effect of ergometrine on serum prolactin levels following delivery. *J Obstet Gynaecol.* 1984;5:36-38.

232. Canales ES et al. Effect of ergonovine on prolactin secretion and milk let-down. *Obstet Gynecol.* 1976;48:228-229.

233. del Pozo E et al. Lack of effect of methyl-ergonovine on postpartum lactation. *Am J Obstet Gynecol.* 1975;123:845-846.

234. Ilett KF et al. Use of nicotine patches in breast-feeding mothers: transfer of nicotine and cotinine into human milk. *Clin Pharmacol Ther.* 2003;74:516-524.

235. Gupta T, Sharma R. An antilactogenic effect of pyridoxine. *J Indian Med Assoc.* 1990;88:336-337.

236. Scaglione D, Vecchione A. Pyridoxine for the suppression of lactation–a clinical trial on 1592 cases. *Acta Vitaminol Enzymol.* 1982;4:207-214.

237. Rollman O, Pihl-Lundin I. Acitretin excretion into human breast milk. *Acta Derm Venereol.* 1990;70:487-490.

238. Akhavan A, Bershad S. Topical acne drugs: review of clinical properties, systemic exposure, and safety. *Am J Clin Dermatol.* 2003;4:473-492.

239. Steiner E et al. Amphetamine secretion in breast milk. *Eur J Clin Pharmacol.* 1984;27:123-124.

240. Ilett KF et al. Transfer of dexamphetamine into breast milk during treatment for attention deficit hyperactivity disorder. *Br J Clin Pharmacol.* 2007;63:371-375.

241. Ayd FJ. Excretion of psychotropic drugs in human breast milk. *Int Drug Ther Newsl.* 1973;8:33-40.

242. Gizurason S. Optimal delivery of vaccines. *Clin Pharmacokinet.* 1996;30:1-15.

243. Anon. Questions and answers about smallpox vaccination while pregnant or breastfeeding. Atlanta, GA: Centers for Disease Control and Prevention. 2009.

244. Cetron MS et al. Yellow fever vaccine. Recommendations of the Advisory Committee on Immunization Practices (ACIP), 2002. *MMWR Recomm Rep.* 2002;51:1-11.

245. Webb JA et al. The use of iodinated and gadolinium contrast media during pregnancy and lactation. *Eur Radiol.* 2005;15:1234-1240.

246. ACR Committee on Drugs and Contrast Media. Administration of contrast medium to breastfeeding mothers. *ACR Bull.* 2001;57:12-13.

247. Mattern J, Mayer PR. Excretion of fluorescein into breast milk [letter]. *Am J Ophthalmol.* 1990;109:598-599.

248. Maguire AM, Bennett J. Fluorescein elimination in human breast milk [letter]. *Arch Ophthalmol.* 1988;106: 718-719.

249. Kubik-Huch RA et al. Gadopentetate dimeglumine excretion into human breast milk during lactation. *Radiology.* 2000;216:555-558.

250. Howe DB et al. Appendix U. Model procedure for release of patients or human research subjects administered radioactive materials. In: NUREG-1556. Consolidated guidance about materials licenses. Program-specific guidance about medical use licenses. Final report. Vol. 9. Rev. 2. US: Nuclear Regulatory Commission Office of Nuclear Material Safety and Safeguards 2008.

251. Stabin MG, Breitz HB. Breast milk excretion of radiopharmaceuticals: mechanisms, findings, and radiation dosimetry. *J Nucl Med.* 2000;41:863-873.

Chapter 71

Pediatric Drug Therapy

William E. Murray

Pediatric drug therapy presents a challenge to the practitioner in many respects. The pediatric population is comprised of a range of patient weights and organ maturity. Often there are no pediatric-specific data in the literature from which to derive appropriate dosage regimens. At times, medications must be used for which data are extrapolated on the basis of limited pharmacokinetic knowledge about the pediatric population. It must be remembered that children should not be treated as "little adults" when designing dosage regimens. Dosage administration nomograms derived from adult data should not be used in the pediatric population. Medication errors including prescribing, dispensing and administration are frequently reported in the pediatric population. The U.S. Food and Drug Administration recommends against the use of cough/cold preparations in young children in part due to dosing errors and medication misadventures. Pharmacodynamic responses for the majority of medications used in children are even less well known. Because of large intrapatient pharmacokinetic/pharmacodynamic differences there may be marked variability in responses to fixed doses of medications. Children can also react much differently from adults to certain medications. Examples are; the use of stimulants such as methylphenidate to control hyperactivity common with attention deficit disorders and paradoxical hyperactivity, which can be observed in children taking phenobarbital. With therapeutically monitored medications, the standard adult therapeutic range is typically used because age-specific, concentration-effect information is scarce. Because of protein binding differences, infants might respond to lower total drug concentrations than those used in adults for certain medications (e.g., phenytoin, theophylline). Free (unbound) drug concentrations are thought to correlate better with pharmacologic effect than total drug concentrations.

Allometric scaling has been studied in children in order to determine appropriate doses in the pediatric population as compared with a known adult dose.[1] One such equation is:

$$\text{Pediatric dose} = \text{Adult dose} \times (\text{weight}/70 \text{ kg})^{0.75}$$

An exponential factor of 0.9 in children <2 y of age may give better estimates of the optimal dose.

One of the problems facing the clinician and caregiver of small children is the administration of medications. Dosage forms are usually designed with the adult population in mind, and the dosage cannot easily be individualized in small patients. This is especially true for most sustained-release products. Most young children cannot swallow tablets and capsules; thus, liquid preparations are generally preferred in this age group. For many drugs, liquid forms are not commercially available and must be extemporaneously compounded. Stability of these preparations is often unknown or of limited duration. Even when appropriate dosage forms suitable for young children are available, palatability, resistance to taking medications and compliance issues can hinder optimal therapy.

■ PHARMACOKINETICS

ABSORPTION

At birth, gastric pH is neutral but falls to values of 1–3 in the first day of life. Subsequently, gastric pH returns toward neutrality because gastric acid secretion is low in the first several weeks to months. Adult values are usually achieved after the age of 2 years.[2,3] Medications that require gastric acidity for absorption can have poor bioavailability in this age group, rendering them ineffective or requiring much higher doses than normal for therapeutic serum concentrations to be reached. Examples of medications in this group are phenytoin, ketoconazole, and itraconazole.[2,4] Alternative agents might have to be used if adequate serum levels cannot be documented when these drugs are administered orally. Certain medications that are acid labile actually might have increased bioavailability in infants, including penicillin G and ampicillin.[5]

Gastric emptying time can be delayed in infants, especially premature infants.[2,4,6] Peak drug concentrations can occur much later in infants than in older children and adults. Other factors that can influence overall bioavailability of a particular medication in infants are the relatively high frequencies of gastroesophageal reflux, which can cause the dose to be spit up or vomited, and acute gastroenteritis (diarrhea), which can considerably shorten intestinal transit time. The oral route must be used with caution in these instances, especially in critically ill patients.

Other routes of administration can pose difficulties in the pediatric population. Overall muscle mass is decreased, and intramuscular administration might not be practical and certainly is not appreciated by most children. Most adults still remember their first injections in the doctor's office when they were children. Also, the dose of drug to be administered might require multiple injections.

Rectal administration may be used in situations where the oral route is not practical or available; however, absorption might be incomplete and erratic. Topical administration of medications can lead to undesired systemic absorption, especially in infants in whom the skin thickness is less and the total skin surface area is proportionally greater than in adults.[2,3,5]

DISTRIBUTION

Rapid changes in body composition can dramatically alter the V_d for many medications during the first several months of life. Newborns have a higher percentage of total body water and extracellular fluid than older children and adults.[2,4,7] Hydrophilic drugs such as the aminoglycosides have a much larger V_d in newborns; this gradually decreases over the first year of life to approach adult values.

Total body fat in newborns (especially premature infants) is much lower than in older children and adults.[7] Medications that are lipophilic might have a lower weight-adjusted V_d in the very young.

Protein binding is an important determinant of the V_d for drugs that are bound by albumin and other plasma proteins. In the neonatal period, the binding affinity of albumin is decreased compared with that in older children and adults (because of the persistence of fetal albumin).[2,4] Highly protein-bound drugs such as phenytoin has higher free fractions in neonates, and there might be an increased pharmacodynamic response at lower concentrations of total drug. The V_d of these drugs is inversely related to the degree of protein binding.

In addition, the clinician must be aware of the potential for highly protein-bound substances to displace bilirubin from binding sites on albumin, particularly in the newborn.[2,4,8] The blood–brain barrier in newborns is more permeable than in older patients, and free bilirubin can readily cross into the CNS and cause kernicterus.

Tissue binding for many medications is unknown but can differ dramatically from that in adults. One example is digoxin, which binds to erythrocytes in pediatric patients to a much greater extent than in adult patients.[3,5] Digoxin has a much larger V_d in pediatric patients, and recommended loading doses in this age group are much larger on a mg/kg basis than in adult patients. In general, drug distribution volumes are larger in neonates and gradually approach adult values (in L/kg) by the first year of life.

METABOLISM

Metabolic processes show dramatic changes in the first weeks to months of life. At birth, most hepatic enzymes are immature and drug-metabolizing capacity is greatly reduced. Phase I reactions (i.e., oxidation) are controlled largely by the mixed-function oxidase system, of which the cytochrome P450 enzymes are the major determinant. These enzymes are largely undeveloped in newborns, especially premature infants, but maturation can take place quickly in the first weeks to months of life. Differences in the rate of maturation of the isoenzymes of the P450 system may account for the variations seen in drug clearance in young infants and children. Phase II reactions (i.e., conjugation) include glucuronidation, sulfation, and acetylation. These reactions also are immature at birth, and drug toxicity has resulted (e.g., with chloramphenicol) because of the absence of knowledge about reduced dosage requirements in newborns.[2,4,7]

The liver size relative to body weight in newborns is much larger than that in adults.[2] Rapid weight gain, with subsequent increases in liver size and metabolic capacity, might require many dosage adjustments to prevent newborns from growing out of their dosages for many medications. When full metabolic capacity is reached in the pediatric patient, the hepatic clearance can greatly exceed that observed in adult patients on a weight-adjusted basis. Pediatric dosages of many medications on a mg/kg basis are often much greater than adult dosages. Figure 71-1 illustrates the change in clearance with age for theophylline.[7] Most medications have similar curves but can be shifted to the left or have different relative peaks compared with adult values. A decrease in hepatic clearance relative to body weight typically begins after a child weighs approximately 30 kg.[9] Thereafter, the increase in total body weight in proportion to liver size becomes greater. Thus, in adolescence, drug dosages typically begin to approach adult values. Drug toxicity can be observed in the adolescent patient if drug dosages on a mg/kg basis (designed for younger patients) are used.

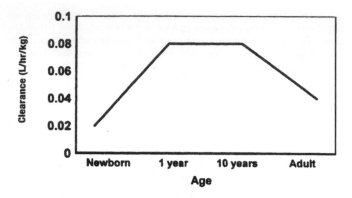

Figure 71-1. Maturation of theophylline metabolism.

RENAL ELIMINATION

The kidneys are the major route of drug elimination for many drugs. The kidneys are functionally immature at birth with regard to glomerular filtration and tubular secretion. Glomerular filtration at birth adjusted for body surface area is only 30%–40% of values in older infants and healthy young adults.[2,4] Premature infants often have even lower values during the first few weeks of life. Dosages of many medications (e.g., aminoglycosides, vancomycin) that are eliminated largely by glomerular filtration must be decreased on the basis of the relative immaturity of the kidneys at birth. Maturation of glomerular filtration occurs over the first several weeks to months of life. The dosages of most medications are similar to those in older children by age 4–6 months. Although the frequency of renal disease in children is much lower than in the adult population, factors that can alter renal function, such as shock, non-steroidal anti-inflammatory drugs, or hypoxia, must be considered when evaluating dosage regimens. Serum creatinine, the usual marker for renal function, is usually lower in young children than in adults because of children's lower muscle mass. Thus, a serum creatinine that indicates normal renal function in an adult might indicate renal impairment in a young child.

Tubular secretion also is diminished in the newborn. Drugs that have a component of tubular secretion (e.g., penicillin) are typically administered at reduced dosages in the newborn. Maturation of tubular secretion occurs somewhat more slowly than glomerular filtration, but approaches adult values by age 8–12 months.[2,4]

EVALUATING DRUG DATA IN CHILDREN

With the numerous maturational changes observed in children from birth through adolescence, results of pediatric drug studies must be used with caution in children whose ages differ from those in the study. Dosages extrapolated only on a weight basis have the potential to underdose or overdose other age groups, depending on the population studied. Consideration of obesity in calculating dosing regimens must be considered especially with the increase in overweight children in the United States over the past several years. Body surface area might correlate better than body weight with total body water and extracellular water and can be useful in certain instances in calculating dosage regimens. With the exception of cancer chemotherapeutic agents, information on drug dosage is more widely available in mg/kg than by body surface area.[6] The ratio of body surface area to body weight changes over time in the pediatric population. In newborns the ratio of BSA/body wt is much greater than in adolescents.[1] The estimation of BSA is also subject to variability depending upon the accuracy of the patients' height and weight and which method is used to calculate BSA. Some medications (e.g. vincristine) are sometimes dosed in terms of mg/kg in infants and in terms of mg/m^2 in older children and adults. Medications with narrow therapeutic ranges should have serum concentrations measured to aid in individualizing drug therapy, especially in critically ill children or those with known decreased renal or hepatic function or other disease states. Therapeutic drug monitoring is most helpful for medications which have a narrow therapeutic range, good correlation between serum drug concentrations and pharmacologic effect, large intrapatient variability, readily available assay and accurate timing of samples.

Pharmacodynamic changes are poorly studied in the pediatric population, and responses to specific drug concentrations might be much different from those in the adult population. Diseases of childhood often differ from those in adults. Medications tolerated by adult patients might be inappropriate for the pediatric population (e.g., aspirin for fever).

Caution must be used in the interpretation of drug levels because there might be much greater fluctuation in serum concentrations because of shorter drug half-lives in children than in adults. Further, the total volume of blood needed for drug level monitoring in small children can limit monitoring. Bayesian methods to help individualize drug therapy have been shown to be useful in designing dosage regimens in infants and pediatric patients for numerous medications. Studies in specific populations designed to help delineate factors known to influence the distribution and elimination of these medications are valuable to help establish initial pharmacokinetic parameters.

Detailed information on specific drugs can be found in the Pediatric Dosage sections of the individual drug monographs or in other specialized dosing handbooks.

■ REFERENCES

1. Mahmood I. *Pediatric Pharmacology and Pharmacokinetics*. Rockville, MD: Pine House Publishers; 2008.
2. Stewart CF, Hampton EM. Effect of maturation on drug disposition in pediatric patients. *Clin Pharm*. 1987;6:548-564.
3. Besunder JB et al. Principles of drug biodisposition in the neonate. A critical evaluation of the pharmacokinetic pharmacodynamic interface (part I). *Clin Pharmacokinet*. 1988;14:189-216.
4. Maples HD et al. Special pharmacokinetic and pharmacodynamic considerations in children. In: Burton ME et al, eds. *Applied Pharmacokinetics and Pharmacodynamics. Principles of Therapeutic Drug Monitoring*. 4th ed. Baltimore, MD: Lippincott Williams & Wilkins; 2006:213-230.
5. Morselli PL et al. Clinical pharmacokinetics in newborns and infants. Age-related differences and therapeutic implications. In: Gibaldi M, Prescott LF, eds. *Handbook of Clinical Pharmacokinetics*. Balgowlah, Australia: ADIS Health Science Press; 1983:98-141.
6. Maxwell GM. Paediatric drug dosing. Body weight versus surface area. *Drugs*. 1989;37:113-115.
7. McLeod HL, Evans WE. Pediatric pharmacokinetics and therapeutic drug monitoring. *Pediatr Rev*. 1992;13:413-421.
8. Morselli PL. Clinical pharmacokinetics in neonates. In: Gibaldi M, Prescott LF, eds. *Handbook of Clinical Pharmacokinetics*. Balgowlah, NSW, Australia: ADIS Health Science Press; 1983:79-97.
9. Rane A, Wilson JT. Clinical pharmacokinetics in infants and children. In: Gibaldi M, Prescott LF, eds. *Handbook of Clinical Pharmacokinetics*. Section II. Balgowlah, Australia: ADIS Health Science Press; 1983:142-168.

Chapter 72

Geriatric Drug Therapy

Emily R. Hajjar

Geriatric drug therapy is an important area of therapeutics and research, because of the growing elderly population, their disproportionately high use of medications, and their increased risk of drug misadventures. Although they represent approximately 12% of the U.S. population, the elderly consume more than 30% of all medications.[1] Trends include increasing numbers of the extreme elderly (older than 85 years), elderly with functional disabilities, and increasing minority populations.[2] It is estimated that the number of elderly who are dependent in their activities of daily living will triple from 1985–2060. Ethical considerations, such as a patient's right to exercise decisions regarding treatment, are particularly relevant to the elderly population.[3–5] As the number of elderly increases and health care resources diminish, cost–benefit considerations will become increasingly important.[6]

The elderly are the most physiologically heterogeneous category of the adult population. The rate of normal aging varies considerably, and comparing data from persons of chronologically similar age can be misleading; health status is probably as important as age. Optimization of drug therapy in the elderly requires an understanding of how aging and concomitant pathology affect the pharmacokinetics and pharmacodynamics of drugs, the need to assess elderly patients individually, and elderly patients' expectations of therapy.[7]

Adherence issues leading to misuse and medication errors can be important in the elderly.[6] The cost of medications, physical difficulty in opening medication containers, swallowing large tablets, consuming multiple medications, reading the prescription label, and the presence of depression or cognitive impairment can contribute to adherence problems.[8,9,10]

Adverse drug reactions are more common in the elderly,[11–13] although the correlation with age alone is debatable.[1,14] Increased medication use, especially medications with greater potential for toxicity, and chronic pathology with intermittent acute exacerbations are thought to contribute to the higher frequency and severity of adverse drug reactions. Most reactions in the elderly are dose related rather than idiosyncratic as a result of changes in pharmacokinetics and/or pharmacodynamics. Given the wide physiologic variability in the elderly population, the contribution of pharmacokinetic and pharmacodynamic changes can vary considerably. Additionally, the elderly are more sensitive to specific adverse reactions. For example, they have an increased sensitivity to anticholinergic side effects, especially central effects such as disorientation and memory impairment. These effects can be additive because many drugs commonly taken by the elderly are centrally active.[15,16] Varying degrees of cognitive impairment or even delirium can be induced by drugs in several classes including benzodiazepines, centrally acting antihypertensive agents, and antidepressants.[15,17] The onset can be insidious and mistakenly attributed solely to the aging process.

■ PHARMACOKINETICS

ABSORPTION

With aging there is some decrease in gastric secretions, acidity, gastric emptying, peristalsis, absorptive surface area, and splanchnic blood flow,[18] although the effect on gastric pH may not be as pronounced as once believed.[19] Taken together, the changes predict an altered extent or rate of absorption of orally administered drugs, yet most formal studies show no difference in oral bioavailability. Some factors might counterbalance each other (e.g., acidity and gastric emptying; decreased absorptive surface; and longer transit time). Some drugs (e.g., digoxin) have shown a clinically unimportant slowed rate of absorption with equivalent quantities absorbed. Drugs with high extraction ratios may have increased bioavailability in the elderly compared with young patients, because of a decreased first-pass effect secondary to reduced hepatic blood flow. Decreased first-pass metabolism in the elderly has been shown for labetalol, propranolol, lidocaine, and verapamil.[20] It is known that the elderly have drier skin with lower lipid content, which is expected to be less permeable to hydrophilic compounds. Although neither conclusively nor well studied, percutaneous drug absorption appears to decrease with age.[21]

DISTRIBUTION

Body weight generally decreases, but more important, body composition changes with age. Total body water and lean body mass decrease, while body fat increases in proportion to total body weight. The percentage of body weight contributed by fat changes ranges from 18% and 33% in young men and women, respectively, to 36% and 45% in their elderly counterparts.[22] These factors can alter the V_d of drugs in the elderly, although other aspects of drug disposition (binding, metabolism, elimination) can be additive or negate the effect. The V_d changes are most marked for highly lipophilic and hydrophilic drugs, and elderly patients are particularly susceptible to overdosage from drugs whose doses should be based on ideal body weight or lean body weight.[23] Theoretically, highly lipid-soluble drugs (e.g., long-acting benzodiazepines, morphine) may have an increased V_d and a prolonged effect if drug clearance remains constant. Conversely, water-soluble drugs (e.g., gentamicin) may have a decreased V_d, and at least transiently increased serum levels, leading to possible toxicity if initial doses are not conservative.[24] Although cardiac output does not appear to decrease with age,[25] some chronic diseases affecting the elderly do contribute to a decrease in cardiac output and regional blood flow. There is some evidence that blood is preferentially shunted away from the liver and kidneys to the brain, heart, and muscles.[15] These changes could explain the slowed elimination of some drugs and the heightened sensitivity to others.

PROTEIN BINDING

The proportion of albumin among total plasma proteins decreases with frailty, catabolic disease states, and immobility seen in many elderly,[26] but it is no longer believed that serum albumin decreases with age alone.[21] Serum albumin determinations should be performed to aid monitoring and dosage adjustment of drugs that are highly protein bound in the chronically immobile or ill elderly. A decrease in serum albumin can increase the percentage of free drug available for pharmacologic effect and elimination. Changes in albumin binding are more important with highly bound (greater than 90%) acidic drugs such as salicylates, phenytoin, and warfarin.[24] Conversely, basic drugs, including lidocaine and propranolol have affinity for α_1-acid glycoprotein, which may increase with age, especially when associated with conditions such as inflammatory diseases and malignancies.[24] Protein binding theoretically may be increased and result in less free drug available, although the clinical relevance of this is unclear.[21] With both types of binding, the net effect on clearance varies, depending on metabolism and elimination. Although not always available, free drug concentration measurements are often desirable in the elderly. There is also some evidence that the elderly may have a greater potential for protein displacement drug interactions.[27]

METABOLISM

Liver size and hepatic blood flow decrease with age and especially with disease. Studies show hepatic blood flow decreases by 35%, and liver volume by 44% and 28% in elderly women and men, respectively, when compared to their younger counterparts.[28] Such a decrease in hepatic blood flow can limit the first-pass effect of drugs with high extraction ratios and markedly reduce their systemic clearance. Studies on phase I drug metabolism (i.e., oxidation) do not consistently show a correlation with age,[21] although most show that the elderly, especially men, have prolonged elimination. Differences may be explained by environmental factors such as smoking habits and genetics. Phase II metabolism (i.e., conjugation) does not appear to be influenced as much by age, although there has been less study in this area.[21,24] The effect of aging on drug acetylation is inconsistent and the importance unclear.[21,24] There does not appear to be any age difference in the degree of inhibition or induction of cytochrome P450 isozymes.[29] Monitoring and management of interactions with drugs such as cimetidine should be handled in the same manner as in younger patients. The changes described in liver size and metabolic function help to explain why certain drugs may have prolonged elimination; however, the variability of data cautions against generalizing about the effect of age alone. The initial dosage of metabolized drugs should be conservative and subsequent dosage adjustments based on careful monitoring of therapeutic and toxic parameters.

RENAL ELIMINATION

The effect of aging on the renal elimination of drugs is probably the most completely understood and important aspect affecting geriatric drug therapy. Glomerular filtration, tubular secretion, and renal blood flow all decrease with age. Creatinine clearance decreases approximately 1% per year after age 40;[30] the effect is variable; and volume depletion, CHF, and renal disease can further decrease organ function. Because creatinine production also decreases with age, serum creatinine may be normal despite a substantial decrease in renal function. It is therefore recommended that Cl_{Cr} be measured or estimated using a method that incorporates age and weight.[31] The dosage of renally excreted drugs with low therapeutic indices should be conservative initially, with subsequent dosage titrated by close clinical and serum drug level monitoring, if applicable.

■ PHARMACODYNAMICS

Heightened drug effects that cannot be explained by altered pharmacokinetic variables alone have been hypothesized to be caused by changes in compensatory homeostasis, drug receptor sensitivity, or complications of chronic diseases that occur in the elderly. There is a gradual decrease in homeostatic reserve with aging. Postural control and orthostatic circulatory response are examples of compensatory mechanisms that are slowed in aging. Adequate postural blood pressure control relies on several factors, including central coordination, muscle tone, and proprioception, all of which can be blunted in the elderly.[15] As a result, side effects that are minimal or absent in a young patient with normal compensatory response can be marked in the elderly. The administration of long-acting anxiolytics, hypnotics, or antipsychotics can further alter these mechanisms and lead to an increased risk of falls in the elderly.[32] Similarly, symptomatic postural hypotension can result from the administration of a variety of antihypertensive agents (especially calcium channel blockers and ACE inhibitors) and other drugs (e.g., antipsychotics, antidepressants) that affect vasomotor tone. Physiologic mechanisms such as vasoconstriction and tachycardia cannot fully compensate for postural hypotension in the elderly.[15] Temperature regulation and intestinal motility are other homeostatic mechanisms that change with aging and can explain heightened effects of certain drugs.

The number and characteristics of drug receptors can change with aging and produce an altered, often heightened, drug response. Research has shown age-related decreases in several autonomic receptors. There is some evidence of increased sensitivity to oral anticoagulants and digoxin, apart from the alterations in pharmacokinetics, which might contribute to the higher frequency of adverse reactions to these two agents in the elderly.[15]

Preliminary data indicate a possible increase in brain sensitivity to certain drugs with aging. It is unknown whether this effect is caused by changes in blood–brain permeability or tissue receptor sensitivity.[24] More research into drug pharmacodynamics in the elderly is needed, especially the interrelationship with pharmacokinetic alterations. The presence and impact of multiple concurrent pathologies and their treatments cannot be overemphasized in their contribution to the various drug effects seen in the elderly.

■ OTHER FACTORS

Cigarette smoking can cause clinically important induction of the metabolism of some drugs to a similar degree in both the elderly and the young.[21,33] This, and the fact that many published studies do not indicate smoking history, could explain some interpatient variability of pharmacokinetic data.

Nutritional intake is sometimes diminished in the elderly and can lead to nutritional and vitamin deficiencies. Nutritional status of the elderly can impact the outcome of drug therapy, and, conversely, drug therapy can affect nutritional status.[18,33]

■ EVALUATING DRUG DATA FOR THE ELDERLY

Because of age-related changes that may impact the outcome of drug therapy as outlined in this chapter, the results of drug studies using young subjects cannot always be extrapolated accurately to the elderly. Studies on diseases and drugs in the elderly do not always include sufficient numbers of elderly, especially extremely aged subjects, to draw appropriate conclusions.[34] Studies that include the elderly do not always separate results by decade of age and health status, two criteria that are helpful in assessing applicability of data in this heterogeneous population. Many studies also do not mention data on nutrition, alcohol, and smoking, which might explain some variability of results.[18] Although single-dose studies in healthy volunteers can be useful, long-term studies in afflicted elderly patients often yield data more applicable to therapeutics. Drugs are often not studied over a wide dosage range, so a minimal effective dosage in the elderly cannot be determined.[35]

When reviewing studies that include the elderly, one should consider the following potential problems: numbers of subjects must be sufficient to allow for high attrition rates and the typically wide variation in this population; study lengths must be sufficient for a chronic disease; concomitant diseases and medications must be acknowledged and their impact assessed; and "normal" values can be different from those of a younger population.[36]

INAPPROPRIATE PRESCRIBING IN THE ELDERLY

Inappropriate prescribing of medications in the elderly can lead to negative health consequences and should be avoided.[37] Tools such as the Beer's criteria can assist providers in finding medications that should not be given to the elderly based on evidence that the medication's risk outweighs the benefit.[38] The Medication Appropriateness Index can also assist providers in determining if medications are clinically relevant for a patient.[39] All efforts should be made to restrict harmful or unnecessary medications in older adults.

Along with inappropriate prescribing, it is also very important to consider the necessity of medications at the end of a patient's life. Patients are often on medications that are appropriate per disease state guidelines, but their usefulness is limited due to the goal of care being shifted from curative to palliative. Factors such as time until onset of medication benefit, goals of treatment, and remaining life expectancy need to be considered when considering starting or continuing medications as a patient nears the end of their life.[5]

■ CONCLUSION

The effects of aging as related to drug therapy illustrate the challenges in caring for the elderly. Clinical practice guidelines have been developed for conditions commonly afflicting the elderly, such as those published by the American Geriatrics Society.[40] Conservative dosage, especially initially, with close clinical monitoring for dose-dependent effects is critical and should be emphasized by all health care practitioners caring for the elderly. For detailed information on specific drugs in the elderly, refer to the Geriatric Dosage section of the individual drug monographs.

■ REFERENCES

1. Gerety MB et al. Adverse events related to drugs and drug withdrawal in nursing home residents. *J Am Geriatr Soc.* 1993;41:1326-1332.
2. Administration on Aging. http://www.aoa.gov/AoARoot/Aging_Statistics/Profile/index.aspx. Accessed November 24, 2008.
3. Faden R, German PS. Quality of life. Considerations in geriatrics. *Clin Geriatr Med.* 1994;10:541-555.
4. Goldstein MK. Ethical considerations in pharmacotherapy of the aged. *Drugs Aging.* 1991;1:91-97.
5. Holmes HM et al. Reconsidering medication appropriateness for patients late in life. *Arch Intern Med.* 2006;166:605-609.
6. Livesley B. Cost-benefit considerations in the treatment of elderly people. *Drugs Aging.* 1991;1:249-253.
7. Tobias DE. Ensuring and documenting the quality of drug therapy in the elderly. *Generations.* 1994;18:40-42.
8. Burns JMA et al. Elderly patients and their medication: a post-discharge follow-up study. *Age Aging.* 1992;21:178-181.
9. Honig PK, Cantilena LR. Polypharmacy. Pharmacokinetic perspectives. *Clin Pharmacokinet.* 1994;26:85-90.
10. Botelho RJ, Dudrak R. Home assessment of adherence to long-term medication in the elderly. *J Fam Pract.* 1992;35:61-65.
11. Hanlon et al. Adverse drug events in high risk older outpatients. *J Am Geriatr Soc.* 1997;45:945-948.
12. Hohl CM et al. Polypharmacy, adverse drug-related events, and potential adverse drug interactions in elderly patients presenting to an emergency department. *Ann Emerg Med.* 2001;38:666-671.
13. Gray SL et al. Adverse drug events in elderly patients receiving home health services following hospital discharge. *Ann Pharmacother.* 1999;33:1147-1153.
14. Walker J, Wynne H. Review: the frequency and severity of adverse drug reactions in elderly people. *Age Ageing.* 1994;23:255-259.
15. Hämmerlein A et al. Pharmacokinetic and pharmacodynamic changes in the elderly. Clinical implications. *Clin Pharmacokinet.* 1998;35:49-64.
16. Feinberg M. The problems of anticholinergic adverse effects in older patients. *Drugs Aging.* 1993;3:335-348.
17. Bowen JD, Larson EB. Drug-induced cognitive impairment. Defining the problem and finding solutions. *Drugs Aging.* 1993;3:349-357.
18. Iber FL et al. Age-related changes in the gastrointestinal system. Effects on drug therapy. *Drugs Aging.* 1994;5:34-48.
19. Gainsborough N et al. The association of age with gastric emptying. *Age Aging.* 1993;22:37-40.
20. Durnas C et al. Hepatic drug metabolism and aging. *Clin Pharmacokinet.* 1990;19:359-389.
21. Roskos KV, Maibach HI. Percutaneous absorption and age. Implications for therapy. *Drugs Aging.* 1992;2:432-449.
22. Novak LP. Aging, total body potassium, fat-free mass, and cell mass in males and females between ages 18 and 85 years. *J Gerontol.* 1972;27:438-443.
23. Morgan DJ, Bray KM. Lean body mass as a predictor of drug dosage. Implications for drug therapy. *Clin Pharmacokinet.* 1994;26:292-307.
24. Tregaskis BF, Stevenson IH. Pharmacokinetics in old age. *Br Med Bull.* 1990;46:9-21.
25. Rodeheffer RJ et al. Exercise cardiac output is maintained with advancing age in healthy human subjects: cardiac dilatation and increased stroke volume compensate for a diminished heart rate. *Circulation.* 1984;69:208-213.
26. Woo J et al. Effect of age and disease on two drug binding proteins: albumin and α-1-acid glycoprotein. *Clin Biochem.* 1994;27:289-292.
27. Ritschel WA. Drug disposition in the elderly: gerontokinetics. *Methods Find Exp Clin Pharmacol.* 1992;14: 555-572.
28. Owens NJ et al. Distinguishing between the fit and frail elderly, and optimizing pharmacotherapy. *Drugs Aging.* 1994;4:47-55.
29. Vestal RE et al. Aging and the response to inhibition and induction of theophylline metabolism. *Exp Gerontol.* 1993;28:421-433.
30. Lindeman RD. Changes in renal function with aging. Implications for treatment. *Drugs Aging.* 1992;2:423-431.
31. Cockcroft DW, Gault MH. Prediction of creatinine clearance from serum creatinine. *Nephron.* 1976;16:31-41.
32. Campbell AJ. Drug treatment as a cause of falls in old age. A review of the offending agents. *Drugs Aging.* 1991;1:289-302.
33. O'Mahony MS, Woodhouse KW. Age, environmental factors and drug metabolism. *Pharmacol Ther.* 1994;61:279-287.
34. Gurwitz JH et al. The exclusion of the elderly and women from clinical trials in acute myocardial infarction. *JAMA.* 1992;268:1417-1422.
35. Kitler ME. Clinical trials and clinical practice in the elderly. A focus on hypertension. *Drugs Aging.* 1992;2: 86-94.

36. Butler RN. The importance of basic research in gerontology. *Age Aging*. 1993;22:S53-S54.
37. Johnson JA, Bootman JL. Drug-related morbidity and mortality: a cost of illness model. *Arch Intern Med*. 1995;155:1949-1956.
38. Fick DM et al. Updating the Beers criteria for potentially inappropriate medication use in older adults: results of a US consensus panel of experts. *Arch Intern Med*. 2003;163:2716-2724.
39. Samsa GP et al. A summated score for the medication appropriateness index; development and assessment of clinimetric properties including content validity. *J Clin Epidemiol*. 1994;47:891-896.
40. Brown AF et al. Guidelines for improving the care of the older person with diabetes mellitus. *J Am Geriatr Soc*. 2003;51:S265-S280.

Chapter 73

Renal Disease

Gary R. Matzke, William E. Dager, and Brett H. Heintz

■ DOSAGE REGIMEN OPTIMIZATION FOR PATIENTS WITH RENAL INSUFFICIENCY

Patients with chronic kidney disease (CKD) often have complicated medication therapy management issues as the result of their need for a multiplicity of medications to slow the progression of their disease and manage the many associated complications as well as concomitant diseases.[1,2] Furthermore, optimization of their pharmacotherapy regimens is challenging because of alterations in protein binding, drug distribution, hepatic and extrahepatic drug metabolism, and finally reduced renal excretion.[3,4] Many medical conditions, termed initiation factors, can contribute to the development of a patient's initial renal injury; yet, hypertension, diabetes mellitus, and glomerulonephritis are the predominant primary diagnoses encountered in patients with severe renal insufficiency, i.e., estimated glomerular filtration rate less than 15 mL/min, which is now designated as stage 5 CKD.[1] These entities often coexist and the rate of the progressive decline in renal function has been noted to be greater in those individuals with multiple risk factors. Patients with stage 5 CKD, i.e., those who are dialysis dependent, are commonly noted to be taking ten or more medications.[2] Thus, CKD patients warrant clinical consultation to individualize their pharmacotherapeutic regimens to optimize therapeutic outcomes and minimize the risk for adverse events.

Acute kidney injury (AKI) is broadly defined as a decrease in glomerular filtration rate (GFR), generally occurring over hours to days, that is associated with an accumulation of urea and creatinine and often with alterations in the volume of distribution, metabolism, and renal excretion of medications.[5] A new classification system for AKI based on GFR and urine output, plus two clinical outcome components which are the key elements in the paradigm, is currently being validated.[5] This relatively abrupt decline in renal function, which is predominantly seen in acutely ill intensive care patients, starkly contrasts with the insidious onset of CKD, which is defined by the presence of proteinuria or albuminuria of at least 3 months' duration, in combination with a GFR greater than 90 mL/min/1.73 m^2 (stage 1 CKD) or a GFR of less than 90 mL/min/1.73 m^2 irrespective of the presence of albuminuria (stage 2–5 CKD).[1,6]

Clinicians who care for CKD or AKI patients must understand and utilize the appropriate methods to individualize drug therapy to ensure that their patients achieve the optimal pharmacotherapeutic outcomes.[3,4] The advent of specific and sensitive methods for measuring drug concentrations in biological fluids has resulted in an extensive literature on drug disposition in each of these patient populations as well as evaluations of the effects of the several renal replacement therapy options which are frequently utilized.[5,7,8]

This chapter provides a brief conceptual discussion of how drug disposition is altered in the presence of AKI and CKD. The primary focus is the presentation of a conceptually sound approach for determining the individual dosage adjustment necessary to achieve the optimal therapeutic outcome with minimal toxicity for the AKI or CKD patient with a given degree of renal function.

The subsequent chapter, Dialysis of Drugs, discusses the concepts of drug removal by hemodialysis in stage 5 CKD patients and continuous renal replacement therapies (CRRTs) that are now frequently used to manage critically ill patients with AKI or CKD. Data on the amount of drug removed by dialysis are tabulated and dosage modification schemes for a number of drugs during dialysis are presented.

THE FOUR BASIC QUESTIONS

A practical approach to guide drug therapy in patients with renal insufficiency can be arrived at if one addresses the following questions:

1. What is the patient's current renal function status?
2. What is the anticipated degree of alteration in the pharmacokinetics or pharmacodynamics of the patient's drug regimen in the presence of renal insufficiency?
3. What method of dosage modification is optimal for each drug?
4. Does the impact of hemodialysis or CRRT on drug disposition warrant further dosage modification or supplementation?

QUANTIFICATION OF RENAL FUNCTION

Several common laboratory tests provide an assessment of a patient's renal function: blood urea nitrogen (BUN), serum creatinine (Cr_s), the ratio of BUN to Cr_s, and creatinine clearance (Cl_{Cr}).[6] The BUN concentration can change because of many factors in addition to changes in renal function. Urea is filtered and reabsorbed by the nephron and its renal excretion is a function of urine flow. Diuretic use, dehydration, and bleeding can increase the BUN concentration even when there is no decline in renal function.[5] These conditions usually result in an increased BUN/Cr_s ratio to values above the normal range of 10–15 and suggest the presence of prerenal AKI.[5]

Creatinine production and elimination in adults are usually constant at approximately 20 mg/kg/d under steady-state conditions.[6] Creatinine is filtered predominantly by the glomerulus and undergoes minimal renal tubular secretion (about 10%) in those with normal renal function. However, secretion becomes an important excretory pathway for patients with a Cl_{Cr} <50 mL/min. In these individuals, accurate measurement of Cl_{Cr} can be obtained by giving cimetidine before initiating the urine collection because cimetidine inhibits the tubular secretion of creatinine.[6]

Because the nonrenal factors that can affect BUN do not alter serum or urine creatinine concentrations, the estimation of creatinine clearance (Cl_{Cr}) or GFR are now the preferred markers of changing renal function. The relationship between Cr_s and Cl_{Cr} is a hyperbolic one: small increases in Cr_s represent a larger absolute decrease in renal function in subjects with normal renal function than do similar increases in Cr_s in individuals with moderate to severe renal insufficiency. For example, an increase in the Cr_s by 1 mg/dL is associated with a halving in Cl_{Cr} (i.e., as Cr_s changes from 1 to 2 mg/dL, the Cl_{Cr} declines from 120 to 60 mL/min), whereas an increase in Cr_s from 2 to 3 mg/dL is indicative of a decrease in Cl_{Cr} from 60 to ~45 mL/min.

Recently a new assay calibration approach has been introduced to standardize and reduce analytical errors associated with serum creatinine assays, and thereby improve the accuracy of Cl_{Cr} and estimated GFR (eGFR) results.[6] This assay calibration technique, called isotope dilution mass spectrometry, which will likely reduce the interlaboratory variability in serum creatinine values has been endorsed by the National Kidney Disease Education Program (NKDEP). The NKDEP also recommends reporting serum creatinine values in mg/dL to two decimal places (e.g., 0.93 mg/dL), and values in μmol/L to the nearest whole number (e.g., 84 μmol/L). This practice will likely reduce rounding errors that in the past contributed to errors in creatinine-based GFR or Cl_{Cr} estimates.

Since it is impractical to measure a patient's Cl_{Cr} or GFR in most clinical settings, either value can be estimated from equations based on the patient's age, height, and weight.[6] The most frequently used equation to estimate Cl_{Cr} for adults with stable renal function was derived by Cockcroft and Gault. The Cl_{Cr} equations are given for men, women, and children in Appendix 2. These equations assume steady-state serum creatinine values and do not provide valid Cl_{Cr} estimates in patients with AKI or those receiving dialysis of any type.

The predominant equation to estimate GFR was derived by Levey and colleagues.[9] Although this group has published several equations for the estimation of GFR, the modified four-variable version of the original modification of diet in renal disease (MDRD) equation (MDRD4) has been shown to provide a similar estimate of GFR results compared to its six-variable predecessor and is now recommended by the NKF and the NKDEP for calculating the eGFR in patients with a history of CKD risk factors and a GFR <60 mL/min/1.73 m².

$$\text{GFR} = 186 \times (\text{Pcr})^{-1.154} \times (\text{Age})^{-0.203} \times 0.742 \text{ (if patient is female)}$$
$$\times 1.210 \text{ (if patient is black)}.$$

■ PHARMACOKINETIC ALTERATIONS OF DRUGS IN THE PRESENCE OF CKD AND AKI

CKD and AKI have been associated with alterations in the absorption, distribution, protein binding, metabolism, and renal excretion of many drugs.[3,4,7] In contrast only rarely have alterations in the pharmacodynamic response to a given concentration of a drug in patients with renal insufficiency been attributed to biochemical or pathophysiologic changes associated with renal disease. The bioavailability of drugs can be altered in patients with severe persistent GI disturbances such as nausea, vomiting, diarrhea, and increased gastric pH because of the ingestion of histamine H2-receptor antagonists or proton pump inhibitors.[4] This can decrease the absorption of ferrous sulfate and other drugs that are best absorbed from an acidic environment. Complexation of a few drugs in the GI tract of patients who routinely take aluminum or calcium antacids has been noted to reduce oral availability. Finally, the bioavailability of dihydrocodeine and some β-blockers is increased because of reduced first-pass metabolism in the gut.[4]

The plasma protein binding of some drugs is altered in patients with severe renal insufficiency. This is most often secondary to hypoalbuminemia, accumulation of acidic byproducts of uremia resulting in competitive displacement of drugs from binding sites, or changes in the structure of albumin resulting in a decreased number of effective binding sites.[4] Weak organic acid drugs, such as cefazolin, phenytoin, salicylate, valproic acid, and warfarin, exhibit decreased plasma protein binding (increased free fraction) while the protein binding of weak organic basic drugs are predominantly unchanged. Propranolol and lidocaine are bound primarily to α_1-acid glycoprotein from which little displacement occurs in renal disease or hypoalbuminemia. Phenytoin protein binding and disposition is altered in the presence of CKD and AKI to a degree that warrants important differences in dosage.[7] The percentage of unbound phenytoin in plasma is normally 10% but increases from 20% to 35%. This results in an increase in the V_d from 0.65 L/kg to 1–1.8 L/kg. Further, the terminal half-life is decreased from 11–16 h to 6–10 h and the apparent plasma clearance increases from 28–41 mL/h/kg to 64–225 mL/h/kg stage 5 CKD patients. These changes in the pharmacokinetics of phenytoin warrant a change in its therapeutic plasma concentration range. In patients with normal kidney function, the usual therapeutic plasma concentration range for total phenytoin (unbound plus bound) is 10–20 mg/L; in those with stage 5 CKD, the range is approximately 4–8 mg/L. Both of these ranges of total drug represent the same concentration range of unbound drug, 1–2 mg/L.

The V_d of drugs tend to be increased in patients with stage 4–5 CKD and those with AKI of non-prerenal origin.[3–5] The increase in V_d is predominantly due to decreased protein binding or fluid overload, secondary to reduced renal excretion or excessive administration of intravenous or oral fluids. Examples of drugs with increased V_d are many cephalosporins, furosemide, all aminoglycosides, naproxen, phenytoin, and vancomycin. Digoxin is the most dramatically impacted agent for which a decrease in V_d has been reported. The rate of distribution may also be slower and require for some drugs such as vancomycin or aminoglycosides, a modification (prolongation) in the time when the "peak concentration" is measured. Drawing peak concentrations too early, at the time typically used for those with normal renal function, after the end of the infusion yields a higher concentration value and thus the calculation of a falsely low volume of distribution.

The degree of reduction in renal clearance depends on the percentage of drug excreted unchanged by the kidney and the relative contribution of tubular secretion and reabsorption to filtration. The renal and systemic clearance of aminoglycosides, cephalosporins, penicillins, vancomycin, acyclovir, lithium, and ranitidine, which are extensively ($>$80%) eliminated renally unchanged are highly dependent on the degree of residual renal function. For many of these drugs, linear correlations have been established between the drug's plasma and renal clearance and Cl_{Cr}.[7] These correlations are often utilized as the foundation for the construction of dosage recommendation tables based on broad categories of renal function.[8,10,11] They can also be used as guides to estimate the drug dosage requirement for individual patients with a given degree of renal function, as outlined later in this chapter.

Drug metabolism typically involves enzymatic conversion of drugs to more water-soluble compounds. These metabolites are formed through the processes of oxidation, reduction, synthesis (e.g., conjugation), or hydrolysis. Once formed, these metabolites often are excreted predominantly by the kidney.[7] Although many metabolites are inactive or have minimal pharmacologic activity, there are several examples where the metabolite is the primary active moiety. Thus in some cases it may be the active metabolites that accumulate and lead to exaggerated pharmacodynamic responses that warrant dosage reduction of the "prodrug" which is administered. Active metabolites that are excreted by the kidney include oxypurinol from allopurinol, which is an active inhibitor of xanthine oxidase; normeperidine from meperidine, which can cause seizures; and N-acetylprocainamide from procainamide, which has its own unique antiarrhythmic properties.[7]

Renal insufficiency also can lead to alterations in drug metabolism.[3,4,7,12–14] The relationship of CKD to cytochrome P450-mediated (CYP-mediated) metabolism in the liver and other organs has recently been reviewed. In rat models of CKD, protein expression in the liver of several CYP enzymes, including CYP3A1 and CYP3A2 (equivalent to human CYP3A4), is reduced by as much as 75%; CYP2C11 and CYP3A2 activity is significantly reduced, whereas CYP1A2 activity is unchanged. In humans, CYP2C19 and CYP3A4 activity is reduced, whereas CYP2D6 and CYP2E1 activity appears to not be affected by the presence of CKD. The reduction of nonrenal clearance (Cl_{nr}) of several drugs in patients with severe CKD supports this premise. Prediction of the effect of renal insufficiency on the metabolism of a particular drug is thus difficult and a general quantitative strategy to adjust drug dosage regimens for extensively metabolized agents is not yet available. However, some insight can be gained if one knows what enzyme(s) are involved in the metabolism of the drug of interest and how the enzyme(s) are affected by the presence of renal insufficiency.

The effect of CKD on the metabolism of a particular drug is, however, difficult to predict even for drugs within the same pharmacologic class. The reductions in Cl_{nr} for those with CKD have frequently been noted to be proportional to the reductions in GFR. In the small number of studies that have evaluated Cl_{nr} in critically ill patients with AKI, residual Cl_{nr} was higher than the values reported in patients with CKD who had a similar Cl_{Cr}. Since a patient with AKI may have a higher Cl_{nr} than a CKD patient, the resultant plasma concentrations will be lower than expected and possibly subtherapeutic if classic CKD-derived dosage guidelines are followed.

DOSAGE ADJUSTMENT APPROACHES THAT ARE USEFUL AND PRACTICAL FOR SPECIFIC DRUGS

The three approaches for maintenance drug dosage adjustments in patients with CKD or stable AKI are to (1) decrease the dose and maintain the usual dosage interval, (2) lengthen the dosage interval and maintain the usual dose, or (3) modify the dose and interval. The primary goal of these approaches is to provide average steady-state plasma concentrations or AUCs in CKD or AKI patients that are similar to those observed in patients with normal kidney function. The choice of approach depends on the drug and the desirability, from a therapeutic or toxic standpoint, of having small or large peak-to-trough fluctuations.[3,4] Other considerations are that the dosage regimen adjustment should be practical and the reduced dose or prolonged dosage interval should be relatively easy to implement. Indeed these principles are utilized by pharmaceutical and biotechnology companies to create the "population or renal function categorical" dosage guidelines that are ultimately approved by regulatory agencies and appear in the official product labeling.[10]

When presented with a patient with renal insufficiency for whom drug dosage regimen decisions must be made, the most practical and efficient approach is to first consult the product labeling or a compendium or internet based sources to access an authoritative reference source for drug dosage in renal failure. Many such resources are available and include, for example "Drug Prescribing in Renal Failure: Dosing Guidelines for Adults"[11] and "Micromedex,"[15] which describe specific pharmacokinetic alterations of drugs in kidney disease and recommended dosage regimens for those with various categories of renal function. The reader also is advised to refer to specific drug monographs in this book and in *AHFS Drug Information*,[16] which briefly describe the effect of renal failure on drug disposition and provide initial dosage recommendations. These sources allow the user to determine whether dosage adjustments are necessary and if there are any important toxicities or precautions that need to be considered regarding the use of a particular drug. These sources, however, usually provide only categorical drug dosing guidelines.

For drugs requiring marked dosage adjustment or for which the achievement of specific therapeutic plasma concentrations is critical, the reader may need to consult the original publications or well-referenced resources, which provide specific data on individual drugs.[16,17] Consulting the original publications or authoritative reviews will often provide details regarding the relationship of renal function to drug elimination and / or a dosage nomogram or specific dosage recommendations and precautions for the use of the drug in patients with various degrees of renal insufficiency.[16,17]

If drug-specific data or guidelines are not available, one can use general dosage equations such as those developed by Rowland and Tozer.[18] Only basic pharmacokinetic information obtained early in the drug development process is needed—the fraction of the bioavailable dose that is normally excreted unchanged in the urine, f_e. The fraction of normal renal function (KF) a given patient has can be calculated as the ratio of the patient's Cl_{Cr} to the "accepted normal" value of 120 mL/min. The patient's Cl_{Cr} can be determined from stable Cr_s values i.e., those at steady state with the method of Cockcroft and Gault.[6] The GFR can also be calculated but its use as a measure of renal function for drug dosage individualization is not currently recommended.[9]

The following equation, which takes into consideration the renal clearance and extrarenal clearance of unbound drug, can be used to determine the dosage adjustment factor, Q:[18]

$$Q = \frac{[(KF \times f_e) + [1-f_e] \times [(140-age) \times \text{weight in kg}^{0.7}]}{160}$$

Q is in essence the ratio of the unbound drug clearance of the patient to that observed in those with a $Cl_{Cr} \geq 120$ mL/min, or [Cl_u (failure)/Cl_u (normal)]. If a drug is minimally protein bound (<25%) and not extensively metabolized ($f_e \geq 70\%$), this equation can be simplified to

$$Q = 1 - [f_e(1 - KF)]$$

Once the value of Q is obtained, a dosage regimen adjustment can be calculated with the following equations based on the desired objectives:

$$D_{RI} = Q \times D_N$$

where D_{RI} is the maintenance dose in the renally insufficient patient that is to be given at the normal dosage interval and D_N is the normal dose for those with $Cl_{Cr} \geq 120$ mL/min.

$$\tau_{RI} = \frac{\tau_N}{Q}$$

where τ_{RI} is the maintenance dosage interval for the renally insufficient patient at which the D_N is the dose to be given and τ_N is the dosage interval for those with $Cl_{Cr} \geq 120$ mL/min.

The final scenario incorporates a modification of D_N and τ_N. This scenario usually is used when the calculated D_{RI} or τ_{RI} are impractical. In that situation, one chooses a clinically relevant "τ_{RI}" and calculates the D_{RI} to be given at that time.

$$D_{RI} = \frac{[D_N \times Q \times \tau_{RI}]}{\tau_N}$$

An example will clarify the use of this approach. An 80-kg, 45-year-old man with a stable Cr_s of 5.4 mg/dL requires treatment with ceftazidime for a pseudomonal infection. This drug is 70% excreted unchanged in the urine, and the usual dosage is 1 g every 8 h IV. The patient's Cl_{Cr}, KF, and Q are calculated as follows:

$$Cl_{Cr} = \frac{(140 - 45) \times 80}{(5.4 \times 72)} = 20 \text{ mL/min}$$

$$KF = \frac{20 \text{ mL/min}}{120 \text{ mL/min}} = 0.17$$

$$\begin{aligned}
Q &= (0.17 \times 0.7) + (1 - 0.7) \\
&= 0.120 + 0.3 \\
&= 0.43
\end{aligned}$$

If the maintenance dose for this patient was reduced and the dosage interval maintained every 8 h, the D_{RI} would be

$$\begin{aligned}
D_{RI} &= 0.43 \times D_N \\
&= 430 \text{ mg q8h}
\end{aligned}$$

This regimen will result in reduced peak and increased trough concentrations relative to subjects with normal renal function receiving the standard dose. The average concentration would, however, be the same.

Alternatively, one might extend the dosage interval and maintain the standard dose size (D_N). This will produce the same postdistribution peak and trough concentrations for the renal patient that one would expect in a patient with Cl_{Cr} ≥120 mL/min. Unfortunately, the use of nonstandard dosage intervals often has been associated with drug administration errors.

$$\tau_{RI} = \frac{\tau_N}{Q} = \frac{8}{0.43} = 18.6 \text{ h}$$

In this example and many patient scenarios, the best individualized dosage adjustment strategy might be to select a feasible prolonged dosage interval (τ_{RI}), e.g., 12 h, and then calculate the D_{RI}.

$$D_{RI} = \frac{[D_N \times Q \times \tau_{RI}]}{\tau_N} = \frac{[1000 \text{ mg} \times 0.43 \times 12]}{8} = 650 \text{ mg}$$

This general approach provides a reasonable initial method for adjusting drug dosage regimens in patients with renal insufficiency until more specific guidelines can be consulted or serum concentrations are measured. This method is based on several assumptions: (1) bioavailability is unchanged in renal failure; (2) metabolites are not therapeutically active or toxic; (3) decreased renal function does not alter metabolism of the drug; (4) metabolism or renal excretion does not exhibit concentration-dependent pharmacokinetics; (5) renal function is constant with time; and (6) the renal clearance of the drug is directly proportional to the renal clearance of the compound used to measure renal function. If any of these assumptions is invalid, the accuracy of the projected dosage regimen will be reduced.

The time to reach steady state is longer for a patient with renal insufficiency than one with normal renal function. Consequently, it is common to initiate therapy for almost all drugs with a loading dose (i.e., at least the D_N and in some cases an even greater dose) to achieve the desired concentration in the expanded V_d. The amount of the loading dose depends on the characteristics of the particular drug, any known alteration in V_d, and the desired therapeutic objectives.

It should be noted that any dosage regimen modification for renally insufficient patients might require plasma concentration determinations of the drug, if available, and close clinical observation for assessment of toxicity and verification of achievement of the desired therapeutic outcomes. One must also be aware that the desired concentration ranges may be in some cases different than those employed for patients with normal renal function (i.e., aminoglycosides and phenytoin).

■ REFERENCES

1. Joy MJ et al. Chronic kidney disease: progression-modifying therapies. In: DiPiro JT et al., eds. *Pharmacotherapy: A Pathophysiologic Approach.* 7th ed. New York, NY: McGraw-Hill; 2008:745-764.

2. Hudson J. Chronic kidney disease: management of complications. In: DiPiro JT et al., eds. *Pharmacotherapy: A Pathophysiologic Approach.* 7th ed. New York, NY: McGraw-Hill; 2008:765-791.

3. Matzke GR, Dowling TD. Dosing concepts in renal dysfunction. In: Murphy JE, ed. *Clinical Pharmacokinetics Pocket Reference.* 4th ed. Bethesda, MD: American Society of Health-System Pharmacists; 2008:427-445.

4. Matzke GR, Comstock TJ. Influence of renal disease and dialysis on pharmacokinetics. In: Burton ME et al., eds. *Applied Pharmacokinetics and Pharmacodynamics: Principles of Therapeutic Drug Monitoring.* 4th ed. Baltimore, MD: Lippincott Williams and Wilkins; 2006:187-212.

5. Dager WE, Spencer A. Acute renal failure. In: DiPiro JT et al., eds. *Pharmacotherapy: A Pathophysiologic Approach.* 7th ed. New York, NY: McGraw-Hill; 2008:723-743.

6. Dowling TC. Quantification of renal function. In: DiPiro JT et al., eds. *Pharmacotherapy: A Pathophysiologic Approach.* 7th ed. New York, NY: McGraw-Hill; 2008:705-722.

7. Matzke GR, Fryc RF. Drug therapy individualization for patients with renal insufficiency. In: DiPiro JT et al., eds. *Pharmacotherapy: A Pathophysiologic Approach.* 7th ed. New York, NY: McGraw-Hill; 2008:833-844.

8. Munar MY, Singh H. Drug dosing adjustments in patients with chronic kidney disease. *Am Fam Physician.* 2007;75:1487-1496.

9. Wargo KA et al. Comparison of the modification of diet in renal disease and Cockroft-Gault equations for antimicrobial dosage adjustments. *Ann Pharmacother.* 2006;40:1248-1253.

10. Guidance for Industry: pharmacokinetics in patients with impaired renal function—study design, data analysis, and impact on dosing and labeling. http://www.fda.gov/Cder/Guidance/1449fnl.pdf. Accessed March 10, 2009.

11. Aronoff GR et al. *Drug Prescribing in Renal Failure: Dosing Guidelines for Adults.* 5th ed. Philadelphia, PA: American College of Physicians; 2007:1-271.

12. Nolin TD et al. Hepatic drug metabolism and transport in patients with kidney disease. *Am J Kidney Dis.* 2003;42:906-925.

13. Michaud J et al. Effect of hemodialysis on hepatic cytochrome P450 functional expression. *J Pharmacol Sci.* 2008;108:157-163.

14. Nolin TD. Altered nonrenal drug clearance in ESRD. *Curr Opin Nephrol Hypertens.* 2008;17:555-559.

15. Micromedex® Healthcare Series - DRUGDEX® System. Greenwood Village, Colorado: Thomson Micromedex; 2009. http://www.micromedex.com/products/drugdex/. Accessed March 10, 2009.

16. McEvoy GK et al. *American Hospital Formulary Service Drug Information.* Bethesda, MD: American Society of Health-System Pharmacists; 2009.

17. Smith HE et al. Appendix II. Design and optimization of dosage regimens: pharmacokinetic data. Brunton LL et al., eds. *Goodman & Gilman's The Pharmacological Basis of Therapeutics.* 11th ed. 2006. http://www.accesspharmacy.com/content.aspx?aID = 956421. Accessed March 10, 2009.

18. Rowland M, Tozer TN. Disease effects. In: *Clinical Pharmacokinetics: Concepts and Applications,* 3rd ed. Philadelphia, PA: Lea and Febiger, 1995:238-254.

Chapter 74

Dialysis of Drugs

Gary R. Matzke, William E. Dager, and Brett H. Heintz

■ DIALYSIS REMOVAL OF DRUGS AND DOSAGE SUPPLEMENTATION

In the United States, more than 350,000 patients with ESRD receive chronic maintenance hemodialysis or peritoneal dialysis.[1] Therapeutic advances in dialysis techniques and medications for the management of anemia, hyperphosphatemia, and the other complications of stage 5 CKD have increased survival, and a reasonable quality of life is now possible for many of these patients. Patients with acute kidney injury (AKI) have also benefited from new approaches for renal replacement therapy, especially when the patient is critically ill. However, there is still considerable debate as to the optimal mode of RRT delivery and a lack of clarity as to the desired intensity of the therapy.[2,3] Although the primary purpose of dialysis is to remove unwanted toxic waste products and excessive fluid, it also enhances the clearance of many pharmacotherapeutic agents. If the extent a drug is removed by dialysis is significant, supplemental doses or a revised dosage regimen might be required to optimize the pharmacological effects and clinical outcome.[4,5] Dialysis procedures, including hemoperfusion, also have been used in drug overdose situations as a means of enhancing drug removal and thereby minimizing adverse outcomes. Therefore, it is important for clinicians especially those who manage critically ill patients to know how effective these procedures are and whether they offer any substantial advantage over conventional means of treating overdoses.[5,6]

The objectives of this chapter are to review those drug and dialysis prescription factors that have an impact on the efficiency of the removal of drugs by dialysis. The impact of hemodialysis on the disposition of a drug can be quantified by direct measurement of the amount of drug recovered in the dialysate, and these data can be used to calculate the rate of appearance of the drug in the dialysate and the drug clearance by the dialyzer (CL_D).[4,5,7] This provides the most accurate assessment of dialyzability. Alternatively one can measure the concentration of the drug of interest in multiple blood samples from the inlet and outflow ports of the dialyzer and use this data to calculate the rate of disappearance (clearance) of drug from the plasma (CL_{pHD}). A minimalist approach is however commonly employed in clinical care settings, which is dependent on the estimation of the total plasma clearance or half-life during dialysis by collecting 2–3 blood samples. These pharmacokinetic data can be used to estimate the fraction of the drug removed by dialysis from the patient during the dialysis procedure.[5]

Peritoneal dialysis is a much less efficient means of removing waste products and drugs than hemodialysis.[8] The additional clearance provided by this mode of dialysis is only of clinical significance for a few agents such as: aminoglycosides, some antifungals, phenobarbital, theophylline, and vancomycin.[9,10] In contrast, the continuous renal replacement therapies, which are frequently used to manage AKI in critically ill patients, can dramatically alter disposition of many drugs used in the acute care setting.[5] These therapies are now widely used and employ hemofilters that are often made of the same materials as hemodialyzers. Thus, the dialyzer filter factors, which influence drug removal, are similar.

DETERMINANTS OF DRUG DIALYZABILITY

The Dialysis Prescription. There have been many improvements in hemodialysis therapy during the last 30 years.[8,11] The blood and dialysate flow rates, two of the primary determinants of the removal of drugs, have increased dramatically, and the utilization of aggressive ultrafiltration to maintain fluid balance has contributed to an increase of 75%–100% in the average delivered dialysis dose. Further, in the 1990s, a major shift in the composition of dialyzer membranes began. The proportion of patients dialyzed with conventional dialyzers composed of cellulose, cuprophane, or slightly modified cellulose filters decreased and by 2007, >80% of stage 5 CKD patients received hemodialysis with semisynthetic or synthetic dialyzers, which were made from substances such as polysulfone, polymethylmethacrylate, polyamide, or cellulose triacetate.[1,12] The clearance of many drugs is now higher than most values reported in the literature during the 70s through the mid to late 90s.[5,11,13,14] In fact, some drugs such as vancomycin, which was not dialyzable with conventional dialyzers, has been demonstrated to be highly dialyzable when these new dialyzers are used.[11] For other agents such as the aminoglycosides and cephalosporins, increases in clearance of 200% are common.[5,11,13,14] In light of these dramatic improvements, if a drug is "dialyzable," it is crucial that clinicians utilize dialyzer and prescription specific information to determine the clearance of the drug of interest and then factor this information into the generation of an individualized dosage regimen design. If the only available dialysis data are generated from experiences with conventional dialyzers and less aggressive delivery of dialysis, the clinician may need to empirically double the literature clearance value as a starting point and strongly consider monitoring plasma concentrations of the drug to assure the desired clinical outcomes are achieved.

Drug Factors. Drugs with low molecular weights, usually <500 daltons, cross conventional dialysis membranes readily. Large-molecular-weight drugs, such as vancomycin (MW 1449) and amphotericin B (MW 924), cross those membranes poorly and are not effectively removed by conventional hemodialysis.[4–6] Semisynthetic and synthetic dialyzers, however, have been associated with marked increases in the clearance of large-molecular-weight agents.

Drugs with high water solubility are removed more readily than lipid-soluble compounds. In addition, the latter usually have a larger V_d that limits the removal by hemodialysis since less of the drug once distributed is in the vascular compartment. Drugs such as digoxin or tricyclic antidepressants, which have $V_d > 5$–7 L/kg, are usually minimally removed by dialysis because the majority of drug is contained in muscle or fat tissue rather than in the vascular compartment, and the drug in these tissues is not as readily accessible for removal. Although one can rapidly clear the blood compartment of a drug, plasma drug concentrations can increase (rebound) as a result of re-distribution of drug from tissue stores back into the plasma.

Plasma protein binding of a drug also impacts how effectively it can be dialyzed.[4] Drugs with a high degree of protein binding, such as propranolol (90%–94%) and warfarin (99%), are poorly removed by dialysis because the drug–protein complex is too large to cross all dialysis membranes. This is not a limitation of hemoperfusion because the drug is removed from plasma proteins as the complex passes through the high surface area absorbent material.[7]

LITERATURE EVALUATION PITFALLS

Several problems are encountered commonly with the literature on removal of drugs by dialysis. First, for some drugs, only anecdotal reports are available. This is primarily true in the overdose setting in which the impact of dialysis on drug removal often is determined primarily by clinical response.[7] For example, a comatose patient awakens during or shortly after dialysis and it is assumed that dialysis removed the drug, accounting for the improved clinical status. Second, the amount of drug ingested and/or the amount of drug recovered in the dialysate often is unknown. Third, the type of dialysis system employed is frequently not specified—this is extremely important when one needs to match the current patient's dialysis prescription with published data. The advances in dialysis technology, discussed above, make much of the data from conventional dialysis inapplicable. Fourth, there often is a lack of patient data, such as weight, hematocrit, and renal and liver function. Fifth, the method used to calculate drug clearance often is unspecified. For example, was clearance determined from the amount of drug recovered in the dialysate or from differences in arterial and venous plasma concentrations across the dialyzer? The optimal methods for dialyzer clearance calculations in various clinical situations are described in several current references.[4,6]

For many drugs, there is a lack of correlation between plasma drug concentration and clinical response. Some drugs have active or toxic metabolites that correlate well with the desired or toxic effects of the drug.[6] Thus to characterize the influence of dialysis on a drug's clinical effects, attention must be given to metabolites as well. Predictions of drug dialyzability, which utilize pharmacokinetic data from healthy subjects or stable stage 5 CKD patients receiving therapeutic dosages, are often fraught with problems because critically ill patients, especially those who have ingested an overdose, may have changes in drug metabolism, V_d, or protein binding.[7] For example, large amounts of drug in the body might saturate plasma protein binding, which in turn might alter drug distribution and metabolism.

ESTIMATION OF THE IMPACT OF DIALYSIS

The impact of dialysis clearance of a drug on total body clearance can be assessed as the fractional increase (F_{inc}) expressed as a percentage in clearance because clearance terms are additive:

$$Cl_{TD} = Cl_T + Cl_D$$
$$F_{inc} = [Cl_D / Cl_T] \times 100$$

where

Cl_{TD} = total body clearance of drug during dialysis
Cl_T = patient's residual total body clearance of drug
Cl_D = dialysis clearance of drug

If dialysis clearance adds substantially to total body clearance then the drug will be eliminated at a faster rate. For example, if the dialysis clearance of a drug is 50 mL/min and the patient's residual total body clearance is 15 mL/min and the drug's V_d is 20L, then the drug would be eliminated from the body five times as fast during the dialysis period. To relate clearance to drug half-life ($t_{1/2}$), the following equations are useful:

$$t_{1/2}. \text{ (off dialysis)} = \frac{0.693 \times V_d}{Cl_T}$$

$$t_{1/2}. \text{ (on dialysis)} = \frac{0.693 \times V_d}{Cl_T + Cl_d}$$

The more the dialysis clearance adds to the patient's residual total body clearance, the shorter the drug half-life will be on dialysis (assuming V_d remains constant). Another extension of this allows one to calculate the fraction of the drug in the body that is lost during a dialysis period.

$$\text{Fraction lost} = 1 - e^{-(Cl + Cl_D)(\tau_d/V_d)}$$

where τ_d is the duration of the dialysis period.

This calculation represents the fraction of drug in the body that is lost during a dialysis period by all routes of elimination (i.e., dialysis, metabolism, and renal excretion). It is necessary to acquire from literature sources (keeping in mind the limitations discussed previously) values for V_d, Cl_T, and Cl_D. If renal or liver function is diminished, this must be taken into consideration because it will result in a lower Cl_T. In addition, changes in V_d in certain disease states (e.g., the decreased V_d of digoxin in renal failure or presence of anasarca) also must be taken into account.

Because drug concentrations in plasma are higher in the distribution phase, especially for intravenously administered drugs, more drug can be removed by dialysis if the procedure is started shortly after drug administration, or as is the case in many chronic dialysis settings, drugs are purposely given intravenously during the last hours of the procedure. As an example, up to 30% of a dose of vancomycin is removed if it is given during the last hour of dialysis.[5,11]

Two examples illustrate the use of pharmacokinetic data to calculate drug clearance during dialysis. Phenobarbital has a V_d of approximately 50 L, a total body clearance of 0.3 L/h, and a conventional hemodialysis clearance of 4.2 L/h. The half-life off dialysis is 115 h and 8 h during dialysis. Approximately 30% of the drug would be removed from the body during 4 h of dialysis. Thus a supplemental dose will be warranted to maintain the desired therapeutic outcomes. In contrast the impact of hemodialysis on digoxin is clinically insignificant. Digoxin has a V_d of about 300 L and total body clearance of 2.4 L/h in an anephric patient, and the hemodialysis clearance of digoxin is 1.2 L/h. Thus the estimated half-lives of digoxin are 86 h off dialysis and 58 h on dialysis. Although this appears to be a substantial decrease in half-life, it means that the patient would have to be dialyzed continuously for 58 h to remove one-half of the digoxin from the body. The fraction of drug lost during a routine hemodialysis period of 4 h would be only 5%. Thus, a supplemental dose of digoxin after hemodialysis is not warranted.

USING THE TABLES

Tables 74–1 through 74–4 provide categorical data on selected commonly utilized drugs in the United States. The drugs are classified on the basis of the reported degree of drug removal by hemodialysis or derived by using pharmacokinetic parameters taken from the literature. Drug removal is intentionally described in a categorical fashion for a number of reasons. First, much of this information changes quite rapidly. Second, a given value for the amount of drug removed or the dialysis clearance determined in one study might differ from that found in another study because of differences in the dialysis prescription or patient population being treated. For example the duration of a maintenance dialysis treatment has decreased from 6+ h, per treatment in the late 1980s to late 1990s to 2.5–3.0 h for many patients now. The information derived from numerous compiled reference sources was utilized to generate the tables. The tabulation of the specific clearance information associated with a given dialyzer is beyond the scope of this review, and the reader is referred to these resources if such information is needed to determine an individualized dosage regimen for a dialysis patient.[5,10,11,13–15]

TABLE 74–1 DRUGS READILY REMOVED BY HEMODIALYSIS[a]

Acyclovir	Flucytosine
Amikacin	Ganciclovir
Amoxicillin	Gentamicin
Cefazolin	Imipenem/cilastatin
Cefepime	Lithium
Cefmetazole	Meropenem
Cefprozil	Methotrexate
Ceftazidime	Mezlocillin
Cidofovir	Oseltamivir
Clavulanic acid	Phenobarbital
Daptomycin	Pregabalin
Doripenem	Theophylline
Famciclovir	Tobramycin

[a]50%–80% removed in a hemodialysis session.

TABLE 74–2 DRUGS MODERATELY REMOVED BY HEMODIALYSIS[a]

Acebutolol	Didanosine	Penicillin G
Allopurinol	Enalapril	Pentoxifylline
Acetaminophen	Ethosuximide	Piperacillin
Ampicillin	Fluconazole	Primidone
Atenolol	Foscarnet	Procainamide
Azathioprine	Gabapentin	Pyrazinamide
Aztreonam	Lenalidomide	Ramipril

(continued)

TABLE 74–2 DRUGS MODERATELY REMOVED BY HEMODIALYSIS[a] (*continued*)

Bretylium	Linezolid	Sotalol
Cefaclor	Lisinopril	Sulbactam
Cefotaxime	Lorazepam	Sulfamethoxazole
Cefoxitin	Metformin	Tenofovir
Cefpodoxime	Methyldopa	Ticarcillin
Ceftizoxime	Metronidazole	Topotecan
Ceftriaxone	Minoxidil	Trimethoprim
Cefuroxime	Nadolol	Vancomycin
Cephalexin	Ofloxacin	
Cyclophosphamide	Omeprazole	

[a]20%–49% within a hemodialysis session.

TABLE 74–3 DRUGS NOT SIGNIFICANTLY REMOVED BY HEMODIALYSIS

Amantadine	Epoetin alfa	Mycophenolate
Amitriptyline	Erythromycin	Metoprolol
Amlodipine	Esmolol	Miconazole
Amphotericin B	Ethambutol	Nafcillin
Bleomycin	Etodolac	Naproxen
Candesartan	Famotidine	Nifedipine
Captopril	Felodipine	Oxacillin
Carbamazepine	Filgrastim	Propranolol
Cefixime	Flecainide	Quinapril
Chloramphenicol	Flurbiprofen	Quinidine
Chloroquine	Furosemide	Ranitidine
Cimetidine	Gemfibrozil	Rifampin
Ciprofloxacin	Glyburide	Rimantadine
Cisplatin	Ibuprofen	Sildenafil
Citalopram	Indinavir	Sulindac
Clindamycin	Indomethacin	Tacrolimus
Clonidine	Isoniazid	Temazepam
Colchicine	Isradipine	Tetracycline
Cyclosporine	Itraconazole	Thiabendazole
Diazepam	Ketoconazole	Timolol
Dicloxacillin	Labetalol	Triazolam
Digoxin	Lamivudine	Valproic acid
Disopyramide	Lidocaine	Verapamil
Doxepin	Methadone	Zidovudine
Doxycycline	Methylprednisolone	

TABLE 74–4 NO DATA REGARDING DRUG REMOVAL BY HEMODIALYSIS

Alprazolam	Clorazepate
Amitriptyline	Clozapine
Amlodipine	Codeine
Azithromycin	Colchicine
Baclofen	Cytarabine
Betaxolol	Dapsone
Bumetanide	Desipramine
Carteolol	Diltiazem
Chlorpheniramine	Dipyridamole
Chlorpromazine	Dopamine
Chlorpropamide	Ethacrynic acid
Cisplatin	Felbamate
Clarithromycin	Fenoprofen
Clofazimine	Fluorouracil
Flurazepam	Penicillamine
Glipizide	Pentamidine
Griseofulvin	Pentazocine
Haloperidol	Phenothiazines
Hydralazine	Phenytoin
Hydrochlorothiazide	Piroxicam
Indinavir	Pravastatin
Indomethacin	Prazosin
Lamivudine	Prednisone
Levodopa	Primaquine
Lovastatin	Probenecid
Melphalan	Rifabutin
Meperidine	Ritonavir
Metolazone	Saquinavir
Midazolam	Sargramostim
Milrinone	Simvastatin
Minocycline	Spironolactone
Misoprostol	Stavudine
Morphine	Sulfisoxazole
Muromonab-CD3	Sulindac
Nelfinavir	Tamoxifen
Nevirapine	Tolmetin
Nitrofurantoin	Triamterene
Norfloxacin	Vinblastine
Nortriptyline	Vincristine
Ondansetron	Warfarin
Paromomycin	

The use of multiple modes of continuous renal replacement therapy in critically ill individuals is increasing.[3] The principles of drug removal for some of the continuous renal replacement therapies are different from those discussed in this section. Therefore, the reader may refer to selected studies that provide an introduction to this topic and tabulations of literature data on drug removal.[5,14,16]

■ REFERENCES

1. U.S. Renal Data System. USRDS 2008 annual data report: atlas of chronic kidney disease and end-stage renal disease in the United States. Bethesda, MD: National Institutes of Health, National Institute of Diabetes and Digestive and Kidney Diseases; 2008. http://www.usrds.org/2008/view/esrd_04.asp. Accessed February 11, 2009.

2. Kellum JA. Renal replacement therapy in critically ill patients with acute renal failure: does a greater dose improve survival? *Nat Clin Pract Nephrol.* 2007;3:128-129. http://www.nature.com/ncpneph/journal/v3/n3/full/ncpneph0398.html. Accessed March 9, 2009.

3. VA/NIH Acute Renal failure trial network. Intensity of renal support in critically ill patients with acute kidney injury. *N Engl J Med.* 2008;359(1):7-20.

4. Matzke GR, Comstock TJ. Influence of renal disease and dialysis on pharmacokinetics. In: Evans WE et al, eds. *Applied Pharmacokinetics: Principles of Therapeutic Drug Monitoring.* 4th ed. Baltimore, MD: Lippincott Williams and Wilkins; 2006:187-212.

5. Heintz BH, Matzke GR, Dager WE. Antimicrobial dosing concepts and recommendations for critically ill adult patients receiving continuous renal replacement therapy or intermittent hemodialysis. *Pharmacotherapy* 2009;29(5):562-577.

6. Matzke GR, Frye RF. Drug therapy individualization for patients with renal insufficiency. In: DiPiro JT et al, eds. *Pharmacotherapy: A Pathophysiological Approach.* 7th ed. New York, NY: McGraw-Hill; 2008:833-844.

7. Chyka PA. Clinical Toxicology. In: DiPiro JT et al, eds. *Pharmacotherapy: A Pathophysiological Approach.* 7th ed. New York, NY: McGraw-Hill; 2008:69-90.

8. Foote EF, Manley HJ. Hemodialysis and peritoneal dialysis. In: DiPiro JT et al, eds. *Pharmacotherapy: A Pathophysiological Approach.* New York, NY: McGraw-Hill Medical; 2008: http://highered.mcgraw-hill.com/sites/dl/free/007147899x/603552/Pharmacotherapy_chap048.pdf. Accessed March 9, 2009.

9. Taylor CA et al. Clinical pharmacokinetics during continuous ambulatory peritoneal dialysis. *Clin Pharmacokinet.* 1996;31:293-308.

10. Piraino B et al. Peritoneal dialysis related infections: 2005 update. *Perit Dial Int.* 2005;25(2):107-131.

11. Matzke GR. Status of hemodialysis of drugs in 2002. *J Pharm Pract.* 2002;15:405-418.

12. Daugirdas JT et al. Hemodialysis apparatus. In: Daugirdas JT et al, eds. *Handbook of Dialysis.* 3rd ed. Philadelphia, PA: Lippincott Williams & Wilkins; 2001:46-66.

13. Matzke GR, Dowling TD. Dosing concepts in renal dysfunction. In: Murphy JE, ed. *Clinical Pharmacokinetics Pocket Reference.* 4th ed. Bethesda, MD: American Society of Health-System Pharmacists; 2008:427-445.

14. Veltri MA et al. Drug dosing during intermittent hemodialysis and continuous renal replacement therapy: Special considerations in pediatric patients. *Pediatr Drugs.* 2004;6:45-65.

15. Smith HE, Thummel KE, Shen DD, et al. Appendix II. Design and optimization of dosage regimens: Pharmacokinetic data. In: Burton LL et al, eds. *Goodman & Gilman's the Pharmacological Basis of Therapeutics.* 11th ed. New York, NY: McGraw-Hill; 2006. http://www.accesspharmacy.com/content.aspx?aID=956421. Accessed March 10, 2009.

16. Aronoff GR et al. *Drug Prescribing in Renal Failure: Dosing Guidelines for Adults.* 5th ed. Philadelphia, PA: American College of Physicians; 2007:1-271.

Immunization 3

Andrea L. McKeever and Heather F. DeBellis

■ INTRODUCTION

Immunization practices aim to protect individuals and society from infectious diseases and to reduce morbidity and mortality associated with these diseases.[1] Public health officials and specialists in clinical and preventative medicine weigh clinical evidence of benefits against potential risks and costs of vaccination for individuals and society. The resulting recommendations account for physiological processes involved in immunity, properties of immunobiologics, and risks for adverse reactions. This chapter summarizes the immunization recommendations practiced in the United States and highlights product-related and administration information to aid in the safe and appropriate use of immunobiologics.

■ VACCINES AND TOXOIDS

Table 1 provides a list of single agent vaccines and toxoids available in the United States. The table columns include brand name, type, FDA-approved age group(s), contraindications, dose, route of administration, storage and handling, excipients, and diluents for reconstitution, if applicable.[2-39] Table 2 shows the individual vaccines and toxoids that comprise combination immunizations, while Table 3 details additional information regarding these agents.[40-54]

TABLE 1. SINGLE AGENT VACCINES AND TOXOIDS AVAILABLE IN THE UNITED STATES

VACCINE/TOXOID	BRAND NAME	TYPE	FDA-APPROVED AGE GROUP	CONTRAINDICATIONS	DOSE AND ROUTE OF ADMINISTRATION	STORAGE AND HANDLING	EXCIPIENTS	DILUENTS
Anthrax[a]	BioThrax[2]	Inactivated avirulent, nonencapsulated bacteria	18–65 y	Hypersensitivity to vaccine/toxoid and excipients	0.5 mL Subcutaneous	Store at 2–8°C; Do not freeze	1.2 mg/mL aluminum, 25 µg/mL benzethonium chloride, 100 µg/mL formaldehyde	None
Haemophilus influenzae type b conjugate	ActHIB[3] (Tetanus Toxoid Conjugate)	Inactivated purified capsular polysaccharide bacteria conjugated to toxoid protein	2–18 mo	Hypersensitivity to vaccine/toxoid and excipients	0.5 mL Intramuscular	Before reconstitution: 2–8°C; Do not freeze After reconstitution: 2–8°C; Discard after 24 h Store supplied diluent at 2–8°C; Do not freeze	Sucrose	Supplied 0.4% sodium chloride May use Tripedia vaccine to make TriHIBit; Refer to Combination Vaccine Table
	HibTITER[4] (Diphtheria CRM197 Protein Conjugate)	Inactivated purified capsular polysaccharide bacteria conjugated to toxoid protein	2–71 mo	Hypersensitivity to vaccine/toxoid	0.5 mL Intramuscular	Store at 2–8°C; Do not freeze	None	None
	Liquid PedvaxHIB[5] (Meningococcal Protein Conjugate)	Inactivated purified capsular polysaccharide bacteria conjugated to protein complex	2–71 mo	Hypersensitivity to vaccine/toxoid and excipients	0.5 mL Intramuscular	Store at 2–8°C; Do not freeze	225 µg aluminum and 0.9% NaCl	None

(continued)

VACCINE/TOXOID	BRAND NAME	TYPE	FDA-APPROVED AGE GROUP[b]	CONTRAINDICATIONS	DOSE AND ROUTE OF ADMINISTRATION	STORAGE AND HANDLING	EXCIPIENTS	DILUENTS
Hepatitis A	HAVRIX[6]	Inactivated virus	≥12 mo	Hypersensitivity to vaccine/toxoid and excipients	≤18 y: 0.5 mL ≥19 y: 1 mL Intramuscular	Store at 2–8°C; Do not freeze	Amino acid supplement in a phosphate buffered saline solution, polysorbate 20, residual MRC-5 cellular proteins, formalin, 0.5 mg of aluminum/mL and neomycin	None
	VAQTA[7]	Inactivated whole virus	≥12 mo	Hypersensitivity to vaccine/toxoid and excipients	≤18 y: 0.5 mL ≥19 y: 1 mL Intramuscular	Store at 2–8°C; Do not freeze	0.45 mg aluminum/mL, 70 μg of sodium borate/mL, 0.9% NaCl, <0.8 μg formaldehyde	None
Hepatitis B	ENGERIX-B[8]	Inactivated recombinant antigen	All age groups	Hypersensitivity to vaccine/toxoid, excipients, and yeast	≤19 y: 0.5 mL ≥20 y: 1 mL Adult hemodialysis: 2 mL Intramuscular	Store at 2–8°C; Do not freeze	0.5 mg aluminum/mL, phosphate buffers, and NaCl	None

(continued)

TABLE 1. SINGLE AGENT VACCINES AND TOXOIDS AVAILABLE IN THE UNITED STATES (*continued*)

VACCINE/TOXOID	BRAND NAME	TYPE	FDA-APPROVED AGE GROUP	CONTRAINDICATIONS	DOSE AND ROUTE OF ADMINISTRATION	STORAGE AND HANDLING	EXCIPIENTS	DILUENTS
	RECOMBIVAX HB[9]	Inactivated recombinant antigen	All age groups	Hypersensitivity to vaccine/toxoid, excipients, and yeast	≤19 y: 0.5 mL pediatric/adolescent formulation 11–15 y: 1 mL adult formulation (2-dose regimen) ≥20 y: 1 mL adult formulation Predialysis & dialysis patients: 1 mL dialysis formulation Intramuscular	Store at 2–8°C; Do not freeze	0.5 mg aluminum/mL	None
Herpes Zoster (Shingles)	ZOSTAVAX[10]	Live attenuated virus	≥60 y	Hypersensitivity to vaccine/toxoid and excipients, immunocompromised[b], pregnancy	0.7 mL Subcutaneous	Before reconstitution: store in freezer at ≤ −15°C; Protect from light After reconstitution: use immediately; Discard after 30 min & do not re-freeze Store diluent at 20–25°C or 2–8°C	Sucrose, gelatin, NaCl, monosodium L-glutamate, sodium phosphate dibasic, potassium phosphate monobasic, KCl, and trace amounts of neomycin and bovine calf serum	Supplied sterile diluent

(continued)

TABLE 1. SINGLE AGENT VACCINES AND TOXOIDS AVAILABLE IN THE UNITED STATES (*continued*)

VACCINE/TOXOID	BRAND NAME	TYPE	FDA-APPROVED AGE GROUP	CONTRAINDICATIONS	DOSE AND ROUTE OF ADMINISTRATION	STORAGE AND HANDLING	EXCIPIENTS	DILUENTS
Human Papillo-mavirus (HPV)	GARDASIL[11]	Inactivated recombinant quadrivalent viruslike particles	Females 9–26 y	Hypersensitivity to vaccine/toxoid and excipients	0.5 mL Intramuscular	Store at 2–8°C or <25 °C for 72 h; Administer promptly after removing from refrigeration; Do not freeze; Protect from light	225 µg aluminum, 9.56 mg of NaCl, 0.78 mg of L-histidine, 50 µg of polysorbate 80, 35 µg of sodium borate, <7 µg of yeast per 0.5 mL dose	None
Influenza	AFLURIA[12]	Inactivated virus	≥18 y	Hypersensitivity to vaccine/toxoid, excipients, and egg or chicken protein	0.5 mL Intramuscular	Store at 2–8°C; Do not freeze; Protect from light	Contains 24.5 µg mercury/dose as thimerosal; thimerosal-free single dose product available	None
	FLUARIX[13]	Inactivated virus	≥18 y	Hypersensitivity to vaccine/toxoid. excipients, and egg or chicken protein	0.5 mL Intramuscular	Store at 2–8°C; Do not freeze; Protect from light	May contain ≤1 µg mercury/dose as thimerosal, ≤0.15 µg gentamicin sulfate, ≤50 µg formaldehyde, ≤0.0016 µg hydrocortisone, ≤1 µg ovalbumin, and ≤50 µg sodium deoxycholate	None

(continued)

TABLE 1. SINGLE AGENT VACCINES AND TOXOIDS AVAILABLE IN THE UNITED STATES (*continued*)

VACCINE/TOXOID	BRAND NAME	TYPE	FDA-APPROVED AGE GROUP	CONTRAINDICATIONS	DOSE AND ROUTE OF ADMINISTRATION	STORAGE AND HANDLING	EXCIPIENTS	DILUENTS
	FLULAVAL[14]	Inactivated virus	≥18 y	Hypersensitivity to vaccine/toxoid, excipients, and egg or chicken protein	0.5 mL Intramuscular	Store at 2–8°C; Do not freeze; Protect from light; Opened multidose vials: discard after 28 d	25 µg mercury/dose as thimerosal	None
	FluMist[15]	Live attenuated trivalent virus	2–49 y	Hypersensitivity to vaccine/toxoid, excipients, and egg or chicken protein, immunocompromised[b], pregnancy, history of Guillain-Barre	0.2 mL (0.1 mL each nostril)[c] Intranasal	Store at 2–8°C; Do not freeze	0.188 mg monosodium glutamate, 2 mg porcine gelatin, 2.42 mg arginine, 13.68 mg sucrose, 2.26 mg dibasic potassium phosphate, 0.96 mg monosodium phosphate, <0.015 µg/mL gentamicin sulfate	None
	FLUVIRIN[16]	Inactivated purified surface antigen	≥4 y	Hypersensitivity to vaccine/toxoid, excipients, and egg or chicken protein	0.5 mL Intramuscular	Store at 2–8°C; Do not freeze	24.5 µg mercury/dose as thimerosal	None

(continued)

TABLE 1. SINGLE AGENT VACCINES AND TOXOIDS AVAILABLE IN THE UNITED STATES (*continued*)

VACCINE/TOXOID	BRAND NAME	TYPE	FDA-APPROVED AGE GROUP	CONTRAINDICATIONS	DOSE AND ROUTE OF ADMINISTRATION	STORAGE AND HANDLING	EXCIPIENTS	DILUENTS
	FLUZONE[17]	Inactivated virus	≥6 mo	Hypersensitivity to vaccine/toxoid, excipients, and egg or chicken protein	6–35 mo: 0.25 mL; ≥3 y: 0.5 mL Intramuscular	Store at 2–8°C; Do not freeze	<100 μg formaldehyde, polyethylene glycol and sucrose, gelatin; Multidose vial contains 25 μg of mercury/0.5 mL dose; thimerosal-free product available	None
Influenza (avian)[a]	H5N1[18]	Inactivated monovalent virus	18–64 y	Hypersensitivity to vaccine/toxoid, excipients, and egg or chicken protein	1 mL Intramuscular	Store at 2–8°C; Do not freeze; Protect from light	50 mcg mercury/dose as thimerosal, ≤200 μg formaldehyde, gelatin, polyethylene glycol, sucrose	None
Japanese Encephalitis[a]	JE-VAX[19]	Inactivated virus	≥1 y	Hypersensitivity to vaccine/toxoid, excipients, and proteins of rodent or neural origin	24–35 mo: 0.5 mL; ≥3 y: 1 mL Subcutaneous	Before reconstitution: 2–8°C; Do not freeze After reconstitution: 2–8°C; Discard after 8 h; Do not freeze	0.007% thimerosal; <100 μg formaldehyde, 500 μg gelatin, <0.0007% polysorbate 80, <50 ng of mouse serum protein	Supplied sterile water

(continued)

1147

VACCINE/TOXOID	BRAND NAME	TYPE	FDA-APPROVED AGE GROUP	CONTRAINDICATIONS	DOSE AND ROUTE OF ADMINISTRATION	STORAGE AND HANDLING	EXCIPIENTS	DILUENTS
Measles	ATTENUVAX[20]	Live virus	≥12 mo	Hypersensitivity to vaccine/toxoid, excipients, and eggs, immunocompromised[b], pregnancy	0.5 mL Subcutaneous	Before reconstitution: 2–8°C or colder; Protect from light After reconstitution: use immediately or store at 2–8°C; Discard after 8 h; Protect from light Store diluent at 20–25°C or 2–8°C	14.5 mg sorbitol, 1.9 mg sucrose, sodium phosphate, NaCl, 14.5 mg gelatin, 0.3 mg human albumin, <1 ppm fetal bovine serum, 25 μg neomycin	Supplied sterile diluent
Meningococcal (Groups A, C, Y, and W-135)	Menactra[21]	Inactivated purified capsular polysaccharide bacteria conjugated to toxoid protein	2–55 y	Hypersensitivity to vaccine/toxoid and excipients	0.5 mL Intramuscular	Store at 2–8°C; Do not freeze	Sodium phosphate, NaCl	None
Polysaccharide	Menomune[22]	Inactivated purified capsular polysaccharide bacteria	≥2 y	Hypersensitivity to vaccine/toxoid and excipients	0.5 mL Subcutaneous	Before reconstitution: 2–8°C After reconstitution: Store at 2–8°C; Use single dose vial immediately or discard after 30 min; Discard multidose vial after 35 d	Multidose vial contains 1:10,000 thimerosal/dose and lactose, thimerosal-free single dose product available	Sterile water

(continued)

TABLE 1. SINGLE AGENT VACCINES AND TOXOIDS AVAILABLE IN THE UNITED STATES (*continued*)

VACCINE/TOXOID	BRAND NAME	TYPE	FDA-APPROVED AGE GROUP	CONTRAINDICATIONS	DOSE AND ROUTE OF ADMINISTRATION	STORAGE AND HANDLING	EXCIPIENTS	DILUENTS
Mumps	MUMPSVAX[23]	Live virus	≥12 mo	Hypersensitivity to vaccine/toxoid, excipients, and eggs, immunocompromised[b], pregnancy	0.5 mL Subcutaneous	Before reconstitution: 2–8°C or colder; Protect from light. After reconstitution: use immediately or store at 2–8°C; Discard after 8 h; Protect from light. Store diluent at 20–25°C or 2–8°C	14.5 mg sorbitol, sodium phosphate, 1.9 mg sucrose, NaCl, 14.5 mg hydrolyzed gelatin, 0.3 mg human albumin, <1ppm fetal bovine serum, 25 μg neomycin, other buffer and media ingredients	Supplied sterile water
Pneumococcal	PNEUMOVAX 23[24]	Inactivated bacterial capsular polysaccharides from 23 pneumococcal types	≥2 y at risk or ≥50 y	Hypersensitivity to vaccine/toxoid and excipients	0.5 mL Intramuscular or subcutaneous	Store at 2–8°C	0.25% phenol	None
	Prevnar[25] (Diphtheria CRM 197 Protein)	Inactivated bacterial capsular polysaccharides from 7 pneumococcal types conjugated to toxoid protein	6 wk up to 10 y	Hypersensitivity to vaccine/toxoid and excipients	0.5 mL Intramuscular	Store at 2–8°C; Do not freeze	0.125 mg aluminum/0.5 mL dose	None

(continued)

TABLE 1. SINGLE AGENT VACCINES AND TOXOIDS AVAILABLE IN THE UNITED STATES (continued)

VACCINE/TOXOID	BRAND NAME	TYPE	FDA-APPROVED AGE GROUP	CONTRAINDICATIONS	DOSE AND ROUTE OF ADMINISTRATION	STORAGE AND HANDLING	EXCIPIENTS	DILUENTS
Poliovirus Vaccine Inactivated	IPOL[26]	Inactivated purified virus of 3 serotypes	≥6 wk	Hypersensitivity to vaccine/toxoid and excipients	0.5 mL Intramuscular or subcutaneous	Store at 2–8°C; Do not freeze	0.5% 2-phenoxyethanol, <0.02% formaldehyde; <5 ng neomycin, 200 ng streptomycin, 25 ng polymyxin B, and <1 ppm calf serum protein per dose	None
Rabies	Imovax[27]	Inactivated virus	At risk age groups pre-exposure; All age groups post exposure	Hypersensitivity to vaccine/toxoid and excipients	1 mL Intramuscular	Before reconstitution: 2–8°C; Do not freeze After reconstitution: use immediately	<150 µg neomycin, <100 mg albumin, <20 µg of phenol red indicator	Supplied sterile water
	RabAvert[28]	Inactivated virus	At risk age groups pre-exposure; All age groups post exposure	Hypersensitivity to vaccine/toxoid and excipients	1 mL Intramuscular	Before reconstitution: 2–8°C; Do not freeze; Protect from light After reconstitution: use immediately	<12 mg bovine gelatin, 1 mg potassium glutamate, 0.3 mg sodium EDTA, <3ng ovalbumin, <1 µg neomycin, <20 ng chlortetracycline, and <2 ng amphotericin B per dose	Supplied sterile water

(continued)

TABLE 1. SINGLE AGENT VACCINES AND TOXOIDS AVAILABLE IN THE UNITED STATES (continued)

VACCINE/TOXOID	BRAND NAME	TYPE	FDA-APPROVED AGE GROUP	CONTRAINDICATIONS	DOSE AND ROUTE OF ADMINISTRATION	STORAGE AND HANDLING	EXCIPIENTS	DILUENTS
Rotavirus	Rotarix[29]	Live, attenuated virus	6–24 wk	Immunocompromised[b], gastrointestinal obstruction	1 dose (~1 mL) Oral[e]	Before reconstitution: 2–8°C; Do not freeze; Protect from light After reconstitution: 2–8°C; Discard after 24 h; Do not freeze; Protect from light	Sucrose, dextran 40, sorbitol, aminoacids, calcium carbonate, xanthian gum, dulbecco's modified eagle medium	Supplied calcium carbonate buffer solvent
	RotaTeq[30]	Live, pentavalent virus	6–32 wk	Immunocompromised[b], gastrointestinal obstruction	2 mL Oral[e]	Store at 2–8°C; Do not freeze; Protect from light	Sucrose, sodium citrate, sodium phosphate monobasic monohydrate, sodium hydroxide, polysorbate 80, cell culture media, trace amounts of fetal bovine serum	None
Rubella	MERUVAX II[31]	Live virus	≥12 mo	Hypersensitivity to vaccine/toxoid and excipients, immunocompromised[b], pregnancy	0.5 mL Subcutaneous	Before reconstitution: 2–8°C or colder; Protect from light After reconstitution: use promptly or store at 2–8°C; Discard after 8 h; Protect from light Store diluent at 2–8°C or 20–25°C	14.5 mg sorbitol, sodium phosphate, 1.9 mg sucrose, NaCl, 14.5 mg gelatin, 0.3 mg human albumin, ≥1ppm fetal bovine serum, 25 μg neomycin, other buffer and media ingredients	Supplied sterile water

(continued)

TABLE 1. SINGLE AGENT VACCINES AND TOXOIDS AVAILABLE IN THE UNITED STATES (*continued*)

VACCINE/TOXOID	BRAND NAME	TYPE	FDA-APPROVED AGE GROUP	CONTRAINDICATIONS	DOSE AND ROUTE OF ADMINISTRATION	STORAGE AND HANDLING	EXCIPIENTS	DILUENTS
Smallpox[a]	ACAM2000[32]	Live virus	High risk patients	Hypersensitivity to vaccine/toxoid and excipients, immuno-compromised[b], pregnancy	1 droplet intro-duced with 15 punctures Percutaneous (scarification)	Before reconstitution: −15 to −25°C; potency remains for 18 mo at 2–8°C; Protect from light Bring to 20–25°C be-fore reconstitution After reconstitution: use within 6–8 h at 20–25°C, use within 30 d at 2–8°C; Protect from light Store diluent at 20–25°C	Human albumin, NaCl, mannitol, and trace amounts of neomycin and polymyxin B	Supplied 50% glycerin, 0.25% phenol in sterile water
	Dryvax[33]	Live virus	High risk patients ≥12 mo	Hypersensitivity to vaccine/toxoid and excipients, immuno-compromised[b], pregnancy	1 droplet intro-duced with 15 punctures Percutaneous (scarification)	Before reconstitution: 2–8°C; Do not freeze; Protect from light After reconstitution: 2–8°C; Protect from light; Discard after 90 d	Neomycin, polymyxin B, dihydrostrepto-mycin, and chlortetra-cycline in trace amounts	Supplied 50% glycerin, 0.25% phenol in sterile water

(continued)

TABLE 1. SINGLE AGENT VACCINES AND TOXOIDS AVAILABLE IN THE UNITED STATES (*continued*)

VACCINE/TOXOID	BRAND NAME	TYPE	FDA-APPROVED AGE GROUP	CONTRAINDICATIONS	DOSE AND ROUTE OF ADMINISTRATION	STORAGE AND HANDLING	EXCIPIENTS	DILUENTS
Tetanus Toxoid Absorbed[34]	None	Inactivated toxoid	≥7 y	Hypersensitivity to vaccine/toxoid and excipients	0.5 mL Intramuscular	Store at 2–8°C; Do not freeze	≤0.25 mg aluminum and ≤0.02% formaldehyde per 0.5 mL dose; ≤0.3 μg mercury per single dose vial and 25 μg mercury/dose from 5 mL multidose vial	None
Tetanus Toxoid (Booster only)[35]	None	Inactivated toxoid	≥7 y	Hypersensitivity to vaccine/toxoid and excipients	0.5 mL Intramuscular or subcutaneous	Store at 2–8°C; Do not freeze	25 μg mercury/dose as thimerosal; <0.02% formaldehyde	None
Typhoid Vi	Typhim Vi[36]	Inactivated polysaccharide bacteria	≥2 y	Hypersensitivity to vaccine/toxoid and excipients	0.5 mL Intramuscular	Store at 2–8°C; Do not freeze	0.25% phenol, phosphate buffered saline, 4.15 mg NaCl, 0.065 mg disodium phosphate, 0.023 mg monosodium phosphate	None
	Vivotif[37]	Live attenuated bacteria (Ty21a)	>6 y	Immunocompromised[b], pregnancy, gastrointestinal obstruction	1 cap × 4 doses (Days 1, 3, 5, & 7)[c] Oral	Store at 2–8°C; Do not freeze; Protect from light	Sucrose, ascorbic acid, amino acid mixture, lactose, magnesium stearate	None

(continued)

TABLE 1. SINGLE AGENT VACCINES AND TOXOIDS AVAILABLE IN THE UNITED STATES (*continued*)

VACCINE/TOXOID	BRAND NAME	TYPE	FDA-APPROVED AGE GROUP	CONTRAINDICATIONS	DOSE AND ROUTE OF ADMINISTRATION	STORAGE AND HANDLING	EXCIPIENTS	DILUENTS
Varicella	VARIVAX[38]	Live attenuated virus	≥12 mo	Hypersensitivity to vaccine/toxoid and excipients, immunocompromised[b], pregnancy	0.5 mL[c] Subcutaneous	Before reconstitution: store in freezer at < −15°C; potency maintained ≤72 hours at 2–8°C; Protect from light. After reconstitution: use immediately; Discard after 30 min; Do not freeze. Store diluent at 20–25°C or 2–8°C	25 mg sucrose, 12.5 mg gelatin, 3.2 mg NaCl, 0.5 mg monosodium L-glutamate, 0.45 mg sodium phosphate dibasic, 0.08 mg potassium phosphate monobasic, 0.08 mg KCl, and trace amounts of sodium phosphate monobasic, EDTA, neomycin and fetal bovine serum	Supplied sterile water
Yellow Fever[a]	YF-VAX[39]	Live virus	≥9 mo	Hypersensitivity to vaccine/toxoid, excipients, and eggs, immunocompromised[b], pregnancy	0.5 mL Subcutaneous	Before reconstitution: 2–8°C; Do not freeze; Protect from light. After reconstitution: Discard after 1 h	Sorbitol, gelatin	Supplied sodium chloride

[a]Limited availability/distribution.

[b]Immunocompromised, includes disease states decreasing immune status (e.g., congenital immunodeficiency, leukemia) and drug-induced decreases in immune function (e.g., corticosteroids with dose equivalent to 20 mg daily or ≥2 mg/kg of prednisone for ≥2 wk); avoid live vaccines until 3 mo after completing chemotherapy or radiation therapy and high-dose extended corticosteroid therapy.

[c]Efficacy may be affected by antimicrobial agents (i.e., antibiotics and mefloquine with oral Ty21a, antivirals with varicella and live-attenuated intranasal influenza vaccines).[1]

[d]Preferred agent(s) within vaccine/toxoid category according to the CDC provided patient's age is appropriate.

[e]If dose is regurgitated, a replacement/repeat dose is not indicated.

TABLE 2. INDIVIDUAL COMPONENTS OF COMBINATION VACCINES/TOXOIDS AVAILABLE IN THE UNITED STATES

BRAND NAME	ACELLULAR PERTUSSIS	DIPHTHERIA TOXOIDS	DIPHTHERIA TOXOID (REDUCED)	HAEMOPHILUS B CONJUGATE	HEPATITIS A INACTIVATED	HEPATITIS B (RECOMBINANT)	INACTIVATED POLIOVIRUS	MEASLES	MUMPS	RUBELLA	TETANUS TOXOIDS	VARICELLA
Adacel[40]	✓		✓								✓	
BOOSTRIX[41]	✓		✓								✓	
COMVAX[42]				✓		✓						
DAPTACEL[43]	✓	✓									✓	
DECAVAC[44]		✓									✓	
Diphtheria and Tetanus Toxoids Adsorbed USP (Pediatric Use)[45]		✓									✓	
INFANRIX[46]	✓	✓									✓	
KINRIX[47]	✓	✓					✓				✓	
M-M-R II[48]								✓	✓	✓		
M-M-VAX[49]								✓	✓			
PEDIARIX[50]	✓	✓				✓	✓				✓	
Pentacel[51]	✓	✓		✓			✓				✓	
ProQuad[52]								✓	✓	✓		✓
TriHIBit[53]	✓	✓		✓							✓	
Tripedia[53]	✓	✓									✓	
TWINRIX[54]					✓	✓						

✓, Present in vaccine/toxoid combination product.

TABLE 3. COMBINATION VACCINES AND TOXOIDS AVAILABLE IN THE UNITED STATES

BRAND NAME	FDA-APPROVED AGE GROUP	CONTRAINDICATIONS	DOSE AND ROUTE OF ADMINISTRATION	STORAGE AND HANDLING	EXCIPIENTS	DILUENTS
Adacel[40]	11–64 y	Hypersensitivity to vaccine/toxoid and excipients, encephalopathy not attributed to another cause within 7 days of previous pertussis containing dose, progressive neurologic disorder[a]	0.5 mL Intramuscular	Store at 2–8°C; Do not freeze	For each 0.5 mL dose: 1.5 mg aluminum phosphate, ≤5 μg residual formaldehyde, ≤50 ng residual glutaraldehyde, and 3.3 mg 2-phenoxyethanol	None
BOOSTRIX[41]	10–18 y	Hypersensitivity to vaccine/toxoid and excipients, encephalopathy not attributed to another cause within 7 days of previous pertussis containing dose, progressive neurologic disorder[a]	0.5 mL Intramuscular	Store at 2–8°C; Do not freeze	For each 0.5 mL dose: 4.5 mg NaCl, <0.39 mg aluminum adjuvant, ≤100 μg residual formaldehyde, ≤100 μg polysorbate 80 (Tween 80)	None
COMVAX[42]	6 wk–15 mo for infants born to HBsAg[b] negative mothers	Hypersensitivity to vaccine/toxoid, excipients, and yeast	0.5 mL Intramuscular	Store at 2–8°C; Do not freeze	For each 0.5 mL dose: 7.5 μg polyribosylribitol phosphate, 125 μg outer membrane protein complex, 225 μg amorphous aluminum hydroxyphosphate sulfate, and 35 μg sodium borate (decahydrate), in 0.9% NaCl, and 0.0004% (w/v) residual formaldehyde	None

(continued)

TABLE 3. COMBINATION VACCINES AND TOXOIDS AVAILABLE IN THE UNITED STATES (*continued*)

BRAND NAME	FDA-APPROVED AGE GROUP	CONTRAINDICATIONS	DOSE AND ROUTE OF ADMINISTRATION	STORAGE AND HANDLING	EXCIPIENTS	DILUENTS
DAPTACEL [43]	6 wk–6 y	Hypersensitivity to vaccine/toxoid and excipients, encephalopathy not attributed to another cause within 7 days of previous pertussis-containing dose, progressive neurologic disorder[a]	0.5 mL Intramuscular	Store at 2–8°C; Do not freeze	For each 0.5 mL dose: 1.5 mg aluminum phosphate, ≤5 μg residual formaldehyde, <50 ng residual glutaraldehyde, and 3.3 mg 2-phenoxyethanol	None
DECAVAC [44]	≥7 y	Hypersensitivity to vaccine/toxoid and excipients	0.5 mL Intramuscular	Store at 2–8°C; Do not freeze	For each 0.5 mL dose: <0.28 mg of aluminum, <100 μg of residual formaldehyde, and ≤0.3 μg mercury	None
Diphtheria and Tetanus Toxoids Adsorbed USP (For Pediatric Use) [45]	6 wk–6 y	Hypersensitivity to vaccine/toxoid and excipients	0.5 mL Intramuscular	Store at 2–8°C; Do not freeze	For each 0.5 mL dose: <0.17 mg aluminum, ≤ 0.3 μg mercury, <0.02% formaldehyde, potassium sulfate, and isotonic sodium chloride	None
INFANRIX [46]	6 wk–7 y	Hypersensitivity to vaccine/toxoid and excipients, encephalopathy not attributed to another cause within 7 days of previous pertussis-containing dose, progressive neurologic disorder[a]	0.5 mL Intramuscular	Store at 2–8°C; Do not freeze	For a 0.5 mL dose: 2.5 mg 2-phenoxyethanol, 4.5 mg NaCl, <0.625 mg aluminum, ≤100 μg formaldehyde, and ≤100 μg polysorbate 80 (Tween 80)	None

(continued)

TABLE 3. COMBINATION VACCINES AND TOXOIDS AVAILABLE IN THE UNITED STATES (continued)

BRAND NAME	FDA-APPROVED AGE GROUP	CONTRAINDICATIONS	DOSE AND ROUTE OF ADMINISTRATION	STORAGE AND HANDLING	EXCIPIENTS	DILUENTS
KINRIX[47]	4–6 y	Hypersensitivity to vaccine/toxoid and excipients, encephalopathy not attributed to another cause within 7 days of previous pertussis containing dose, progressive neurologic disorder[a]	0.5 mL Intramuscular	Store at 2–8°C; Do not freeze	For a 0.5 mL dose: 4.5 mg NaCl, <0.6 mg aluminum, ≤100 μg formaldehyde, ≤100 μg polysorbate 80 (Tween 80), ≤0.05 ng neomycin, and ≤0.01 ng polymyxin	None
M-M-R II[48]	≥12 mo	Hypersensitivity to vaccine/ toxoid, excipients, and eggs, immunocompromised[c], pregnancy	0.5 mL Subcutaneous	Before reconstitution, store the vial at 2–8°C or colder After reconstitution, store at 2–8°C and protect from light; Discard if not used within 8 h Store diluent at 20–25 °C or 2–8 °C; Do not freeze	For a single dose vial: 14.5 mg sorbitol, sodium phosphate, sodium chloride, 1.9 mg sucrose, 14.5 mg hydrolyzed gelatin, ≤0.3 mg recombinant human albumin, <1 ppm fetal bovine serum, and 25 μg neomycin	Supplied sterile water

(continued)

TABLE 3. COMBINATION VACCINES AND TOXOIDS AVAILABLE IN THE UNITED STATES *(continued)*

BRAND NAME	FDA-APPROVED AGE GROUP	CONTRAINDICATIONS	DOSE AND ROUTE OF ADMINISTRATION	STORAGE AND HANDLING	EXCIPIENTS	DILUENTS
M-M-VAX[49]	≥12 mo	Hypersensitivity to vaccine/toxoid, excipients, and eggs; immunocompromised[c]; pregnancy	0.5 mL Subcutaneous	Before reconstitution, store the vial at 2–8°C or colder After reconstitution, store at 2–8°C and protect from light; Discard if not used within 8 h Store diluent at 20–25 °C or 2–8 °C; Do not freeze	For a single dose vial: 14.5 mg sorbitol, sodium phosphate, sodium chloride, 1.9 mg sucrose, 14.5 mg hydrolyzed gelatin, ≤0.3 mg recombinant human albumin, <1 ppm fetal bovine serum, and 25 µg neomycin	Supplied diluents
PEDIARIX[50]	6 wk–7 y	Hypersensitivity to vaccine/toxoid and excipients, encephalopathy not attributed to another cause within 7 days of previous pertussis containing dose, progressive neurologic disorder[a]	0.5 mL Intramuscular	Store at 2–8°C; Do not freeze	For a 0.5 mL dose: 4.5 mg NaCl, <0.85 mg aluminum, ≤100 µg formaldehyde, ≤100 µg polysorbate 80 (Tween 80), ≤0.05 ng neomycin, ≤0.01 ng polymyxin B, and ≤5% yeast protein	None

(continued)

TABLE 3. COMBINATION VACCINES AND TOXOIDS AVAILABLE IN THE UNITED STATES (*continued*)

BRAND NAME	FDA-APPROVED AGE GROUP	CONTRAINDICATIONS	DOSE AND ROUTE OF ADMINISTRATION	STORAGE AND HANDLING	EXCIPIENTS	DILUENTS
Pentacel[51]	6 wk–4 y	Hypersensitivity to vaccine/toxoid and excipients, encephalopathy not attributed to another cause within 7 days of previous pertussis-containing dose, progressive neurologic disorder[a]	0.5 mL Intramuscular	Store at 2–8°C; Do not freeze; Use immediately after reconstitution	For a 0.5 mL dose: 0.33 aluminum, 10 ppm polysorbate 80, ≤5 µg formaldehyde, <50 ng glutaraldehyde, ≤50 ng bovine serum albumin, 3.3 mg 2-phenoxyethanol, <4 pg of neomycin and <4 pg polymyxin B sulfate	Supplied vial of DTaP-IPV component
ProQuad[52]	12 mo–12 y	Hypersensitivity to vaccine/ toxoid, excipients, and eggs, immunocompromised[c], pregnancy	0.5 mL Subcutaneous	Before reconstitution, store in freezer at 5 °F (−15 °C) for up to 18 mo; may be stored at 2–8°C for 72 h prior to reconstitution; Protect from light After reconstituting, discard if not used within 30 min; Protect from light; Do not freeze reconstituted vaccine Store diluent at 20–25 °C or 2–8 °C	For a 0.5 mL dose: ≤21 mg sucrose, ≤11 mg hydrolyzed gelatin, ≤2.4 mg NaCl, ≤1.8 sorbitol, ≤0.4 mg monosodium L-glutamate, ≤0.34 mg sodium phosphate dibasic, ≤0.31 mg human albumin, ≤0.17 mg sodium bicarbonate, ≤72 µg potassium phosphate monobasic, ≤60 µg potassium chloride, ≤36 µg potassium phosphate dibasic, ≤16 µg neomycin, and 0.5 µg bovine calf serum.	Supplied sterile water

(continued)

TABLE 3. COMBINATION VACCINES AND TOXOIDS AVAILABLE IN THE UNITED STATES (*continued*)

BRAND NAME	FDA-APPROVED AGE GROUP	CONTRAINDICATIONS	DOSE AND ROUTE OF ADMINISTRATION	STORAGE AND HANDLING	EXCIPIENTS	DILUENTS
TriHIBit[3,53]	15–18 mo	Hypersensitivity to vaccine/toxoid and excipients, encephalopathy not attributed to another cause within 7 days of previous pertussis-containing dose, progressive neurologic disorder[a]	0.5 mL Intramuscular	Refer to ActHIB in Table 1 and Tripedia below; Use within 30 min after reconstitution	Refer to ActHIB in Table 1 and Tripedia below	Reconstitute ActHIB with Tripedia
Tripedia[53]	6 wk–7 y	Hypersensitivity to vaccine/toxoid and excipients, encephalopathy not attributed to another cause within 7 days of previous pertussis-containing dose, progressive neurologic disorder[a]	0.5 mL Intramuscular	Store at 2–8°C; Do not freeze	Phosphate-buffered saline, gelatin, polysorbate 80 (Tween-80), aluminum ≤0.170 mg/0.5 mL dose, formaldehyde ≤100 µg (0.02%)/0.5 mL dose. Single dose vial (0.5 mL) ≤0.3 µg mercury; multidose vial (7.5 mL) ≤25 µg mercury/dose.	None
TWINRIX[54]	≧18 y	Hypersensitivity to vaccine/toxoid and excipients	1 mL Intramuscular	Store at 2–8°C; Do not freeze	For a dose of 1 mL: 0.45 mg aluminum, amino acids, NaCl, phosphate buffer, polysorbate 20, ≤0.1 mg formalin, ≤2.5 µg MRC-5 cellular proteins, <20 ng neomycin, and <5% yeast protein	None

[a]Includes infantile spasms, uncontrolled epilepsy, and progressive encephalopathy.

[b]Hepatitis B surface antigen.

[c]Immunocompromised, includes disease states decreasing immune status (e.g., congenital immunodeficiency, leukemia) and drug-induced decreases in immune function (e.g., corticosteroids with dose equivalent to 20 mg daily or ≥2 mg/kg of prednisone for ≥2 wk); avoid live vaccines until 3 mo after completing chemotherapy or radiation therapy and high-dose extended corticosteroid therapy.

Contraindications listed in the tables are regarded as true or absolute, meaning the vaccine or toxoid should be avoided.[1] Relative contraindications and precautions are omitted, as the benefit for immunization administration may outweigh the potential risk in certain situations. Temperature specifications for storage and handling ensure ideal conditions for maximum potency of the product. Fluctuations in temperature may affect efficacy; therefore, immunobiologics must be stored at recommended temperatures from procurement until administration. If improper storage or handling occurs, the immunobiologic should not be used until the manufacturer is consulted. Excipients are additional ingredients added to immunobiologics and include suspending fluids used during manufacturing (e.g., sterile water, saline, serum proteins, egg antigen), preservatives, stabilizers, and antibiotics added for increased stability (e.g., thimerosal, phenols, albumin, glycerine, neomycin), and adjuvants used to improve immunogenicity (e.g., aluminum). Patients may exhibit allergies to excipients contained in vaccines or toxoids; therefore, knowledge of immunization excipients is important.

■ GUIDELINES

The Center for Disease Control and Prevention (CDC) publishes recommendations for immunizing infants/children, adolescents (7–18 years old), and adults (see Tables 4–6).[55–57] Refer to these immunization schedules to determine age-appropriate immunizations and their administration frequency. Written documentation of vaccination history that includes date and age of vaccine/toxoid administration and complies with the CDC guidelines is acceptable proof.[1] Serum titers, although not always predictive, may be drawn in the absence of written immunization history to determine level of protection. Otherwise, assume patients are not adequately protected and vaccinate accordingly.[1] Catch-up schedules are available for children and adolescents missing or delayed in receiving immunizations or when a vaccination history cannot be established (see Table 7).[58]

United States citizens traveling abroad may require additional vaccinations beyond the general immunization schedules.[59] Several vaccines/toxoids listed in Table 1 are primarily for travelers and include yellow fever, Japanese encephalitis, and typhoid. Booster doses of immunization series that have been completed may be necessary. Travelers should consult their health care provider regarding travel plans, including airplane flight layovers, at least four to six weeks prior to leaving. The CDC's Yellow Book provides guidance for travelers' immunizations and is available at www.cdc.gov/travel.

TABLE 4. RECOMMENDED IMMUNIZATION SCHEDULE, AGES 0–6 YEARS, UNITED STATES, 2009[55]

Vaccine ▼ Age ►	Birth	1 month	2 months	4 months	6 months	12 months	15 months	18 months	19–23 months	2–3 years	4–6 years
Hepatitis B[a]	HepB	HepB			HepB						
Rotavirus[b]			RV	RV	RV[b]						
Diphtheria, Tetanus, Pertussis[c]			DTaP	DTaP	DTaP	see footnote c	DTaP	DTaP			DTaP
Haemophilus influenzae type b[d]			Hib	Hib	Hib[d]	Hib	Hib				
Pneumococcal[e]			PCV	PCV	PCV	PCV	PCV			PPSV	
Inactivated Poliovirus			IPV	IPV		IPV	IPV				IPV
Influenza[f]						Influenza (Yearly)					
Measles, Mumps, Rubella[g]						MMR	MMR		see footnote g		MMR
Varicella[h]						Varicella	Varicella		see footnote h		Varicella
Hepatitis A[i]						HepA (2 doses)	HepA (2 doses)			HepA Series	
Meningococcal[j]										MCV	MCV

Range of recommended ages

Certain high-risk groups

(continued)

TABLE 4. RECOMMENDED IMMUNIZATION SCHEDULE, AGES 0–6 YEARS, UNITED STATES, 2009[55] *(continued)*

a **Hepatitis B vaccine (HepB).** *(Minimum age: birth)*

At birth:
- Administer monovalent HepB to all newborns before hospital discharge.
- If mother is hepatitis B surface antigen (HBsAg)-positive, administer HepB and 0.5 mL of hepatitis B immune globulin (HBIG) within 12 hours of birth.
- If mother's HBsAg status is unknown, administer HepB within 12 hours of birth. Determine mother's HBsAg status as soon as possible and, if HBsAg-positive, administer HBIG (no later than age 1 week).

After the birth dose:
- The HepB series should be completed with either monovalent HepB or a combination vaccine containing HepB. The second dose should be administered at age 1 or 2 months. The final dose should be administered no earlier than age 24 weeks.
- Infants born to HBsAg-positive mothers should be tested for HBsAg and antibody to HBsAg (anti-HBs) after completion of at least 3 doses of the HepB series, at age 9 through 18 months (generally at the next well-child visit).

4-month dose:
- Administration of 4 doses of HepB to infants is permissible when combination vaccines containing HepB are administered after the birth dose.

b **Rotavirus vaccine (RV).** *(Minimum age: 6 weeks)*
- Administer the first dose at age 6 through 14 weeks (maximum age: 14 weeks 6 days). Vaccination should not be initiated for infants aged 15 weeks or older (i.e., 15 weeks 0 days or older).
- Administer the final dose in the series by age 8 months 0 days.
- If Rotarix® is administered at ages 2 and 4 months, a dose at 6 months is not indicated.

c **Diphtheria and tetanus toxoids and acellular pertussis vaccine (DTaP).** *(Minimum age: 6 weeks)*
- The fourth dose may be administered as early as age 12 months, provided at least 6 months have elapsed since the third dose.
- Administer the final dose in the series at age 4 through 6 years.

d **Haemophilus influenzae type b conjugate vaccine (Hib).** *(Minimum age: 6 weeks)*
- If PRP-OMP (PedvaxHIB® or Comvax® [HepB-Hib]) is administered at ages 2 and 4 months, a dose at age 6 months is not indicated.
- TriHiBit® (DTaP/Hib) should not be used for doses at ages 2, 4, or 6 months but can be used as the final dose in children aged 12 months or older.

(continued)

1164

TABLE 4. RECOMMENDED IMMUNIZATION SCHEDULE, AGES 0–6 YEARS, UNITED STATES, 2009[55] (continued)

e **Pneumococcal vaccine. (Minimum age: 6 weeks for pneumococcal conjugate vaccine [PCV]; 2 years for pneumococcal polysaccharide vaccine [PPSV])**
- PCV is recommended for all children aged younger than 5 years. Administer 1 dose of PCV to all healthy children aged 24 through 59 months who are not completely vaccinated for their age.
- Administer PPSV to children aged 2 years or older with certain underlying medical conditions, including a cochlear implant.

f **Influenza vaccine. (Minimum age: 6 months for trivalent inactivated influenza vaccine [TIV]; 2 years for live, attenuated influenza vaccine [LAIV])**
- Administer annually to children aged 6 months through 18 years.
- For healthy nonpregnant persons (i.e., those who do not have underlying medical conditions that predispose them to influenza complications) aged 2 through 49 years, either LAIV or TIV may be used.
- Children receiving TIV should receive 0.25 mL if aged 6 through 35 months or 0.5 mL if aged 3 years or older.
- Administer 2 doses (separated by at least 4 weeks) to children aged younger than 9 years who are receiving influenza vaccine for the first time or who were vaccinated for the first time during the previous influenza season but only received 1 dose.

g **Measles, mumps, and rubella vaccine (MMR). (Minimum age: 12 months)**
- Administer the second dose at age 4 through 6 years. However, the second dose may be administered before age 4, provided at least 28 days have elapsed since the first dose.

h **Varicella vaccine. (Minimum age: 12 months)**
- Administer the second dose at age 4 through 6 years. However, the second dose may be administered before age 4, provided at least 3 months have elapsed since the first dose.
- For children aged 12 months through 12 years the minimum interval between doses is 3 months. However, if the second dose was administered at least 28 days after the first dose, it can be accepted as valid.

i **Hepatitis A vaccine (HepA). (Minimum age: 12 months)**
- Administer to all children aged 1 year (i.e., aged 12 months through 23 months). Administer 2 doses at least 6 months apart.
- Children not fully vaccinated by age 2 years can be vaccinated at subsequent visits.
- HepA also is recommended for children older than 1 year who live in areas where vaccination programs target older children or who are at increased risk of infection.

j **Meningococcal vaccine. (Minimum age: 2 years for meningococcal conjugate vaccine [MCV] and for meningococcal polysaccharide vaccine [MPSV])**
- Administer MCV to children aged 2 through 10 years with terminal complement component deficiency, anatomic or functional asplenia, and certain other high-risk groups.
- Persons who received MPSV 3 or more years previously and who remain at increased risk for meningococcal disease should be revaccinated with MCV.

TABLE 5. RECOMMENDED IMMUNIZATION SCHEDULE, AGES 7–18 YEARS, UNITED STATES, 2009[56]

Vaccine ▼	Age ▶	7–10 years	11–12 years	13–18 years
Tetanus, Diphtheria, Pertussis[a]		see footnote a	Tdap	Tdap
Human Papillomavirus[b]		see footnote b	HPV (3 doses)	HPV Series
Meningococcal[c]		MCV	MCV	MCV
Influenza[d]		Influenza (Yearly)		
Pneumococcal[e]		PPSV		
Hepatitis A[f]		HepA Series		
Hepatitis B[g]		HepB Series		
Inactivated Poliovirus[h]		IPV Series		
Measles, Mumps, Rubella[i]		MMR Series		
Varicella[j]		Varicella Series		

Range of recommended ages

Catch-up immunization

Certain high-risk groups

(continued)

1166

TABLE 5. RECOMMENDED IMMUNIZATION SCHEDULE, AGES 7–18 YEARS, UNITED STATES, 2009[56] (*continued*)

a **Tetanus and diphtheria toxoids and acellular pertussis vaccine (Tdap).** *(Minimum age: 10 years for BOOSTRIX® and 11 years for ADACEL®)*
- Administer at age 11 or 12 years for those who have completed the recommended childhood DTP/DTaP vaccination series and have not received a tetanus and diphtheria toxoid (Td) booster dose.
- Persons aged 13 through 18 years who have not received Tdap should receive a dose.
- A 5-year interval from the last Td dose is encouraged when Tdap is used as a booster dose; however, a shorter interval may be used if pertussis immunity is needed.

b **Human papillomavirus vaccine (HPV).** *(Minimum age: 9 years)*
- Administer the first dose to females at age 11 or 12 years.
- Administer the second dose 2 months after the first dose and the third dose 6 months after the first dose (at least 24 weeks after the first dose).
- Administer the series to females at age 13 through 18 years if not previously vaccinated.

c **Meningococcal conjugate vaccine (MCV).**
- Administer at age 11 or 12 years, or at age 13 through 18 years if not previously vaccinated.
- Administer to previously unvaccinated college freshmen living in a dormitory.
- MCV is recommended for children aged 2 through 10 years with terminal complement component deficiency, anatomic or functional asplenia, and certain other groups at high risk.
- Persons who received MPSV 5 or more years previously and remain at increased risk for meningococcal disease should be revaccinated with MCV.

d **Influenza vaccine.**
- Administer annually to children aged 6 months through 18 years.
- For healthy nonpregnant persons (i.e., those who do not have underlying medical conditions that predispose them to influenza complications) aged 2 through 49 years, either LAIV or TIV may be used.
- Administer 2 doses (separated by at least 4 weeks) to children aged younger than 9 years who are receiving influenza vaccine for the first time or who were vaccinated for the first time during the previous influenza season but only received 1 dose.

e **Pneumococcal polysaccharide vaccine (PPSV).**
- Administer to children with certain underlying medical conditions, including a cochlear implant. A single revaccination should be administered to children with functional or anatomic asplenia or other immunocompromising condition after 5 years.

(continued)

TABLE 5. RECOMMENDED IMMUNIZATION SCHEDULE AGES 7–18 YEARS, UNITED STATES, 2009[56] (continued)

f Hepatitis A vaccine (HepA).

- Administer 2 doses at least 6 months apart.
- HepA is recommended for children older than 1 year who live in areas where vaccination programs target older children or who are at increased risk of infection.

g Hepatitis B vaccine (HepB).

- Administer the 3-dose series to those not previously vaccinated.
- A 2-dose series (separated by at least 4 months) of adult formulation Recombivax HB® is licensed for children aged 11 through 15 years.

h Inactivated poliovirus vaccine (IPV).

- For children who received an all-IPV or all-oral poliovirus (OPV) series, a fourth dose is not necessary if the third dose was administered at age 4 years or older.
- If both OPV and IPV were administered as part of a series, a total of 4 doses should be administered, regardless of the child's current age.

i Measles, mumps, and rubella vaccine (MMR).

- If not previously vaccinated, administer 2 doses or the second dose for those who have received only 1 dose, with at least 28 days between doses.

j Varicella vaccine.

- For persons aged 7 through 18 years without evidence of immunity, administer 2 doses if not previously vaccinated or the second dose if they have received only 1 dose.
- For persons aged 7 through 12 years, the minimum interval between doses is 3 months. However, if the second dose was administered at least 28 days after the first dose, it can be accepted as valid.
- For persons aged 13 years and older, the minimum interval between doses is 28 days.

TABLE 6. RECOMMENDED IMMUNIZATION SCHEDULE, ADULTS, UNITED STATES, 2009[57]

VACCINE ▼ / AGE GROUP ▶	19–26 years	27–49 years	50–59 years	60–64 years	≥65 years
Tetanus, diphtheria, pertussis (Td/Tdap)[a]	Substitute 1-time dose of Tdap for Td booster; then boost with Td every 10 yr				Td booster every 10 yrs
Human papillomavirus (HPV)[b]	3 doses (females)				
Varicella[c]	2 doses				
Zoster[d]				1 dose	1 dose
Measles, mumps, rubella (MMR)[e]	1 or 2 doses		1 dose		
Influenza[f]			1 dose annually		
Pneumococcal (polysaccharide)[g,h]	1 or 2 doses				1 dose
Hepatitis A[i]	2 doses				
Hepatitis B[j]	3 doses				
Meningococcal[k]	1 or more doses				

For all persons in this category who meet the age requirements and who lack evidence of immunity (e.g., lack documentation of vaccination or have no evidence of prior infection)

Recommended if some other risk factor is present (e.g., on the basis of medical, occupational, lifestyle, or other indications)

No recommendation

(continued)

TABLE 6. RECOMMENDED IMMUNIZATION SCHEDULE, ADULTS, UNITED STATES, 2009[57] *(continued)*

a Tetanus, diphtheria, and acellular pertussis (Td/Tdap) vaccination

Tdap should replace a single dose of Td for adults aged 19 through 64 years who have not received a dose of Tdap previously.

Adults with uncertain or incomplete history of primary vaccination series with tetanus and diphtheria toxoid–containing vaccines should begin or complete a primary vaccination series. A primary series for adults is 3 doses of tetanus and diphtheria toxoid–containing vaccines; administer the first 2 doses at least 4 weeks apart and the third dose 6–12 months after the second. However, Tdap can substitute for any one of the doses of Td in the 3-dose primary series. The booster dose of tetanus and diphtheria toxoid–containing vaccine should be administered to adults who have completed a primary series and if the last vaccination was received 10 or more years previously. Tdap or Td vaccine may be used, as indicated.

If a woman is pregnant and received the last Td vaccination 10 or more years previously, administer Td during the second or third trimester. If the woman received the last Td vaccination less than 10 years previously, administer Tdap during the immediate postpartum period. A dose of Tdap is recommended for postpartum women, close contacts of infants aged less than 12 months, and all health-care personnel with direct patient contact if they have not previously received Tdap. An interval as short as 2 years from the last Td is suggested; shorter intervals can be used. Td may be deferred during pregnancy and Tdap substituted in the immediate postpartum period, or Tdap may be administered instead of Td to a pregnant woman after an informed discussion with the woman.

Consult the ACIP statement for recommendations for administering Td as prophylaxis in wound management.

b Human papillomavirus (HPV) vaccination

HPV vaccination is recommended for all females aged 11 through 26 years (and may begin at age 9 years) who have not completed the vaccine series. History of genital warts, abnormal Papanicolaou test, or positive HPV DNA test is not evidence of prior infection with all vaccine HPV types; HPV vaccination is recommended for persons with such histories.

Ideally, vaccine should be administered before potential exposure to HPV through sexual activity; however, females who are sexually active should still be vaccinated consistent with age-based recommendations. Sexually active females who have not been infected with any of the four HPV vaccine types receive the full benefit of the vaccination. Vaccination is less beneficial for females who have already been infected with one or more of the HPV vaccine types.

A complete series consists of 3 doses. The second dose should be administered 2 months after the first dose; the third dose should be administered 6 months after the first dose.

c Varicella vaccination

All adults without evidence of immunity to varicella should receive 2 doses of single-antigen varicella vaccine if not previously vaccinated or the second dose if they have received only one dose, unless they have a medical contraindication. Special consideration should be given to those who 1) have close contact with persons at high risk for severe disease (e.g., health-care personnel and family contacts of persons with immunocompromising conditions) or 2) are at high risk for exposure or transmission (e.g., teachers; child care employees; residents and staff members of institutional settings, including correctional institutions; college students; military personnel; adolescents and adults living in households with children; nonpregnant women of childbearing age; and international travelers).

(continued)

TABLE 6. RECOMMENDED IMMUNIZATION SCHEDULE ADULTS, UNITED STATES, 2009[57] (*continued*)

Evidence of immunity to varicella in adults includes any of the following: 1) documentation of 2 doses of varicella vaccine at least 4 weeks apart; 2) U.S.-born before 1980 (although for health-care personnel and pregnant women, birth before 1980 should not be considered evidence of immunity; 3) history of varicella based on diagnosis or verification of varicella by a health-care provider (for a patient reporting a history of or presenting with an atypical case, a mild case, or both, health-care providers should seek either an epidemiologic link to a typical varicella case or to a laboratory-confirmed case or evidence of laboratory confirmation, if it was performed at the time of acute disease); 4) history of herpes zoster based on health-care provider diagnosis or verification of herpes zoster by a health-care provider; or 5) laboratory evidence of immunity or laboratory confirmation of disease.

Pregnant women should be assessed for evidence of varicella immunity. Women who do not have evidence of immunity should receive the first dose of varicella vaccine upon completion or termination of pregnancy and before discharge from the health-care facility. The second dose should be administered 4–8 weeks after the first dose.

d Herpes zoster vaccination

A single dose of zoster vaccine is recommended for adults aged 60 years and older regardless of whether they report a prior episode of herpes zoster. Persons with chronic medical conditions may be vaccinated unless their condition constitutes a contraindication.

e Measles, mumps, rubella (MMR) vaccination

Measles component: Adults born before 1957 generally are considered immune to measles. Adults born during or after 1957 should receive 1 or more doses of MMR unless they have a medical contraindication, documentation of 1 or more doses, history of measles based on health-care provider diagnosis, or laboratory evidence of immunity.

A second dose of MMR is recommended for adults who 1) have been recently exposed to measles or are in an outbreak setting; 2) have been vaccinated previously with killed measles vaccine; 3) have been vaccinated with an unknown type of measles vaccine during 1963–1967; 4) are students in postsecondary educational institutions; 5) work in a health-care facility; or 6) plan to travel internationally.

Mumps component: Adults born before 1957 generally are considered immune to mumps. Adults born during or after 1957 should receive 1 dose of MMR unless they have a medical contraindication, history of mumps based on health-care provider diagnosis, or laboratory evidence of immunity.

A second dose of MMR is recommended for adults who 1) live in a community experiencing a mumps outbreak and are in an affected age group; 2) are students in postsecondary educational institutions; 3) work in a health-care facility; or 4) plan to travel internationally. For unvaccinated health-care personnel born before 1957 who do not have other evidence of mumps immunity, administering 1 dose on a routine basis should be considered and administering a second dose during an outbreak should be strongly considered.

Rubella component: 1 dose of MMR vaccine is recommended for women whose rubella vaccination history is unreliable or who lack laboratory evidence of immunity. For women of childbearing age, regardless of birth year, rubella immunity should be determined and women should be counseled regarding congenital rubella syndrome. Women who do not have evidence of immunity should receive MMR vaccine upon completion or termination of pregnancy and before discharge from the health-care facility.

(continued)

TABLE 6. RECOMMENDED IMMUNIZATION SCHEDULE ADULTS, UNITED STATES, 2009[57] (*continued*)

f Influenza vaccination

Medical indications: Chronic disorders of the cardiovascular or pulmonary systems, including asthma; chronic metabolic diseases, including diabetes mellitus, renal or hepatic dysfunction, hemoglobinopathies, or immunocompromising conditions (including immunocompromising conditions caused by medications or human immunodeficiency virus [HIV]); any condition that compromises respiratory function or the handling of respiratory secretions or that can increase the risk of aspiration (e.g., cognitive dysfunction, spinal cord injury, or seizure disorder or other neuromuscular disorder); and pregnancy during the influenza season. No data exist on the risk for severe or complicated influenza disease among persons with asplenia; however, influenza is a risk factor for secondary bacterial infections that can cause severe disease among persons with asplenia.

Occupational indications: All health-care personnel, including those employed by long-term care and assisted-living facilities, and caregivers of children less than 5 years old.

Other indications: Residents of nursing homes and other long-term care and assisted-living facilities; persons likely to transmit influenza to persons at high risk (e.g., in-home household contacts and caregivers of children aged less than 5 years old, persons 65 years old and older and persons of all ages with high-risk condition[s]); and anyone who would like to decrease their risk of getting influenza. Healthy, nonpregnant adults aged less than 50 years without high-risk medical conditions who are not contacts of severely immunocompromised persons in special care units can receive either intranasally administered live, attenuated influenza vaccine (FluMist®) or inactivated vaccine. Other persons should receive the inactivated vaccine.

g Pneumococcal polysaccharide (PPSV) vaccination

Medical indications: Chronic lung disease (including asthma); chronic cardiovascular diseases; diabetes mellitus; chronic liver diseases; cirrhosis; chronic alcoholism, chronic renal failure or nephrotic syndrome; functional or anatomic asplenia (e.g., sickle cell disease or splenectomy [if elective splenectomy is planned, vaccinate at least 2 weeks before surgery]); immunocompromising conditions; and cochlear implants and cerebrospinal fluid leaks. Vaccinate as close to HIV diagnosis as possible.

Other indications: Residents of nursing homes or other long-term care facilities and persons who smoke cigarettes. Routine use of PPSV is not recommended for Alaska Native or American Indian persons younger than 65 years unless they have underlying medical conditions that are PPSV indications. However, public health authorities may consider recommending PPSV for Alaska Natives and American Indians aged 50 through 64 years who are living in areas in which the risk of invasive pneumococcal disease is increased.

h Revaccination with PPSV

One-time revaccination after 5 years is recommended for persons with chronic renal failure or nephrotic syndrome; functional or anatomic asplenia (e.g., sickle cell disease or splenectomy); and for persons with immunocompromising conditions. For persons aged 65 years and older, one-time revaccination if they were vaccinated 5 or more years previously and were aged less than 65 years at the time of primary vaccination.

i Hepatitis A vaccination

Medical indications: Persons with chronic liver disease and persons who receive clotting factor concentrates.

Behavioral indications: Men who have sex with men and persons who use illegal drugs.

Occupational indications: Persons working with hepatitis A virus (HAV)–infected primates or with HAV in a research laboratory setting.

(continued)

TABLE 6. RECOMMENDED IMMUNIZATION SCHEDULE ADULTS, UNITED STATES, 2009[57] (*continued*)

Other indications: Persons traveling to or working in countries that have high or intermediate endemicity of hepatitis A and any person seeking protection from HAV infection.

Single-antigen vaccine formulations should be administered in a 2-dose schedule at either 0 and 6–12 months (Havrix®), or 0 and 6–18 months (Vaqta®). If the combined hepatitis A and hepatitis B vaccine (Twinrix®) is used administer 3 doses at 0, 1 and 6 months; alternatively, a 4-dose schedule, administered on days 0, 7, and 21 to 30 followed by a booster dose at month 12 may be used.

j Hepatitis B vaccination

Medical indications: Persons with end-stage renal disease, including patients receiving hemodialysis; persons with HIV infection; and persons with chronic liver disease.

Occupational indications: Health-care personnel and public-safety workers who are exposed to blood or other potentially infectious body fluids.

Behavioral indications: Sexually active persons who are not in a long-term, mutually monogamous relationship (e.g., persons with more than 1 sex partner during the previous 6 months); persons seeking evaluation or treatment for a sexually transmitted disease (STD);current or recent injection-drug users; and men who have sex with men.

Other indications: Household contacts and sex partners of persons with chronic hepatitis B virus (HBV) infection; clients and staff members of institutions for persons with developmental disabilities; international travelers to countries with high or intermediate prevalence of chronic HBV infection and any adult seeking protection from HBV infection.

Hepatitis B vaccination is recommended for all adults in the following settings: STD treatment facilities; HIV testing and treatment facilities; facilities providing drug-abuse treatment and prevention services; health-care settings targeting services to injection-drug users or men who have sex with men; correctional facilities; end-stage renal disease programs and facilities for chronic hemodialysis patients; and institutions and nonresidential daycare facilities for persons with developmental disabilities.

If the combined hepatitis A and hepatitis B vaccine (Twinrix®) is used, administer 3 doses at 0, 1, and 6 months; alternatively, a 4-dose schedule, administered on days 0, 7, and 21 to 30 followed by a booster dose at month 12 may be used.

Special formulation indications: For adult patients receiving hemodialysis or with other immunocompromising conditions, 1 dose of 40 μg/mL (Recombivax HB®) administered on a 3-dose schedule or 2 doses of 20 μg/mL (Engerix-B®) administered simultaneously on a 4-dose schedule at 0, 1, 2 and 6 months.

k Meningococcal vaccination

Medical indications: Adults with anatomic or functional asplenia, or terminal complement component deficiencies.

Other indications: First-year college students living in dormitories; microbiologists routinely exposed to isolates of Neisseria meningitidis; military recruits; and persons who travel to or live in countries in which meningococcal disease is hyperendemic or epidemic (e.g., the "meningitis belt" of sub-Saharan Africa during the dry season [December–June]), particularly if their contact with local populations will be prolonged. Vaccination is required by the government of Saudi Arabia for all travelers to Mecca during the annual Hajj.

Meningococcal conjugate vaccine (MCV) is preferred for adults with any of the preceding indications who are aged 55 years or younger, although meningococcal polysaccharide vaccine (MPSV) is an acceptable alternative. Revaccination with MCV after 5 years might be indicated for adults previously vaccinated with MPSV who remain at increased risk for infection (e.g., persons residing in areas in which disease is epidemic).

TABLE 7. IMMUNIZATION CATCH-UP SCHEDULE, AGES 4 MONTHS THROUGH 18 YEARS, UNITED STATES, 2009[58]

CATCH-UP SCHEDULE FOR PERSONS AGED 4 MONTHS THROUGH 6 YEARS

Vaccine	Minimum Age for Dose 1	Minimum Interval Between Doses			
		Dose 1 to Dose 2	Dose 2 to Dose 3	Dose 3 to Dose 4	Dose 4 to Dose 5
Hepatitis B[a]	Birth	4 weeks	8 weeks (and at least 16 weeks after first dose)		
Rotavirus[b]	6 wks	4 weeks	4 weeks[b]		
Diphtheria, Tetanus, Pertussis[c]	6 wks	4 weeks	4 weeks	6 months	6 months[c]
Haemophilus influenzae type b[d]	6 wks	4 weeks if first dose administered at younger than age 12 months 8 weeks (as final dose) if first dose administered at age 12-14 months No further doses needed if first dose administered at age 15 months or older	4 weeks[d] if current age is younger than 12 months 8 weeks (as final dose)[d] if current age is 12 months or older and second dose administered at younger than age 15 months No further doses needed if previous dose administered at age 15 months or older	8 weeks (as final dose) This dose only necessary for children aged 12 months through 59 months who received 3 doses before age 12 months	
Pneumococcal[e]	6 wks	4 weeks if first dose administered at younger than age 12 months 8 weeks (as final dose for healthy children) if first dose administered at age 12 months or older or current age 24 through 59 months No further doses needed for healthy children if first dose administered at age 24 months or older	4 weeks if current age is younger than 12 months 8 weeks (as final dose for healthy children) if current age is 12 months or older No further doses needed for healthy children if previous dose administered at age 24 months or older	8 weeks (as final dose) This dose only necessary for children aged 12 months through 59 months who received 3 doses before age 12 months or for high-risk children who received 3 doses at any age	
Inactivated Poliovirus[f]	6 wks	4 weeks	4 weeks	4 weeks[f]	
Measles, Mumps, Rubella[g]	12 mos	4 weeks			
Varicella[h]	12 mos	3 months			
Hepatitis A[i]	12 mos	6 months			

(continued)

TABLE 7. IMMUNIZATION CATCH-UP SCHEDULE, AGES 4 MONTHS THROUGH 18 YEARS, UNITED STATES, 2009[58] (*continued*)

CATCH-UP SCHEDULE FOR PERSONS AGED 7 THROUGH 18 YEARS					
Tetanus, Diphtheria/ Tetanus, Diphtheria, Pertussis[j]	**7 yrs**[j]	**4 weeks**	**4 weeks** if first dose administered at younger than age 12 months **6 months** if first dose administered at age 12 months or older	**6 months** if first dose administered at younger than age 12 months	
Human Papillomavirus[k]	**9 yrs**	**Routine dosing intervals are recommended**[k]			
Hepatitis A[i]	**12 mos**	**6 months**			
Hepatitis B[a]	**Birth**	**4 weeks**	**8 weeks** (and at least 16 weeks after first dose)		
Inactivated Poliovirus[f]	**6 wks**	**4 weeks**	**4 weeks**	**4 weeks**[f]	
Measles, Mumps, Rubella[g]	**12 mos**	**4 weeks**			
Varicella[h]	**12 mos**	**3 months** if the person is younger than age 13 years **4 weeks** if the person is aged 13 years or older			

[a] **Hepatitis B vaccine (HepB).**

- Administer the 3-dose series to those not previously vaccinated.
- A 2-dose series (separated by at least 4 months) of adult formulation Recombivax HB® is licensed for children aged 11 through 15 years.

[b] **Rotavirus vaccine (RV).**

- The maximum age for the first dose is 14 weeks 6 days. Vaccination should not be initiated for infants aged 15 weeks or older (i.e., 15 weeks 0 days or older).
- Administer the final dose in the series by age 8 months 0 days.
- If Rotarix® was administered for the first and second doses, a third dose is not indicated.

[c] **Diphtheria and tetanus toxoids and acellular pertussis vaccine (DTaP).**

- The fifth dose is not necessary if the fourth dose was administered at age 4 years or older.

(continued)

TABLE 7. IMMUNIZATION CATCH-UP SCHEDULE, AGES 4 MONTHS THROUGH 18 YEARS, UNITED STATES, 2009[58] (*continued*)

d *Haemophilus influenzae* type b conjugate vaccine (Hib).

- Hib vaccine is not generally recommended for persons aged 5 years or older. No efficacy data are available on which to base a recommendation concerning use of Hib vaccine for older children and adults. However, studies suggest good immunogenicity in persons who have sickle cell disease, leukemia, or HIV infection, or who have had a splenectomy; administering 1 dose of Hib vaccine to these persons is not contraindicated.
- If the first 2 doses were PRP-OMP (PedvaxHIB® or Comvax®), and administered at age 11 months or younger, the third (and final) dose should be administered at age 12 through 15 months and at least 8 weeks after the second dose.
- If the first dose was administered at age 7 through 11 months, administer 2 doses separated by 4 weeks and a final dose at age 12 through 15 months.

e Pneumococcal vaccine.

- Administer 1 dose of pneumococcal conjugate vaccine (PCV) to all healthy children aged 24 through 59 months who have not received at least 1 dose of PCV on or after age 12 months.
- For children aged 24 through 59 months with underlying medical conditions, administer 1 dose of PCV if 3 doses were received previously or administer 2 doses of PCV at least 8 weeks apart if fewer than 3 doses were received previously.
- Administer pneumococcal polysaccharide vaccine (PPSV) to children aged 2 years or older with certain underlying medical conditions, including a cochlear implant, at least 8 weeks after the last dose of PCV.

f Inactivated poliovirus vaccine (IPV).

- For children who received an all-IPV or all-oral poliovirus (OPV) series, a fourth dose is not necessary if the third dose was administered at age 4 years or older.
- If both OPV and IPV were administered as part of a series, a total of 4 doses should be administered, regardless of the child's current age.

g Measles, mumps, and rubella vaccine (MMR).

- Administer the second dose at age 4 through 6 years. However, the second dose may be administered before age 4, provided at least 28 days have elapsed since the first dose.
- If not previously vaccinated, administer 2 doses with at least 28 days between doses.

(continued)

TABLE 7. IMMUNIZATION CATCH-UP SCHEDULE, AGES 4 MONTHS THROUGH 18 YEARS, UNITED STATES, 2009[58] *(continued)*

h **Varicella vaccine.**
- Administer the second dose at age 4 through 6 years. However, the second dose may be administered before age 4, provided at least 3 months have elapsed since the first dose.
- For persons aged 12 months through 12 years, the minimum interval between doses is 3 months. However, if the second dose was administered at least 28 days after the first dose, it can be accepted as valid.
- For persons aged 13 years and older, the minimum interval between doses is 28 days.

i **Hepatitis A vaccine (HepA).**
- HepA is recommended for children older than 1 year who live in areas where vaccination programs target older children or who are at increased risk of infection.

j **Tetanus and diphtheria toxoids vaccine (Td) and tetanus and diphtheria toxoids and acellular pertussis vaccine (Tdap).**
- Doses of DTaP are counted as part of the Td/Tdap series.
- Tdap should be substituted for a single dose of Td in the catch-up series or as a booster for children aged 10 through 18 years; use Td for other doses.

k **Human papillomavirus vaccine (HPV).**
- Administer the series to females at age 13 through 18 years if not previously vaccinated.
- Use recommended routine dosing intervals for series catch-up (i.e., the second and third doses should be administered at 2 and 6 months after the first dose). However, the minimum interval between the first and second doses is 4 weeks. The minimum interval between the second and third doses is 12 weeks, and the third dose should be given at least 24 weeks after the first dose.

1177

■ ADMINISTRATION

Frequency of immunization administration is provided for the respective age groups in Tables 4–7.[55-58] Time intervals for vaccines/toxoids administered in a series may be extended in appropriate situations (e.g., febrile illness) but preferably not shortened, unless recommended on the Catch-up Schedule (Table 7) or if travel is impending.[1] Administration of two or more inactivated or an inactivated and live vaccine/toxoid can occur concomitantly or at any interval between doses. Live antigens (intranasal or injectable) may also be administered simultaneously; however, they must be separated by at least 4 weeks if not given concomitantly. Exceptions apply to oral live vaccines (e.g., rotavirus), which can be administered concomitantly or at any interval around inactivated or live antigens.

Route of administration differs with each immunization, and site of injection varies among age groups.[1] Appropriate doses and routes of administration are provided in Tables 1 and 3.[2-54] For intramuscular injections in newborns through 12 months of age, the anterolateral thigh is the preferred administration site; the deltoid muscle of the arm may be used for toddlers (1–2 years old) as an alternative and is preferred for all patients 3 years of age and older.[1] Likewise, the anterolateral thigh may be used as an alternative intramuscular injection site for patients 3–18 years of age. All intramuscular injections are administered at a 90-degree angle as compared to a 45-degree angle for subcutaneous injections. Sites of administration for subcutaneous injections include the thigh for infants less than 12 months of age and the upper-outer triceps area for all other age groups; administration into the upper-outer triceps area of infants may be necessary in certain situations. To minimize inflammation, different anatomical sites are recommended if vaccinations are administered simultaneously. If administration via different anatomical sites is not possible, the thigh may be used for multiple injections (separated by at least one inch) in infants and young children and the deltoid muscle in older children and adults. Table 8 lists potential injection sites and suggested needle sizes by age group and weight.

TABLE 8. INTRAMUSCULAR AND SUBCUTANEOUS INJECTION SITES AND SUGGESTED NEEDLE SIZE BY AGE GROUP AND WEIGHT

	NEWBORN (<28 D)	INFANT (1–12 MO)	TODDLER (1–2 Y)	CHILD/ADOLESCENT (3–18 Y)	ADULT[a] MALE & FEMALE <60 kg	ADULT[a] FEMALE 60–90 kg	ADULT[a] FEMALE >90 kg	ADULT[a] MALE 60–118 kg	ADULT[a] MALE >118 kg
Intramuscular									
Needle length	5/8"[b] (16 mm)	1" (25 mm)	1"–11/4" (25–32 mm)	1"–11/4" (25–32 mm)	5/8"[b]–1" (16–25 mm)	1" (25 mm)[d]	1"–11/2" (25–38 mm)	11/2" (38 mm)	
Injection site	90-degree angle into anterolateral thigh	90-degree angle into anterolateral thigh	90-degree angle into anterolateral thigh[c]	90-degree angle into anterolateral thigh	90-degree angle into deltoid muscle of the arm[c]	90-degree angle into deltoid muscle of the arm			
			90-degree angle into deltoid muscle of the arm						
Subcutaneous									
Injection site	45-degree angle into thigh; upper-outer triceps area may be used in infants	45-degree angle into thigh; upper-outer triceps area may be used in infants	45-degree angle into upper-outer triceps area	45-degree angle into upper-outer triceps area					
Needle length	5/8" (23–25 gauge)								

Reprinted with additions/modifications and permission from MMWR.[1]

[a]Age ≥19 years.
[b] Skin is stretched tight and subcutaneous tissue is not bunched.
[c]Preferred site.
[d]Certain experts recommend a 5/8" (16 mm) needle for males and females who weigh <60 kg (130 lbs).
Adapted from Ref. 60.

■ ACTIVE VERSUS PASSIVE IMMUNIZATION

Vaccines and toxoids provide active immunity by introducing inactivated or weakened disease organisms into the body.[61] The immune system response uses B and T cells that possess memory capabilities to combat the foreign antigen and defend against future exposures. By evoking these cells, the immunity is lengthened and potentially life-long. Passive immunity is utilized when infectious exposure has recently occurred or is expected in the immediate future and employs the transfer of immune globulins or antitoxins from a donor to the host needing protection. Limitations of passive immunity that restrict its frequent utility include increased risk of adverse reactions (e.g., serum sickness, anaphylaxis), if nonhuman derived, and shortened duration of immunity (weeks to months).

■ IMMUNE GLOBULINS AND ANTITOXINS

Table 9 provides a list of immune globulins and antitoxins available in the United States for treatment and/or prophylaxis of certain infectious diseases.[62–84] Table columns include brand name, type/source, FDA-approved indication(s), contraindications, and route of administration. Criteria for administration of these immune globulins and antitoxins differ with each disease; therefore, the CDC or the local health department should be consulted to determine appropriate use and whether the immune globulin/antitoxin is indicated.

■ EDUCATION

The National Childhood Vaccine Injury Act of 1986 (42 U.S.C. § 300aa-26) requires distribution of Vaccine Information Statements (VIS), which serve as educational consent forms for patients and guardians/caregivers.[1,85] VIS forms review the infectious disease and corresponding vaccine/toxoid, benefits of immunization, and potential risks. Current VIS forms are available at http://www.cdc.gov/nip/publications/VIS/default.htm and are required to be disseminated prior to administration for the following vaccines/toxoids: (1) diphtheria, tetanus, and acellular pertussis (DTaP), (2) tetanus and diphtheria toxoids (Td), (3) measles, mumps, and rubella (MMR), (4) polio, (5) hepatitis A, (6) hepatitis B, (7) *Haemophilus influenzae* type b (Hib), (8) influenza, (9) pneumococcal conjugate, and (10) varicella (chickenpox) vaccine. Other VIS forms are available and are encouraged, but not required, for distribution prior to vaccination.

■ ADVERSE REACTIONS AND REPORTING

Adverse reactions can occur following vaccination and range from minor, local reactions to severe, life-threatening systemic reactions.[1] If an adverse reaction occurs, it can be reported through the Vaccine Adverse Event Reporting System (VAERS), which is accessible at http://www.cdc.gov/vaccines/vac-gen/safety/default.htm. Severe reactions should be reported and are required for compliance with the National Childhood Vaccine Injury Compensation Program (VICP) Act. VICP provides monetary compensation to patients for certain vaccine-associated adverse reactions (e.g., thrombocytopenic purpura after measles vaccine), removing liability from the manufacturer and provider, except in cases of negligence.

TABLE 9. IMMUNE GLOBULINS AND ANTITOXINS IN THE UNITED STATES

IMMUNE GLOBULIN/ANTITOXIN	*BRAND NAME	TYPE	PROPHYLAXIS[a]	TREATMENT	FDA-APPROVED INDICATIONS	CONTRAINDICATIONS	ROUTE OF ADMINISTRATION
Botulism immune globulin	BabyBIG[62]	Human IgG		✓	Treatment of infant (<1 year of age) botulism caused by toxin type A or B	Previous anaphylaxis to other human immunoglobulin products; selective immunoglobulin A deficiency[b]	Intravenous
Cytomegalovirus immune globulin (CMV-IGIV)	CytoGam[63]	Human IgG	✓		Prophylaxis of CMV disease associated with kidney, lung, liver, pancreas, and heart transplantation	Previous anaphylaxis to other human immunoglobulin products; selective immunoglobulin A deficiency[b]	Intravenous
Diphtheria antitoxin[64] (DAT)	None	Equine, polyclonal IgG	✓	✓	Treatment of probable or confirmed respiratory diphtheria; postexposure prophylaxis to known or suspected toxigenic C. diphtheria	None – Patients with hypersensitivity reactions will undergo desensitization	Intravenous preferred, especially in severe cases; intramuscular acceptable for mild/moderate cases

(continued)

TABLE 9. IMMUNE GLOBULINS AND ANTITOXINS IN THE UNITED STATES (*continued*)

IMMUNE GLOBULIN/ANTITOXIN	*BRAND NAME	TYPE	PROPHYLAXIS[a]	TREATMENT	FDA-APPROVED INDICATIONS	CONTRAINDICATIONS	ROUTE OF ADMINISTRATION
Hepatitis B Immune Globulin (HBIG)	HepaGam B[65]	Human IgG	✓	✓	Prevention of Hepatitis B recurrence following liver transplantation in HBsAg-positive liver transplant patients; postexposure prophylaxis following acute exposure to blood containing HBsAg, perinatal exposure of infants born to HBsAg positive mothers, sexual exposure to HBsAg positive persons, and household exposure to persons with acute HBV infection	Previous anaphylaxis to other human immunoglobulin products; selective immunoglobulin A deficiency[b]	Intravenous (prevention of recurrence) Intramuscular (postexposure prophylaxis)
	HyperHEP B S/D[66]	Human IgG	✓		Postexposure prophylaxis of acute exposure to blood containing HBsAg, perinatal exposure of infants born to HBsAg positive mothers, sexual exposure to HBsAg positive persons, and household exposure to persons with acute HBV infection	Previous anaphylaxis to other human immunoglobulin products	Intramuscular

(continued)

TABLE 9. IMMUNE GLOBULINS AND ANTITOXINS IN THE UNITED STATES (*continued*)

IMMUNE GLOBULIN/ANTITOXIN	*BRAND NAME	TYPE	PROPHYLAXIS[a]	TREATMENT	FDA-APPROVED INDICATIONS	CONTRAINDICATIONS	ROUTE OF ADMINISTRATION
	Nabi-HB[67]	Human IgG	✓		Postexposure prophylaxis of acute exposure to blood containing HBsAg, perinatal exposure of infants born to HBsAg positive mothers, sexual exposure to HBsAg positive persons, and household exposure to persons with acute HBV infection	Previous anaphylaxis to other human immunoglobulin products; selective immunoglobulin A deficiency[b]	Intramuscular
Immune globulin (IVIG)	Carimune NF[68]	Human IgG		✓	Treatment of primary immunodeficiency[d] and immune thrombocytopenic purpura (ITP)	Previous anaphylaxis to other human immunoglobulin products; selective immunoglobulin A deficiency[b]	Intravenous
	Flebogamma 5%[69]	Human IgG		✓	Treatment of primary[d] and secondary immunodeficiency	Previous anaphylaxis to other human immunoglobulin products; selective immunoglobulin A deficiency[b]	Intravenous
	GAMMAGARD LIQUID[70]	Human IgG		✓	Treatment of primary immunodeficiency[d]	Previous anaphylaxis to other human immunoglobulin products; selective immunoglobulin A deficiency[b]	Intravenous

(continued)

TABLE 9. IMMUNE GLOBULINS AND ANTITOXINS IN THE UNITED STATES (*continued*)

IMMUNE GLOBULIN/ANTITOXIN	*BRAND NAME	TYPE	PROPHYLAXIS[a]	TREATMENT	FDA-APPROVED INDICATIONS	CONTRAINDICATIONS	ROUTE OF ADMINISTRATION
	GAMMAGARD S/D[71]	Human IgG		✓	Treatment of primary immunodeficiency[d], immune thrombocytopenic purpura (ITP), Kawasaki Disease, and B-cell Chronic Lymphocytic Leukemia (CLL)	Previous anaphylaxis to other human immunoglobulin products; selective immunoglobulin A deficiency[b]	Intravenous
	Gammar-P IV[72]	Human IgG		✓	Treatment of primary immunodeficiency[d]	Previous anaphylaxis to other human immunoglobulin products; selective immunoglobulin A deficiency[b]	Intravenous
	Gamunex[73]	Human IgG		✓	Treatment of primary immunodeficiency[d] and immune thrombocytopenic purpura (ITP)	Previous anaphylaxis to other human immunoglobulin products; selective immunoglobulin A deficiency[b]	Intravenous
	IVEEGAM EN[74]	Human IgG		✓	Treatment of primary immunodeficiency[d] and Kawasaki Disease	Previous anaphylaxis to other human immunoglobulin products; selective immunoglobulin A deficiency[b]	Intravenous
	OCTAGAM[75]	Human IgG		✓	Treatment of primary immunodeficiency[d]	Previous anaphylaxis to other human immunoglobulin products; selective immunoglobulin A deficiency[b]	Intravenous

(continued)

IMMUNE GLOBULIN/ANTITOXIN	*BRAND NAME	TYPE	PROPHYLAXIS[a]	TREATMENT	FDA-APPROVED INDICATIONS	CONTRAINDICATIONS	ROUTE OF ADMINISTRATION
Immune globulin	Privigen[76]	Human IgG		✓	Treatment of primary immunodeficiency[d] and immune thrombocytopenic purpura (ITP)	Previous anaphylaxis to other human immunoglobulin products; selective immunoglobulin A deficiency[b]; hyperprolinemia	Intravenous
Immune globulin (IGIM)	GamaSTAN S/D[77]	Human IgG	✓	✓	Treatment of immunodeficiency; Postexposure prophylaxis for hepatitis A, measles, rubella, and varicella (if VZIG unavailable)	Previous anaphylaxis to other human immunoglobulin products; selective immunoglobulin A deficiency[b]; severe thrombocytopenia	Intramuscular
Immune globulin (IGSC)	Vivaglobin[78]	Human IgG		✓	Treatment of primary immunodeficiency[d]	Previous anaphylaxis to other human immunoglobulin products; selective immunoglobulin A deficiency[b]	Subcutaneous
Palivizumab	Synagis[79]	Human IgG1κ Murine Monoclonal Antibody	✓		Prevention of serious lower respiratory tract disease caused by respiratory syncytial virus in high-risk pediatric patients	History of severe reactions to this vaccine or any of it components	Intramuscular

(continued)

TABLE 9. IMMUNE GLOBULINS AND ANTITOXINS IN THE UNITED STATES (*continued*)

IMMUNE GLOBULIN/ANTITOXIN	*BRAND NAME	TYPE	PROPHYLAXIS[a]	TREATMENT	FDA-APPROVED INDICATIONS	CONTRAINDICATIONS	ROUTE OF ADMINISTRATION
Rabies immune globulin	HyperRAB S/D[80]	Human IgG	✓		Preexposure prophylaxis for high risk patients and postexposure prophylaxis in suspected or documented rabies cases	Previous anaphylaxis to other human immunoglobulin products; Active rabies infection	Intramuscular and at bite site
	Imogam Rabies-HT[81]	Human IgG	✓		Preexposure prophylaxis for high risk patients and postexposure prophylaxis in suspected or documented rabies cases	Previous anaphylaxis to other human immunoglobulin products; Active rabies infection	Intramuscular and at bite site
Tetanus immune globulin	HyperTET S/D[82]	Human IgG	✓	✓	Postexposure prophylaxis in unimmunized patients; treatment of active tetanus, although limited evidence	Previous anaphylaxis to other human immunoglobulin products	Intramuscular

(continued)

TABLE 9. IMMUNE GLOBULINS AND ANTITOXINS IN THE UNITED STATES (*continued*)

IMMUNE GLOBULIN/ANTITOXIN	*BRAND NAME	TYPE	PROPHYLAXIS[a]	TREATMENT	FDA-APPROVED INDICATIONS	CONTRAINDICATIONS	ROUTE OF ADMINISTRATION
Vaccinia immune globulin (VIGIV)[83]	None	Human IgG		✓	Treatment of eczema vaccinatum, progressive vaccinia, severe generalized vaccinia, infections induced by vaccinia by accidental implantation in the eyes, mouth, or other exposed areas that would be especially harmful, and vaccinia infections in patients with burns, impetigo, varicella-zoster, or poison ivy	Previous anaphylaxis to other human immunoglobulin products; selective immunoglobulin A deficiency[b]; presence of isolated vaccinia keratitis	Intravenous
Varicella-Zoster immune globulin (VZIG)[84]	None	Human IgG	✓		Postexposure prophylaxis for exposed, susceptible individuals who are at greater risk of complications from varicella	Previous anaphylaxis to other human immunoglobulin products; selective immunoglobulin A deficiency[b]; severe thrombocytopenia	Intramuscular

[a]Includes pre- and postexposure prophylaxis. Preexposure prophylaxis occurs if exposure to the infectious agent is expected in the immediate future; postexposure prophylaxis occurs if exposure to the infectious agent recently occurred.
[b]Selective immunoglobulin A deficient patients may develop antibodies to immunoglobulin A and react to subsequent blood products containing immunoglobulin A.
[c]Limited availability/distribution.
[d]Primary immunodeficiency disorders are associated with humoral immunity and include, but are not limited to congenital X-linked agammaglobulinemia, common variable immunodeficiency, Wiskott-Aldrich syndrome, and congenital agammaglobulinemia.
HBsAg, Hepatitis B surface antigen.

■ REFERENCES

1. General recommendations on immunization. Recommendations of the Advisory Committee on Immunization Practices (ACIP). *MMWR Recomm Rep.* 2006;55(RR15):1-48.
2. Product Information: BioThrax™, anthrax vaccine adsorbed. Lansing, MI: Bioport Corporation; 2002.
3. Product Information: ActHIB®, haemophilus b conjugate vaccine. Swiftwater, PA: Sanofi Pasteur Incorporated; 2005.
4. Product Information: HibTITER®, haemophilus b conjugate vaccine. Philadelphia, PA: Wyeth Pharmaceuticals; 2007.
5. Product Information: Liquid PedvaxHIB®, hemophilus b conjugate vaccine. West Point, PA: Merck & Company Incorporated; 2001.
6. Product Information: HAVRIX®, hepatitis A vaccine. Research Triangle Park, NC: GlaxoSmithKline; 2008.
7. Product Information: VAQTA®, hepatitis A vaccine inactivated. Whitehouse Station, NJ: Merck & Company Incorporated; 2007.
8. Product Information: ENGERIX-B®, hepatitis B vaccine (recombinant). Research Triangle Park, NC: Glaxo-SmithKline; 2006.
9. Product Information: RECOMBIVAX HB®, hepatitis B vaccine (recombinant). Whitehouse Station, NJ: Merck & Company Incorporated; 2007.
10. Product Information: ZOSTAVAX®, zoster vaccine live. Whitehouse Station, NJ: Merck & Company Incorporated; 2008.
11. Product Information: GARDASIL®, human papillomavirus quadrivalent vaccine (recombinant). Whitehouse Station, NJ: Merck & Company Incorporated; 2006.
12. Product Information: AFLURIA®, influenza virus vaccine. King of Prussia, PA: CSL Biotherapies Incorporated; 2007.
13. Product Information: FLUARIX®, influenza virus vaccine. Research Triangle Park, NC: GlaxoSmithKline; 2008.
14. Product Information: FLULAVAL®, influenza virus vaccine. Research Triangle Park, NC: GlaxoSmithKline; 2008.
15. Product Information: FluMist®, influenza virus vaccine live intranasal. Gaithersburg, MD: MedImmune Vaccines; 2008.
16. Product Information: FLUVIRIN®, influenza virus vaccine. Emeryville, CA: Novartis Vaccines and Diagnostics Incorporated; 2006.
17. Product Information: Fluzone®, influenza virus vaccine. Swiftwater, PA: Sanofi Pasteur Incorporated; 2008.
18. Product Information: H5N1 avian influenza virus vaccine. Swiftwater, PA: Sanofi Pasteur Incorporated; 2007.
19. Product Information: JE-VAX®, Japanese encephalitis virus vaccine inactivated. Swiftwater, PA: Sanofi Pasteur Incorporated; 2005.
20. Product Information: ATTENUVAX®, measles virus vaccine live. Whitehouse Station, NJ: Merck & Company Incorporated; 1999.
21. Product Information: Menactra®, meningococcal polysaccharide diphtheria toxoid conjugate vaccine. Swiftwater, PA: Sanofi Pasteur Incorporated; 2007.
22. Product Information: Menomune®, meningococcal polysaccharide vaccine. Swiftwater, PA: Sanofi Pasteur Incorporated; 2005.
23. Product Information: MUMPSVAX®, mumps virus vaccine live. Whitehouse Station, NJ: Merck & Company Incorporated; 1999.
24. Product Information: PNEUMOVAX® 23, pneumococcal vaccine polyvalent. Whitehouse Station, NJ: Merck & Company Incorporated; 2007.
25. Product Information: Prevnar®, pneumococcal 7-valent conjugate vaccine. Philadelphia, PA: Wyeth Pharmaceuticals; 2007.
26. Product Information: IPOL®, poliovirus vaccine inactivated. Swiftwater, PA: Sanofi Pasteur Incorporated; 2005.
27. Product Information: IMOVAX®, rabies vaccine. Swiftwater, PA: Sanofi Pasteur Incorporated; 2005.
28. Product Information: RabAvert™, rabies vaccine. Emeryville, CA: Chiron Corporation; 1997.
29. Product Information: ROTARIX®, rotavirus vaccine live attenuated oral. Research Triangle Park, NC: Glaxo-SmithKline; 2006.
30. Product Information: RotaTeq®, rotavirus vaccine live oral pentavalent. Whitehouse Station, NJ: Merck & Company Incorporated; 2008.
31. Product Information: MERUVAX® II, rubella virus vaccine live. Whitehouse Station, NJ: Merck & Company Incorporated; 1999.
32. Product Information: ACAM2000™, smallpox (vaccinia) live vaccine. Cambridge, MA: Acambis Incorporated; 2007.
33. Product Information: Dryvax®, smallpox vaccine live. Philadelphia, PA: Wyeth Pharmaceuticals; 2007.
34. Product Information: Tetanus toxoid adsorbed. Swiftwater, PA: Aventis Pasteur Incorporated; 2005.
35. Product Information: Tetanus toxoid for booster use only. Swiftwater, PA: Sanofi Pasteur Incorporated; 2005.

36. Product Information: Typhim Vi®, typhoid Vi polysaccharide vaccine. Swiftwater, PA: Sanofi Pasteur Incorporated; 2005.

37. Product Information: Vivotif®, typhoid vaccine live oral Ty21a. Coral Gables, FL: Berna Products; 2006.

38. Product Information: VARIVAX®, varicella virus vaccine live. Whitehouse Station, NJ: Merck & Company Incorporated; 2001.

39. Product Information: YF-VAX®, yellow fever vaccine. Swiftwater, PA: Sanofi Pasteur Incorporated; 2008.

40. Product Information: Adacel®, tetanus toxoid, reduced diphtheria toxoid, and acellular pertussis vaccine adsorbed. Swiftwater, PA: Sanofi Pasteur Incorporated; 2008.

41. Product Information: BOOSTRIX®, tetanus toxoid, reduced diphtheria toxoid, and acellular pertussis vaccine adsorbed. Research Triangle Park, NC: GlaxoSmithKline; 2008.

42. Product Information: COMVAX®, haemophilus b conjugate (meningococcal protein conjugate) and hepatitis b (recombinant) vaccine. Whitehouse Station, NJ: Merck & Company Incorporated; 2004.

43. Product Information: DAPTACEL®, diphtheria and tetanus toxoids and acellular pertussis vaccine adsorbed. Swiftwater, PA: Sanofi Pasteur Incorporated; 2008.

44. Product Information: DECAVAC®, tetanus and diphtheria toxoids adsorbed. Swiftwater, PA: Sanofi Pasteur Incorporated; 2005.

45. Product Information: Diphtheria and tetanus toxoids adsorbed USP. Swiftwater, PA: Sanofi Pasteur Incorporated; 2005.

46. Product Information: INFANRIX®, diphtheria and tetanus toxoids and acellular pertussis vaccine adsorbed. Philadelphia, PA: SmithKline Beecham Pharmaceuticals; 2003.

47. Product Information: KINRIX™, diphtheria and tetanus toxoids and acellular pertussis adsorbed and inactivated poliovirus vaccine. Research Triangle Park, NC: GlaxoSmithKline; 2008.

48. Product Information: M-M-R® II, measles, mumps, and rubella virus vaccine live. Whitehouse Station, NJ: Merck & Company Incorporated; 2007.

49. Product Information: M-M-VAX™, measles and mumps virus vaccine live. Whitehouse Station, NJ: Merck & Company Incorporated; 2002.

50. Product Information: PEDIARIX®, diphtheria and tetanus toxoids and acellular pertussis adsorbed, hepatitis B (recombinant) and inactivated poliovirus vaccine combined. Research Triangle Park, NC: GlaxoSmithKline; 2007.

51. Product Information: Pentacel®, diphtheria and tetanus toxoids and acellular pertussis adsorbed, inactivated poliovirus and haemophilus b conjugate (tetanus toxoid conjugate) vaccine. Swiftwater, PA: Sanofi Pasteur Incorporated; 2008.

52. Product Information: ProQuad®, measles, mumps, rubella, and varicella virus vaccine live. Whitehouse Station, NJ: Merck & Company Incorporated; 2008.

53. Product Information: Tripedia®, diphtheria and tetanus toxoids and acellular pertussis vaccine adsorbed. Swiftwater, PA: Aventis Pasteur Incorporated; 2000.

54. Product Information: TWINRIX®, hepatitis A inactivated and hepatitis B (recombinant) vaccine. Research Triangle Park, NC: GlaxoSmithKline; 2007.

55. Centers for Disease Control and Prevention. Recommended immunization schedule for persons aged 0 through 6 years – United States 2009. www.cdc.gov/vaccines/recs/schedules. Accessed February 6, 2009.

56. Centers for Disease Control and Prevention. Recommended immunization schedule for persons aged 7 through 18 years – United States 2009. www.cdc.gov/vaccines/recs/schedules. Accessed February 6, 2009.

57. Centers for Disease Control and Prevention. Recommended adult immunization schedule – United States 2009. www.cdc.gov/vaccines/recs/schedules. Accessed February 6, 2009.

58. Centers for Disease Control and Prevention. Catch-up immunization schedule for persons aged 4 months through 18 years who start late or who are more than 1 month behind – United States 2009. www.cdc.gov/vaccines/recs/schedules. Accessed February 6, 2009.

59. Centers for Disease Control and Prevention Travelers' Health. www.cdc.gov/travel. Accessed February 6, 2009.

60. Poland GA, Borrud A, Jacobsen RM, et al. Determination of deltoid fat pad thickness: Implications for needle length in adult immunization. *JAMA*. 1997;277:1709-1711.

61. Centers for Disease Control and Prevention Immunity Types. www.cdc.gov/vaccines/vac-gen/immunity-types. Accessed February 6, 2009.

62. Product Information: BabyBIG®, botulism immune globulin intravenous. Temecula, CA: FFF Enterprises; 2008.

63. Product Information: Cytogam®, cytomegalovirus immune globulin intravenous. Melville, NY: Precision Pharma Services; 2007.

64. Centers for Disease Control and Prevention. Diphtheria Antitoxin IND Protocol 2008. http://www.cdc.gov/vaccines/vpd-vac/diphtheria/dat/downloads/protocol_032504.pdf. Accessed October 6, 2009.

65. Product Information: HepaGam B™, hepatitis B immune globulin intravenous. Weston, FL: Apotex Corporation; 2007.

66. Product Information: HyperHEP B™ S/D, hepatitis B immune globulin. Research Triangle Park, NC: Talecris Biotherapeutics; 2007.

67. Product Information: Nabi-HB®, hepatitis B immune globulin. Boca Raton, FL: Nabi Biopharmaceuticals; 2003.
68. Product Information: Carimune® NF, immune globulin intravenous (human). Kankakee, IL: ZLB Behring LLC; 2005.
69. Product Information: Flebogamma® 5%, immune globulin intravenous (human). Los Angeles, CA: Grifols USA; 2003.
70. Product Information: GAMMAGARD® LIQUID, immune globulin intravenous (human). Westlake Village, CA: Baxter Healthcare Corporation; 2005.
71. Product Information: GAMMAGARD® S/D, immune globulin intravenous (human). Westlake Village, CA: Baxter Healthcare Corporation; 2008.
72. Product Information: Gammar®-P I.V., immune globulin intravenous (human). Kankakee, IL: ZLB Behring LLC; 2004.
73. Product Information: GAMUNEX®, immune globulin intravenous (human). Research Triangle Park, NC: Talecris Biotherapeutics; 2005.
74. Product Information: IVEEGAM EN®, immune globulin intravenous (human). Westlake Village, CA: Baxter Healthcare Corporation; 2005.
75. Product Information: OCTAGAM®, immune globulin intravenous (human). Centreville, VA: Octapharma USA Incorporated; 2006.
76. Product Information: Privigen®, immune globulin intravenous (human). Kankakee, IL: CSL Behring LLC; 2008.
77. Product Information: GamaSTAN™ S/D, immune globulin (human). Research Triangle Park, NC: Talecris Biotherapeutics; 2008.
78. Product Information: Vivaglobin®, immune globulin subcutaneous (human). Kankakee, IL: CSL Behring LLC; 2007.
79. Product Information: SYNAGIS®, palivizumab. Gaithersburg, MD: MedImmune; 2007.
80. Product Information: HyperRAB™ S/D, rabies immune globulin (human). Research Triangle Park, NC: Talecris Biotherapeutics; 2008.
81. Product Information: Imogam® Rabies – HT, rabies immune globulin (human). Swiftwater, PA: Aventis Pasteur; 1999.
82. Product Information: HyperTET™ S/D, tetanus immune globulin (human). Research Triangle Park, NC: Talecris Biotherapeutics; 2008.
83. Product Information: Vaccinia immune globulin intravenous (human). Atlanta, GA: Centers for Disease Control and Prevention; 2005.
84. Product Information: Varicella-Zoster immune globulin (human). Boston, MA: Public Health Biologic Laboratories; 2000.
85. Centers for Disease Control and Prevention. Fact Sheet for Vaccine Information Statements. www.cdc.gov/vaccines/pubs/vis/vis-facts. Accessed February 6, 2009.

Medical Emergencies: Anaphylaxis, Cardiac Arrest, Poisoning, Status Epilepticus

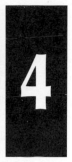

Kelly M. Smith

Anaphylaxis is a serious, acute, and potentially fatal clinical emergency. Management requires rapid identification, diagnosis, and administration of medications. The incidence of anaphylaxis in the United States has been increasing, particularly in children and among cases involving foodborne allergens.

Chapter 75

Anaphylaxis

Frank Romanelli

Anaphylaxis is defined as an acute systemic and extreme allergic reaction, which occurs following exposure to an allergen. The individual who experiences anaphylaxis must either have been previously exposed to the allergen (sensitized) or must be in contact with the allergen for a prolonged period of time. Anaphylaxis is mediated by an IgE-induced release of histamine and other proinflammatory chemicals. Anaphylactoid reactions, which are clinically indistinguishable from anaphylactic reactions, can occur without sensitization and are caused by the direct allergen-induced release of histaminergic and other inflammatory chemicals. Following exposure to an allergen, symptoms often develop within seconds or minutes and may include urticaria, bronchospasm, angioedema, and hypotension. Upper airway obstruction and cardiovascular collapse are the most common causes of death in anaphylaxis. Treatment consists of basic life support interventions and the emergent administration of medications aimed at reversing bronchospasm and cardiovascular manifestations.

GENERAL THERAPY

1. Removal of suspected allergen or trigger.

2. Epinephrine 0.3–0.5 mg IM (children 0.01 mg/kg) administered in the anterolateral thigh. If no response, prepare for epinephrine IV infusion (2–10 µg/min).

3. Place patient in a recumbent position with lower extremities elevated; supplemental oxygen up to 100% may be administered.

4. IV access should be a priority and in the event that fluid resuscitation is necessary normal saline 1–2 L (children 20 mL/kg boluses over 5–10 min with monitoring of urine output) as needed should be administered.

5. Other agents, which may be considered, include:
   - nebulized albuterol 2.55 mg in 3 ml of normal saline repeated as needed for resistant bronchospasm,
   - antihistaminic agents such as diphenhydramine 25–50 mg IV (not to exceed 5 mg/kg in children) followed by ranitidine 50 mg (children 1 mg/kg) IV, and
   - methylprednisolone 125 mg IV (not to exceed 0.5 mg/kg/d in children).

6. Concurrent administration of certain medications may make the reversal of anaphylaxis more difficult by either blunting compensatory mechanisms or interfering with the effects of treatment (e.g., angiotensin inhibitors, beta-blockers, alpha-adrenergic antagonists).

7. For refractory symptoms, epinephrine by IV infusion may be administered (2–20 µg/min) and titrated to effect. Dopamine may be added for additional vasopressor activity (5–10 µg/kg/min IV) and glucagon 1–2 mg slow IVP (children 20–30 µg/kg to a maximum of 1 mg) may provide some benefit in patients not responding to epinephrine secondary to beta-blocker therapy.

8. Hemodynamic monitoring and pulse oximetry should be performed and assessed continuously.

9. Long-term management of anaphylactic risk should include the avoidance of known allergens and the prescription of epinephrine auto-injection devices (e.g., EpiPen®).

■ REFERENCES

1. Nurmatov U, Worth A, Sheikh A. Anaphylaxis management plans for the acute and long-term management of anaphylaxis: a systematic review. *J Allergy Clin Immunol.* 2008;122:353-361.
2. Jevon P. Severe allergic reaction: management of anaphylaxis in hospital. *Br J Nurs.* 2008;17:104-108.
3. Estelle F, Simmons R. Anaphylaxis. *J Allergy Clin Immunol.* 2008;121:S402-S407.

Chapter 76

Cardiac Arrest

Heather M. Schumann and Krysta A. Zack

Cardiac arrest is a medical emergency requiring a systematic approach. Early recognition must be followed by prompt, effective application of Basic Life Support (BLS) techniques to sustain the patient until Advanced Cardiac Life Support (ACLS) capabilities are available. The management of cardiac arrest is a 4-step approach:

- **Recognition and Assessment**
- **Basic Life Support (BLS)**
- **Advanced Cardiovascular Life Support (ACLS)**
- **Postresuscitation Care**

■ RECOGNITION AND ASSESSMENT

Verify that respiration and circulation have ceased:

1. Loss of consciousness.
2. Loss of functional ventilation (respiratory arrest or inadequate respiratory effort).
3. Loss of functional perfusion (no pulse).

Without assessing the respiratory or perfusion status of the patient, lay rescuers should summon help and obtain an automated external defibrillator (AED) if the patient is unconscious.[1]

■ BASIC LIFE SUPPORT (BLS)

The findings listed above are sufficient to justify the immediate application of BLS techniques. The goal of a **rescuer** in cardiac arrest is the restoration of spontaneous circulation (ROSC). The first step toward achieving ROSC is prompt initiation of BLS, including chest compressions, to rapidly and effectively perfuse the tissues with oxygenated blood. Management has changed, focusing on earlier initiation with fewer interruptions in chest compressions. Early initiation of BLS including chest compressions can greatly increase the patient's survival rate.

1. Summon help and resuscitation equipment.
2. Establish an adequate airway using the head tilt-chin lift maneuver.
3. Provide rescue breathing by delivering two breaths. Ventilate by mouth-to-mouth, mouth-to-mask, or bag-valve-mask techniques. Lay rescuers concerned about disease transmission may utilize a barrier device, if available, to prevent disease transmission. Lay rescuers may also forgo

the administration of rescue breaths if they are unwilling or unable to perform them and proceed straight to the initiation of chest compressions, which emphasizes the importance of providing chest compressions (class IIa).

4. Check for pulse and other signs of circulation for ≤10 s. Lay persons are not expected to perform a pulse check. Rather, they are instructed to look for other signs of circulation such as normal breathing, coughing or movement. If no pulse or other signs of circulation are present, initiate rescue breathing and chest compressions.
   - For rescue breathing:
     – Give each breath over one second, looking for the patient's chest to rise (class IIa).
     – Deliver 8–10 breaths per min.
   - For external chest compressions:
     – Position patient supine on a firm surface.
     – Ensure proper placement of hands on sternum.
     – Depress sternum at rate of 100 cycles per min, allowing the chest to completely recoil after each compression.
     – For every 30 chest compressions, give 2 breaths. Chest compressions and rescue breathing should continue for 5 cycles, or approximately 2 min, before reassessing the patient.

5. When available, assess the heart rhythm with an AED, or monophasic/biphasic defibrillator. AEDs are computerized devices, available in many public areas, that provide visual and audio instructions to the rescuer and analyze the victim's cardiac rhythm. AEDs are easy to operate, and generally require the rescuer to turn the device on and apply defibrillator pads to the victim's bare chest. The device will provide commands to the rescuer to guide compressions and/or defibrillation. Lay person rescuers may administer 5 cycles of chest compressions and rescue breathing prior to assessing the heart rhythm with an AED (class IIb).
   - If ventricular tachycardia or ventricular fibrillation is documented, defibrillate with 120–200 J of direct current shock if using a biphasic defibrillator or 360 J if using a monophasic defibrillator.
   - Five cycles of chest compressions and rescue breathing should immediately follow defibrillation.

6. Reassess cardiac rhythm and check for a pulse.[1]

■ ADVANCED CARDIOVASCULAR LIFE SUPPORT (ACLS)

Note: Only adult dosages are given in this section.
Trained personnel should attempt to maintain an advanced patent airway, establish vascular access for administration of fluids and drugs, establish an electrocardiographic diagnosis, and apply specific treatments to correct any recognized electrical and/or mechanical abnormalities. Drug therapy may be administered via the IV, intraosseous (IO), and in some cases, via the endotracheal (ET) route.[1–3] If attempts at obtaining IV access are unsuccessful, intraosseous access may be established in pediatric and adult patients (class IIa).[1,2]

DRUG THERAPY IN ACLS
Ventricular Tachyarrhythmias. Ventricular tachyarrhythmias, which are managed in the same fashion, include: unstable ventricular flutter; ventricular tachycardia (VT), including pulseless VT; and ventricular fibrillation (VF). All are associated with decreased cardiac output and hypotension. The most important early interventions for management of these arrhythmias are early initiation of chest compressions with minimal interruptions and early defibrillation (class I).

1. **Electrical defibrillation** with 120–200 J if using a biphasic defibrillator and 360 J if using a monophasic defibrillator. Defibrillation should immediately be followed by 5 cycles of chest compressions and rescue breathing, representing a change from the previous guidelines (class I).
   - The rescuer should then immediately resume chest compressions and rescue breathing for five cycles without reassessing the rhythm or pulse (class IIa).
2. For pulseless VT/VF refractory to 1 or 2 cycles of chest compressions and defibrillation, **administration of medications** should begin. Chest compressions should not be interrupted during administration of medications. Medications should be administered as soon as possible after rhythm assessment, and can be given either before or after defibrillation following the sequence below:
   - **Epinephrine HCL, 1 mg IV push/IO** (10 mL of 1:10,000 solution) every 3–5 min until the ROSC *or* **vasopressin 40 units** (2 mL of 20 units/mL vial) IV or IO times 1 dose. If after 5–10 min there is no response to vasopressin, administer epinephrine as instructed
   - If IV access has not been established or has been lost, consider administering **epinephrine HCL** *or* **vasopressin via endotracheal tube,** (2–2.5 times the intravenous dose, *See* Special Considerations) followed by 3 or 4 rapid ventilations to aerosolize the drug (class—indeterminate for epinephrine and vasopressin)
     - Epinephrine is used to increase perfusion and sustain blood pressure. Stimulation of alpha receptors causes vasoconstriction, increasing systemic vascular resistance (SVR) and blood pressure. However, the beta agonist activity of epinephrine increases heart rate and contractility, increasing myocardial oxygen demand in resuscitated patients, which may precipitate or worsen myocardial ischemia.
     - Vasopressin is an initial alternative to epinephrine. It is an endogenous antidiuretic hormone that, at high doses (e.g., ACLS doses), possesses considerable vasoconstrictor activity. Unlike epinephrine, vasopressin has no beta agonist activity and does not increase myocardial oxygen demand.[1]
3. If pulseless VT/VF persists the next step is to initiate antiarrhythmic drug therapy. Amiodarone is the initial antiarrhythmic of choice as it has been shown to increase survival to hospital admission.
   - **Amiodarone, 300 mg IV push/IO** (6 mL of 50 mg/mL ampule, may be diluted to 20–30 mL of NS or D5W). If pulseless VT/VF persists,

give an additional 150 mg IV push/IO. Initiate an intravenous infusion (450 mg in 250 mL NS, 1.8 mg/mL) at 1 mg/min for 6 h then decrease to 0.5 mg/min if a response is seen to either initial loading dose. Maximum dose is 2.2 g in 24 h (class IIb).

- Amiodarone, in addition to its sodium, potassium, and calcium channel blocking activity, also possesses alpha and beta antagonistic properties. The short-term side effects of amiodarone include bradycardia, hypotension, and QT prolongation. Associated hypotension, which was thought to be due to the diluents polysorbate 80 and benzyl alcohol, has been minimized with a newer aqueous formulation of amiodarone. If hypotension develops, the infusion rate should be slowed.

- Intravenous infusions of amiodarone lasting longer than 2 h should be admixed in glass bottles or polyolefin containers as drug adsorption to plastic containers is likely with prolonged exposure. However, traditional PVC tubing for administration is acceptable.[1,4]

4. If amiodarone fails to control the arrhythmia, consider:

   • **Lidocaine HCL, 1.0–1.5 mg/kg IV push.** If the arrhythmia persists the drug may be given at 0.5–0.75 mg/kg IV push/IO in 5–10 min to a cumulative maximum dose of 3 mg/kg. If the arrhythmia is controlled, initiate an intravenous infusion (1 g/250 mL D5W, 4 mg/mL) at 1–4 mg/min.

   • If IV access has not been established or has been lost, consider administering **lidocaine HCL via endotracheal tube,** (2–2.5 times the intravenous dose, *see* Special Considerations) followed by 3 or 4 rapid ventilations to aerosolize the drug.

      - Class recommendation: Indeterminate (insufficient data to support class recommendation).

      - Lidocaine is a class Ib antiarrhythmic agent, which blocks cellular sodium ion channels and increases the electrical stimulation threshold of the heart. Lidocaine inhibits its own hepatic metabolism after 24–48 h of therapy; therefore it should be used with caution in the elderly and in patients with hepatic dysfunction. Signs of toxicity include mental status changes, muscle twitching, seizures, and bradycardia. If prolonged administration is likely, monitoring of blood levels may be helpful.[1]

5. If amiodarone- and lidocaine-resistant dysrhythmias persist, previous guidelines considered the use of procainamide, a class Ia antiarrhythmic. Use of procainamide in pulseless ventricular arrhythmias in currently limited by slow infusion and questionable efficacy and is no longer routinely recommended.[1]

6. If the rhythm is documented polymorphic VT (Torsades de Pointes) or secondary to hypomagnesemia, administer:

   • **magnesium sulfate, 1–2 g IV infusion/IO** over 5–20 min. Rapid IV push administration can lead to significant hypotension, bradycardia, and asystole; therefore it is not recommended. Consider a maintenance infusion of 0.5–1 g/h if arrhythmia successfully terminates with magnesium (class IIa).[1]

7. Administering sodium bicarbonate during cardiac arrest has traditionally been a controversial issue. Commonly in practice this medication is used in VT/VF arrests only after other accepted interventions (e.g., defibrillation, intubation/ventilation, chest compressions, and vasopressors) have been ineffective.
   - **Sodium bicarbonate, 1 mEq/kg slow IV push** (50 mL of 8.4% solution, 1 mEq/mL)[1].
8. During management of the arrest the provider should also consider the presence of reversible causes of the arrest or factors that may be interfering with successful resuscitation, referred to in the next section as the "H's and T's."[1]

Asystole and Pulseless Electrical Activity (PEA). Asystole is characterized by the lack of cardiac muscular and electrical activity. Survival rates from asystole are extremely poor, as this rhythm is frequently associated with irreversible cardiac damage. PEA was previously known as electromechanical dissociation and is characterized by ineffective cardiac output (hypotension) in the face of ECG evidence of electrical myocardial activity. Etiologies of asystole and PEA are often reversible and can be remembered by the 5 "H's and 5 T's":

Hypovolemia	**T**ablets (drugs)
Hypoxia	**T**amponade (cardiac)
Hydrogen ions (acidosis)	**T**ension pneumothorax
Hypo/ hyperkalemia	**T**hrombosis, coronary
Hypothermia	**T**hrombosis, pulmonary (embolism)

The most effective method to treat asystole and PEA is to correct the underlying cause. These two arrhythmias share similar etiologies and management, thus the treatment algorithms have been combined in the most recent guidelines. The methods discussed below are temporizing measures until the causative etiology is found and remedied. Assume chest compressions and rescue breathing, or the placement of an advanced airway, are already underway. Efforts should be made to minimize interruption in chest compressions.

1. Non-specific treatment measures include administration of:
   - **Epinephrine HCL, 1 mg IV push/IO** (10 mL of 1:10,000 solution) every 3–5 min. A single dose of **vasopressin 40 units IV push/IO** may be administered in place of the first or second dose of epinephrine.
   - If bradycardic, give **atropine sulfate, 1 mg IV push** (10 mL of 0.1 mg/mL solution) every 3–5 min to a maximum dose of 3 mg or 0.04 mg/kg. Atropine can be given via the endotracheal tube at 2–2.5 times the intravenous dose (2–2.5 mg, *See* Special Considerations) followed by 3 or 4 rapid ventilations to aerosolize the drug.
2. Again, the use of buffering agents is controversial. When clinical situations arise where alkalinization is considered necessary (e.g,. hyperkalemia), administer:
   - **Sodium bicarbonate, 1–2 mEq/kg slow IV push over 5 minutes,** (50 mL of 8.4% solution, 1 mEq/mL)

    – In addition to sodium bicarbonate, calcium is also indicated for hyperkalemia with ECG changes. Calcium acts as a cardioprotectant and offsets the arrhythmogenic potential of excessive potassium levels. Administer **calcium chloride, 0.5–1 g slow IV push over 2–5 min** (5–10 mL of 10% solution = 6.8–13.6 mEq).

    – **Glucose 25 g IV** *and* **10 units of regular insulin IV** are also recommended for management of moderate and severe hyperkalemia

    Sodium bicarbonate boluses 1–2 mEq/kg IV repeated to maintain an arterial pH ranging from 7.45–7.55. This treatment is recommended when treating arrhythmias and hypotension related to sodium channel blocking agents and tricyclic antidepressants. (class IIa).

3. Hypovolemia is the most common underlying cause of PEA; therefore, a rapid assessment of fluid status is crucial. In hypovolemic patients, fluid resuscitation using crystalloid (NS or Lactated Ringer's solution) or colloid (hetastarch or human albumin) products should be initiated immediately.

4. If volume is adequate and there is no evidence of cardiac tamponade, consider vasopressors for vasoconstrictor and inotropic/chronotropic effects.

    • **Dopamine HCL, start at 5 μg/kg/min IV infusion** (400 mg/500 mL D5W, 800 μg/mL or 800 mg/500 mL D5W, 1600 μg/mL) and titrate to effect (blood pressure and heart rate). Maximum dose is 20 μg/kg/min. Doses above 20 μg/kg/min have no increased effect on blood pressure and increase the risk for drug-induced tachyarrhythmias.

    – Dopamine possesses dopaminergic, beta and alpha activity. At doses less than 5 μg/kg/min, dopaminergic receptor activation causes an increase in renal and mesenteric blood flow. At doses between 5–10 μg/kg/min, beta-adrenergic receptor stimulation (beta-1 > beta-2) occurs, increasing heart rate and contractility. At doses greater than 10 μg/kg/min, alpha receptor stimulation leads to an increase in systemic vascular resistance (SVR) and elevation in blood pressure.

    • **Norepinephrine bitartrate, start at 0.5–1.0 μg/min IV infusion** (4 mg/250 mL D5W, 16 μg/mL or 8 mg/250 mL D5W, 32 μg/mL) and titrate to effect (blood pressure and heart rate). No maximum dose is noted.

    – Norepinephrine stimulates both alpha- and beta-adrenergic receptors, increasing blood pressure (secondary to increased SVR), heart rate, and contractility.

    – Because increased doses of norepinephrine enhance beta agonist activity (especially in patients with prior cardiac disease), patients are at increased risk for drug-induced tachyarrhythmias.[1]

Bradyarrhythmias. Bradycardia is defined as a heart rate <60 beats per minute. All bradyarrhythmias, which are managed similarly, include: first, second, and third degree heart block, slow ventricular focus, sinus bradycardia, and agonal rhythm. In dealing with any of these symptomatic arrhythmias, cardiac pacing is the best long-term approach (class I). Initial efforts should focus on starting transcutaneous or transvenous pacing for unstable patients. Drugs are used to enhance or initiate cardiac activity, until transcutaneous or transvenous pacing capabilities are available.

1. If symptomatic bradycardia occurs, initiate drug management with:
   - **Atropine sulfate, 0.5 mg IV push** (10 mL of 0.1 mg/mL solution) every 3–5 min to a maximum dose of 3 mg or 0.04 mg/kg.
     - Patients with denervated transplanted hearts will not respond to atropine; therefore, proceed immediately to transcutaneous pacing, administration of catecholamines, or both.
2. If capabilities are available attempt:
   - **Transcutaneous pacing** to capture the slow rhythm and increase heart rate to a level where symptoms disappear. If continued pacing is necessary, continue transcutaneous pacing until a transvenous pacer can be placed.
3. Alternative drug therapy may be considered when response to atropine fails as a temporary measure until transcutaneous pacing can be initiated.
   - **Epinephrine infusion** initiated at **2–10 μg/min IV** and titrated to patient response for patients with bradycardia and hypotension (class IIb).
   - **Dopamine HCl infusion** initiated at **2–10 μg/kg/min** titrated to patient response.
   - **Glucagon 3 mg IV push** followed by an infusion at **3 mg/h** in patients with bradycardia secondary to an overdose of beta blocker or calcium channel blocker agents.[1]

SUPPORTIVE THERAPY

Management of Acidosis. Severe acidosis can develop within 5 min after cardiac arrest and will continue unless BLS is provided. Acidosis can be respiratory and/or (to a lesser extent) metabolic in etiology.

1. Respiratory Acidosis
   - Secondary to hypoventilation and an accumulation of CO_2.
   - Treat by providing adequate ventilation. There is no role for sodium bicarbonate in this situation.
2. Metabolic Acidosis
   - Due to tissue hypoxia and subsequent anaerobic metabolism, which results in slow accumulation of lactic acid.
   - Treat by adequate tissue perfusion and return to aerobic metabolism. Sodium bicarbonate administration is not indicated unless there is evidence of a preexisting metabolic acidosis, hyperkalemia, or tricyclic antidepressant overdose. There is no evidence supporting routine use of bicarbonate and it should be limited to specific clinical situations.
   - If sodium bicarbonate is to be given, the following guidelines are recommended:
     - If an arterial blood gas (ABG) is not available, empirically administer **sodium bicarbonate, 1 mEq/kg IV push over 5 min** (50 mL of 8.4% solution, 1 mEq/mL).
     - If an ABG is available, the sodium bicarbonate dose may be calculated from the base deficit although complete correction of the base deficit should be avoided to prevent unintentional induction of alkalosis.[1]

■ POSTRESUSCITATION CARE

With the ROSC after cardiac arrest, cardiovascular and hemodynamic compromises are often significant and can manifest in the different types of shock (hypovolemic, cardiogenic, and vasodilatory associated with systemic inflammatory response syndrome). If the patient is not already in an intensive care setting, transport to an intensive care unit should occur as soon as possible. Continuous monitoring, resuscitation equipment, and skilled nursing care are needed. Providers should focus on:

- Optimizing perfusion and cardiopulmonary and neurologic function;
- Identifying and treating reversible causes of arrest;
- Monitoring and regulating temperature and metabolism.[1]

THERAPEUTIC HYPOTHERMIA

Therapeutic hypothermia is an induced mild cooling of a patient after cardiac arrest in order to improve neurologic outcomes and survival. It is designed to suppress many of the chemical reactions that occur once reperfusion is established in cardiac arrest survivors to prevent further cerebral injury. The leading cause of disability after cardiac arrest is brain injury, despite the advances in cardiopulmonary management. Though therapeutic hypothermia was included in the 2005 American Heart Association's Guidelines for CPR and Emergency Cardiovascular Care Guidelines, utilization still remains low.[5]

The 2005 American Heart Association's Guidelines for CPR and Emergency Cardiovascular Care include specific treatment recommendations for therapeutic hypothermia:

- Unconscious adult patients resuscitated after out-of-hospital cardiac arrest with an initial rhythm of ventricular fibrillation should be cooled to a **core body temperature of 32°C to 34°C for 12–24 h** (class IIa).
  - Similar therapy may be beneficial for adult patients with in-hospital cardiac arrest or out-of-hospital cardiac arrest associated with an initial rhythm other than ventricular fibrillation (class IIb).

Cooling methods to achieve the goal core body temperature of 32°C to 34°C vary and include use of ice packs, cooling blankets, cold intravenous fluids, and specific devices for inducing, maintaining, and reversing hypothermia. No one method/device is preferred, as none have shown to be superior. When deciding which cooling method to use, several factors need to be considered including:

- Location of the patient undergoing hypothermia (e.g., cooling in the field, emergency department, or intensive care unit)
- Availability of methods/devices to promote cooling at that location.[1]

The optimal timing of initiating hypothermia after resuscitation has not been determined. However, most studies suggest initiation of cooling measures as soon as possible after the resuscitation.[6–8] In previous studies, the time interval between the completion of the resuscitation and cooling ranges from 4 to 16 h.[6–10]

The patient's temperature needs to be closely monitored throughout the process using a bladder, swan, or rectal probe.[1] Continuous electrocardiopulmonary and neurologic monitoring is needed the entire time the patient is being cooled or re-warmed.[1] Once indicated, re-warming should be performed slowly in order to avoid worsening neurologic injury, sudden vasodilation, and shock.[1,11,12]

■ SPECIAL CONSIDERATIONS

- Time to drug effect
  - Systemic circulation times are grossly prolonged during external chest compressions. Remember to allow 1–2 min between the time of peripheral injection and anticipated response. To enhance the onset and activity of peripherally administered medications, give as rapid bolus injections, followed by 20 mL NS flushes and, if possible, elevate the extremity for 10–20 s after administration.[1]
- High-dose epinephrine
  - It was once believed high-dose epinephrine may be more effective than standard ACLS doses. However, more recent studies have found no improvement in survival-to-discharge rates or in neurological outcomes and therefore use of high-dose epinephrine is not recommended.[1]
- Endotracheal administration
  - Administration of epinephrine, lidocaine, vasopressin, and atropine can be accomplished via the endotracheal tube if IV or IO access has not been established or has been lost. Doses are 2–2.5 times the IV dose. Undiluted drug (e.g., epinephrine 1:1000) can be given, but it must be diluted to 10 mL with NS or followed by a 10 mL NS or sterile water flush. Some studies have shown that dilution with sterile water as opposed to NS results in better drug absorption. After administration of medications via the endotracheal route, three or four rapid ventilations should be performed to aerosolize the drug and maximize absorption. This route of administration may not be as effective as IV.[1,3]
- Intraosseous administration
  - Epinephrine, atropine, sodium bicarbonate, lidocaine, vasopressin, vasopressors, or calcium via the distal tibia or the sternum can be used in situations in which IV access and endotracheal intubation have not been established. This route of administration is often reserved for the pediatric population, but may be attempted in adults in whom establishing IV access is difficult.[1,2]
- Intracardiac administration
  - Administration of medication directly in to the myocardium has *no role* in the modern management of cardiac arrest. Drugs do not work within the chambers of the heart, but rather at the cellular level after delivery via coronary circulation. Stopping BLS to attempt intracardiac injections only serves to interrupt vital CNS perfusion.[1]

- Physical Incompatibilities
  - With many medications being given during a cardiac arrest (often through the same IV access site), it is important to recognize the likelihood of physical incompatibilities. Sodium bicarbonate inactivates catecholamines and may form a precipitate when mixed with calcium containing solutions. If possible, concomitant administration should be avoided. If sodium bicarbonate is administered through the same vascular access site, the line must be flushed both before and after bicarbonate administration.[1]

■ REFERENCES

1. American Heart Association in collaboration with the International Liaison Committee on Resuscitation (ILCOR). Guidelines 2005 for cardiopulmonary resuscitation and emergency cardiovascular care: an international consensus on science. *Circulation* 2005;112:IV1-IV203.
2. Iserson KV. Intraosseous infusions in adults. *J Emerg Med.* 1989;7:587-591.
3. Schwab S et al. Moderate hypothermia in the treatment of patients with severe middle cerebral artery infarction. *Stroke.* 1998;29:2461-2466.
4. Package insert. Amiodarone hydrochloride injection. Bedford, OH: Bedford Laboratories. May 2005.
5. Merchant RM et al. Therapeutic hypothermia utilization among physicians after resuscitation from cardiac arrest. *Crit Care Med.* 2006;34:1935-1940.
6. Bernard SA et al. Treatment of comatose survivors of out-of-hospital cardiac arrest with induced hypothermia. *N Engl J Med.* 2002;346(8):557-563.
7. Geocadin RG et al. Management of brain injury after resuscitation from cardiac arrest. *Neurol Clin.* 2008;26: 487-506.
8. Hypothermia after cardiac arrest study group. Mild hypothermia to improve the neurologic outcome after cardiac arrest. *N Engl J Med.* 2002;346:549-556.
9. Bernard SA et al. Clinical trial of induced hypothermia in comatose survivors of out-of-hospital cardiac arrest. *Ann Emerg Med.* 1997;30:146-153.
10. Yanagawa Y et al. Preliminary clinical outcome study of mild resuscitative hypothermia after out-of-hospital cardiopulmonary arrest. *Resuscitation.* 1998;39:61-66.
11. Felberg RA, Krieger DW, Chuang R et al. Hypothermia after cardiac arrest: feasibility and safety of an external cooling protocol. *Circulation.* 2001;104:1799-1804.
12. Raehl CL. Endotracheal drug therapy in cardiopulmonary resuscitation. *Clin Pharm.* 1986;572-579.

Chapter 77

Poisoning

F. Lee Cantrell

Management of the poisoned patient involves procedures designed to prevent the absorption, minimize the toxicity, and hasten the elimination of the suspected toxin. The prompt employment of appropriate emergency management procedures often can prevent unnecessary morbidity and mortality.

A regional poison center is a practitioner's best source of definitive treatment information and should be consulted in all poisoning cases. Consider contacting your regional poison to learn of its staffing, resources, and capabilities before a need for its services arises. Well-qualified regional poison centers are certified by the American Association of Poison Control Centers.

In all cases, every attempt should be made to accurately identify the toxin, estimate the quantity involved, and determine the time that has passed since the exposure. These data, plus patient-specific parameters such as age, weight, sex, clinical status and underlying medical conditions or drug/medication use, will assist you and the regional poison center in designing an appropriate therapeutic plan for the patient.

The techniques described below are intended for the initial management of the poisoned patient with the use of materials that should be readily available.

■ DERMAL EXPOSURES

1. Immediately irrigate affected areas with a copious amount of water; a mild detergent may be used if a stubborn, oily substance is the contaminant. Skin should be gently washed, not scrubbed, and special attention should be given to the hair, skin folds, umbilicus, and other areas where the contaminant might be trapped.
2. If the patient's clothes have been contaminated, remove them during the irrigation and clean them before they are worn again. Clothing can interfere with the irrigation process and serve as a reservoir of toxic material.
3. Do not attempt to "neutralize" the contaminant with another chemical (e.g., acids and alkalis). Attempts at neutralization waste valuable time, are of no benefit, and might be harmful.
4. Do not cover the affected area with emollients. These can trap unremoved contaminant against the skin. Severely damaged skin may be temporarily covered with a light, dry dressing.
5. Protect yourself from contamination. Protective gowns, goggles, face shields and nitrile gloves will minimize the risk of secondary exposure.
6. After the irrigation is complete, contact a regional poison center for specific treatment information.

■ EYE EXPOSURES

1. Immediately irrigate the eye; damage can occur within seconds. The stream of tap water or normal saline should strike the patient on the bridge of the nose and then flow into the eye.
2. The eyelids should be open, with frequent blinking during the irrigation.
3. The irrigation should continue for at least 15 min (by the clock) to ensure adequate removal of the contaminant and normalization of the conjunctival pH.
4. After the irrigation is complete, contact a regional poison center for specific treatment information.

■ INHALATION EXPOSURES

1. Remove the patient from the suspected contaminated area, regardless of its apparent safety. Some inhaled toxins, such as carbon monoxide, cannot be detected by sight, smell, or taste.
2. Institute artificial ventilation, if necessary, and provide supplementary humidified oxygen, if available and needed.
3. Protect yourself from contamination at all times.
4. Contact a regional poison center for specific treatment information.

■ INGESTIONS

1. Remove any remaining contaminant from inside and around the mouth of the patient.
2. Contact a regional poison center for specific treatment information.
3. In many cases, it will not be necessary to take additional steps. The following information can be used if additional care is recommended by the regional poison center.

■ GASTROINTESTINAL DECONTAMINATION

Gastrointestinal (GI) decontamination can be accomplished by the administration of activated charcoal, gastric lavage or whole-bowel irrigation. GI decontamination may be useful with ingestions of a potentially toxic amount of a substance or of an unknown dose of a toxic substance. None of these techniques should be presumed to provide complete removal or binding of the ingested toxin(s). Comparative experimental studies have shown only limited success with these techniques, and there is considerable interpatient variability in the results.[1] For all methods of GI decontamination, efficacy diminishes rapidly with time. Scientific data suggest that GI decontamination is most effective if instituted within 1 h after ingestion. In general, activated charcoal is the most useful agent for preventing absorption of ingested toxic substances. Other methods of GI decontamination may be considered if the ingested contaminant is not adsorbed by activated charcoal or if the benefits of the interventions outweigh the risks involved.

ACTIVATED CHARCOAL

Activated charcoal is a nonspecific adsorbent that binds unabsorbed toxins within the GI tract. There is limited experience using activated charcoal in the home setting.[2]

Activated charcoal is not effective for adsorbing strong acids and alkalis, ethanol, methanol, ethylene glycol, or elemental substances such as iron and lithium.

1. Activated charcoal is administered orally or by gastric tube. Typical doses are 50–100 g in adults and 1 g/kg in children.
2. Activated charcoal is commercially supplied as a slurry in water or a powder for dispersion in a liquid vehicle. Gentle encouragement may be needed to make children swallow the charcoal. Mixing the activated charcoal in an enjoyable beverage (e.g., juice, milk, soda) and having the child take the liquid through a drinking straw is sometimes helpful.
3. In decades previous, activated charcoal administration had either been combined with or followed by the administration of a cathartic (e.g., sorbitol, magnesium citrate, or magnesium sulfate) to hasten the elimination of the activated charcoal–toxin complex. To date, there is no scientific evidence to support the use of cathartics in poisonings.
4. Alert the patient that charcoal will cause the stools to turn black.
5. Repeated oral doses of activated charcoal (e.g., 25 g q2–4h) have been used to enhance the elimination of some drugs, most notably carbamazepine, dapsone, phenobarbital, quinine, and theophylline. While controlled studies have shown that multiple-dose activated charcoal can decrease drug concentrations in the serum, positive effects of this intervention on patient outcome have not been clearly demonstrated. Multiple-dose activated charcoal is only suitable for patients with active bowel sounds.

GASTRIC LAVAGE

Gastric lavage has declined in popularity over the last decade due to little available clinical evidence to support its use.[3] Situations in which it may be considered include recent massive ingestions or with ingestions of extremely toxic substances (e.g., paraquat). Lavage is contraindicated for patients who have ingested corrosives or hydrocarbons (i.e., gasoline) and for patients at risk for esophageal or gastric perforation due to underlying medical conditions (e.g., esophageal varices).

1. The patient should be placed in the left lateral decubitus position to prevent ingested material from being pushed into the duodenum. If the patient's gag reflex is weak or absent, the airway must be protected by the use of a cuffed endotracheal tube.
2. The largest possible orogastric tube should be used (26–28 F for children and 34–42 F for adults): the larger the tube diameter, the more efficient the lavage. The tube should be introduced through the mouth with the aid of a water-soluble lubricant. Nasogastric passage is not recommended.
3. Gastric lavage may be performed with water, but a solution such as 0.45% NaCl may be used to minimize the risk of dilutional hyponatremia, especially in children. Aliquots of fluid up to 100 mL in children and 200 mL in adults are introduced through the tube and then removed by gravity or suction-assisted drainage. The lavage should be continued until the returning fluid is clear. Warming the lavage fluid reduces the risk of hypothermia.

INDUCTION OF EMESIS

While employed for centuries as a method of gastric emptying, routine induction of emesis in potentially poisoned patients is no longer advocated.[4] The induction of emesis should only be considered following specific recommendations from a poison control center, an emergency department physician, or other qualified medical personnel.

Do not induce emesis if the patient is experiencing or is at risk for CNS depression, seizures, or loss of gag reflex, or if the patient has ingested a caustic substance or a hydrocarbon with high aspiration potential (e.g., gasoline).

1. Induce emesis only with **syrup of ipecac.** Salt water, mustard water, other "home remedies," or gagging have no place in the management of the poisoned patient. These techniques are ineffective and can be dangerous.
2. The usual initial dose of syrup of ipecac is 30 mL in persons older than 12 years, 15 mL in children 1–12 years old, and 10 mL in children between 6 months and 1 year.
3. Give the patient additional water to drink: 125–250 mL (4–8 fluid ounces) in children, 250–500 mL (8–16 fluid ounces) in adults. Activated charcoal should not be given until after ipecac-induced emesis has occurred.
4. Emesis usually occurs within 15–20 min. If 30 min have passed without emesis, administer an additional dose of syrup of ipecac and more water.
5. Have the patient vomit into a bowl or other container so that the vomitus can be inspected for the presence of the ingested toxin.

WHOLE-BOWEL IRRIGATION

Whole-bowel irrigation with an orally administered **polyethylene glycol electrolyte solution** (e.g., GoLYTELY or CoLyte) is commonly used before bowel procedures. It is used as an alternative to or in conjunction with activated charcoal administration in the management of acute poison ingestions. Results of studies are mixed but the technique may have value in cases of ingestions involving substances poorly adsorbed to activated charcoal, enteric-coated or sustained-release products, foreign bodies,[5] and drug smuggling packets. Instillation rates range from 500 mL/h in children to 2 L/h in adults. The endpoint of therapy is clearing of the rectal effluent or 10 L total volume. Contraindications to whole-bowel irrigation are persistent vomiting, adynamic ileus, bowel obstruction or perforation, and GI hemorrhage.

■ REFERENCES

1. Heard K. Gastrointestinal decontamination. *Med Clin North Am.* 2005;89:1067-1078.
2. Eldridge DL et al. Pediatric toxicology. *Emerg Med Clin North Am.* 2007;25:283-308.
3. Greene S et al. Gastrointestinal decontamination of the poisoned patient. *Pediatr Emerg Care.* 2008;24:176-186.
4. Manoguerra AS, Cobaugh DJ; Guidelines for the Management of Poisoning Consensus Panel. Guideline on the use of ipecac syrup in the out-of-hospital management of ingested poisons. *Clin Toxicol.* 2005;43(1):1-10.
5. Greene SL et al. Acute poisoning: understanding 90% of cases in a nutshell. *Postgrad Med J.* 2005;81:204-216.

Chapter 78

Status Epilepticus

April D. Miller

Status epilepticus is a medical emergency in which prompt recognition and effective medical intervention are required to reduce the risk of permanent sequelae and death. Status epilepticus is defined as continuous seizures lasting at least 5 min, or two or more sequential seizures without full recovery of consciousness between seizures.

Status epilepticus can be categorized into two major types: convulsive and nonconvulsive. Convulsive status epilepticus is associated with the highest risk of morbidity and mortality, so this section focuses on the clinical features and management of this form of status epilepticus.

In about one-half of patients, status epilepticus is the first manifestation of seizures. The causes of status epilepticus are similar to those for new-onset seizures and include CNS infection, cerebral tumor, trauma, stroke, metabolic disorders, cardiopulmonary arrest with cerebral anoxia, and drug toxicity. In the remainder of patients, status epilepticus occurs in the setting of a preexisting seizure disorder. Among persons with a history of epilepsy, antiepileptic drug withdrawal (usually noncompliance with prescribed therapy) is the most common cause of status epilepticus.

The primary determinant of patient outcome after status epilepticus is the underlying cause of the episode. In general, patients with status caused by an acute or progressive neurologic insult (e.g., cardiopulmonary arrest, stroke) have poorer outcomes than patients in whom status epilepticus occurs in the setting of a more chronic or stable underlying condition (e.g., antiepileptic drug withdrawal or medically refractory epilepsy). Nonetheless, aggressive medical intervention and administration of effective antiepileptic drug therapy are important to reduce status-related morbidity and mortality, regardless of the etiology.

Status epilepticus should be managed in an emergency department or an environment where continuous skilled medical and nursing support are available. The emergency management of status epilepticus should include the following:

- Ensure airway patency and adequate oxygenation.
- Obtain blood specimens for baseline laboratory measurements, including CBC, serum electrolytes (including calcium and magnesium), toxicology, screen, and anticonvulsant serum levels.
- Establish IV access.
- Administer IV glucose (100 mg thiamine followed by 50 mL of 50% dextrose in adult patients at risk for nutritional deficiencies).
- Administer IV antiepileptic drugs.
- Monitor BP, respiratory rate, and temperature. Treat hyperthermia with passive cooling.
- Obtain other diagnostic studies as needed.
- Treat precipitating factors.

■ DRUG THERAPY OF STATUS EPILEPTICUS

Only adult doses are given in this section.

If a treatable cause of status epilepticus can be identified rapidly, then drug therapy to terminate seizures might be unnecessary. In these situations, treatment of the underlying cause might be sufficient to stop status. Examples are status caused by an acute metabolic derangement (where correction of the underlying abnormality often stops seizures) or status after isoniazid overdose (where IV pyridoxine is usually effective). However, when a treatable cause is not known, drug therapy should begin immediately. The goal of drug treatment is to terminate seizures as rapidly as possible. Evidence from animal and human studies indicates that 60–120 min of status epilepticus is associated with neurologic sequelae and that the risk increases as status continues. Thus, it is important to have a clear, stepwise plan for the administration of effective drug therapy. Figure 78-1 shows an example of a status epilepticus treatment protocol. In addition, adequate support should be available to manage cardiac and respiratory complications that might occur during drug administration.

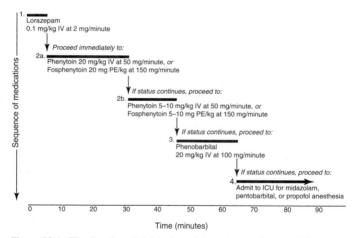

Figure 78-1. Timeline for administration of drug therapy for convulsive status epilepticus. Heavy bars (—) indicate duration (in minutes) of intravenous drug administration. PE = phenytoin equivalents.

1. For rapid termination of seizures
   - **Lorazepam, IV, 0.1 mg/kg (4–8 mg) at rate of 2 mg/min;** may repeat in 10 min if seizures continue (to maximum of 0.2 mg/kg). Lorazepam has a longer duration of anticonvulsant effect than diazepam and is often preferred for this reason.
   or
   - **Diazepam, IV, 0.2 mg/kg (maximum initial dose 10 mg) at rate of 5 mg/min;** may repeat in 10 min if seizures continue (to maximum

of 20 mg). Diazepam has a short duration of anticonvulsant effect (15–60 min) and must be immediately followed by a long-acting agent (e.g., phenytoin).

2a. After benzodiazepine administration, give:
- **Phenytoin, IV infusion, 20 mg/kg at rate of 50 mg/min** or **fosphenytoin 20 mg/kg phenytoin equivalents IV at a rate of 150 mg/min.** Monitor BP and ECG during administration of phenytoin or fosphenytoin loading dose. Elderly and severely ill patients are predisposed to phenytoin-related hypotension and arrhythmias. Fosphenytoin may also be administered intramuscularly at the same dose. However, this route is associated with delayed peak concentrations and should only be used when IV access cannot be obtained.

2b. If status continues, then give up to 2 additional doses of 5 mg/kg to a total dose of phenytoin/fosphenytoin of 30 mg/kg. If status is terminated, then begin maintenance phenytoin or fosphenytoin therapy.

3. If seizures are not terminated after administration of phenytoin or fosphenytoin 30 mg/kg, *then:*
- **Phenobarbital, IV, 20 mg/kg at rate of 100 mg/min.** The risk of hypoventilation is increased markedly when phenobarbital is administered after a benzodiazepine; respiratory support is often required. Phenobarbital use in status epilepticus is controversial because of a high risk of respiratory depression.

4. For patients who continue in status epilepticus despite the above recommendations, anesthetic doses of a benzodiazepine, barbiturate, or propofol are often required to suppress seizure activity. Ventilatory assistance and vasopressor drug therapy are often required; therefore, the patient should be admitted to the ICU and the following therapies considered:

3a. **Midazolam, IV slow push, 0.2 mg/kg,** *then maintenance:*
- **Midazolam, IV infusion, 0.05–2 mg/kg/h.** High-dose midazolam is probably associated with a lower risk of hypotension than high-dose pentobarbital; however, there is less experience with its use.

3b. **Propofol, IV slow push, 1–2 mg/kg, max 10mg/kg,** *then maintenance:*
- **Propofol, IV infusion 2–10 mg/kg/h.** Reduce dosage by one-half in elderly or hemodynamically unstable patients.

The EEG should be monitored continuously during the first 1–2 h of therapy, and infusion rates should be adjusted until suppression of electrographic seizures is evident. After seizures are terminated, the rate of the maintenance infusion can be slowed periodically to determine if status has remitted.

3c. **Pentobarbital, IV slow push 10–15 mg/kg, *then maintenance:***
- **Pentobarbital, IV infusion, 0.5–1 mg/kg/h.** Hypotension is a frequent complication of high-dose pentobarbital therapy; a vasopressor (e.g., dopamine) may be required.

There is also limited evidence for newer parenteral antiepileptic agents in the treatment of refractory status epilepticus that do not appear in algorithms. These include valproic acid and levetiracetam.

■ REFERENCES

1. Kalviainen R. Status epilepticus treatment guidelines. *Epilepsia*. 2007;48(suppl 8):99-102.
2. Prasad K et al. Anticonvulsant therapy for status epilepticus (Review). *Cochrane Database Syst Rev.* 2005;CD003723.
3. Prasad K et al. Anticonvulsant therapy for status epilepticus. *Br J Clin Pharmacol.* 2007; 63:640-647.
4. Rosenow F, Knake S. Recent and future advances in the treatment of status epilepticus. Ther Adv Neurol Disord 2008;1:25-32.

Drug Interactions and Interferences

5

Kelly M. Smith

Chapter 79

Cytochrome P450 Enzyme Interactions

John R. Horn

Cytochrome P450 enzymes are found throughout the body and play an important role in the metabolism of many drugs by catalyzing α-hydroxylation, N-demethylation, ring oxidation, and more.[1,2] Most substrates are metabolized by a specific enzyme, whereas each cytochrome P450 enzyme is generally capable of metabolizing many different compounds.[2,3] Induction or inhibition of these enzymes can dramatically affect the outcome of drug therapy.

Cytochrome P450 enzymes are identified by the prefix "CYP" followed by an Arabic number identifying the family. The three important enzyme families in humans are CYP1, CYP2, and CYP3. Subfamilies are given letters (e.g., CYP2B, CYP2C) that are followed by numbers identifying the specific enzyme (e.g., CYP2C9).[4]

Although most concentrated in the liver, cytochrome P450 enzymes exist in all tissues of the human body.[2,3] Intestinal mucosal cytochrome P450 enzymes appear to be generally from the CYP3A family, primarily CYP3A4 in humans.[3] These enzymes can markedly affect the bioavailability of some drugs.

■ INDUCTION AND INHIBITION

When the amount of enzyme present in the body is increased by a drug or chemical, the enzyme is said to be "induced." Although most inducers are P450 substrates, this is not always the case. Induction can increase the rate of clearance of a drug, decreasing its efficacy. It also can increase the rate of formation of an active or toxic metabolite, resulting in exaggeration of therapeutic effect or increased toxicity.

Theoretically, all substrates metabolized by a specific enzyme can compete for the same binding site, causing competitive inhibition. However, the clinical relevance of competitive inhibition depends on the concentrations, relative affinities, and the presence of other elimination pathways of each substrate. Like inducers, not all inhibitors are enzyme substrates. Some drugs or their metabolites can form an inactive complex with a cytochrome P450 enzyme or its heme group resulting in enzyme inhibition that persists after the drug's plasma concentrations have declined. Inhibition can lead to increased toxic effects by causing drug accumulation, or it can lower toxic or therapeutic effects by decreasing the amount of toxic or active metabolite(s).

■ DRUG INTERACTIONS

Knowing which drugs are metabolized by each cytochrome P450 enzyme and the drugs that influence those enzymes can help in predicting drug–drug interactions. However, there are additional points to consider when predicting drug interactions.

The effect of inhibition on drug elimination depends partly on whether a substrate has alternate elimination pathways. Inhibition of an enzyme might not be clinically important if there are alternative metabolic pathways. However, phenytoin, which is metabolized by CYP2C9 and CYP2C19, can interact with CYP2C9 and CYP2C19 inhibitors, resulting in phenytoin toxicity.

Therapeutic range also is important. If a drug has a wide therapeutic range, factors such as induction or inhibition might be clinically unimportant. The opposite is true for drugs with a narrow therapeutic range, such as warfarin and antiarrhythmics.

Last, consider metabolites. Not only does inhibition and induction of cytochrome P450 enzymes influence the formation of active metabolites, the formation of active metabolites can enhance inhibition or induction. Fluoxetine, an inhibitor of CYP2D6, has an active metabolite norfluoxetine that also inhibits CYP2D6.

The following table is meant to serve as an aid in the prediction of drug–drug interactions. However, it is also important to consider many other parameters: whether the patient is a poor or extensive metabolizer, the affinity of the drug for the binding site, the concentration of drug in the liver, the presence of alternate elimination pathways, and the therapeutic range of the drug. Because research on P450 metabolism is currently being published at a rapid rate, the table is not complete. The absence of a drug from the table does not necessarily imply that it is not metabolized by one of the P450 enzymes. When using the table, consider the following principles:

- Inhibition of drug metabolism tends to be substrate independent. That is, a potent inhibitor of CYP2D6 is likely to inhibit the metabolism of any drug metabolized by CYP2D6.
- The magnitude of cytochrome P450 enzyme inhibition is usually dose-related over the dosage range of the inhibitor. For example, fluconazole 100 mg/d is usually a modest inhibitor of CYP3A4, but at 400 mg/d it can substantially inhibit the isozyme.
- Some cytochrome P450 inhibitors affect more than one enzyme. For example, ritonavir inhibits both CYP2D6 and CYP3A4.
- Drug enantiomers can be metabolized by different cytochrome P450 isozymes. For example, (R)-warfarin is metabolized by CYP1A2 and CYP3A4, and the more potent (S)-warfarin is metabolized primarily by CYP2C9. Thus, CYP1A2 or CYP3A4 inhibitors tend to produce only small increases in the hypoprothrombinemic response to warfarin, and CYP2C9 inhibitors produce large increases in warfarin effect.

COMMON DRUGS THAT INTERACT WITH P450 ENZYMES

SUBFAMILY SUBSTRATES		INDUCERS	INHIBITORS
1A2	acetaminophen, amitriptyline, caffeine, clomipramine, clozapine, frovatriptan, imipramine, olanzapine, ondansetron, tacrine, theophylline, (R)-warfarin, zileuton	barbiturates, charcoal-broiled food, carbamazepine, rifampin, smoking	atazanavir, ciprofloxacin, clarithromycin, enoxacin, erythromycin, fluvoxamine, mexiletine, tacrine, zileuton
2B6	bupropion, cyclophosphamide, ifosfamide	phenobarbital, phenytoin	clopidogrel, thiotepa, ticlopidine
2C8	benzphetamine, cerivastatin, diazepam, diclofenac, (R)-mephenytoin, paclitaxel, pioglitazone, rosiglitazone, zopiclone		gemfibrozil, trimethoprim
2C9	celecoxib, diclofenac, dronabinol, flurbiprofen, hexobarbital, ibuprofen, losartan, (R)-mephenytoin, montelukast, naproxen, phenytoin, piroxicam, tolbutamide, torsemide, (S)-warfarin	barbiturates, carbamazepine, phenytoin, primidone, rifampin, rifapentine	amiodarone, clopidogrel, disulfiram, efavirenz, fluconazole, fluoxetine, fluvastatin, imatinib, metronidazole, ritonavir, sulfamethoxazole, sulfinpyrazone, voriconazole, zafirlukast
2C19	amitriptyline, clomipramine, diazepam, esomeprazole, hexobarbital, imipramine, lansoprazole, mephenytoin, mephoomeprazole, omeprazole, pantoprazole, phenytoin, propranolol, vorcorazole	carbamazepine, rifampin, St. John's wort	efavirenz, esomeprazole, felbamate, fluoxetine, fluvoxamine, omeprazole, ticlopidine, voriconazole
2D6	amitriptyline, carvedilol, chorpheniramine, clomipramine, codeine, debrisoquine, desipramine, dextromethorphan, diphenhydramine, flecainide, fluoxetine, galantamine, haloperidol, hydrocodone, imipramine, loratadine, metoprolol, mexiletine, paroxetine, perphenazine, propafenone, propranolol, risperidone, thioridazine, timolol, tramadol, trazodone, venlafaxine		amiodarone, bupropion, chloroquine, cimetidine, diphenhydramine, fluoxetine, haloperidol, paroxetine, perphenazine, propoxyphene, quinidine, ritonavir, SSRIs,[a] terbinafine, thioridazine
2E1	acetaminophen, alcohol, chlorzoxazone, dapsone, halothane, isoflurane, methoxyflurane, sevoflurane	alcohol (chronic), isoniazid	alcohol (acute intoxication), disulfiram

(continued)

COMMON DRUGS THAT INTERACT WITH P450 ENZYMES (continued)

	SUBFAMILY SUBSTRATES	INDUCERS	INHIBITORS
3A4	alfentanil, alprazolam, amiodarone, [b] amitriptyline, amlodipine, androgens, atorvastatin, benzphetamine, bromocriptine, buspirone, carbamazepine, cilostazol, cisapride, clomipramine, clonazepam, cocaine, corticosteroids, cyclosporine, [b,c] dapsone, dexamethasone, [c] diazepam, diltiazem, [b,c] disopyramide, doxorubicin, [c] ergotamine, erythromycin, [b] ethinyl estradiol, ethosuximide, etoposide, [c] felodipine, [b] fentanyl, fexofenadine, finasteride, galantamine, hydrocortisone, [b,c] ifosfamide, imatinib, imipramine, indinavir, isradipine, itraconazole, [b] ketoconazole, [b] lidocaine, [b] losartan, lovastatin, miconazole, midazolam, mifepristone, [b] montelukast, nefazodone, nelfinavir, [b,c] nicardipine, [b,c] nifedipine, [b] nimodipine, nisoldipine, nitrendipine, [b] omeprazole, paclitaxel, [c] pimozide, pioglitazone, progesterone, propafenone, quinidine, [b] quinine, rifabutin, ritonavir, [b,c] saquinavir, [b,c] sertraline, sibutramine, sildenafil, simvastatin, sirolimus, [c] tacrolimus, [b,c] tamoxifen, teniposide, testosterone, [b] theophylline, triazolam, troleandomycin, verapamil, [b,c] vinca alkaloids, [c] voriconazole, (R)-warfarin, zolpidem	aminoglutethimide, barbiturates, bosentan, carbamazepine, corticosteroids, [c] efavirenz, griseofulvin, phenytoin, primidone, rifabutin, rifampin, St. John's wort, sulfinpyrazone	conivaptan, [b] cyclophosphamide, cyclosporine, [b,c] darunavir, delavirdine, diltiazem, [b,c] fluconazole, fluvoxamine, grapefruit juice, ifosfamide, indinavir, [b,c] itraconazole, [b] ketoconazole, [b] macrolides, [d] miconazole (IV), nefazodone, nelfinavir, [b,c] nicardipine, [b,c] quinupristin, ritonavir, [b,c] verapamil, [b,c] zafirlukast

[a] CYP2D6 enzyme inhibition by SSRI varies by drug: paroxetine = fluoxetine >> sertraline > citalopram > fluvoxamine.

[b] Also an inhibitor of P-glycoprotein.[7]

[c] Also a substrate of P-glycoprotein.[7]

[d] CYP3A4 enzyme inhibition by macrolide antibiotics varies by drug: troleandomycin > erythromycin > clarithromycin > azithromycin = dirithromycin = 0.

Compiled from Refs. 5–7.

■ REFERENCES

1. Correia M. Drug biotransformation. In: Katzung BG, ed. *Basic and Clinical Pharmacology*. New York, NY: The McGraw-Hill Companies, Inc; 2007:50-64.
2. Watkins PB. Role of cytochromes P450 in drug metabolism and hepatotoxicity. *Semin Liver Dis*. 1990;10:235-250.
3. Watkins PB. Drug metabolism by cytochromes P450 in the liver and small bowel. *Gastroenterol Clin North Am*. 1992;21:511-526.
4. Anzenbacher P, Anzenbacherova E. Cytochromes P450 and metabolism of xenobiotics. *Cell Mol Life Sci*. 2001;58:737-747.
5. Tatro DS, ed. *Drug Interactions Facts*. St. Louis, MO: Facts and Comparisons; 2007.
6. Hansten PD, Horn JR. *Drug Interactions Analysis and Management*. St. Louis, MO.: Facts and Comparisons; 2008.
7. Hansten PD, Horn JR. *The Top 100 Drug Interactions: A Guide To Patient Management*. Freeland, WA: H&H Publications; 2008.

Chapter 80

Drug-Induced Discoloration of Feces and Urine

Annette T. McFarland and Amy Sutton Peak

Medications, foods, dyes, chemicals, and various medical conditions can lead to discolored urine or feces. In many instances, drug-induced discoloration of urine or feces is harmless and transient. There is no specific treatment for discolored urine or feces. Identifying the underlying cause of the discoloration will guide treatment. Nontoxic discoloration caused by some medications does not necessitate drug discontinuation. It is important to differentiate innocuous drug-induced discolorations from more serious conditions/adverse effects that could be related to drug therapy. For example, when feces color changes to black or red or becomes tarry in consistency, consider blood loss. Similarly, heme tests should be considered when urine appears pink, red, or brown. This is especially important when evaluating patients receiving medications that may cause bleeding (e.g., anticoagulants, antiplatelets, corticosteroids, NSAIDS). The tables below outline a myriad of medications that have been reported to cause discoloration of urine or feces.

DRUGS THAT CAN DISCOLOR FECES	
DRUG/DRUG CLASS	COLOR PRODUCED
Acetazolamide	black
Aloe/aloin	black[a]
Aminophylline	black
Aminosalicylic acid	black[a]
Amphetamine	black
Amphotericin B	black
Antacids (aluminum hydroxide types)	white/speckling or black
Antibiotics, Oral	greenish gray or white/speckling or black
Anticoagulants (i.e. heparin or warfarin)	pink to red or black[a]
Bismuth Salts	green-black
Carbamazepine + Thioridazine	orange
Cefdinir	red
Charcoal	black
Chloramphenicol	blue or black
Chlorpropamide	black
Chlorophyll	green

(continued)

DRUGS THAT CAN DISCOLOR FECES (*continued*)

DRUG/DRUG CLASS	COLOR PRODUCED
Clindamycin	black
Clofazimine	red to brown-black
Colchicine	gray-white
Copper	black
Corticosteroids	black[a]
Cyclophosphamide	black
Cytarabine	black
Deferoxamine	black
Digitalis	black
Ergot preparations	tarry
Ethacrynic acid	black
Fats/lipids	black or clay/putty or yellow
Ferrous salts	black or green
Floxuridine	black
Fluorides	black
Fluorouracil	black
Gold	yellow green
Halothane	black
Histamine	black
Hydralazine	black
Indocyanine Green	green or white/speckling
Indomethacin	green (due to biliverdinemia) or black[a]
Iodine-containing drugs	black
Isopropanol	black
Laxatives (e.g., senna)	green or yellow
Levodopa	black
Lincomycin	black
Manganese	black or blue or pink or dark brown
Mefenamic acid	black
Melphalan	black
Mercury	black or tan
Methotrexate	black
Methylene blue	black or blue
Nitrates	black
NSAIDs	pink to red or tarry or black[a]
Omeprazole	discoloration
Orlistat	yellow

(*continued*)

DRUGS THAT CAN DISCOLOR FECES (*continued*)

DRUG/DRUG CLASS	COLOR PRODUCED
Phenazopyridine	orange-red
Phenylephrine	black
Phosphorous	black
Potassium salts	black
Procarbazine	black
Reserpine	black
Rifampin	red-orange
Rifabutin	red or orange
Risperidone	discoloration
Salicylates (especially aspirin)	pink to red or tarry or black[a]
Silver	black
Sulfonamides	black
Tetracycline	red (syrup) or black
Theophylline	black
Thiotepa	black

[a]Can indicate intestinal bleeding.

DRUGS THAT CAN DISCOLOR URINE

DRUG/DRUG CLASS	COLOR PRODUCED
Acetaminophen	dark brown (with overdose)
Aloe/aloin	red-brown or yellow-brown or rust or pink (in alkaline urine)
Aminosalicylic Acid (ASA; aspirin)	yellow-brown red in hypochlorite solution[a]
Amitriptyline	blue-green
Anthraquinones (i.e. cascara & senna)	yellow-brown or brown-black (in acidic urine) green or blue or violet or red or pink (in alkaline urine)
Bismuth	yellow-brown
Cadmium	dark
Chlorophyll	blue or green
Chloroquine	rust yellow to brown or red or black
Chlorpromazine	red
Chlorzoxazone	orange or purplish red
Choline salicylate	pink
Cimetidine (injection)	green[b]
Clofazimine	red to brown-black

(*continued*)

DRUGS THAT CAN DISCOLOR URINE (*continued*)

DRUG/DRUG CLASS	COLOR PRODUCED
Cotrimoxazole (TMP/SMZ)	black
Cyanokit®	red
Daunorubicin	red
Deferoxamine	red-brown or pink
DeWitts Pills®	blue
Dihydroergotamine mesylate	orange or red
Doan's Pills®	blue-green
Doxorubicin	red
Entacapone	brown-orange
Erythrityl tetranitrate	brown or red or pink
Ferrous Salts	dark or black or red
Flutamide	amber or yellow-green or blue-green
Gandolinium texaphyrin	green
Heparin	red-brown[c]
Ibuprofen	red-purple
Idarubicin	red
Imipenem/cilastatin	discoloration
Indomethacin	green (due to biliverdinemia)
Isosorbide	brown-black
Laxatives	red or orange
Levodopa	red-brown (in acidic urine) dark brown black or red (in hypochlorite solution[a])
Loratadine	discoloration
Magnesium salicylate	blue-green
Methocarbamol	dark brown or black or blue-green (on standing)
Methyldopa	dark brown-black or red (in hypochlorite solution[a])
Methylene blue	blue or green
Metronidazole	dark or rust or yellow-brown or brown black
Mitoxantrone	blue-green
Niacin	dark
Nitrates	brown-black
Nitrofurantoin	rust yellow to brown-black
Oxyphenbutazone	red-brown
Phenazopyridine	orange to red-brown (in acidic urine)
Phenothiazines	pink to red or red-brown
Phenytoin	pink to red or red-brown
Primaquine	rust yellow to brown

(*continued*)

DRUGS THAT CAN DISCOLOR URINE (*continued*)

DRUG/DRUG CLASS	COLOR PRODUCED
Promethazine (injection)	green[b]
Propofol (injection)	blue-green or white or pink or brown or red-brown
Quinine	brown or black or dark or red-brown[c]
Resorcinol	dark or green or blue (on standing)
Rifabutin	brown-orange
Rifampin	red-orange or pink
Rifapentine	red-orange
Salicylates (i.e., aspirin)	pink[c]
Sulfasalazine	orange-yellow (in alkaline urine)
Sulfonamides, antibacterial	black or rust yellow to brown[c]
Sulindac	discoloration
Thioridazine	red
Tiopronin	brown
Tolcapone	bright yellow
Triamterene	pale blue fluorescence
Vitamin A (retinoids & β-carotene)	yellow-orange
Vitamin B₂ (riboflavin)	yellow fluorescence or rust or dark or red or brown or orange
Vitamin C (ascorbic acid)	orange
Warfarin	orange or red-brown[c]

[a]Hypochlorite solution in toilet bowl from prior use of chlorine bleach
[b]Caused by phenol as a preservative in the injectable formulation
[c]Could be a sign of bleeding

■ REFERENCES

1. Allen J, Burson SC. Drug discoloration of the urine. Detail document 150907. Pharmacist's Letter Online. Stockton, CA: Therapeutic Research Center. http://www.pharmacistsletter.com/. Accessed September 15, 2008.
2. Baran RB, Rowles B. Factors affecting coloration of urine and feces. *J Am Pharm Assoc*. 1973;NS13:139-142.
3. Blakey SA, Hixson-Wallace JA. Clinical significance of rare and benign side effects: propofol and green urine. *Pharmacotherapy*. 2000;20:1120-1122.
4. Bodenham A et al. Propofol infusion and green urine [letter]. *Lancet*. 1987;2:740.
5. Bowling P et al. Intravenous medications and green urine [letter]. *JAMA*. 1981;246:216.
6. Brooks DJ. Safety and tolerability of COMT inhibitors. *Neurology*. 2004;62(1)(suppl 1):S39-S46.
7. Chong BS, Mersfelder TL. Entacapone. *Ann Pharmacother*. 2000;34(9):1056-1065.
8. Clark PM, Clark JD, Wheatley T. Urine discoloration after acetaminophen overdose. *Clin Chem*. 1986;32(9):1777-1778.
9. Cohen BA, Mikol DD. Mitoxantrone treatment of multiple sclerosis: safety considerations. *Neurology*. 2004;63(suppl 6):S28-S32.
10. Package insert. Cyanokit. Napa, CA: Dey, L.P.; 2007.
11. Devereaux MW, Mancall EL. Brown urine, bleach, and L-DOPA [letter]. *N Engl J Med*. 1974;291:1142.
12. DiPalma JR. Drugs that induce changes in urine color. *RN*. 1977;40(1):34-35.
13. Fecal Discoloration Induced by Drugs, Chemicals, and Disease States. Drugdex Consults. Greenwood Village, CO. Thomson Micromedex. http://www.thomsonhc.com/hcs/librarian. Accessed November 13, 2008.

14. Gastroenterology. *Pharmacist's Let.* 2007;23(11). http://www.pharamcistsletter.com/. Accessed September 15, 2008.
15. Getting GK, Roberts JR. Urine discoloration secondary to metronidazole. *Am J Emerg Med.* 2001;19(4):322.
16. Keung AC et al. Single-dose pharmacokinetics of rifapentine in women. *J Pharmacokinet Biopharm.* 1998;26(1):75-85.
17. Koller W et al. Randomized trial of tolcapone versus pergolide as add-on to levodopa therapy in Parkinson's disease patients with motor fluctuations [abstract]. *Mov Disord.* 2001;16(5):858-866.
18. Michaels RM, ed. Discolored urine. *Phys Drug Alert.* 1981;2(9):71.
19. Nalin DR et al. Imipenem/cilastatin for pediatric infections in hospitalized patients [abstract]. *Scand J Infect Dis Suppl.* 1987;52:56-64.
20. Nates J et al. Appearance of white urine during propofol anesthesia [letter]. *Anesth Analg.* 1995;81:204-13.
21. Oral R et al. Neonatal *Klebsiella pneumonia* sepsis and imipenem/cilastatin [abstract]. *Indian J Pediatr.* 1998;65(1):121-129.
22. *Physicians' Desk Reference.* 49th ed. Montvale, NJ: Medical Economics Data Production; 1995.
23. Raymond JR, Yarger WE. Abnormal urine color: differential diagnosis. *South Med J.* 1988;81:837-841.
24. Slawson M. Thirty-three drugs that discolor urine and/or stools. *RN.* 1980;43(1):40-41.
25. Wallach J. *Interpretation of diagnostic tests.* 6th ed. Boston: Little, Brown; 1996:867-868, 879.
26. *Urine Discoloration—Drug and Disease Induced.* Drugdex Consults. Greenwood Village, CO: Thomson Micromedex. http://www.thomsonhc.com/hcs/librarian. Accessed November 13, 2008.

Nutrition Support | 6

Phil Ayers

The American Society for Parenteral and Enteral Nutrition (A.S.P.E.N) defines nutrition support therapy as the provision of oral, enteral, or parenteral nutrients to treat or prevent malnutrition. This includes provision as total enteral or parenteral nutrition along with therapeutic nutrients to maintain or restore health.[1] Enteral nutrition implies the delivery of a regimen via some region of the gastrointestinal tract. Parenteral nutrition refers to regimens delivered by the intravenous route. It is imperative that the nutrition support practitioner understands the importance of nutrition assessment, fluid/acid–base balance, electrolytes and appropriate monitoring in the care of patients requiring specialized nutrition support.

■ NUTRITION ASSESSMENT

Nutrition assessment involves a comprehensive approach that includes the use of diet/medical histories, physical examination, anthropometric measurements, and laboratory data. Severity of the illness and nutritional status are important components of the assessment. Trauma, sepsis, cancer, and other diagnoses associated with high mortality affect metabolism and nutrient ingestion.[2]

Important elements of a dietary history such as appetite, bowel habits, changes in taste, food allergies, weight changes, and medications should be noted.

Anthropometric measurements include height and weight, as well as composition of fat and lean body mass. Skin fold and arm circumference measurement devices, bioelectric impedance analysis devices, and imaging technologies may also be utilized, but may not be relevant in the clinical setting.[3]

Body mass index (BMI) is a weight-stature index used as a measure of obesity and malnutrition.

$$BMI = weight\ (kg)/height\ (m^2)$$

BMI INTERPRETATION[3]	
18.5–25	Normal
25.1–29.9	Overweight
30–34.9	Obesity grade I
35–39.9	Obesity grade II
≥ 40	Obesity grade III
17–18.4	Protein–energy malnutrition grade I
16–16.9	Protein–energy malnutrition grade II
<16	Protein–energy malnutrition grade III

■ VISCERAL PROTEINS

The current nutritional status of the patient can be assessed by the patient's weight and by the use of the visceral protein status of the patient. Classification of malnutrition as mild, moderate or severe may be accomplished by measuring the patient's albumin, prealbumin, and serum transferrin. The hydration, renal, and hepatic status of the patient should be assessed along with these parameters to ensure accuracy. Nonhepatic causes of hypoalbuminemia include protein malnutrition, malabsorption, nephrotic syndrome, ascites, and overhydration. Prealbumin has a half-life of 2 days compared to 20 days for albumin and is more sensitive to protein malnutrition.[3] Prealbumin may be increased in renal insufficiency and acute alcohol intoxication or decreased by inflammation, major surgery, or zinc deficiency. Guidelines for assessment are listed below:[4]

VISCERAL PROTEIN	MILD	MODERATE	SEVERE
Albumin (g/dL)	2.8–3.5	2.1–2.7	<2.1
Prealbumin (mg/dL)	—	11–17	<10
Transferrin (mg/dL)	150–200	100–150 (149)	<100

Nitrogen balance (NB), another method used for assessment of changes in body nitrogen and protein turnover, is calculated using the following equation:

$$\begin{aligned} NB &= \text{Nitrogen intake (daily protein intake/6.25)} - \text{Nitrogen output (g/day)} \\ &= \text{Urinary urea nitrogen (mg/100 mL)} \times \text{urinary volume (L/day)/100} \\ &\quad + 20\% \text{ of urinary urea loss} + 2 \text{ g.}^5 \end{aligned}$$

A 24-h collection is required for urinary urea nitrogen measurement. Critically ill patients will often remain in a negative nitrogen balance.

■ ESTIMATING CALORIC NEEDS

The calculation of energy requirements using the kcal/kg method is widely accepted in practice. The A.S.P.E.N guidelines recommend 20–35 kcal/kg for the adult patient.[2] Table 1 provides guidelines for caloric needs in the pediatric patient.[2] In 1919, Harris and Benedict described in equation format an estimation of energy expenditure. The formulas listed below are used in practice, but may overestimate requirements in many patients.[6]

Men: Energy expenditure = 66 + 13.75 (wt in kg) + 5 (ht in cm) − 6.8 (age)

Women: Energy expenditure = 655 + 9.6 (wt in kg) + 1.8 (ht in cm) − 4.7 (age)

TABLE 1. CALORIC REQUIREMENTS FOR THE PEDIATRIC PATIENT[7]

Preterm neonate	90–120 kcal/kg
<6 mo	85–105 kcal/kg
6–12 mo	80–100 kcal/kg
1–7 y	75–90 kcal/kg
7–12 y	50–75 kcal/kg
>12–18 y	30–50 kcal/kg

Indirect calorimetry provides another method for calculating energy needs. Indirect calorimetry calculates resting energy expenditure (REE) and respiratory quotient (RQ) by measuring whole body oxygen (V_{O_2}) and carbon dioxide (V_{CO_2}).[8] The abbreviated Weir equation is used in indirect calorimetry (energy expenditure = $(3.94 \times V_{O_2}) + (1.11 \times V_{CO_2})$).[9] Indirect calorimetry may be performed on mechanically ventilated patients as well as patients breathing spontaneously. The resting energy expenditure (REE) expressed in kcal/day should be met with total calories and a carbohydrate:lipid:protein ratio of 50%:20–30%: 15–20%.[8]

A number of factors may decrease indirect calorimetry accuracy such as Fi_{O_2} >60, mechanical ventilation with positive end expiratory pressure (PEEP) >12 cm H_2O, and a leak in the sampling system.[10] This is by no means an all-inclusive list and the reader is encouraged to engage in further research. The RQ is used as an indirect measurement of substrate utilization. Fat, protein, and carbohydrate have RQ values of 0.7, 0.8, and 1, respectively. An RQ of <0.7 may indicate underfeeding or lipid catabolism, whereas an RQ value of >1 may indicate overfeeding or excessive CO_2 production.[8] The RQ value of 0.85 would imply a mixed substrate utilization or optimal nutrition regimen.[10] Other equations used to estimate energy requirements include the Owen equation, Mifflin-St. Jeor equation, and the Ireton-Jones equation.[3]

■ ESTIMATING PROTEIN NEEDS

Daily protein requirements are dependent on the renal function of the patient and the metabolic status. Protein requirements for maintenance are in the range of 0.8–1 g/kg for the adult patient. The catabolic patient requires 1.2–2 g/kg of protein.[7] Guidelines for the renal failure (RF) patient are:[2,7]

Chronic RF, no dialysis	0.6–0.8 g/kg
Chronic RF, hemodialysis, or peritoneal dialysis	1.2–1.3 g/kg
RF, continuous hemofiltration	1 g/kg
Acute RF with severe malnutrition or hypercatabolic state	1.5–1.8 g/kg

Protein requirements for the pediatric patient are listed in Table 2.[7]

TABLE 2. PROTEIN REQUIREMENTS FOR THE PEDIATRIC PATIENT[7]	
Preterm neonates	3–4 g/kg
1–12 mo	2–3 g/kg
1–10 y	1–2 g/kg
11–17 y	0.8–1.5 g/kg

■ PARENTERAL NUTRITION (PN)

Parenteral nutrition formulations are complex products intended for use via the intravenous route. Compounding errors have led to serious harm and the clinician must consider the doses, stability, and limits of all the components of the PN regimen.

The practitioner is referred to "Safe Practices for Parenteral Nutrition" published in the November–December 2004 *Journal of Parenteral and Enteral Nutrition* supplement for in-depth recommendations concerning the PN label/order, compounding, stability, and administration.[7]

The candidate for parenteral nutrition must be selected based on stringent criteria. The gastrointestinal tract along with enteral nutrition should be utilized if at all possible. Enteral nutrition improves nutritional status, decreases length of stay in the critical care patient and is associated with fewer complications versus parenteral nutrition.[11] Characteristics of patients in which PN may be indicated include the following:[2]

1. Patients who are unable to receive all nutrient requirements through the oral or enteral route.
2. Patients who are unable to absorb nutrients through the gastrointestinal tract because of:
   extensive small-bowel resection;
   small-bowel disease;
   radiation enteritis;
   severe diarrhea;
   intractable vomiting;
   major trauma;
   major surgery;
   closed head injury.
3. Malnourished high-dose chemotherapy patients, radiation, or bone marrow transplant patients.
4. Severe necrotizing pancreatitis when enteral feeding is not tolerated or feasible.
5. AIDS/HIV patients with intractable diarrhea.

■ PARENTERAL NUTRITION (PN) DELIVERY

The PN formula can be delivered via a peripheral or central vein. The use of peripheral parenteral nutrition (PPN) limits the practitioner in terms of provision of adequate calories. The maximum osmolality tolerated by a peripheral vein is 900 mOsm/L.[12] Table 3 provides information for calculation of osmolality.[7] The PPN typically requires larger volumes and higher fat content for calories. The majority of total parenteral nutrition (TPN) patients will require infusions via a central line.[12] Examples of central access devices include subclavian central venous catheters, peripherally inserted central catheters (PICC), or implanted ports. Midline or midclavicular catheters may not be utilized for infusions requiring central access. Appropriate care including flushing, dressing changes, and proper cleaning of the central venous catheter is imperative for decreasing the risk of infection.[13]

TABLE 3. OSMOLALITY[7]

PN COMPONENT	mOsm
Dextrose	5 per gram
Amino acid	10 per gram
Fat emulsion	1.3–1.5 per gram
Electrolytes	1 per mEq

■ PARENTERAL NUTRITION MICRONUTRIENTS

The macronutrient components of parenteral nutrition include protein, carbohydrate, and fat. The protein component is delivered by infusing commercially available crystalline amino acids. These products will provide 4 kcal/g of energy and 6.25 g protein = 1 g nitrogen for nitrogen balance studies.[13] Table 4 provides a listing of some commercially available amino acid/amino acid–dextrose solutions.[14–16] Dextrose is the most commonly used carbohydrate energy source.

TABLE 4. SELECTED AMINO ACID/AMINO ACID COMBINATIONS[14–16]

BRAND	CONCENTRATION
Travasol (Baxter)	10%
Clinisol (Baxter)	15%
Aminosyn PF (Hospira)	7%, 10%
Aminosyn (Hospira)	8.5%
HepatAmine (B. Braun)	8%
Hepatasol (Baxter)	8%
FreAmine HBC (B. Braun)	6.9%
Aminosyn II Nutrimix (Hospira)	5/25, 3.5/5, 3.5/25
Amino Acid/Dextrose Clinimix (Baxter)	2.75/5, 4.25/25, 4.25/20, 4.25/10, 4.25/5
Amino Acid/Dextrose	5/15, 5/20, 5/25

Concentrations of commercially available products range from 2.5% to 70%. Dextrose provides 3.4 kcal/g and concentrations above 10% are reserved for central venous administration.[13] Intravenous fat emulsion (IVFE) should provide approximately 20%–30% of the total calories. IVFE in the United States comprises solely long-chain triglycerides. Currently there are 3 strengths available in the United States: 10%, 20%, and 30%.[13]

The 10% fat emulsion provides 1.1 kcal/mL, the 20% 2 kcal/mL, and the 30% 3 kcal/mL.[14] The 10% and 20% may be infused peripherally and the 30% should be used for compounding purposes only. IVFE may be administered separately or as a total nutrient admixture (TNA) commonly referred to as 3:1. If infused separately the infusion time for lipids should not exceed 12 hours per CDC guidelines.[17]

■ WRITING THE PRESCRIPTION

PN admixtures may be prepared in two forms, the dextrose-amino acid (2:1) or the dextrose-amino acid-fat emulsion (3:1 or TNA). The prescriber is encouraged to use a standard parenteral nutrition form for clarity and to reduce the possibility of an error of omission. The nutrition support practitioner should evaluate the electrolyte, acid-base, fluid, and hemodynamic status of the patient before initiating therapy. In order to avoid refeeding syndrome, it is prudent to initiate PN at 15–20 kcal/kg and advance to goal only when electrolytes, fluid status, and glycemic control are achieved.[18]

Example of TNA for 65 kg patient:

Write a TPN to provide 25 kcal/kg and 1.5 g/kg protein using 10% A.A. solution, 70% dextrose, and 20% IVFE; 30% of calories from IVFE

$$\text{Calories: 65 kg} \times 25 \text{ kcal/kg} = 1625 \text{ kcal}$$

$$\text{Protein: 65 kg} \times 1.5 \text{ g/kg} = 97.5 \text{ g}$$

Amino acid 10%: 10 g/100 mL = 97.5 g/x mL $\boxed{\text{975 mL 10% amino acid}}$

20% IVFE (2 kcal/mL): 1625 × 30% = 487.5 kcal/2 kcal/mL $\boxed{\text{244 mL 20% IVFE}}$

Remainder of the calories from dextrose 1625 kcal – 487.5 kcal (IVFE) – 390 kcal (protein 4 kcal/g × 97.5 g) = 747.5 kcal.

$$747.5 \text{ kcal}/3.4 \text{ kcal/g} = 219.9 \text{ g}/x \text{ mL} = 70 \text{ g}/100 \text{ mL (70% dextrose)}$$
$$\boxed{\text{314 mL 70% dextrose}}$$

These components would be admixed into a single bag and administered at 64 mL/h to deliver a 24-h supply.

The TPN should be admixed in accordance to The United States Pharmacopeia (USP) 797 guidelines for sterile compounding. Labeling of the PN should contain the amount per day or quantity per liter of all components and dosing weight.[7] The PN label should be compared to the order before administration to the patient.

■ ELECTROLYTES

Electrolytes are added to the parenteral nutrition regimen for maintenance and therapeutic purposes. Standard daily ranges for adults are listed below:[7]

Sodium	1–2 mEq/kg	(chloride, acetate, phosphate)
Potassium	1–2 mEq/kg	(chloride, acetate, phosphate)
Calcium	10–15 mEq	(gluconate, gluceptate)
Magnesium	8–20 mEq	(sulfate, chloride)
Phosphorous	20–40 mol	

Electrolyte requirements for the pediatric patient are listed in Table 5.[7]

TABLE 5. DAILY ELECTROLYTE REQUIREMENTS FOR PEDIATRIC PATIENTS[7]

ELECTROLYTE	PRETERM NEONATE	INFANTS/CHILDREN	ADOLESCENTS/ CHILDREN > 50 kg
Sodium	2–5 mEq/kg	2–5 mEq/kg	1–2 mEq/kg
Potassium	2–4 mEq/kg	2–4 mEq/kg	1–2 mEq/kg
Calcium	2–4 mEq/kg	0.5–4 mEq/kg	10–20 mEq/d
Phosphorus	1–2 mmol/kg	0.5–2 mmol/kg	10–40 mmol/d
Magnesium	0.3–0.5 mEq/kg	0.3–0.5 mEq/kg	10–30 mEq/d
Acetate/Chloride	maintain acid/base	maintain acid/base	maintain acid/base

Acetate and chloride salts are adjusted in the PN solution to maintain acid–base balance. Patients with a metabolic acidosis may benefit from a PN solution higher in acetate (converted to bicarbonate), whereas patients in a metabolic alkalosis would benefit from PN enriched with chloride salts. Calcium gluconate and magnesium sulfate are the preferred forms for PN because they are less likely to produce physicochemical incompatibilities.[19] The nutrition support practitioner must be aware of the incompatibility associated with the use of calcium and phosphorus in amounts that exceed upper limits. In 1994 the Food and Drug Administration released a safety alert concerning reports of two deaths and at least two cases of respiratory distress associated with insoluble PN formulations (calcium/phosphate crystals).[20]

Factors that may influence calcium phosphate solubility include amino acid concentration, phosphate in amino acid solutions, calcium/phosphate concentrations, pH of PN formulation, temperature of the PN and order of mixing.[13] Resources are available to assist in determining appropriate calcium and phosphate concentrations. They include product-specific curves and the use of automated compounding devices.

TRACE ELEMENTS

Trace elements commonly used in PN include chromium, copper, manganese, selenium, and zinc. These products are available as single entity or as combinations of multiple trace elements (MTE). Other trace elements that may be supplemented are iodine, molybdenum, and iron. Iron is available in an injectable form, but only iron dextran is approved and may be used only in the 2:1 (dextrose–amino acid) formulation. In patients with an elevated bilirubin, manganese should be used with caution as accumulation may result in neurologic toxicity.[13] Table 6 provides guidance for trace element dosing in adult and pediatric patients.[7]

**TABLE 6. DAILY TRACE ELEMENT SUPPLEMENTATION:
ADULT AND PEDIATRIC PATIENTS[7]**

TRACE ELEMENT	PRETERM NEONATE <3 kg	TERM NEONATE 3–10 kg	CHILDREN 10–40 kg	ADOLESCENTS >40 kg	ADULTS
Chromium	0.05–0.2 μg/kg	0.2 μg/kg	0.14–0.2 μg/kg	5–15 μg	10–15 μg
Copper	20 μg/kg	20 μg/kg	5–20 μg/kg	200–500 μg	0.3–0.5 mg
Iron	–	–	–	–	Not routinely added
Manganese	1 μg/kg	1 μg/kg	1 μg/kg	40–100 μg	60–100 μg
Selenium	1.5–2 μg/kg	2 μg/kg	1–2 μg/kg	40–60 μg	20–60 μg
Zinc	400 μg/kg	50–250 μg/kg	50–125 μg/kg	2–5 mg	2.5–5 mg

Aluminum is a trace element found as a contaminant in many of the large-volume (LVP) and small-volume parenterals (SVP) used to compound PN. Federal regulations regarding labeling and aluminum content indicate that the maximum aluminum load permitted in LVP is 25 μg/L. Labels on pharmacy bulk packaging and SVP must include the following statement, "not more than 25 μg/L" or provide the aluminum content in μg/L.[21]

■ MULTIVITAMINS

Vitamin supplementation is achieved by providing products that contain both fat-soluble and water-soluble vitamins. Some formulations of parenteral multivitamins may contain Vitamin K and patients on warfarin therapy should be monitored for changes if different products are used.

These multivitamin products are not stable when added more than 24 h in advance and require addition to the PN premixed products and home TPN.[13] Tables 7 and 8 provide guidance regarding vitamin supplementation.[7]

TABLE 7. ADULT DAILY REQUIREMENTS FOR PARENTERAL VITAMINS[7]

VITAMIN	REQUIREMENT
Thiamin (B_1)	6 mg
Riboflavin (B_2)	3.6 mg
Niacin (B_3)	40 mg
Folic acid	600 μg
Pantothenic acid	15 mg
Pyridoxine	6 mg
Cyanocobalamin (B_{12})	5 μg
Biotin	60 μg
Ascorbic Acid (C)	200 mg
Vitamin A	3300 IU
Vitamin D	200 IU
Vitamin E	10 IU
Vitamin K	150 μg

TABLE 8. PEDIATRIC MULTIVITAMIN DAILY DOSE RECOMMENDATION[7]

WEIGHT (kg)	DOSE (mL)
<1	1.5
1–3	3.25
>3	5

Pediatric multiple vitamin formulation 5 mL (A, 2300 IU; D, 400 IU; E, 7 IU; K, 200 μg; C, 80 mg; B_1, 1.2 mg; B_2, 1.4 mg; B_3, 17 mg; B_5, 5 mg; B_6, 1 mg; B_{12}, 1 μg; Biotin, 20 μg; folic acid, 140 μg).

■ FILTRATION/TUBING

A 0.22 micron filter is recommended for use with the 2:1 formulations while a 3:1 (TNA) requires a 1.2 micron filter. Alternatively, a 1.2 micron filter may be used for all PN formulations. Administration sets in patients receiving TNA should be changed every 24 h. In the 2:1 formulations, the administration sets may be changed every 72 h.[13]

■ MONITORING

PN patients require monitoring in the hospital and home care settings. Suggested monitoring for patients receiving PN at baseline include: CBC with differential, PT, PTT, serum glucose, Na, K, Cl, CO_2, Mg, Phosphorus, BUN, CR, triglycerides, albumin, prealbumin, AST, ALT, ALP, total bilirubin, weight, and intake and output. In the critically ill/hospitalized patient, recommended monitoring includes: daily intake/output, electrolytes, BUN, CR, serum glucoses with capillary glucoses

3–4 times a day. Weekly monitoring should include CBC, triglycerides, LFTs, prealbumin, PT, and PTT. Home care or stable patients can be maintained with weekly laboratory and LFTs checked monthly.[12]

■ ENTERAL NUTRITION ACCESS

The enteral route is preferred for specialized nutrition support.[2] Numerous factors assist in determining whether to feed the patient via the enteral route, including risk, ethics, concomitant disease states, bowel function, length of therapy, and long/short term goals.[2] Nasogastric and nasoenteric tubes are generally considered short-term devices, whereas percutaneous endoscopic gastrostomy (PEG), gastrostomy (G), and jejunostomy (J) are considered more long-term devices. Complications associated with enteral devices include occlusion, sinusitis, aspiration, site infections, leakage, and fistulas. Table 9 provides an overview of nasoenteric and enterostomy tube sizes.[22]

TABLE 9. NASOENTERIC AND ENTEROSTOMY TUBE SIZES[23]

TUBE TYPE	SIZE (FRENCH)
Nasogastric	8–12
Nasoenteric	8–12
Gastrostomy	18–28
Gastrojejunal	8–12 jejunal lumen; 9–22
Jejunostomy	8–14

ENTERAL NUTRITION FORMULATIONS

Enteral nutrition is the preferred method of specialized nutrition support compared to parenteral nutrition.[24] Enteral formulations are considered medical foods by the Food and Drug Administration. Common terms and definitions associated with enteral formulations include:[25]

Polymeric	Formula containing intact nutrients
Elemental/Semi-elemental	Contains partially or completely hydrolyzed nutrients
Disease-specific	Used in organ dysfunction or specific metabolic conditions
Modular	Used for supplementation to create a formula or add to nutrient

Table 10 lists common enteral nutrition products and classification.

TABLE 10. ENTERAL PRODUCTS[26,27]

PRODUCT	kcal/mL
Standard	——
Jevity (Abbott)	1
Jevity 1.2 (Abbott)	1.2
Jevity 1.5 (Abbott)	1.5

(*continued*)

TABLE 10. ENTERAL PRODUCTS[26,27] (*continued*)

PRODUCT	kcal/mL
Isosource (Nestle)	1.2
Isosource 1.5 (Nestle)	1.5
Elemental	—
Optimental (Abbott)	1
Crucial (Nestle)	1.5
Peptamen (Nestle)	1
Peptamen 1.5 (Nestle)	1.5
Diabetic	—
Glucerna (Abbott)	1
Glucerna 1.2 (Abbott)	1.2
Diabetisource AC (Nestle)	1.2
Pulmonary	—
Oxepa (Abbott)	1.5
Pulmocare (Abbott)	1.5
Nutren Pulmonary (Nestle)	1.5
Hepatic	—
Nutril lep (Nestle)	1.5
Renal	—
Nepro (Abbott)	1.8
Suplena (Abbott)	1.8
Novasource Renal (Nestle)	2
Renacal (Nestle)	2
Metabolic Stress	—
Perative (Abbott)	1.3
Pivot (Abbott)	1.5
Impact (Nestle)	1
Impact 1.5 (Nestle)	1.5

ENTERAL NUTRITION COMPLICATIONS

From 12% to 20% of patients receiving enteral nutrition experience nausea and vomiting. Delayed gastric emptying is the most common cause identified. Potential reasons for delayed gastric emptying include: hypotension, sepsis, stress, gastric neoplasms, autoimmune diseases, vagotomy, opiate analgesics, anticholinergics, and rapid infusion of formula.[28]

Diarrhea is the most common gastrointestinal effect reported in enterally fed patients. Common causes of diarrhea include sorbitol-containing liquids, antibiotics, prokinetic agents, infection, and intolerance because of formula characteristics (e.g., osmolality, fat content).

Other complications include: abdominal distension, malabsorption, constipation, aspiration, fluid/electrolyte imbalances, and hyperglycemia (see Table 11).[29]

TABLE 11. METABOLIC COMPLICATIONS OF NUTRITION SUPPORT AND MANAGEMENT[7,13,30]

COMPLICATION	POTENTIAL CAUSES	MANAGEMENT
Hyperglycemia	diabetes, overfeeding, dextrose-containing fluids, steroids	reduce dextrose load, add insulin (SQ, added to TPN bag or infusion)
Hyponatremia	SIADH, adrenal insufficiency, overhydration, GI loss, medications	fluid restriction, addition of sodium, review medications
Hypernatremia	diabetes insipidus, dehydration, exogenous sodium load, medications	desmopressin, volume resuscitation, decrease sodium load, review medications
Hypokalemia	alkalosis, alcoholism, vomiting, diarrhea, fistula, diuretics, amphotericin B, hypomagnesemia	correct acid–base status, replace magnesium and potassium
Hyperkalemia	acidosis, renal failure, hemolysis, potassium-sparing diuretics, trimethoprim	correct acid–base status, reduce potassium load
Hypomagnesemia	GI loss, renal loss, diuretics, alcoholism	replace magnesium (may require IV replacement in severe cases)
Hypophosphatemia	refeeding syndrome, phosphate binders	appropriate replacement, advance nutrition slowly, d/c phosphate binders
Hyperphosphatemia	renal failure, propofol, IV clindamycin	discontinue phosphate sources, phosphate binders
Hypocalcemia	hyperphosphatemia, hypoalbuminemia, hypomagnesemia, Vit D deficiency, hypoparathyroidism	correct for low albumin, check ionized calcium, replace magnesium, check vitamin D, PTH
Hypertriglyceridemia	impaired clearance, sepsis, propofol	decrease lipids, change sedation medication
Elevated Liver Function Tests	overfeeding, lack of GI tract use	enteral feedings, decrease caloric load, limit dextrose to 3–5 mg/kg/min
Metabolic Acidosis	renal failure, diarrhea, chloride salts in TPN	volume resuscitation, maximize acetate salts in TPN
Metabolic Alkalosis	emesis, NG suction, bicarbonate administration	volume resuscitation, maximize chloride salts in TPN

■ DISEASE-SPECIFIC FORMULAS

Enteral formulas are available for specific diseases or conditions such as diabetes, hepatic failure, and pulmonary disease. Routine use of these products could lead to higher cost, and each patient should be assessed to determine possible benefit. There is a need for further prospective, randomized controlled trials to determine the role of the formulas in the diabetic and pulmonary patient. The use of immune-enhancing formulations remains a controversial area. Large and well-designed trials are needed to establish the patient populations that may benefit, type of nutrients, and length of therapy. The use of hepatic formulas enriched with branched-chain amino acids (BCAA) may benefit encephalopathic patients unresponsive to pharmacotherapy in conjunction with standard enteral regimens.[23]

■ REFERENCES

1. American Society for Parenteral and Enteral Nutrition. http://www.nutritioncare.org./Index.aspx?id = 108 Accessed December 5, 2008.
2. American Society for Parenteral and Enteral Nutrition Board of Directors and the Clinical Guidelines Task Force. Guidelines for the use of parenteral and enteral nutrition in the adult and pediatric patients. *JPEN J Parenter Enteral Nutr.* 2002;26(suppl 1):1SA-138SA.
3. Russell MK, Mueller C. Nutrition screening and assessment. In: Gottschlich MM, DeLegge MH, Mattox T, Mueller C, Worthington P, eds. *The A.S.P.E.N. Nutrition Support Core Curriculum: A Case Based Approach-the Adult Patient* Silver Springs, MD: American Society for Parenteral and Enteral Nutrition; 2007:163-186.
4. Blackburn GL et al. Nutrition and metabolic assessment of the hospitalized patient. *JPEN J Parenter Enteral Nutr.* 1977;1(1):11-22.
5. Wilmore DW. *Metabolic Management of the Critically Ill.* New York, NY: Plenum; 1977:193.
6. Harris JA, Benedict FG. *A Biometric Study of Basal Metabolism in Man.* Washington DC: Carnegie Institute; 1919. Publication No. 279.
7. Mirtallo J et al., for the Task Force for the Revision of Safe Practices for Parenteral Nutrition. Safe practices for parenteral nutrition. *JPEN J Parenter Enteral Nutr.* 2004;28(6 suppl):S39-S70
8. Matarese LE. Indirect calorimetry in clinical aspects. *J Am Diet Assoc.* 1997;10(suppl):S154-S160.
9. Weir JB. New methods for calculating metabolic rate with special reference to protein metabolism. *J Physiol.* 1949;109:1-14.
10. Wooley JA, Sax HC. Indirect calorimetry: applications to practice. *Nutr Clin Pract.* 2003;18:434-439.
11. Braunschweig CL et al. Enteral compared with parenteral nutrition: a meta-analysis. *Am J Clin Nutr.* 2001;74:534-542.
12. Mirtallo J. Overview of parenteral nutrition. In: Gottschlich MM, DeLegge MH, Mattox T, Mueller C, Worthington P, eds. *The A.S.P.E.N. Nutrition Support Core Curriculum: A Case Based Approach-the Adult Patient.* Silver Springs, MD: American Society for Parenteral and Enteral Nutrition; 2007:264-276.
13. Barber JR et al. Parenteral nutrition formulations. In: Gottschlich MM, DeLegge MH, Mattox T, Mueller C, Worthington P, eds. *The A.S.P.E.N. Nutrition Support Core Curriculum: A Case Based Approach-the Adult Patient.* Silver Springs, MD: American Society for Parenteral and Enteral Nutrition; 2007:277-299.
14. Baxter Healthcare. http://www.baxter.com. Accessed December 5, 2008.
15. Hospira, Inc. http://www.hospira.com. Accessed December 5, 2008.
16. B. Braun Medical Inc. http://www.bbraunusa.com. Accessed December 5, 2008.
17. Center for Disease Control and Prevention. Guidelines for the management of intravascular catheter-related infections [erratum 2002;51:711]. *MMWR Morb Mortal Wkly Rep.* 2002;51(N0. RR-10):1-28.
18. Kraft MD et al. Review of the refeeding syndrome. *Nutr Clin Pract.* 2005;20:625-633.
19. Driscoll DF et al. Precipitation of calcium phosphate from parenteral nutrition fluids. *Am J Hosp Pharm.* 1994;51:2834-2836.
20. Knowles JB et al. Pulmonary deposition of calcium phosphate crystals as a complication of home parenteral nutrition. *JPEN J Parenter Enteral Nutr.* 1989;13:209-213.
21. Department of Health and Human Services (HHS). Food and Drug Administration (FDA). Aluminum in large and small volume parenterals used in total parenteral nutrition. *Fed Regist.* 200;65:4103-4111.

22. Bankhead RR, Fang JC. Enteral access devices. In: Gottschlich MM, DeLegge MH, Mattox T, Mueller C, Worthington P, eds. *The A.S.P.E.N. Nutrition Support Core Curriculum: A Case Based Approach-the Adult Patient.* Silver Springs, MD: American Society for Parenteral and Enteral Nutrition; 2007:233-245.

23. Lefton J et al. Enteral formulations. In: Gottschlich MM, DeLegge MH, Mattox T, Mueller C, Worthington P, eds. *The A.S.P.E.N. Nutrition Support Core Curriculum: A Case Based Approach-the Adult Patient.* Silver Springs, MD: American Society for Parenteral and Enteral Nutrition; 2007:209-232.

24. Farber MS et al. Reducing costs and patient morbidity in the enterally fed intensive care unit patient. *JPEN J Parentr Enteral Nutr.* 2005;29:S562-S569.

25. Matarese LE. Enteral nutrition. In: Lysen LK ed. *Quick Reference to Clinical Dietetics.* Gaithersburg, MD: Aspen Publishers; 1997.

26. Abbott Nutrition. http://www.abbottnutrition.com. Accessed December 5, 2008.

27. Nestle Healthcare Nutrition. http://nestlenutrition.com/us. Accessed December 5, 2008.

28. Montejo JC. Enteral nutrition related gastrointestinal complications in critically ill patients: a multicenter study. *Critical Care Med.* 1992;27:1447-1453.

29. Lefton J. Management of common gastrointestinal complications in tube fed patients. *Support Line.* 2002;24:19-25.

30. Btaiche IF, Khalidi N. Metabolic complication of parenteral nutrition in adults, part 1. *Am J Health Syst Pharm.* 2004;61:1938-1949.

PART III

Appendices

Principal Editor: Kelly M. Smith

Conversion Factors | 1

Kelly M. Smith

■ SI UNITS

SI units (*le Système International d'Unités*) are used internationally to express clinical laboratory and serum drug concentration data. Instead of employing units of mass (such as micrograms), the SI system uses moles (mol) to represent the amount of a substance. A molar solution contains 1 mole (the molecular weight of the substance in grams) of the solute in 1 liter of solution. The following formula is used to convert units of mass to moles (μg/mL to μmol/L or, by substitution of terms, mg/mL to mmol/L or ng/mL to nmol/L).

Micromoles per liter (μmol/L)

$$\mu mol/L = \frac{Drug\ concentration\ (\mu g/mL) \times 1000}{Molecular\ weight\ of\ drug\ (g/mol)}$$

■ MILLIEQUIVALENTS

An equivalent weight of a substance is that weight which will combine with or replace 1 g of hydrogen; a milliequivalent is 1/1000 of an equivalent weight.

Milliequivalents per liter (mEq/L)

$$mEq/L = \frac{Weight\ of\ salt\ (g) \times Valence\ of\ ion \times 1000}{Molecular\ weight\ of\ salt}$$

$$Weight\ of\ salt\ (g) = \frac{mEq/L \times Molecular\ weight\ of\ salt}{Valence\ of\ ion \times 1000}$$

APPROXIMATE MILLIEQUIVALENTS: WEIGHTS OF SELECTED IONS

SALT	mEq/g SALT	mg SALT/mEq
Calcium carbonate ($CaCO_3$)	20.0	50.0
Calcium chloride ($CaCl_2 \cdot 2H_2O$)	13.6	73.5
Calcium gluceptate ($Ca[C_7H_{13}O_8]_2$)	4.1	245.2
Calcium gluconate ($Ca[C_6H_{11}O_7]_2 \cdot H_2O$)	4.5	224.1

(continued)

APPROXIMATE MILLIEQUIVALENTS: WEIGHTS OF SELECTED IONS (*continued*)

SALT	mEq/g SALT	mg SALT/mEq
Calcium lactate (Ca[C$_3$H$_5$O$_3$]$_2$ · 5H$_2$O)	6.5	154.1
Magnesium gluconate (Mg[C$_6$H$_{11}$O$_7$]$_2$ · H$_2$O)	4.6	216.3
Magnesium oxide (MgO)	49.6	20.2
Magnesium sulfate (MgSO$_4$ · 7H$_2$O)	8.1	123.2
Potassium acetate (K[C$_2$H$_3$O$_2$])	10.2	98.1
Potassium chloride (KCl)	13.4	74.6
Potassium citrate (K$_3$[C$_6$H$_5$O$_7$] · H$_2$O)	9.2	108.1
Potassium iodide (KI)	6.0	166.0
Sodium acetate (Na[C$_2$H$_3$O$_2$] · 3H$_2$O)	7.3	136.1
Sodium bicarbonate (NaHCO$_3$)	11.9	84.0
Sodium chloride (NaCl)	17.1	58.4
Sodium citrate (Na$_3$[C$_6$H$_5$O$_7$] · 2H$_2$O)	10.2	98.0
Sodium iodide (NaI)	6.7	149.9
Sodium lactate (Na[C$_3$H$_5$O$_3$])	8.9	112.1
Zinc sulfate (ZnSO$_4$ · 7H$_2$O)	7.0	143.8

VALENCES AND ATOMIC WEIGHTS OF SELECTED IONS

SUBSTANCE	ELECTROLYTE	VALENCY	MOLECULAR WEIGHT
Calcium	Ca^{++}	2	40.1
Chloride	Cl$^-$	1	35.5
Magnesium	Mg^{++}	2	24.3
Phosphate	HPO$_4^{--}$ (80%)	1.8	96.0[a]
(pH = 7.4)	H$_2$PO$_4^-$ (20%)		
Potassium	K$^+$	1	39.1
Sodium	Na$^+$	1	23.0
Sulfate	SO$_4^-$	2	96.0[a]

[a]The molecular weight of phosphorus only is 31; that of sulfur only is 32.1.

■ ANION GAP

The anion gap is the concentration of plasma anions not routinely measured by laboratory screening. It is useful in the evaluation of acid–base disorders. The anion gap is greater with increased plasma concentrations of endogenous (e.g., phosphate, sulfate, lactate, ketoacids) or exogenous (e.g., salicylate, penicillin, ethylene glycol, ethanol, methanol) species. The formulas for calculating the anion gap follow:

$$\text{(A) Anion gap} = (Na^+ + K^+) - (Cl^- + HCO_3^{--})$$

or

$$\text{(B) Anion gap} = Na^+ - (Cl^- + HCO_3^{--})$$

where:

the expected normal value for A is 11–20 μmol/L;
the expected normal value for B is 7–16 μmol/L. (Note that there is variation at the upper and lower limits of the normal range.)

■ TEMPERATURE

Fahrenheit to Centigrade: ($°F - 32$) $\times$ 5/9 = $°C$
Centigrade to Fahrenheit: ($°C \times 9/5$) + 32 = $°F$
Centigrade to Kelvin: $°C$ + 273 = $°K$

■ WEIGHTS AND MEASURES

Metric Weight Equivalents

1 kilogram (kg) = 1000 grams
1 gram (g) = 1000 milligrams
1 milligram (mg) = 0.001 gram
1 microgram (mcg, μg) = 0.001 milligram
1 nanogram (ng) = 0.001 microgram
1 picogram (pg) = 0.001 nanogram
1 femtogram (fg) = 0.001 picogram

Metric Volume Equivalents

1 liter (L) = 1000 milliliters
1 deciliter (dL) = 100 milliliters
1 milliliter (mL) = 0.001 liter
1 microliter (μL) = 0.001 milliliter
1 nanoliter (nL) = 0.001 microliter
1 picoliter (pL) = 0.001 nanoliter
1 femtoliter (fL) = 0.001 picoliter

Apothecary Weight Equivalents

1 scruple (Э) = 20 grains (gr)
60 grains (gr) = 1 dram (ʒ)
8 drams (ʒ) = 1 ounce (℥)
1 ounce (℥) = 480 grains
12 ounces (℥) = 1 pound (lb)

Apothecary Volume Equivalents
60 minims (m) = 1 fluidram (fl ℨ)
8 fluidrams (fl ℨ) = 1 fluid ounce (fl ℥)
1 fluid ounce (fl ℥) = 480 minims
16 fluid ounces (fl ℥) = 1 pint (pt)

Avoirdupois Equivalents
1 ounce (oz) = 437.5 grains
16 ounces (oz) = 1 pound (lb)

Weight/Volume Equivalents
1 mg/dL = 10 μg/mL
1 mg/dL = 1 mg%
1 ppm = 1 mg/L

Conversion Equivalents
1 gram (g) = 15.43 grains
1 grain (gr) = 64.8 milligrams
1 ounce (ℨ) = 31.1 grams
1 ounce (oz) = 28.35 grams
1 pound (lb) = 453.6 grams
1 kilogram (kg) = 2.2 pounds
1 milliliter (mL) = 16.23 minims
1 minim (m) = 0.06 milliliter
1 fluid ounce (fl oz) = 29.57 mL
1 pint (pt) = 473.2 mL
0.1 mg = 1/600 gr
0.12 mg = 1/500 gr
0.15 mg = 1/400 gr
0.2 mg = 1/300 gr
0.3 mg = 1/200 gr
0.4 mg = 1/150 gr
0.5 mg = 1/120 gr
0.6 mg = 1/100 gr
0.8 mg = 1/80 gr
1 mg = 1/65 gr

Anthropometrics | **2**

Kelly M. Smith

■ CREATININE CLEARANCE FORMULAS

FORMULAS FOR ESTIMATING CREATININE CLEARANCE IN PATIENTS WITH STABLE RENAL FUNCTION

Adults [Age 18 years and older][1]

$$Cl_{Cr} = \frac{(140 - Age) \times (Weight)}{Cr_s \times 72}$$

$$Cl_{Cr} \text{ (Females)} = 0.85 \times \text{Above value}^b$$

where:

Cl_{Cr} = creatinine clearance in mL/m
Cr_s = serum creatinine in mg/dL
age is in years
weight is in kilograms.

Note that some studies suggest that the predictive accuracy of this formula for women is better *without* the correction factor of 0.85.

Children [Age 1–18 years][2]

$$Cl_{Cr} = \frac{0.48 \times (height) \times (BSA)}{Cr_s \times 1.73}$$

where:

BSA = body surface area in m^2
Cl_{Cr} = creatinine clearance in mL/m
Cr_s = serum creatinine in mg/dL
height is in centimeters.

FORMULA FOR ESTIMATING CREATININE CLEARANCE FROM A MEASURED URINE COLLECTION

$$Cl_{Cr}(ml/m) = \frac{U \times V}{P \times t}$$

where:

U = concentration of creatinine in a urine specimen (in same units as P)
V = volume of urine in mL

1243

P = concentration of creatinine in serum at the midpoint of the urine collection period (in same units as U)

t = time of the urine collection period in minutes (e.g., 6 h = 360 m; 24 h = 1440 m).

Note that the product of $U \times V$ equals the production of creatinine during the collection period and, at steady state, should equal 20–25 mg/kg/d ideal body weight (IBW) in males and 15–20 mg/kg/d IBW in females. If it is less than this, inadequate urine collection may have occurred and Cl_{Cr} will be underestimated.

■ IDEAL BODY WEIGHT

IBW is the weight expected for a nonobese person of a given height. The IBW formulas below and various life insurance tables can be used to estimate IBW. Most dosing methods described in the literature use IBW as a method in dosing obese patients.

Adults [Age 18 years and older][3]

IBW (males) = 50 + (2.3 × height in inches over 5 ft)

IBW (females) = 45.5 + (2.3 × height in inches over 5 ft)

where IBW is in kilograms.

Children [Age 1–18 years][2]

Height under 5 ft:

$$IBW = \frac{(Height^2 \times 1.65)}{1000}$$

where:

IBW is in kilograms
height is in centimeters

5 ft or Taller:

IBW (males) = 39 + (2.27 × height in inches over 5 ft)

IBW (females) = 42.2 + (2.27 × Height in inches over 5 ft)

where IBW is in kilograms.

■ SURFACE AREA NOMOGRAMS

Nomograms represent the relationship between height, weight, and body surface area in infants and adults. To use a nomogram, a ruler is aligned with the height and weight on the two lateral axes. The point at which the centerline is intersected provides the corresponding value for body surface area.

NOMOGRAM FOR DETERMINATION OF BODY SURFACE AREA FROM HEIGHT AND WEIGHT (INFANTS)[4]

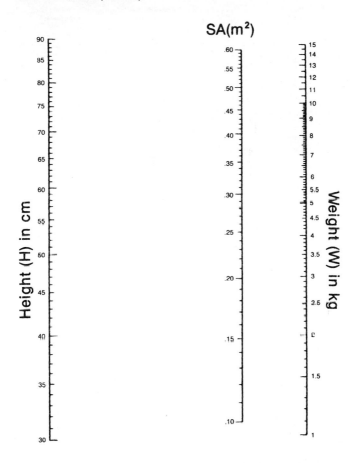

$$SA = W^{0.5378} \times H^{0.3964} \times 0.024265$$

where:

SA is in m^2
height (H) is in centimeters
Weight (W) is in kilograms.

Note that the above formula has been reproduced from Ref 4, with permission.

NOMOGRAM FOR DETERMINATION OF BODY SURFACE AREA
FROM HEIGHT AND WEIGHT (ADULTS)[5]

Height	Body surface area	Weight

$$SA = W^{0.425} \times H^{0.725} \times 71.84$$

where:

SA is in m^2
height (H) is in centimeters
Weight (W) is in kilograms:

Note that the above formula has been reproduced from Ref. 5, with permission.

■ REFERENCES

1. Cockcroft DW, Gault MH. Prediction of creatinine clearance from serum creatinine. *Nephron.* 1976;16:31-41.
2. Traub SL, Johnson CE. Comparison of methods of estimating creatinine clearance in children. *Am J Hosp Pharm.* 1980;37:195-201.
3. Devine BJ. Gentamicin therapy. *Drug Intell Clin Pharm.* 1974;8:650-655.
4. Haycock GB et al. Geometric method for measuring body surface area: a height-weight formula validated in infants, children, and adults. *J Pediatr.* 1978;93:62-66.
5. DuBois and DuBois. *Arch Intern Med.* 1916;17:863.

Laboratory Indices | 3

Blood, Serum, Plasma Chemistry; Urine, Renal Function Tests; Hematology

Kelly M. Smith

The following table lists typical reference ranges for clinical laboratory tests in common use. Reference ranges for laboratory tests vary widely among testing facilities, often as a result of methodologic differences. It is therefore always advisable to obtain reference ranges from the laboratory performing the analyses. Laboratory test results should never be accepted without correct identification of the units of measurement because most tests can be reported in several systems of measurement. The table presents conventional and international (usually the same as *Système International*, or SI) units. Unless otherwise indicated, values reflect those generally accepted for adult patients.

COMMON LABORATORY REFERENCE VALUES

		REFERENCE RANGE	
TEST/SPECIMEN	SPECIAL CHARACTERISTIC	*Conventional*	*International Units*
Absolute Neutrophil Count (ANC)	ANC = (% Sogo + % Bands) × Leukocyte Count		
Acid Phosphatase (S)		0.11–0.60 units/L	0.11–0.60 units/L
Alanine		*units/L*	*units/L*
Aminotransferase (S)	M	10–40	10–40
(ALT, SGPT)	F	8–35	8–35
Albumin		3.4–4.7 mg/dL	3.4–4.7 mg/dL
Alkaline Phosphatase (S)		30–120 units/L	30–120 units/L
Ammonia (S,P)		15–45 mg/dL	11–32 μmol/L
Amylase (S)		25–125 units/L	25–125 units/L
Anion Gap	(Na + K) − (Cl + HCO₃)	8–16 mEq/L	8–16 mmol/L
Aspartate Aminotransferase (S)		*units/L*	*units/L*
(AST, SGOT)	M	20–40	20–40
	F	15–30	15–30

(continued)

COMMON LABORATORY REFERENCE VALUES (*continued*)

TEST/SPECIMEN	SPECIAL CHARACTERISTIC	REFERENCE RANGE	
		Conventional	*International Units*
Bicarbonate (S)		*mEq/L*	*mmol/L*
	Arterial	21–28	21–28
	Venous	22–29	22–29
(WB, art)		18–23	18–23
Bilirubin (S)		*mg/dL*	*mmol/L*
Total	Child, Adult	0.3–1.0	5–17
Conjugated (direct)	Child, Adult	<0.4	<0.7
Bleeding time		3–9 min	180–540 sec
Calcium (S)		*mg/dL*	*mmol/L*
Ionized		4.64–5.28	1.16–1.32
Total	Child	8.8–10.8	2.20–2.70
	Adult	8.6–10.0	2.15–2.55
Carbon Dioxide, Partial Pressure (WB, art) (pCO_2)		35–45 mm Hg	35–45 mm Hg
Chloride (S,P)		98–106 mEq/L	98–106 mmol/L
Cholesterol, Total (S,P)	Desired	<200 mg/dL	<6.0 mmol/L
Cortisol (S,P)		*μg/dL*	*nmol/L*
	08:00 h	5–25	138–690
	16:00 h	3–16	83–442
	20:00 h	≤ 50% of 08:00 h	≤ 50% of 08:00 h
Creatine Kinase, total (CK) (S)		*units/L*	*units/L*
	M	38–174	38–174
	F	26–140	26–140
Creatinine (S,P)		*mg/dL*	*μmol/L*
	Child	0.3–0.7	27–62
	Adolescent	0.5–1.0	44–88
	Adult, M	0.7–1.3	62–115
	Adult, F	0.6–1.1	53–97
Erythrocyte Count (WB)		$4.7–6.1 \times 10^6/\mu L$	$4.7–6.1 \times 10^{12}/L$
Erythrocyte Sedimentation Rate (WB)		*mm/h*	*mm/h*
	M	1–15	1–15
	F	1–25	1–25
Fibrinogen (P)		175–433 mg/dL	1.75–4.3 g/L

(continued)

COMMON LABORATORY REFERENCE VALUES (*continued*)

TEST/SPECIMEN	SPECIAL CHARACTERISTIC	REFERENCE RANGE	
		Conventional	*International Units*
Hematocrit (WB)		% Packed RBC Volume	Volume Fraction
	2–9 yr	33–43	33–43
	10–17 yr, M	36–47	36–47
	10–17 yr, F	35–45	35–45
	Adult, M	42–52	42–52
	Adult, F	37–47	37–47
Hemoglobin (WB)		*g/dL*	*mmol/L*
	2–9 yr	11.5–14.5	7.14–9.0
	10–17 yr, M	12.5–16.1	7.76–9.99
	10–17 yr, F	12.0–15.0	7.44–9.31
	Adult, M	13.5–18.0	8.38–11.17
	Adult, F	12.5–16.0	7.76–9.93
Hemoglobin A$_{1c}$ (WB)		3.9–6.9%	3.9–6.9%
(γ-Glutamyltransferase (S)		*units/L*	*μkat/L*
(GGT)	M	2–30	0.03–0.51
	F	1–24	0.02–0.41
Glucose, Fasting (S) (Oral)		60–109 mg/dL	3.3–6.0 mmol/L
Glucose Tolerance Test (S)		*mg/dL*	*mmol/L*
	Normal	<100 <140	<5.6 <7.8
	Impaired glucose tolerance	100–125 140–199	5.6–6.9 7.8–11.0
	Diabetic	≥ 126 ≥ 200	≥ 7.0 ≥ 11.1
HDL-Cholesterol (S,P)		30–80 mg/dL	0.8–2.5 mmol/L
	M	27–67	0.7–1.73
	F	34–88	0.88–2.28
Iron (S)		*μg/dL*	*μmol/L*
	Child	50–120	9–21
	Adult	50–175	9–31
Iron-Binding Capacity, Total (S) (TIBC)		250–460 μg/dL	45–82 μmol/L
Lactate Dehydrogenase (S)		110–220 units/L	110–220 units/L
LDL Cholesterol (S)		<130 mg/dL	<3.37 mmol/L
Lead (WB)		*μg/dL*	*μmol/L*
	Child	<25	<1.21
	Adult	<40	<1.93

(continued)

COMMON LABORATORY REFERENCE VALUES (*continued*)

TEST/SPECIMEN	SPECIAL CHARACTERISTIC	REFERENCE RANGE	
		Conventional	*International Units*
Leukocyte Count (WB)		4.8–10.8 × 10³/μL	4.8–10.8 × 10⁹/L
	Segs	31–71%	31–71%
	Bands	0–12%	0–12%
	Lymphocytes	15–50%	15–50%
	Monocytes	0–12%	0–12%
	Eosinophils	0–5%	0–5%
	Basophils	0–2%	0–2%
Lipase (S)		0–160 units/L	0–2.66 μkat/L
Magnesium (S)		1.8–3.0 mEq/L	0.75–1.25 mmol/L
Mean Corpuscular Hemoglobin (WB)		26–34 pg	26–34 pg
Mean Corpuscular Volume (WB)		78–100 μm³	78–100 fL
Osmolality (S)	Child, Adult	275–295 mOsmol/kg	275–295 mOsmol/kg
Oxygen, Partial Pressure (WB, art)) (pO2)		83–108 mm Hg	11.04–14.36 kPa
Partial Thromboplastin Time, Activated (WB) (aPTT)		25–37 sec	25–37 sec
pH (U)		5–8	5–8
pH (WB, art)		7.35–7.45	7.35–7.45
Phosphorus, Inorganic (S)		*mg/dL*	*mmol/L*
	Child	4.5–5.5	1.45–1.78
	Adult	2.5–4.5	0.8–1.45
Platelets (WB)		150–450 × 10³/μL	0.15–0.45 × 10¹²/L
Potassium (S,P)		*mEq/L*	*mmol/L*
	Child	3.4–4.7	3.4–4.7
	Adult	3.5–5.0	3.5–5.0
Prealbumin		19.5–35.8 mg/dL	195–358 g/L
Protein, Total (S)		6–8 g/dL	60–80 g/L
Protein, Total (U)		1–14 mg/dL	10–140 mg/L
	At Rest	50–80 mg/day	50–80 mg/day
Prothrombin Time (WB)		Less than 2-s deviation from control.	

(continued)

COMMON LABORATORY REFERENCE VALUES (*continued*)

TEST/SPECIMEN	SPECIAL CHARACTERISTIC	REFERENCE RANGE	
		Conventional	*International Units*
Reticulocytes (WB)		$33-137 \times 10^3 \, \mu L$	$33-137 \times 10^9 /L$
Specific Gravity, Random (U)		1.001–1.035	1.001–1.035
Sodium (S,P)		*mEq/L*	*mmol/L*
	Child	138–145	138–145
	Adult	135–145	135–145
Thyroid-Stimulating Hormone (S,P) (TSH)		$< 10 \, \mu units/mL$	$< 10 \, \mu units/L$
Thyroxine, Total (T_4) (S)		$5-11 \, \mu g/dL$	64–142 nmol/L
Transferrin (S)		190–375 mg/dL	1.9–3.75 g/L
Triglycerides, Fasting (S)		40–150 mg/dL	0.4–15 mmol/L
Triiodothyronine, Total (S) (T_3)		95–190 ng/dL	1.5–2.9 nmol/L
Urea Nitrogen (BUN) (S)		8–20 mg/dL	2.9–7.1 mmol/L
Uric Acid (S)		*mg/dL*	*mmol/L*
	M	2.2–8.0	150–480
	F	2.7–7.0	130–420
Uric Acid, 24-h (U)		250–750 mg	1.48–4.43 mmol

F, Female; M, Male; P, Plasma; S, Serum; U, Urine; WB, Whole Blood; WB, art, Whole Blood Arterial.

■ REFERENCES

1. Burtis CA, Ashwood ER, eds. *Tietz Textbook of Clinical chemistry*. 2nd ed. Philadelphia: WB Saunders; 1994.
2. Henry JB, ed. *Clinical Diagnosis and Management by Laboratory Methods*. 18th ed. Philadelphia: WB Saunders; 1991.
3. Preventing lead poisoning in young children: a statement by the Centers for Disease Control. 4th rev. ed. Atlanta: Centers for Disease Control; 1991.
4. Système International (SI) units conversion table for common laboratory tests. *Ann Pharmacother*. 1995;29:100-7.
5. Tietz NW, ed. *Clinical Guide to Laboratory Tests*. 2nd ed. Philadelphia: WB Saunders; 1990.
6. Wallach J. *Interpretation of Diagnostic Tests: a Synopsis of Laboratory Medicine*. 6th ed. Boston: Little, Brown; 1996.

Drug-Laboratory Test Interferences 4

Linda Sobeski Farho

Drugs can interfere with laboratory tests through pharmacological or toxic effects or through actual chemical interference with the testing process. Either effect can lead to an altered value of the laboratory test, resulting in an inappropriate diagnosis or treatment. It is therefore essential that clinicians recognize possible drug-laboratory interactions and use this information in the overall assessment of a patient's clinical status.

The following table lists common clinical laboratory tests and commonly used drugs that can interfere with those tests. For detailed information on laboratory tests not covered here, see Refs. 1–3 at the end of this section. Also, it should be noted that drugs can interfere with laboratory tests by many different mechanisms, and that interference may vary depending on the specific methodology used. The reader should refer to the references cited in the table and other relevant sources to obtain more information about a specific test.

The following abbreviations are used in the table:

(B)	Blood
(I)	Analytical Interference of Drug
(P)	Pharmacological/Toxic Effect of Drug
(S)	Serum

■ DRUGS THAT CAN AFFECT RESULTS AND CAUSE OF INTERFERENCE

BLOOD, SERUM, & PLASMA CHEMISTRY

Albumin (S). *Decreased by* L-asparaginase (P), clofibric acid (I), cisplatin (P), dapsone (P), estrogen (P), ethanol (P), heroin (P), ibuprofen (P), isoniazid (P), nitrofurantoin (P), oral contraceptives (P), phenylbutazone (I), tamoxifen (P), valproic acid (P).[1,2]

Alkaline Phosphatase (S). *Elevated by* acetaminophen (P), acebutolol (P), acetohexamide (P), albumin (I), alitretinoin (P), allopurinol (P), aluminum salts (P), aminoglycosides (P), amiodarone (P), amitriptyline (P), amphotericin B (P), anabolic steroids (P), androgens (P), vitamin C (I), asparaginase (P), azathioprine (P), barbiturates (P), bromocriptine (P), captopril (P), carbamazepine (P), carboplatin (P), cephalosporins (P), chenodiol (P), chlorambucil (P), chloramphenicol (P), chlorpropamide (P), cimetidine (P), clindamycin (P), clofibrate (P), clotrimazole

(P), colchicine (P), cyclophosphamide (P), cyclosporine (P), cytarabine (P), danazol (P), dantrolene (P), dapsone (P), desipramine (P), didanosine (P), disopyramide (P), disulfiram (P), docetaxel (P), enalapril (P), erythromycin (P), estrogens
(P), ethambutol (P), ethanol (P), ethionamide (P), etoposide (P), etretinate (P),
filgrastim (P), fluconazole (P), flucytosine (P), foscarnet (P), ganciclovir (P), glycopyrrolate (P), gold salts (P), griseofulvin (P), haloperidol (P), halothane (P),
hepatotoxic drugs (P), HMG-CoA reductase inhibitors (P), hydralazine (P), ibuprofen (I,P), imipramine (P), interferon (P), isoniazid (P), isotretinoin (P),
ketoconazole (P), labetalol (P), levamisole (P), lincomycin (P), lithium salts (P),
magnesium (I), MAO inhibitors (P), mebendazole (P), meprobamate (P), mercaptopurine (P), methotrexate (P), methyldopa (P), mitomycin (P), morphine (P),
nafarelin (P), nifedipine (P), niacin (P), nicotinic acid (P), nitrofurantoin (P), nonsteroidal anti-inflammatory drugs (P), omeprazole (P), ondansetron (P), oral contraceptives (P), papaverine (P), paramethadione (P), penicillamine (P), penicillins
(P), phenazopyridine (P), phenobarbital (P), phenothiazines (P), phenytoin (P),
pindolol (I), plicamycin (P), probenecid (P), procainamide (P), propoxyphene (P),
propylthiouracil (P), protriptyline (P), pyrazinamide (P), quinidine (P), rifampin
(P), salicylates (P), streptozosin (P), sulfasalazine (P), sulfonamides (P), sulfonylureas (P), tamoxifen (P), tetracyclines (P), thiabendazole (P), thioguanine (P),
ticlopidine (P), topotecan (P), trimethadione (P), trimethoprim (P), troleandomycin (P), valproic acid (P), verapamil (P), vitamin A (P), zidovudine (P).[1-5]

Decreased by azathioprine (P), bisphosphonates (P), calcitriol (P), carvedilol
(P), citrate salts (I), clofibrate (I), cyclosporine (P), danazol (P), EDTA (I), estrogens (P), fluoride salts (I), oral contraceptives (P), phosphate salts (I), prednisolone (P), prednisone (P), tamoxifen (P), theophylline (I), tricyclic antidepressants (P), ursodiol (P), zinc (I).[2-4]

Aminotransferases (ALT [SGOT] or AST [SGPT]) (S). *Elevated* by abacavir (P),
acarbose (P), acebutolol (P), acetaminophen (I,P), acetohexamide (P), acyclovir
(P), albendazole (P), alitretinoin (P), allopurinol (P), aminoglycosides (P), amiodarone (P), amitriptyline (P), ampicillin (I), anabolic steroids (P), androgens (P),
anastrozole (P), vitamin C (P), asparaginase (P), azathioprine (P), azithromycin
(P), aztreonam (P), barbiturates (P), benzodiazepines (P), bromocriptine (P), captopril (P), carbamazepine (P), carboplatin (P), carmustine (P), cephalosporins (P),
chenodiol (P), chloral hydrate (P), chlorambucil (P), chloramphenicol (P), chlordiazepoxide (I,P), chlorothiazide (P), chlorpropamide (P), cholestyramine (P),
cholinergic agents (P), cimetidine (P), clarithromycin (P), clavulanic acid (P),
clindamycin (P), clofibrate (P), clopidogrel (P), clotrimazole (P), COX-2 inhibitors (P), cyclophosphamide (P), cyclosporine (P), cytarabine (P), dacarbazine
(P), danazol (P), dantrolene (P), dapsone (P), delavirdine (P), denileukin diftitox
(P), didanosine (P), disopyramide (P), disulfiram (P), diuretics (thiazide) (P), docetaxel (P), efavirenz (P), enflurane (P), erythromycin (I,P), estrogens (P), ethacrynic
acid (P), ethambutol (P), ethanol (P), ethionamide (P), etoposide (P), etretinate
(P), fenofibrate (P), fluconazole (P), flucytosine (P), fluoroquinolones (P), flutamide (P), fomepizole (P), foscarnet (P), ganciclovir (P), gemcitabine (P), gemtuzumab ozogamicin (P), gentamicin (I,P), glyburide (P), glycopyrrolate (P), gold
salts (P), griseofulvin (P), haloperidol (P), halothane (P), heparin (I,P), hepatotoxic

drugs (P), HMG-CoA reductase inhibitors (P), hydralazine (P), IM injections (P), idarubicin (P), imipramine (P), indinavir (P), interferon alfa-2a (P), interferon beta-1a (P), interferon beta-1b (P), interleukin 2 (P), irinotecan (P), iron salts (I), isoniazid (P), isoproterenol (I), isotretinoin (P), ketoconazole (P), labetalol (P), leflunomide (P), levamisole (P), levodopa (I,P), lincomycin (P), MAO inhibitors (P), mebendazole (P), mefloquine (P), meprobamate (P), mercaptopurine (P), methimazole (P), methotrexate (P), methoxyflurane (P), methyldopa (I), metoprolol (P), mexiletine (P), mirtazapine (P), mitoxantrone (P), nafarelin (P), naltrexone (P), nevirapine (P), niacin (P), nicotinic acid (P), nifedipine (P), nilutamide (P), nitrofurantoin (P), nonsteroidal anti-inflammatory drugs (P), olanzapine (P), omeprazole (P), ondansetron (P), opiates (I,P), oral contraceptives (P), papaverine (P), paramethadione (P), penicillamine (P), penicillins (I,P), pentamidine (P), pentosan polysulfate sodium (P), phenazopyridine (P), phenobarbital (P), phenothiazines (P), phenytoin (P), pindolol (P), plicamycin (P), porfimer (P), probenecid (P), procainamide (P), progestins (P), propoxyphene (P), propylthiouracil (P), protriptyline (P), pyrazinamide (P), pyridoxine (P), quetiapine (P), quinidine (P), quinine (P), quinupristin/dalfopristin (P), ranitidine (P), retinol (P), rifabutin (P), rifampin (P), rifapentine (P), riluzole (P), ritodrine (P), ritonavir (P), salicylates (I,P), sargramostim (P), streptozosin (P), sulfasalazine (P), sulfonamides (P), sulfones (P), sulfonylureas (P), tacrine (P), tamoxifen (P), temozolomide (P), tetracyclines (P), thiabendazole (P), thioguanine (P), ticlopidine (P), tolbutamide (P), tolcapone (P), topotecan (P), parenteral nutrition (P), tretinoin (P), trimethadione (P), troleandomycin (P), valproic acid (P), verapamil (P), vidarabine (P), vinorelbine (P), vitamin A (P), zafirlukast (P), zalcitabine (P), zidovudine (P).[1-7]

Decreased by acetaminophen (I), acetazolamide (I), vitamin C (I), aspirin (I), cyclosporine (P), dopamine (I), fluoride salts (I), interferon (I), isoniazid (I), methyldopa (I), metronidazole (I), naltrexone (P), opiates (P), penicillamine (I), pindolol (I), rifampin (I), succinate salts (I), tartrate salts (I), tricyclic antidepressants (P), ursodiol (P).[2,3]

Ammonia (B). *Elevated* by acetazolamide (P), alcohol (P), ammonium salts (P), asparaginase (P), barbiturates (P), carbamazepine (P), diuretics (loop, thiazide) (P), fluorides (I), isoniazid (P), parenteral nutrition (P), tobacco (P), valproic acid.[1-3,5,6]

Decreased by cefotaxime (I), diphenhydramine (P), kanamycin (P), *Lactobacillus acidophilus* (P), lactulose (P), levodopa (P), MAO inhibitors (P), neomycin (P), phosphate salts (I), potassium salts (P), tetracycline (P), tobacco (P).[2,3,5,6]

Amylase (S). *Elevated* by alcohol (P), angiotensin II receptor blockers (P), ACE inhibitors (P), asparaginase (P), azathioprine (P), bethanechol (P), captopril (P), chloride salts (I), cholinergic agents (P), cimetidine (P), cisplatin (P), clofibrate (P), corticosteroids (P), cyproheptadine (P), denileukin diftitox (P), didanosine (P), diphenoxylate (P), diuretics (loop, thiazide) (P), erythromycin (P), estrogens (P), fluorescein (I), fluoride salts (I), ibuprofen (P), indinavir (P), indomethacin (P), lamivudine (P), methyldopa (P), metronidazole (P), narcotics (P), nitrofurantoin (P), opiates (P), oral contraceptives (P), pentamidine (P), potassium iodide (P), rifampin (P), ritonavir (P), secretin (P), sulfonamides (P), sulindac (P), tetracycline (P), diuretics (thiazide) (P), valproic acid (P), vinorelbine (P).[1-4,8]

Decreased by anabolic steroids (P), cefotaxime (I), citrate salts (P), EDTA (I), fluoride salts (I), somatostatin (P).[2,3]

Bilirubin, Total (S). *Elevated* by acarbose (P), acetaminophen (P), acetohexamide (P), allopurinol (P), amiodarone (P), amitriptyline (P), amphotericin B (I,P), anabolic steroids (P), androgens (P), vitamin C (I,P), asparaginase (P), azathioprine (P), barbiturates (P), benzodiazepines (P), capecitabine (P), captopril (P), carbamazepine (P), carbarsone (P), cephalosporins (P), chenodiol (P), chlorambucil (P), chloramphenicol (P), chloroquine (P), chlorpropamide (P), cholinergics (P), cimetidine (P), clavulanic acid (P), colchicine (P), cyclophosphamide (P), cyclosporine (P), cytarabine (P), danazol (P), dantrolene (P), dapsone (P), dextran (I), dimercaprol (P), disulfiram (P), diuretics (thiazide, loop) (P), docetaxel (P), epinephrine (I), erythromycin (P), estrogens (P), ethanol (P), ethionamide (P), etoposide (P), etretinate (P), fluconazole (P), flutamide (P), gemtuzumab ozogamicin (P), glyburide (P), glycopyrrolate (P), gold salts (P), haloperidol (P), halothane (P), hemolytic agents (P), hepatotoxic drugs (P), HMG-CoA reductase inhibitors (P), hydralazine (P), imipramine (P), indinavir (P), interferon beta-1b (P), irinotecan (P), iron salts (P), isoniazid (P), isoproterenol (I), isotretinoin (P), ketoconazole (P), levodopa (I,P), MAO inhibitors (P), meprobamate (P), mercaptopurine (P), methimazole (P), methotrexate (I,P), methyldopa (I,P), mitoxantrone (P), niacin (P), nicotinic acid (P), nitrofurantoin (I,P), nonsteroidal anti-inflammatory drugs (P), opiates (I), oral contraceptives (P), papaverine (P), paramethadione (P), penicillamine (P), penicillins (P), phenazopyridine (I,P), phenelzine (I), phenobarbital (P), phenothiazines (P), phenytoin (P), plicamycin (P), primaquine (P), probenecid (P), procainamide (P), progestins (P), propoxyphene (P), propranolol (I), propylthiouracil (P), pyrazinamide (P), pyrimethamine (P), quinidine (P), quinine (P), quinupristin/dalfopristin (P), rifampin (I,P), rifapentine (P), riluzole (P), salicylates (I,P), sulfasalazine (P), sulfonamides (P), sulfones (P), sulfonylureas (P), tamoxifen (P), tetracyclines (P), theophylline (I), thiabendazole (P), tolbutamide (P), topotecan (P), trimethadione (P), troleandomycin (P), valproic acid (P), vitamin A (P), zafirlukast (P), zidovudine (P).[2–4,6,8]

Decreased by amikacin (I), barbiturates (especially in newborns) (P), carbamazepine (P), corticosteroids (P), cyclosporine (P), fexofenadine (P), isotretinoin (P), levodopa (I), nitrofurantoin (I), oral contraceptives (P), phenazopyridine (I), phenytoin (P), pindolol (I), sulfonamides (P), temozolomide (P), tobacco (P), theophylline (I), ursodiol (P), vitamin C (I).[1,2,4,5]

Calcium, Total (S). *Elevated* by alitretinoin (P), amifostine (P), anabolic steroids (P), androgens (P), antacids (alkaline) (P), basiliximab (P), calcitriol (P), calcium salts (P), cefotaxime (I), chlorpropamide (I), danazol (P), diuretics (thiazide, loop) (P), estrogens (P), hydralazine (I), interferon (I), iron salts (I), isotretinoin (P), lithium salts (P), magnesium salts (I), phenobarbital (P), progestins (P), PTH (P), sevelamer (P), tamoxifen (P), toremifene (P), thyroid (P), vitamin A (P), vitamin D (P).[1–6,8,9]

Decreased by acetazolamide (P), albuterol (P), alprostadil (P), aminoglycosides (P), asparaginase (P), aspirin (I), barbiturates (P), bisphosphonates (P), calcitonin (P), carbamazepine (P), carboplatin (P), cisplatin (P), citrate salts (P), corticosteroids (P), diuretics (loop) (P), EDTA (I), ergocalciferol (P), ethanol (P), fluoride salts (I,P), foscarnet (P), glucagon (P), heparin (I), indapamide (P), insulin (P), isoniazid (P), laxatives (P), magnesium salts (P), methicillin (P), oral contraceptives (P), phenobarbital (P), phenytoin (P), phosphate salts (P), plicamycin (P), sodium polystyrene sulfonate (P), sulfate salts (I), sulfisoxazole (I).[1–6,8,9]

Carbon Dioxide, Total (B). *Elevated* by aldosterone (P), bicarbonate salts (P), carbenicillin (P), corticosteroids (P), diuretics (loop, thiazide) (P), respiratory depressants (P).[3,4,6]

Decreased by acetazolamide (P), ammonium chloride (P), aspirin (overdose) (P), methicillin (P), nephrotoxic drugs (P), nitrofurantoin (P), tetracyclines (P), theophylline (P), triamterene (P).[2–4,6]

Chloride (S). *Elevated* by acetazolamide (P), ammonium carbonate (I), anabolic steroids (P), androgens (P), vitamin C (I), aspirin (I,P), cannabinoids (P), carbamazepine (I), cefotaxime (I), cholestyramine (P), corticosteroids (by salt retention) (P), corticotropin (P), COX-2 inhibitors (P), cyclosporine (P), diuretics, carbonic anhydrase inhibitor, thiazide (chronically by alkalosis) (P), estrogens (P), guanethidine (P), halogens (e.g., bromides, fluorides, iodides) (I), methyldopa (P), N-acetylcysteine (I), nonsteroidal anti-inflammatory drugs (P), procainamide (I), triamterene (P).[1–4]

Decreased by allopurinol (I), bicarbonates (P), cefotaxime (metabolite) (I), chlorpropamide (P), corticosteroids (by alkalosis) (P), diuretics (loop, thiazide) (by acute diuresis) (P), fluoride salts (I), laxatives, long-term use (P), mannitol (P), mineralocorticoids (by alkalosis) (P), theophylline (P), triamterene (P), trimethoprim (P).[2–4]

Cholesterol, Total (S). *Elevated* by ACTH (P), acetohexamide (P), β-adrenergic blocking agents (P), amiodarone (P), amphotericin B (I), amprenavir (P), anabolic steroids (by cholestasis) (P), androgens (P), aspirin (I), basiliximab (P), carbamazepine (P), cefotaxime (I), chenodiol (P), clopidogrel (P), oral contraceptives (P), corticosteroids (I,P), cyclosporine (P), danazol (P), dextran (I), diclofenac (P), disulfiram (P), diuretics (loop, thiazide) (P), ethanol (P), fibrates (P), gold salts (P), hepatotoxic drugs (cholestatic effect) (P), heroin (P), ibuprofen (P), imipramine (P), isotretinoin (P), levodopa (P), meprobamate (P), methotrexate (I), mirtazapine (P), mycophenolate (P), nafarelin (P), phenobarbital (P), phenothiazines (I,P), phenytoin (I,P), protease inhibitors (P), quetiapine (P), retinoids (P), ritonavir (P), rosiglitazone (P), sirolimus (P), sorbitol (P), sotalol (P), spironolactone (P), sulfadiazine (P), tamoxifen (P), tetracycline (I), thiabendazole (P), ticlopidine (P), tobacco (P), vitamin A (I), vitamin C (I,P), vitamin D (I,P).[1–3,8]

Decreased by acarbose (P), acebutolol (P), α-adrenergic blocking agents (P), allopurinol (I,P), aluminum salts (P), amiloride (P), amiodarone (P), ampicillin (I), anabolic steroids (by inhibiting synthesis) (P), ACE inhibitors (P), vitamin C (I,P), asparaginase (P), azathioprine (P), bile acid sequestrants (P), calcium channel blockers (P), carvedilol (P), chlorpropamide (P), citrate salts (I), clofibrate (P), clomiphene (P), colchicine (P), diuretics (thiazide) (P), estrogens (P), ethanol (chronic use) (P), fenofibrate (P), fibrates (P), fluoride salts (I), haloperidol (P), heparin (P), hepatotoxic drugs (decreased synthesis) (P), HMG-CoA reductase inhibitors (P), hydroxychloroquine (P), insulin (P), isoniazid (P), isotretinoin (P), kanamycin (oral) (P), ketoconazole (P), levothyroxine (P), MAO inhibitors (P), metformin (P), methyldopa (I,P), metronidazole (P), neomycin (P), niacin (P), nitrates (I), orlistat (P), penicillamine (I), pentamidine (P), phenytoin (P), pindolol (P), probucol (P), psyllium (P), raloxifene (P), rifampin (I), sevelamer (P), tacrolimus (P), tamoxifen (P), tetracyclines (P), thyroid (P), ursodiol (P), valproic acid (P). [2–6,8]

Creatine Kinase (S). *Elevated* by aminocaproic acid (P), amphotericin B (P), barbiturates (P), captopril (P), carbon monoxide (poisoning) (P), carteolol (P), cefotaxime (I), chlorpromazine (P), clofibrate (P), clonidine (P), cocaine (P), colchicine (P), cyclopropane (P), cyclosporine (P), danazol (P), diethyl ether (P), ethanol (chronic) (P), ethchlorvynol (P), fenofibrate (P), gemfibrozil (P), haloperidol (P), halothane (P), HMG-CoA reductase inhibitors (P), isotretinoin (P), labetalol (P), lidocaine (P), lithium salts (P), lysergide (LSD) (P), niacin (P), D-penicillamine (P), perphenazine (P), phencyclidine (PCP) (P), pindolol (P), prochlorperazine (P), propranolol (P), quinidine (P), succimer (I), saquinavir (P), succinylcholine + halothane (during anesthesia) (P), tricyclic antidepressants (P), zidovudine (P). [1–3,5,6,8]

Decreased by amikacin (I), anesthetic agents (P), vitamin C (I), aspirin (I), dantrolene (P), phenothiazines (P), pindolol (I), succinylcholine (P), sulfamethoxazole (P). [2,3]

Creatinine (S). *Elevated* by acebutolol (P), acetaminophen (I,P), acetazolamide (P), acetohexamide (I), acyclovir (P), amiloride (P), aminocaproic acid (P), aminoglycosides (P), amiodarone (P), amphotericin B (P), ACE inhibitors (P), antacids (P), vitamin C (I), asparaginase (P), aztreonam (P), capreomycin (P), carvedilol (P), cephalosporins (Jaffe method) (I,P), chloroquine (P), cidofovir (P), cimetidine (P), carboplatin (P), cisplatin (P), clofibrate (P), colistin (P), corticosteroids (P), cotrimoxazole (P), creatine (I), cyclophosphamide (P), cyclosporine (P), demeclocycline (P), denileukin diftitox (P), dextran (P), digoxin (P), diuretics (thiazide, potassium-sparing) (P), dopamine (I), doxycycline (P), flucytosine (I,P), foscarnet (P), furosemide (I,P), ifosfamide (P), ganciclovir (P), hydroxychloroquine (P), lactulose (I), levodopa (I), lidocaine (I,P), lithium (I,P), mannitol (P), methicillin (P), methotrexate (P), methoxyflurane (P), methyldopa (I), mitomycin (P), nalidixic acid (P), nephrotoxic drugs (P), nifedipine (P), nitrofurantoin (I), nitrosoureas (P), nonsteroidal anti-inflammatory drugs (I,P), penicillamine (P), penicillins (I), pentamidine (P), phosphate salts (P), plicamycin (P), polymyxin B (P), probenecid (P), pyrimethamine (P), quinine (P), radiographic contrast media [ionic, nonionic] (P), rifampin (P), ritonavir (P), salicylates (P), sirolimus (P), streptozosin (P), sulbactam (I), sulfamethoxazole (I), sulfonamides (P), tacrolimus (P), tetracyclines (P), triamterene (P), trimethoprim (P), vancomycin (P), vitamin D (P). [1–6,9]

Decreased by N-acetylcysteine (I), amikacin (I), anabolic steroids (P), androgens (P), vitamin C (I), cannabinoids (P), cephalosporins (I), citrate salts (I), diuretics (thiazide) (P), dobutamine (I), dopamine (I), ibuprofen (P), interferon alfa-2a (P), methyldopa (I), sulfonylureas (P). [1–3,8,9]

Glucose (S). *Elevated* by abacavir (P), ACTH (P), acetaminophen (SMA 12/60 method) (I), acetazolamide (P), β-adrenergic agonists (P), β-adrenergic blocking agents (also mask hypoglycemia) (P), albuterol (P), amiodarone (P), heterocyclic antidepressants (P), vitamin C (glucose oxidase method) (I), asparaginase (P), basiliximab (P), bicalutamide (P), caffeine (P), calcitonin (salmon) (P), cefotaxime (I), cholestyramine (P), citrate salts (I), clonidine (P), clozapine (P), corticosteroids (P), cyclosporine (P), daclizumab (P), dextran (I), dextroamphetamine (P), diazoxide (P), diclofenac (I), diltiazem (P), diuretics (loop, thiazide) (P), epinephrine (I,P), ephedrine (P), estrogens (P), fosphenytoin (P), gemfibrozil (P), glucagon (P), interferon alfa-2a (P), iron dextran (I), indomethacin (P), isoniazid (P), isoproterenol (I), labetalol (I), lactose (I), levodopa (SMA 12/60 method) (I), lipids (P), lithium salts (P), mercaptopurine (I), methyldopa (I), metronidazole (I), morphine (P), mycophenolate (P), nalidixic acid (I), niacin (I,P), nicotinic acid (P), nifedipine (P), octreotide (P), olanzapine (P), oral contraceptives (P), pentamidine (IV) (paradoxical effect) (P), perphenazine (P), phenothiazines (P), phenytoin (P), pravastatin (P), progestins (P), propranolol (P), propylthiouracil (I), protease inhibitors (P), reserpine (P), rifampin (I,P), salicylates (acute toxicity) (I), somatostatin (P), sorbitol (P), streptozosin (P), tacrolimus (P), terbutaline (P), tetracyclines (P), thiabendazole (P), thyroid (P), tolbutamide (P), triamterene (P), vitamin C (neocuproine method) (I).[1–6,8]

Decreased by acarbose (P), acetaminophen (GOD-Perid method) (I,P), acetazolamide (P), β-adrenergic blocking agents (nonselective) (P), alcohol (P), allopurinol (P), amikacin (I), anabolic steroids (P), antihistamines (P), cannabinoids (P), chloroquine (P), chlorpropamide (I), captopril (P), cimetidine (P), clofibrate (P), cyproterone (P), disopyramide (P), doxazosin (P), erythromycin (P), estrogens (P), ethanol (P), fenfluramine (P), gemfibrozil (P), glutathione (hexokinase method) (I), guanethidine (P), interferon beta-1b (P), hydralazine (I), indomethacin (P), insulin (P), isoniazid (I), levodopa (glucose oxidase and other methods) (I), lipids (I), MAO inhibitors (P), metformin (P), methyldopa (I), metronidazole (I), miglitol (P), niacin (P), octreotide (P), pentamidine (IV) (P), phenazopyridine (I), phosphorus (P), psyllium (P), repaglinide (P), salicylates (acute and chronic toxicity) (P), saquinavir (P), spironolactone (P), SSRIs (P), sulfonamides (P), sulfonylureas (P), tetracyclines (I), thiabendazole (P), tolazamide (I), tolbutamide (I,P), tromethamine (P), verapamil (P), vitamin C (GOD-Perid method) (I,P).[2–4,6,7,]

Hemoglobin, Glycosylated (B). *Elevated* by hydrochlorothiazide (P), indapamide (P), morphine (P), propranolol (P).[2]

Iron (S). *Elevated* by cefotaxime (I), chloramphenicol (P), cisplatin (P), oral contraceptives (P), estrogens (P), ethanol (P), ferrous salts (I), iron (parenteral) (I,P), methyldopa (P), methotrexate (P), miglitol (P), oral contraceptives (P), rifampin (I).[2–4,8]

Decreased by allopurinol (P), aspirin (large doses) (P), anabolic steroids (P), cholestyramine (P), colchicine (P), corticotropin (P), corticosteroids (P), deferoxamine (I,P), entacapone (P), metformin (P), penicillamine (P), pyrazinamide (I,P).[2–4,8]

Iron Binding Capacity, Total (S). *Elevated* by estrogens (P), oral contraceptives (P), propylthiouracil (P).[2–4,8]

    Decreased by asparaginase (P), chloramphenicol (P), corticotropin (P), corticosteroids (P), testosterone (P).[2–4,8]

Lipoprotein, High-density (S). *Elevated* by carbamazepine (P), estrogens (P), ethanol (moderate intake) (P), fibrates (P), HMG-CoA reductase inhibitors (P), bile acid sequestrants (P), niacin (P), phenobarbital (P), phenytoin (P).[2]

    Decreased by anabolic steroids (P), androgens (P), β-adrenergic blocking agents (P), cyclosporine (P), diuretics (thiazides) (P), glucocorticoids (P), retinoids (P), interferon (P), interleukin (P), probucol (P), progestins (P), protease inhibitors (P), tobacco (P).[1,2]

Lipoprotein, Low-density (S). *Elevated* by androgens (P), β-adrenergic blocking agents (P), cyclosporine (P), danazol (P), diuretics (thiazide) (P), corticosteroids (P), progestins (P), retinoids (P).[1,2]

    Decreased by α-adrenergic blocking agents (P), bile acid sequestrants (P), cyproterone (P), estrogens (P), fibrates (P), HMG-CoA reductase inhibitors (P), interferon (P), interleukin (P), ketoconazole (P), neomycin (P), niacin (P), probucol (P), thyroxine (P).[2]

Magnesium (S). *Elevated* by aspirin (chronic therapy) (P), cefotaxime (I), diuretics (potassium-sparing) (P), lithium salts (P), magnesium salts (P), pentamidine (P), progestins (P), vitamin D (chronic renal failure) (P).[2–5,7]

    Decreased by albuterol (P), amifostine (P), aminoglycosides (P), amphotericin B (P), bisphosphonates (P), calcium salts (I), cefotaxime (I), cisplatin (P), citrate salts (I,P), cyclosporine (P), digitalis (toxic concentrations) (P), diuretics (loop, thiazide) (P), ethanol (P), foscarnet (P), glucagon (P), insulin (P), laxatives (P), oral contraceptives (P), pentamidine (P), phenytoin (P), tacrolimus (P).[2–5,7]

Osmolality (S). *Elevated* by alcohol (ADH suppression) (P), citrate salts (I), corticosteroids (P), demeclocycline (ADH inhibition) (P), glucose (I), glycerin (P), insulin (P), lithium salts (ADH inhibition) (P), mannitol (I,P), methoxyflurane (P).[2,3,5]

    Decreased by tricyclic antidepressants (P), carbamazepine (P), chlorpropamide (P), clonidine (P), cisplatin (P), cyclophosphamide (P), cytarabine (P), diuretics (thiazide) (P), fluoxetine (P), haloperidol (P), interferon alfa (I), MAO inhibitors (P), phenothiazines (P), SSRIs (P), sulfonylureas (P), vasopressin (P), vinca alkaloids (P).[2,3,5]

Phosphate (S). *Elevated* by androgens (P), β-adrenergic blocking agents (P), basiliximab (P), cefotaxime (I), ethanol (P), etidronate (P), ergocalciferol (P), foscarnet (P), furosemide (P), growth hormone (P), hydrochlorothiazide (P), mannitol (I), methicillin (I,P), methotrexate (I), oral contraceptives (P), phosphate salts (P), pindolol (P), rifampin (I,P), tetracycline (P), vitamin D (excessive) (P).[2,3,5,9]

    Decreased by acetazolamide (P), β-adrenergic agonists (P), amino acids (P), anesthetic agents (P), antacids (phosphate binding; e.g., aluminum, calcium, and magnesium salts) (P), bisphosphonates (P), calcitonin (P), carbamazepine (P), cidofovir (P), citrate salts (I), diuretics (loop, thiazide) (P), epinephrine (P), estrogens (P), glucagon (P), glucocorticoids (P), foscarnet (P), hydrochlorothiazide (chronic use) (P), ifosfamide (P), insulin (P), isoniazid (P), oral contraceptives (P), lithium salts (P), mannitol (I), mycophenolate (P), parenteral nutrition (P), phenobarbital (P), phenothiazines (I,P), phenytoin (P), sevelamer (P), sirolimus (P), sorbitol (P), sucralfate (P), tacrolimus (P), tartrate salts (I).[1–3,5,7,8]

Potassium (S). *Elevated* by aminocaproic acid (P), angiotensin II receptor blockers (P), ACE inhibitors (P), arginine (P), β-adrenergic blocking agents (P), antineoplastic agents (cytotoxic effect) (P), basiliximab (P), cannabinoids (P), cefotaxime (I), cisplatin (I), cyclosporine (P), COX-2 inhibitors (P), digoxin (toxicity) (P), diuretics (potassium-sparing) (P), epinephrine (initial effect) (P), fluconazole (P), fluoride salts (I), foscarnet (P), heparin (P), heroin (P), iodide salts (I), isoniazid (P), levodopa (I), lithium salts (I,P), low-molecular-weight heparins (P), mannitol (P), mycophenolate (P), nephrotoxic drugs (P), nonsteroidal anti-inflammatory drugs (primarily indomethacin) (P), pentamidine (P), potassium penicillin (P), procainamide (I), salt substitutes (P), succinylcholine (P), tacrolimus (P), tetracycline (P), trimethoprim (P), tromethamine (P).[1–9]

Decreased by acetazolamide (P), aspirin (I), β-adrenergic agonists (P), aminoglycosides (P), ammonium chloride (P), amphotericin B (P), azlocillin (P), basiliximab (P), bicarbonate salts (P), bisacodyl (P), bisphosphonates (P), capreomycin (P), cholestyramine (P), cisplatin (P), corticosteroids (P), corticotropin (P), cyanocobalamin (P), diuretics (loop, thiazide) (P), fenoldopam (P), fluconazole (P), foscarnet (P), glucagon (P), glucose (P), ifosfamide (P), insulin (P), laxatives (P), levodopa (P), mineralocorticoids (P), mycophenolate (P), ondansetron (P), penicillin G (sodium salt) (P), penicillins (extended-spectrum) (P), phosphate salts (P), polymyxin B (P), salicylates (P), sirolimus (P), sorbitol (P), sodium bicarbonate (P), sodium chloride (P), sodium polystyrene sulfonate (P), sodium phenylbutyrate (P), sulfasalazine (P), tacrolimus (P), theophylline (P).[1–9]

Protein, Total (S). *Elevated* by androgens (P), aspirin (I), chloramphenicol (I), clofibrate (P), corticosteroids (P), corticotropin (P), dextran (biuret method) (I), epinephrine (P), imipramine (I), insulin (P), lidocaine (I), mannitol (I), methotrexate (I), penicillins (I), phenazopyridine (I), phenothiazines [CSF] (I), progestins (I,P), radiocontrast agents [ionic, nonionic] (I), rifampin (I), sulfonamides (I), tetracyclines (I), thyroid (P), vancomycin (I), vitamin C (I).[2–4,6]

Decreased by acetaminophen (P), allopurinol (P), cefotaxime (I), oral contraceptives (from estrogen) (P), cytarabine (I,P), dexamethasone (P), dextran (I,P), estrogens (P), hepatotoxic drugs (P), pyrazinamide (P), rifampin (P), sulfasalazine (I).[2–4,6]

Sodium (S). *Elevated* by acetohexamide (P), ACTH (P), amphotericin B (P), androgens (P), bicarbonate salts (P), cannabinoids (P), carbamazepine (I,P), carbenicillin (P), cefotaxime (I), cisplatin (I), clonidine (P), colchicine (P), corticosteroids (P), COX-2 inhibitors (P), demeclocycline (P), diazoxide (P), diuretics (loop, osmotic, thiazide) (P), estrogens (P), ethanol (I), foscarnet (P), gentamicin (P), glyburide (P), guanethidine (P), fluoride salts (I), lactulose (P), lithium salts (P), mannitol (P), methicillin (P), methoxyflurane (P), methyldopa (P), mineralocorticoids (P), nitrofurantoin (P), nonsteroidal anti-inflammatory drugs (P), norepinephrine (P), oral contraceptives (P), propoxyphene (P), radiographic contrast media [ionic, nonionic] (P), reserpine (P), sodium bicarbonate (P), tetracycline (P), tolazamide (P), vinblastine (P).[1-4,8,9]

Decreased by ACE inhibitors (P), acetaminophen (P), acetazolamide (P), aminoglycosides (P), ammonium chloride (P), amphotericin B (P), tricyclic antidepressants (P), bicarbonate salts (I), carbamazepine (P), carboplatin (P), chlorpropamide (P), cholestyramine (P), cisplatin (P), clofibrate (P), clonidine (P), cyclophosphamide (P), cytarabine (P), diuretics (loop, thiazide, potassium-sparing) (P), fluoxetine (P), glucose (P), haloperidol (P), heparin (I,P), indomethacin (P), interferon (P), ketoconazole (P), laxatives (P), lithium salts (P), mannitol (P), MAO inhibitors (P), miconazole (P), nifedipine (P), nonsteroidal anti-inflammatory drugs (P), opiates (P), oxytocin (P), phenothiazines (P), SSRIs (P), somatostatin (P), spironolactone (P), sulfonylureas (P), vasopressin and analogues (P), tobacco (P), tolbutamide (P), tricyclic antidepressants (P), trimethoprim (P), vinca alkaloids (P).[1-5,8,9]

Thyroxine, Total (T4) (S). *Elevated* by amiodarone (I,P), amphetamines (P), clofibrate (P), estrogens (P), fluorouracil (P), heparin (I), heroin (P), insulin (P), levodopa (P), methadone (P), oral contraceptives (P), prazosin (P), propranolol (P), propylthiouracil (P), prostaglandins (P), radiographic contrast media, [ionic] (I,P), tamoxifen (P), thyroid agents (P).[2-8]

Decreased by amiodarone (P), androgens (P), asparaginase (P), barbiturates (P), carbamazepine (P), chlorpropamide (P), cholestyramine (P), clofibrate (P), colestipol (P), corticosteroids (P), corticotropin (P), danazol (I,P), diazepam (P), furosemide (P), growth hormone (P), heparin (I), heroin (P), interferon alfa-2a (P), iodide salts (P), iron salts (P), isotretinoin (P), lithium salts (P), methimazole (P), penicillamine (P), phenytoin (P), propylthiouracil (P), reserpine (P), rifampin (P), salicylates (P), somatotropin (P), sulfonamides (P), sulfonylureas (P), thyroid (P), triiodothyronine (P), valproic acid (P).[1-6,8]

Triglycerides (S). *Elevated* by β-adrenergic blocking agents (P), amiodarone (P), amprenavir (P), vitamin C (I), aspirin (I,P), bile acid sequestrants (P), corticosteroids (P), cyclosporine (P), danazol (P), didanosine (P), diuretics (loop, thiazide) (P), estrogens (P), ethanol (P), fomepizole (P), protease inhibitors (P), interferon (P), itraconazole (P), lipids (P), low-molecular-weight heparins (P), HMG-CoA reductase inhibitors (P), mirtazapine (P), nitroglycerin (I), olanzapine (P), oral contraceptives (P), quinidine (P), retinoids (P), sirolimus (P), tamoxifen (P), tobacco (P).[2,4-6,8]

Decreased by acarbose (P), α-adrenergic blocking agents (P), aminocaproic acid (P), aminosalicylic acid (P), amiodarone (P), ACE inhibitors (P), ascorbic acid (P), asparaginase (P), aspirin (I), chenodiol (P), citrate salts (I), clofibrate (P), danazol (P), fibrates (P), heparin (P), HMG-CoA reductase inhibitors (P), hydroxychloroquine (P), hydroxyurea (I), ketoconazole (P), metformin (P), methotrexate (I), methyldopa (I), naproxen (I), niacin (P), nifedipine (P), omega-3 fatty acids (P), orlistat (P), probucol (P), psyllium (P), rifampin (I), spironolactone (P), sulfonylureas (P), verapamil (P).[2-6]

Urea Nitrogen (S). *Elevated* by ACE inhibitors (P), acetaminophen (overdose) (P), acetazolamide (P), acetohexamide (I), aminoglycosides (P), amphotericin B (P), anabolic steroids (P), antacids (prolonged use) (P), asparaginase (P), busulfan (P), cannabinoids (P), carbamazepine (P), capreomycin (P), carboplatin (P), cephalosporins (P), chloral hydrate (I), chloramphenicol (Nesslerization method) (I), cisplatin (P), clonidine (P), colistin (P), corticosteroids (P), cotrimoxazole (P), cyclophosphamide (P), cyclosporine (P), dexamethasone (P), dextran (I,P), diuretics (loop, thiazide) (P), foscarnet (P), flucytosine (P), gold salts (P), hydralazine (P), hydroxyurea (P), ifosfamide (P), iron salts (P), lithium (P), mannitol (P), methotrexate (P), methoxyflurane (P), methyldopa (P), mitomycin (P), nalidixic acid (P), nephrotoxic drugs (P), nitrofurantoin (P), nitrosoureas (P), nonsteroidal anti-inflammatory drugs (P), penicillamine (P), penicillins (P), pentamidine (P), plicamycin (P), polymyxin B (P), quinine (P), radiographic contrast media [ionic, nonionic] (P), rifampin (P), salicylates (P), streptozosin (P), sulfonamides (I), tacrolimus (P), tetracyclines (I,P), thyroid agents (P), triamterene (P), vancomycin (P), vitamin D (P).[1–5,8]

Decreased by amikacin (I), vitamin C (I), cefotaxime (I), chloramphenicol (Berthelot method) (I), citrate salts (I), fluoride salts (I), growth hormone (P), levodopa (P), phenothiazines (P), streptomycin (I).[2–5,8]

Uric Acid (S). *Elevated* by acetaminophen (I), β-adrenergic blocking agents (P), anabolic steroids (P), antineoplastics (P), vitamin C (I), azathioprine (P), basiliximab (P), caffeine (I), cisplatin (P), citrate salts (P), corticosteroids (in acute leukemias) (P), cyclosporine (P), cytarabine (P), diazoxide (P), didanosine (P), diuretics (carbonic anhydrase inhibitor, loop, thiazide) (P), epinephrine (I,P), ethanol (P), ethambutol (P), filgrastim (P), hydralazine (I), isoniazid (I), levodopa (I,P), mercaptopurine (P), methyldopa (I), niacin (P), norepinephrine (P), phenytoin (P), pyrazinamide (P), propranolol (P), propylthiouracil (P), rifampin (I), ritonavir (P), salicylates (low doses) (I,P), sodium phenylbutyrate (P), spironolactone (P), tacrolimus (P), theophylline (I,P), triamterene (P) .[1,2,4–6,8]

Decreased by acetohexamide (P), allopurinol (P), vitamin C (by Seralyzer) (I,P), azathioprine (P), cannabinoids (P), cefotaxime (I), cidofovir (P), corticosteroids (P), diflunisal (P), diuretics (IV loop) (P), fibrates (P), glucose infusions (P), griseofulvin (P), guaifenesin (P), hydralazine (I), indomethacin (P), levodopa (I), lithium (P), losartan (P), mannitol (P), methyldopa (I), nonsteroidal anti-inflammatory drugs (P), phenothiazines (P), radiographic contrast media [ionic] (P), rasburicase (P), salicylates (large doses) (P), spironolactone (P), sulfonamides (P), uricosurics (e.g., probenecid, sulfinpyrazone) (P), verapamil (P). [1,2,4–6,8]

■ URINE CHEMISTRY

Bilirubin. *Elevated* by acetohexamide (P), etodolac (I), hepatotoxic drugs (P), phenazopyridine (I), phenothiazines (I,P), salicylates (I).[2,3,8]

Decreased by vitamin C (large amounts) (I).[2]

Color. *See* Drug-Induced Discoloration of Feces and Urine, page 1216

Creatinine. *Elevated* by ACE inhibitors (P), anabolic steroids (increased muscle mass) (P), vitamin C (I), asparaginase (I), cephalosporins (except cefotaxime and ceftazidime) (Jaffe method) (I), corticosteroids (P), levodopa (I), methotrexate

(P), methyldopa (I), nephrotoxic drugs (P), nitrofurantoin (I), reserpine (P), vitamin C (I).[2,3,5,8]

Decreased by aspirin (P), anabolic steroids (anabolic effect) (P), captopril (P), cimetidine (P), diuretics (thiazide, potassium-sparing) (P), probenecid (P), pyrimethamine (P), trimethoprim (P).[3,5,8,9]

Glucose. *Elevated or False Positive* by acetazolamide (P), aspirin (copper reduction) (I,P), aminosalicylic acid (copper reduction) (I), carbamazepine (P), cephalosporins (except cefotaxime) (copper reduction) (I), chloral hydrate (copper reduction) (I), cidofovir (P), corticosteroids (P), dextroamphetamine (P), diuretics (loop, thiazide) (P), glucagon (P), isoniazid (P), levodopa (copper reduction) (I), lithium salts (P), niacin (P), penicillins (I), pentamidine (P), phenazopyridine (Tes-Tape) (I), phenothiazines (P), probenecid (I), reserpine (P), sulfonamides (I), vitamin C (copper reduction).[1–8]

Decreased or False Negative by aspirin (glucose oxidase) (I,P), bisacodyl (I), chloral hydrate (glucose oxidase) (I), diazepam (I), digoxin (I), ferrous salts (I), flurazepam (I), furosemide (I), insulin (P), levodopa (glucose oxidase) (I), phenazopyridine (glucose oxidase) (I), phenobarbital (P), prednisone (glucose oxidase) (I), secobarbital (I), tetracycline (I), vitamin C (glucose oxidase) (I).[3–8]

Gonadotropins (Pregnancy Test). *False Positive* by methadone (I), phenothiazines (I).[3,8]

Ketones. *Elevated* by acetylcysteine (I), albuterol (P), captopril (I), cephalosporins (I), dimercaprol (I), insulin (P), isoniazid (P), levodopa (Labstix) (I), mesna (I), metformin (I), methyldopa (I), niacin (P), penicillamine (I), phenazopyridine (I), phenothiazines (I), pyrazinamide (I), salicylates (acidotic effect) (I,P), succimer (I), valproic acid (I).[3,5,6,8]

Decreased by aspirin (oxidation of ketone bodies) (P), phenazopyridine (I).[3]

Protein, Total. *Elevated* by acetaminophen (P), acetazolamide (I), aminoglycosides (I,P), amphotericin B (P), asparaginase (P), bacitracin (P), bicarbonate salts (I), bismuth salts (P), capreomycin (P), captopril (P), carbamazepine (P), cephalosporins (I,P), chlorpromazine (I), chlorpropamide (P), cidofovir (P), cisplatin (P), colistin (P), corticosteroids (P), cotrimoxazole (P), cyclosporine (P), delavirdine (P), dihydrotachysterol (I,P), diuretics (thiazide) (P), enalapril (P), gemcitabine (P), gold salts (P), griseofulvin (P), hydralazine (P), interferon (P), iron salts (P), isoniazid (P), lithium salts (P), mitomycin (P), nephrotoxic drugs (P), nonsteroidal anti-inflammatory drugs (P), penicillamine (P), penicillins (I), pentamidine (P), phenazopyridine (I), polymyxin B (P), radiographic contrast media [ionic, nonionic] (I), rifapentine (P), salicylates (I), sulfonamides (I), sulfones (P), tetracycline (P), tolbutamide (I), vancomycin (P), vitamin C (I).[2,3,8]

Decreased by ACE inhibitors (P), cyclosporine (P), diltiazem (P), indomethacin (in nephrotic syndrome) (P), interferon alfa-2a (P), prednisolone (P).[2,3]

Specific Gravity. *Elevated* by dextran (I,P), diuretics (P), isotretinoin (P), mannitol (P), radiographic contrast media [ionic, nonionic] (I,P), sucrose (P).[2,3,5,8]

Decreased by aminoglycosides (P), colistin (P), cyclosporine (P), lithium (P), methoxyflurane (P).[2,3]

■ HEMATOLOGY

Coombs' [Direct] (S). *Positive* by aztreonam (P), captopril (P), cephalosporins (P), chlorpromazine (P), chlorpropamide (P), ethosuximide (P), hemolytic agents (P), hydralazine (P), imipenem/cilastatin (P), indomethacin (P), isoniazid (P), levodopa (P), melphalan (P), methyldopa (P), nitrofurantoin (P), penicillamine (P), penicillins (P), phenytoin (P), procainamide (P), quinidine (P), quinine (P), rifampin (P), sulfasalazine (P), sulfonamides (P), sulfonylureas (P), tetracyclines (P), tolmetin (I).[3–5,7]

Erythrocyte Sedimentation Rate (B). *Elevated* by oral contraceptives (P), cyclosporine (P), dextran (P), fluoride salts (I), isotretinoin (P), methyldopa (P), methysergide (P), nitrofurantoin (P), procainamide (P), quinine (I), theophylline (P), vitamin A (P).[2,3,8]

Decreased by corticosteroids (P), corticotropin (P), cyclophosphamide (P), infliximab (P), fluoride salts (I), gold salts (P), methotrexate (P), nonsteroidal anti-inflammatory drugs (P), penicillamine (P), quinine (P), salicylates (P), sulfasalazine (P), tamoxifen (P), trimethoprim (P), drugs that cause hyperglycemia (P).[2,3,8]

Prothrombin Time (B) [Does not include anticoagulants or drugs which potentiate or antagonize them]. *Elevated* by acetaminophen (toxicity) (P), acetohexamide (P), allopurinol (P), amiodarone (P), anabolic steroids (P), antibiotics (gut sterilizing) (P), anticoagulants (oral) (P), asparaginase (P), bile acid sequestrants (P), carbenicillin (P), cephalosporins (P), chloramphenicol (P), chloral hydrate (P), chlorpromazine (P), chlorpropamide (P), cimetidine (P), clofibrate (P), cyclophosphamide (P), disulfiram (P), diuretics (thiazide) (I), erythromycin (P), ethacrynic acid (P), ethanol (toxicity, alcoholism) (P), glucagon (P), halothane (P), heparin (P), hetastarch (P), hepatotoxic drugs (P), interferon (I), laxatives (P), mercaptopurine (P), methotrexate (P), metronidazole (P), miconazole (P), nalidixic acid (P), niacin (P), nonsteroidal anti-inflammatory drugs (P), phenytoin (P), plicamycin (P), propylthiouracil (P), pyrazinamide (P), quinidine (P), quinine (P), salicylates (P), sulfonamides (P), tamoxifen (P), ticarcillin (P), tolazamide (P), tolbutamide (P).[1–3,5,8]

Decreased by anabolic steroids (P), azathioprine (P), estrogens (P), ethanol (chronic use) (P), mercaptopurine (P), oral contraceptives (P), phytonadione (P).[2–4,8]

■ REFERENCES

1. Burtis CA, Ashwood ER, eds. *Tietz Textbook of Clinical Chemistry*. 4th ed. Philadelphia, PA: WB Saunders; 2005.
2. Wu A, ed. *Tietz Clinical Guide to Laboratory Tests*. 4th ed. St Louis, MO: Saunders Elsevier; 2006.
3. Young DS. *Effects of Drugs on Clinical Laboratory Tests*. 5th ed. Washington, DC: AACC Press; 2000.
4. Sher PP. Drug interferences with clinical laboratory tests. *Drugs*. 1982;24:24-63.
5. McEvoy GK, ed. *AHFS Drug Information* 2008. Bethesda, MD: American Society of Health-System Pharmacists; 2008.
6. Salway JG, ed. *Drug-test Interaction Handbook*. 1st ed. New York, NY: Raven Press; 1990.
7. Aronson JK ed. *Side Effects of Drugs, Annual*. 22nd ed. Amsterdam: Elsevier; 1999.
8. Wallach J. *Interpretation of Diagnostic Tests*. 8th ed. Philadelphia, PA: Lippincott, Williams, & Brown; 2006.
9. Lee M, ed. *Basic Skills in Interpreting Laboratory Data*. 3rd ed. Bethesda, MD: American Society of Health-System Pharmacists; 2004.

Pharmacokinetic Equations 5

Gary Theilman

$Alb_{measured}$ = measured serum albumin
Alb_{normal} = normal serum albumin
$C_{effective}$ = effective (or normalized) serum concentration
Cl = serum drug clearance
C_{meas} = measured serum concentration
C_{ss} = steady-state serum concentration
C_0 = initial serum concentration
D = dose
F = fraction of dose absorbed (bioavailability)
f_u = fraction of drug unbound to albumin
K_0 = infusion rate (dose/t_{inf})
k_{el} = elimination rate constant
K_m = Michaelis-Menten constant
S = salt fraction
τ = dosage interval
$t_{90\%}$ = time to reach 90% of steady state
$t_{1/2}$ = elimination half-life
t_{inf} = duration of infusion
t_{wait} = time one has waited following the end of an infusion before obtaining a serum concentration
V_d = apparent volume of distribution
V_{max} = maximum rate of metabolism

■ FIRST-ORDER, ONE COMPARTMENT

Concentration immediately after an intravenous bolus and same equation rearranged to estimate dose needed to increase concentration from C_0 to C:

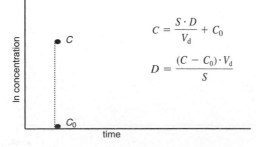

$$C = \frac{S \cdot D}{V_d} + C_0$$

$$D = \frac{(C - C_0) \cdot V_d}{S}$$

Concentration at time t following an intravenous bolus:

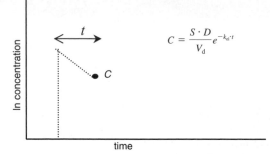

$$C = \frac{S \cdot D}{V_d} e^{-k_{el} \cdot t}$$

Concentration immediately after an intravenous infusion administered over time t:

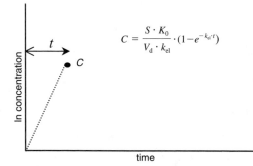

$$C = \frac{S \cdot K_0}{V_d \cdot k_{el}} \cdot (1 - e^{-k_{el} \cdot t})$$

Concentration immediately following an intravenous infusion when patient already has a concentration of C_0 and the same equation rearranged to estimate the dose needed to raise concentration from C_0 to C:

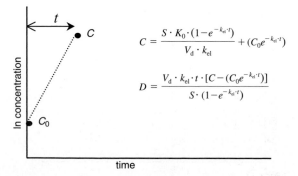

$$C = \frac{S \cdot K_0 \cdot (1 - e^{-k_{el} \cdot t})}{V_d \cdot k_{el}} + (C_0 e^{-k_{el} \cdot t})$$

$$D = \frac{V_d \cdot k_{el} \cdot t \cdot [C - (C_0 e^{-k_{el} \cdot t})]}{S \cdot (1 - e^{-k_{el} \cdot t})}$$

Concentration at time t following the start of a continuous intravenous infusion:

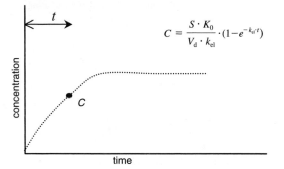

$$C = \frac{S \cdot K_0}{V_d \cdot k_{el}} \cdot (1 - e^{-k_{el} \cdot t})$$

In concentration at time t_{wait} after the end of an intravenous infusion administered over time t:

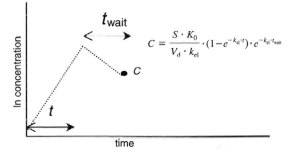

$$C = \frac{S \cdot K_0}{V_d \cdot k_{el}} \cdot (1 - e^{-k_{el} \cdot t}) \cdot e^{-k_{el} \cdot t_{wait}}$$

Elimination rate constant (k_{el}) given two concentrations:

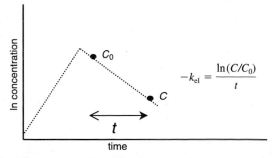

$$-k_{el} = \frac{\ln(C/C_0)}{t}$$

Other elimination rate constant (k_{el}) relationships:

$$k_{el} = \frac{Cl}{V_d} \qquad t_{1/2.} = \frac{0.693}{k_{el}}$$

Steady-state concentration of a first-order drug given by intermittent infusion (e.g., gentamicin) immediately following the end of the infusion:

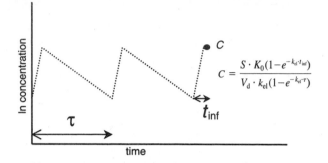

$$C = \frac{S \cdot K_0(1 - e^{-k_{el} \cdot t_{inf}})}{V_d \cdot k_{el}(1 - e^{-k_{el} \cdot \tau})}$$

Steady-state concentration of a first-order drug given by intermittent infusion (e.g., gentamicin) at some time (t_{wait}) following the end of the infusion:

$$C = \frac{S \cdot K_0(1 - e^{-k_{el} \cdot t_{inf}})}{V_d \cdot k_{el}(1 - e^{-k_{el} \cdot \tau})} \, e^{-k_{el} \cdot t_{wait}}$$

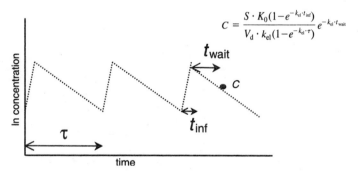

Concentration at some time following a known concentration (C_0) and the same equation rearranged to estimate time needed for concentration to fall from C_0 to C:

$$C = C_0 e^{-k_{el} \cdot t}$$

$$t = \frac{\ln(C/C_0)}{-k_{el}}$$

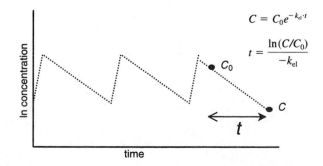

Dosage interval (τ) needed for new regimen with a desired steady-state peak (C_0), trough (C) and a known elimination rate constant (k_{el}):

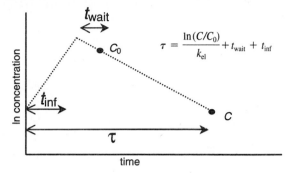

$$\tau = \frac{\ln(C/C_0)}{k_{el}} + t_{wait} + t_{inf}$$

■ NONLINEAR PHARMACOKINETICS

Daily dose of a Michaelis-Menten drug (e.g., phenytoin) needed to achieve an average steady-state concentration (C_{ss}):

$$\text{Daily dose} = \frac{V_{max}\, C_{ss}}{S \times F(K_m + C_{ss})}$$

Average steady-state concentration (C_{ss}) of a Michaelis-Menten drug achieved when giving a particular daily dose:

$$C_{ss} = \frac{S \times F \times \text{daily dose} \cdot K_m}{V_{max} - (S \times F \times \text{daily dose})}$$

Time to reach 90% of steady-state concentration:

$$t_{90\%} = \frac{K_m \cdot V_d}{[V_{max} - (S \times F \times \text{daily dose})]^2} \times [2.3 V_{max} - (0.9 \times S \times F \times \text{daily dose})]$$

Michaelis Constant (K_m) when one has two **steady-state** concentrations at two **different** daily doses:

$$-K_m = \frac{\text{Dose}_1 - \text{Dose}_2}{\dfrac{\text{Dose}_1}{\text{Conc}_1} - \dfrac{\text{Dose}_2}{\text{Conc}_2}}$$

V_{max} once one knows K_m:

$$V_{max} = \frac{(\text{Daily dose} \times S \times F)(K_m + C_{ss})}{C_{ss}}$$

"Effective" (or "normalized") concentration of phenytoin in a patient with hypoalbuminemia. *Note that this equation is inaccurate in some patient populations.*

Actual unbound ("free") concentrations should be directly measured whenever possible.

$$C_{\text{effective}} = \frac{C_{\text{measured}}}{\left[(1 - f_u) \cdot \dfrac{\text{Alb}_{\text{measured}}}{\text{Alb}_{\text{normal}}} \right] + f_u}$$

Index